Diagnostic Radiology

Diagnostic Radiology
An Anglo-American Textbook of Imaging

EDITED BY

Ronald G. Grainger
MD, FRCP, DMRD, FRCR, FACR(Hon), FRACR(Hon)
Professor of Diagnostic Radiology, University of Sheffield;
Consultant Radiologist, Royal Hallamshire Hospital and
Northern General Hospital, Sheffield, UK

David J. Allison
BSc, MD, DMRD, FRCR
Professor and Director, Department of Diagnostic Radiology,
Royal Postgraduate Medical School, Hammersmith Hospital,
London, UK

VOLUME THREE

CHURCHILL LIVINGSTONE
EDINBURGH LONDON MELBOURNE AND NEW YORK 1986

CHURCHILL LIVINGSTONE
Medical Division of Longman Group Limited

Distributed in the United States of America by Churchill Livingstone
Inc., 1560 Broadway, New York, N.Y. 10036 and by associated
companies, branches and representatives throughout the world.

First published 1986

ISBN 0 443 02443 X (3 volumes)

British Library Cataloguing in Publication Data
Diagnostic radiology : an Anglo-American textbook
of imaging.
  1. Diagnosis, Radioscopic
  I. Grainger, Ronald G II. Allison, D.J.
  616.07'57 RC78

Library of Congress Cataloging in Publication Data
Main entry under title:
Diagnostic radiology.
  Includes index.
  1. Diagnostic imaging. I. Graiger, Ronald G.
II. Allison, David J. [DNLM: 1. Nuclear Magnetic
Resonance——diagnostic use. 2. Radiology——methods.
3. Radionuclide Imaging. 4. Tomography, X-Ray
Computed. 5. Ultrasonic Diagnosis. WN 100 D536]
RC78.7.D52D53   1986   616.07'5   85—15162

Printed in Great Britain by B.A.S. Printers Ltd., Over Wallop.
Bound by William Clowes Limited, Beccles and London.

Preface

This completely new, authoritative, Anglo-American, integrated text of organ imaging is designed to help the radiologist throughout the various stages of his professional career. It is particularly orientated towards the radiological trainee, resident or registrar and to facilitate this purpose many of the contributing authors have had experience as examiners for the American Boards, Royal College of Radiologists and other examining bodies. For the trainee, a rather didactic style has been adopted, the examination syllabi have been covered and special attention has been paid to favourite examination topics. An additional Multiple Choice Question volume based on this textbook is in an advanced stage of preparation.

This book is also designed for the working bench in the reading (reporting) room and is well illustrated and indexed to facilitate rapid reference to the appropriate subject. Each chapter carries an extensive updated bibliography and a further list of classic papers and monographs to encourage further reading, should more detail be required. It is therefore hoped that these volumes will continue to serve as an illustrated text and as an entry to the literature, long after the early formal years of radiological training.

We believe that this is the first attempt at producing a comprehensive and integrated text of the several modalities of organ imaging, written by a large and distinguished international group of teachers, authors, practitioners and research workers. About one half of the contributors are from either side of the Atlantic, equal prominence being given to American and British practice.

Probably no field of medicine is advancing so rapidly at the present time as organ imaging. The last 10–15 years have seen the introduction and development of completely new technologies such as computer assisted tomography, digital imaging, isotope studies, ultrasound and magnetic resonance imaging. All of these and other techniques are discussed in this book, both in separate and specific technical chapters written by recognized authorities, and also by integration with conventional radiology in the general text where appropriate. Despite the great success of the alternative systems of organ imaging, conventional film radiology remains the major system in Departments of Radiology in the mid-1980s and this is reflected by the emphasis given in this text.

Radiology has become increasingly interventional and therapeutic as well as diagnostic, and good coverage of these procedures is presented by internationally acknowledged practising experts.

Imaging technology is developing so rapidly and so expensively that the major problems are those of providing the finances for the necessary technical and clinical developments, and in selecting the optimal imaging technique. As Dr Margulis points out in the opening chapter, the allocation of the necessary finance and resources is a matter for society in general, and for the medical profession in particular.

The editors wish to thank the Section and Advisory Editors and all of the many contributors to this work for their conscientious collaboration despite the many other demands on their valuable time and expertise.

We wish to thank Dr Anne Hemingway, Dr C. R. Merrill and Dr A. Adam for their major assistance in preparing the text for publication and in proof-reading, our secretaries Ms N. Moorcraft, Mrs V. Morris, Miss H. Pybus, Miss S. Smith and Mrs Y. Steel for typing and organisational assistance, and the photographic and illustration departments of our hospitals for their ever-willing and high-quality contributions.

Sheffield and London   R.G.G.
1986   D.J.A.

*This work is dedicated
with our love
to*

our dear wives

Ruth   *Deirdre*

*and
our dear children*

David Nicholas,   *Catherine,*
Jonathan Peter   *Helen,*
                                         Richard

R.G.G.   *D.J.A.*

Acknowledgements

Anyone who has participated in writing or publishing a book will know that the project is not viable without the co-operation and contributions of very many people.

To publish a completely new integrated textbook of a rapidly changing subject in which major technological advances are being made every year, with over 100 authors, writing in two different languages (American English and British English), with over 2000 pages and several thousand illustrations is absolutely impossible without the help, support, co-operation and advice of an army of several hundred people involved in the writing, illustrating, typing, editing, designing, typesetting, proofreading, printing, etc., etc.

It is obviously impossible to thank individually in print everyone who has endeavoured to secure the success of this book. The editors and publishers wish most sincerely to thank them collectively for the magnificent co-operation which we have received throughout this major project over its 5-year gestation.

The editors are particularly grateful to the Fleischner Society for permission to publish, at the end of Section Two, the 'Glossary of "Chest" Radiological Terms' suggested by their Terminology Committee.

Dr Nolan would like to thank his secretary, Miss Susan Dyson, for the preparation of his own chapters, 44 and 46, and for preparing the final manuscripts for all the other chapters in Section Four. The illustrations for Chapters 44 and 46 were prepared by the Department of Medical Illustration, John Radcliffe Hospital, Oxford, UK.

Dr Zegal and Dr Pollack wish to thank Paul S. Ellis, MD, and Linda Di Sandro, without whose invaluable assistance Chapter 60 could not have been prepared.

Dr Harris acknowledges with grateful appreciation the invaluable assistance of Ellen Cruz and Sally Auberg, Editorial Associates, and Roz Vecchio, Medical Photographer, in the preparation of Chapter 68.

Professor Allison is grateful to Dr A. Leung and to Mr Doig Simmonds and Mr David Hawtin, from the Department of Medical Illustration at the Royal Postgraduate Medical School, London, UK, for their help with the illustrations for Chapters 94, 97 and 98.

Professor Grainger is most grateful to the radiographic, nursing and office staff of the Royal Hallamshire and Northern General Hospitals, Sheffield, to the Department of Medical Illustration and to Mr P. M. Elliott, Medical Artist for their ever-willing help in the preparation of Chapters 28–31. Several members of the Department of Radiology in Sheffield are thanked for their help in proofreading at various manuscript stages.

Contributors

Bennett A. Alford MD
Associate Professor of Radiology and Pediatrics and
Director of Pediatric Radiology, University of Virginia
School of Medicine, Charlottesville, Virginia, USA

David J. Allison BSc, MD, DMRD, FRCR
Professor and Director, Department of Diagnostic
Radiology, Royal Postgraduate Medical School,
London, UK

John D. Armstrong II MD
Professor, Diagnostic Radiology, University of Utah
School of Medicine, Salt Lake City, Utah, USA

Peter Armstrong FRCR
Professor and Vice Chairman, Department of
Radiology, University of Virginia, Charlottesville,
Virginia, USA

M.L. Aubin MD
Associate Chief of Department, Department of
Radiology, Fondation Adolphe de Rothschild, Paris,
France

A.B. Ayers MD, FRCR
Consultant Radiologist, St Thomas' Hospital, London,
UK

Clive I. Bartram MRCP, FRCR
Consultant Radiologist, St Mark's and St Bartholomew's
Hospitals, London, UK

Olivier Bergès MD
Assistant, Department of Radiology, Fondation Adolphe
de Rothschild, Paris, France

Frank H. Boehm MD
Professor of Obstetrics and Gynecology; Director,
Division of Maternal/Fetal Medicine, Vanderbilt
University Hospital, Nashville, Tennessee, USA

J. Bonavita MD
Department of Radiology, Hospital of the University of
Pennsylvania, Philadelphia, Pennsylvania, USA

N.B. Bowley DMRD, FRCR
Consultant Radiologist, Queen Victoria Hospital, East
Grinstead, E. Sussex; formerly Senior Lecturer, Royal
Postgraduate Medical School, Hammersmith Hospital,
London, UK

Jan Brismar MD
Associate Professor of Radiology, University Hospital,
Lund, Sweden

Graham M. Bydder MRCP
Senior Lecturer, Royal Postgraduate Medical School,
London, UK

M. Paul Capp MD
Professor and Chairman, Department of Radiology,
University of Arizona College of Medicine, Tucson,
Arizona, USA

E. Chadrycki
Assistant à titre étranger du Fondation Adolphe de
Rothschild, Rio de Janeiro, Brazil

David O. Cosgrove MA, MSc, MRCP
Consultant in Nuclear Medicine and Ultrasound, Royal
Marsden Hospital, London, UK

P.B. Cotton MD, FRCP
Consultant Physician, Department of Gastroenterology,
The Middlesex Hospital, London, UK

Keith C. Dewbury FRCR
Consultant Radiologist, Southampton University
Hospitals, Southampton, UK

Robert Dick MB, BS, FRACR, FRCR
Consultant in Radiology, Royal Free Hospital; Teacher
in Radiology, Royal Free Hospital School of Medicine,
London, UK

Richard M. Donner BA, MD
Associate Professor of Pediatrics, Temple University
School of Medicine; Director, Echocardiography
Laboratory, St Christopher's Hospital for Children,
Philadelphia, Pennsylvania, USA

Stephen A. Feig MD
Professor of Radiology, Thomas Jefferson Medical
College, Philadelphia, Pennsylvania, USA

Stuart Field MA, FRCR, DMRD
Consultant Radiologist, Kent and Thanet Health
Authority, Kent and Canterbury Hospital, Canterbury,
Kent, UK

Arthur C. Fleischer MD
Associate Professor of Radiology; Assistant Professor of Obstetrics and Gynecology, Vanderbilt University Medical Center, Nashville, Tennessee, USA

C.D.R. Flower FRCP(Can), FRCR
Consultant Radiologist, Addenbrooke's Hospital, Cambridge, UK

David W. Gelfand MD, FACR
Professor and Chief of Gastrointestinal Radiology, Bowman-Gray School of Medicine, of Wake-Forrest University, Winston-Salem, North Carolina, USA

Harry K. Genant BS, MD
Professor of Radiology, Medicine and Orthopedic Surgery and Chief, Skeletal Section, Department of Radiology, University of California, San Francisco, California, USA

Julian Gibbs BDS, PhD
Associate Professor of Radiology, Vanderbilt University Medical Center, Nashville, Tennessee, USA

D.G. Gibson MA, MB, FRCP
Consultant Cardiologist, Brompton Hospital, London, UK

Lawrence R. Goodman MD
Professor of Radiology and Head, Chest Radiology Section, Medical College of Wisconsin, Milwaukee, Wisconsin, USA

Ronald G. Grainger MD, FRCP, DMRD, FRCR, FACR(Hon), FRACR(Hon)
Professor of Diagnostic Radiology, University of Sheffield; Consultant Radiologist, Royal Hallamshire Hospital and Northern General Hospital, Sheffield, UK

N. David Greyson BSc, MD, FRCP(C)
Associate Professor of Radiological Sciences, University of Toronto; Director, Department of Nuclear Medicine, St Michael's Hospital; Associate Professor of Diagnostic Radiology, University of Toronto, Toronto, Ontario, Canada

John C. Harbert MD
Professor of Medicine and Radiology, Georgetown University Medical School, Washington, DC, USA

H. Theodore Harcke MD
Director, Department of Medical Imaging, Alfred I. duPont Institute, Wilmington, Delaware; Associate Professor of Radiology and Pediatrics, Temple University School of Medicine, Philadelphia, Pennsylvania, USA

George S. Harell MD
Director of Radiology, East Jefferson General Hospital, Metairie, Louisiana, USA

John H. Harris Jr. MD
Professor of Radiology, University of Texas Health Center, Houston, Texas, USA

Anne P. Hemingway MRCP, DMRD, FRCR
Senior Lecturer (Honorary Consultant Radiologist), Royal Postgraduate Medical School, Hammersmith Hospital, London, UK

Hans Herlinger MD, FRCR
Professor of Radiology, University of Pennsylvania, Philadelphia, Pennsylvania, USA

Charles B. Higgins MD
Professor of Radiology and Chief, Magnetic Resonance Imaging, University of California Medical Center, San Francisco, California, USA

Alan D. Hoffman MD
Assistant Professor of Radiology, Mayo Medical School, Rochester, Minnesota, USA

Janet E. Husband MRCP, FRCR
Consultant Radiologist, Royal Marsden Hospital, London; Honorary Senior Lecturer, Institute of Cancer Research, Sutton, Surrey, UK

A. Everette James Jr. AB, LIB, ScM, JD, MD
Professor and Chairman, Department of Radiology and Radiological Sciences, Vanderbilt University, Nashville, Tennessee; Consultant, Smithsonian Institutions, Washington, DC, USA

William D. Kaplan MD
Associate Professor of Radiology, Harvard Medical School; Chief, Oncologic Nuclear Medicine, Dana-Farber Cancer Institute, Boston, Massachusetts, USA

Theodore E. Keats BS, MD
Professor and Chairman, Department of Radiology, University of Virginia School of Medicine, Charlottesville, Virginia, USA

Michael J. Kellett MA, FRCR
Consultant Radiologist, St Peter's Hospitals and the Institute of Urology, London, UK

Ian Kelsey Fry DM, FRCP, FRCR
Consultant Radiologist, St Bartholomew's Hospital, London, UK

Louis Kreel MD, FRCP, FRCR
Director of Radiology, Newham Health Authority; Senior Lecturer, London Hospital Medical School, London, UK

Barton Lane BA, MD
Associate Chief of Radiology, Mount Zion Hospital, San Francisco; Associate Clinical Professor, University of California, San Francisco; Clinical Associate Professor, Stanford University, Stanford, California, USA

Martin J. Lipton MD
Professor of Radiology and Medicine and Chief, Cardiovascular Imaging Section, Department of Radiology, University of California Medical Center, San Francisco, California, USA

Anders Lunderquist MD
Head of Gastrointestinal and Interventional Radiology,
University Hospital, Lund, Sweden

V. L. McAllister LRCP, MRCS, FRCR, DMRD
Consultant Neuroradiologist, Regional Neurological
Centre, Newcastle General Hospital, Newcastle upon
Tyne, UK

James McIvor FDSRCS, DMRD, FRCR
Senior Lecturer in Radiology, Institute of Dental
Surgery; Consultant Radiologist, Charing Cross
Hospital, London, UK

Michael Maisey, MD, FRCP, FRCR
Professor of Radiological Sciences and Director,
Department of Nuclear Medicine, Guy's Hospital,
London, UK

Leon S. Malmud MD, BSinEE, MD
Chairman, Department of Diagnostic Imaging and
Associate Dean for Clinical Affairs, Temple University
Hospital, Philadelphia, Pennsylvania, USA

Alexander R. Margulis MD
Professor and Chairman, Department of Radiology,
University of California School of Medicine, San
Francisco, California, USA

Alan H. Maurer AB, ScB (Elect Eng), MS (Biomedical
Eng) Assistant Professor of Diagnostic Imaging and
Internal Medicine, Temple University, Philadelphia,
Pennsylvania, USA

Thomas F. Meaney MD
Chairman, Division of Radiology, Cleveland Clinic
Foundation, Cleveland, Ohio, USA

H. Meire FRCR, DMRD
Consultant Radiologist (Ultrasound), King's College
Hospital, London, UK

Constantine Metreweli MA, MRCP, FRCR
Professor of Diagnostic Radiology and Organ Imaging,
The Chinese University of Hong Kong, Shatin, Hong
Kong

J. Millis MD
Department of Radiology and Radiological Sciences,
Vanderbilt University, Nashville, Tennessee, USA

Gary S. Mintz MD
Director, Cardiac Ultrasound Laboratory; Attending
Cardiologist, Cardiac Catheterization Laboratories and
Echocardiography Laboratory, Hahnemann University
Hospital, Philadelphia, Pennsylvania, USA

Ivan F. Moseley BSc, MD, MRCP, FRCR
Consultant Radiologist, National Hospital for Nervous
Diseases, London, UK

William A. Murphy MD, FACR
Professor of Radiology, Washington University School
of Medicine; Codirector, Musculoskeletal Section,
Mallinckrodt Institute of Radiology, St Louis, Missouri,
USA

Daniel J. Nolan MD, MRCP, FRCR
Consultant Radiologist, John Radcliffe Hospital,
Headington; Clinical Lecturer, University of Oxford,
Oxford, UK

Théron W. Ovitt MD
Professor of Radiology, University of Arizona College
of Medicine, Tucson, Arizona, USA

C.M. Parks FRCR, DMRD
Consultant Radiologist, St Peter's Group of Hospitals,
London, UK

Colin Parsons FRCS, FRCR
Consultant Radiologist, Royal Marsden Hospital,
London, UK

J. Terence Patton FRCR
Consultant Radiologist, Manchester Royal Infirmary,
Manchester, UK

Howard M. Pollack MD
Professor of Radiology, University of Pennsylvania
School of Medicine and Hospital, Philadelphia,
Pennsylvania, USA

Thomas Powell FRCR, FRCP
Consultant Neuroradiologist, Royal Hallamshire
Hospital, Sheffield, UK

Vijay M. Rao MD
Associate Professor of Radiology, Jefferson Medical
College, Thomas Jefferson University Hospital,
Philadelphia, Pennsylvania, USA

M.J. Raphael MD, FRCP, FRCR
Consultant Radiologist, National Heart Hospital,
London, UK

P.S. Robbins MD
Department of Diagnostic Imaging, Temple University
School of Medicine, Philadelphia, Pennsylvania, USA

Hans Roehrig MS, PhD
Research Associate Professor, Department of Radiology,
University of Arizona College of Medicine, Tucson,
Arizona, USA

Max I. Shaff MD
Associate Professor of Radiology and Radiological
Sciences, Vanderbilt University, Nashville, Tennessee,
USA

James F. Silverman MD
Professor of Radiology, Stanford University School of
Medicine, Stanford, California, USA

Renate L. Soulen MD
Professor of Radiology, Associate Professor of Medicine
(Cardiology), Chief, Section of Cardiovascular
Radiology and Vice-Chairman, Department of
Diagnostic Imaging, Temple University Health Sciences
Center, Philadelphia, Pennsylvania, USA

Robert E. Steiner MD, FRCR, FRCP
Emeritus Professor of Diagnostic Radiology, Royal
Postgraduate Medical School, Hammersmith Hospital,
London, UK

Robert M. Steiner MD, FACC
Professor of Radiology and Associate Professor of
Medicine, Thomas Jefferson University Hospital,
Philadelphia, Pennsylvania, USA

Dennis J. Stoker FRCP, FRCR
Consultant Radiologist, Royal National Orthopaedic
Hospital and St George's Hospital, London, UK

Lee B. Talner MD
Professor of Radiology and Chief, Diagnostic
Radiology, University of California Medical Center, San
Diego and Veterans Administration Hospital, La Jolla,
California, USA

Charles J. Tegtmeyer MD
Professor of Radiology, Associate Professor of Anatomy
and Chief, Interventional Radiology, University of
Virginia School of Medicine, Charlottesville, Virginia,
USA

Jacques Théron MD
Chief, Department of Neuroradiology, University
Hospital, Caen, France

J. Vignaud MD
Chef de Service, Department of Radiology, Fondation
Adolphe de Rothschild, Paris, France

James B. Vogler MD
Chief of Skeletal Radiology, Department of Radiology,
David Grant Medical Center, Travis AFB, California,
USA

Judith A.W. Webb MD, MRCP, FRCR
Consultant Radiologist, St Bartholomew's Hospital,
London, UK

Richard J. Wechsler MD
Associate Professor of Radiology, Thomas Jefferson
University Hospital, Philadelphia, Pennsylvania, USA

Meredith A. Weinstein MD
Staff Neuroradiologist and Head, Section of
Neuroradiological Nuclear Magnetic Resonance,
Cleveland Clinic Foundation, Cleveland, Ohio, USA

G.H. Whitehouse FRCP, FRCR, DMRD
Professor of Diagnostic Radiology, University of
Liverpool; Honorary Consultant Radiologist, Royal
Liverpool Hospital, Liverpool Maternity Hospital and
the Women's Hospital, Liverpool, UK

C. Williams FRCP
Consultant Physician, St Mark's Hospital, London, UK

A.G. Wilson MB, MRCP, FRCR
Consultant Radiologist, St George's Hospital; Honorary
Senior Lecturer, University of London, UK

A.C. Winfield MD
Department of Radiology and Radiological Sciences,
Vanderbilt University, Nashville, Tennessee, USA

B.S. Worthington BSc, LIMA, DMRD, FRCR
Professor of Diagnostic Radiology, University of
Nottingham, Nottingham, UK

C.H. Wright DMRD, FRCR
Consultant Radiologist, Glan Clwyd Hospital, North
Wales, UK

Harry G. Zegal MD
Clinical Assistant Professor of Radiology, Hahnemann
University; Staff Radiologist, St Agnes Medical Center,
Philadelphia, Pennsylvania, USA

Contents of Volume Three

Section Eight
THE FEMALE REPRODUCTIVE SYSTEM
Editor: *Ronald G. Grainger*

80 Obstetrics 1551
A.C. Fleischer, F.H. Boehm, A.C. Winfield,
J. Millis, M.I. Shaff, A.E. James, J. Gibbs

81 Gynaecology 1593
G.H. Whitehouse, C.H. Wright

82 The breast 1631
Stephen A. Feig

Section Nine
THE CENTRAL NERVOUS SYSTEM
Editor: *Ivan F. Moseley*

83 The skull and brain: Methods of examination;
diagnostic approach 1671
J. Brismar, B. Lane, I.F. Moseley, J. Theron

84 Cranial pathology (1) 1705
J. Brismar, B. Lane, I.F. Moseley, J. Theron

85 Cranial pathology (2) 1739
J. Brismar, B. Lane, I.F. Moseley, J. Theron

86 Cranial pathology (3) 1769
J. Brismar, B. Lane, I.F. Moseley, J. Theron

87 The spine: Methods of examination; diagnostic
approach 1797
V.L. McAllister, I.F. Moseley, J. Theron

88 Spinal pathology 1821
V.L. McAllister, I.F. Moseley, J. Theron

89 Radionuclide scanning 1857
John C. Harbert

Section Ten
THE FACE: ORBIT; TEETH; ENT
Editor: *Ronald G. Grainger*

90 The orbit 1875
J. Vignaud, O. Bergès, M.L. Aubin,
E. Chadrycki, I.F. Moseley

91 Maxillofacial radiology 1899
James McIvor

92 Dental radiology 1925
James McIvor

93 The ear, nose and throat 1937
Thomas Powell

Section Eleven
ANGIOGRAPHY, INTERVENTIONAL RADIOLOGY
AND OTHER TECHNIQUES
Editor: *David J. Allison*

94 Arteriography 1987
David J. Allison

95 Venography 2061
Anne P. Hemingway

96 Digital subtraction angiography 2099
Thomas F. Meaney, Meredith A. Weinstein

97 Vascular ultrasound 2113
H. Meire

98 Interventional radiology 2121
David J. Allison

99 Radiology in oncology 2167
Colin Parsons

100 Nuclear medicine in oncology 2183
William D. Kaplan

101 Paediatric nuclear medicine 2197
H. Theodore Harcke

102 Paediatric ultrasonography 2213
Constantine Metreweli

103 Ultrasonography of the infant brain 2229
Keith Dewbury

Index I1

Contents of Volumes One and Two

VOLUME 1
Section One
TECHNIQUES AND IMAGING MODALITIES
Editor: *Ronald G. Grainger*

1 Introduction *Alexander R. Margulis;* 2 Radionuclide imaging *Alan H. Maurer, Leon S. Malmud;* 3 Ultrasound *David O. Cosgrove;* 4 Whole body computed tomography *Janet E. Husband;* 5 Magnetic resonance imaging *G.M. Bydder, R.E. Steiner, B.S. Worthington;* 6 Digital radiography *M.P. Capp, H. Roehrig, T. W. Ovitt;* 7 Intravascular contrast media *Ronald G. Grainger*

Section Two
THE RESPIRATORY SYSTEM
Editor: *C.D.R. Flower*

8 The normal chest *Peter Armstrong;* 9 Techniques *C.D.R. Flower, Peter Armstrong;* 10 Interpreting the chest radiograph *A.G. Wilson;* 11 The chest wall and pleura *A.G. Wilson;* 12 The diaphragm *C.D.R. Flower;* 13 The mediastinum *Peter Armstrong;* 14 Pulmonary infection *A.G. Wilson, C.D.R. Flower, P. Armstrong;* 15 Large airway obstruction *A.G. Wilson;* 16 Asthma and emphysema *C.D.R. Flower;* 17 Pulmonary neoplasms *Peter Armstrong, C.D.R. Flower;* 18 Diffuse pulmonary disease *C.D.R. Flower, J.D. Armstrong II, A.G. Wilson;* 19 Pulmonary thromboembolism *John D. Armstrong II;* 20 Chest trauma *C.D.R. Flower* 21 The postoperative and critically ill patient *Lawrence R. Goodman;* 22 The infant and young child *Bennett A. Alford, Theodore E. Keats;* 23 Congenital pulmonary anomalies *Peter Armstrong, Bennett A. Alford;* Glossary of 'chest' radiological terms

Section Three
THE HEART AND GREAT VESSELS
Editor: *Ronald G. Grainger*

Part 1: Techniques — 24 Cardiac radiology: techniques: normal appearances *M.J. Raphael;* 25 Echocardiography *R.M. Donner, Renate L. Soulen;* 26 Nuclear cardiology *A.H. Maurer, P.S. Robbins, L.S. Malmud;* 27 Cardiovascular imaging: CT, MRI, DSA *Martin J. Lipton, Charles B. Higgins.*

Part 2: Congenital heart disease — 28 General principles *Ronald G. Grainger;* 29 Left to right shunts *Ronald G. Grainger, R.M. Donner;* 30 Central cyanosis *Ronald G. Grainger, R.M. Donner;* 31 Other congenital lesions *Ronald G. Grainger, R.M. Donner*

Part 3: Acquired heart disease — 32 Cardiac enlargement *M.J. Raphael, D.G. Gibson;* 33 Pulmonary circulation *Charles B. Higgins, Martin J. Lipton;* 34 Acquired valvular heart disease *M.J. Raphael, D.G. Gibson;* 35 Ischaemic heart disease *M.J. Raphael, J.F. Silverman, D.G. Gibson;* 36 Miscellaneous cardiac disorders *M.J. Raphael, D.G. Gibson;* 37 Cardiac pacemakers *Robert M. Steiner, Charles J. Tegtmeyer;* 38 Prosthetic cardiac valves *Robert M. Steiner, Gary S. Mintz;* 39 The pericardium *Robert M. Steiner, Vijay M. Rao;* 40 The thoracic aorta *R.M. Steiner, R.J. Wechsler, R.G. Grainger*

VOLUME 2
Section Four
THE GASTROINTESTINAL TRACT
Editor: *Daniel J. Nolan* with contributions on radioisotope imaging by *Leon S. Malmud*

41 The acute abdomen — the plain radiograph *Stuart Field;* 42 The oesophagus *G.S. Harell;* 43 The stomach *David W. Gelfand, Leon S. Malmud;* 44 The duodenum *Daniel J. Nolan;* 45 Upper gastrointestinal endoscopy *P.B. Cotton;* 46 The small intestine *Daniel J. Nolan;* 47 The large bowel *Clive I. Bartram;* 48 Lower gastrointestinal endoscopy *Christopher B. Williams;* 49 The newborn and young infant *Bennett A. Alford, Theodore E. Keats*

Section Five
THE LIVER, BILIARY TRACT, PANCREAS AND ENDOCRINE SYSTEM   Editor: *David J. Allison*

50 The liver *H. Herlinger, L.S. Malmud, D.O. Cosgrove, J.E. Husband, D.J. Allison;* 51 The gallbladder and biliary system *N.B. Bowley, Leon S. Malmud;* 52 Interventional techniques in the hepatobiliary system *Robert Dick;* 53 The pancreas *Anders Lunderquist, P.B. Cotton;* 54 The spleen *A.B. Ayers;* 55 Endocrine disease *Louis Kreel*

Section Six
THE GENITOURINARY TRACT
Editor: *Michael J. Kellett*

56 Methods of investigation *Michael J. Kellett, Ian Kelsey Fry;* 57 Nuclear medicine *Michael Maisey;* 58 Calculus disease *Michael J. Kellett;* 59 Urinary obstruction *Lee B. Talner;* 60 Renal masses *Harry G. Zegal, Howard M. Pollack;* 61 Urothelial lesions *Michael J. Kellett;* 62 Renal parenchymal disease *Ian Kelsey Fry;* 63 Renal failure and renal

transplantation *Judith A.W. Webb*; 64 Hypertension and other vascular disorders *Judith A.W. Webb, Michael Maisey*; 65 Injuries to the genitourinary tract *J. Bonavita, Howard M. Pollack*; 66 Paediatric uroradiology *Alan D. Hoffman*; 67 Urodynamics *C.M. Parks*

Section Seven
THE SKELETAL SYSTEM   Editor: *J. Terence Patton*
68 Skeletal trauma *John H. Harris Jr*; 69 Bone tumours (1) *Dennis J. Stoker*; 70 Bone tumours (2) *Dennis J. Stoker*; 71 Myeloproliferative and similar syndromes *Dennis J. Stoker*; 72 Bone and joint infection *J. Terence Patton*; 73 Metabolic and endocrine diseases *James B. Vogler, Harry K. Genant*; 74 Skeletal dysplasia *J. Terence Patton*; 75 The musculoskeletal system in children *Theodore E. Keats, Bennett A. Alford*; 76 Joint disease *William A. Murphy*; 77 Soft tissues *J. Terence Patton*; 78 CT scanning *Harry K. Genant*; 79 Radionuclide bone scanning *N. David Greyson*

8

The Female
Reproductive System

Editor: Ronald G. Grainger

Contents
80 Obstetrics *A. C. Fleischer, F. H. Boem, A. C. Winfield, J. Millis, M. I. Shaff, A. E. James, J. Gibbs*
81 Gynaecology *G. H. Whitehouse, C. H. Wright*
82 The breast *Stephen A. Feig*

80 Obstetrics

A. C. Fleischer, F. H. Boehm, A. C. Winfield, J. Millis, M. I. Shaff, A. E. James and J. Gibbs

Obstetric sonography
  Scanning methods and patient preparation
  General applications throughout pregnancy
    Date-size discrepancy or unknown dates
    Localization and evaluation of the placenta
    Evaluation of fetal position
    Evaluation of fetal viability
  First trimester
    Normal features and scanning techniques
    Abortion
    Ectopic pregnancy
    Molar pregnancy
    Pregnancy with IUCDs (Intrauterine contraceptive device)
  Second trimester
    Normal features and scanning techniques
    Placental localization prior to amniocentesis
    Multiple gestation
    Pelvic masses occurring during pregnancy
    Intrauterine growth retardation (IUGR)
    Fetal anomalies which can be detected in the second trimester
  Third trimester
    Normal features and scanning techniques
    Placenta praevia and placental abruption
    Fetal anomalies that can be detected in the third trimester
    Conditions affecting labour and delivery
    Assessment of fetal condition
  Maternal disorders which may occur during pregnancy
  Postpartum disorders

Obstetric radiology
  Amniography
  Pelvimetry
  Radiography of the maternal abdomen
  Radiation hazards in utero

Obstetric sonography

Sonographic imaging has, and will continue to have, one of its most significant impacts in medicine in the field of obstetrics (see suggestions for further reading). This chapter will emphasize the most common applications of diagnostic sonography in obstetrical disorders (Table 80.1). Other less frequently employed radiographic procedures such as amniography and pelvimetry will also be mentioned.

Table 80.1 Indications for obstetric sonography

A. *General*
  1. Estimate gestational duration (menstrual age)
  2. Confirm presence of intrauterine pregnancy and viability
  3. Localization and textural evaluation of placenta
  4. Detection of multiple gestation
  5. Evaluation of pelvic masses occurring during pregnancy
  6. Detection of certain anatomical and functional anomalies of the fetus

B. *First trimester*
  1. Evaluation of uterine bleeding occurring in first trimester
  2. Evaluation for suspected blighted ovum, threatened, incomplete or missed abortion
  3. Distinguish intrauterine from ectopic pregnancy (combined with laboratory determinations)
  4. Evaluation for suspected molar pregnancy
  5. Confirm pregnancy associated with intrauterine contraceptive device

C. *Second trimester*
  1. Localization and evaluation of the placenta prior to amniocentesis
  2. Evaluation of fetal growth
  3. Detection and differentiation of disorders associated with abnormal amounts of amniotic fluid

D. *Third trimester*
  1. Confirm or exclude presence of placenta praevia
  2. Determination of optimal time and mode of delivery

E. *Maternal disorders occurring during pregnancy*
  1. Evaluation for suspected calculus cholecystitis
  2. Evaluate for suspected pancreatitis
  3. Evaluate for suspected hydro- or pyonephrosis of pregnancy
  4. Evaluate for suspected ascites
  5. Screening for large vascular aneurysms

F. *Postpartum*
  1. Evaluation for retained products of conception

Scanning methods and patient preparation

Two general types of scanning devices are available for the obstetric patient; (a) scanners that have the transducer mounted on an articulated arm that produce 'static' images, and (b) those scanning devices, that by their immediate processing of data, allow dynamic depiction of structures, called 'real-time' scanners. Articulated arm scanners are valuable in that a series of tomographic images allows for a global depiction of the area of interest. The images obtained with a real-time scanner depict only a relatively limited region of interest at any one time. Real-time imaging allows for flexible imaging of structures within the body, due to its dynamic portrayal of regions of interest and its capability to alter the scanning plane.

A series of static images may augment the real-time examination when an overall appreciation of a large area of interest or structure is desired. For example, precise localization of the placenta may require serial tomographic static images. Because the field of view is limited in some real-time scanners, an articulated arm scanner is usually needed for an assessment of uterine size, e.g. for total intrauterine volume calculation. Static scanning is also helpful in evaluation of possible fetal anomalies since it can 'map out' regions of the fetus in a tomographic manner.

There are several types of transducer configurations for real-time scanners. *Linear array transducers* allow depiction of a large region of interest but have limited manipulative flexibility due to the relatively large size of the transducer head. The smaller scanning surface of the *mechanical sector real-time devices* allows more flexibility and is the preferred method of real-time examination in the first trimester, for pelvic masses that are present during pregnancy, and for some congenital anomalies.

Real-time scanning can be documented by multiple still frames with recording of selected views on a multi-image format camera, or by videotape recording. We prefer recording of certain routine 'views' on transparent film and only use videotaping in difficult and/or unusual cases. Videotaping is usually necessary when a moving structure such as the heart is being studied, or to document lack of fetal heart motion in intrauterine fetal demise.

Distension of the urinary bladder is most important in evaluating the patient in the first trimester and those patients who are suspected of having a placenta praevia. This is best accomplished by having the patient drink 250 to 350 ml of water or tea approximately 45 minutes prior to the examination. If the patient is under fluid intake restriction, distension of the urinary bladder can be achieved by intravenous administration of fluid or by introduction of a Foley catheter into the bladder, but the latter involves a slight risk of ascending infection. Distension of the urinary bladder displaces gas containing bowel out of the pelvis and, most important, brings the anteflexed uterus perpendicular to the incident beam which allows better depiction of the uterine texture by utilizing the axial resolution properties of the scanning device.

After the second trimester, and if a placenta praevia is not suspected clinically, we do not require the patient to be scanned with a fully distended bladder. If a low lying placenta is encountered on the initial scans, additional examinations can be performed utilizing the full bladder technique.

GENERAL APPLICATIONS THROUGHOUT PREGNANCY

Date-size discrepancy or unknown dates

One of the most frequent indications for sonography in obstetrics is to estimate gestational age, which is usually expressed from the first day of the last menstrual cycle (menstrual age). This problem is most frequently encountered in the patient who cannot accurately recollect her last menstrual period, has recently discontinued ovulation suppression contraception, who may have not had a regular menstrual cycle or may not have been menstruating, (such as patients who were breast feeding). Estimation of gestational duration during the first trimester of pregnancy can be achieved by sonography (Fig. 80.1) by recognition and/or measurement of certain anatomic structures and features characteristic of an early pregnancy (Table 80.2).

Table 80.2 Sonographic developmental features in pregnancy

Weeks (± 2 weeks)	Feature
3–4 weeks	Rim of choriodecidual tissue surrounding gestational sac
4–5 weeks	Chorion frondosum develops
5–6 weeks	Embryo, umbilical stalk, yolk sac identifiable
6–8 weeks	Fetal heart motion discernible by real-time scanning
10 weeks to term	Biparietal diameter measurable
12–27 weeks	Placental growth maximal
25–36 weeks	Uterine growth maximal
20 weeks to term	Major fetal viscera discernible

These features are discussed and illustrated in more detail in the section concerning normal sonographic features of the first trimester. Since differentiation and development of the major fetal organs occur between 9 and 15 weeks, we recommend restricting scan time to the minimum [1]. Although there is little evidence, it is possible that ultrasound may harm the developing fetus.

The choriodecidua forms an echogenic ring around the gestational sac at 3 to 4 weeks of pregnancy (Fig. 80.1B). At about 5 weeks of pregnancy, the choriodecidua becomes localized, forming the chorion frondosum (Fig. 80.1C) which appears as a localized echogenic region around the gestational sac. At approximately 6 to 7 weeks, the developing embryo as well as the umbilical stalk and yolk sac may be identified within the gestational sac adjacent to the chorion frondosum (Fig. 80.1D). From 8 to 12 weeks, an estimation of the length of the fetus (crown to rump length) can be used to assess accurately gestation duration (Table 80.3 & Fig. 80.1E). Estimation of gestational age by fetal length is accurate to within plus or minus 1 week. This anatomical method of 'dating' the pregnancy is preferable to measurement of gestational sac size alone since that par-

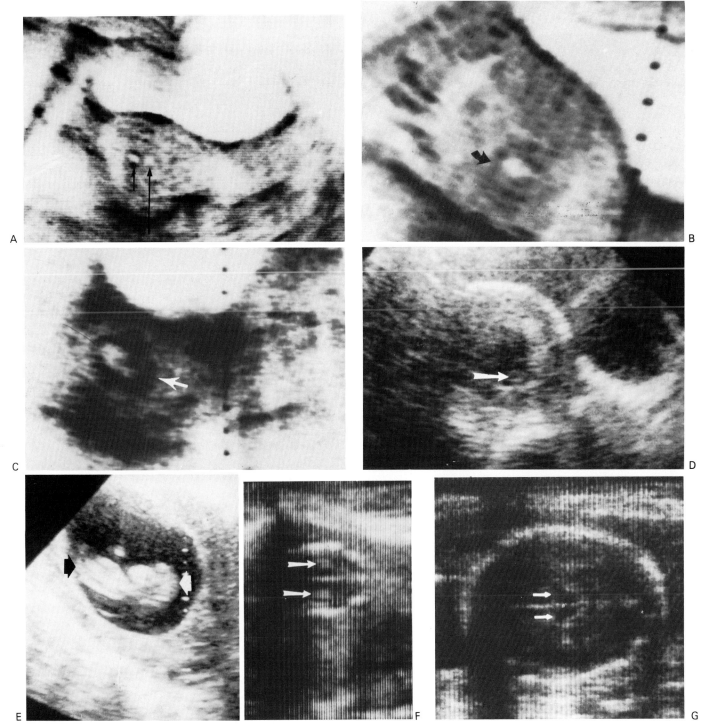

Fig. 80.1A-G Sonographic determination of gestational age.

(A) 3 week (1 week postconception) pregnancy (static longitudinal sonogram). The developing amniotic cavity [short arrow] yolk sac [long arrow] and embryonic plate can be identified within the uterus. Early pregnancy was clinically unsuspected but confirmed by beta-HCG radioimmunoassay.

(B) 3 to 4 week intrauterine pregnancy (longitudinal static sonogram). There is a concentric ring of echogenicity in the upper portion of the uterus corresponding to the choriodecidua [arrow].

(C) 5 to 6 week intrauterine pregnancy (transverse static sonogram). At this stage in pregnancy, there is located thickening of the chorion [arrow] representing the chorion frondosum. Adjacent to this area is the developing embryo and umbilical stalk.

*(D) 5 to 6 week pregnancy (longitudinal real-time sonogram, white-on-black format). There is a 5 mm rounded structure [arrow] connected to the umbilical stalk representing the yolk sac [arrow]. The yolk sac has a role in development of the haematopoietic system.

*(E) 6 to 7 week fetus (real-time sonogram). At this stage in pregnancy the fetus can be identified and the fetal length (between arrows) is an accurate parameter of gestational duration.

*(F) Sonographic features of fetal head at 12 weeks (transverse real-time sonogram). The lateral ventricles, falx cerebri and choroid plexus [arrow] can be identified within the head of this 12 week fetus.

*(G) Biparietal dimension. This transverse real time sonogram demonstrates the appropriate level to obtain a biparietal dimension. The quadrigeminal plate cistern and cerebral peduncles [arrow] form an echogenic V-shaped structure along the posterior aspect of the fetal head. The distance from the falx cerebri is equidistant to both tables of the skull.

In this, and subsequent illustrations an asterisk * indicates a white ultrasonic display on a black background.

ameter can be altered by varying degrees of bladder filling and the shape and consistency of the uterus.

After 12 weeks the gestational age can be estimated accurately using the transverse measurement of the head at the level of the parietal bones, the biparietal diameter (BPD) (Fig. 80.1F). It is important that the BPD measurement is obtained in a plane at right angles to the fetal cerebral midline and across the maximum head diameter. When obtaining a measurement, one must first locate the fetal head and assess its degree of lateral flexion with respect to the fetal trunk. Visualizing the orbits often gives a valuable clue. The scan plane must then be orientated at a right angles to the fetal cerebral midline and also, if possible, along the long axis of the fetal head. One should be sure that the midline echo is truly centred between the cranial tables. (In more mature fetuses, the delineation of cerebral landmarks becomes possible and improves confidence that the correct measurement has been made. Landmarks include the thalami and cerebral peduncles as well as a 'V-shaped' echogenic region thought to be due to the quadrigeminal plate cistern [2]. The transducer position should then be altered slowly whilst viewing the image in order to obtain a scan through the maximum transverse diameter. When this is judged to have been achieved, the image should be frozen and the BPD measured from the outer surface of the proximal cranial table to the inner surface of the distal using the electronic calipers: ideally the swept gain characteristics of the scanner should be adjusted so that the proximal and distal echoes are of equal amplitude. If they are substantially different, the stronger echo will appear inappropriately wide on the image and may give rise to an underestimate of the BPD. The echo amplitude is easier to judge on an 'A' mode display and measurements from the leading edges of the two echoes are accurate to ±0.3 mm. The 'B' mode calipers on most static and real-time scanners only measure in increments of 1 mm, but this is quite adequate for routine clinical use.

Measurement of the BPD permits assessment of the gestational age to within ±5 days at 15 weeks because growth of the fetal head is rapid and is subject to little biological variation. However head growth subsequently slows down and the range of biological variation increases so that the uncertainty increases to ±10 days by 28 weeks, and is too great to be clinically useful in the third trimester [3]. Other measurements which can be used to assess gestational age include femur length (see Fig. 80.13B) [4].

Localization and evaluation of the placenta

Sonographic imaging allows evaluation of the position and texture of the placenta from its formation at about 10 weeks up to the time of labour. Changes in position of the placenta relative to the internal cervical os can be documented as can changes in texture of the placenta associated with placental ageing.

The placenta begins to develop after fusion of the chorionic and decidual tissue into a functional unit at about 10 weeks (Fig. 80.2A). Placental growth is at a maximum during the second trimester whereas uterine growth is greatest early in the third trimester of pregnancy. These factors influence the relative uterine surface area that the placenta occupies. For example, during the early second trimester, when placental growth is maximal, the placenta may cover up to three fourths of the entire uterine surface, whereas in later pregnancy, the placenta covers only about one third to two thirds of the uterine surface.

Changes in configuration of the uterus also influence apparent relative changes in position of the placenta (Figs. 80.2B & C). Early in the third trimester, the majority of uterine growth occurs in the fundus. This fundal growth contributes to apparent upward (fundal) change in position of the placenta out of the lower uterine segment. The thinning and stretching of the lower uterine segment during the third trimester also contribute to this apparent change in position of the placenta. Arteriographic studies of the placenta have demonstrated minor changes in placental implantation along the periphery of the placenta, which probably is a response to changes in placental position resulting from the uterine forces of fundic growth and thinning of the lower uterine segment [5].

The dynamics of placentation as portrayed by sonography have important clinical implications. It is not uncommon to observe the placenta near the lower uterine segment during the second trimester of pregnancy, but only a few of these placentas remain in the lower uterine segment as pregnancy approaches term (Figs. 80.2A & 2B) [6,7].

Serial sonographic evaluation has demonstrated textural changes in the placenta as it matures. Premature senescence of the placenta may have clinical implications in patients suspected of having uteroplacental insufficiency [7]. The textural changes in the placenta include fibrin deposition in the subchorionic region, hydropic changes in the midportion of the placenta secondary to intervillous thrombosis, and calcification of the basal plate and septa (Figs. 80.2D, E & F). Fibrin deposition is thought to be the result of thrombosis due to stasis within the more venous area of the placenta near the chorionic plate (Fig. 80.2D). Hydropic degeneration or sonolucent irregular areas within the midportion of the placenta on histological examination are devoid of villous structures and are also attributed to intervillous thrombosis (Fig. 80.2E). Calcification can be observed in the senescent placenta along the basal plate and septa, probably due to vascular and metabolic changes (Fig. 80.2F).

The clinical implications of these textural changes are still uncertain since they are commonly encountered in uncomplicated pregnancies. Calcification appears to be most closely related to the level of serum calcium in the mother and increases in incidence with decreased parity. Textural changes of the placenta have been correlated to fetal pulmonary maturity, with the more 'mature' placenta associated with functionally mature fetal lungs [8].

Determination of fetal position

Although engagement of the presenting part occurs late in pregnancy, it may be important to determine the position of the fetus prior to term. Sonography can assist in determining

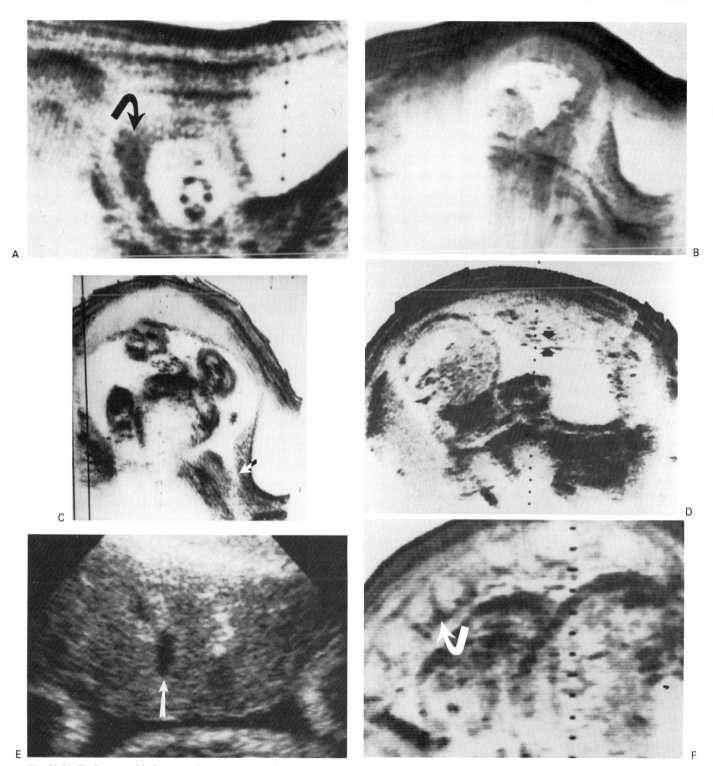

Fig. 80.2A-F Sonographic features of normal placental development.

*(A) Placental development at 10 weeks (longitudinal static sonogram). The placenta [arrow] becomes a functional unit around 10 to 11 weeks and appears as an echogenic thickened area within the fundus of the uterus.

(B) Anterior placenta at 16 weeks (longitudinal static sonogram). The placenta occupies the lower uterine segment at this stage in pregnancy.

(C) Placental ascension at 37 weeks (longitudinal static sonogram). Same pregnancy as 80.2B. The placenta now occupies more fundal portion of the uterus having ascended out of the lower uterine segment due to fundic growth and stretching of the lower uterine segment (arrow).

(D) Subchorionic fibrin deposition (transverse static sonogram). Fibrin deposition is present immediately beneath the chorionic plate and appears a sonolucent region [arrows]. Fibrin deposition is thought to be the result of thrombosis within the placenta.

*(E) Hydropic changes (longitudinal real-time sonogram). There are several sonolucent areas [arrow] within the placenta, probably resulting from intervillous thrombosis.

(F) Calcification of basal plate and septa (transverse static sonogram). The basal plate and septa [arrow] are echogenic due to calcium deposits in the mature placenta.

fetal position and the exact location of the umbilical cord about the presenting part. Sonographic determination of fetal position and the exact situation of the umbilical cord are indicated immediately prior to an attempt at external version. If the cord is wrapped around the fetal neck, this is a contraindication to a version attempt.

Evaluation of fetal viability

Real-time sonography can reliably detect fetal heart motion as early as 7 weeks. The absence of fetal heart motion in a first trimester pregnancy should be taken as an ominous sign, since most of these pregnancies will end in abortion [9]. Real-time sonography is more accurate than Doppler assessment in determining fetal viability, since the appropriate area is visualized and the examination is not hampered by obesity. When examining a fetus for intrauterine fetal demise, the operator should carefully examine the area of the thorax in the long and short axes. An observation period of at least 2 minutes with videotape documentation is recommended. One of the most common causes of intrauterine fetal demise is extensive placental abruption that can occur spontaneously or secondary to abdominal trauma. The sonographic signs of fetal death are presented on page 1587.

FIRST TRIMESTER

The most common indication for sonography during the first trimester of pregnancy is to evaluate bleeding. The clinical possibilities with this presentation include threatened or incomplete abortions, ectopic pregnancy and molar pregnancy. Sonography is helpful in distinguishing these entities. Another complication that may be encountered in the first trimester of pregnancy is the unsuspected pregnancy occurring in a patient with an intrauterine contraceptive device in place.

Normal features and scanning techniques

Urinary bladder distension is needed for adequate sonographic evaluation of patients in the first trimester. Because of the overall body contour in the lower abdomen and pelvis, a mechanical sector scanner with small contact surface allows more flexible delineation of structures within the pelvis and along the pelvic side wall and the enlarged gravid uterus of first trimester pregnancy. In order to detect accurately fetal heart motion and detail, real-time scanners should operate above 30 frames per second, but lower rates will detect cardiac pulsation (Table 80.2).

Sonography allows detailed depiction of the morphological changes in the developing pregnancy. One of the earliest features that can be detected sonographically is formation of the ring of choriodecidual tissue around the developing amniotic cavity yolk sac and embryo (see Figs. 80.1A & B).

Table 80.3 Estimation of gestational duration in the first trimester

Menstrual age (weeks)	Gestational sac* (mm) (SD ± 1–2 weeks)	Crown-rump length (mm) (SD ± 1–4 days)	Biparietal skull diameter (mm) (SD ± 1 week)
3			
4			
5	10		
6	20		
7	30	10	
8	45	17	10
9	60	25	12
10	70	32	14
11		40	17
12		55	21
13		65	25
14		80	29
15		100	33

* Measured by greatest diameter of gestational sac

The choriodecidual tissue is depicted as an echogenic ring of tissue surrounding a relatively sonolucent area in the upper portion of the uterine lumen. This feature is present from 3 to 4 weeks menstrual age. Between 4 and 5 weeks menstrual age, the choriodecidua becomes localized and thickened and forms the chorion frondosum (see Fig. 80.1C). Small crescent-shaped sonolucent areas may be present around the gestational sac itself representing 'implantation bleeds' that occur around the gestational sac as it imbeds within the endometrium (Fig. 80.3A). These sonolucent areas are most frequently observed at 3 to 4 weeks, as opposed to sonolucent areas which occur around the choriodecidual tissue at 8 to 9 weeks with a threatened or incomplete abortion, which represents areas of bleeding due to separations of the choriodecidua from the uterus (Fig. 80.3B). In addition, sonolucent areas may be encountered around the gestational sac which represent a portion of the unobliterated uterine lumen that remains slightly effaced. More than one gestational sac may be present [10,11].

At 5 to 6 weeks, an embryo, umbilical stalk and, occasionally, a yolk sac can be depicted sonographically (see Fig. 80.1D). The embryo and umbilical stalk have been termed the 'embryonic or fetal pole' and are always located near the chorion frondosum. The yolk sac is a rounded structure of about 5 mm diameter that can be demonstrated in most early pregnancies around 6 weeks and is attached to the umbilical stalk. It is involved in early haematopoiesis [12].

At 7 to 8 weeks, the fetus itself can be detected sonographically (see Fig. 80.1D). Real-time scanning can demonstrate fetal heart motion as early as 7 to 8 weeks. The absence of fetal heart motion in a patient who had bled and demonstrates separation of the choriodecidual tissue is a probable indication of lack of fetal viability and impending abortion [9]. Estimation of gestational duration can be achieved by measuring the fetal length: the standard deviation for fetal length measurements is plus or minus 1 week [13].

At 10 to 12 weeks, the fetal head assumes a configuration similar to the more mature fetus with a central echogenic interface representing the falx cerebri and interhemispheric fissure (see Fig. 80.1F). The lateral ventricles are large at this stage of cranial development and the choroid plexuses often appear prominent. From 12 weeks onward, the fetal BPD

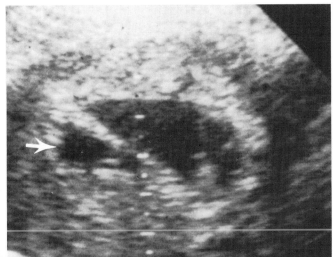

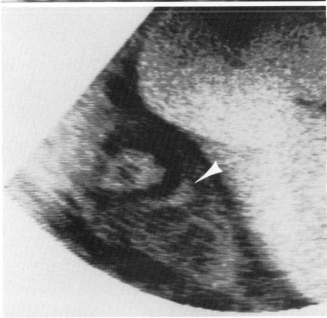

Fig. 80.3A & B Bleeding in the 1st trimester.
*(A) Implantation bleeding (transverse real-time sonogram). There is a sonolucent area [arrow] on the periphery of the gestational sac representing bleeding associated with implantation. This is a normal finding at 3 to 4 weeks.

(B) Marginal separation (longitudinal real-time sonogram). The sonolucent area [arrow] inferior to the gestational sac represents bleeding from a separation of the developing placenta and uterine wall.

can be obtained and compared to standard growth charts for evaluation of gestational age.

Abortion (Fig. 80.4)

Sonography is the most precise diagnostic method to confirm the viability of pregnancy during the early stages of the first trimester after the patient has experienced bleeding [9].

Although the sonographic findings in a patient who experienced first trimester bleeding are frequently conclusive, it is recommended that the fetus be given 'the benefit of the doubt' and the patient be re-examined after a 1 to 2 week interval to confirm the initial findings.

The clinical presentation of patients with a *threatened abortion* include uterine bleeding without evidence of passage of tissue. Bleeding associated with abortion most commonly occurs in the tenth to twelfth weeks, later than so called implantation bleeding that occurs at 3 to 4 weeks of pregnancy. In threatened abortions, there is bleeding but no passage of either the fetus or gestational tissue.

Sonographically, threatened abortions demonstrate a grossly intact gestational sac complex with a viable fetus (Fig. 80.4A). Separations of the choriodecidual tissue from the uterine surface may be detected as relatively small sonolucent areas between the echogenic choriodecidual tissue and the uterus itself (Fig. 80.4A). In some patients, the sonolucent rim represents the remnant of a gestational sac of a blighted twin [10,11]. It appears as a sonolucent space delineated by a thin interface between the viable sac and the maldeveloped second gestational sac and contents.

An incomplete abortion can occasionally be distinguished clinically from a threatened abortion in that the patient may recognize vaginal passage of tissue mixed with blood. The term 'incomplete abortion' implies that a portion of the products of conception have been passed, such as the fetus itself or portions of the placenta and membranes.

Sonographically, incomplete abortions usually demonstrate a lack of a definable embryo or fetus within the remnants of the gestational sac as well as disruption in the normally smooth choriodecidual tissue (Fig. 80.4B). The gestional sac itself is usually distorted. Echogenic interfaces representing tissue may be seen within the lower uterine segment if the patient is examined during the abortion process.

A missed abortion describes retention of the products of conception within the uterus and a dead fetus. Lack of fetal heart motion can be detected by real-time scanning as well as retention of the fetus and the embryo within the uterus (Fig. 80.4C). Usually the amniotic fluid is markedly diminished, resulting in overall small size of the gestational sac.

Blighted ovum refers to termination of development of the ovum in the very early stages of pregnancy. Sonographically, a gestational sac may be present within the uterus, but an embryro will not be demonstrated. These patients may or may not experience vaginal bleeding but all demonstrate a lack of fetal development and a lack of progression in pregnancy when re-examined over a 1 to 2 week period.

Ectopic pregnancy (Fig. 80.5)

The potential complications of a ruptured ectopic pregnancy emphasize the importance of its diagnosis by sonography (Table 80.4) and laboratory tests [14]. Ectopic pregnancies most frequently occur in the ampullary portion of the Fallopian tube but may occur within the interstitial portion of the tube or intra-abdominally. They are associated with inflammatory disease of the tube but can be encountered in patients who do not have a previous history of salpingitis. It has been

Table 80.4 Sonographic findings in ectopic pregnancy

Unruptured	Ruptured
1. Absence of intrauterine gestational sac	1. Absence of intrauterine gestational sac
2. Complex or solid adnexal mass	2. Complex or solid adnexal mass
3. No blood in cul-de-sac or paracolic recesses	3. Unclotted or clotted blood in cul-de-sac or paracolic recesses
4. Decidual cyst	4. Decidual cyst

suggested that antibiotic treatment of pelvic inflammatory disease may eradicate the bacteriological cause of the disease but may leave the tube with abnormal peristaltic activity which inhibits migration of the fertilized egg within the tube. Patients with previous tubal surgery are more likely to develop ectopic pregnancy.

These patients may present with first trimester bleeding, nonspecific pelvic pain, and an adnexal mass. The bleeding is due to sloughing of the decidua because of lack of normal progestational hormonal support.

Once the fertilized egg implants within the tube, a gestational sac is formed but because the muscular lining of the tube is very thin, it can be stretched, and rupture frequently occurs with intraperitoneal bleeding. Attempts at abortion of the gestational sac and membranes usually occur producing uterine cramps. The products of conception may occasionally pass into the peritoneum. If adequate vascular

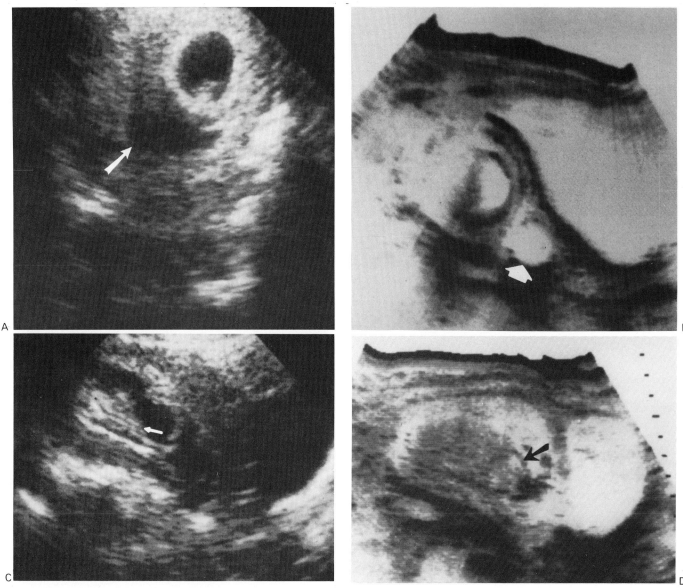

Fig. 80.4A-D Sonographic features of abortion.
  *(A) Imminent abortion (longitudinal real-time sonogram). Although fetal heart motion was present, there is a large separation between the choriodecidua and uterine wall [arrow] indicative of an imminent abortion.
  (B) Blighted twin (longitudinal static sonogram). Two gestational sacs were present in this patient; the lower one [arrow] is in the process of decompression per vaginum.
  *(C) Incomplete abortion (longitudinal real-time sonogram). There has been passage of the fetus. The umbilical cord [arrow] and a portion of the choriodecidua remains within the uterus.
  (D) Missed abortion (longitudinal static sonograms). Real-time sonography failed to demonstrate fetal heart motion. Since the fetus remained within the uterus after an episode of bleeding, this represented a missed abortion, also note hydropic swelling of the placenta [arrow] which mimics a molar pregnancy.

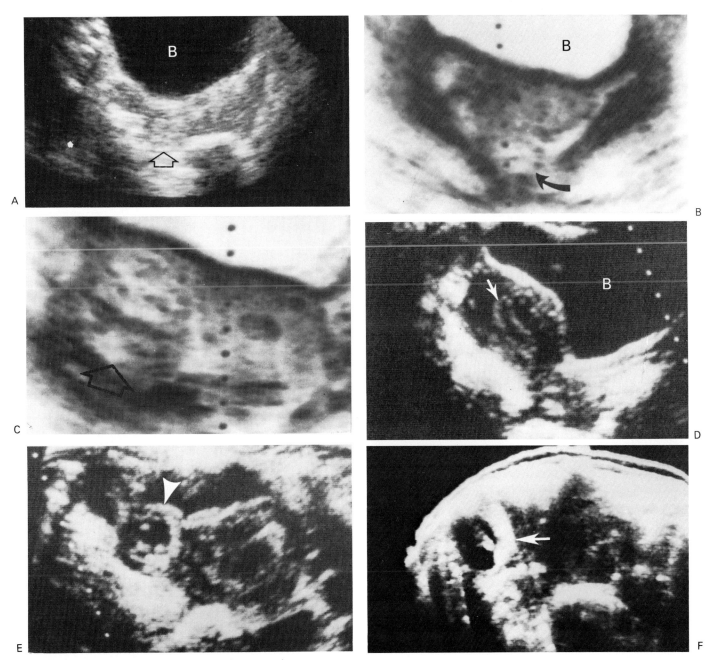

Fig. 80.5A-F Sonographic features of ectopic pregnancies.

*(A) Unruptured ectopic pregnancy (transverse real-time sonogram). An unruptured ectopic pregnancy [open arrow] is present within the right tube between the ovary and the uterus.

(B) Ruptured ectopic pregnancy (transverse real-time sonogram). There is blood [arrow] in the cul-de-sac posterior to the nongravid uterus.

(C) Ruptured ectopic pregnancy with organized haematoma (transverse static sonogram). The organized haematoma [arrow] resulting from rupture of ectopic pregnancy has a similar echogenicity to the uterus.

*(D) Decidual cast associated with an interstitial ectopic pregnancy (longitudinal sonogram). There is thickening of the decidua [arrow] associated with this ectopic pregnancy, also shown in Fig. 80.5F.

*(E) Interstitial ectopic pregnancy (transverse static sonogram). This gestational sac (arrow) could be identified within the outline but very eccentric within the uterus. (Courtesy of Tom Lawson, MD.)

*(F) Abdominal ectopic pregnancy (transverse static sonogram). The uterus was devoid of gestational sac or demonstrable decidual cast. A gestational sac and viable fetus were identified in the right lower quadrant of the abdomen [arrow].

support is achieved by attachment to mesentery, omentum or peritoneum, an intra-abdominal ectopic pregnancy may develop.

It is helpful to have results of the pregnancy tests, especially the beta subunit of HCG (human chorionic gonadotropin) radioimmunoassay. The serum β-HCG level can be quantitated and correlated with the stage of early pregnancy. Its presence above a defined level is conclusive proof of a pregnancy but does not accurately discriminate intra- from extrauterine pregnancy, or viable from abortive pregnancies. In a normal intrauterine pregnancy, the beta subunit level should double every 2 days during the first trimester. If the pregnancy is intrauterine, a definite gestational sac with a viable embryo or fetus should be present within the uterus if the level of HCG is 6500 mIU/ml or greater [15]. This test may require a day's laboratory time and may not be available at the initial sonographic evaluation of the patient with suspected ectopic pregnancy.

One of the most important sonographic determinations that can be made in patients with suspected ectopic pregnancy is to exclude intrauterine pregnancy. One should be aware that decidual proliferation within the uterus can occur with ectopic pregnancies and can simulate choriodecidual reactions associated with a normal intrauterine pregnancy. However, after 5 weeks, a normal intrauterine pregnancy should demonstrate a developing embryo (see Fig. 80.1C). An embryonic pole is not present in the uterine decidual cast present with ectopic pregnancy.

The spectrum of sonographic findings associated with ectopic pregnancies are summarized in Table 80.4. The findings will depend upon whether rupture of the ectopic has occurred before sonographic examination. Most frequently, in either an unruptured or ruptured ectopic pregnancy, an adnexal mass either solid or complex with a cystic component will be demonstrated (Figs. 80.5A-F). Due to the relatively small size of the gestational sac, definitive sonographic detection of an adnexal mass in patients with an ectopic pregnancy may be difficult. If rupture of the ectopic pregnancy has occurred, fluid within the cul-de-sac can be detected. If it is unorganized blood, it will be sonolucent (Fig. 80.5B) but when the blood begins to organize, the collection becomes moderately echogenic (Fig. 80.5C). This may result in difficulty in outlining definitively the posterior aspect of the uterus relative to the area of organized haematoma since their echogenicity is very similar.

One of the most frequent uterine changes observed in patients with an ectopic pregnancy is increased echogenicity of the endometrium due to decidual transformation (Fig.

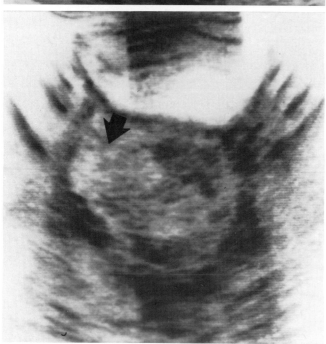

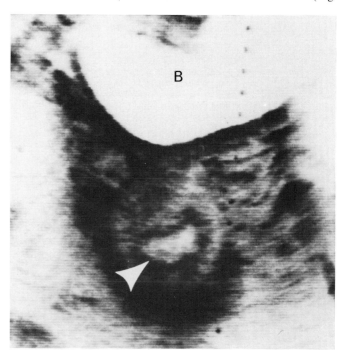

Fig. 80.6A-C Conditions which can sonographically mimic ectopic pregnancy.

(A) Haemorrhagic corpus luteum cysts (transverse static sonogram). There is a hypoechoic mass [arrow] associated with a first trimester pregnancy which represented a corpus luteum cysts of pregnancy.

(B) Regression of corpus luteum cysts (arrow) seen in Fig. 80.6A (transverse static sonogram). This cyst regressed and seemed more echogenic as pregnancy progressed.

(C) Intrauterine pregnancy in a retroverted uterus (longitudinal static sonogram). This condition may sonographically mimic an ectopic pregnancy. However, with careful sonographic examination, the gestational sac [arrow head] was identified within the upper portion of the retroverted uterus.

80.5D). Bleeding may occur within the uterine lumen and thus simulate the sonographic appearance of an early gestational sac. In addition, the thickened decidua observed in ectopic pregnancies may mimic thickening of the endometrium which is normally observed in the later phases of the menstrual cycle, prior to menstruation.

Abdominal (peritoneal) ectopic pregnancies are associated with overall enlargement of the uterus which however is devoid of a normally formed gestational sac. In abdominal ectopic pregnancies, the gestational sac itself may be ident-

ified as extrauterine and is located intraperitoneally in the lower abdomen (Fig. 80.5F).

Other unusual forms of ectopic pregnancies include the *interstitial ectopic pregnancy* (Figs. 80.5D & E) in which the gestational sac forms within the interstitial portion of the tube within the uterine cornu. If rupture of this type of ectopic pregnancy occurs, it usually involves the uterine artery and vein which course along the lateral aspect of the uterus. Haemorrhage from these vessels results in profound blood loss.

Sonographically, an interstitial ectopic pregnancy should be considered when a gestational sac appears to have an abnormally eccentric location but seems to be within the

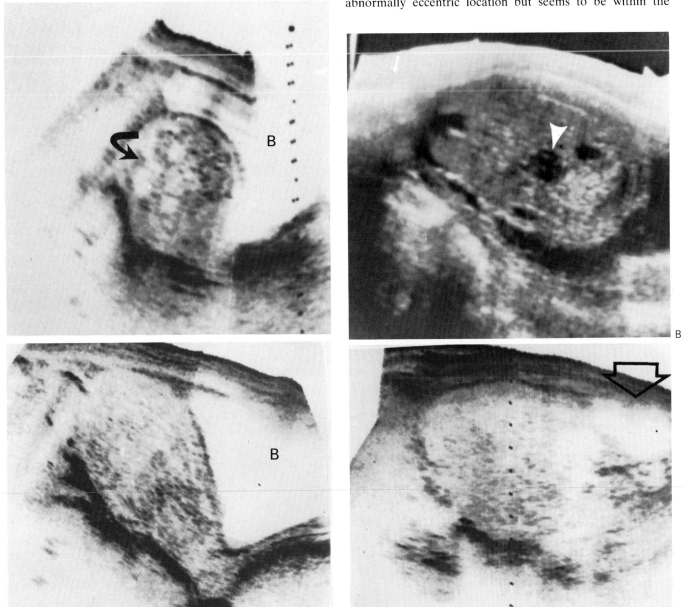

Fig. 80.7A-D Molar pregnancies.

(A) Hydatidiform mole at 13 weeks (longitudinal static sonogram). Early molar degeneration was depicted within the uterus as irregular hypoechoic areas [arrow] within this 10 to 12 week size uterus.

*(B) Hydatidiform mole at 25 weeks (longitudinal static sonogram, white on black format). The typical vesicular appearance of haemorrhagic degeneration [arrow] are seen within this hydatidiform mole.

(C) Retained trophoblastic tissue (longitudinal static sonogram). Within this enlarged uterus is a tissue has a vesicular texture. This patient also had a theca lutein cyst in the left adnexa.

(D) Theca lutein cyst (transverse static scan). These cysts generally appear as anechoic pelvic masses (arrow). Same patient as in Fig. 80.7C.

uterine outline (Fig. 80.5E). An early intrauterine pregnancy within one horn of a bicornuate uterus could simulate an interstitial pregnancy but multiple scans of a bicornuate uterus should demonstrate the characteristic bilobulated outline.

The most common entity that may simulate the sonographic and clinical features of an ectopic pregnancy is the haemorrhagic corpus luteum cyst (Fig. 80.6A). In this condition, continued bleeding occurs within the corpus luteum producing a sonolucent or mildly echogenic adnexal mass (Fig. 80.6B). Assuming that a corpus luteum cyst is not associated with intrauterine pregnancy, one way which may differentiate from ectopic pregnancy is a pregnancy test, preferably the beta subunit of HCG assay. It has been shown however, that ectopic pregnancies may be associated with negative urinary pregnancy tests which are relatively insensitive at the lower levels of HCG production. An intrauterine pregnancy within a retroverted uterus might also simulate an ectopic pregnancy but careful sonographic examination will demonstrate that the gestational sac is within the uterus (Fig. 80.6C).

Molar pregnancy (Fig. 80.7)

Definitive diagnoses of hydatidiform molar pregnancies can be made by sonography [16]. Molar pregnancies probably result from degeneration of a blighted ovum [17]. These patients usually present with vaginal bleeding, hypertension, and a uterus that is too large for dates. Only a few patients will describe the characteristic and diagnostic passage of grape-like vesicles per vaginum. One third of these patients will have palpable adnexal cystic masses representing theca lutein cysts which enlarge under the influence of human chorionic gonadotropin (HCG) which is elaborated by the trophoblastic cells of the mole. 2% of molar pregnancies will have coexistent fetal growth. Recurrent and invasive trophoblastic disease may occur after dilatation and evacuation of the uterus for hydatidiform mole.

The characteristic hydropic villi present within molar tissue give rise to the typical sonographic pattern of multiple small sonolucencies within tissue that has a texture similar to placenta (Fig. 80.7A). Larger sonolucent areas within the molar tissue itself represent areas of haemorrhage (Fig. 80.7B). Bilateral multiloculated cysts may be present with a molar pregnancy, representing theca lutein cysts.

It may be difficult to distinguish the sonographic appearance of an early intrauterine pregnancy from early molar

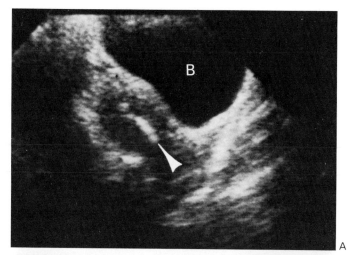

A

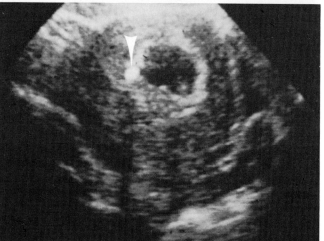

B

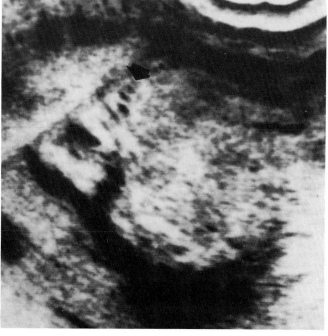

C

Fig. 80.8A-C Sonographic features of intrauterine contraceptive devices.
*(A) Normal appearance of copper-7 device within the uterus (longitudinal real-time sonogram). The metal around the shaft of the copper-7 device is echogenic [arrow]. The IUCD is in normal position within the lumen of the fundic portion of the uterus.
*(B) 8 week intrauterine pregnancy with intrauterine contraceptive device (longitudinal real-time sonogram). Cephalic to this gestational sac is an echogenic focus [arrow] with distal shadowing corresponding to the copper-7 intrauterine device.
(C) Lippes loop imbedded within the uterus (transverse static sonogram). The multiple interfaces of the Lippes loop (arrow) can be identified within the wall of the uterus.

pregnancy [18] due to the variable extent of thickening of the surrounding uterine tissue in normal pregnancy. It has been reported that the gestational sac contents will not be as distinct in an early molar pregnancy as in an early normal intrauterine pregnancy in the first trimester period (Fig. 80.7A) [18].

If the overall texture of the intrauterine contents suggests the presence of a hydatidiform mole, the rest of the intraluminal contents should be examined for a concomitant second gestational sac or fetus. The prognosis for completing to term a pregnancy with a fetus coexistent with hydatidiform mole is usually poor due to the frequent complication of severe eclampsia.

Retained trophoblastic tissue produces textural abnormalities within the uterus (Fig. 80.7C). Retained molar tissue appears as an overall echogenic pattern that has multiple small sonolucencies within it. Retained, recurrent, or invasive disease may be associated with the presence of theca lutein cysts (Fig. 80.7D). Serial sonographic examinations should be combined with serial radioimmunoassay of HCG for monitoring of the response of recurrent or invasive trophoblastic disease to therapeutic measures [19].

Pregnancy with IUCDs (Fig. 80.8)

Sonography can detect pregnancies that occur when an intrauterine contraceptive device is in place (Fig. 80.8B). The IUCD is usually peripheral to the developing gestational sac. Except for the 'Progestosert' which does not contain any metallic wire, most metallic IUCDs can be identified by their highly echogenic appearance (Fig. 80.8A). The IUCD within an intrauterine pregnancy may be difficult to identify and a pelvic radiograph may be necessary. Sonographic examination has a higher likelihood of identifying an IUCD within the uterine lumen but can occasionally locate the IUCD that is imbedded within the uterine wall or is intraperitoneal (Fig. 80.8C). The presence of an IUCD does not always result in early termination of the pregnancy.

SECOND TRIMESTER

There are certain obstetric disorders that usually become manifest clinically during the second trimester. Those that are particularly amenable to sonographic evaluation include placental localization prior to amniocentesis, evaluation of pelvic masses that occur with pregnancy, evaluation for intrauterine growth retardation, detection of some structural anomalies of the fetus and evaluation of patients who are too large for dates.

Normal features and scanning techniques

In the second trimester pregnancy, the uterus has enlarged to displace gas-containing bowel loops out of the pelvis.

Therefore, in a patient without a history of uterine bleeding, the examination can be performed with only a moderately distended urinary bladder. If a low lying placenta is detected on initial scans, re-examination can be performed once the bladder is fully distended.

Since the uterus is larger in the second trimester, it can be easily examined using either linear array or mechanical sector real-time scanners. For evaluation of the patient for suspected fetal anomalies, placental localization, pelvic masses, or a patient who is too large for dates, we prefer a series of static images to accompany real-time sonography since this allows for complete documentation of the location of the placenta as well as the tomographic anatomy of the fetus.

Placental localization prior to amniocentesis
(Fig. 80.9)

Localization of the placenta becomes important before amniocentesis. Amniocentesis for detection of fetal abnormalities is ideally performed between 16 and 19 weeks since it takes up to 4 weeks for successful culturing of fibroblasts derived from amniotic fluid for analysis of chromosomal composition. We prefer a series of static images for precise localization of the position of the placenta and fetus, which is very helpful prior to amniocentesis.

At our institution, amniocentesis is frequently performed in the second trimester for genetic evaluation, as well as the detection of amnionitis in patients with premature rupture of membranes. In most cases, the location of the fetus as well as the umbilical cord can be determined by static and real-time sonography. The site for amniocentesis should be away from areas of umbilical cord insertion, thick portions of the placenta, or the fetus. The umbilical cord appears as a series of parallel echogenic interfaces which is suspended within the amniotic fluid. Occasionally the vein and two arteries which comprise the normal umbilical cord can be resolved. 1% of singleton pregnancies will have a cord with a single artery. Of these, 15% have a congenital anomaly. 6% of twin gestations will have a single artery cord. Therefore, sonographic examination of the umbilical cord may be helpful in the in utero evaluation for fetal anomalies.

Precise localization of the placenta is imperative in patients who bleed in the late second trimester. Placental bleeding that occurs during this period is most commonly a result of separation of the placenta from the myometrium, either due to partial abruption, or to displacement of the placenta due to changes in configuration of the uterus and particularly the lower uterine segment. Hypoechoic areas may be encountered behind the placenta, usually representing areas of 'unstretched' uterus, since they typically are not present on repeat scans after 20 to 30 minutes (Fig. 80.9A) [20]. Retroplacental haematomas produce bulging of the chorionic plate (Fig. 80.9B) [21].

Over distension of the bladder may displace an anteriorly located placenta to simulate the findings of a placenta praevia (Figs. 80.9C & D) [22]. We therefore suggest re-evaluating these patients after partial bladder voiding. Real-

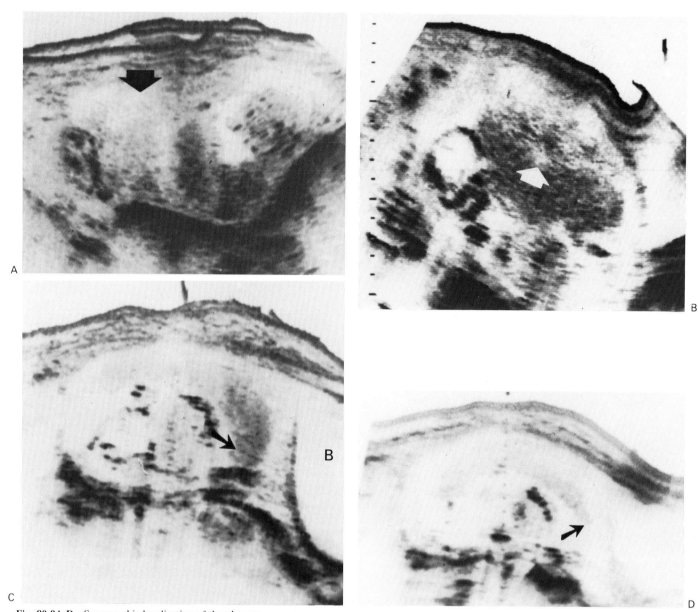

Fig. 80.9A-D   Sonographic localization of the placenta.

(A) The placenta at 16 weeks of pregnancy (transverse static sonogram). At this stage in pregnancy, the placenta is echogenic. To the right of the placenta is an unsoftened portion of the uterus [arrow] which is frequently encountered during the second trimester of pregnancy.

(B) Retroplacental haematoma (longitudinal static sonogram). This patient experienced an episode of blunt abdominal trauma and bleeding. There is bulging of the chorionic plate in an area of moderate echogenicity corresponding to a retroplacental haematoma [arrow].

(C) Effect of various degrees of bladder distension on placenta localization (longitudinal static sonogram). When the bladder is fully distended, this anterior placenta appears to lie in the region of the internal cervical os.

(D) Same patient as in 80.9C. After voiding, this anterior placenta does not extend into the region of the internal cervical os.

time sonography is helpful to locate the precise region of the internal cervical os relative to the placenta (see later).

Multiple gestation (Fig. 80.10)

Sonography can determine the number of developing embryos or fetuses as early as 5 to 6 weeks (Fig. 80.10A). It has been observed that 5 to 10% of pregnancies begin with more than one gestational sac [10,11]. Not all of these pregnancies result in delivery of more than one fetus since one of the sacs can be aborted. *Multiple gestation* occurs frequently when the patient has received hormonal ovulation induction. Many women with twin pregnancies have a familial history of twins. Twin pregnancies are also more common in the older pregnant patient. In the second trimester, the patient with a possible multiple gestation will present with a uterus too large for dates (Figs. 80.10B & C).

Hydramnios is another cause of a gravid patient with uterus too large for dates. Although maternal diabetes is one of the most common causes of hydramnios, there are some sonographically detectable fetal anomalies that can be associated with hydramnios. These include fetuses with impaired swallowing due to a brainstem dysfunction and fetuses with gastrointestinal tract obstructions from atresias. Twin pregnancy should also be considered in acute hydramnios (Fig. 80.10D).

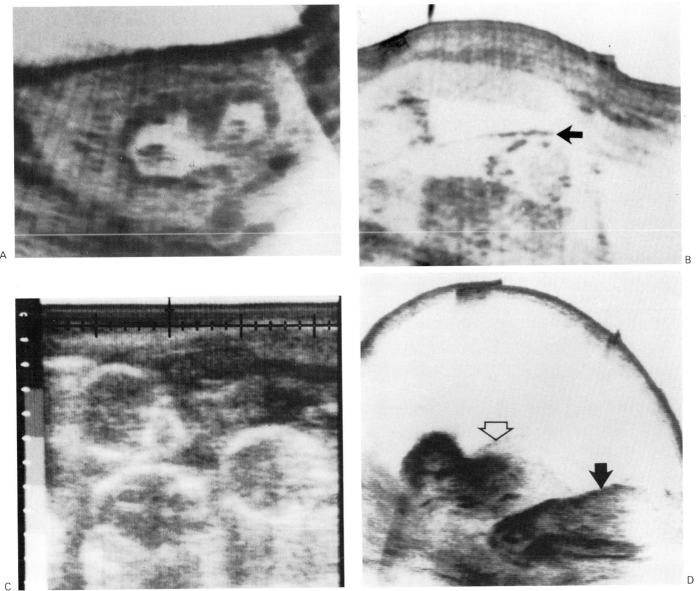

Fig. 80.10A-D Sonographic demonstration of multiple gestation.
(A) Twin pregnancy at 6 weeks (transverse static sonogram). There are two gestational sacs in the uterus at 6 weeks pregnancy.
(B) 19 week diamniotic pregnancy demonstrating presence of membrane [arrow] between two amniotic cavities (longitudinal static sonogram).
*(C) Triplet pregnancy at 19 weeks (longitudinal real-time sonogram). Three fetal heads can be identified.
(D) Hydramnios associated with twin pregnancy (longitudinal static sonogram). Marked hydramnios present within the upper [open arrow = fetus] amniotic cavity. The lower twin [solid arrow] was difficult to identify due to rupture of the amniotic cavity of this twin.

Sonographically, it is important to be aware of the two types of twin pregnancies, since certain complications are more frequent in one type. The most common type of twin pregnancy results from fertilization of two zygotes (dizygotic). *Dizygotic twinning* is more common in older pregnant patients and always results in the formation of two separate amniotic cavities. *Monozygotic twinning* is not as common as dizygotic: there is a possibility of both fetuses forming in only one amniotic sac, which may be associated with umbilical cord torsion. It is, therefore, important to establish the presence of a membrane covering both fetuses (Fig. 80.10B) by sonography or amniography (see Fig. 80.22).

In twin gestation, one fetus may have more placental blood supply than the other. The fetus whose placental supply is disproportionately large can become polycythaemic while the other fetus becomes anaemic. Hydramnios may be present in the amniotic cavity of the polycythaemic fetus.

Fetuses of twin or multiple pregnancies are usually smaller in size than their singleton counterparts. Therefore, we use a different BPD chart for estimation of their gestational duration in the third trimester [23].

Pelvic masses occurring during pregnancy
(Fig. 80.11)

The presence of a pelvic mass associated with pregnancy may first become clinically evident during the second trimester

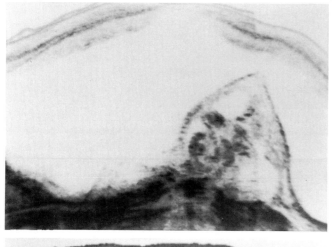

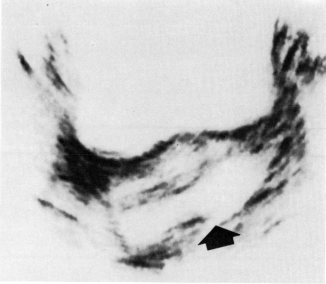

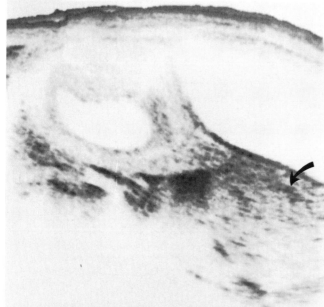

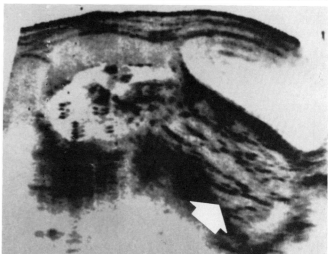

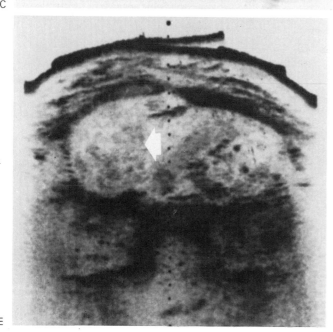

Fig. 80.11A-E Sonographic appearances of pelvic mass occuring during intrauterine pregnancy.

(A) Large paraovarian cyst associated with second trimester pregnancy (longitudinal static sonogram). There is a huge cystic mass superior to the fundus of the uterus. This was successfully excised during second trimester.

(B) Paraovarian cyst occuring during second trimester of pregnancy (transverse static sonogram). This fusiform cystic mass [arrow] also represents a paraovarian cyst.

(C) Dermoid cyst occuring during second trimester of pregnancy (longitudinal static sonogram). Dermoid cyst [arrow] demonstrated moderate echogenicity and was located posterior to the lower uterine segment.

(D) Cystadenoma associated with second trimester of pregnancy (longitudinal static sonogram). The sonographic appearance of this multiloculated mass [arrow] allowed its specific characterization as a cystadenoma.

(E) Leiomyoma associated with second trimester pregnancy (transverse static sonogram). This moderately echogenic fibroid [arrow] was contiguous with the wall of the uterus.

when it is displaced out of the pelvis by the enlarging uterus. This is particularly true with pelvic masses that are on a pedicle, e.g. a pedunculated dermoid cyst. However in our experience, dermoid cysts associated with pregnancy tend to be posterior to the lower uterine segment (Fig. 80.11C).

Masses that may be encountered during the second trimester include the *corpus luteum cyst* of pregnancy, *uterine leiomyoma*, and *demoid cysts* (Table 80.5). It is

Table 80.5 Sonographic features of some common pelvic masses occurring during pregnancy

Mass	Sonographic features
Uterine	
Leiomyoma	Variable echogenicity depending on composition, type of degeneration
Extrauterine	
Dermoid cyst	Cystic to complex appearance, depending upon composition
Cystadenoma	Unilocular or septated
Corpus luteum cyst	Sonolucent, echogenic if contains organized clot
Theca lutein cyst	Multilocular, bilateral; associated with hydatidiform mole
Para-ovarian cyst	Sonolucent adnexal mass
Other	
Pelvic kidney	Reniform configuration

important to establish the origin of the pelvic mass as well as its size or enlargement during this period of pregnancy. In general, masses larger than 5 cm should be followed sonographically for possible enlargement. Another important factor is its mobility or fixation within the pelvis. A mass that is fixed in proximity to the lower uterine segment may rupture during labour and/or may obstruct the progress of labour. In the rare case of a malignant mass encountered during pregnancy, it is important to assess the presence or absence of associated findings such as maternal ascites. Maternal ascites may however be encountered without an associated pelvic mass, as in severe maternal toxaemia.

Indications for surgical removal of a pelvic mass during pregnancy include significant enlargement of the pelvic mass, intractable pain, or the possibility of obstruction of labour. The preferred time for surgical removal of such a pelvic mass is in the second trimester since this has the least likelihood of premature labour or untoward effects of the pregnancy itself.

Corpus luteum cysts of pregnancy are pelvic masses that are encountered in up to a third of normal, uncomplicated pregnancies. These cysts enlarge from remnants of the corpus luteum but usually regress after 16 to 18 weeks when the production of HCG gradually decreases. They appear as anechoic or mildly echogenic adnexal masses.

Other cystic masses that may simulate the sonographic appearance of a corpus luteum cyst include *paraovarian cysts* (Figs. 80.11A & B) and some cystic ovarian tumours such as *dermoid cysts* and *cystadenomas* (Fig. 80.11C). Cystadenomas are predominantly cystic masses and usually contain several thin internal septa (Fig. 80.11D). Those occurring in pregnancy have similar characteristics as in the nongravid patient (Fig. 80.11D). Serous cystadenomas tend to be unilocular, whereas mucinous cystadenomas tend to be septated. *Paraovarian cysts* arise from the meso-ovarium adjacent to the

ovary from the remnant of Gartner's duct. They appear as cystic, oblong-shaped masses which originate from the adnexa (Figs. 80.11A & B).

Complex masses that can be encountered in pregnancy include dermoid cysts and septated cystic *ovarian epithelial tumours*. Dermoid cysts demonstrate a spectrum of sonographic findings ranging from completely anechoic to markedly echogenic. In our experience, the most common sonographic appearance of a dermoid cyst is a homogeneously hyperechoic mass (Fig. 80.11C). Dermoid cysts arise from the ovary and are commonly located superior to the uterine fundus but may lie posterior to the lower uterine segment (Fig. 80.11C). Dermoid cysts are often pedunculated, and may undergo torsion, producing abdominal pain.

Solid masses associated with pregnancy are most commonly uterine *leiomyomas* (fibroids). Leiomyomas also have a spectrum of sonographic appearances ranging from relatively hypoechoic masses to moderately echogenic masses with areas of high level echoes corresponding to areas of calcification (Fig. 80.11E). Early in the second trimester, leiomyomas have similar sonographic features to the unsoftened portion of the uterus since most uterine leiomyomas are intramural. Leiomyomas often enlarge during pregnancy presumably due to the high levels of oestrogen production. They may exhibit areas of hyaline and cystic degeneration which appear as irregular anechoic areas within the masses. Their sonographic texture probably depends on the relative amount of smooth muscle and connective tissue within the tumour as well as their vascularity. The vascular masses tend to be more hyperechoic.

Intrauterine growth retardation (IUGR)
(Fig. 80.12)

Detection of fetal growth retardation depends on an understanding of normal growth patterns. Measurements of the circumference of the fetal head and abdomen have proved useful and are best obtained by tracing the perimeter using a light pen or digitizing tablet [24]. Nomograms for the normal abdominal circumference are available [25,26]. Linear measurements of the abdomen are simpler to perform but are less accurate (Fig. 80.12A).

The detection of growth retardation is clinically important for several reasons. The growth retarded fetus has a higher incidence of fetal distress during labour as well as neonatal complications such as hypoglycaemia, hypocalcaemia, and failure to thrive. Long-term follow up of these individuals has suggested their overall learning ability may also be impaired.

Intrauterine growth retardation is usually of two basic types. The more common type *asymmetrical growth retardation* (or 'head spared' growth retardation) is most commonly the result of uteroplacental insufficiency, which may be associated with a variety of maternal disorders such as pregnancy induced hypertension and severe diabetes and the postmature syndrome (Fig. 80.12C). In these growth retarded babies, the fetal liver is small and subcutaneous fat is markedly reduced (Fig. 80.12B).

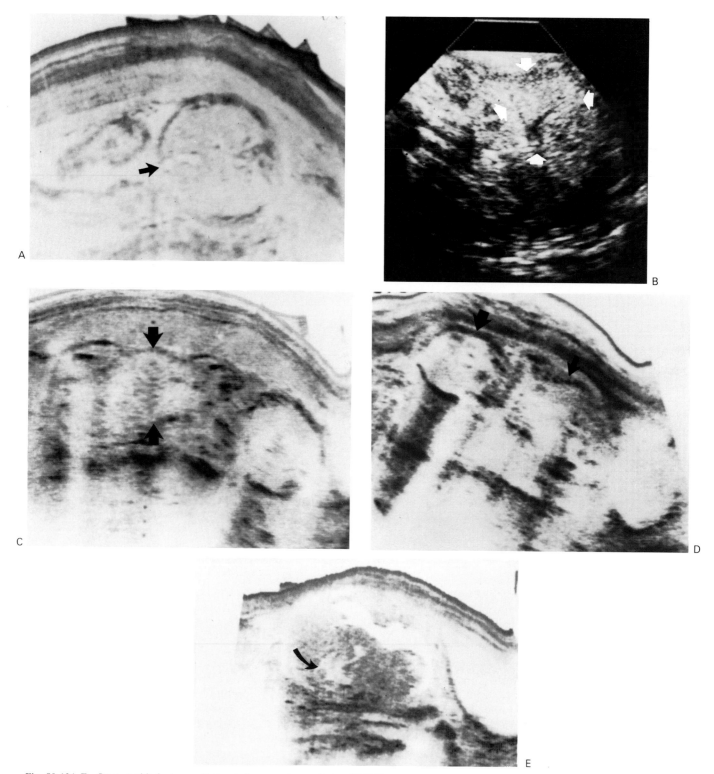

Fig. 80.12A-E   Sonographic features of intrauterine growth retardation (IUGR).

(A) Measurement of the abdominal circumference (transverse sonogram obtained through the level of the mid abdomen of the fetus). Measurement of the abdominal circumference should be made at the level of the short segment of the umbilical vein [arrow].

*(B) Normal fetal liver at 25 weeks (coronal scan obtained through fetal liver). The fetal liver [outlined by arrows] can be identified on this scan obtained in a coronal section through the fetus.

(C) Asymmetrical intrauterine growth retardation (longitudinal static sonogram). The fetal body was much smaller than the fetal head. This patient was on medication for heart disease.

(D) Symmetrical growth retardation associated with microcephaly (longitudinal sonogram). Both fetal head and body [arrows] are reduced in size.

(E) Premature senescence of the placenta associated with intrauterine growth retardation (longitudinal sonogram). There is a large area of hydropic degeneration [arrow] within the placenta. The fetus was born growth retarded.

On the other hand, *symmetrically growth retarded* babies have a higher incidence of congenital defects (Fig. 80.12D) such as those due to chromosomal abnormalities [23,27]. It is thought that their growth derangement occurs early in pregnancy and leads to overall reduction in body weight and organ size.

The controversy over which sonographic parameters to use to detect intrauterine growth retardation reflects the complexity of this disorder. Measurement of total intrauterine volume has been advocated by some groups as an accurate parameter to detect intrauterine growth retardation [28]. Total intrauterine volume (TIUV) is obtained by measuring the long axis of the uterus from the bladder dome to the fundus, the greatest transverse dimension of the uterus and the anteroposterior dimension of the uterus through the plane that is perpendicular to the greatest transverse dimension. These dimensions are multiplied by 0.523, as the geometric approximation of the uterus is the prolate ellipsoid. Since the total intrauterine volume reflects fetal size, placental volume and the amount of amniotic fluid, it is a nonspecific measurement. This is particularly evident in the patients with oligohydramnios who have a reduced overall amount of amniotic fluid but do not necessarily have a growth retarded fetus [28,29].

Since the amount of subcutaneous fat and the liver size is always below normal in asymmetrical growth retarded fetuses, we advocate precise measurement of the fetus itself in attempts to detect IUGR. The abdominal circumference is measured on scans taken at the level of the long segment of the umbilical vein. It is an anatomical parameter of fetal weight and can be charted according to percentile group [26]. The growth retarded fetus will have an abnormally low fetal weight compared to menstrual age as determined by patient dates or by biparietal diameter.

In the symmetrically growth retarded fetus, however, both head size and body size may be diminished. Therefore, the assessment of gestational age and weight by biparietal dimension can be misleading. Reduction of head size may also occur in microcephaly (Fig. 80.12D) but head size is markedly reduced compared to body size in true microcephaly [31].

Pathological examination in growth retardation has demonstrated that the placenta is usually diminished in volume and may demonstrate areas of thrombosis and/or infarction (Fig. 80.12E). Therefore, the presence of extensive degenerative changes in the placenta occurring in the late second trimester or early third trimester should be considered abnormal, and coupled with a small-for-dates fetus, should be taken as highly suggestive of intrauterine growth retardation.

Structural anomalies of the fetus that can be detected in the second trimester

Detection of structural abnormalities of the fetus has implications not only for the parents and fetus but for the obstetrician [32,33]. The management of the patient and fetus once a congenital defect is identified by sonography is influenced by medical and legal restrictions. In most cases, even when a congenital anomaly is detected, the therapeutic alternatives are limited to either conservative management or termination of pregnancy. Therefore, it is quite important to be able to identify certain congenital anomalies by sonography prior to 24 weeks' gestation. With the resolution of currently available scanners, it may be difficult definitively to diagnose some fetal anomalies at this stage. Once an anomaly is detected, it may be difficult to assess confidently the degree of functional impairment by sonography. For example, even though moderate to severe cerebral ventricular dilatation is detected in utero, some of these hydrocephalic fetuses may have near normal sized ventricles if successfully treated ex utero [34].

Evaluation of the parents who have had a genetically malformed fetus with a definable chromosomal defect includes amniocentesis and analysis of chromosomes obtained by fibroblast cell culture. Other biochemical substances such as alpha fetoprotein can also be analysed from amniotic fluid samples. Detection of fetal anomalies also becomes important during the third trimester and has immediate implications concerning the optimal mode of delivery of the defective fetus.

One of the most common congenital anomalies that the ultrasonographer may be asked to evaluate is that of a neural tube defect. *Neural tube defect* is a general term describing abnormalities arising from the neural axis, including cranial malformations such as *anencephaly*, and in the spine and central nervous system, such as *spina bifida* and *meningomyelocele*. Most commonly, these patients will present for sonographic evaluation and amniocentesis due to an elevated serum alpha fetoprotein level, hydramnios or with a history of a previously affected fetus.

Maternal serum and amniotic fluid samples will be obtained for quantification of alpha fetoprotein. It is exceedingly important to assess accurately the gestational age by biparietal diameter since the range of normal values of alpha fetoprotein depends on gestational age. The neural tube defect must be 'open' or communicating with the amniotic fluid for the alpha fetoprotein to be elevated. Elevation of alpha fetoprotein may be encountered in several other conditions including fetomaternal blood admixture during amniocentesis, twin gestation, intrauterine fetal demise, gastrochisis or omphalocele and, rarely, congenital nephrosis (Table 80.6). Sonography has an important role in

Table 80.6 Causes of elevated amniotic fluid alpha fetoprotein

Craniospinal defect (open neural tube defect)
Omphalocele
Gastrochisis
Duodenal atresia
Congenital nephrosis
Cystic hygroma (Turner's syndrome)
Unbalanced D/G dislocation
Pilonidal sinus
Rh disease
Fetal demise
Incorrect dates
Multiple pregnancy

differentiating these entities from one another once the patient is shown to have an elevated alpha fetoprotein level. Additional specificity of neural tube defects with alpha

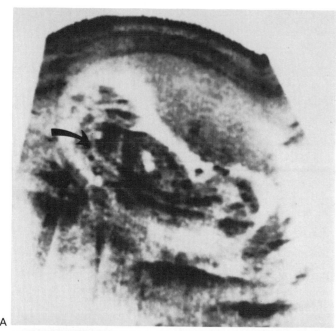

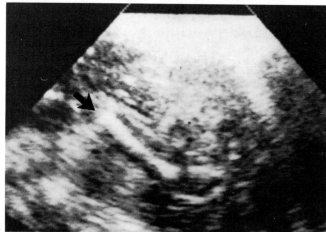

Fig. 80.13A & B Sonographic features of normal second trimester fetus. (A) Normal fetal spine (static sonogram obtained down long axis of fetal spine). Echogenic interfaces are noted to arise from the pedicles of the fetal spine [arrow]. Very minimal flaring is noted of the row of echogenicities noted in the cervical and lumbosacral region (black on white format).

*(B) Normal femur at 20 weeks (real-time sonography). Sonography can be utilized to measure the fetal osseous structures such as femur [arrow]. (white on black format)

fetoprotein can be obtained utilizing an assay for acetylcholinesterase.

Real-time sonography can be used for evaluation of the spine of the fetus during the second trimester. The normal spine appears as a parallel row of echogenic interfaces (Fig. 80.13A), each arising from a pedicle of a vertebral body. Very slight flaring (1 to 2 mm) can be detected as normal in the region of the cervical spine and in the lumbosacral area. Excessive separation of the echogenic interfaces arising from the pedicles may be an indication of spinal dysraphism and meningomyelocele (Fig. 80.14A). If the meninges and nerves are contained within a cystic space, a sonolucent structure protruding from the back will be observed (Fig. 80.14F).

The most common location for a meningomyelocele is in the lumbosacral area (see Fig. 80.18C). Once a meningomyelocele is suspected, the ventricular system of the fetal head should be closely evaluated for possible hydrocephalus. In our experience, however, severe hydrocephalus that is associated with a meningomyelocele may be difficult to distinguish from the normally prominent lateral ventricles in a fetus prior to the third trimester (see p. 1583–1584 and Table 80.8).

Cystic hygromas typically arise from the posterior aspect of the neck and could mimic a cervical meningomyelocele (Fig. 80.14F) but cystic hygroma is usually a component of widespread lymphatic dysplasia with abdominal lymphangiectasia and ascites.

Anencephaly describes severe underdevelopment of the cranium and malformation of the fetal brain. Although the base of the cranium is usually formed, the brain may be exposed (Fig. 80.14B). This condition can be associated with an excessive amount of amniotic fluid since in the later stages of pregnancy, the fetal swallowing mechanism is thought to be impaired due to midbrain dysfunction. Not all anencephalic fetuses will be associated with hydramnios. Amniography can be used to confirm the sonographic impression of anencephaly or an encephalocele (Figs. 80.14C & 80.25).

Less severe forms of fetal cranial malformation such as *microcephaly* may be difficult to diagnose since the configuration of the head may be normal but only small in size relative to the estimated gestational age or fetal body size. Microcephaly is very difficult to distinguish from symmetrical growth retardation (Fig. 80.12D) but in most cases of microcephaly, a significant discrepancy can be detected between the fetal body and the small head, and the BPD is much less than expected by dates.

Another abnormality that may be present in the second trimester is *oligohydramnios* associated with *renal agenesis* of the fetus (Fig. 80.14D). In most fetuses, the kidneys can be identified late in the second trimester [37]. In complete renal agenesis, the fetal kidneys and bladder cannot be detected but, with partial development of the fetal kidneys, there may be a small quantity of urine which partially distends the urinary bladder [36]. Relative to the kidneys, the adrenals of the fetus are large compared to the adult and may simulate the sonographic appearance of the fetal kidneys (see Fig. 80.15A).

Distension of the renal collecting system, ureter or bladder can be identified by sonography from the late second trimester. A male fetus with distended urinary bladder, hydroureter and hydronephrosis should be suspected of having posterior ureteral valves. If only moderate distension is present and a normal amount of amniotic fluid is seen, this condition may be treatable in utero [33,37], but if associated with oligohydramnios, severe lung hypoplasia is usually present. Bilateral massive hydroureters may also be encountered in the *prune-belly syndrome.*

Cystic abdominal masses arising from the kidneys or other abdominal organs such as the liver or mesentery can also be detected (Fig. 80.14E). These masses may be so large as to make determination of their organ of origin difficult by prenatal sonography.

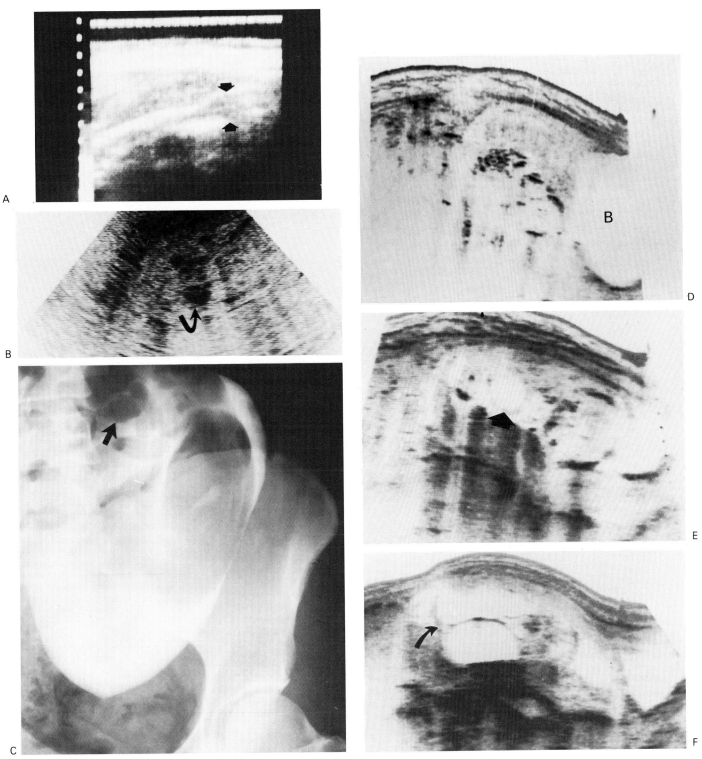

Fig. 80.14A & B Fetal anomalies that can be detected sonographically

(A) Lumbar meningomyelocele (real-time sonogram taken from videotape down long axis of fetal spine). There is abnormal bulging in the lumbosacral region [arrow]. This corresponds to a lumbar meningomyelocele. The amniotic fluid alpha-fetoprotein was markedly abnormal.

(B) Encephalocele at 22 weeks (real-time sonogram). There is maldevelopment of the fetal cranium (arrow) in this 22 week fetus.

(C) Fetoamniogram of same patient demonstrating encephalocele [arrow] and maldevelopment of fetal head.

(D) Renal agenesis (longitudinal static sonogram). There is marked oligohydramnios associated with renal agenesis.

(E) Hepatic cyst in 21 week fetus (longitudinal static sonogram). There is a large cyst [arrow] which occupies the majority of the fetal abdomen which corresponds to a hepatic cyst.

(F) Cystic hygroma (longitudinal static sonogram). There is a cystic mass [arrow] arising from the posterior aspect of the neck which represented a collection of lymphatic fluid.

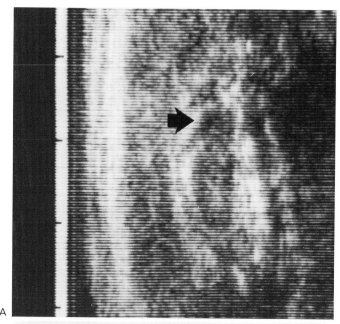

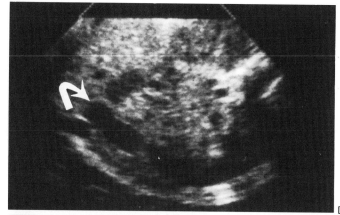

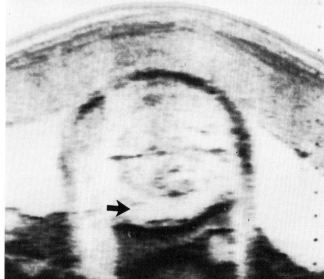

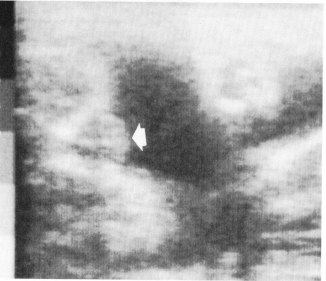

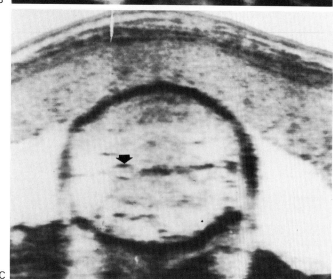

Fig. 80.15A-E Normal sonographic features of third trimester fetus.

*(A) Fetal kidney and adrenal at 32 weeks (real-time sonography obtained along coronal section of the fetus). The fetal kidney and adrenal [arrow] are identified. The fetal adrenal is 30 to 40% the size of the fetal kidney at this stage in development.

(B) Sonolucent area of brain parenchyma of 32 week fetus (transverse static sonogram). A sonolucent area of brain parenchyma [arrow] is frequently identified in fetuses in this stage of development probably due to the non-myelinated brain normally seen at this stage in development.

(C) Normal fetal head demonstrating trunk of corpus callosum (transverse sonogram). The trunk of the corpus callosum [arrow] can be identified by two parallel echogenic interfaces in the anterior aspect of the fetal brain.

*(D) Fetal large bowel (transverse real-time sonography). Since the fetus swallows amniotic fluid in utero, the fetal bowel can be readily identified [arrow].

(E) Fetal scrotum (longitudinal sonogram). The fetal scrotum [arrow] can be identified between the legs in male fetuses particularly when surrounded by amniotic fluid.

THIRD TRIMESTER

Sonography is most important in the evaluation of those patients with bleeding for the first time during the third trimester as well as in the detection of some structural fetal anomalies that may impede labour and delivery.

Normal features and scanning techniques
(Fig. 80.15)

Most patients in the third trimester can be examined sonographically utilizing a moderately distended bladder, but in suspected placenta praevia a fully distended bladder is imperative.

We prefer a combination of both static and real-time evaluation of the patient in the third trimester. Static imaging allows overall documentation of the location of the placenta and fetus, whereas real-time scanning can be used for closer examination of particular areas of interest.

By the third trimester of pregnancy, many of the major viscera of the fetus can be routinely identified. The fetal kidneys can be delineated to either side of the aorta and inferior vena cava. The fetal urinary bladder is usually apparent, particularly when the mother ingests water to distend the urinary bladder prior to her sonographic examination. Since the fetus swallows amniotic fluid, the stomach and a few loops of bowel can be identified as sonolucent tubular structures that demonstrate configurational changes corresponding to peristaltic contractions (Fig. 80.15D). The cardiac chambers and valves are readily apparent on real-time examination and pulsation of some of the major intracranial arteries may be identified.

The placenta may exhibit sonographic features which correspond to maturational changes. These include sonolucent areas near the chorionic plate resulting from fibrin deposition, irregular sonolucent areas within the midportion of the placenta corresponding to areas of hydropic degeneration, and echogenic interfaces arising from the basal plate and septa that occur with calcification. As discussed earlier, the pathophysiological significance of these changes remains unsettled since they are frequently encountered in uncomplicated pregnancies near term.

As the pregnancy approaches term, the uterus assumes a more globular shape. When the fetal head engages within the lower uterine segment, ballooning of this portion of the uterus can be observed. Within the amniotic fluid, low level echoes that tend to collect in the dependent portion of the amniotic cavity can be observed arising from fetal vernix, or desquamated skin, another sonographic sign of a near term pregnancy.

Placenta praevia and placental abruption
(Fig. 80.16)

One of the most important applications of sonography is in the detection of a placenta praevia prior to the onset of labour. Because the placenta and myometrium are so richly perfused during the second and third trimesters, short periods of bleeding may have drastic implications for both fetus and mother. Most commonly, the mother experiences only a limited amount of bleeding initially. Placenta praevia is most commonly encountered in patients with numerous previous pregnancies and history of previous Caesarian section or induced abortion [39]. It has been proposed that the placenta praevia occurs as a result of abnormal attachment of the placenta in the lower uterine segment and failure of it to ascend with uterine fundic growth and the thinning of the lower uterine segment that occurs in the late second and early third trimester [40].

It is of the utmost importance to document the location of the placenta relative to the lower uterine segment and the approximate area of the endocervical canal [41]. We classify the abnormally low location of the placenta into (a) the *low lying* placenta which extends into the lower uterine segment but not near the internal cervical os; (b) the *partial* or *marginal* placenta praevia, which appears to extend to, but not entirely cover the internal cervical os region; and (c) the *complete placenta praevia* which covers the entire area of the lower uterine segment (Fig. 80.16A).

The exact location of the lower extent of the placenta can be determined by real-time scanning after a series of static images. Although the initial examination of the patient with a placenta praevia should occur with a distended bladder, over distension of the bladder may compress the normal anteriorly located placenta and create a sonographic appearance similar to placenta praevia as the lower uterine segment is displaced toward the internal cervical os [41]. For this reason, we examine most patients who appear to have a low lying placenta on initial scans, both with a distended bladder and also with a partially distended bladder (see Figs. 80.9C & 80.9D).

Areas of *placental abruption* may appear as sonolucent regions if the blood is unclotted, and mildly echogenic regions if organization of the blood has occurred (Fig. 80.16C). Placental abruption may occur secondary to abdominal trauma. Small areas of abruption can be detected in patients with placenta praevia as sonolucent areas along the periphery of the placenta. Areas of placental abruption have a different appearance from the normal vasculature that occurs along the basal plate side of the placenta. The veins in the decidua basalis and myometrium appear as tubular structures as opposed to areas of abruption which may be diffusely sonolucent or moderately echogenic, depending on the state of organization of blood (Fig. 80.16C) [42].

Slight degrees of placental abruption along the edge of the placenta may be present in normal pregnancies and have little or no obstetric consequence. The patient with more extensive placental abruption (40 to 50% of the basal plate surface of the placenta) usually presents a tender and contracted uterus. Placental abruption may extend down into the lower uterine segment and cause uterine bleeding, or may be confined to the retroplacental area and not be associated with bleeding.

The fetus should be examined closely under real-time scanning in those patients where placental abruption is suspected. Since real-time devices can detect abnormally slow fetal

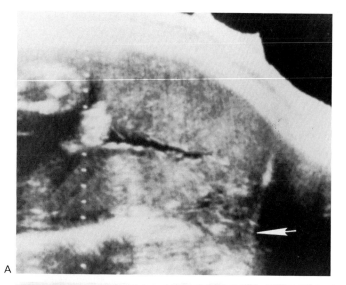

A

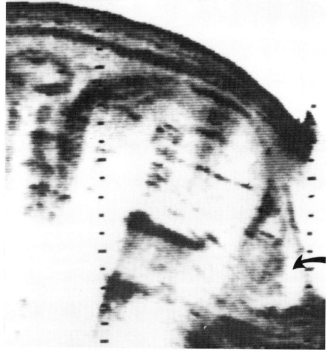

B

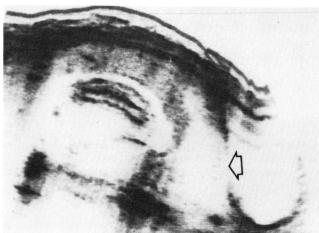

C

Fig. 80.16A-C Sonographic feature of placenta praevia and placental abruption.

*(A) Complete placenta praevia (longitudinal static sonogram white on black format). Sonolucent areas correspond to haemorrhage [arrow]. The placenta covers the entire area of the internal cervical os.

(B) Partial placenta praevia (longitudinal static sonogram). The placenta extends over the internal cervical os. A marginal sinus rupture [arrow] is also present.

(C) Placental abruption (longitudinal static sonogram). There is a sonolucent area [open arrow] between the placenta and uterine wall representing an area of placental abruption.

heart rate or a distressed fetus by a lack of fetal breathing motion, movement and tone, it is an important modality for assessment of fetal condition.

The management of patients with placental abruption is critical since acute placental abruptions may lead to disseminated intravascular coagulation in the mother and also to fetal death. Fetal death can be detected by lack of fetal heart motion on real-time scanning (Fig. 80.17A). When death has been present for 1 to 2 weeks, there usually is oligohydramnios, overlapping of fetal sutures (Spalding's sign) and oedema of soft tissue (Figs. 80.17B & C). Oligohydramnios is probably the result of a cessation of amniotic fluid production by the fetal kidney.

Fetal anomalies detectable in the third trimester

Sonographic detection of the fetal anomaly affects decisions concerning the optimal time and mode of delivery of the fetus. Surgical intervention of the malformed fetus in utero may be limited due to the inability to stop labour which may be precipitated by the procedure itself. The presence and extent of structural anomalies should be assessed as completely as possible since it will affect the decision whether or not to subject the patient to Caesarian section. This is not a trivial decision, since there is operative risk despite which the fetus may not be salvaged.

Sonographic evaluation of the fetus should be directed toward assessment of the nature of and severity of the congenital anomaly. Management decisions can be based on

Table 80.7 Some common causes of hydramnios and oligohydramnios

Hydramnios
Idiopathic (normal variant, transient)
Maternal diabetes
Depressed fetal swallowing
   anencephaly
   hydrocephaly
   hydranencephaly
Gastrointestinal tract obstructions
   atresias (oesophageal, duodenal)
   obstruction (diaphragmatic hernia, malrotation)
Twin gestation

Oligohydramnios
Premature rupture of membranes
Pre-eclampsia, intrauterine growth retardation
Renal agenesis
Intrauterine fetal demise

whether the anomaly is potentially correctable or uniformly fatal. In most cases, this is not an easy determination since some disorders such as hydrocephalus or hydronephrosis may be reversible to some degree, even if severe.

Patients with a congenitally malformed fetus may first seek medical attention due to either a previous history of delivery of a malformed fetus or a uterus whose size is too large or too small for dates (Table 80.7).

An excessive amount of amniotic fluid (*hydramnios*) is associated with several fetal disorders, including *hydrocephaly*, *hydranencephaly*, and *anencephaly* and *gastrointestinal tract obstructions* or *atresias*. About one half of

patients with hydramnios will not have an associated fetal anomaly and hydramnios is then commonly due to maternal disorders such as diabetes. When hydramnios is encountered, one should carefully examine the uterus for twins (see Fig. 80.10D).

A diminished amount of amniotic fluid (*oligohydramnios*) is associated with fetuses that have *renal agenesis, growth retardation*, or are chronically *stressed*. It is thought that diminished blood flow to the fetal kidneys in pre-eclamptic patients may decrease the amount of amniotic fluid production leading to oligohydramnios [29]. Amniotic fluid kinetics is still an area that is incompletely understood [43].

Hydramnios is defined as greater than 1500 ml amniotic fluid in the third trimester. It can be detected as an excessive amount of amniotic fluid, allowing for easy extension of fetal extremities within the enlarged amniotic cavity. In the later stages of hydramnios, the placenta may be excessively thin

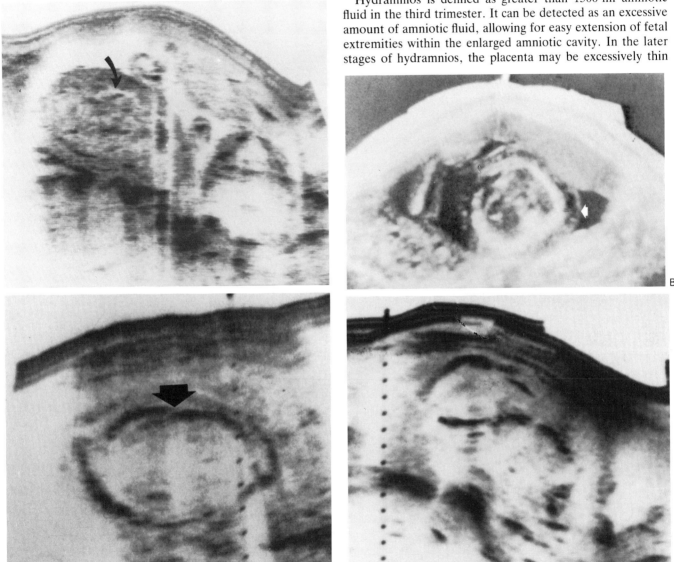

A   B

C   D

Fig. 80.17A-D Sonographic features of intrauterine fetal death.
(A) Hyperextension of the fetal head relative to the body (longitudinal static sonogram). This fetus died due to massive placental abruption [arrow]. Demise had occured within the hour of this examination.
*(B) Fetal anasarca due to intrauterine fetal demise (transverse static sonogram) [arrow].
(C) Overlapping of cranial sutures associated with fetal demise (longitudinal static sonogram). Overlapping of the cranial sutures [arrow] occurs 1 to 2 weeks after fetal demise. (Equivalent of Spalding's sign)
(D) Oligohydramnios secondary to intrauterine fetal demise (longitudinal static sonogram). There is a paucity of amniotic fluid, a result of long standing intrauterine fetal death.

(less than 2 to 3 cm). If the amount of amniotic fluid is greater than the estimated fetal volume, hydramnios may be present. Oligohydramnios, on the other hand, results in crowding of the fetus in the amniotic cavity (see Fig. 80.14D). One should be aware that the volume of amniotic fluid varies from patient to patient and in different periods of pregnancy, making difficult the sonographic definitive diagnosis of excessive or diminished amount of amniotic fluid.

Structural abnormalities of the head and spine that can be detected sonographically include *hydrocephalus, hydranencephaly, porencephaly, encephaloceles,* and *meningomyelocele* (Fig. 80.18). Measurement of the distance from the falx cerebri to the lateral aspect to the body of the lateral ventricle compared to the distance from the falx cerebri to the inner table of the skull (lateral ventricular/hemispheric width ratio index) has been used to assess the presence of

hydrocephalus in the fetus (Fig. 80.18A & Table 80.8) [44]. Early in development, however, the fetal lateral ventricles and choroid plexuses are prominent (See Fig. 80.1F). In the late second and third trimesters the lateral ventricles should not be clearly outlinable unless they are dilated. Sonolucent areas within the fetal brain are usually the result of brain infarction and liquefaction. One should also be aware that a sonolucent band of the parenchyma along the periphery of the brain may be present, which represents areas of non-myelinated brain. (see Figs. 80.15B & C).

Hydranencephaly is thought to be the result of complete occlusion of the carotid arteries. If only a portion of the brain

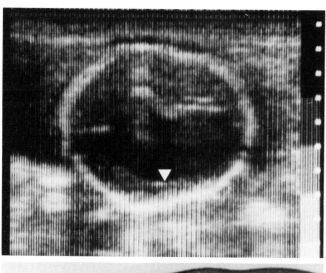

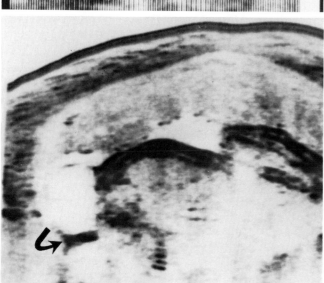

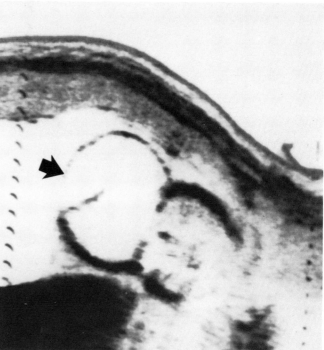

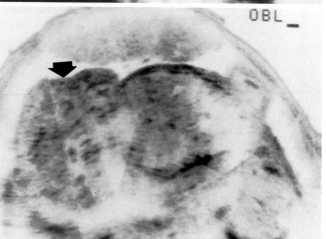

Fig. 80.18A-D Sonographic appearance of fetal anomalies which may be encountered during third trimester

(A) Hydrocephalus (transverse real-time sonogram). There is marked dilatation of the lateral ventricles of the fetus with only 5 mm of brain parenchyma [arrow head] remaining.

(B) Encephalocele (longitudinal static sonogram). There is a cystic mass protruding from the posterior aspect of the cranium [arrow]. On real-time scanning, it was shown that a portion of the fetal brain was contained within this cystic mass.

(C) Meningomyelocele (longitudinal static sonogram). There is a cystic mass [arrow] along the posterior aspect of the fetal spine corresponding to a large meningomyelocele.

(D) Sacrococcygeal teratoma (longitudinal static sonogram). There is a large solid mass [arrow] extending along the posterior aspect of the sacrum in this fetus. This corresponded to a large sacrococcygeal teratoma [arrow].

is affected, *porencephalic* regions may develop. Extensive ventricular dilatation in the fetus is most commonly associated with Chiari malformation associated with a meningomyelocele or aqueduct stenosis but can also be observed in fetuses with viral infection of the brain. Discontinuity in the skull and herniation of brain tissue can be detected in patients with encephaloceles (Fig. 80.18B).

Real-time sonography is helpful in detailed evaluation of fetal brain [45]. The sonolucent brain mantle seen in the third trimester as the result of highly cellular and proliferative brain cortex can be clearly distinguished from enlarged lateral ventricles (see Figs. 80.15B & C). Two short parallel echogenic interfaces may be present in the anterior aspect of the midline corresponding to the trunk of the corpus callosum (see Fig. 80.15C). This is distinguished from the third ventricle of the fetus which is not normally seen. One should be aware that the relative size of the ventricles compared to the brain cortex varies with brain development. The ratio of the size of the lateral ventricle to hemispheric width is a useful parameter to assess ventricular size. This ratio can be determined when the brain is imaged in an axial plane which portrays the lateral wall of the bodies of the lateral ventricle as a linear interface parallel to the falx cerebri interhemispheric fissure interfaces (Table 80.8).

Table 80.8 Lateral ventricular/hemispheric width ratio [48]

Menstrual age (weeks)	Lat. vent width (LVW) (cm)	Hemispheric width (HW) (cm)	Ratio (LVW/HW) (% ± 2 S.D.)
15	0.75	1.4	56 (40–71)
16	0.86	1.5	57 (45–69)
17	0.85	1.5	52 (42–62)
18	0.83	1.8	46 (40–52)
19	–	–	–
20	0.82	1.9	43 (29–57)
21	0.76	2.2	35 (27–43)
22	0.82	2.6	32 (26–38)
23	0.83	2.5	33 (24–42)
24	0.83	2.7	31 (23–39)
25	1.1	3.0	34 (26–42)
26	0.9	3.0	30 (24–36)
27	0.9	3.0	28 (23–34)
28	1.1	3.3	31 (18–45)
29	1.0	3.4	29 (22–37)
30	1.0	3.4	30 (26–34)
31	1.0	3.4	29 (23–36)
32	1.1	3.6	31 (26–36)
33	1.1	3.4	31 (25–37)
34	1.1	3.8	28 (23–33)
35	1.1	3.8	29 (26–31)
36	1.1	3.9	28 (23–34)
37	1.2	4.1	29 (24–34)
Term	1.2	4.3	28 (22–33)

From Johnson et al [48]

Dilatation of the ventricular system first involves the posterior aspect such as the atria and occipital horns of the lateral ventricles. Ventricular dilatation is most frequently the result of congenital malformation of the ventricular system such as those associated with meningomyoceles or secondary to aqueduct stenosis.

Real-time sonography allows detection of *cardiac arrhythmias* of the fetus as well as conduction abnormalities. High output cardiac failure may result in fetal ascites and anasarca (fetal hydrops). Some cardiac arrhythmias may be amenable to medical treatment, both in utero and after the fetus has been delivered [46]. Bradycardia may be associated with a malformed heart. Disassociation of contraction of the cardiac atria and ventricle may be observed in mothers who have connective tissue disorders, such as systemic lupus erythematosus. This is thought to be the result of transplacental transfer of antibodies to fetal cardiac conductive tissue.

Hydrops fetalis describes a neonate with extensive soft tissue swelling, usually associated with ascites, pleural and/or pericardial effusion. Hydrops usually indicates that the fetus is severely compromised. Before the extensive use of hyperimmune globulin, Rh-isoimmunization was the most common cause. Now, however, it is most commonly associated with a variety of nonimmunological causes and fetal malformations such as lymphatic dysplasia. Hydrops can be encountered secondary to disorders such as tachyarrhythmia that are potentially treatable and, on the other extreme, conditions such as thanatropic dwarfism which is uniformly fatal (Table 80.9). Anasarca can be diagnosed when the skin is greater

Table 80.9 Some common anatomical and functional abnormalities which may be associated with fetal hydrops

	Fetus
Head	Arteriovenous malformation
	Ventricular dilatation secondary to viraemia
Neck	Lymphatic dysplasia (cystic hygroma)
Thorax	High output failure secondary to haemolytic anaemia or arrhythmia
	Diaphragmatic hernia
	Dwarfism
Abdomen	Tumours
	Gastro intestinal tract obstructions
Retroperitoneum	Obstructive uropathy
Extremities	Dwarfism
	Placenta
	Chorioangioma
	Twin-twin transfusion
	Umbilical cord
	Umbilical cord torsion

than 5 mm in thickness. Fetal intra-abdominal ascites will be present and collects in certain areas depending upon the position of the fetus. The presence of oligohydramnios may be an indication of severe fetal compromise. An excessively thick placenta (> 6 cm) may be a contraindication to vaginal delivery since it may not support the fetus through those vigours.

Bowel obstruction can be diagnosed sonographically. *Atresia* of the duodenum produces two cystic upper abdominal masses, one in the stomach and the second C-shaped tubular sonolucent structure in the duodenum. This condition is usually associated with maternal hydramnios. Because of the high association of duodenal atresia with Down's syndrome, one should examine the fetal heart for atrioventricular canal defects.

Although a few loops of fluid-filled bowel can be recognized in some normal near-term fetuses, persistently dilated bowel may be the result of *meconium ileus* (Fig. 80.15D). *Protrusion* of bowel loops can be identified sonographically. *Omphaloceles* which result from herniation of bowel into the umbilical stalk appear as midline masses as opposed to *gastrochisis* which results from eccentric herniation of bowel contents and has a more guarded prognosis.

It is hoped that as experience is gained, in utero therapeutics may permit effective treatment of some of these congenital anomalies (Table 80.10). Sonography can now be used for some types of intrauterine interventional techniques such as intrauterine transfusions (Fig. 80.19). Once the mechanisms of labour are better understood and premature labour consistently controlled, in utero treatment of some of the fetal anomalies mentioned above may become feasible [33].

Table 80.10 Sonographically detectable fetal anomalies

Head
Ancephaly
Encephalocele
Hydrocephalus
Microcephaly

Neck
Cystic hygroma

Thorax
Cardiac arrhythmias
Diaphragmatic herniations
Pleural effusions
Mediastinal lung tumours

Abdomen
Bowel atresias, obstruction

Retroperitoneum
Hydronephrosis
Renal agenesis

Spine
Meningocele

Extremities
Dwarfism
Osteogenesis imperfecta

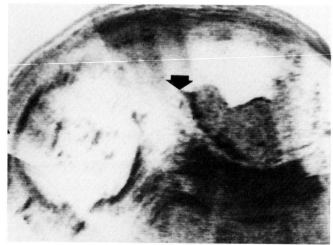

A

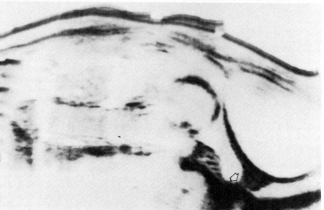

B

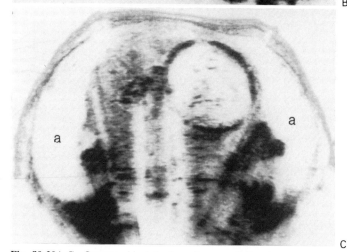

C

Fig. 80.20A-C Sonographic detection of maternal disorders which may occur during pregnancy.

(A) Uterine subseptus. (transverse static sonogram). The fetal head is on the right side of the uterine fundus while the placenta is on the left. A septum arising from the posterior aspect of the uterus can also be seen [arrow].

(B) Ruptured membranes (longitudinal static sonogram). There is a dilatation of the endocervical canal [arrow] and fluid within the upper vagina resulting from premature rupture of membranes secondary to an incomplete cervix.

(C) Maternal ascites (transverse static sonogram). Ascites [a] was due to liver failure in this patient who was pregnant.

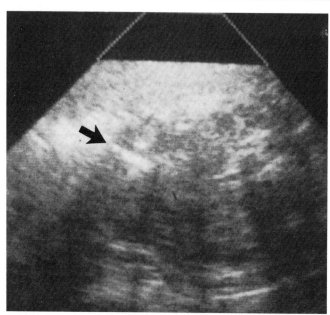

*Fig. 80.19 Intrauterine transfusion (still frame taken during real-time guidance for passage of needle into fetal peritoneum). The needle appears as an echogenic interface that could be identified within the peritoneal cavity of the fetus prior to the injection of blood.

Conditions affecting labour and delivery

The abnormally bulging lower uterine segment and incompetent cervix can be determined sonographically by extensive ballooning of the lower uterine segment and opening of the endocervical canal (Fig. 80.20B). The lower uterine segment normally becomes effaced as the result of engagement of the fetal head (Fig. 80.20B). In some patients, the umbilical cord can be identified prolapsing into the lower uterine segment and endocervical canal [47]. This has important obstetric implications since the prolonged compression of the umbilical cord may lead to extensive fetal distress and demise during labour or delivery.

Uterine malformations may have implications in later stages of pregnancy. Sonography can be helpful in detection of uterine septation as a linear echogenic interface along the midportion of the uterus, usually arising from the posterior wall (Fig. 80.20A). It should be suspected when the placenta appears on one side of the uterus with the fetus on the other. As previously mentioned, sonography is helpful in detection of pelvic masses which may impair normal labour.

Sonographic localization of the placenta prior to a Caesarian section can be helpful in determining the appropriate location for uterine incision. Sonography has an important role in the decision to allow vaginal delivery or perform a Caesarian section in those patients in whom a fetal anomaly is detected, e.g. if the mass or abnormal portion of the fetus is greater than 10 cm in dimension, vaginal delivery may be contraindicated (see Fig. 80.18C).

Assessment of fetal condition

Real-time sonography can be used to assess the condition of the fetus in the third trimester. Besides assessment of fetal heart rate and contraction regularity, 10 to 15 minutes of real-time sonography can be used to determine the presence or absence of fetal thoracic movements, extension and flexion of the limbs and trunk and fetal tone. These features combined with assessment of amniotic fluid volume and placenta maturity have been coupled with the results of the nonstress test to derive an overall assessment of fetal well-being [47,48].

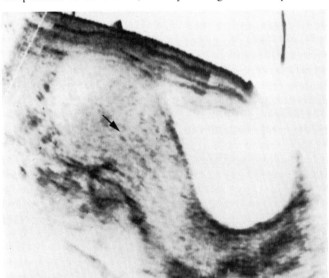

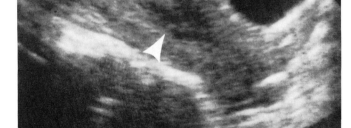

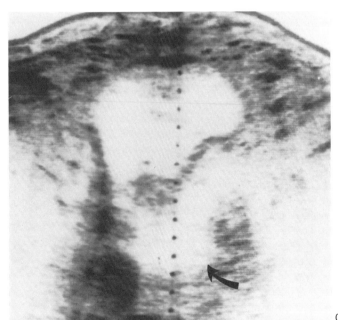

Fig. 80.21A-C Sonography in post partum disorders.

(A) Normal involuted uterus — 2 weeks post partum (longitudinal static sonogram). The uterine lumen is closely opposed and the texture of the uterus is homogeneous.

*(B) Retained products of conception (longitudinal real-time sonogram). The lower uterine segment contains retained placental tissue [arrow] and haematoma.

(C) Pelvic abscess associated with involuting uterus (transverse static sonogram). This patient has a post partum fever and an adnexal mass was identified [arrow] which corresponded to a tubo-ovarian abscess.

MATERNAL DISORDERS WHICH MAY OCCUR DURING PREGNANCY

Since it does not involve ionizing radiation, sonography should be the first diagnostic modality for evaluation of some maternal disorders that may accompany pregnancy [49]. For example, sonography can be effectively utilized to detect gallbladder calculi that may be found within the gravid patient. Hydro- or pyonephrosis can be detected by sonography, pus within the renal pelvis appearing as mobile low level echoes.

It may be difficult completely to delineate the maternal pancreas in the third trimester because of enlarged gravid uterus. Pancreatitis may be detected in the mother by documenting an enlarged and oedematous pancreas. Maternal ascites or abscesses not related to the pregnancy can also be detected sonographically (Fig. 80.20C). Sonography can be used to screen the major arteries such as the aortic, splenic, renal and hepatic arteries for the presence of aneurysms but angiography may be necessary for confirmation. Aneurysms are prone to rupture and massive bleeding in the gravid patient due to the added cardiovascular stress of the pregnancy and labour.

POSTPARTUM DISORDERS (Fig. 80.21)

Sonography is most commonly used in the patient after delivery for evaluation of the uterus that fails to involute or in the patient who remains febrile after delivery [50]. Most commonly, this is due to *retained placental* tissue within the uterus, or inflammatory processes occurring within the parametrium. Retained placental tissue effaces the normally completely collapsed endometrial cavity of the involuting uterus. The placental tissue itself is moderately echogenic compared to the less echogenic myometrium (Figs. 80.21A & 80.21B).

Another cause of postpartum fever that can be diagnosed by sonography is an *adnexal or pelvic abscess*. These abscesses may be the result of a tubo-ovarian abscess (TOA) which was present prior to and during pregnancy (Fig. 80.21C). If rupture of a TOA occurs, a loculated pattern of intraperitoneal fluid collection is usually present [51].

Obstetric radiology

AMNIOGRAPHY (*M. I. Shaff*)

Amniography refers to the opacification of the amniotic fluid by intrauterine injection of water soluble contrast agents. The procedure is complementary to sonography and amniotic fluid analysis in detecting fetal defects at an early gestational age. The accurate diagnosis of specific malformations has an effect on fetal and neonatal prognosis and is essential for the prenatal counselling of parents.

Fetography is the term applied to the opacification of the vernix caseosa and fetal skin with oil soluble contrast Pantopaque (Myodil). Its use is limited to the last trimester of pregnancy and it presents the additional hazard of fetal inhalation of oil droplets. Its advantage is excellent delineation of the fetal skin. The areas of skin coated by the contrast medium will depend on the fetal maturity. The distribution of Pantopaque (Myodil) on the fetal body and limbs has unreliably been used as a measure of fetal maturity. Pantopaque will not coat neural tube defects that are lined by meninges. A number of cases of skin sloughing after subcutaneous injection of contrast medium (oily or aqueous) have been reported. This complication should be avoided by attention to technique. Fetography has been discontinued in most diagnostic centres. Fetoamniography applies to the combination of the two procedures [52].

Indications

Neural tube defects

The risk of recurrent neural tube defects in the fetus of a woman with a previously affected child is about 5%. Amniotic fluid alpha-fetoprotein (AFP) values have been used to predict the presence of these defects but there are inaccuracies in both serum and amniotic fluid AFP determination.

AFP is a normal fetal serum protein synthesized by embryonal liver and yolk sac cells. In addition to neural tube defects, AFP is elevated in other fetal anomalies as diverse as Down's, Tay-Sachs, Klinefelter's and Turner's syndromes, high GI obstruction, congenital nephrosis, hydrocephalus, epidermolysis bullosa and fetal tumours. In addition, elevated AFP levels are found in some pregnancies without demonstrable cause or where no fetal anomaly is present.

To overcome these deficiencies in a single diagnostic test, serum AFP levels should be determined early in the middle trimester and if elevated, patients should be examined by ultrasound. Amniotic AFP levels are determined if ultrasound fails to reveal an obvious cause. Amniography is considered if AFP levels are elevated +3 standard deviations and the ultrasound examination is normal or equivocal.

Atresia of upper alimentary tract

Oesophageal atresia will prevent fetal swallowing of amniotic fluid. The dilated stomach and duodenum proximal to an area of *duodenal atresia* may be detected by ultrasound. The diagnosis may be confirmed by amniography which will demonstrate inability of the fetus to swallow opacified amniotic fluid and the absence of opacified small intestine on delayed radiographs. Hydrops fetalis and incipient fetal death are the only other fetal abnormalities that prevent swallowing in a fetus with an intact, unobstructed upper GI tract.

Monoamniotic twins

Ultrasound may be unable to detect the membrane separating diamniotic twins (Fig. 80.22). Since the prognosis of diamniotic twins is so much better than monoamniotic twins, it may be necessary to introduce contrast into the amniotic sac to delineate the boundaries between two sacs.

Miscellaneous conditions

Amniography may confirm or elucidate suspected anomalies detected by ultrasound such as *prune belly, gastroschisis, iniencephaly*. It may also be used in late trimester pregnancy

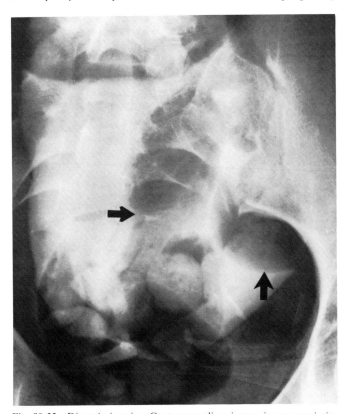

Fig. 80.22 Diamniotic twins. Contrast medium is seen in one amniotic sac only with the fetus appearing as a lucency within the surrounding contrast (horizontal arrow). The head of the second fetus is seen invaginating the opacified sac [vertical arrow]. The second sac does not contain contrast. Ultrasound had raised the possibility of monamniotic twins.

to opacify bowel in order to choose an appropriate site for intraperitoneal exchange transfusion. It has been used from time to time at this period to investigate a variety of obstetrical problems such as unusual fetal position, polyhydramnios, fetal foregut and midgut atresia and soft tissue abnormalities. In the absence of ultrasonic facilities, intrauterine injection of water-soluble contrast may be used to demonstrate the presence of hydatidiform mole.

Technique

Amniography is performed at the time of amniocentesis and ideally 15 to 20 weeks after the last menstrual period. A 20 gauge spinal needle is inserted into the amniotic sac under ultrasonic guidance. *Fetography* or fetoamniography done in the last trimester should be performed with a needle equipped with a soft teflon outer core (e.g., B. D. Longdwell). After correct placement, the rigid inner needle is removed and the soft outer sheath is retained in place. This precaution prevents a moving fetus from impaling itself on the sharp, rigid needle tip with subsequent injury or subcutaneous injection of contrast [53]. For fetography 9 ml of Pantopaque is injected through the soft teflon outer core using a 10 ml syringe to obtain the maximal hydrostatic advantage. Pantopaque is extremely viscous and does not mix with water soluble contrast. Larger doses of Pantopaque (Myodil) inhibit fetal swallowing.

For amniography, meglumine diatrizoate or iothalamate is used because high sodium preparations may induce abortion. Preparations such as Conray 280 or Renografin 76 have been found suitable. (The role of non-ionic contrast media is currently being evaluated.) After aspiration of amniotic fluid for examination. 1.5 ml per gestational week of the contrast medium is introduced. The patient is allowed to walk around to promote mixing of amniotic fluid and contrast and is then taken to a radiographic room.

Great care should be exercised in obtaining radiographic images, under the control of an experienced technologist and radiologist. The patient is placed supine on the radiographic table and the uterine fundus palpated and marked on the skin with a marking pen. The height of the uterine fundus from the pubic symphysis indicates the area to be examined and determines the coordinates of the coned field. The patient is then placed in a prone and slightly obliqued position to displace fetal parts away from the maternal spine. A compression band is placed loosely over the maternal back and the field is coned to the smallest possible dimensions (Fig. 80.23). Rare earth screens and a low kV, high mAs technique are used. Shortly before the exposure is made, the compression band is tightened as much as possible in order to decrease maternal soft tissue and reduce the incident X–ray dose required for the required exit dose. The compression band is released immediately after the exposure and the mother remains in this position until the film has been developed. The film is examined and if nondiagnostic, the procedure is repeated with the patient in the opposite obliquity.

Alternatively, the procedure can be performed by direct fluoroscopy. The maternal abdomen is fluoroscoped and the

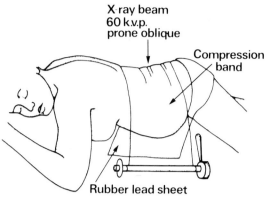

Fig. 80.23 The patient is positioned in the prone oblique and compression band is applied. A radiographic technique involving low kV, high mAs and reduction of scatter is used.

patient is rotated until the fetus is a perfect lateral projection. Spot amniograms of the fetus are taken which allows for evaluation of the fetal spine region [54]. This method is of particular value in the diagnosis of neural tube defects as the fetal spine cannot be evaluated unless it is seen in profile.

Risks and radiation exposure

Amniography, if done at the time of amniocentesis carries the same risk as amniocentesis to which must be added the dangers of exposure to ionizing radiation. The risk of spontaneous abortion following amniocentesis is 1%. The risk of injury to the fetus from the needle is reduced by using ultrasound. As previously stated, a teflon sheath may be left in situ after removal of the rigid needle and this will prevent injury to the fetus secondary to sudden fetal movement. Pantopaque (Myodil) injected subcutaneously produces skin sloughing. In addition, Pantopaque inhalation may cause lipoid pulmonary granulomas and partly for this reason, its use has been largely discontinued.

The radiation risk to a 2nd trimester fetus is obvious and amniography should not be used unless ultrasound and amniotic fluid analysis predict a strong likelihood of fetal abnormality.

The fetal dose from amniography is approximately 1 Rad (1 cGy) which falls within the acceptable range of 5 Rads. Fetal thyroid function has not been shown to be affected by contrast material.

Radiographic interpretation

In a well performed amniogram, the amniotic fluid becomes homogeneously opacified. The fetus appears as a nonopacified lucent body bathed by the opaque amnion. The placental site is usually identifiable as a peripheral semilunar lucency indenting the smooth amniotic contour. Parts of the umbilical cord are seen traversing the amnion. With a little practice, fetal limbs, thorax, spine, face and head are easily recognized.

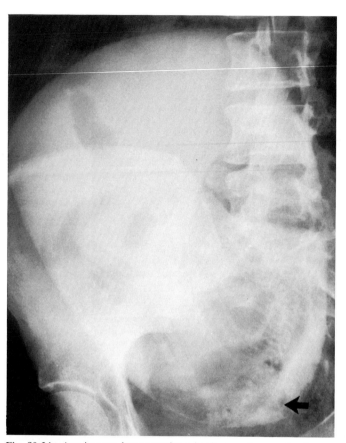

Fig. 80.24 Amniogram demonstrating a lumbar meningomyelocele [horizontal arrow]. Ultrasound was equivocal and the alpha-fetoprotein only slightly elevated at this stage.

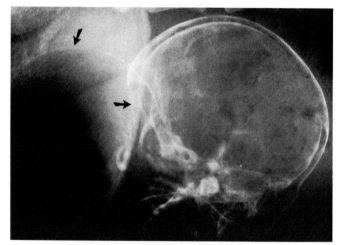

Fig. 80.25 Occipital encephalocele. The encephalocele which was covered with skin is outlined by Pantopaque (Myodil) [vertical arrow]. The calvarial defect is shown [horizontal arrow]. The alpha-fetoprotein was not raised.

As previously mentioned, the fetal spine must be seen in profile for evaluation. Attention should be paid to the vertebral anatomy. Meningocele and encephaloceles are seen as rounded lucent masses arising from the spine and surrounded by opaque amnion (Figs. 80.24 & 80.25). They are often small and require careful scrutiny. Every centimetre of fetal contour must be examined and explained in anatomical terms. Spina bifida and lesser forms of dysraphism present as a niche in the region of the fetal back which traps contrast (Fig. 80.26).

Attention should be given to fetal abdominal and thoracic girth. A large abdomen and small chest suggest gastroschisis prune belly or renal cysts (Fig. 80.27). Abnormalities of position suggest hypotonia as in Down's, IUGR, impaired fetal well-being or a displacement by fetal masses.

In the diagnostic triad of ultrasound, amniotic fluid analysis and amniography, it is amniography that should be left until last. It is undoubtedly a test that is best performed when the presence of fetal anomaly is strongly suspected. It is, however, of great help in resolving the diagnostic dilemma of retaining a grossly abnormal pregnancy or aborting a normal fetus. Physicians and patients often benefit greatly by the anatomically exquisite and readily understandable information that amniography provides in confirmation of evidence previously provided by ultrasound and amniotic fluid analysis (Figs. 80.28A & B).

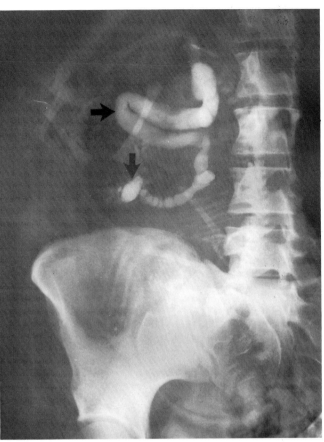

Fig. 80.27 Amniogram demonstrating the protuberant abdomen and displaced fetal bowel containing contrast material. The caecum [vertical arrow] and splenic flexure [horizontal arrow] are in markedly abnormal positions. Diagnosis is prune belly syndrome.

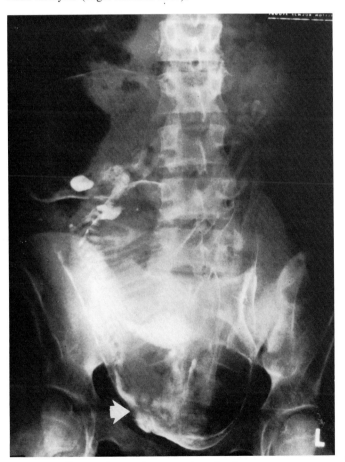

Fig. 80.26 Fetoamniogram demonstrating a lumbar meningomyelocele (horizontal arrow). This is an underlying abnormality of the lumbar spine. Pantopaque (Myodil) has pooled in a niche.

PELVIMETRY (A. C. Winfield)

Indications

Controversy exists and approaches differ among workers in this field. As recently as 1967 Bean et al [55] presented a list of 20 'prime indications' which he felt were self-explanatory. Most of these would no longer be considered as appropriate reasons to proceed with the study. More recently, numerous authors [56,57,58] have attempted to evaluate the place of pelvimetry in management of the labouring mother. Despite their work there is still no uniformity as to the appropriate indications and there is marked variance in the frequency of the study from institution to institution.

Data complied by Kelly from 1960–70, reflect a pelvimetry use rate in those hospitals surveyed of 6.9% of all deliveries [56]. Similar statistics issued by the US Public Health Service in 1963 showed a 5.1% frequency [59]. There has, since these data were collected, been a general tendency to reduce significantly the frequency of the examination. The chief reason for such a trend has been the appreciation of the

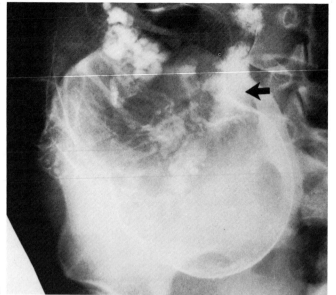

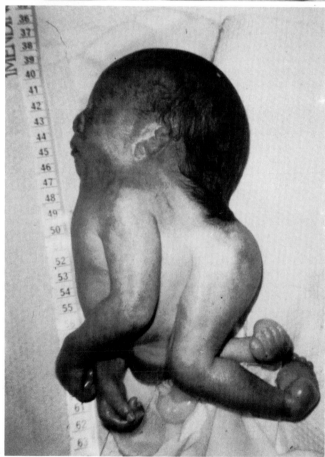

Fig. 80.28 (A) Fetoamniogram demonstrating iniencephaly [arrow]. (B) The dead fetus, post-delivery.

potential harm of radiation exposure, no matter how small, to the fetus.

The United Nation Scientific Committee on the Effects of Atomic Energy (1977 Report) estimated a mean fetal whole body dose of 620 mrad (0.62 cGy) from an average pelvimetry examination [59]. Pelvimetry in the United States in the major single source of ionizing radiation to the fetus [58]. Since no threshold danger dose has been established, it is mandatory that the examination be utilized only for logical and appropriate indications. It is clear however, that in some patients the clinical assessment of the size of the maternal pelvis is indefinite, especially in the primigravida, whose pelvis is unproven by previous delivery. This lack of assurance of the adequacy of the birth canal may well alter management of the parturient patient, particularly if compounded by an atypical fetal presentation. Under these circumstances there is little doubt that pelvimetry is indicated.

At Vanderbilt University Hospital our utilization of pelvimetry is approximately 20% of obstetric patients. Indications for the procedure are not absolute, but vary with the clinical assessment by the attending physician and the past obstetrical history of the patient. The most frequent indication for pelvimetry is abnormal fetal presentation, usually breech, in a primigravida, but all such patients do not need the study. If ultrasound examination shows a small or normal sized fetal head with an associated ample maternal pelvis by clinical evaluation, then pelvimetry is not employed. If any doubt exists as to the adequacy of the pelvis we do not hesitate to radiograph the patient.

Other indications, all relative and dependent upon clinical assessment, include previous caesarean section, unusual fetal attitude, abnormal pelvic configuration and abnormal progress of labour. On occasions, the clinical question presented can be answered by a single film of the abdomen rather than a one or two film pelvimetry study. The examination is used promptly whenever we believe that the results of the study will affect positively the management of the patient and her labour.

Technique

Once it has been determined to proceed with pelvimetry, all consideration should be directed to keeping radiation dosage to a minimum without compromising radiographic quality or information. One must be sure that the technical staff can perform the examination without repeated exposures and regular instruction to the technologists is appropriate. Radiographic factors are important; increasing the kilovoltage to the 90 to 100 kVp range, with corresponding attenuation of milliamperage and/or time, will reduce radiation dosage without significantly compromising radiographic contrast. A combination of high speed film and high speed cassette screens are used. Rare earth intensifying screens reduce exposure by 50%. Beam filtration of 2 to 3 mm Al is suggested and meticulous collimation is urged. Fastidious attention to these details will permit good pelvimetry and still maintain fetal radiation exposure to less than 0.5 (0.5 cGy) rad for the two projection examination.

Most of the methods in current use are acceptable with careful technique. Meticulous positioning, appropriate exposure factors, and careful concern for the details of the examination are more important in obtaining consistent results than the choice of one technique over another.

Numerous methods for pelvimetry are now available. All are based on the need to measure the critical areas of the maternal bony pelvis, correcting for distortion due to magnification. Our technique is a modification of the Colcher-Sussman method described originally in 1944 [60] This method has been chosen because it has a minimum of error potential, is reproducible, quick to learn and easy to perform. With the advent of ultrasound examinations of the gravid patient, there is no longer need to measure the fetal head on radiographs. The ultrasound study is clearly superior for cranial measurements and recognition of fetal abnormality. To pelvimetry is left the task of measuring the maternal pelvis.

Films are obtained in both lateral and (usually) anteroposterior projections. The lateral projection is nearly always the more important film and is obtained with care to assure that the positioning is ideal (Fig. 80.29). The accuracy of the lateral position is checked by noting how closely the two femoral heads superimpose. A perforated metal rule is placed at the level of the buttocks crease, with the rule parallel to the film in the midsagittal plane. Since all diameters of interest in the lateral projection are presumed to be midline, measurements can be read directly from the rule and are depicted in Fig. 80.29. Measurements of the antero-

posterior diameter (conjugate diameter) of the pelvic inlet (AB), the midpelvis (AC), and the pelvic outlet (DE) are recorded and compared to known normals. The degree of concavity of the sacrum is assessed as is the attitude of the presenting fetal part. Engagement is evaluated in cephalic presentations by noting the relationships of the occiput to the ischial spine (F).

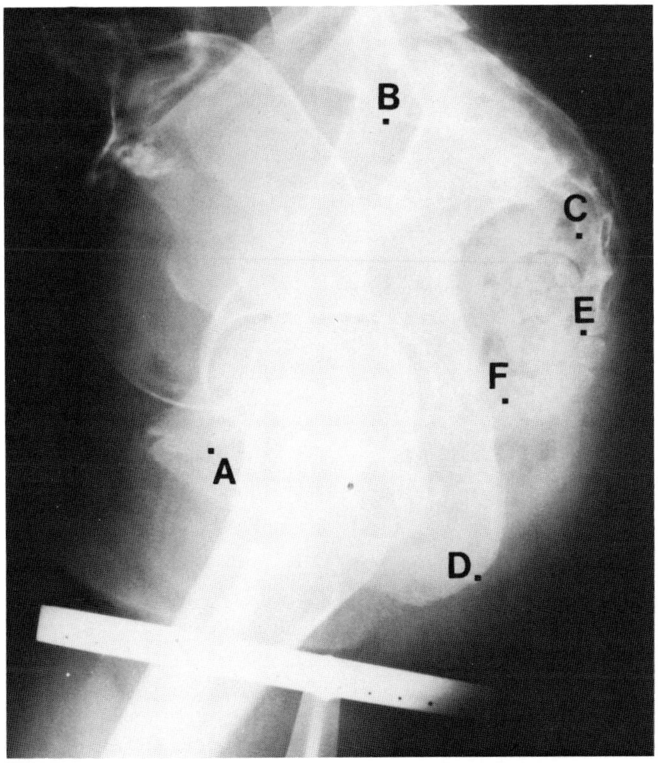

Transverse pelvic diameters are determined by the orthometric method described by Schwartz in 1956 [61]. This technique permits the measuring of the transverse diameters directly from the film with no correction factors necessary. The results of the lateral projection are not needed to assist in measurement of the anteroposterior film. This technique is based upon the use of a perpendicular X–ray beam through the plane of interest. Two exposures are obtained, each covering one half of the pelvis. This first exposure is taken of the right half of the true pelvis with the central beam 5.5 cm (average distance of the ischial spine from midline) to the right of the midline. The left hemipelvis is protected with a lead shield. Then, without moving the patient, a second exposure is made including only the left half of the pelvis, and with the central ray shifted 5.5 cm to the left of midline. The right hemipelvis is masked. This results in a single exposure of each of the two sides of the pelvis with virtually no beam divergence (Fig. 80.30).

This technique has proven most accurate for the true transverse diameter of the inlet and the bi-ischial (interspinous) diameters. One can measure directly the transverse diameter of the inlet (AA), the bi-ischial or interspinous diameter of the midpelvis (BB), and the intertuberous or transverse diameter of the outlet (CC) (Fig. 80.30).

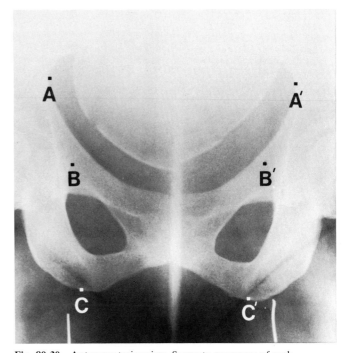

Fig. 80.29 Lateral view. Anatomic landmarks identified include posterior margin of symphysis [A], sacral promontory [B], anterior margin of sacral hollow 2 cm above level of ischial spine [C], ischial tuberosity [D], sacrococcygeal articulation [E], and ischial spine [F]. Note perforated metal ruler in midsagittal plane for measurements.

Fig. 80.30 Anteroposterior view. Separate exposures of each hemipelvis, with central ray approximating plane of ischial spine. Designated landmarks are lateral-most margins of pelvic inlet [A,A], ischial spines [B,B'], ischial tuberosities [C,C']. Measurements are taken directly without correction factor.

Although the above describes the technique employed by the author, the examiner has a choice of several alternative methods. Any of these may offer equally satisfactory results if meticulous attention to technique is employed. Ball and Golden [62] describe a triangulation method using films in anteroposterior and lateral projections with the patient in the erect position. The significant measurements are made on the films and corrected for geometric error by a published nomogram or a special slide rule devised for this purpose. One may also obtain both anteroposterior and lateral films at 72 inches permitting direct measurements with no correction factors and having an inherent magnification of less than 5%.

Fully 50 years ago, H. Thoms described a method whereby films in both projections are employed [63]. A metal rule in the midsagittal plane is used for the lateral projection. The anteroposterior view is obtained and is followed by exposure of a perforated grid placed at the height of the pelvic inlet on the same film.

The anteroposterior view of Thoms is obtained in a semisitting position, using a back rest at about 45°. It is believed that this results in placing the plane of the pelvic inlet parallel to the film. Although this may seem anatomically more sound than a supine film, it is a slower, clumsier technique. There is no evidence to suggest that any statistical gain is achieved by this technique which involves high fetal radiation and it is seldom used today.

Similarly, several authors have described techniques to measure the pelvic outlet. All tend to employ cephalad tube angulation in the supine position. Measurements of the pelvic outlet are now generally considered of little clinical value and are rarely employed.

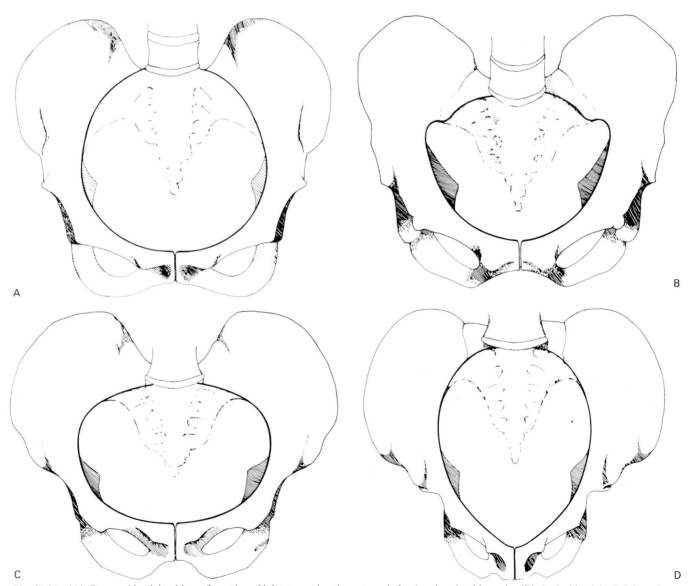

Fig. 80.31 (A) Gynaecoid pelvis with configuration of inlet approximating a true circle. Ample subpubic angle. (B) Android pelvis. Pelvic outlet triangular in contour; ischial spines are prominent. (C) Platypelloid pelvis. Ovoid inlet with narrow anteroposterior diameter. (D) Anthropoid pelvis. Pelvic inlet elongated in anteroposterior diameter but transverse diameter is narrow.

Interpretation

During the many years in which pelvimetry has been employed, a myriad of measurements have been extracted from the examination. Average diameters for the measured parameters are found in Table 80.11. Similarly, attempts have been made to classify the pelvic architecture into four basic types; gynaecoid, android, anthropoid, and platypelloid (Fig. 80.31).

The *gynaecoid* pelvis demonstrates a relatively round inlet with the widest transverse measurement near its centre. The *anthropoid* pelvis is ovoid with the transverse diameter narrower than the anteroposterior measurement. Conversely the *platypelloid* pelvis is ovoid with its long axis in the transverse plane. Finally the *android* pelvis is triangular or wedge shaped with a narrow anterior and a shallow broad posterior segment.

Although statistical data reveals that most complications of delivery occur with platypelloid and/or android configuration[55], such information is of little use in the individual case.

Specific pelvic deformities have been described in the past. The *Roberts* pelvis shows extreme transverse contraction and the *Naegele* pelvis with its marked asymmetry and unilateral contraction were once thought to be developmental. It seems more likely that these abnormalities, now rarely seen in the western world, were probably secondary to childhood rickets or other underlying bone disease.

Many diameters and combinations of measurements have been recorded and calculated, but it is believed today that most of these measurements are unnecessary and of little value.

Two measurements seem significant and valuable from a prognostic viewpoint. Borell and Femstrom[64], in a careful analysis of pelvic mensuration and its significance, have found that the AP diameter of the inlet is the single most important measurement, with the bi-ischial diameter of somewhat lesser importance. The remainder of the measurements obtained are of little value except under most unusual circumstances.

The AP diameter of the inlet (the true or obstetric conjugate) is the most important single measurement. It is that line connecting the posterior margin of the symphysis

Table 80.11 Average pelvic diameters in cm

	Average diameter in cm
Pelvic inlet	
Anteroposterior	12.5
Transverse	13.0
Midpelvis	
Anteroposterior	12.5
Transverse (Interspinous)	11.0
Pelvis outlet	
Anteroposterior (post sagittal)	7.5
Transverse (Intertuberous)	10.5

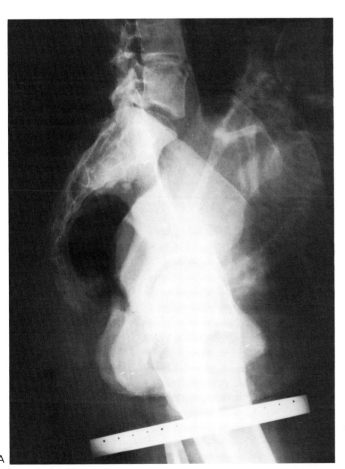

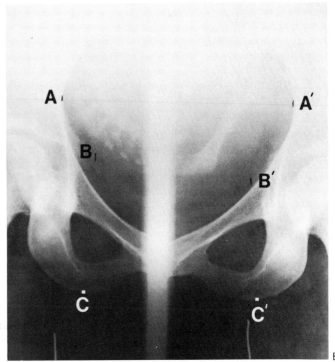

Fig. 80.32 (A) Lateral view of pelvimetry-breech presentation. Pelvic measurements in the anteroposterior plane are ample (conjugate diameter 13 cm). The sacral hollow is deep.

(B) Anteroposterior view reveals that the transverse measurements are significantly smaller than average. The ischial diameter is less than 9 cm and the spines are moderately prominent. Caesarean section was necessary.

pubis and the anterosuperior angle of the sacrum as seen in a true lateral projection. More properly it is the shortest inlet measurement between sacrum and symphysis and on occasion may be located below the anterosuperior sacral margin, expecially if the sacrum is straight and shows little or no concavity (see Fig. 80.29). The average range of this parameter is 11.0 to 12.5 cm. Bean [55] and Dyer [65] both state that values of less than 10.5 cm relate to increased difficulty in vaginal delivery. Joyce et al [57] present data to suggest than an obstetric conjugate of 11.7 cm or more is needed to predict safe vaginal delivery for a term infant in breech presentation. With an occipital presentation, a diameter of 10 cm may be sufficient to permit a trial of labour.

Less statistical evidence is available as regards the value of the interspinous (bi-ischial) diameter which is the transverse measurement in the midpelvis. Dyer [65] has shown that the likelihood of caesarean section is increased when the bi-ischial diameter is less than 10 cm and we use this level as a guide. Although other measurements are usually obtained as seen in Figures 80.29 and 80.30, they have much less significance in guiding the management of the patient in labour. Measurements of the pelvic outlet (intertuberous and posterior sagittal diameters) have little value in patient management. On the other hand the degree of concavity of the sacral curve, the prominence of the ischial spines, and the attitude of the fetal presenting part are all noted and provide additional qualitative data. Several of these features can be seen in Figure 80.32, a pelvimetry examination of a primigravida patient with a complete breech presentation. Although we can recognize ample measurements of the conjugate (anteroposterior) diameter of the pelvis and a deep sacral concavity, we are also made aware of the narrow transverse measurements. The bi-ischial diameter of less than 9 cm is significantly reduced and associated with prominent ischial spines. Difficulty in the fetus negotiating the midpelvis can be anticipated and delivery via caesarean section should be chosen.

Moulding of the fetal head is a necessary part of the passage of the fetus through the birth canal. This is not the result of impingement of the fetal head on the maternal bony pelvis as originally thought, but rather is caused by pressure of the maternal soft tissue while the head traverses the lower uterine segment.

The pattern of moulding will vary with the attitude of the fetal head. During descent of a flexed head through the maternal pelvis a characteristic cranial contour develops with elevation of the parietal bones in reference to the occipital and frontal bones and depression of the temporal bones in the region of the temporoparietal sutures (Fig. 80.33). This permits a desired reduction in both the anteroposterior and transverse cranial diameters.

With a brow or face presentation, on the other hand, the parietal bones are depressed along the sagittal suture. This alteration results in increased occipitofrontal and diminished submentobregmatic diameters, a desirable feature in the delivery of a deflexed or extended fetal head. The altered alignment of the bones of fetal calvarium may be mistaken for the marked over riding seen after fetal demise (Spalding sign), particularly during a prolonged labour but fortunately other criteria are readily available.

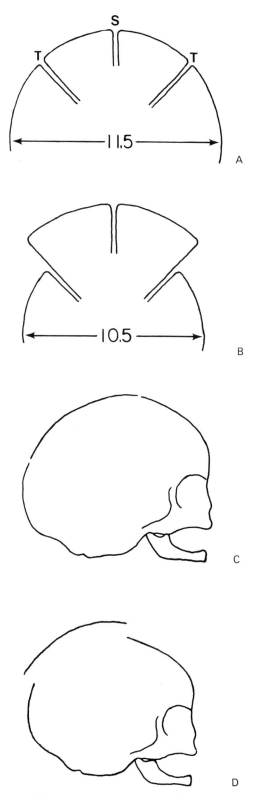

Fig. 80.33A-D Effect of moulding on normally flexed fetal skull [S = sagittal suture; T = temporo-parietal suture].
(A) Coronal diagram of skull with no displacement at sagittal and temporo-parietal sutures. (B) During moulding the parietal bones are elevated and the transverse diameter is reduced. (C) Sagittal plane of skull prior to moulding, bony alignment is regular at frontoparietal and temporoparietal sutures. (D) During moulding, the parietal bone elevation causes a decrease in the anteroposterior dimension.

Conclusion

The role of pelvimetry in the management of labour has changed over the years. Indications and utilization have both diminished. It is clearly recognized that normal pelvimetry cannot itself predict the safe culmination of delivery via the vaginal route. Abnormal measurements do not necessarily exclude vaginal delivery, but, in selected cases, the information obtained from a carefully performed pelvimetry may provide sufficient supplemental data to influence the clinical decision to initiate, continue or terminate a trial of labour via the vaginal route.

RADIOGRAPHY OF THE MATERNAL ABDOMEN

Until about 1960, radiography was employed fairly extensively during mid and late pregnancy to assess fetal maturity, fetal abnormalities, placental localization and suspected maternal disease. In the last 2 or 3 decades there has been an increasing awareness of the dangers of X–irradiation to both mother and particularly to the fetus. Some previously utilized radiographic projections involved considerable irradiation to sensitive fetal parts, e.g. the fetal gonads receive very high irradiation during the Thom's inlet projection (p. 1594) if the fetus is vertex presentation.

Fortunately, ultrasonography (particularly real-time) provides remarkable information especially of fetal maturity, abnormality and placental localization. Estimation of maternal alpha-fetoprotein (p. 1577) provides an excellent forecast of the possibility of fetal open neural tube defects. Amniocentesis with chromosome analysis of fetal cells provides good evidence of some fetal genetic disorders, e.g. Mongolism.

These relatively new diagnostic techniques have almost completely replaced conventional radiology of the maternal abdomen. It is now universal practice to try and avoid this irradiation during pregnancy. Pelvimetry is often delayed until after the birth of the child if the information is thought likely to be of value in future pregnancies.

Conventional radiography of the pregnant abdomen is occasionally still utilized especially in one of three circumstances, but only if other methods have been carefully considered and the irradiation can be justified.
1. Suspected disease of the mother requiring urgent investigation.
2. To determine fetal maturity if ultrasonography is unsatisfactory or the mother presents too late in pregnancy to permit construction of ultrasonic fetal growth charts. The most valuable radiological indicator of fetal age is the state of ossification of the knee (Fig. 80.34). The lower femoral epiphysis is seen to ossify at 36 weeks and the upper tibial epiphysis can be seen radiologically at 38 weeks. If these epiphyses can be seen on the radiograph of the maternal abdomen, then the fetus is near term and

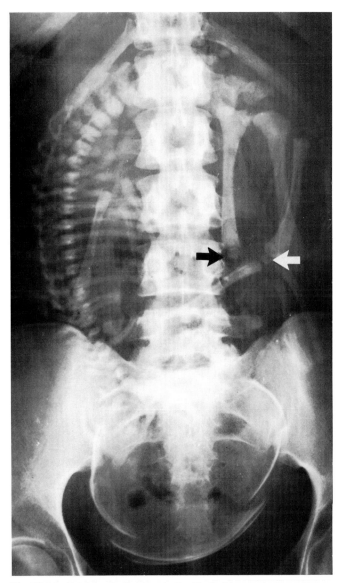

Fig. 80.34 Fetal death. Fetal maturity. Single fetus, vertex presentation. The extensive ossification of the lower femoral epiphysis [→] and the upper tibial epiphysis [←] indicates that the fetus is at full term. There is gross overlapping by the parietal bones of the frontal and occipital bones. The mother is not in labour. This marked malalignment of fetal skull bones is a certain sign of fetal death — Spalding's sign.

most unlikely to develop diseases of immaturity, e.g. respiratory distress syndrome.
3. To confirm or to demonstrate (particularly to the parents) the presence, type and extent of fetal abnormality or death (Fig. 80.34) suspected from clinical, ultrasonic, cytological, genetic or alpha-fetoprotein studies.

THE RISKS OF EXPOSURE IN UTERO TO X–RADIATION (*J. Gibbs*)

It has been recognized for many years that the mammalian embryo is more sensitive to biological effects of radiation than is the adult [66,67]. For purposes of radiation effects, it is convenient to divide intrauterine life into three periods: *preimplantation*, *organogenesis*, and *fetal*. The biological effects of radiation of concern are *prenatal death*, *teratogenesis* and *carcinogensis*.

Human experience and animal experiments have indicated that *prenatal death* is a function of exposure to sufficient doses of radiation during the preimplantation period. In experimental animals, the results are resorption; in man, the most likely result would be early, unrecognizable abortion. The approximate threshold dose for this effect in man is currently estimated as 10 rads (10 cGy) [68].

Congenital abnormalities are the result of radiation exposure during the period of organogenesis. The abnormalities induced by radiation are in no way different from those arising from other causes. Thus, in an irradiated population, the only clue is excess incidence of abnormalities. For a teratogenic effect in a specific organ or tissue, the exposure must occur during a critical period of growth and development of that organ or tissue. Consensus of published recommendations indicates a practical threshold of approximately 10 rads (10 cGy) for this effect [68].

Several retrospective epidemiologic studies have indicated statistically significant associations between exposure to diagnostic doses of X-ray in utero and subsequent incidence of childhood *cancer* [67,68]. However, other studies have found no significant effect. One major prospective study performed in the eastern United States found an association in white but not in black children [69]. A major study at the University of Chicago found no effect when the exposure was 'routine' [70]. No excess cancer has been found in Japanese atomic bomb survivors exposed in utero. With this conflicting evidence, it is not possible to draw firm conclusions at this time.

In theory, *genetic effects* should be possible from *in utero* exposure. However, we have no data dealing with this subject from man or experimental animals.

Because of the known embryonic radiosensitivity, it appears prudent to avoid, when possible, diagnostic procedures on pregnant females that include the pelvic region in the primary beam. When such a procedure is deemed medically necessary, consultation with the radiologist should allow modified procedures so as to answer the specific diagnostic questions, while minimizing exposure to the uterine contents.

In some countries, the '*10 day rule*' is in effect for female patients of childbearing age. This rule states that diagnostic procedures involving the pelvic region of females of childbearing age shall be limited to the 10 day period following the onset of menstruation. It is aimed at preventing exposure during an unrecognized early pregnancy. It has not been adopted in the United States, on the grounds that management of current disease should take precedence over the possibility of radiation exposure of an embryo. The United States National Council on Radiation Protection and Measurements recommends only postponement of those diagnostic procedures which could be postponed to term in case the patient is pregnant — such as follow up or employment examinations [67].

Occasionally, a patient who has been exposed to diagnostic radiation procedures involving the lower abdomen and pelvis is subsequently determined to have been pregnant at the time of exposure. The attending physician is then faced with the problem of counsel for possible therapeutic abortion. Before doing so, it is recommended that he consult with the radiologist, or a radiological physicist or radiobiologist in his community for determination of the dose to the embryo

Current consensus of expert (US) opinions suggest that there is no real reason to express concern if the dose to the embryo was less than 1 rad (1 cGy). With exposure less than 1 rad, current evidence suggests that the risk of adverse effects is extremely small, especially when compared to the spontaneous incidence of congenital abnormalities.

If the dose to the embryo was in the 1 to 10 rad (cGy) range, radiation risk alone should not be considered as grounds for recommending therapeutic abortion. Only if the dose to the embryo was greater than 10 rads (10 cGy) should therapeutic abortion be recommended on grounds of X-ray exposure alone. With modern practice, it is extremely rare that a patient receives sufficient radiation, even from multiple procedures, to deliver 10 rads (10 cGy) to the embryo. Therefore, recommendation for therapeutic abortion of grounds of X-ray exposure is quite rare in the US.

In summary, it is prudent practice to avoid any unnecessary radiation exposure to any patient. It is especially necessary to do so for the highly radiosensitive embryo and in any female who may possibly be pregnant.

BIBLIOGRAPHY

REFERENCES

1. Baker M, Dalrymple G 1978 Biological effects of diagnostic ultrasound: a review. Radiology 126:479–483
2. Young G 1980 'The arrow' pattern: a new 'anatomical' fetal biparietal diameter. Radiology 137:445–449
3. Campbell S, Newman G 1971 Growth of fetal biparietal diameter during normal pregnancy. Br J Obstet Gynaecol 78:513–519
4. Hohler C, Quetel T 1981 Comparison of ultrasound femur length and biparietal diameter in late pregnancy. Am J Obstet Gynecol 141:759–762
5. Young G 1978 The peripatetic placenta. Radiology 128:183–188
6. Mittlestadt C, Partain C, Boyce I 1979 Placenta praevia: significance in the second trimester. Radiology 131:465–468
7. Spirit B, Kagen E, Rosanski R 1978 Placenta: sonographic and pathologic correlation. Am J Roentgenol 131:961–965
8. Grannum P, Berkowitz R, Hobbins J 1979 The ultrasonic changes in maturing placenta and their relation to fetal pulmonic maturity. Am J Obstet Gynecol 133:915–922
9. Anderson S 1981 Management of threatened abortion with real-time sonography Obstet Gynecol 55(2):259–262
10. Finberg H, Birnholz J 1979 Ultrasound observation in multiple gestation with first trimester bleeding: the blighted twin. Radiology 132:137–140
11. Levi S 1977 Ultrasonic assessment of the high rate of human multiple pregnancy in the first trimester. J Clin Ultrasound 413–519

12. Mantoni M, Pederson J 1979 Ultrasonic visualization of human yolk sac. J Clin Ultra 7:459–460

13. Robinson H 1973 Sonar measurement of fetal crown rump length as means of assessing maturity of the first trimester of pregnancy. Br Med J 4:28–31

14. Fleischer A, Boehm F, James A 1980 Sonographic evaluation of ectopic pregnancy. In: Sanders R, James A E Jr (eds) Principles and practice of ultrasonography in obstetrics and gynecology, 2nd edn. Appleton-Century-Crofts, New York 227–290

15. Kadar N, DeVore G, Romero R 1980 Discriminatory HCG zone: its use in the sonographic evaluation for ectopic pregnancy. Obstet Gynecol 58(2):156–160

16. Fleischer A, James A, Krause D, Millis J 1978 Sonographic patterns of trophoblastic disease. Radiology 126:215–220

17. Hertig A, Edmonson W 1947 Hydatidiform mole: a patho-clinical correlation. Am J Obstet Gynecol 53:1–9

18. Whittman B, Fulton L, Cooperburg P 1981 Molar pregnancy: early diagnosis by ultrasound. J Clin Ultra 9:153–156

19. Requard C, Mettler F 1980 The use of ultrasound in evaluation of trophoblastic disease and its response to therapy. Radiology 135:419–422

20. Sample W 1978 The unsoftened portion of the uterus. Radiology 126:227–231

21. Spirit B, Kagan G, Aubry R 1981 Clinically silent retroplacental hematoma: sonographic and pathologic correlation: a case report. J Clin Ultra 9:203–205

22. Zemlyn S 1978 The effects of the urinary bladder on obstetrical sonography. Radiology 128:169–175

23. Laveno K, Santos Rhamos, Duenhoelter J, Whally P 1978 Sonar cephalometry in twins: a comparison with single fetus and in evaluation of twin disordancy. Presented at meeting of American Institute of Ultrasound in Medicine, San Diego, California, 1978

24. Sabagga R (ed) 1980 Intrauterine growth retardation. In: Diagnostic ultrasound applied to obstetrics and gynecology. New York; Harper and Row, New York 1980:103–110

25. Sarti D 1981 Correlation of fetal body diameter to BPD for 12 to 26 weeks gestation. Am J Roentgenol 137:87–92

26. Metreweli C 1978 Practical clinical ultrasound. Heinemann, Chicago

27. Miller H, Merritt T 1979 Fetal growth in humans. Yearbook, Chicago pp. 99

28. Chinn D, Filly R, Allen P 1981 Prediction of intra-uterine growth retardation by sonographic estimation of TIUV. J Clin Ultra 9:175–179

29. Carroll B 1980 Ultrasonic features of pre-eclampsia. J Clin Ultra 8:483–488

30. Tamura R, Sabagga R 1980 Percentile ranks of fetal abdominal circumference measurements. Am J Obstet Gynecol 138(5):475–479

31. Kurtz A, Wayne R, Rubin C, Cole-Beuglet C, Ross D, Goldey B 1980 Ultrasound criteria for in utero diagnosis of microcephaly. J Clin Ultra 8:11–16

32. Fletcher J 1981 The fetus as patient: ethical issues (editorial). JAMA 246(7):772–773

33. Harrison H, Golbus M, Filly R 1981 Management of the fetus with a correctable congenital defect. JAMA 246(7):774–777

34. Haber K 1981 Automated water delay head scanning. In: Babcock D, Han B (eds) Cranial ultrasonography of infants. Williams and Wilkins, Baltimore 105–111

35. Lawson T, Foley W, Berland L 1981 Ultrasonic evaluation of fetal kidneys: an analysis of normal size and frequency of visualization as related to stage of pregnancy. Radiology 138:155–156

36. Dubbins P, Kurtz A, Wapner R, Goldberg B 1981 Renal agenesis: a spectrum of in utero findings. J Clin Ultra 9:189–193

37. Hadlock F, Deter R, Carpenter R Gonzalez E, Park S 1981 Sonography of fetal urinary tract anomalies: a review. Am J Roentgenol 137:261–267

38. Filly R, Golbus M, Carey J 1981 Short-limbed dwarfism: ultrasonic diagnosis by measuration of fetal femoral length. Radiology 138:653–656

39. Barrett J, Boehm F Placenta praevia in induced abortion (paper in preparation)

40. Hohler C, Quetel T 1981 Comparison of ultrasound femur length and biparietal diameter in late pregnancy. Am J Obstet Gynecol 141:759–762

41. Jeffrey R, Laing F 1981 Sonography of the low-lying placenta value of Trendelenberg and traction scans. Am J Roentgenol 137:547–549

42. Hadlock F, Deter R, Carpenter R Park S, Athey P 1980 Hypervascularity of the uterine wall during pregnancy: incidence, sonographic appearance and obstetric implications. J Clin Ultra 8(5):399–404

43. Wallenberg H, Wladimeroff J 1977 Polyhydramnios and oligohydramnios. J Prenatal Med 6:233–242

44. Johnson M, Dunne M, Mach L, Rashbaum C 1980 Evaluation of fetal intracranial anatomy by static and real-time sonography. J Clin Ultra 8:311–318

45. Hadlock F, Deter R, Park S 1981 Real-time sonography: ventricular and vascular anatomy of the fetal brain in utero. Am J Roentgenol 136:133–137

46. Fleischer A, Killam A, Boehm F Hutchison A, Jones T, Shaff Metal 1981 Hydrops fetalis: sonographic detection and clinical implications. Radiology 141:163–168

47. Fried A 1981 Bulging amnion in premature labor: a spectrum of sonographic findings. Am J Roentgenol 136:181–185

48. Manning Ff, Platt L, Spos L 1981 Antepartum fetal evaluation: development of fetal biophysical profile. Am J Obstet Gynecol 136:787–795

49. Fleischer A, Boehm F, James A E Sonography and radiology of maternal disorders that occur during pregnancy and the puerperium. Seminars in Roentgenology (in preparation)

50. VanRees D, Bernstein R, Crawford W 1981 Involution of the post-partum uterus, an ultrasonic study. J Clin Ultra 9:55–57

51. Edell S, Gefler W 1979 Ultrasonic differentiation of types of ascitic fluid. Am J Roentgenol 133:111–114

52. Russell J G B 1973 Radiology in obstetrics and antenatal pediatrics. Butterworth, London

53. Shaff M I, 1977 Fetal complications in amniography. Br J Radiol 50:841

54. Balsam D, Weiss R 1981 Amniography in prenatal diagnosis. Radiology 141(2):379–385

55. Bean K M, Cook R T, Eavenson L W, Bristol L J 1967 Pelvimetry. Radiol Clin North Am 5:29–46

56. Kelly K M, Madden D A, Arcorese J S, Barnett M, Brown R F 1975 The utilization and efficacy of pelvimetry. Am J Roentgenol 125:66–74

57. Joyce D N, Giwa-Osagie F, Stevenson G W 1975 Role of pelvimetry in active management of labour. Br Med J 4:505–507

58. Campbell J A 1976 X-ray pelvimetry: useful procedure or medical nonsense. J Nat Med Assn 68:514–520

59. The pelvimetry examination 1980 US Department of Health and Human Services, July 1980

60. Colcher A E, Sussman W 1944 Practical technique for roentgen pelvimetry with new positioning. Am J Roentgenol 51:207–214

61. Schwartz G S 1956 An orthometric radiograph for obstetrical roentgenometry. Radiology 66:753–766

62. Ball R P, Golden R 1943 Roentgenographic obstetric pelvicephalometry in erect posture. Am J Roentgenol 49:731–737

63. Thoms H 1930 Fetal cephalometry in utero. JAMA 95:21–24

64. Borell U, Femstrom I 1960 Radiologic pelvimetry. Acta Radiol (Suppl) 191

65. Dyer I 1950 Clinical evaluation of X-ray pelvimetry. Am J Obstet Gynec 60:302–314

66. Brent R L, Gorson R O 1972 Radiation exposure in pregnancy. Current problems in radiology 2:1–48

67. National Council on Radiation Protection and Measurements 1977 Medical radiation exposure of pregnant and potentially pregnant women. NCRP Report No. 54. NCRP Publications, Washington DC

68. Gibbs S J 1981 Approaches to radiation risks estimation. In: Coulam C M, Erickson J J, Rollo F D, James A E Jr (eds) The physical basis of medical imaging. Appleton-Century-Crofts, New York. pp 329–342

69. Diamond E L, Schmerler H, Lilienfeld A M 1973 The relationship of intrauterine radiation to subsequent mortality and development of leukemia in children. Am J Epidemiol 97:282–313

70. Oppenheim B E, Griem M L, Meier P 1974 Effects of low-dose prenatal irradiation in humans: Analysis of Chicago lying-in data and comparison with other studies. Radiat Res 57:508–544

SUGGESTIONS FOR FURTHER READING.

Callen P (ed) 1982 Obstetrical and gynecologic ultrasonography. In: Radiol Clin North Am. W. B. Saunders Co, New York.

Felson B (ed) 1982 Obstetrical radiology. In: Seminars in Roentgenology. Grune & Stratton, New York.

Fleischer A, James A E 1980 Introduction to diagnostic sonography. John Wiley & Sons, New York.

Sabbagha R (ed) 1980 Diagnostic ultrasound applied to obstetrical gynecology. Harper & Row, New York.

Sanders R, James A E (eds) 1980 Principles and practice of ultrasonography in obstetrics and gynecology, 2nd edn. Appleton-Century-Crofts, New York.

Ultrasonography in obstetrics and gynecology. Radiol Clin North Am. June 1982, Multiple Authors.

81 Gynaecology

G. H. Whitehouse and C. H. Wright

Imaging techniques
Congenital abnormalities of the female genital tract
Inflammatory disease of the female genital tract
Uterine tumours
Cysts and tumours of the ovary
The vulva
The vagina
Miscellaneous conditions of the uterus
Miscellaneous conditions of the Fallopian tubes
Contraception
Abortion
Complications of radiotherapy
Stress incontinence

IMAGING TECHNIQUES

Plain radiography

ABDOMEN

An abdominal radiograph in gynaecological practice is usually taken in the supine position, especial care being taken to show all the pelvic cavity. A radiograph in the erect position is indicated when there is a suspicion of intestinal obstruction, pneumoperitoneum, or ascites. A full bladder may mimic a gynaecological mass lesion, so it is important that the bladder is empty.

An anteroposterior radiograph of the pelvic cavity normally shows the empty bladder and the uterus as soft tissue ovoid densities separated by a fat plane. A contracted sigmoid colon is sometimes seen end on as a rounded soft tissue mass on the left side of the pelvic cavity.

Abnormal appearances

A rounded soft tissue *pelvic mass* may be due to a distended bladder, an ovarian cystic lesion or a fibroid uterus, although the latter may have a lobulated margin. Pelvic infection sometimes obscures the normal pelvic fat planes, giving a homogenous soft tissue density, with extraluminal gas being an occasional feature. Vaginal tampons have a radiolucent rectangular appearance. Gas bubbles in the wall of the vagina occur in emphysematous vaginitis.

Pelvic phleboliths are present in 25 to 33% of European adults and tend to increase in number with age. Phleboliths may be displaced by pelvic masses, best evaluated on serial radiographs. Uterine artery calcification is especially common in diabetic women.

Uterine fibroids sometimes undergo *calcification*, especially after the menopause. Ovarian lesions which undergo calcification include cystadenoma, cystadenocarcinoma, cystic teratoma and gonadoblastoma. Calcification is sometimes visible in corpora albicantia and amputated ovaries. Tuberculous disease causes calcification within the Fallopian tubes, in the region of the ovaries, and in pelvi-abdominal lymph nodes.

Contraceptive devices and *radio-opaque foreign bodies*, especially in the vagina of children, are identifiable on plain radiographs.

Ascites is frequently associated with ovarian carcinoma, but may be present in benign ovarian conditions. *Paralytic ileus* secondary to pelvic infection is usually localized, but a generalized peritonitis, perhaps from a ruptured tubo-ovarian abscess, will cause a widespread paralytic ileus. *Haemoperitoneum*, with radiological evidence of free peritoneal fluid and sometimes paralytic ileus, occurs as a result of rupture of a corpus luteum in the second half of the menstrual cycle, ruptured ectopic pregnancy and, rarely, torsion and infarction of an ovarian cyst.

Pneumoperitoneum is a frequent sequel to abdominal surgery, usually disappearing within ten days. Peritoneal gas also results from diagnostic pneumography, laparoscopy, tubal insufflation, vaginal douche, and occasionally from a patulous genital tract in the postpartum state, or in multigravid women when in the knee-elbow position.

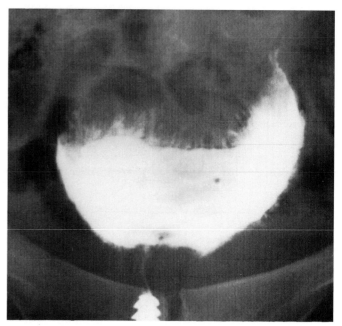

Fig. 81.1 Hysterogram in early pregnancy shows 'shaggy' outline to a large, rounded uterine cavity with a filling defect due to the trophoblast.

Chest radiography

Indications for chest radiography in the gynaecological patient include:
1. The detection of pleural or pulmonary metastases in pelvic malignant disease.
2. Postoperative chest complications.
3. To exclude pulmonary tuberculosis in infertility.
4. The assessment of congenital cardiac abnormalities which may be associated with severe anomalies of the genital tract.

The pituitary fossa

Raised levels of serum prolactin are associated with secondary amenorrhoea and infertility, and sometimes with galactorrhoea, because of inhibition of progesterone production by the ovarian granulosa cells. Some pituitary adenomas, which are often very small, will secrete abnormally high levels of prolactin. The normal mechanism for inhibition of prolactin may be impaired either by a pituitary chromophobe adenoma or a craniopharyngioma, or sometimes by the 'empty sella syndrome' in which the subarachnoid space penetrates through an incomplete sellar diaphragm into the fossa and flattens the pituitary gland. All these conditions are capable of causing sellar enlargement. Tumours may also erode the bony margins of the fossa.

High quality plain radiographs in four views (lateral, Caldwell inclined PA, half axial PA and submentovertical) will show abnormalities of the pituitary fossa in some patients with hyperprolactinaemia. Hypocycloidal tomography some-

times demonstrates a localized bulging with attenuation of the lamina dura caused by small prolactin secreting adenomas [1]. In general, however, there are very few patients with hyperprolactinaemia in whom tomography will show an abnormal pituitary fossa which was not appreciated on high quality plain radiographs [2,3]. Cisternography using a non-ionic contrast medium is useful in selected cases to demonstrate the 'empty sella syndrome' and suprasellar extension of pituitary tumours.

Computed tomography (CT) is valuable not only in identifying pituitary adenomas, but in documenting the degree of suprasellar extension. A significant percentage of pituitary adenomas demonstrate contrast enhancement, although the tumour may be isodense. Parasellar and suprasellar lesions may also be readily identified by CT. Coronal sections of the pituitary fossa are mandatory in the evaluation of a suspected sellar abnormality [4]. Metrizamide cisternography is of value in identifying the empty sella and contour abnormalities caused by the tumour [5].

Skeleton

Bone metastases are occasionally found in malignant tumours of the female genital tract, especially from carcinoma of the cervix.

Generalized skeletal growth retardation occurs with hypogonadism, e.g. in Turner's syndrome and hypopituitarism. Accelerated skeletal maturation may be seen in the adrenogenital syndrome, in oestrogen and androgen secreting gonadal tumours, occasionally with ectopic gonadotrophin production from a variety of tumours including teratoma, and in Albright's syndrome.

Hysterosalpingography

Technique

The optimal time to perform hysterosalpingography is towards the end of the first week after the menstrual period, when the isthmus is at its most distensible and the Fallopian tubes are most readily filled by contrast medium. The bladder is emptied immediately before the investigation. Premedication is not required in most cases, but 5 to 10 mg of intravenous diazepam may be given to nervous patients. Morphia and pethidine are contraindicated because they contract the smooth muscle of the Fallopian tubes.

The patient is placed in the lithotomy position on the screening table. The external os is then visualized through a vaginal speculum and is swabbed with a mild antiseptic solution. The anterior lip of the cervix is grasped by vulsellum forceps and a cannula is then inserted into the cervical canal. Contrast medium which has been warmed to body temperature is then slowly and steadily injected under image intensifier control. The contrast medium may be introduced into the uterine cavity by various methods:

1. *Metal cannulae*, such as the Green-Armytage and Jarcho types, which have a rubber acorn towards the distal end of the cannula.

2. *The Malström-Westerman vacuum uterine cannula* incorporates a plastic or aluminum cup which is placed over the cervix and is then evacuated by a vacuum pump [6]. A central cannula runs through the cup and contrast medium is then injected through it into the cervical canal. The advantages of this method are that a water-tight junction is provided, traction may be performed, and there is no need for vulsellum forceps. The technique cannot be used when there is severe cervical laceration.

3. *A No. 8 or 10 paediatric Foley catheter* is inserted through the cervical canal. Vulsellum forceps are not applied to the cervix. The catheter balloon is inflated by 1 to 1.5 ml of water and lies in the lower part of the uterine cavity. Traction is applied to the catheter. The lower uterine segment and cervical canal are not well seen, unless the balloon is gradually deflated while traction is applied to the catheter.

Non-filling of the Fallopian tubes is sometimes due to cornual spasm, which is differentiated from organic obstruction by the smooth muscle relaxation induced by i.v. glucagon [7].

Water soluble contrast medium is injected until either bilateral peritoneal spill or tubal blockage has been shown. Radiographs are taken during uterine filling, and after the uterus and Fallopian tubes have been delineated with early peritoneal spill. A further radiograph is taken 20 minutes later to determine the spillage pattern.

It is important for hysterosalpingographic contrast media to have adequate contrast density, but sufficient viscosity to diminish leakage into the vagina and rapid transit through the Fallopian tubes with resultant flooding of the peritoneal cavity. Viscosity is increased either by using contrast agents with large molecular sizes and high concentration (e.g. Hexabrix 320 or Urografin 370), or by adding 'thickeners' to the contrast medium (e.g. Diaginol Viscous which includes dextran). All water soluble contrast media disappear within one hour, except in cases of hydrosalpinx where opacification of the occluded tubes may persist for several hours. Low osmolar contrast media are being assessed and early reports suggest that they may cause less peritoneal irritation [8].

Indications

1. *Infertility*. Congenital abnormalities of the uterus and tubal occlusion.

2. *Abnormal uterine bleeding*. Hysterosalpingography complements curettage in the investigation of menstrual disorders e.g. fibroids, endometrial polyps and adenomyosis.

3. *Recurrent abortion*. The width and configuration of the internal os and cervical canal may be determined in cases of mid trimester abortion. Cervical incompetence is likely when the diameter of the internal os is more than 7 mm. Distortion of the uterine cavity by congenital abnormalities or fibroids may cause early abortion.

4. *Post Caesarean section*. The integrity of the uterine scar following Caesarean section is accurately shown by hysterography.

5. *After laparoscopic sterilisation* for assessment of Fallopian tube obstruction or patency.

6. *Before artificial insemination* for exclusion of structural abnormalities of the genital tract.

7. *Malignant uterine neoplasms*. Hysterography will accurately depict the location and extent of the tumour if necessary.

Contraindications

1. *Pregnancy*. Care must be taken to exclude pregnancy as abortion may occur. Hysterography during the first two months of pregnancy reveals an enlarged, atonic and globular uterus with thickened endometrium and the ovum as a filling defect (Fig. 81.1).

The manipulation and the injection of contrast medium in ectopic pregnancy makes dislodgement of the mole and haemorrhage a potential hazard. Ultrasonography is the investigation of choice in suspected ectopic pregnancy.

2. *Pelvic infection*. A history of salpingitis within the preceeding 6 months precludes hysterosalpingography unless a course of antibiotics has been given with a subsequent clinical assessment of successful treatment. Acute vaginitis and cervicitis are also contraindications.

3. *Immediate pre- and postmenstrual phases*. The thickened or denuded endothelium, which is respectively present before and after the menstrual period, increases the chance of intravasation. This does not put the patient at any additional risk, but may obscure adnexal detail.

4. *Sensitivity to contrast medium*. Other procedures, such as laparoscopy, should be considered as an alternative. Antihistamine cover should be given to those with a strong history of allergy.

Complications

1. *Pain*. The passage of the speculum and injection cannula often cause transient lower abdominal discomfort. A brief episode of pain is usually experienced when the cervix is grasped by the vulsellum. Distention of the uterus and Fallopian tubes, especially with rapid injection or tubal occlusion, causes central abdominal discomfort or pain. Water soluble contrast media are associated with pain on peritoneal spillage, often lasting for about one hour, but occasionally up to 24 hours.

2. *Pelvic infection*. The incidence of pelvic infection after hysterosalpingography has been estimated as 0.25 to 3%, usually as an acute exacerbation of pre-existing chronic pelvic infection, but occassionally de novo.

3. *Haemorrhage*. Slight bleeding often occurs when the cervix is grasped by the vulsellum. Bleeding after the investigation suggests the presence of an organic lesion, such as a polyp or carcinoma, or endometrial damage by the tip of the injection cannula.

4. *Allergic phenomena*. These include urticaria, asthma and laryngeal oedema as a reaction to the contrast medium.

5. *Vasovagal attacks*. Syncopal attacks are an unusual but transient occurrence.

6. *Venous intravasation* (Fig. 81.2) Delineation by contrast medium of the uterine venous network and the pelvic veins results from direct trauma to the endometrium, especially when the endometrium is thick or is denuded by recent menstruation or currettage. A high intraluminal pressure during contrast injection with tubal occlusion or excessive injection pressure, or abnormalities such as tuberculosis, uterine carcinoma or fibroids are other causes of intravasation.

Radiological anatomy (Fig. 81.3)

The cervical canal, which is best shown on hysterography with the vacuum injector, is usually 3 to 4 cm long and tends to become shorter after childbirth. The cervical canal is about one third the entire length of the uterus, and is often spindle shape. Longitudinal ridges run on the anterior and posterior wall of the cervix and have lateral branchings, the plicae palmatae, which often disappear after childbirth.

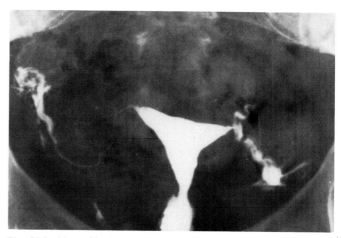

Fig. 81.3   Normal hysterosalpingogram. Isthmus and uterine body are delineated by contrast medium. Both Fallopian tubes are shown, with early peritoneal spill.

Glandular filling often occurs in the normal cervix. The isthmus is seen as a distinct segment, narrower than the uterine body and cervical canal, in only half of all normal hysterograms. The internal os appears as a short constriction of the lumen in many cases.

The cavity of the uterine body is triangular in shape, its walls being normally regular and straight or concave, although the fundal surface is occasionally convex. Both the average length and the intercornual diameters are 3.5 cm. The cornual sphincters are pear or spindle shaped and are often separated from the uterine body by a short dark line. The apex of each cornu is continuous with the tubal lumen.

The Fallopian tubes are about 5 or 6 cm in length, with a variable degree of tortuosity, the isthmic portion being of uniform diameter and opening into the wide ampulla.

Normal variants

1. A fine saw tooth pattern, giving a spiculated outline, is commonest in premenopausal women and is due to glandular filling in an atrophic endometrium [6].

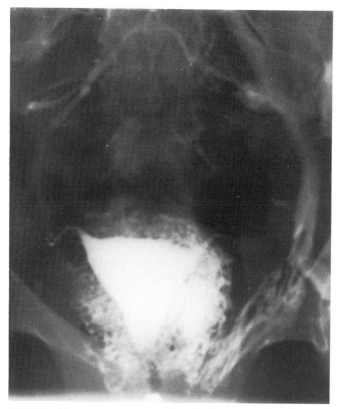

Fig. 81.2   Hysterosalpingogram with marked venous intravasation. The myometrial venous network, pelvic and iliac veins show contrast opacification.

2. Broad longitudinal uterine folds, usually 5 to 10 mm wide and parallel to the lateral borders of the uterine cavity are probably remnants of Müllerian ducts [10].
3. A double outline to the uterine cavity is due to penetration of endometrial glands, usually in the secretory phase of the menstrual cycle [11].
4. Polypoidal filling defects, usually in the secretory phase, may be associated with a normal endometrium and the absence of abnormal uterine bleeding [12].
5. Cystic spaces within the uterine wall in the upper half of the uterus are often due to adenomyosis. Dilated cervical glands and cystic cavities within the isthmus are regarded as being normal variants [13].

Pelvic pneumography

Pelvic pneumography is the visualization of the female pelvic cavity by establishing a pneumoperitoneum with carbon dioxide and then radiographing the pelvic cavity with the patient in the prone, head down position (Fig. 81.4). This technique has been rendered obsolete by ultrasonography and laparoscopy.

Vaginography

Technique

A Foley catheter is inserted into the vagina and its balloon is distended by 20 to 30 ml air to provide a snug fit just above the introitus. A water soluble contrast medium is then injected through the catheter into the vagina.

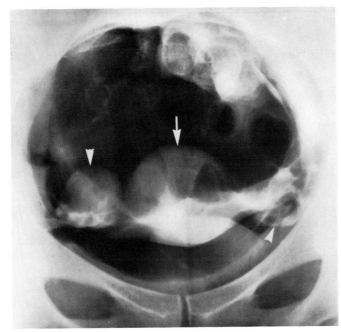

Fig. 81.4 Normal pelvic pneumogram. The uterus, [arrow] broad ligaments and ovaries [arrow heads], are clearly shown.

Indications

1. To demonstrate fistulae between the vagina and ureter, bladder or rectum.
2. Congenital or acquired abnormalities of the vagina, such as diverticula.
3. To localize, by reflux, an ectopic ureter opening into the vagina.

Gastrointestinal Studies

Barium meal and small bowel series

Gastric carcinoma occasionally metastasizes to the ovaries, giving rise to Krukenberg tumours. Fistulae between the small intestine and vagina are uncommon but may be associated with appendicectomy, pelvic abscess, operative injury and foreign bodies left at pelvic surgery. Peritoneal spread from uterine and ovarian carcinoma may distort and obstruct segments of small intestine. Adhesions from pelvic surgery or radiotherapy, pelvic inflammatory disease and endometriosis are potential causes of ileal obstruction.

Barium enema

A barium enema may be used in:
1. The evaluation of large pelvic masses
2. The assessment of spread from pelvic malignant disease
3. Diverticular disease, which may have sigmoidovaginal or, rarely, sigmoidouterine fistulae as sequelae.

Intravenous urography

Radiological assessment of the urinary tract is useful:
1. When the ureters may be deviated or compressed by large pelvic masses, possibly causing hydronephrosis. Tomography of the pelvic cavity soon after the rapid intravenous injection of contrast medium sometimes detects, and discriminates between, inflammatory pelvic masses, uterine masses, and solid and cystic ovarian masses [14].
2. Before and after gynaecological surgery. Suspected damage to the urinary tract is a definite indication for i.v. urography [15]. The presence of urinary tract symptoms before gynaecological surgery merits preoperative urographic evaluation.
3. In cases of uterine or ovarian malignancy where unsuspected neoplastic involvement of the urinary tract may be revealed, with a base line being provided for comparison with post-treatment urography.
4. In extensive pelvic endometriosis, which is associated with a high incidence of ureteric obstruction.
5. In procidentia, which sometimes causes ureteric obstruction.
6. With severe congenital abnormalities of the genital tract, which are associated with a high incidence of urinary tract anomalies.

Arteriography

The arterial supply to the uterus and adnexa is demonstrated by aortography or internal iliac arteriography, but CT scanning and ultrasonography have largely replaced gynaecological angiography.

Uterine fibroids. Angiography is especially helpful when there is a suspicion of sarcomatous change.

Carcinoma of the cervix. It has been claimed [16] that arteriography is helpful in staging carcinoma of the cervix, although coexistent inflammatory disease may give similar angiographic appearances.

Carcinoma of the endometrium may present a neoplastic circulation.

Trophoblastic tumours. Arteriography is of value where the ultrasonic findings are equivocal and where there is a suspicion of local invasion or metastasis[17].

Ovarian tumours. The blood supply of ovarian tumours is derived from the adnexal branch of the uterine artery and from the ovarian artery. Angiography, especially in combination with ultrasonography, has been found to be helpful in diagnosing the presence of ovarian tumours and for differentiating benignity from malignancy [18].

Uterine haemorrhage. The site and cause of heavy uterine bleeding may be determined by arteriography. Uterine arteriovenous malformations are especially amenable to angiographic demonstration [19]. Transcatheter embolization of the anterior division of internal iliac artery has been successfully used in the treatment of haemorrhage from advanced or recurrent carcinoma of the cervix [20].

Venography

Pelvic venography will demonstrate iliac vein thrombosis which may follow gynaecological surgery. Direct spread from uterine carcinoma and ovarian malignancies may compress the iliac veins, and cause secondary venous thrombosis.

Uterine phlebography

Contrast medium is directly injected into the fundal myometrium via a special metal cannula. Intravasation of contrast medium into the venous plexus of the uterine wall is followed by visualisation of the uterovaginal and ovarian venous plexi. Intrauterine phlebography is used to demonstrate pelvic varicoceles [21].

Lymphography

The inguinal, iliac and para-aortic lymph nodes are delineated by bipedal lymphography. It is impossible to show the hypogastric, paracervical, obturator and presacral lymph nodes. These node groups directly drain the uterine cervix and will be included in radiation portals.

Preoperative lymphography will assist in determining the feasibility and extent of proposed surgery in pelvic malignancy, while the completeness of dissection or the presence of recurrence may be determined after the operation.

Ultrasonography

An ultrasonic examination of the female pelvis is a simple non-invasive examination. The ready availability of static scanners, or high quality real-time scanners, in most departments provides an initial means of confirming and localizing a clinically suspected pelvic mass and, often, a definite diagnosis.

A full bladder is essential for the investigation, as bowel gas precludes a satisfactory pelvic examination. If necessary, the bladder is filled via a catheter. Following the initial scan, it may be useful to empty the bladder and re-examine the patient when there is difficulty in differentiating the bladder from a cystic mass. This is also useful in demonstrating fixity of the pelvic structures.

Whether real-time or static scanning is used, the gain setting should be set to show uniform diffuse echoes from within the uterus. The examination should be conducted in both sagittal and transverse planes, and an adequate hard copy record of the scan should be made at 1 to 2 cm intervals. Angulation of the transducer probe on transverse sections is useful in separating the uterus from the adnexa, while angled scans to survey the pelvic side walls are also of value in assessing the adnexal areas, and identifying the ovaries [22].

In sagittal section, the vaginal canal appears as a uniform echogenic line. The uterus lies posterior to the bladder and shows a uniformly fine echo pattern. The presence or absence of the endometrial echo is variable, but it is most frequently seen at the time of menstruation [23].

The normal uterus measures approximately $7.5 \times 5 \times 2$ cm. The Fallopian tubes and adnexal structures extend from the lateral margins of the uterus as a thin sonolucent region. The normal Fallopian tube cannot be identified as a separate structure.

The normal ovaries are visualized in a high percentage of cases. The ovaries normally measure $1 \times 2 \times 3$ cm, and are more easily defined on transverse scans than on the sagittal scans. Follicular and luteal cysts may be visualised within the ovary and assessment of follicular development and its response to hormone therapy indicates the optimum time for the induction of ovulation and conception [24].

Fluid filled loops of bowel may simulate a complex adnexal mass, but re-examination of the patient after an interval will usually show significant change in the appearances.

Computed tomography

The role of computed tomography (CT) has yet to be fully established in the assessment of the pelvic cavity. Both CT and ultrasonography may provide similar information [25]. Ultrasonography remains the initial, noninvasive imaging procedure of choice in the assessment of a gynaecological pelvic mass, but CT may provide further useful information on an unusual pelvic mass [26].

The majority of CT pelvic scans are performed in the assessment and staging of neoplasms of the pelvic organs, or in the detection of nodal involvement in lymphoma and other neoplasms [27,28]. CT is valuable in identifying the presence and extent of a pelvic tumour, both for biopsy and radiotherapy [29]. It is also useful in the identification and localization of a pelvic mass when the bladder is surgically absent or indistensible. CT is of value in the staging of bladder neoplasms and in identifying the level and nature of a ureteric obstruction. Abnormalities of the extragenital soft tissues and bony pelvis are also demonstrated accurately by CT.

Before using CT it is essential to exclude the possibility of pregnancy. The scan technique, collimation, slice-spacing and patient preparation depend on the equipment and on the suspected abnormality. 15 mm cuts with a 10 cm collimator will usually provide sufficient anatomical detail in the evaluation of a pelvic mass. Overlapping cuts are obtained if necessary. In the assessment of neoplastic disease the scans should be continued to include the para-aortic, liver and renal areas.

The patient is scanned in the supine position. A vaginal tampon assists in localizing the vagina. 500 ml of 2% oral Gastrografin 3 hours and half an hour prior to the examination is frequently sufficient to identify both the small and large bowel, while a limited enema using a similar concentration of water soluble contrast agent may be necessary to fully define the pelvic anatomy. Intravenous contrast medium delineates the ureters and vascular pelvic structures. Residual barium in the distal bowel will result in considerable scan artefacts and, if possible, the examination should be deferred until the bowel is clear.

CONGENITAL ABNORMALITIES OF THE FEMALE GENITAL TRACT

Uterine hypoplasia

Uterine agenesis is rare, and is usually associated with other severe anomalies of the genitourinary tract. The *'fetal' uterus*, which consists of a solid knob of fibrous tissue is the grossest form of hypoplasia and may be associated with absence of the vagina. Less severe forms of hypoplasia are found on hysterography in about 8% of cases of primary infertility [30]. The *'infantile' uterus* has a small body and a cervical canal which is twice the length of the uterine body. The cervical canal in the *'pubescent' uterus* is the same length as the uterine body cavity. The least severe form of hypoplasia is the *'small adult' uterus* in which there is a small capacity uterine cavity

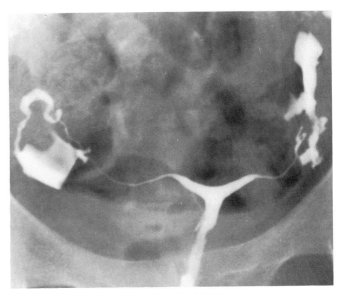

Fig. 81.5 Uterine hypoplasia of 'small adult' type.

with a slender cervical canal and perhaps relatively long Fallopian tubes (Fig. 81.5). Bicornuate or arcuate deformities (see Fig. 81.35) are sometimes seen with uterine hypoplasia. Exposure in utero to diethylstilboestrol may result in a T-shaped hypoplastic uterus in adults [31].

Failure of Müllerian duct fusion

The embryologically paired Müllerian duct systems may partially or totally fail to undergo fusion, resulting in a spectrum of congenital abnormalities in the uterus and vagina.

Uterus didelphys comprises duplication of the vagina, cervix and uterus (Fig. 81.6). In the *uterus bicornis bicollis* there are two separate uterine horns, each with its own cervix, but a single vagina. In the *bicornuate uterus* (Fig. 81.7) the two separate uterine horns are joined above the cervix, hystero-

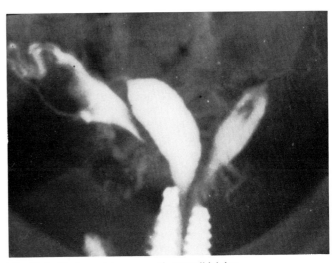

Fig. 81.6 Hysterosalpingogram of uterus didelphys.

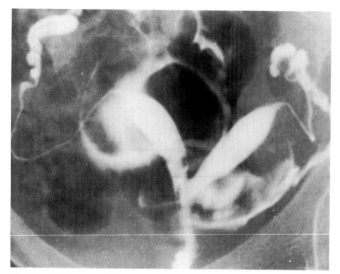

Fig. 81.7   Hysterosalpingogram of bicornuate uterus.

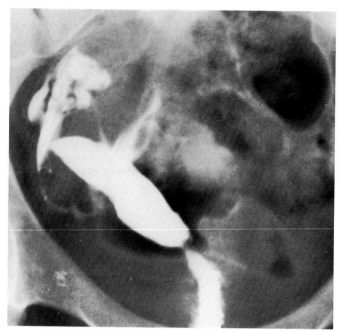

Fig. 81.8   Unicornuate uterus

graphy showing the two opacified horns to be typically separated by a wide angle. Renal agenesis or ectopia may be found in patients with bicornuate uteri. The *septate uterus* has a septum which is often thin, dividing the uterine cavity into two compartments down to the level of the isthmus. A *subseptate .uterus* is commoner than the septate type, with the septum extending only partly down the uterine body. Differentiation between a bicornuate and a septate uterus may be difficult when there is an acute angle between the two horns. A bicornuate uterus is more likely when the point of cleavage lies in the isthmus, but separation at a higher level may be seen in both bicornuate and septate uteri. Convexity of the lateral borders of the opacified bifid uterine cavity is more suggestive of bicornuate uterus, a subseptate uterus generally having straight borders.

An **arcuate uterus** shows a rounded indentation of the fundal cavity contour on hysterography and is a common uterine anomaly (see Fig. 81.35). Slight fundal concavity is common, but a true arcuate uterus has a depth of concavity of at least one fifth of the height of the uterine body. The hysterographic appearances may be mimicked by a fundal fibroid.

Unicornuate uterus represents failure of development of one half of the uterus (Fig. 81.8). One uterine horn may be absent or rudimentary and communicates with the uterine cavity or cervix in only 20% of cases. It will, therefore, not usually be demonstrated by hysterography. Haematometra may occur in an occluded rudimentary horn. Unilateral renal agenesis and ectopia often occur on the same side as the deficient or absent horn.

Congenital abnormalities of the vagina

Vaginal aplasia. Complete absence of the vagina is usually associated with an absent uterus or severe uterine anomalies.

Renal agenesis, renal ectopia and major congenital vertebral abnormalities are common associated anomalies.

Vaginal atresia and imperforate hymen. The atretic segment is usually at the junction of the upper two thirds and lower third of the vagina, where the Müllerian duct system merges with the urogenital sinus. Vaginal atresia and imperforate hymen may present with an abdominal mass, due to *hydrometrocolpos*, in the first week of life. Intravenous urography shows bilateral hydronephrosis and hydroureter due to ureteral compression by the mass in 70% of cases [32]. Fistulous connections may occur between the vagina and rectum above rectal atresia, in which case gas may be seen in the abdominal mass, or may be demonstrated between the bladder and vagina on cystography.

Haematocolpos and *haematometrocolpos* due to congenital vaginal occlusion may also present as an abdominal mass, associated with amenorrhoea, in teenagers. Vesical compression and ureteric dilatation in the presence of a pelviabdominal mass are demonstrable on intravenous urography in this older group.

Disorders of the Wolffian duct remnants

The ureters and vestibule both develop from the Wolffian duct. Occasionally an ectopic ureter opens into the vestibule or, more rarely, into the vagina. Atrophic Wolffian duct remnants form Gartner's duct and rarely protrude upon the bladder base when they are situated in the vaginal fornix [33]. The proximal portions of Gartner's duct may be delineated lateral to the uterus on hysterography when they communicate with the uterine cervix, extending upwards to the cornua or downwards to the level of the lower vagina.

The persistent urogenital sinus and intersex states

The urogenital sinus arises as the confluence of the urethra and the internal genitalia of Müllerian duct origin. The urinary and genital tracts share a common passage to the exterior when there is persistence of the urogenital sinus.

Genitography (the radiological investigation of the urogenital sinus and its communicating structures) is performed by inserting a French 8 balloon catheter into the perineal orifice, inflating the balloon and injecting contrast medium under fluoroscopic control in the left lateral position [34]. As well as the urogenital sinus, the urethra and vagina will also be delineated, and sometimes also the uterine cavity and Fallopian tubes. The urogenital sinus may be probed with a soft rubber catheter, and the urethra and bladder defined by the subsequent careful injection of contrast medium.

In the female pseudohermaphrodite, there is masculinization of the external genitalia, often with an enlarged phallus with a single perineal opening at its base. Genitography is useful in assessing the anatomy prior to plastic surgery. The perineal orifice is continuous with the urogenital sinus and there is a normal sized vagina, the urethra entering the superior part of the sinus.

The persistent cloaca

The urorectal septum may partially or totally fail to descend and divide the cloaca. A single perineal opening is found in the female infant with a *persistent cloaca*. The retrograde injection of contrast medium into the cloaca will show communications with the rectum, vagina and urethra, and often vesicoureteral reflux [35].

Ultrasonographic evaluation of congenital abnormalities of the genital tract

Abnormalities of development in the uterus and vagina are difficult to identify by ultrasound in the prepubertal patient unless they are gross. In the adolescent or adult patient, the presence of a unicornuate uterus may be suspected from its eccentric location and small size. A bicornuate uterus has a bilobed appearance with an increase in the transverse diameter. Septation abnormalities of the vagina are similarly difficult to identify ultrasonically unless obstruction is present [36]. A bifid vagina may be suspected from an increased AP diameter of the vaginal image.

The clinical history and findings of an *imperforate hymen* are characteristic in the adolescent patient. When there is obstruction of one of the septal elements of a bifid vagina, a palpable paravaginal mass is associated with painful menses. In both these circumstances, the distended vagina is identified ultrasonically by its midline position posterior to the bladder and by its elongated shape (Fig. 81.9). A *haematocolpos* has a transonic appearance with posterior echo

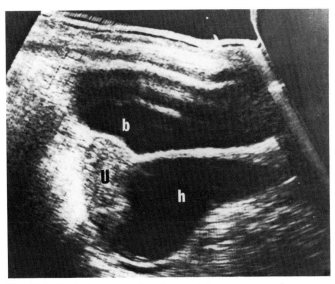

Fig. 81.9 Sagittal scan showing characteristic appearance of a haematocolpos posterior to the bladder. The uterus is not distended. [b = bladder; h = haematocolpos; u = uterus].

enhancement. A fine diffuse echo pattern may be noted due to the altered blood contents. Ultrasonography not only confirms the clinical diagnosis and assesses the extent of involvement of the uterus and Fallopian tubes, but also shows whether or not there is a hydronephrosis or other renal abnormalities.

The ultrasonographic evaluation of a developmental genital abnormality should routinely include a scan of the renal areas. Renal atresia and ectopia may be identified,

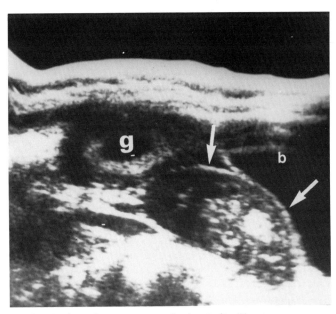

Fig. 81.10 A routine scan to assess fetal maturity. The uterus was considered to be large for dates but the presence of a pelvic mass was suspected. A uterus containing a normal gestational sac [g] lies cephalad to a pelvic kidney (arrows) which is cephalad to the bladder [b].

while the pelvic kidney demonstrates a characteristic appearance on ultrasonography (Fig. 81.10). A pelvic kidney may be an incidental finding, as in the routine obstetric scan illustrated, or may have presented clinically as a pelvic mass. The dense central sinus echo pattern, uniform parenchymal echo and characteristic reniform shape are readily identifiable features.

INFLAMMATORY DISEASE OF THE FEMALE GENITAL TRACT

Acute salpingitis

Acute inflammation of the Fallopian tubes may be due to a variety of organisms, including gonococci, staphylococci and coliforms. Most organisms enter via the vagina, but infection often occurs in combination with uterine and peritoneal inflammation. Adhesions may form after acute salpingitis, especially at the fimbriated ends of the Fallopian tubes, resulting in a distended tube which may either be filled with clear fluid (*hydrosalpinx*) or with pus (*pyosalpinx*). A *tubo-ovarian abscess* is another possible complication.

Plain radiography

The normal pelvic fat lines are obliterated by inflammatory exudate. Moderately dilated loops of small intestine with fluid levels are sometimes seen in the lower part of the abdomen and represent local ileus. A generalised paralytic ileus and free peritoneal fluid may result from widespread peritonitis in more severe cases. Peritoneal adhesions occasionally result in mechanical intestinal obstruction. An intrauterine contraceptive device is associated with acute pelvic inflammatory disease in about 34% of cases [37].

Ultrasonography of acute pelvic inflammatory disease

There are characteristic ultrasonographic appearances of acute pelvic inflammatory disease (Fig. 81.11). The uterus appears slightly enlarged and more transonic than normal. The endometrial echo becomes prominent, with a sonolucent margin due to the associated endometritis. The adnexa appear prominent and have a complex echo pattern. The appearance is usually symmetrical [38]. The uterine margins are not clearly defined, and small amounts of fluid may be present in the cul-de-sac and adnexal areas. Complete resolution of these appearances may occur, although the adnexa may subsequently show a little thickening. The changes in uterine echogenicity usually show rapid resolution.

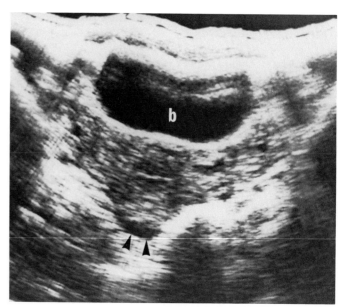

Fig. 81.11 Acute pelvic inflammatory disease. Transverse scan. The adnexa are markedly thickened and the ovaries cannot be identified as separate structures. There is an overall increase in transonicity of the pelvic structures and a small amount of fluid is seen in the cul-de-sac [arrows]. [b = bladder].

Hydrosalpinx

Hysterosalpingography

Hysterosalpingography shows tubal dilatation, especially of the ampullary portion, with loculation and absent or limited

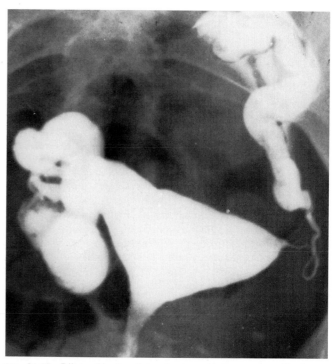

Fig. 81.12 Bilateral hydrosalpinx due to past inflammatory adhesions. Slight peritoneal spill from the left Fallopian tube outlines ampulla.

peritoneal spillage of contrast medium (Fig. 81.12). Tubal dilatation, however, is not inevitable in the presence of periampullary adhesions. The Fallopian tubes may be fixed, or in an abnormal position, due to adhesions. Contrast medium will still be present in the obstructed tubes 1 hour after the examination. Convolution of both the isthmus and ampulla is common in the presence of peritubal adhesions [39]. Agreement between laparoscopic findings and hysterosalpingography in regard to tubal patency is found in 70 to 76% of cases [40,41], with laparoscopy giving the better appraisal of tubal structure and the state of the pelvic peritoneum.

Ultrasonography

A hydrosalpinx may be ultrasonically indistinguishable from an ovarian cyst. Adhesions within the hydrosalpinx may be thicker than commonly encountered with a simple ovarian cyst (Fig. 81.13).

Pyosalpinx, tubo-ovarian and ovarian abscess

An adnexal abscess is rarely due to primary gonococcal infection, being usually caused by reinfection or secondary bacterial invasion by other organisms. Septic abortion, intra-uterine manipulations and pelvic operations may also provoke a pyogenic adnexal abscess. In one series [42], over half the cases of tubo-ovarian abscess were found in women with intrauterine contraceptive devices.

A tubo-ovarian abscess shows radiographically as a soft tissue mass in most cases. Occasionally, small radiolucent gas bubbles are visible within the abscess. Adnexal abscesses may rupture, causing a generalized peritonitis, and sometimes perforate into the intestine, bladder or vagina.

Ureteric dilatation, with obstruction at or just below pelvic brim level, occurs in 80% of tubo-ovarian abscesses [43]. The ureter may be deviated in either a lateral or a medial direction. Periureteric scarring leads to failure of regression of the ureteral obstruction in many cases even after successful treatment of the abscess. Adhesions may also cause recto-sigmoid narrowing seen on barium enema.

Ultrasonography of chronic pelvic inflammatory disease and abscess

No significant uterine changes are identified in the presence of chronic pelvic inflammatory disease. The adnexal findings show a variable appearance. Abscess formation may be unilateral or bilateral. A tubo-ovarian abscess usually shows an irregular thickened echogenic wall with a transonic centre [44]. Faint echoes may be seen within the transonic cystic area due to cellular debris, and may show gravity-dependent layering (Fig. 81.14). Septation is sometimes identified within the abscess and frequently has a thickened and irregular appearance.

Pelvic inflammatory disease of extragenital origin

Diverticulitis. Adnexal inflammatory disease may be mimicked by acute diverticulitis with or without abscess formation. A diverticular abscess sometimes causes vagino-colic fistula, demonstrable on barium enema examination.

Appendicitis. Right sided acute salpingitis, or hydrosalpinx, may be caused by the spread of infection from adjacent appendicitis.

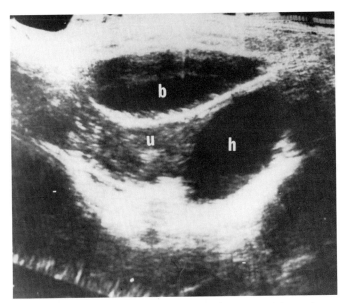

Fig. 81.13 Hydrosalpinx showing characteristic elongated shape. A little residual debris is present. [h = hydrosalpinx; b = bladder u = uterus].

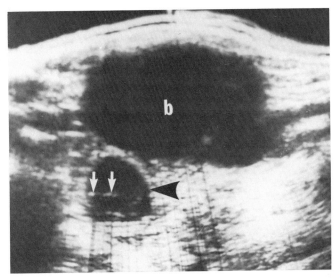

Fig. 81.14 Pelvic inflammatory disease. Adnexal abscess [black arrow] showing faint gravity dependent echoes and layering of debris [white arrows]. [b = bladder].

Crohn's disease. Salpingitis, usually unilateral, and tubo-ovarian abscess may be due to direct involvement of the adnexa from the adjacent rectosigmoid or terminal ileum when these are affected by Crohn's disease. Rectovaginal fistula is another possible sequel. Crohn's disease occasionally presents as an acute salpingitis.

Ultrasonography

Abscess formation ultrasonically presents a thick wall appearance with internal echoes due to the debris and pus. More commonly, a complex ill defined mass is identified with dense echogenic areas due to the inflamed and adherent loops of bowel. Both a gallium isotope scan and a CT scan may provide a definitive diagnosis where the ultrasound findings are inconclusive or at variance with the clinical findings [45].

Diverticulosis of the Fallopian Tubes (salpingitis isthmica nodosa)

Hysterosalpingography shows multiple small diverticula of the Fallopian tubes. The diverticula are up to 2 mm in diameter and are usually situated on a 1 to 2 cm long segment of the proximal portions of the Fallopian tubes (Fig. 81.15). Both Fallopian tubes are often involved, with tubal obstruction being present in many cases [46]. Inflammatory changes are often found on pathological examination, but infection may not be the sole cause and could be a secondary effect. The consistently nodular and uniform appearance of the diverticula is the main feature which distinguishes the condition from tuberculous salpingitis.

Uterine infections

Gas gangrene. Uterine gas gangrene is due to clostridial infection and usually follows septic abortion. Bubbles of gas may be seen within either the cavity or wall of the uterus, sometimes extending into the surrounding tissues.

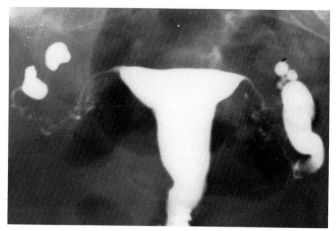

Fig. 81.15 Diverticulosis of Fallopian tubes.

Physopyometra. Cervical stenosis, especially when due to carcinoma of the cervix or following radiotherapy, predisposes to physopyometra. A large rounded pelvic mass which contains gas and a fluid level is sometimes seen on radiographs.

Cervicitis

Gross dilatation of cervical (Nabothian) glands and ulceration of the endocervix are found on hysterography in cases of endocervicitis, but the diagnosis of cervicitis cannot be made from hysterographic appearances alone [47]. Nonspecific inflammatory changes may be found in curettings even when the cervical contours are smooth or only slightly irregular on hysterography. A normal microscopic appearance may be associated with a very irregular and protruberant cervical contour.

Vaginitis

Vaginal foreign bodies are a cause of vaginitis in the paediatric age group, being identified and localized on pelvic radiographs if they are radio-opaque or by vaginography if they are radiolucent.

Emphysematous vaginitis is a benign, self-limiting condition in which gas filled cysts are present in the lamina propria of the vaginal wall and cervix. Trichomonas infection is the cause of emphysematous vaginitis, which often occurs in pregnant patients. Small gas bubbles are seen behind and above the symphysis pubis on plain radiographs.

Tuberculosis

Tuberculosis of the female genital tract tends to be a latent disease with few symptoms and often no abnormality on physical examination, although it is a cause of infertility and amenorrhoea. Initially, tuberculosis involves the muscle component of the Fallopian tubes, from whence it spreads to involve the serosal and mucosal layers. The uterus is secondarily affected in only about half the cases of tuberculous salpingitis, so that a negative culture from uterine curettings does not exclude the diagnosis of genital tuberculosis. 10% of patients with genital tuberculosis have renal involvement.

Tuberculous salpingitis

Plain radiographs of the pelvic cavity may show calcification in the region of the Fallopian tubes and ovaries. Tubal occlusion, usually bilateral, is often seen on hysterosalpingography, although the Fallopian tubes may remain patent. Tubal dilatation is usually moderate or slight in degree, with a club-like appearance to the ampullae [48] (Fig. 81.16). The tubal occlusion may be in the isthmic or ampullary portions. Gross thickening of the longitudinal mucosal folds of the

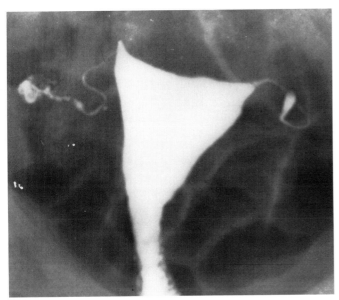

Fig. 81.16 Tuberculous salpingitis. Bilateral tubal occlusion. Irregularity and beading of right Fallopian tube.

Fallopian tube is suggestive of tuberculosis. Although the tubal contours are often smooth, tuberculous salpingitis may cause an irregular or ragged outline, the presence of cavities, and multiple tubal strictures which give a beaded or 'rosary' appearance (Fig. 81.16). Small sinus tracts or irregular recesses may fill during salpingography from the diseased Fallopian tubes. Sometimes the Fallopian tubes are rigid and straight, giving a 'pipe stem' appearance [49], or are fixed in an abnormal situation. Tubointestinal and tubo-vesical fistulae sometimes communicate with tuberculous pyosalpinges.

Uterine tuberculosis

Tubal changes are to be anticipated in all cases of uterine tuberculosis. Hysterography shows polypoidal lesions, a hyperplastic endometrium and a ragged sawtoothed uterine contour [50]. Sinus tracks may extend into the myometrium. Eventually, fibrosis results in a shrivelled and deformed uterus (Fig. 81.17). Venous and sometimes lymphatic intravasation are associated hysterographic features.

UTERINE TUMOURS

Fibroids (Fibromyomata)

Plain radiographic findings

Multiple and large fibroids may show as a soft tissue pelvic mass, the outline of which tends to be lobulated. Calcification within fibroids either follows necrosis in pregnancy or is secondary to postmenopausal degeneration. Small scattered calcifications are initially seen, increasing in size and number and eventually coalescing to form coarse aggregations. Less commonly, a peripheral rim of calcification is apparent (Fig. 81.18).

Hysterosalpingography

Submucosal fibroids are especially likely to cause distortion of the uterine cavity, while subserosal and small intramural

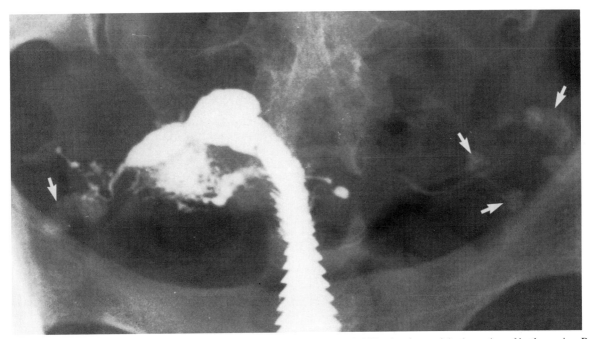

Fig. 81.17 Tuberculous metritis with deformed uterus and venous intravasation. Calcification (arrows) in the region of both ovaries. Both Fallopian tubes occluded.

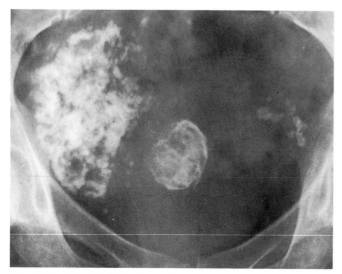

Fig. 81.18 Fibroid calcification, both sponge-like and curvilinear in type.

fibroids are often associated with a normal hysterogram appearance. A single fibroid will cause a smooth and rounded filling defect on the uterine contour, while multiple submucosal fibroids are associated with separate filling defects and sometimes gross distortion of the uterine cavity (Fig. 81.19). Large fibroids may cause a crescentic or spindle

shaped elongation of the cavity. Submucosal intramural fibroids are often associated with globular enlargement of the uterine cavity [51]. Asymmetry and blunting of the cornua, and sometimes obstruction to tubal filling may be caused by fibroids.

Small sessile, polypoidal submucosal fibroids may be difficult to distinguish from endometrial polyps, but tend to be more regular in outline. Pedunculated fibroids may occupy most of the uterine cavity, sometimes descending into a dilated and elongated cervical canal. Fibroids arising from the cervix itself tend to elongate and distort its outline.

Subserous fibroids usually give no hysterosalpingographic signs, but are occasionally large enough to deform the uterine cavity or compress and deviate a Fallopian tube. Peritoneal spillage of contrast medium may delineate subserous fibroids.

Hysterography will show the extent of uterine deformity after myomectomy.

I.V. Urography

Uterine fibroids have been demonstrated in 85% of cases by pelvic tomography during the vascular phase of i.v. urography [52]. Large fibroid masses often cause ureteric obstruction and hydronephrosis, with restoration to normal after hysterectomy. The bladder dome is sometimes concave, or shows multiple pressure defects, due to an enlarged and lobulated fibroid uterus. Cervical fibroids, or a retroverted fibroid uterus, may cause bladder neck obstruction.

Barium enema

The sigmoid segment is sometimes compressed and/or stretched by a fibroid uterus at pelvic inlet and may be deviated upwards or downwards.

Angiography

Arteriography is seldom performed, but is occasionally helpful in cases of suspected malignant change in fibroids. Large fibroids straighten and laterally displace the marginal segment of the uterine artery. The intramural vessels adjacent to the fibroids are also straightened and there is opacification of the capsular vessels of the tumour. Fibroids are often very vascular, contain numerous small intercommunicating vessels, and give a tumour blush in the capillary phase.

Ultrasonography

Ultrasonography is very accurate in distinguishing a uterine fibroid from extrauterine pathology. The uterus usually shows some increase in size and the outline is a little irregular or lobular, although still showing good definition. The commonest appearance is that of a well defined transonic area within the uterine outline (Fig. 81.20). Uniform low level echoes are present throughout the tumour, but there

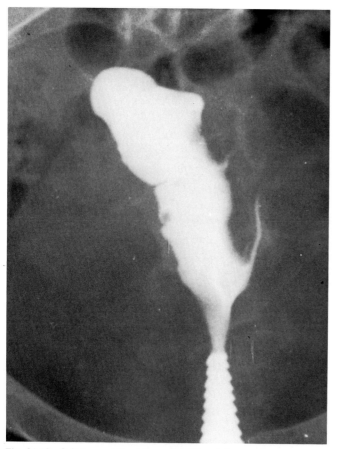

Fig. 81.19 Submucosal fibroids causing filling defects on hysterogram.

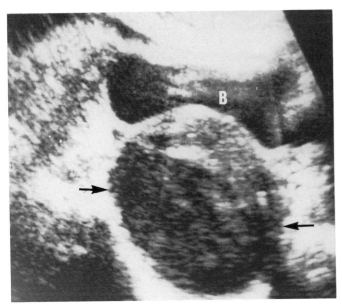

Fig. 81.20 A large uterine fibroid [arrows] showing diffuse low level echoes, with small areas of degeneration present. [B = bladder].

may be small areas of increased echogenicity due to degeneration. Calcification is demonstrated as dense echogenic areas which may show acoustic shadowing[53]. The tumour may have a well defined margin, while an incomplete echogenic line may be identified at the tumour margin due to a pseudocapsule.

Distortion of the endometrial cavity echo may occur and is helpful in identifying smaller submucous fibroids. Associated menorrhagia may cause a prominent uterine cavity echo.

Less commonly, extensive degeneration occurs within fibroids, giving a bizarre appearance with extensive echogenic areas and poor internal definition of the margins, difficult to distinguish from endometrial carcinoma or leiomyosarcoma. A pendunculated fibroid has to be distinguished from a solid extrauterine tumour, but careful scanning will usually reveal its uterine attachment and origin. Ascites may be present in association with the uterine fibroid. Careful evaluation of the ovaries and adnexa is indicated to exclude other pelvic pathology.

Care should be taken to exclude a pregnancy within a fibroid uterus in a woman of childbearing age (Fig. 81.21), as an early gestational sac may be missed in a uterus containing multiple fibroids. Fibroids are said to commonly increase in size during pregnancy[54], but an apparent decrease in size may be due to the concomitant growth of the uterus. Sequential pre- and postpartum scans are indicated because of the known complications of fibroids in pregnancy.

Carcinoma of the cervix

Carcinoma of the uterine cervix, after breast cancer, is the second most common malignancy in women and accounts for two thirds of malignant tumours found in the female genital tract. Most cases of cervical carcinoma occur between the late thirties and the middle of the sixth decade.

Absence of a defining capsule to the cervix and a rich lymphatic network contribute to spread of the tumour to parametrial tissues and pelvic lymph nodes. Extension to the vagina, and thence to the bladder, may cause vesicovaginal fistula although direct spread from the supravaginal portion of the cervix may also reach the bladder. The ureters often become obstructed when there is parametrial spread. The rectum is not often directly involved, because of its separation from the cervix by the pouch of Douglas. Distant metastases reach the lungs or skeleton.

Lymphography

Initial lymphatic spread is to the nodes in parametrium, and to the obturator, internal and external iliac groups of nodes. Later on, the disease spreads to the common iliac and to the para-aortic lymph nodes. The internal iliac and obturator lymph nodes are not shown on bipedal lymphography, but will be included in standard radiotherapy fields. Lymph node metastases cause filling defects within the nodes, sometimes with enlargement, displacement or matting of nodes. Extensive lymph node involvement causes their obliteration, with stasis in lymph vessels and the formation of collateral lymphatic flow.

In one series[55], pedal lymphography had a diagnostic accuracy of 85% in carcinoma of the cervix, the frequency of positive lymphograms being 10% in clinical Stage I disease, 19% in Stage II and 39% in Stage III disease. In comparison[56], pedal lymphography has been considered to be too unreliable in determining treatment in Stage I and Stage II disease, while being of value in combination with operative findings when the aim was to remove nodes which had been classified as positive or equivocal for metastasis. Increase in size of a nodal defect over a six week period is the most reliable sign of metastasis, and differentiates from reactive hyperplasia, infection and fibrous or fatty defects[56]. Follow-up radiographs also allow assessment of response to radiotherapy.

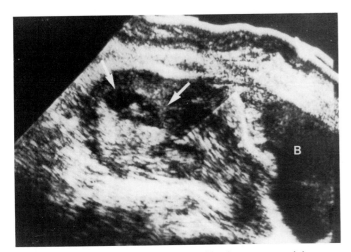

Fig. 81.21 Scan 3 cm to the left of the midline in uterus containing multiple fibroids and containing an early gestational sac [arrows] [B = Bladder].

Urography

The pelvic portion of the ureter is vulnerable to extension of cervical carcinoma to the parametrium. The incidence of ureteric obstruction from spread of cervical carcinoma increases with each clinical stage of the disease. An overall incidence of 7.4% of ureteric obstruction has been found before treatment [57]. Ureteric involvement has a grave prognostic significance, only 41.7% of patients surviving one year, while 77.8% with normal urograms survived one year post radiotherapy in one series [58]. Ureteric obstruction persisting or developing after radiotherapy is associated with tumour recurrence in the great majority of cases, only rarely being caused by the direct effects of radiotherapy. While vesicovaginal fistula is sometimes due to direct spread of the tumour, in most cases of cervical carcinoma the fistula is likely to be a complication of hysterectomy or irradiation.

Pelvic venography

Iliac vein obstruction is sometimes caused by tumour spread, but large pelvic lymph node masses may not be associated with any iliac vein abnormality.

Pelvic arteriography

Arteriography has been found to be accurate in the staging of cervical carcinoma [16]. Most cervical carcinomas have a tumour blush in the capillary phase, often with abnormal corkscrew-like arteries and sometimes arteriovenous fistulae. Vascular cervical carcinomas tend to be more radiosensitive than avascular tumours. Unfortunately, coincidental inflammatory disease may mimic cervical carcinoma on arteriography.

Barium enema

Spread of cervical carcinoma to the rectosigmoid may cause a smooth long stenosis, usually with an intact mucosa.

Distant metastases

Lung metastases are usually multiple and may show cavitation. Mediastinal and hilar lymphadenopathy are sometimes seen, with lymphangitis carcinomatosa as an occasional manifestation.

Bone metastases are usually osteolytic. The lumbosacral spine and pelvis are the most frequent sites of bone involvement, in many cases due to direct invasion from iliac and para-aortic lymph node metastases.

Isotope imaging

Isotope scanning of patients who have received Indium III attached to bleomycin shows a high level of accuracy in determining the site and extent of cervical carcinoma [59].

Ultrasonography and computed tomography

Neither ultrasonography nor computed tomography has been shown to be useful in the diagnosis of Stage I or II carcinoma of the cervix. CT has proved disappointing in the evaluation of lymph node metastases from pelvic tumour. In one series [28], 40% of false negatives were encountered, principally due to lack of nodal enlargement and the inability of CT to detect micronodular involvement. The presence of lymph node enlargement is readily demonstrated by CT (Fig. 81.22), which is more accurate than ultrasonography in the detection of pelvic and para-aortic lymph node involvement. Both modalities are very accurate in the detection of liver metastases and both will demonstrate hydronephrosis due to ureteric obstruction.

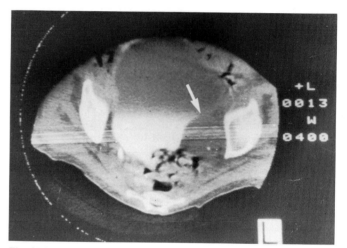

Fig. 81.22 CT scan showing involvement of internal iliac lymph nodes [arrow] with metastases from carcinoma of the cervix. Both ureters are seen and are of normal calibre.

Carcinoma of the endometrium

Endometrial carcinoma is one third as common as cervical carcinoma and usually presents with postmenopausal bleeding.

Hysterosalpingography

It has been claimed [60] that the presence and extent of endometrial carcinoma is accurately diagnosed by hysterography, sometimes more reliably than by curettage. The appearances are those of a focal mass or diffuse irregularity of outline.

Lymphography

Lymph node metastases have been found in 19% of patients with endometrial carcinoma [61], para-aortic lymph node involvement being demonstrated in 90% of positive cases. Uterine body tumours spread directly to para-aortic lymph nodes, while those low down in the uterus metastasize to internal iliac nodes.

Urography

Ureteric obstruction may result from spread of endometrial carcinoma.

Angiography

Hypervascularity with tumour vessels, arteriovenous shunts and venous lakes are angiographic features of endometrial carcinoma [62].

Distant metastases

As in cervical carcinoma, invasion of the pelvic bones and lumbar vertebrae sometimes occur as a result of iliac and para-aortic lymph node metastases. The incidence of bone metastases is low and lung metastases are less frequent than in cervical carcinoma.

Ultrasound and computed tomography

As in cervical carcinoma, similar reservations apply to the ability of both ultrasound and CT to detect early endometrial neoplasms. CT may demonstrate a central low density area with irregular margins, and the ultrasound examination occasionally shows central markedly irregular high density echoes. The normal uterine outline is lost if there is local invasion. Ascites, if present, may readily be demonstrated by ultrasonography.

Sarcoma of the uterus

Leiomyosarcomas represent malignant degeneration of uterine fibroids. These tumours, including their lung and lymph node metastases, are sometimes well differentiated and slow growing in nature. Mixed mesenchymal tumours sometimes have an osteosarcomatous element which may show calcification.

Choriocarcinoma

Choriocarcinoma is preceeded by hydatidiform mole in 50% of cases, and by a normal pregnancy or abortion in about equal proportions in the rest.

Angiography (Fig. 81.23)

Arteriography is helpful in distinguishing between hydatidiform mole and choriocarcinoma in problem cases, and provides a means of early detection of choriocarcinoma in those patients whose chorionic gonadotrophin levels remain elevated after molar pregnancy. The uterine arteries are usually much increased in size, with associated dilatation of intramural arteries. Vascular spaces of irregular size and

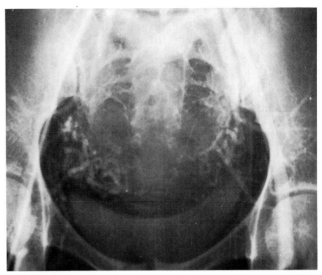
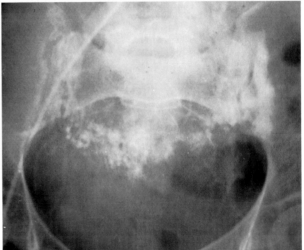

Fig. 81.23 Choriocarcinoma (A) Arterial phase showing dilatation and tortuosity of uterine and ovarian arteries (B) Later arterial phase with irregular tumour vessels, vascular spaces within uterine cavity and arteriovenous shunting.

shape are seen, with shunting of contrast medium into draining veins. Areas of abnormal vascularity often show central avascular areas due to blood clot or fibrinoid material [63]. The position of these abnormal vascular changes reflect tumour spread within and beyond the uterine wall. The differential diagnosis of choriocarcinoma and invasive mole may be difficult and relies on subtle distinctions [64]. Arteriovenous shunting within the uterus may persist after successful chemotherapy [65].

Metastases

Occasionally there is ureteric obstruction and bladder involvement by choriocarcinoma. Lung metastases occur in 45% of cases [66]. The metastases are usually multiple and well defined, although they may be ill defined and infiltrative in appearance. Calcification occasionally develops at sites of pulmonary metastases which have been successfully treated by chemotherapy. Malignant pleural effusion may develop.

Ultrasonography of uterine sarcomas and choriocarcinomas

Both leiomyosarcoma and choriocarcinoma may show an extremely bizarre ultrasonographic configuration. The tumour is often extremely large and it may be difficult to determine the origin of the mass. Leiomyosarcomas show a marked propensity to necrosis and large cystic areas may be demonstrated within the tumour.

Ultrasonography has been found [17] to be as sensitive, and perhaps more specific, than angiography in the detection of choriocarcinoma, with the advantages of being noninvasive and easily repeatable. Arteriography still has a role in cases in which ultrasonography is equivocal and where there is a suspicion of local invasion.

The diagnosis of choriocarcinoma may be suspected on ultrasonography because of the presence of multiple theca lutein cysts. Liver metastases are often necrotic in both leiomyosarcoma and choriocarcinoma.

CYSTS AND TUMOURS OF THE OVARY

Non-neoplastic cysts of the ovaries

Follicular cysts

A follicular cyst results from fluid distention of an atretic ovarian follicle and is usually 3 to 10 cm in diameter. Follicular cysts may undergo torsion and rupture, but often undergo spontaneous regression.

Lutein cysts

Granulosa lutein cysts. Resorption of blood after haemorrhage into a corpus luteum may initiate the accumulation of fluid and result in a granulosa lutein cyst which is usually 1 to 4 cm in diameter. Rupture of the cyst sometimes occurs, resulting in intraperitoneal haemorrhage.

Theca lutein cysts. Luteinization of theca cells of atretic follicles causes the formation of theca lutein cysts, associated with excessive gonadotrophin production in cases of hydatidiform mole and choriocarcinoma. The ovaries are polycystic and vary in size from slight enlargement to large pelviabdominal masses.

Radiology

Benign ovarian cysts are seen on plain radiographs as well defined, rounded soft tissue masses within the pelvic cavity, sometimes rising into the abdomen (Fig. 81.24), but distinct

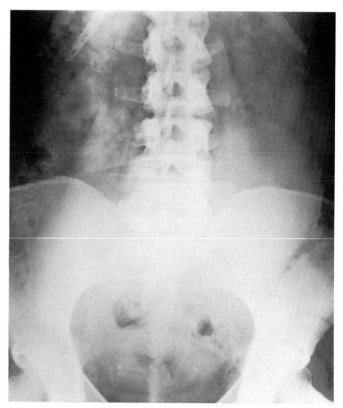

Fig. 81.24 Large lobulated soft tissue mass due to ovarian cyst.

from the urinary bladder and uterus. Large ovarian cysts often appear as midline masses. The intestines are displaced in superior and lateral directions by large cysts.

Urography

Tomography of an ovarian cyst during the injection of urographic contrast medium shows the cyst to be avascular, although a thin curvilinear rim of opacification is present in at least half of the cases [52]. The bladder is flattened and concave due to extrinsic pressure from large cysts which may displace and obstruct the ureters causing hydronephrosis.

Hysterosalpingography

Large ovarian cysts cause displacement of the uterus, the ipsilateral Fallopian tube being stretched around the mass.

Barium enema

Compression of the sigmoid colon may occur at pelvic brim level. Very large cysts displace other parts of the colon.

Angiography

Ovarian cysts are avascular with displacement of the tuboovarian branches of the uterine artery. Ultrasonography is more useful than arteriography.

Ultrasonography of ovarian cysts

The dimensions and identification of the normal ovaries have been described previously. Although the normal ovaries may be routinely identified with careful scanning, failure to visualize them should not be considered abnormal. An ovarian cyst is readily identified, the cyst showing a transonic appearance with posterior echo enhancement and well defined margins (Fig. 81.25). Faint internal echoes are present, depending on the content of the cyst, and are caused by thick mucin or long standing haemorrhage within the cyst. A follicular cyst may be up to 10 cm in diameter.

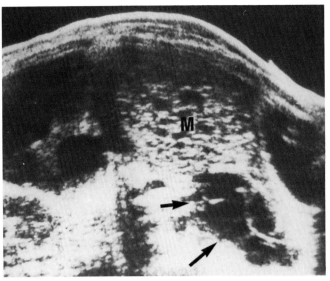

Fig. 81.27 Multiple theca-lutein cysts [arrows] associated with a hydatidiform mole [M].

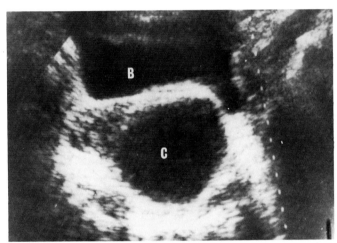

Fig. 81.25 Transverse scan showing a simple, well defined ovarian cyst. Faint echoes within the cyst are due to the mucin content. [C = cyst; B = bladder].

It may be impossible to distinguish from a serous cystadenoma or hydrosalpinx unless serial scans are obtained, in which case there is demonstrable regression of the follicular cyst. A luteal cyst shows a similar transonic appearance (Fig. 81.26). Haemorrhage within a luteal cyst may cause quite marked enlargement and may clinically mimic the symptoms and signs of ectopic pregnancy, but there are usually characteristic ultrasonic appearances. Theca lutein cysts, which are usually multiple and lateral, occur with hydatidiform mole and choriocarcinoma (Fig. 81.27).

Stein-Leventhal syndrome

The Stein-Leventhal syndrome consists of amenorrhoea and sterility, with hirsuitism in 50% of patients and obesity in 10% of cases [67]. The breasts are either hypoplastic or show normal development. Multiple follicular cysts and capsular thickening are found in the ovaries.

Pelvic pneumography

Pelvic pneumography was originally used to demonstrate polycystic ovaries. The size and shape of the ovaries in the Stein-Leventhal syndrome show much inconsistency, having a tendency to enlargement but often being of normal size.

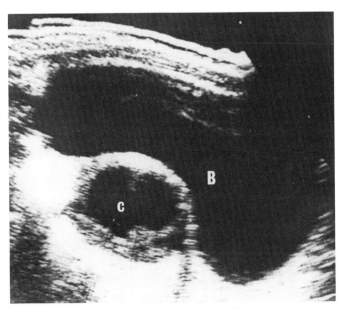

Fig. 81.26 Sagittal scan through the right ovary in a patient presenting clinically with suspected ectopic gestation. The ultrasonographic diagnosis of a haemorrhagic luteal cyst was confirmed by laparoscopy. [C = cyst, B, bladder].

Ultrasonography

This readily identifies the enlarged, bilateral polycystic ovaries and multiple small cysts are found in those cases where ovarian enlargement is not a feature. Laparoscopy is a more accurate method of demonstrating the polycystic ovaries. Uterine hypoplasia occurs in long standing cases [67].

Epithelial tumours

Epithelial tumours comprise over half of all ovarian neoplasms and occur as mucinous or serous types, which are either benign or malignant, or as solid carcinomas.

Serous cystadenoma and cystadenocarcinoma

Serous cystadenomas are benign and are mainly cystic in nature while cystadenocarcinomas, which comprise a quarter of all serous ovarian tumours, have a larger solid component. Serous tumours vary in size from a few centimetres in diameter to enormous dimensions. Papillary masses are found on the external and internal surfaces. Psammoma bodies are present in both benign and malignant types. The tumours are bilateral in nearly half the cases.

Mucinous cystadenoma and cystadenocarcinoma

Only 5% of mucinous cystic ovarian tumours are malignant, being bilateral in 5%. The surface is usually smooth and papillary excrescences are much less frequent than in the serous types. Rupture of benign or malignant tumours gives pseudomyxoma peritonei.

Solid carcinoma

Some solid carcinomas are undifferentiated while others are derived from cystadenomatous and granulosa cell tumours.

Radiology

Plain radiography

Soft tissue pelvic masses, often extending into the abdomen, are present. Psammoma body calcification is often visible in serous cystadenomas and in 12% of serous cystadenocarcinomas [68] (Fig. 81.28). Aggregations of psammoma bodies give a granular, hazy calcification. Metastases also show this same pattern of calcification and may be visible within the peritoneum, liver, abdominal lymph nodes, lungs and other organs. Serosal metastases are often distributed along the course of the colon and could be mistaken for previously ingested barium.

A high uptake of technetium diphosphonate has been demonstrated on isotope scanning in the calcified abdominal metastases [69]. Bizarre, dense and well defined calcifications are sometimes visible within serous cystadenocarcinomas. Mucinous cystic ovarian tumours rarely calcify, but curvilinear calcifications may develop in pseudomyxoma peritonei.

Ascites is common in ovarian carcinoma. Pleural effusions are usually due to pleural metastases, although sometimes ascites and pleural effusions are not related to metastasis but resolve spontaneously when the ovarian tumour is removed, being examples of pseudo-Meigs syndrome (vide infra).

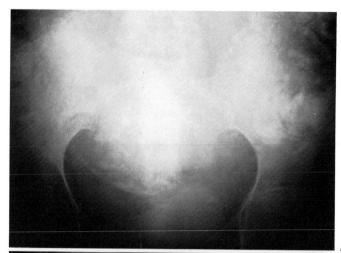

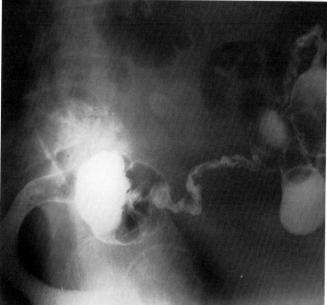

Fig. 81.28 Papillary cystadenocarcinoma of ovary (A) calcification (B) barium enema shows stricture of sigmoid colon and anterior rectal mass due to carcinoma.

Urography

Some large ovarian tumours are delineated by the total body opacification effect during i.v.u. Ovarian carcinomas cause ureteral obstruction in up to 70% of cases [70].

Barium studies

Malignant ovarian masses may stretch, indent and narrow the rectosigmoid and cause nodular defects on the luminal aspect. Elsewhere in the intestinal tract, strictures and fixation with alteration of mucosal pattern develop when peritoneal metastases invade the bowel wall (Fig. 81.28B).

Lymphography

Ovarian carcinomas metastasize in about 46% of patients [71] to para-aortic and iliac lymph nodes, while tumours which have spread to adjacent pelvic viscera and peritoneum metastasize to iliac lymph nodes. Serous cystadenocarcinomas spread more frequently to lymph nodes than do mucinous tumours.

Angiography

Ovarian tumours derive their blood supply from the adnexal branch of the uterine artery. They may be relatively avascular or very vascular overall or in part.

Ultrasound and computed tomography in the evaluation of the ovarian cyst

Ultrasound very accurately defines the location of a pelvic mass, and provides relevant information as to its internal consistency (cyst, solid or complex), but the ultrasonic findings have always to be considered in the light of the clinical history in order to obtain a specific diagnosis. The appearance of physiological and pathophysiological cysts and cystic ovarian tumours may be indistinguishable. Fimbrial and paraovarian cysts are seen as well defined, unilocular cysts. Faint internal echoes may be present within the cyst from mucin, altered blood or cellular debris from infection.

Serous cystadenomas may show a considerable variation in size, commonly being less than 20 cm diameter, but occasionally being extremely large, displacing the intestines upwards and laterally, so enabling differentiation from massive ascites. The tumours are frequently bilateral, (Fig. 81.29), and may then be mistaken for a single lobulated tumour because thin septa are sometimes present in a serous cystadenoma. The tumour is thin walled with well defined margins.

Serous cystadenocarcinomas show loss of the well defined outline, which is seen with their benign counterpart, and solid elements are identified within the tumour. Lymph node

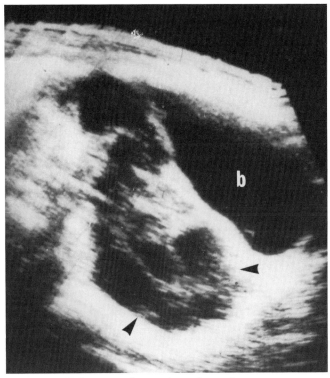

Fig. 81.30 Mucinous cystadenocarcinoma [arrows]. Extensive solid elements are present in the tumour and there is loss of marginal definition [b = bladder].

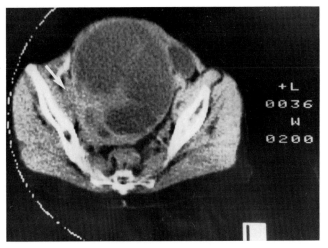

Fig. 81.31 Mucinous cystadenocarcinoma. The ultrasound findings were equivocal, but a CT scan shows loss of marginal definition [arrow] of the tumour, indicating its malignant nature.

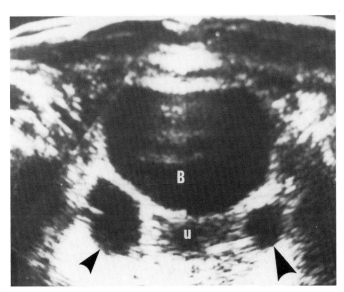

Fig. 81.29 Bilateral serous cystadenoma. Well defined unilocular ovarian cysts are identified [arrows]. [B = bladder; u = uterus].

involvement occurs early and scans should routinely include the para-aortic areas.

The mucinous cystadenocarcinoma shows a highly specific, well defined multilocular appearance on ultrasonography [72]. Solid elements may be present within a benign tumour and lead

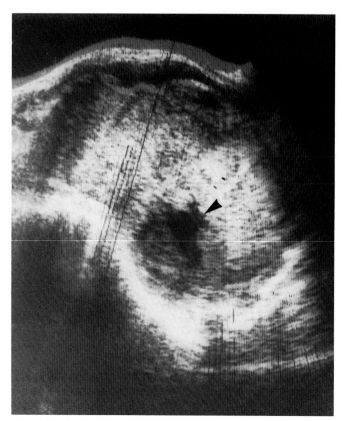

Fig. 81.32 Undifferentiated ovarian carcinoma. A large, essentially solid, pelvic tumour containing a small posterior cystic area [arrow]. The malignant and undifferentiated nature of the tumour was suspected from its large size and acoustic characteristics.

to difficulty in deciding if the tumour is benign or malignant. Loss of marginal definition of the tumour aids in establishing a final diagnosis (Fig. 81.30). Confirmatory features are bilaterality of the tumour, and the presence of ascites [73]. Computed tomography may be of value in evaluating the marginal characteristics of the tumour, and assessing the occurrence of local spread (Fig. 81.31).

Solid malignant ovarian tumours are usually large at the time of presentation. The normal pelvic anatomy is obliterated and areas of necrosis may be present within the tumour (Fig. 81.32). Although high level echoes are frequently present within the tumour, little attenuation is present and there is good acoustic transmission.

Teratoid tumours

Teratomas contain elements of all three germ layers and comprise 10% of all ovarian tumours. Over 96% are benign cystic teratomas while the rest are malignant in nature.

Benign cystic teratomas (Dermoid cysts)

Benign cystic teratomas are asymptomatic in 23% of cases [74], while the rest present with pain or, less often, an abdominal

mass or abnormal uterine bleeding. 18% are bilateral, 80% being 10 cm or less in diameter.

Radiology

A benign cystic teratoma is typically seen as a rounded, soft tissue mass in the pelvic cavity or lower abdomen, with a sharply defined capsule and containing dental or osseous structures. The mass may show some translucency (Fig. 81.33) due to sebaceous material, often mottled because of an admixture with hair. Occasionally, there is a rim of peripheral calcification. Teeth have been found in 31% and bone in 41% of cystic teratomas [75]. Diagnostic radiological signs are present in two thirds of cases [74]. Necrosis secondary to torsion may be associated with a homogenous calcific density to the tumour.

Thyroid tissue, which may be functional, is present in some cystic teratomas — the 'struma ovarii'. An isotope scan may show increased uptake of radioactive iodine by the teratoma.

Complications of cystic teratomas include torsion, rupture and inflammation. A fistula occasionally develops into the bladder or rectum following infection of the tumour.

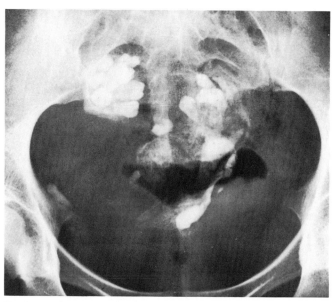

Fig. 81.33 Osseous and dental structures in large benign cystic teratoma of ovary.

Ultrasonography

The ultrasonographic appearances of ovarian teratomas, although often bizarre, may be highly specific with three features which assist in the diagnosis. Layering of hair, fat and sebum occur within the tumour. There may be inverse layering whereby the solid elements 'float' on the cystic elements (Fig. 81.34). Acoustic shadowing is frequently demonstrated, more commonly associated with the hair and sebum within the tumour rather than the calcific or osseous elements [76]. The outline may be obscured by the acoustic

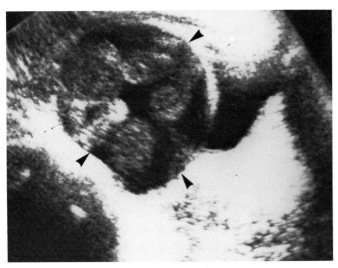

Fig. 81.34 Cystic teratoma of ovary [arrow], showing solid elements due to hair and sebum floating within the tumour.

shadowing and tumour contents but usually shows good definition. The tumour is poorly defined if malignancy has occurred, when there is often demonstrable lymphadenopathy. Due to the markedly different densities of the material within the tumour, ovarian teratomas should be readily diagnosable by computed tomography.

Malignant teratoma

Malignant transformation occurs in 2% of benign cystic teratomas. The majority of solid teratomas are highly malignant, usually occur in childhood or adolescence, and sometimes contain calcification in the form of linear and branching spicules. Recognisable teeth and bone are rare.

Other tumours

Meigs' Syndrome. There are four criteria of Meigs' syndrome. (1) A benign and solid ovarian tumour with the gross appearance of a fibroma. Thecomas, granulosa cell tumours and Brenner's tumour, which also have large fibrous elements are included in this category. (2) Ascites, small to enormous in amount. (3) Pleural effusion, usually on the right but occasionally on the left and rarely bilateral. (4) Spontaneous disappearance of the ascites and pleural fluid on removal of the ovarian tumour.

Fluid exudes from the tumour into the peritoneal cavity. Widening of interstices in the diaphragm, due to distention of the peritoneal cavity which allows ascitic fluid to permeate into the pleural cavity, is a plausible explanation for the syndrome. Occasionally, other ovarian tumours have satisfied the last three criteria, when the condition is known as pseudo-Meigs syndrome.

Fibroma. Apart from Meigs' syndrome, other radiological manifestations of ovarian fibromas are calcification and ossi-

fication of the tumour. The calcification has a diffuse stippled or mottled appearance and results from necrosis.

Thecoma. A thecoma rarely contains fine granular calcification.

Gonadoblastoma. Circumscribed, mottled or punctate calcification is found in half the cases of gonadoblastoma [72]. The fibroma-thecoma tumours are solid on ultrasonography but may show different degrees of internal echogenicity, as is seen with a uterine fibroid. Lack of posterior acoustic enhancement indicates the presence of a solid tumour. The tumour margins should be carefully scanned to exclude the possibility of a pedunculated uterine fibroid. Ascites is often present.

Dysgerminoma is a malignant ovarian neoplasm which tends to spread to other pelvic structures. Metastases sometimes spread to the peritoneal cavity, but metastases to iliac and para-aortic lymph nodes are seen on lymphography in one third of cases [78].

Sclerosing stromal cell tumour of ovary, a very rare ovarian tumour, has appeared as a calcified mass with a whorled pattern, mimicking a calcified fibroid, on plain radiographs [79]. Gonadoblastomas and dysgerminomas appear on ultrasonography as solid tumours with no distinguishing characteristics.

Krukenberg tumours are adenocarcinomas found in the ovary, usually bilaterally. Most are metastases from carcinoma of the stomach, while others arise from the colon and breast. Ascites may be present, together with peritoneal metastases. Secondary ovarian tumours are usually seen to be solid and bilateral on ultrasonography but cystic metastases are occasionally encountered. It is not possible to identify the metastatic nature of the tumour ultrasonographically, but evidence of other intra-abdominal and nodal deposits, in conjunction with the clinical and radiological findings, may serve to confirm the secondary nature of the tumour.

THE VULVA

Carcinoma

Metastases from carcinoma of the vulva spread to the superficial inguinal lymph nodes and subsequently to the deep inguinal and external iliac groups. Lymphography is of uncertain value.

Vulval varices

Varices of the vulva usually occur in multiparous women, often with varicose veins of the legs. Contrast medium may be injected directly into vulvar varicose veins to show their connections, but they may also be opacified by intraosseous pelvic phlebography [80].

THE VAGINA

Congenital abnormalities and vaginitis have been described in previous sections.

Foreign bodies

The presence of a foreign body in the vagina is usually manifested by a blood stained or foul discharge. Radio-opaque foreign bodies are localised by AP and lateral radiographs. Vaginography is occasionally helpful in demonstrating nonopaque foreign bodies. Radio-opaque suppositories are sometimes confused with bladder calculi on AP radiographs.

Vaginal calculi

Urine in the vagina from an ectopic ureter, a urinary fistula or as a result of urinary incontinence, may cause vaginal calculi to form by the deposition of urinary salts. A vaginal calculus sometimes results from the deposition of organic salts around foreign bodies in the vagina. Vaginal strictures also predispose to the formation of vaginal calculi. A vaginal calculus is often radio-opaque and sometimes shows lamination.

Vaginal fistulae

Ureterovaginal fistula. The causes of ureterovaginal fistula are ureteric severence or vascular compromise during hysterectomy, and radiotherapy for uterine malignancy.

Vesicovaginal fistula. Gynaecological surgery is responsible for 80% of vesicovaginal fistulae [81], hysterectomy and colporraphy accounting for two thirds of these cases. The rest are obstetric in origin, and Caesarean section is a potential cause. I.V. urography and cystography demonstrate most vesicovaginal fistulae. A tampon inserted into the vagina before urography and then radiographed after its removal will become radio-opaque from the contrast medium which enters the vagina if a vesicovaginal fistula is present [82].

Urethrovaginal fistula is usually due to ischaemic necrosis of the vaginal and urethral walls following anterior colporraphy, or to infection after excision of a urethral diverticulum.

Rectovaginal and sigmoidovaginal fistulae. Most cases of sigmoidovaginal fistulae are due to diverticular disease, other causes being granulomatous colitis and irradiation for carcinoma of the cervix. Rectovaginal fistula occurs secondary to carcinoma of the vagina, granulomatous proctitis and obstetric injury. A careful enema examination using dilute barium, with particular regard to the lateral radiograph of the rectum before and after evacuation, will demonstrate most cases. Vaginography is sometimes a helpful investigation.

Fibromyoma of the vagina

A fibromyoma of the vagina which enlarges in the midline resembles prostatic hypertrophy in males on urography, with bladder neck obstruction and an extrinsic bladder mass. Vaginal fibromyomas probably arise from embryonal rests.

MISCELLANEOUS CONDITIONS OF THE UTERUS

Endometrial polyps

Endometrial polyps are smooth, sessile or pedunculated, localized areas of endometrial hyperplasia. They are rarely larger than 1 cm in diameter, occur anywhere in the uterine

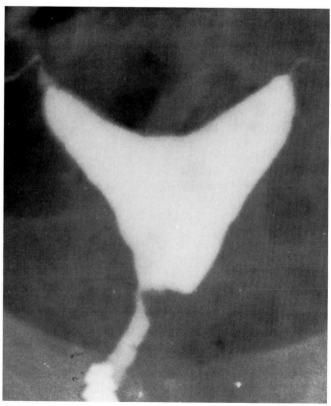

Fig. 81.35 Endometrial polyp in hysterography. The uterus is of the arcuate variety.

cavity (Fig. 81.35) and are sometimes multiple. Only 8% of polypoidal filling defects seen on hysterograms are endometrial polyps [12]. The differential diagnosis. includes air bubbles, which change in size and position, and blood clots which are irregular and have a poorly defined outline. It may be difficult to differentiate endometrial polyps from submucosal fibroids on hysterography.

Retained products of conception

Hysterography generally shows the uterine cavity to be enlarged in cases of missed abortion or retained products of conception. Multiple and very irregular filling defects may be present, or there may be fairly well circumscribed single or multiple defects.

In the postpartum period or following a therapeutic abortion, ultrasonography may be helpful in establishing whether or not retained products of conception are present. The postpartum uterus should have returned to normal size within three months [83], but is enlarged due to hypertrophied uterine muscle in the presence of retained products, with a prominent endometrial echo due to residual blood clot within the uterine cavity (Fig. 81.36). A definitive diagnosis of retained products is made if recognizable placental or fetal structures are identified within the uterine cavity. If the findings are not so specific, the diagnosis is less reliable and indicates a conservative approach to treatment [82].

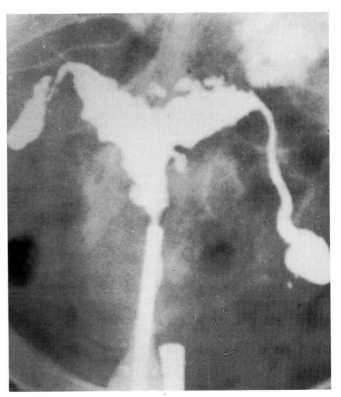

Fig. 81.37 Adenomyosis shown on hysterosalpingography.

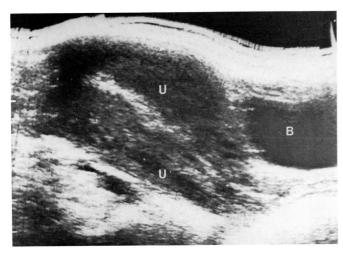

Fig. 81.36 Postpartum uterus showing normal appearances. The endometrial echo is prominent but there is no ultrasonographic evidence of retained products of conception. (B = Bladder U = Uterus).

Adenomyosis

Glandular tissue, often containing blood, and surrounding stroma penetrates into the myometrium in adenomyosis. Pelvic endometriosis and uterine fibroids occur fairly often in cases of adenomyosis. On hysterography, the uterus is usually enlarged and, in 25% of cases, spicules project from the uterine cavity for up to 5 mm or, occasionally, to a

deeper extent. The spicules terminate in small rounded sacs, (Fig. 81.37), 2 to 4 mm in diameter in 30% of cases. Other cases of adenomyosis show only irregularity of the endometrium or localized filling defects which mimic submucosal fibroids. A spiculated outline or small cavities in the wall of the uterus are regarded as normal variants in the majority of cases [13].

Ultrasonography sometimes demonstrates small cystic areas in the myometrium and may show associated extra-uterine endometriosis [25].

Metropathia haemorrhagica

Endometrial cystic hyperplasia, caused by oestrogen activity in the absence of progesterone, and associated with prolonged uterine bleeding preceded by amenorrhoea, is found in metropathia haemorrhagica. More than half the cases have normal hysterographic appearances, while the rest show a hypertrophic, ragged endometrial outline with a polypoidal tendency. These prominences may give an irregular criss-cross appearance resembling a Swiss cheese.

Intrauterine adhesions (synechiae)

Asherman [85], described the presence of single or multiple intrauterine adhesions, tending to occur especially after repeated curettage, in association with amenorrhoea. In practice, most cases have followed puerperal curettage, and to a lesser extent postabortal curettage and instrumental

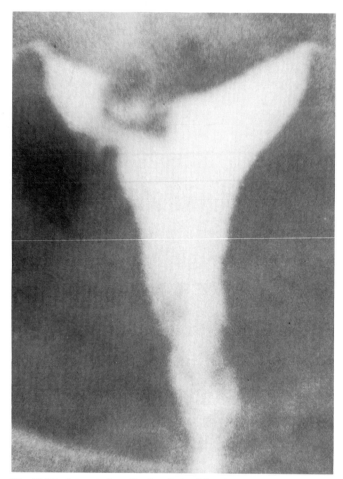

Fig. 81.38 Intrauterine adhesions in fundal region seen on hysterography.

abortion, rather than repeated curettage of the nonpregnant uterus. Filling defects are seen on hysterography and are very variable in shape (Fig. 81.38). They may be rounded, ovoid, linear, branch-like, angulated or generally bizarre in configuration, occupying a variable extent of the uterine cavity. Venous intravasation and cornual blockage are fairly common associated conditions.

Changes following lower segment Caesarean section

The hysterographic appearances of the uterus after Caesarean section are best shown on lateral radiographs. Usually, a localised wedge-shaped or convex protrusion lies on the ventral aspect at the level of the isthmus and upper part of the cervical canal at the site of the uterine scar, for a depth and width of less than 5 mm. Larger deformities tend to have a more saccular contour and indicate a weaker, dehiscent scar. Vesicouterine fistula occasionally occurs as a result of breakdown of the Caesarean section scar.

Uterine fistulae

Uterovesical fistula

Apart from Caesarean section (see above) and other obstetric and gynaecological operations, other causes of uterovesical fistula include malignant and inflammatory disease of the bladder and uterus, radiotherapy and urological procedures.

Enterouterine fistula

Fistula formation between the sigmoid colon and uterus is usually the result of carcinoma in either structure. Diverticulitis is a less frequent cause. Enterouterine fistula is usually demonstrable on barium enema examination.

Incompetence of the uterine isthmus

Incompetence of the internal os causes miscarriage during the second trimester. Incompetence is suspected if the internal os is 6 mm or more in width on hysterography (Fig. 81.39), with an imperceptible merging of the cervical canal and the cavity of the uterine body.

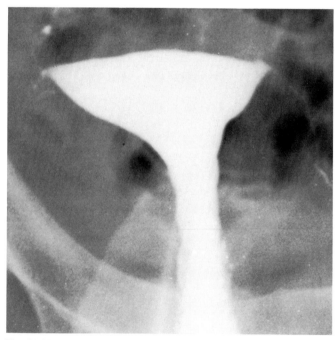

Fig. 81.39 Incompetence of uterine isthmus. Wide cervical canal and internal os on hysterography.

Arteriovenous malformations of the uterus

Arteriovenous malformations of the uterus present with heavy vaginal bleeding. The uterus is found to be enlarged and pulsatile, often with a bruit. These vascular abnormalities are probably congenital and are often circoid in type.

Arteriography is very useful in demonstrating the presence and extent of uterine arteriovenous malformations, together with their vascular connections [19]. The uterine arteries are shown to be enlarged and supply a plexus of convoluted vessels within the uterus and parametrium through which blood is rapidly shunted to draining veins (Fig. 81.40). Retained placenta, Caesarean section, hysterectomy and treated choriocarcinoma are other causes of arteriovenous shunts within the female pelvic cavity.

MISCELLANEOUS CONDITIONS OF THE FALLOPIAN TUBES

Tumours

Polyps. Rounded endometrial polyps, 1 mm or more in diameter, are occasionally found in the intramural and ampullary portions of the Fallopian tubes.

Teratoma. Teratomas of the Fallopian tubes are uncommon and are on average 6 cm in diameter. Bone occurs in one third of tubal teratomas, but tooth formation is found in only 7%.

Carcinoma. Primary adenocarcinoma of the Fallopian tubes is not common. Hydrosalpinx is a frequent complication. Irregular, polypoidal masses within dilated and obstructed tubes are occasionally found on hysterosalpingography.

Tubal pregnancy

Hysterosalpingography is contraindicated in suspected ectopic pregnancy because of the risk of dislodgement and haemorrhage, although contrast medium will delineate the mole and intervillous spaces within the occluded tube. Hysterosalpingography should be performed after resection of a Fallopian tube for ectopic pregnancy, to ensure that the remaining tube is patent.

Ultrasonography in the diagnosis of ectopic pregnancy

The various pathological entities involving the adnexa may show very similar sonographic appearances. A full clinical history is essential but it may only be possible to give a differential diagnosis with an indication as to which is the most likely entity [73,87].

The early diagnosis of ectopic pregnancy by ultrasound has remained difficult and reports vary as to its accuracy. Despite the relative infrequency of the condition, this important diagnosis should be considered in any patient with a complex adnexal mass. The incidence of ectopic pregnancy has recently increased, probably due to an increased occurrence

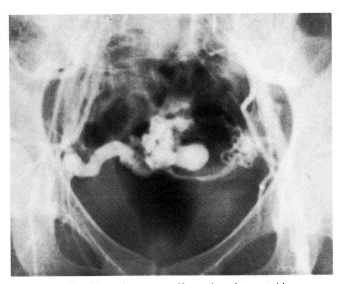

Fig. 81.40 Circoid arteriovenous malformation of uterus with arteriovenous shunting.

of pelvic inflammatory disease and the use of the intrauterine device, which does not protect the patient from ectopic gestation [88] (Fig. 81.41).

The criteria of an unruptured tubal pregnancy are:
1. The demonstration of a gestation sac or foetus in an extra-uterine location.
2. An oval or elongated fluid-filled adnexal mass, due to a distended Fallopian tube, and containing an echodense and ring-like structure which represents the gestational sac.

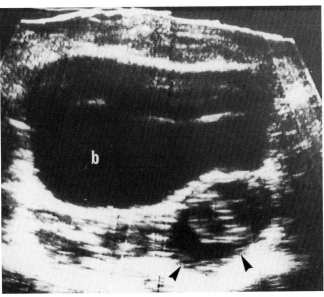

Fig. 81.41 Unruptured tubal pregnancy showing the fluid-distended Fallopian tube [arrows], containing a dense ring-like structure [b = bladder].

3. Moderate uterine enlargement with prominence of the endometrial echo.
4. Fetal heart motion is rarely seen, being demonstrated only if the fetus is viable and the duration of the gestation is at least 10 weeks.

These signs apply to an *unruptured* tubal ectopic pregnancy. A *ruptured* interstitial or tubal pregnancy or a pelvic ectopic gestation may not be identified so readily. An *interstitial* pregnancy should be suspected from its eccentric location in relation to the uterus. A ruptured tubal pregnancy is associated with a complex mass due to haematoma, which may extend to involve the contralateral adnexal area. The gestational sac may not be as easily identified and often has a fragmented appearance. The ultrasonographic appearance may be very similar to pelvic inflammatory disease with early abscess formation.

Plastic operations on the Fallopian tubes

Hysterosalpingography is important in the preoperative assessment and postoperative evaluation of surgical procedures designed to restore patency to occluded Fallopian tubes. These operations include salpingolysis, salpingostomy, resection and anastomosis, and cornual resection and reimplantation.

Tubal sterilization techniques

There are a variety of methods for occluding the Fallopian tubes as a means of contraception, including ligation of the tube with or without excision of a segment, detachment of the tube from the uterus by cornual excision, and excision or burying of the fimbrial ends of the tubes. Occlusive metallic, plastic or silicone clips and rings may be applied to the isthmus; or the Fallopian tubes may be divided by electrocoagulation during laparotomy or through a laparoscope. The latter is occasionally associated with damage to the small intestine and this method, which causes much tissue destruction, is now losing favour. Hysterosalpingography is useful in assessing the results of clip application and electrocoagulation but should be performed no less than twelve weeks later, by which time fibrosis should be complete. A hysterosalpingogram prior to tubal reconstruction after surgical occlusion is also a useful investigation.

Endometriosis

Endometriosis is the occurrence of endometrial tissue (epithelial, glandular and stromal elements) in sites other than the lining of the uterine cavity. It occurs between menarche and menopause, usually presenting in the fourth decade. The pelvic cavity is the main situation for endometriosis, the ectopic endometrial tissue being associated with bleeding and subsequent fibrosis. 'Chocolate cysts' of the ovary and dense pelvic adhesions are typical features.

Hysterosalpingography. Severe pelvic endometriosis results in fixity of the uterus, usually in retroflexion. Periampullary adhesions cause ampullary dilatation with loculation and limited peritoneal spillage of contrast medium. The appearances are indistinguishable from pelvic inflammatory disease.

The urinary tract. The ureter is involved either by extrinsic compression from pelvic endometrial tissue and fibrosis or, less commonly, by endometriotic foci within the ureteral wall. Both types cause a smoothly tapering stenosis in the pelvic portion of the ureter, with proximal hydroureter and hydronephrosis.

Ultrasonography. A spectrum of appearances may be seen in a patient with endometriosis [25]. The cysts present are often multiple and are usually 2 to 5 cm in size. They may appear completely sonolucent, or contain internal echoes due to the altered blood content. Loss of the uterine outline may be seen and the ovaries frequently cannot be identified as separate structures. Fixity of the pelvic organs occurs due to the fibrosis and adhesions. Occasionally, clot-formation and inspissation of the contents of the cyst may produce an extremely bizarre configuration (Fig. 81.42).

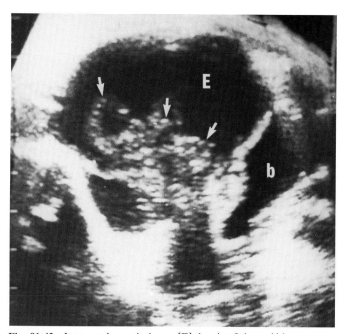

Fig. 81.42 Large endometriotic cyst [E] showing fixity and bizarre echoes [arrows] due to clot formation within the cyst.

CONTRACEPTION

Intrauterine contraceptive devices

Types of IUCD

Lippes Loop (Fig. 81.43) and the *Saf-T-Coil* are two popular devices, both being made of polyethylene and impregnated

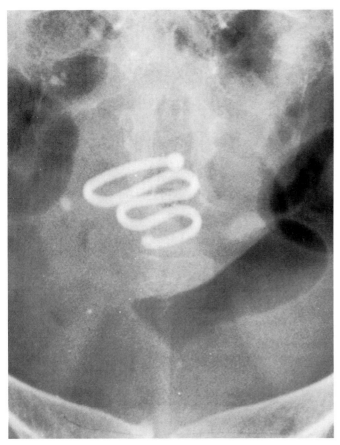

Fig. 81.43 Lippes loop.

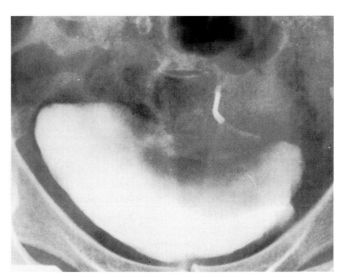

Fig. 81.44 Copper 7 device shown on i.v. urogram.

with barium sulphate to give radiographic visualisation. The *Gravigard (Copper 7)* (Fig. 81.44) is another commonly used IUCD, being composed of a polypropylene carrier impregnated with barium and coated with copper. The *Gyne T (Copper T)* is a similar device.

The *Dalkon Shield* is of low radiographic density and consists of a series of lateral fins surrounding a central membrane. This device has been withdrawn because of the associated high incidence of septic abortions. Another device which has been abandoned is the *Majzlin spring* which is difficult to remove and is associated with a high risk of pelvic infection.

The *Progestasert* is a T-shaped radio-opaque unit which contains progesterone in a hollow stem. The *Birnberg bow*, *Antigon*, and *Margulies coil* are other ring-like devices.

Complications

Missing threads

The causes of missing threads include expulsion, the incidence of which varies from 2 to 20% depending on the type of device, and translocation which occurs in 0.05 to 13 per thousand insertions. Pregnancy will cause the threads to retract into the enlarged uterus. In most cases of missing threads, the IUCD is within a nonpregnant uterus.

Ultrasonography is the most reliable and safest method for investigating missing threads. A plain radiograph will help to differentiate between expulsion and translocation through the uterine wall if ultrasonography fails to demonstrate the device within the uterus.

Pregnancy

The pregnancy rate with a correctly positioned IUCD is 1 to 4% in the first year of insertion, becoming lower in succeeding years except in the case of copper devices where it rises after the second year. There is a relationship between extrauterine pregnancies, and also spontaneous abortions, and the use of IUCDs. In many cases, however, the IUCD does not impede the otherwise normal pregnancy.

Infection

Pelvic infection is four to five times more likely among IUCD users than in other women and is the main cause of mortality and severe morbidity associated with IUCDs. The inflammation may range from a mild incident to a tubo-ovarian abscess. The resulting tubal damage may cause infertility.

Malposition and distortion of IUCDs

Distortion of an IUCD within the uterine cavity, especially the Lippes loop, may affect all or part of the device. The presence of distortion raises the possibility of uterine perforation. The IUCD may lie upside down or on its side within the uterine cavity.

Uterine perforation

Translocation of an IUCD with perforation of the uterine wall may occur at the time of its insertion. In most cases, the IUCD is completely extruded into the peritoneal cavity, less often being partly embedded in the uterine wall. The patient is usually symptomless, but abscesses may develop in the pelvic cavity. In the case of a translocated Lippes loop, the separation of approximately 1 cm between the bulbous tip and the second loop is very suggestive of uterine perforation, as these two points lie in close apposition in a correctly inserted device [89].

The role of ultrasonography in the management of intrauterine contraceptive devices

The more commonly used intrauterine devices are recognised by their configuration on the ultrasound scan [90]. A Lippes loop shows a series of dense, equally spaced echoes in the sagittal axis of the uterus, with a central echo within the uterine cavity on transverse section. The *Saf-T-Coil* is more difficult to delineate, but adjacent scans should demonstrate the continuous echo of the central arm in the sagittal axis and interrupted echoes on the transverse scans. The *Dalkon shield* appears as a dense linear echo. The *Copper 7* and *Copper T* devices demonstrate a linear echo where the scan axis coincides with the axis of the arms of the device in both sagittal and transverse section, and as a single dense echo where the scan axis passes perpendicular to the device.

Ultrasonography should now be the preliminary investigation in the assessment of a lost intrauterine device. If a thread has been detached, the device may still be present within the uterus and will be readily identified. Uptake of the device may have occurred in association with pregnancy in which case radiography is an undesirable initial investigation. If the device cannot be identified by ultrasound within the uterus, it may have been expelled or may be lying within the pelvic cavity. It is this circumstance which necessitates an AP radiograph of the pelvis. If the device is extrinsic to the uterus it cannot be reliably demonstrated by ultrasonography. If pregnancy has occurred and the device is still present within the uterus, then it cannot be reliably identified after 10 to 12 weeks gestation.

Ultrasonography demonstrates the position of the device following insertion. Penetration of the uterine myometrium is identified by the eccentric location of the device, an AP radiograph confirming complete perforation.

Oral contraception

Circulatory disorders

The increased risk of myocardial ischaemia, hypertension, cerebrovascular disorders and venous thrombosis in women on the Pill is now well established [91], these complications being most likely in older women and smokers. The risk of developing venous thrombosis and pulmonary embolism, as well as other circulatory disorders, is related to the amount of oestrogen in the Pill.

Liver tumours

There is an increased incidence of hepatic adenomas and focal nodular hyperplasia in women on the Pill, the preva-

lence being rather higher in the USA than in the UK. In some cases, the benign lesions may progress to malignant change in the form of hepatocellular carcinoma. Pain and haemoperitoneum are the commonest presenting features of hepatic adenomas. Hepatic angiography shows these hepatic adenomas to be highly vascular and supplied by a large number of arteries, with malignant tumours having indistinguishable appearances.

ABORTION

Criminal abortion

Blunt objects, such as urethral catheters, or long pointed instruments such as knitting needles, are sometimes used to produce an abortion. All such objects may perforate the uterine wall. The urinary bladder may also be damaged by a sharp instrument.

Air embolism is a life threatening hazard of criminal abortion, air being introduced through a tube or nozzle inadvertently inserted into the friable vessels of the vascular pregnant uterus.

Surgical abortion

The intra-amniotic injection of hypertonic saline via an abdominal amniocentesis is a popular method of abortion after the first trimester. The injection of contrast medium prior to the hypertonic saline ensures that an intravascular injection is not made, shock and sometimes death resulting from the installation of hypertonic saline into the circulatory system.

Bladder laceration and ureteric damage are rare complications of elective abortion. Colonic dilatation sometimes follows termination of pregnancy.

COMPLICATIONS OF HYSTERECTOMY

Haematoma

The usual site for haematoma formation is between the suture line of the vagina and the pelvic peritoneum. Plain radiographs show a soft tissue pelvic mass. I.V. urography may show the mass to be obstructing or deviating the ureters or compressing the bladder. Ultrasonographically, the haematoma is demonstrated as a cystic, transonic mass. Serial scans may be used to assess resolution. If the haematoma becomes infected, internal echoes are seen and there is thickening and irregularity of the wall.

Pelvic sepsis

Pelvic suppuration sometimes develops in a postoperative pelvic haematoma. The abscess may discharge spontaneously into the vagina or rectum, or through the abdominal incision. Pelvic abscesses have the same radiological signs as haematomas, in addition to causing a loss of definition of pelvic structures and local paralytic ileus.

Urinary tract complications

These are most likely to occur after radical hysterectomy [15].

Ureteric complications

Direct injury to the pelvic portion of the ureter, or deprivation of its nerve or blood supply due to stripping the ureter from the peritoneum or Waldeyer's sheath, may cause flank and loin pain, pyrexia, urinary infection and leakage of urine in the postoperative period.

Transient hydroureter and hydronephrosis. A high incidence of upper urinary tract dilatation is found on routine i.v. urography within three weeks of radical hysterectomy, usually resolving completely within three months. The incidence of this transient ureteric obstruction is much lower after nonradical hysterectomy. Local mural and periureteral oedema, together with separation of Waldeyer's sheath account for this reversible change.

Ureteric stricture. Irreversible denervation and devascularization of the distal ureter with subsequent fibrosis account for the majority of cases of ureteric stricture after hysterectomy. Ureteric stricture is especially common when radical hysterectomy is combined with radiotherapy.

Ureterovaginal fistula. Ureteric severence or vascular compromise are causes of a ureterovaginal fistula. i.v. urography demonstrates the fistula, which is often associated with ipsilateral ureteric obstruction.

Ureteric severence. Ureterovaginal fistula, ureteric obstruction or a urinary collection in the pelvis are postoperative manifestations of ureteric severence during hysterectomy. Extravasation of urine may cause a large soft tissue retroperitoneal mass on plain radiographs, while i.v. urography sometimes shows extravasation of contrast medium at the level of severence (Fig. 81.45).

Bladder complications

Vesicovaginal fistula. Damage to the bladder base may lead to the formation of a vesicovaginal fistula; radiotherapy and

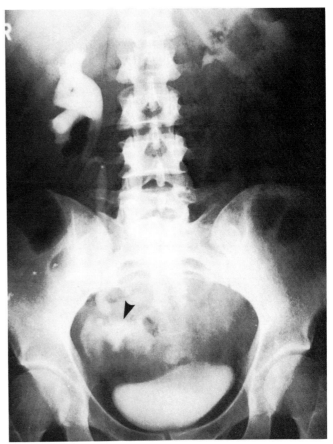

Fig. 81.45 Severence of right ureter at hysterectomy and bilateral salpingo-oophorectomy for carcinoma of the cervix. Extravasation [arrow] of contrast medium from dilated right ureter.

recurrence of carcinoma are other causes. The vagina is seen to communicate with the bladder on i.v. urography, cystography and vaginography.

Postoperative bladder calculi. Denervation of the bladder, the high incidence of urinary infection and postoperative indwelling urinary catheters predispose to the increased incidence of vesical calculi which occurs after radical hysterectomy.

Urinary retention and other postoperative bladder symptoms. Urinary retention is common after hysterectomy, especially the radical operation, but is usually a transient phenomenon.

The so-called 'urethral syndrome', with dysuria and retropubic discomfort, sometimes develops after hysterectomy and seems to be related to periurethral fibrosis and oestrogen deficiency. Cystography sometimes shows an elevated bladder base with bladder neck hypertrophy, paraurethral glandular hyperplasia and periurethral calcification [92].

Arteriovenous fistula

Transfixion of the uterine artery and vein by a needle at the time of ligation is likely to be the cause of an arteriovenous fistula between these vessels after hysterectomy.

Lymphocysts

The continued flow of lymph from transected lymphatic vessels leads to the development of lymphocysts after radical hysterectomy. A soft tissue pelvic mass, usually with compression or deviation of the ureters and impingement on the bladder, is visible on i.v. urography. Compression of pelvic veins, demonstrable by venography, sometimes causes leg oedema. Ultrasonographically, the lymphocyst is identified as a well defined cystic mass.

COMPLICATIONS OF RADIOTHERAPY

The development of ureteric stricture after radiotherapy for carcinoma of the cervix is due to recurrence of the tumour in the vast majority of cases, being secondary to irradiation fibrosis in only 1% of cases [93]. The fibrous ureteric stricture from radiotherapy is smoothly tapered and develops about three years after treatment. Transient hydronephrosis, due to oedema which is secondary to irradiation, sometimes occurs three weeks after radium application for cervical carcinoma.

Radiological evidence of *bladder* damage following radiotherapy is rare. I.V. urography in chronic radiation reaction shows a thick walled, small volume bladder, sometimes with bilateral ureteric obstruction. Vesical fistulae rarely develop after radiotherapy, except in cases of direct involvement of the bladder by cancer.

Damage to the *intestine* is infrequent, while radionecrosis of *bone* is now an unusual complication of radiotherapy for uterine and cervical carcinoma.

STRESS INCONTINENCE

Stress incontinence is an involuntary loss of urine which occurs when the intravesical pressure exceeds the maximum urethral pressure in the absence of detrusor activity. Genuine stress incontinence is associated with a deficient urethral closure mechanism, usually with an insufficient suspension of the bladder neck and proximal urethra, in contradistinction to urge incontinence which is usually due to detrusor hyperreflexia or instability. Obstetric injury and postmenopausal soft tissue atrophy are prime factors in the development of stress incontinence, often with obesity and chronic pulmonary disease as other exacerbating factors.

Radiological investigation

I.V. urography should be performed in the presence of suspected outflow obstruction, continuous incontinence, recurrent urinary infection and procidentia.

Cystourethrography. While information on urethral distorsion and the demonstration of prolapse is provided by a lateral cystourethrogram at rest, on straining and during micturition, this investigation does not demonstrate bladder function which will dictate the line of treatment.

Videocystourethrography [94,95] is a combination of supine cystometry and radiographic screening of the bladder and urethra during voiding, recorded on videotape. It is a functional investigation used in the diagnosis of urinary incontinence, voiding difficulties and retention. Intravesical pressures and rectal (abdominal) pressures are measured by fluid filled catheters attached to transducers. The electronic subtraction of these two pressure readings gives the detrusor pressure, which is an exact index of detrusor activity. The peak flow rate and volume voided during micturition are recorded by a uroflowmeter.

Ureteric obstruction associated with uterine prolapse

Severe degrees of uterine prolapse are associated with ureteric obstruction in many cases. The obstruction is usually bilateral and is accentuated in the prone and erect positions. The lower ureters are kinked and compressed, probably due to the caudal displacement of the trigone [96].

Urethral diverticula

Urethral diverticula arise secondary to infection and obstruction of a urethral gland which subsequently ruptures into the urethral lumen, the patients presenting with dysuria or occasionally dyspareunia. The majority arise on the vaginal aspect of the middle third of the urethra and are usually 1 to 2.5 cm in diameter. Micturating cystourethrography will often delineate the diverticulum, but retrograde urethrography has its advocates. Calculi and occasionally carcinomas may arise within a urethral diverticulum.

COMPUTED TOMOGRAPHY (CT) IN GYNAECOLOGY
Janet E. Husband

In the assessment of pelvic masses, both ultrasound and CT may provide similar information [97] but ultrasound remains the initial, noninvasive imaging technique of choice in the assessment of gynaecological disorders [98].

The majority of pelvic CT examinations are performed for the assessment and staging of neoplasms [99,100,101]. The CT technique shows the presence and extent of primary and recurrent tumours, as well as localizing masses for biopsy and radiotherapy planning [102,103].

Pelvic lymph node involvement from primary pelvic cancers or lymphoma may also be detected with CT [104,105].

Before the CT examination is carried out, it is essential to be certain that no possibility of pregnancy exists. The scan technique and patient preparation depends on the suspected abnormality. Collimation and slice spacing depend on the scanner available, but in general, 10 mm collimation with a slice interval of 10 to 15 mm provides sufficient anatomical detail in the evaluation of pelvic masses. Following the initial series of scans, overlapping slices can be obtained if necessary. In the assessment of neoplastic disease, scans should be continued to include the para-aortic and renal areas and the liver.

The patient is scanned in the supine position. A full baldder is essential as it clarifies the pelvic anatomy and a vaginal tampon assists in localizing the vagina. Oral contrast medium (2% Gastrografin 600 to 900 ml) should be given at least 1½ hours before the examination and rectal contrast medium is useful for delineating the rectum and sigmoid colon (Gastrografin 2% 100 ml). Intravenous contrast medium will show the line of the ureters and their relationship to any abnormality present; it also helps to identify the pelvic vascular structures. If residual barium is present in the distal bowel from a recent barium study, considerable scan artefacts will occur and the examination should be deferred until the bowel is clear.

Ultrasound and computed tomography in the assessment of carcinoma of the cervix

Neither ultrasound nor CT have been shown to be clinically useful in the diagnosis of Stage I and early Stage II disease, that is, tumour confined within the cervix (Stage I) or early parametrial involvement (Stage II). In more advanced disease when tumour extends to the pelvic side wall (Stage III) or involve pelvic organs, such as the bladder and rectum (Stage IV), CT is more effective. Overall, comparisons of CT staging with surgery have shown an accuracy of 64 to 88% [99,106] but a 92% accuracy in advanced disease [107].

Tumours of the cervix are seen on CT as solid masses of soft tissue density (Fig. 81.46). Extension to the pelvic side wall is seen as soft tissue strands extending to the obturator internus muscle and/or pyriformis muscle (Fig. 81.47). In extensive disease, the tumour is inseparable from adjacent structures, such as the rectum, sigmoid colon and pelvic side wall.

CT may also show hydronephrosis, dilatation of the ureters due to obstruction by the pelvic mass, and enlargement of para-aortic and pelvic lymph nodes (vide infra).

In patients with suspected recurrence, CT is valuable for showing central pelvic masses and recurrent lymph node disease, but one of the limitations of the technique is the difficulty in distinguishing radiation fibrosis from early recurrent disease [107]

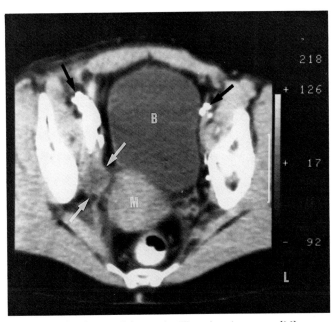

Fig. 81.46 Carcinoma of the cervix. There is a 4 cm mass [M] occupying the cervix but there is no evidence of parametrial spread. The patient has had a lymphogram. Note opacified nodes on both sides of the pelvis [black arrows]. The nodes on the patient's right are enlarged. In addition, there is an enlarged unopacified right internal iliac node [white arrows].

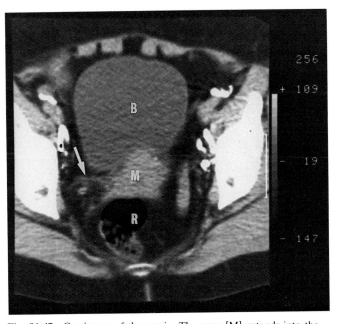

Fig. 81.47 Carcinoma of the cervix. The mass [M] extends into the right parametrium [arrow].
[B = bladder; R = rectum]

Carcinoma of the endometrium

As in cervical carcinoma, similar reservations apply to the ability of both ultrasound and CT to detect early endometrial neoplastic disease. However, in more advanced disease, the accuracy of CT staging is in the region of approximately 85% [108]. With CT, the tumour may appear as a central low density area with irregular margins, and with ultrasound as a region of markedly irregular high density echoes. If local extrauterine invasion has occurred, the normal uterine outline is lost.

CT cannot distinguish a fibroid uterus from uterine cancer unless there is extensive extrauterine spread [109]. Hypodense areas within the uterine corpus also occur with intrauterine fluid collections (hydrometra or pyometra).

Sarcoma of the uterus

Both leiomyosarcoma and choriocarcinoma may show an extremely bizarre ultrasound configuration. The tumour is frequently extremely large at the time of the examination and it is difficult to determine the origin of the mass (Fig. 81.48). Leiomyosarcomas show a marked propensity to necrosis and large cystic areas may be demonstrated within the tumour by ultrasound and CT. The diagnosis of choriocarcinoma may be suspected from the presence of multiple theca lutein cysts. If liver metastases are present, these are often necrotic in both leiomyosarcoma and choriocarcinoma.

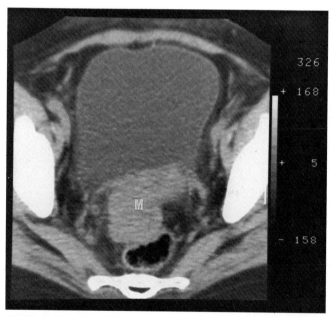

Fig. 81.48 Sarcoma of the uterus. The body of the uterus is replaced by a large irregular mass [M].

Carcinoma of the ovary

CT has a role in the diagnosis and staging of ovarian cancer as well as monitoring response to treatment [110,111]. The characteristic CT findings of ovarian cancer are variable. The mass may be either solid or cystic with thick, irregular walls and septa, but on occasions a simple thin-walled cyst may be present. In the latter situation it is impossible to distinguish a benign simple cyst from cancer. Calcification

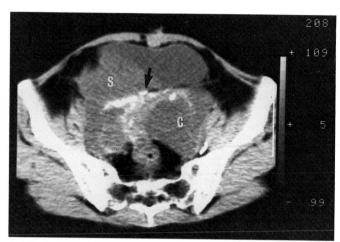

Fig. 81.49 Carcinoma of the ovary containing solid areas [S], cystic areas [C] and calcified septa [arrow].

may be seen either in the cyst wall or within the solid areas (Fig. 81.49).

Ovarian cancers characteristically spread transcoelomically producing peritoneal and mesenteric metastases. One of the major limitations of CT in assessment of carcinoma of the ovary is the inability to detect small peritoneal and mesenteric deposits [112] but large tumour masses (greater than 2 cm in diameter) can be easily detected. Other findings, such as ascites and liver metastases, are readily identified. CT has an important role in monitoring response to chemotherapy in patients with advanced disease and also in the detection of recurrence [113].

Lymph node involvement from pelvic cancer

One of the main disadvantages of CT in the assessment of primary pelvic tumours is the inability to identify metastases in normal or minimally enlarged nodes [114]. With CT, the criteria for an enlarged node is a transverse diameter greater than 1.5 cm. In evaluating pelvic lymph node metastases from carcinoma of the cervix, in one study CT had an overall accuracy of 74% with a true positive rate of 70% and a false negative rate of 30%. The true negative rate was 78% and the false positive rate 22% [99].

Lymphography has the advantage over CT that it demonstrates the internal architecture of the node and metastases can therefore be identified in nodes that are not enlarged. Occasionally CT can demonstrate enlarged nodes in sites which are unopacified at lymphography, such as the internal iliac group (Fig. 81.46).

BIBLIOGRAPHY

REFERENCES

1. Vezina J L, Sutton T J 1974 Prolactin-secreting pituitary microadenomas. Am J Roentgenol 120:46–54
2. Swanson J A, Jacoby C G, Sherman B H, Dolan K D, Chapler

F K, 1978 Evaluation of the pituitary. Patients with suspected prolactin-producing tumours. Obstet Gynecol 52:52–72

3. Marrs R P, Kletzky O A, Teal J, Kavajan V, March C, Mishell D R 1979 Comparison of serum prolactin, plain radiography and hypocycloidal tomography of the sella tunica in patients with galactorrhea. Am J Obstet Gynecol 135:467–469

4. Sylvester A, Haughton V M, Williams A L, Cusick J F 1979 The computed tomographic appearance of the normal pituitary gland and pituitary microadenomas. Radiology 133:385–391

5. Drayer B, Kaltah J, Rosenbaum A, Kennerdell J, Maroon J 1979 Diagnostic approaches to pituitary adenomas. Neurology 29:161–169

6. Wright J T 1961 A new method of hysterosalpingography. Br J Radiol 34:465–467

7. Gerlock A J, Hooser C W 1976 Oviduct response to glucagon during hysterosalpingography. Radiology 119:727–728

8. Stiris G, Andrew E 1979 Hysterosalpingography with Amipaque. Radiology 130:795–796

9. Slezak P, Tillinger K G 1973 The significance of the spiculated outline of the uterine cavity in hysterography. Radiology 107:527–531

10. Slezak P, Tillinger K G 1973 Broad longitudinal folds in the uterine cavity in hysterography. Radiology 106:87–90

11. Slezak P, Tillinger K G 1968 The occurrence and significance of a double outlined uterine cavity in the hysterographic picture. Radiology 90:756–760

12. Slezak P, Tillinger K G 1978 Hysterographic evidence of polypoid filling defects in the uterine cavity. Radiology 115:79–83

13. Slezak P, Tillinger K G 1976 The incidence and clinical importance of hysterographic evidence of cavities in the uterine wall. Radiology 118:581–586

14. Peck A G, Yoder I C, Pfister R C 1975 Tomography of pelvic abdominal masses during intravenous urography. Am J Roentgenol 125:322–330

15. Whitehouse G H 1977 The radiology of urinary tract abnormalities associated with hysterectomy. Clin Radiol 28:201–210

16. Lang E K 1980 Angiography in the diagnosis and staging of pelvic neoplasms. Radiology 134:353–358

17. Levin D C, Stains S, Schneider M, Becker J A 1975 Sonography and arteriography in the management of uterine choriocarcinoma. Am J Roentgenol 125:462–468

18. Karlsson S, Persson P H 1979 Angiography, ultrasound and fine-needle aspiration biopsy in the evaluation of gynaecological tumours. Acta Radiol Diagn 10:779–788

19. Bottomley J P, Whitehouse G H 1975 Congenital arteriovenous malformations of uterus demonstrated by angiography. Acta Radiol (Diagn) 16:43–48

20. Lang E K 1979 Current and future applications of angiography in the abdomen. Radiol Clin North Amer 17:55–76

21. Murray E, Comparato M R 1968 Uterine phlebography. Am J Obstet Gynecol 102:1088–1093

22. Sample W F, Lippe B M, Gyepes M T 1977 Grey scale ultrasonography of the normal female pelvis. Radiology 125:477–483

23. Hall D B, Hann L E, Ferrucci J T et al 1979 Sonographic morphology of the normal menstrual cycle. Radiology 113:185–188

24. Hackeloer B J 1977 The ultrasonic demonstration of follicular development during the normal menstrual cycle and after hormone stimulation. In: Recent advances in ultrasonic diagnosis. Churchill Livingstone, Edinburgh pp 122–128

25. Walsh W J, Rosenfield A T, Jaffe C C et al 1978 Prospective comparison of ultrasound and computed tomography in the evaluation of gynecologic pelvic masses. Am J Roentgenol 131:955–960

26. Carter B L, Kahn P C, Wolpert S M, Hammerschlag S B, Schwartz Am, Scott R M 1976 Unusual pelvic masses. A comparison of computed tomographic scanning and ultrasonography. Radiology 121:383–386

27. Lee J K T, Stanley R J, Sagel S S, Levitt R G 1978 Accuracy of computed tomography in detecting intra-abdominal and pelvic lymphadenopathy in lymphoma. Am J Roentgenol 131:311–315

28. Lee J K T, Stanley R J, Sagel S S, McLennan B 1978 Accuracy of C T in detecting intra-abdominal and pelvic lymph node metastases from pelvic cancer. Am J Roentgenol 131:675–679

29. Jacques P F, Staab E, Richey W, Photopulos G, Swanson M 1978 C T assisted pelvic and abdominal biopsy in gynecological lesions. Radiology 128:651–655

30. Pontifex G, Trichopoulus D, Karpathios S 1972 Hysterosalpingography in the diagnosis of infertility (statistical analysis of 3437 cases). Fertil Steril 23:829–833

31. Rennell C L 1979 T-shaped uterus in diethylstilboestrol (DES) exposure. Am J Roentgenol 132:979–980

32. Cook G T, Marshall V F 1964 Hydrocolpos causing urinary obstruction. J Urol 92:127–132

33. Rhamme R C, Derrick F C 1973 Gartner's duct involving urinary tract. J Urol 109:60; 61

34. Cremin B J 1974 Intersex states in young children. The importance of radiology in making a correct diagnosis. Clin Radiol 25:63–73

35. Cheng G K, Fisher J H, O'Hara K G, Retik A B, Darling D B 1974 Anomaly of the persistent cloaca in female infants. Am J Roentgenol 120:413–423

36. Haller J, Schneider M, Kassner G, Staiano S, Nayes M et al 1977 Ultrasonography in pediatric gynecology and obstetrics. Am J Roentgenol 128:423–429

37. Scott R B 1968 A survey of deaths and critical illnesses in association with the use of intrauterine devices. Internat J Fertil 13:297–300

38. Sample W F 1977 Pelvic inflammatory disease. In: Saunders R C, James A C (eds) Ultrasonography in obstetrics and gynecology. 2nd ed.: Appleton Century Crofts, New York pp 357–385

39. Horwitz R C, Morton P C, Shaff M I, Hugo P 1979 A radiological approach to infertility-hysterosalpingography. Br J Radiol 52:255–262

40. Keirse M J N C, Vandervellen R 1973 A comparison of hysterosalpingography and laparoscopy in the investigation of infertility. Obstet Gynecol 41:685–688

41. Ladipo O A 1979 Tests of tubal patency. Comparison of laparoscopy and hysterosalpingography. Br Med J 2:1297–1298

42. Golde S H, Israel R, Leger W J 1977 Unilateral tubo-ovarian abscess: a difficult entity. Am J Obstet Gynecol 127:807–810

43. Phillips J C 1974 A spectrum of radiologic abnormalities due to tubo-ovarian abscess. Radiology 110:307–331

44. Ulrich P C, Saunders R C 1976 Ultrasonic characteristics of pelvic inflammatory disease. J Clin Ultrasound 4:199–204

45. Levitt R G, Sagel S S, Stanley R J, Evans R G 1978 Computed tomography of the pelvis. Seminars Roentgenol 13:

46. Freakley G, Norman W J, Ennis J T, Davies E R 1974 Diverticulosis of the Fallopian tubes. Clin Radiol 25:535–542

47. Asplund J 1952 The uterine cervix and isthmus under normal and pathological conditions. Acta Radiol Suppl 91

48. Madsen V 1947 Hysterograms in genital tuberculosis in women. Acta Radiol 28:812–823

49. Magnusson W 1947 Further experiences in the roentgen diagnosis of tuberculous salpingitis. Acta Radiol 28:824–823

50. Ekengren K, Ryden A B V 1951 Roentgen diagnosis of tuberculous endometritis. Acta Radiol 36:485–494

51. Pietilä K 1969 Hysterography in the diagnosis of uterine myoma. Acta Obstet Gynecol Scandinav 48: Suppl 5

52. Imray T J 1975 Evaluation of pelvic masses during infusion excretory urography. Am J Roentgenol 125:60–65

53. Wright C H 1981 Ultrasound in gynaecological diagnosis. In: Whitehouse G H (ed)Gynaecological radiology. Blackwell Scientific Publications Oxford, pp 208–225

54. Von Micksky L I 1974 Gynecologic sonography. In: King D L (ed) Diagnostic ultrasound. Mosby, St Louis pp 207–241

55. Fuchs W A, Seiler-Rosenberg G 1975 Lymphography in carcinoma of the uterine cervix. Acta Radiol Diagn 16:353–361

56. Kolbenstvedt A 1975 Lymphography in the diagnosis of metastases from carcinoma of the uterine cervix stages I and II. Acta Radiol Diagn 16:81–97

57. Griffin J W, Parker R G, Taylor W J 1976 An evaluation of procedures used in staging carcinoma of the cervix. Am J Roentgenol 127:825–827

58. Stander R W, Rhamy R K, Henderson W R, Lansford K G, Piercy M 1961 The intravenous pyelogram and carcinoma of the cervix. Obstet Gynecol 17:26–29

59. Wolfenden J M, Waxman A D, Disaia P J, Siemsen J K 1975 Evaluation of carcinoma of the cervix using ^{111}In bleomycin Obstet Gynecol 46:347–352

60. Norman O 1950 Hysterography in cancer of the corpus of the uterus. Acta Radiol; Suppl 79

61. Douglas B, Macdonald J S, Baker J W 1972 Lymphography in carcinoma of the uterus. Clin Radiol 23:286–294

62. Lang E K 1967 Arteriography in gynecology Radiol Clin North Amer 5:133–149
63. Brewis R A L, Bagshawe K D 1968 Pelvic arteriography in invasive trophoblastic neoplasia. Br J Radiol 41:581–495
64. Takahashi M, Nagata Y 1971 Angiography of trophoblastic tumours. Am J Roentgenol 112:779–787
65. Cockshott W P, Hendrickse J P de V 1967 Persistent arterio-venous fistulae following chemotherapy of malignant trophoblastic disease. Radiology 88:329–334
66. Libsbitz H I, Collins C, Baber E, Hammond C B 1977 The pulmonary metastases of choriocarcinoma. Obst Gynec 49:412–416
67. Stein I F 1945 Bilateral polycystic ovaries. Am J Obstet Gynecol 50:385–398
68. Castro J R, Klein E W 1962 The incidence and appearance of roentgenologically visible psammomatous calcifications of the papillary cystadenocarcinomas of the ovaries. Am J Roetgenol 88:861–891
69. Teplick J G, Haskin M E, Alvi A 1976 Calcified intraperitoneal metastases from ovarian carcinoma. Am J Roentgenol 127:1003–1006
70. Lond J P, Montgomery J B 1952 The incidence of ureteral obstruction in benign and malignant gynecologic lesions. Am J Obstet Gynecol 59:552–562
71. Athey P A, Wallace S, Jing B S, Gallagher H S, Smith J P 1975 Lymphangiography in ovarian cancer. Am J Roentgenol 123:106–113
72. Fleischer A C, James A E, Mills J B, Julian C 1978 Differential diagnosis of pelvic masses by grey scale sonography. Am J Roentgenol 131:469–476
73. Morley P, Barrett E 1977 The ovarian mass. In: Sanders R C, James A E, ed. Ultrasonography in obstetrics and gynecology, 2nd edn Appleton Century Crofts, New York 333–335
74. Peterson W F, Provost E D, Edmunds F T, Hundley J M, Morris F K 1955 Benign cystic teratomas of the ovary. Am J Obstet Gynecol 10:368–382
75. Blackwell W J, Dockerty M B, Masson J C, Masey R D 1946 Dermoid cyst of the ovary: their clinical and pathological significance. Am J Obstet Gynecol 1946; 5:151–172
76. Guttman P H 1977 In search of the elusive benign cystic ovarian teratoma. Application of the ultrasound 'tip of the iceberg' sign. J Clin Ultrasound 5:403–406
77. Seymour E Q, Hood J B, Underwood P B, Williamson H O 1976 Gonadoblastoma: an ovarian tumour with characteristic pelvic calcification. Am J Roentgenol 127:1001–1002
78. Markovits P, Bergiron C, Chauvel C, Castellino R A 1977 Lymphography in the staging, treatment planning, and surveillance of ovarian dysgerminomas. Am J Roentgenol 128:835–838
79. Rosenberg R F, Hausner M M 1979 Sclerosing stromal tumour of ovary. Radiology 132:70
80. Lea Thomas M, Fletcher E W L, Andress M R, Cockett F B 1967 The venous connection of vulvar varices. Clin Radiol 18:313–317
81. Chassar Moir J 1973 Vesico-vaginal fistulae as seen in Britain. J *Obst Gynaec Br Cwth 80:598–602
82. Wesolowski D P, Meaney T F 1977 The use of a vaginal tampon in the diagnosis of vesicovaginal fistulae. Radiology 122:263
83. Sanders R C 1977 Postpartum diagnostic ultrasound. In: Sanders R C, James A E (eds) Ultrasonography in obstetrics and gynecology 2nd, Appleton Century Crofts, New York 285–295
84. Marshak R H, Eliasoph J 1955 The roentgen findings in adenomyosis. Radiology 57:892–896
85. Asherman J G 1950 Traumatic intrauterine adhesions. J Obstet Gynaecol Br Emp 57:892–896
86. Mazzonella P Okagaki T, Richant R M 1972 Teratoma of the uterine tube. Obstet Gynecol 39:381–388
87. Lawson T L, Albarelli J N 1977 Diagnosis of pelvic masses by grey scale ultrasonography. Analysis of specifity and accuracy. Am J Roentgenol 128:1003–1006
88. Maklad N F, Wright C H 1978 Grey scale ultrasonography in the diagnosis of ectopic pregnancy. Radiology 126:221–225
89. Eisenberg R L 1972 The widened loop sign of Lippe's loop perforations. Am J Roentgenol 116:487–852
90. Cochrane W J, Thomas M A 1977 The value of ultrasound in the management of intrauterine devices. In: Sanders R C and James A E (eds) Ultrasonography in obstetrics and gynaecology. 2nd edn Appleton Century Crofts, New York pp 387–400

91. Vessey M P, McPherson K, Johnson B 1977 Mortality among women particularly in the Oxford/Family Planning Association contraceptive study. Lancet 2:731–733
92. Jackson E A 1976 Urethral syndrome in women. Radiology 119:287–291
93. Kaplan A L 1977 Postradiation ureteral obstruction. Obstet Gynecol Survey 32:1–8
94. Bates P, Whiteside C G, Turner-Warwick R 1970 Synchronous cine/pressure/flow/cystometry with special reference to stress and urge incontinence. Br J Urol 42:714–723
95. Stanton S L 1978 Postoperative investigation and diagnosis. Clin Obstet Gynecol 21:207–721
96. Elkin M, Goldman S M, Meng C H 1974 Ureteric obstruction in patients with uterine prolapse. Radiology 110:289–294
97. Walsh J W 1979 Comparison of ultrasound and computed tomography in the evaluation of pelvic masses. Clin Diagn Ultrasound 2:229–242
98. Carter B L, Kahn P C, Wolpert S M et al 1976 Unusual pelvic masses. A comparison of computed tomographic scanning and ultrasonography. Radiology 121:383–390
99. Walsh J W, Goplerud D R 1981 Prospective comparison between clinical and CT staging in primary cervical carcinoma. Am J Roentgenol 137:997–1003
100. Ginaldi S, Wallace S, Jing B-S, Bernadino M E 1981 Carcinoma of the cervix: lymphangiography and computed tomography. Am J Roentgenol 136:1087–109
101. Johnson R J, Blackledge G, Eddleston B, Crowther D 1983 Abdomino-pelvic computed tomography in the management of ovarian carcinoma. Radiology 146:447–452
102. Lee K R, Mansfield C M, Dwyer S J et al 1980 CT for intracavitary radiotherapy planning. Am J Roentgenol 135:809–813
103. Jaques P F, Staab E, Rickey W et al 1978 CT-assisted pelvic and abdominal aspiration biopsies in gynecological malignancy. Radiology 128:651–655
104. Lee J K T, Stanley R J, Sagel S S, Levitt R R 1978a Accuracy of computed tomography in detecting intra-abdominal and pelvic adenopathy in lymphoma Am J Roentgenol 131:311–315
105. Lee J K T, Stanley R J, Sagel S S, McClennan B L 1978b Accuracy of CT in detecting intra-abdominal and pelvic lymph node metastases from pelvic cancers. Am J Roentgenol 131:675–679
106. Whitley N O, Brenner D E, Francis A et al 1982 Computed tomographic evaluation of carcinoma of the cervix. Radiology 142:439–446
107. Walsh J W, Amendola M A, Hall D J et al 1981 Recurrent carcinoma of the cervix: CT diagnosis. Am J Roentgenol 136: 117–122
108. Walsh J W, Goplerud D R 1983 A critical evaluation of computed tomography in primary, persistent and recurrent endometrial malignancy. Am J Roentgenol 139:1149–51
109. Seidelmann F E, Cohen W N 1978 Pelvis. In: Haaga J, Reich N E (eds) Computed tomography of abdominal abnormalities. Mosby, St Louis. pp 221–276
110. Amendola M A, Walsh J W, Amendola B E et al 1981 Computed tomography in the evaluation of carcinoma of the ovary. J Comput Assist Tomogr 5:179–186
111. Whitley N, Brenner D, Francis A et al 1981 Use of the computed tomographic whole body scanner to stage and follow patients with advanced ovarian carcinoma. Invest Radiol 16:479–486
112. Chen S S, Kumari S, Lee L 1980 Contributions of abdominal computed tomography (CT) in the management of gynecologic cancer: correlated study of CT image and gross surgical pathology. Gynecol Oncol 10:167–172
113. Blaquiere R M, Husband J E 1983 Conventional radiology and computed tomography (CT) in ovarian cancer. J Royal Soc Med (in press)
114. Husband J E, Fry I K 1981 Lymph node disease of the abdomen and pelvis. In computed tomography of the body — A radiological and clinical approach. Macmillan Press, London, pp 132–145

SUGGESTIONS FOR FURTHER READING

Asplund J 1952 The uterine cervix and isthmus under normal and pathological conditions. Acta Radiol Suppl 91

Bryk D 1966 Roentgen evaluation of large uterine and ovarian masses. Obstet Gynecol 28:630–636

Deutsch A L and Gosink B B 1982 Non-neoplastic gynaecologic disorders. Semin Roentgenol 17:269–283

Foda M S, Youssef A F, Shafeek M A, Kassen K A 1962 Hysterographic diagnosis of abnormalities of the uterus. I. Congenital abnormalities, Br J Radiol 35:115–121

Foda M S, Youssef A F, Shafeek M A, Kassen K A 1962 Hysterographic diagnosis of abnormalities of the uterus. Br J Radiol 35:783–795

Fullenlove T H 1969 Experience with over 2000 uterosalpingographies. Am J Roentgenol 106:463–471

Griffin T W, Parker R G, Taylor W S 1976 An evaluation of procedures used in staging carcinoma of the cervix. Am J Roentgenol 127:825–827

Keirse M H N G, Vandervellen R 1973 A comparison of hysterosalpingography and laparoscopy in the investigation of infertility. Obstet Gynecol 41:685–688

Lang E K 1967 Arteriography in gynecology. Radiol Clin N Amer 5:133–149

Lawson T L, Albarelli J N 1972 Diagnosis of pelvic masses by grey scale ultrasonography. Analysis of specificity and accuracy. Am J Roentgenol 128:1003–1006

Lewis E, Zornoza J, Jing B S, Chuang V P, Wallace S 1982 Radiologic contributions to the diagnosis and management of gynaecologic neoplasms. Semin Roentgenol 17:251–268

Noonan C D 1965 Primary and secondary malignancy of female reproductive tract. Radiol Clin N Amer 3:375–387

Pontiflex G, Trichopoulos D, Karpathios S 1972 Hysterosalpingography in the diagnosis of infertility (statistical analysis of 3437 cases). Fertil Steril 23:829–833

Rozin S 1952 The X-ray diagnosis of genital tuberculosis. J Obst Gynaec Br Emp 59:59–63

Sample W F, Lippe B M, Gypes M T 1977 Grey scale ultrasonography of the normal female pelvis. Radiology 125:477–483

Sanders R C, James A E (ed) 1977 Ultrasonography in obstetrics and gynecology, 2nd edn Appleton Century Crofts, New York

Shopfner C E 1967 Radiology in pediatric gynecology. Radiol Clin N Amer 5:151–167

Stephens F D 1966 Urethrovaginal malformations. Austral NZ J Obst Gynaec 5:64–73

Stern W Z, Wilson L 1973 Radiologic aspects of an abortion program. Am J Roetgenol 119:841–851

Tietze C 1966 Contraception with intrauterine devices. Am J Obstet Gynecol 96:1040–1054

Whitehouse G H 1981 Gynaecological radiology. Blackwell Scientific Publications. Oxford.

Ultrasonography in obstetrics and gynecology. Radiol clin North Am June 1982 Multiple Authors.

82 The breast

Stephen A. Feig

Normal anatomy
Benign dysplasias
    Adenosis
    Fibroadenoma
    Papillomatosis
    Papilloma
    Cyst
Parenchymal patterns and breast cancer risk
Breast carcinoma
    Scirrhous carcinoma
    Circumscribed carcinoma
    Malignant calcifications
Mammography
    Accuracy
    Mammography versus physical examination
    — Indications for mammography
    Biopsy method for nonpalpable lesions
    Technical requirements for mammography
    Direct film mammography
    Screen-film mammography
    Dedicated mammography units
    Xeromammography
    Xeromammography versus screen-film mammography
    Risk from mammography
Breast cancer screening
    Criteria for benefit
    Evidence of benefit
    Benefit/risk comparison
Thermography
Telethermography
Other methods
Limitations
Breast ultrasound
    Equipment
    Diagnostic criteria
    Accuracy
    Indications
Breast computerized tomography
Magnetic resonance imaging
Transillumination lightscanning

NORMAL ANATOMY

The breast contains 15 to 20 lobes. Each lobe is comprised of a variable number of lobules, which consist of 10 to 100 acini or blind ending sacs (Fig. 82.1). The breast ducts form a branching structure, which conveys milk from the acini to the nipple. The various sized ducts can be described on the basis of their location as *intralobular*, *interlobular*, *intralobar* and *interlobar*. The acini are lined by a single layer of cuboidal epithelium, which merges into the columnar epithelium of the smaller ducts and finally into the stratified squamous epithelium of the major (interlobar) lactiferous ducts. Thus, each lobe may be defined as a collection of glandular tissue which is drained by a single major lactiferous duct. Since some of the major ducts merge prior to their termination on the nipple, the number of duct openings is less than the number of major ducts.

The glandular and ductal tissue constitute the parenchyma. The fatty and fibrotic tissue, which both surrounds and extends into the lobules, constitutes the stroma. Both are contained within a sac formed when the superficial pectoral fascia splits into anterior (superficial) and posterior (deep) layers. *Cooper's ligaments* are tentlike projections of the superficial layer of the superficial fascia through the subcutaneous tissue to the skin. They also form a connective tissue skeleton between the two layers of superficial fascia.

The number of lobules per lobe and the number of acini per lobule vary according to age, parity, and other individual factors. During adolescence, the breast undergoes both growth and differentiation. With pregnancy, the number of acini is increased; the breast is converted into an almost solid glandular structure. If breast feeding occurs, these changes persist into the period of lactation. Following pregnancy and/or lactation, there is a marked decrease in the number of acini so that the breast will be less glandular than it was prior to pregnancy. The breast of a parous woman will usually be less glandular than that of a nulliparous woman of similar age.

Mammographic studies [1] show that parenchymal atrophy begins in the early twenties or after the first pregnancy,

1631

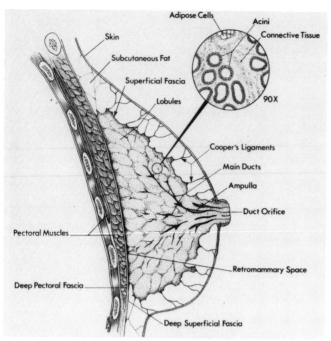

Fig. 82.1 Anatomy of the female breast. (Reproduced with permission from Feig S. A. 1980 Crit Rev Diag Imag 13:229–248)

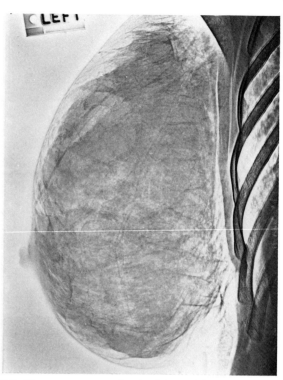

Fig. 82.2 Xeromammogram of a glandular and fibrotic breast (DY parenchymal pattern) is generally dense except for lucent areas of subcutaneous and retromammary fat.

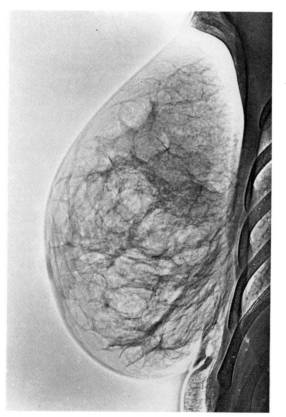

Fig. 82.3 Intermediate density breast. Most glandular tissue is in the upper outer quadrant. Other quadrants are largely fatty but traversed by fibrotic strands (Cooper's ligaments).

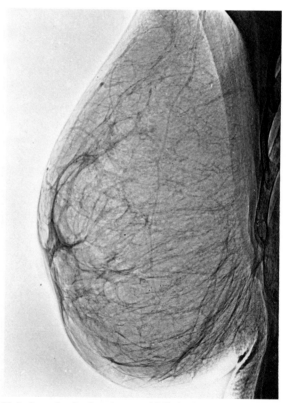

Fig. 82.4 Low density fatty breast with little glandular or ductal tissue (N-1 parenchymal pattern). Cooper's ligaments are seen as thin, straight fibrotic structures. Veins are broader, longer, curved and branching. A few scattered benign microcalcifications are noted. Pectoralis major muscle overlies the rib cage.

whichever comes earlier. It continues with advancing age and accelerates at menopause. Because of this decrease in the number of lobules and acini, the breasts of older women contain relatively more fatty tissue and less glandular tissue than those of younger women of the same parity (Figs. 82.2–82.4).

BENIGN DYSPLASIAS

Benign dysplasias [2-7] are hyperplastic breast conditions; there is more glandular and fibrotic tissue than expected for the patient's age and parity. The tissue is also morphologically abnormal. There are five main types: *adenosis* — *epithelial hyperplasia* of the lobules, *papillomatosis* — *epithelial hyperplasia* of the ducts, *fibroadenoma, papilloma*, and *fibrocystic* disease. These five types never occur as pure forms. Although one may predominate, they always coexist.

Adenosis

On mammography, adenosis [2-7] may be seen as patchy or homogeneous areas of increased density. The breasts appear denser than expected for the patient's age and parity. These areas may contain punctate adenosic calcifications (Fig. 82.5) which may represent the only mammographic abnormality. Calcifications are usually rounded or oval in shape and have smooth margins. Because most of them measure 1 mm or less, they are referred to as *microcalcifications*. In adenosis, the distribution of both soft tissue densities and calcifications should be generally similar between the two breasts. Any significant asymmetry which cannot be accounted for by previous surgery, i.e. removal of calcifications or soft tissues from one breast, should be further evaluated by means of biopsy.

Histologically, adenosis represents an increase in the number of lobules and number of acini within each lobule. These acini show epithelial proliferation and dilatation. The microcalcifications represent calcified debris within the lumina of these acini. Adenosis tends to regress with age, especially after the menopause.

The term *sclerosing adenosis* refers to a specific type of adenosis, where connective tissue proliferation is predominant. It is thought to represent a late stage where the epithelial elements have regressed and are replaced by fibrosis. On mammography, sclerosing adenosis is characterized by smooth and well demarcated margins which may be straight, curved, or even rounded so as to appear as a discrete mass on mammography.

Fibroadenoma

This lesion [2-7] represents the most common benign tumour

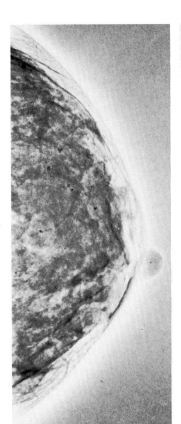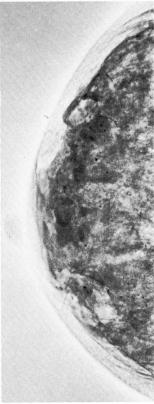

Fig. 82.5 Adenosis. Both breasts are radiographically dense due to glandular and/or fibrotic tissue. Punctate microcalcifications are scattered in both breasts.

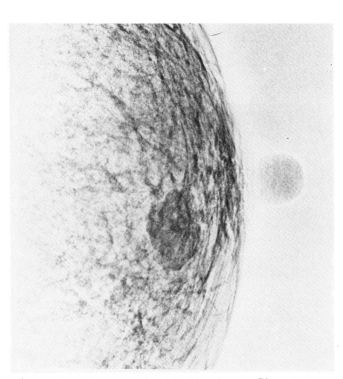

Fig. 82.6 Well circumscribed nodular fibroadenoma. Biopsy was performed since a mass with this appearance may represent carcinoma.

of the breast. It is thought to arise from adenosis. Fibroadenomas may be seen as well circumscribed masses on mammography. Their borders are round, oval or nodular (Fig. 82.6). They are frequently multiple and bilateral and rarely exceed 3 cm in size. They generally arise in younger women and never develop or grow after the menopause. On physical examination, they are firm but relatively moveable since they do not induce proliferation of fibroblasts in the surrounding breast tissue. On histological section, they contain both fibrotic and glandular tissue in varying proportions so that some pathologists prefer to designate them as either fibroadenoma or adenofibroma. Long clefts lined by one or two layers of epithelium may be present.

Considering their glandular composition, it is not surprising that fibroadenomas regress with age. Necrosis within the tumour is seen as coarse conglomerate calcifications on mammography. These calcifications are much larger than those in benign adenosis. Their peripheral distribution within the tumour is a characteristic feature (Fig. 82.7). Ultimately, the soft tissue components may completely disappear so that only calcification remains.

Papilloma

When the intraductal proliferation reaches macroscopic size, the condition is termed *intraductal papilloma*. This lesion usually occurs in the retroareolar region and is a frequent cause of serous or sanguineous nipple discharge. Usually the lesion is only several millimetres in size so that the mammogram may show slight bulging of a retroareolar duct or may appear normal (Fig. 82.8). In a woman with unilateral nipple discharge and a normal mammogram, contrast ductography (galactography) may demonstrate the presence of an intraductal filling defect. This finding is nonspecific and does not distinguish a benign intraductal papilloma from an intraductal papillary carcinoma. Occasionally, the lesion may reach a size of 2 to 3 cm and can be seen as an oval circumscribed mass in the retroareolar area.

Solitary papillomas are frequent and have no malignant potential, whereas multiple papillomas are infrequent and are associated with an increased risk of malignancy. Multiple papillomas are sometimes referred to as *papillomatosis* but here the term is used in a different sense from the microscopic description of papillomatosis previously discussed.

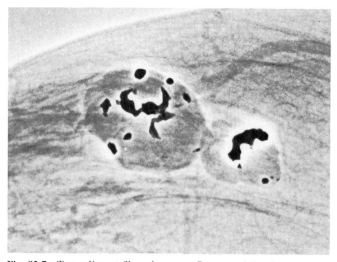

Fig. 82.7 Two adjacent fibroadenomas. Coarse peripheral calcification is pathognomonic. Centrally located and/or smaller calcifications, frequently seen in other fibroadenomas, may also occur in other conditions.

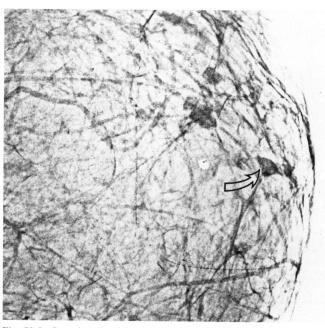

Fig. 82.8 Intraductal papilloma. Bulging of a retroareolar duct from a 0.8 × 0.3 cm lesion.

Papillomatosis

Microscopic papillary proliferation in the large and small lactiferous ducts is common and may be referred to as papillomatosis [2-7]. It is often associated histologically with benign adenosis and may have similar mammographic characteristics i.e. microcalcifications and patchy areas of increased density. When papillomatosis is found in the large ducts, the microcalcifications are closer to the nipple and tend to be more linearly arrayed than those seen in adenosis.

Cyst

Breast cysts [2-7] also arise from adenosis when the lumina of the ducts and acini become dilated and lined by atrophic epithelium. They also appear as round or oval well circumscribed masses on mammography, however, a multiloculated cyst or a cluster of several adjacent cysts may have a nodular shape. Although some cysts may attain a larger size than fibroadenomas, they usually cannot be distinguished from noncalcified fibroadenomas on mammography. Cysts frequently disappear or subside following menopause. Neither cysts nor fibroadenomas grow after menopause so that any increase in size of a mass during that period should be suspect for carcinoma.

Like fibroadenomas, cysts are often multiple and bilateral. Calcification is infrequent, but may be seen as a thin peripheral egg shell (Fig. 82.9), different from the coarse peripheral calcification of fibroadenomas. Cysts may rarely contain milk of calcium fluid, which on an erect lateral mammogram layers out on the floor of the cyst. Fibrocystic breasts often contain increased fibrotic tissue so that fibrocystic disease may be sub-classified as predominantly cystic, fibrotic or indeterminate.

Although cystic disease often produces no symptoms, it may be severely painful and tender. These symptoms may be continuous or may appear only in the premenstrual phase of the menstrual cycle, and are related to fluid tension within the cyst. Aspiration may be therapeutic as well as diagnostic. Another clinical feature which helps to differentiate cysts from carcinoma is that cysts may develop quickly, often prior to menses and diminish in size just as rapidly. The consistency of cysts depends on their fluid pressure. When the pressure is low, they are soft, but when it is high, the cysts are firm.

PARENCHYMAL PATTERNS AND BREAST CANCER RISK

Some investigators believe that a patient's future risk of breast cancer can be predicted from the parenchymal pattern seen on her baseline mammographic examination [8,9]. These patterns can be defined by the distribution and relative amount of ductal tissue, fatty tissue, fibrotic and/or glandular tissue seen on mammography.

Ducts on mammography appear as serpiginous structures fanning out from the nipple, most often towards the upper outer quadrant. Ducts are visualized because of the collagen tissue or periductal collagenosis which envelops them. The proportion of breast volume occupied by ducts varies among patients from 0 to 100. The most commonly used system of parenchymal classification was devised by Wolfe [9]. There are four main patterns. The *N1* breast (See Fig. 82.4) is primarily fat with no visible ducts and little or no dysplasia. In the *P1* breast (Fig. 82.10), ducts comprise 10–25% of the breast volume, and in the *P2* breast (Fig. 82.11) greater than 25% of volume. The *DY* breast (See Fig. 82.2) contains more

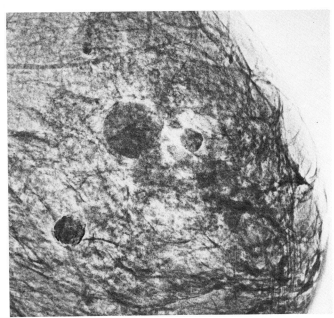

Fig. 82.9 Multiple cysts. Thin curvilinear calcifications are present in the wall of the lower left cyst. The other cysts are round noncalcified masses which are indistinguishable from noncalcified fibroadenomas.

Cystic disease is thought to be stimulated by a hormonal imbalance. Its response to treatment by Danocrine which results in decrease in circulating oestrogen is well documented. Although some investigators have stated that fibrocystic disease decreases following abstinence from caffeine, this claim has not been supported by others. Many authors believe that women with gross cystic disease are at a high risk for carcinoma [7]. This does not imply that carcinoma evolves from cysts, but rather that both have a common aetiological factor.

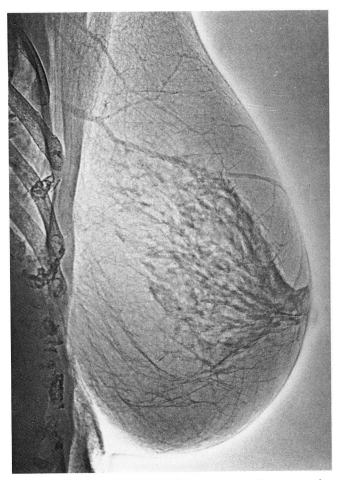

Fig. 82.10 P-1 parenchymal pattern. In this patient, ducts occupy less than 25% of breast volume and are seen as rope-like structures fanning out from the nipple.

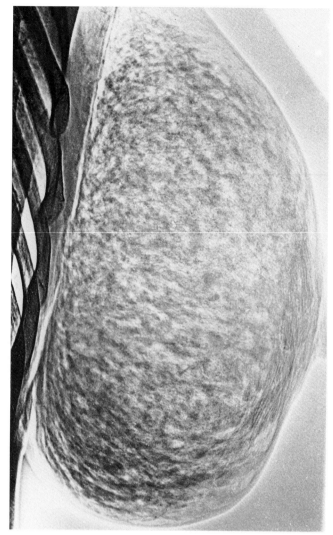

Fig. 82.11 P-2 parenchymal pattern. In this patient, ducts extend throughout the entire breast.

fibrotic and glandular tissue than ductal tissue. Ducts may be present, but they are obscured by these surrounding tissue elements.

Based on their studies, Wolfe and others contend that women with P2 and DY patterns have a greater risk of subsequent breast cancer than those with N1 or P1 patterns. Specifically, Wolfe described the following relative risks of breast cancer [9] when patients from 21 to 83 years of age with each of these four parenchymal patterns were followed for less than 48 months: N1 (1.0), P1 (2.0), P2 (7.2), DY (10.7); and for 48 plus months: N1 (1.0), P1 (1.4), P2 (9.0), DY (24.0). Although the relative risk from DY and, to a lesser extent, P2 was diminished after age 50, both of these patterns continued to convey an excess breast cancer risk regardless of patient age.

To understand why certain parenchymal patterns might be expected to convey an increased risk, a brief discussion of breast cancer development would be in order. Breast cancer is thought to arise as the final step in a sequence of histo-logical changes from normal tissue to dysplasia to cellular atypia and finally to anaplasia. Dysplasia and cellular atypia are nonobligate precursors of anaplasia. They do not necessarily progress to cancer; only a few cases do. They may, in fact, regress to normal tissue, but they do represent necessary intermediate stages. This discussion implies that the amount of dysplastic tissue present should correlate with subsequent breast cancer risk.

Evidence that parenchymal patterns do indicate the amount of dysplasia and atypia may be found in a study [10] which compared breast biopsy results with mammographic images. Histological specimens were graded as normal (0), hyperplasia (1), mild atypia (2), moderate atypia (3), severe atypia (4), and ductal carcinoma in situ (5). A positive correlation was found between the mean grade of ductal epithelial proliferation and the mammographic parenchymal pattern. These were as follows: N1 (0.5), P1 (1.3), P2 (2.2) and DY (3.0).

A significant predictive value of the Wolfe classification has not been confirmed by all investigators. Some believe that more breast cancers show up in P2 and DY breasts on follow-up studies because these cancers were originally present on baseline examination, but were obscured by the surrounding glandular tissues. [11] Other studies [12,13] indicate that if P2 and DY women are at excess risk, it is not sufficiently great to justify preferential screening of these patients. In one study [13], women with P2 or DY breasts constituted 51% of the population but accounted for only 63% of all cancers on short term follow-up. Moreover, there was no significant correlation between mammographic parenchymal patterns and high risk pathological markers. These results are in contrast to those of Wolfe, where, by means of parenchymal patterns, 93% of cancers could be found in 57% of the population [9].

A recent review [8] of the literature concludes that P2 and DY patterns do confer increased breast cancer risk, but one which is much smaller than that stated by Wolfe. One problem may be reader variability i.e. difference in classification among radiologists. Until more definitive data are obtained, the following practical conclusions would seem warranted:

1. Mammographic parenchymal patterns should not exclude a woman from screening mammography, especially when performed with present low dose technique.
2. All women above the age 50 years should received annual mammographic screening regardless of their parenchymal pattern.
3. For women below age 50, mammographic parenchymal patterns along with other risk factors could determine the age at which screening should begin as well as the subsequent screening frequency e.g. baseline mammogram at age 35 and annual mammography thereafter versus baseline mammogram at age 40 and screening every 2 years until age 50.
4. Mammographic parenchymal patterns should not be an indication for prophylactic mastectomy.

BREAST CARCINOMA

Histology

Ductal carcinoma, which arises from the epithelium of the breast ducts, accounts for nearly 94% of all breast cancers [14]. Lobular carcinoma, which arises from the acini of breast lobules, accounts for 5.5% of cases. Less than 1% of breast malignancies are of sarcomatous or other mesenchymal origin.

Ductal and lobular carcinomas may be further subdivided by histological type and stage of invasion. Noninfiltrating lesions are still confined to the ducts and acini. Infiltrating lesions have broken through the basement membrane and invaded the breast stroma. Of those breast cancers encountered in clinical practice (nonscreening situation), 95% are infiltrating and 5% are noninfiltrating (*in situ*) [15]. Among infiltrating ductal carcinomas, approximately 95% are ductal NOS (not otherwise specified) or ductal with fibrosis (scirrhous). The remaining ductal carcinomas may be characterized by a specific histological feature, such as large reticular cells and lymphoid infiltrate (*medullary carcinoma*), production of colloid or mucinous material (*colloid carcinoma*), papillary growth (*papillary carcinoma*), well defined ductal tubular structures (*tubular carcinoma*) or occurrence near the nipple with appearance of Paget's cells (*Paget's carcinoma*) [14].

Location

Since the upper outer quadrant usually contains more glandular tissue than any other section of the breast, it is not surprising that 50% of all breast cancers originate there. The next most common site is the retroareolar region (18%) on which ducts from the entire breast converge. Only 15% of breast cancers arise from the upper inner quadrant, 11% from the lower outer quadrant, and 6% from the lower inner quadrant [16].

Scirrhous carcinoma

The most common mammographic appearance of carcinoma is a stellate or spiculated mass (Fig. 82.12). Corresponding to the irregular border seen on mammography, a desmoplastic response extending into the surrounding tissue is observed on microscopic examination [17]. These cancers may be referred to as *scirrhous carcinomas*, a descriptive term for any invasive ductal carcinoma which provokes such connective tissue proliferation. In most instances, these fibrotic extensions do not contain tumour cells, so that the size of the neoplasm is best measured as that of the central mass. However, with extensive spread, even these hyalinized bands may be invaded by tumour cells. Thus far, there is no satisfactory explanation why this stellate reaction is produced by some invasive ductal carcinomas but not by others. The cells of the central tumour mass may exhibit any degree of anaplasia. A small minority of scirrhous carcinomas may

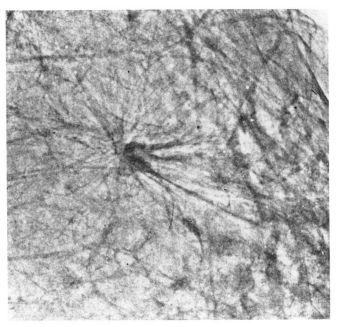

Fig. 82.12 Infiltrating ductal carcinoma. Fibrotic spiculations and malignant microcalcifications extend beyond the 1 cm tumour mass into the surrounding tissue.

contain a sufficient proportion of well differentiated ductal structures to be further classified as *tubular carcinomas* [18].

In addition to these features, **microcalcifications** may be seen on mammography in approximately 30% of cases and on histological examination in 70% of cases [19]. These calcifications represent necrotic debris.

On physical examination, scirrhous carcinoma is firm or hard, frequently nonmoveable. Secondary signs of flattening, thickening, and retraction of the overlying skin or nipple may be present, but these are nonspecific findings, which may also be caused by previous biopsy, fat necrosis, breast inflammation and radiation therapy. Benign nipple retraction is a common phenomenon which is frequently bilateral in older women. It may be due to previous abscess, secretory disease with fat necrosis, or may occur on an idiopathic basis.

A large scirrhous carcinoma in a fatty breast can be easily identified on mammography. Its sunburst appearance readily distinguishes it from benign masses. Recognition of smaller scirrhous carcinomas or those occurring in denser breasts may be considerably more difficult (Fig. 82.13). Smaller cancers may pass unnoticed or may be mistaken for cysts, fibroadenomas, or normal breast trabeculae by observers without sufficient training and experience. Even larger lesions may be partially or completely masked by surrounding glandular, fibrotic, and ductal tissue.

Often, the tumour mass itself may not be visible so that the only evidence of carcinoma is the presence of abnormal trabecular markings i.e. 'architectural distortion'. One must consciously search the mammogram for straight spiculations that do not follow the same path as that of normal breast trabeculae, which follow a gentle arc-like course toward the nipple. In contrast, spiculations due to carcinoma radiate from another point within the breast. Normal breast trabe-

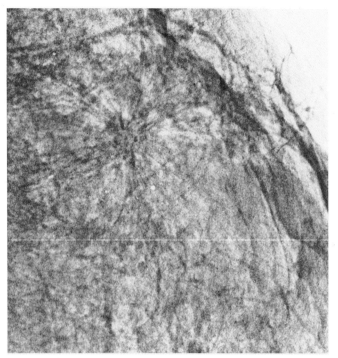

Fig. 82.13 Stellate reaction aids recognition of a 1 cm carcinoma in a dense breast.

culae are usually parallel to each other. Carcinoma spiculations are oriented at some other angle to themselves and to normal breast markings. Each mass, even the tiniest one of 0.5 cm or less, should be scrutinized for any irregular border characteristics which may distinguish it from a small cyst or fibroadenoma.

It is also helpful to interpret the mammogram with the comparable images placed side by side. The two lateral and craniocaudal views should be mirror images. They do not have to be completely symmetric but departure from symmetry should be viewed with suspicion. The following types of asymmetry may indicate carcinoma: disposition of trabeculae; quantity, distribution, and contour of parenchymal tissue. (Fig. 82.14).

Differential diagnosis

Several benign breast conditions can produce a stellate shaped density, which may be indistinguishable on mammography from carcinoma [20]. For example, breast biopsy may cause *parenchymal scarring* as well as overlying skin thickening and retraction [21] (Fig. 82.15). Some radiologists have their technician tape a row of metallic pellets over the skin scar for identification on mammography, however, this author prefers a simple diagrammatic notation on the X-ray

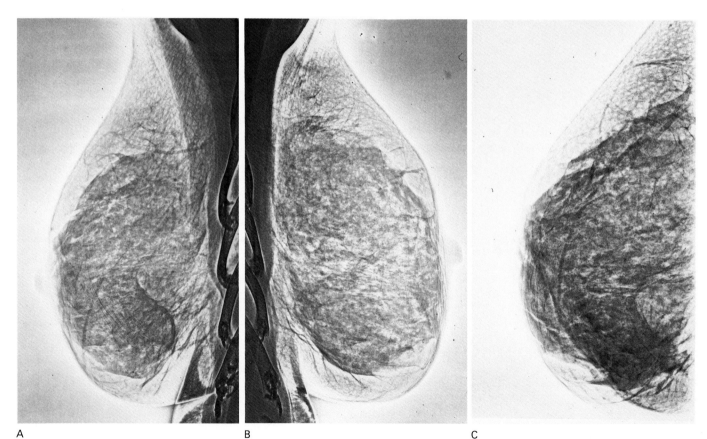

A   B   C

Fig. 82.14 Chest wall lateral projections of both breasts (A, B) show an asymmetrical density in the lower left breast (A) which on the contact lateral view (C) appears as an irregular mass partially obscured by surrounding glandular tissue. An infiltrating ductal carcinoma was found at biopsy. Compared to the standard chest wall lateral view (A), the contact lateral view (C) includes less breast tissue but may show greater detail.

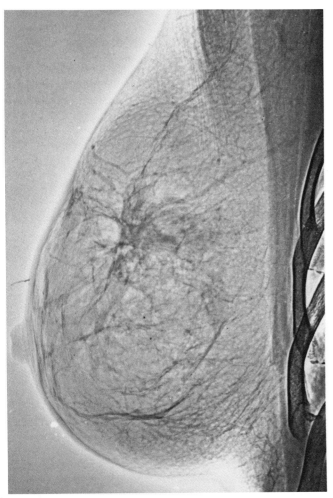

Fig. 82.15 Post-biopsy scarring. The irregular stellate mass with overlying skin thickening and retraction mimics a carcinoma.

request sheet. Most excisional scars can be easily differentiated from carcinoma on the basis of such history, lack of change from a previous mammogram, or absence of an associated mass. Nevertheless, if there is any significant possibility that the parenchymal density might be due to carcinoma, it is best to biopsy the patient again. Also, all parenchymal scars should be compared with those seen on the previous mammogram to determine if any change has occurred. Carcinoma may develop adjacent to a scar, but the alteration in mammographic appearance may be subtle.

Traumatic fat necrosis may assume any of several mammographic appearances: stellate mass, circumscribed mass, amorphous density, calcification [22]. Many cases appear indistinguishable from carcinoma on mammography. Only 30 to 40% of patients with biopsy proven fat necrosis can recall a specific injury. Skin retraction may be seen in 50% of patients, pain and/or tenderness in 35% [23]. Physical examination and history are often helpful, but a history of trauma may occasionally be misleading, since some patients first notice a carcinoma on examining their breasts following an

injury. Early histological findings include haemorrhage, fat, and histiocytes or foam cells. Fibrosis occurs at a later stage.

Breast abscess is usually retroareolar and occurs in young primiparous women during lactation. It is usually due to a staphylococcal infection. There is also pain, swelling and erythema, so that the clinical diagnosis is usually clear, although the mammographic appearance may resemble carcinoma. Rarely, abscess may occur in a patient who is not post-partum or in another location in the breast.

Stellate densities caused by *sclerosing adenosis* and *fibrous mastopathy* usually cannot be differentiated on the mammogram from carcinoma. On histological examination, fibrous mastopathy (radial scar) usually measures less than 1 cm and consists of a sclerotic centre surrounded by dilated radiating tubules. Sclerosing adenosis may be larger. In addition to these, normal breast trabeculae may, if superimposed, form a summation shadow which resembles a tiny carcinoma.

A *hyalinized fibroadenoma*, a rare lesion, may also be seen as a stellate shaped density. It is produced when the fibroadenoma shrinks down and becomes surrounded by radiating fibrous bands.

Except for post-biopsy scarring, all of the above entities are considerably less common than scirrhous carcinoma. Suspicious stellate masses should be considered to represent carcinoma until proven otherwise by biopsy. Lack of change in appearance of a stellate mass over long periods supports the diagnosis of benign disease, but does not totally exclude the possibility of carcinoma. Some slow growing cancers may show little change in mammographic appearance over periods of 6 to 12 months [24].

Circumscribed carcinoma

Carcinoma may also present as a circumscribed mass, where spiculation is absent or less prominent than in scirrhous carcinoma. Circumscribed carcinoma is a descriptive term which includes all medullary, papillary, and gelatinous carcinomas as well as some ductal carcinomas. The latter appearance of ductal carcinoma has been described as 'knobby carcinoma' or 'carcinoma simplex'. Compared to scirrhous carcinoma, its contour is more nodular and less spiculated. (Figs. 82.16, 82.17).

Medullary carcinoma [14] has a distinctive microscopic appearance. The tumour cells are large, hyperchromatic, and form broadly anastomosing bands or masses. A heavy lymphocytic infiltrate is common. On mammography, the tumour is round, oval, or lobular. Margins may be finely spiculated, partially obscured, or completely sharp. Since it may be soft on palpation and well marginated on mammography, it can be mistaken for a cyst.

Papillary carcinoma [14] is recognized pathologically by the presence of papillary processes or a cribriform (cartwheel-like) pattern of growth. Even when invasive, it produces

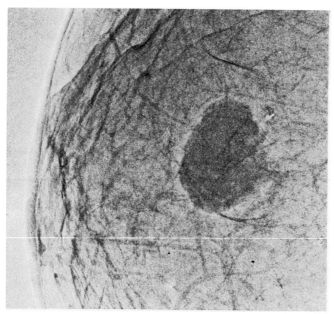

Fig. 82.16 Circumscribed ductal carcinoma with infiltration along its posterior border. Its other margins are well defined. A cyst or fibroadenoma may have a similar appearance if one border is obscured by adjacent glandular or fibrotic tissue. The absence of such tissue in this fatty breast makes malignant infiltration a more likely explanation.

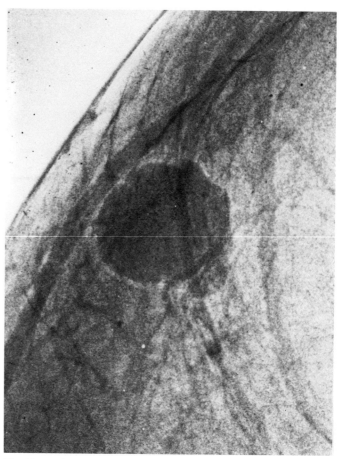

Fig. 82.17 Circumscribed ductal carcinoma with no obvious infiltration. Its slightly lobulated but well defined contour may be identical to that of a cyst or fibroadenoma.

little fibrotic response so that it is seen on mammography as a smoothly contoured mass. In its earliest stage, as an intraductal tumour of a few millimetres in size, papillary carcinoma may produce sanguineous or serous nipple discharge in the absence of a palpable mass or any mammographic abnormality. Rarely, a single dilated retroareolar duct is seen on mammography, but in most cases, ductography is the only X–ray method of identifying a lesion [25]. Intracystic papillary carcinoma is a rare type of papillary carcinoma, where the tumour mass is found on the inner wall of the cyst.

The term *mucinous, colloid,* or *gelatinous carcinoma* refers to one which produces a sufficient amount of mucoid material to be visible grossly. Many mucoid carcinomas on physical examination may be well delineated and soft, so that they may be mistaken for a cyst.

Differential diagnosis

Since the vast majority of circumscribed masses are benign, yet not always distinguishable on mammography from those which are malignant, determination of the need for biopsy can be a difficult practical problem. Cysts and fibroadenomas are so common that it is neither feasible nor desirable to advise biopsy on all circumscribed masses. However, if no circumscribed masses were biopsied, a significant proportion of breast cancers would be undetected until a later stage. Several factors can help determine if biopsy is necessary:

1. *Shape.* A nodular mass is more suspicious for malignancy than one which is round or oval.

2. *Margins.* The presence of spiculation usually indicates carcinoma. Irregular, ill-defined margins increase the possibility of malignancy, since they may indicate invasion of surrounding tissue. However, fibrotic or glandular tissue adjacent to a benign lesion can also obscure its borders.

3. *Calcification.* Coarse calcification (more than 1 mm thickness) located within the margin of a mass indicates a calcified fibroadenoma. A thin (1 mm or less) curvilinear calcification at the rim of a mass indicates a benign lesion such as a cyst, fat necrosis or fibroadenoma; most of these, especially long, thin, arc-like calcifications are cysts or fat necrosis. Coarse calcification within the body of a well circumscribed mass usually indicates a fibroadenoma, but may at times be seen in carcinoma.

4. *Solitary mass vs. multiple masses.* In the absence of typical 'benign' type calcifications, the possibility of malignancy should be considered for any solitary circumscribed mass regardless of size. Biopsy should be performed unless

it is found to be a cyst on aspiration or ultrasound. For example, although a solitary 1 cm nodular mass with well defined margins is probably a fibroadenoma, it should be further investigated.

On the other hand, if a well circumscribed mass is part of a generalized process, the likelihood that it is benign increases. Multiple round or oval masses of similar size and appearance in one or both breasts, or a single such mass in each breast are probably cysts or fibroadenomas, even if some borders are obscured. However, this presumptive diagnosis should be confirmed by physical examination, history, comparison to previous mammography, and if necessary aspiration, ultrasound and follow-up mammography.

In a breast with multiple masses, any mass which is dominant should be further evaluated. A mass may be dominant if it is significantly larger, denser, or has suspicious borders when compared to other masses.

Even a solitary, well circumscribed mass of 0.5 cm, should be biopsied unless it is unchanged from a previous mammogram. Lesions of this size are difficult to aspirate and cannot be reliably evaluated by ultrasound. Adherence to this rule will result in improved detection of early cancers. Contrary to expectations, this policy does not lead to an excessive biopsy rate. Careful observation of the mammogram shows that such small lesions are rarely solitary. One or more similar masses can nearly always be found in the opposite breast or elsewhere in the same breast to support the diagnosis of benign disease and obviate the need for immediate biopsy so that follow-up mammography and physical examination is sufficient.

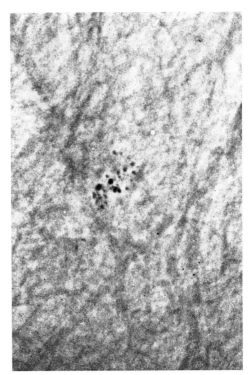

Fig. 82.18 In-situ ductal carcinoma seen as a cluster of 20 round and oval microcalcifications. This 0.5 cm lesion was nonpalpable.

Malignant calcifications

Microcalcifications range from microscopic size to 2 mm and are a frequent finding in both benign and malignant breast disease. Where no mass is present, they may represent the only evidence of such disease. Certain aspects of their appearance should suggest the possibility of malignancy [26–29].

An isolated cluster of microcalcifications with few or none elsewhere in the breast may represent either carcinoma or a benign process such as adenosis or papillomatosis (Fig. 82.18). The likelihood of carcinoma is proportional to the concentration of calcific particles. Therefore, one should consider biopsy of any focus of three or more microcalcifications if no other calcifications are present elsewhere in the breast or in the opposite breast. The chance of malignancy also depends on other factors such as the appearance and deployment of the calcifications.

Some features such as linear distribution along the course of a duct, or a thin splinter-like microlinear shape strongly suggest carcinoma (Fig. 82.19). Branching microlinear calcifications shaped like the letter 'Y' or 'U' are found histologically at the bifurcation of a duct and usually indicate carcinoma. When the branching is so extensive that the calcifications form a lace-like or reticular pattern, it is virtually pathognomonic of carcinoma.

Carcinoma may also be indicated by a crystalline or rhomboidal shape of calcifications. Variability in shape and size of

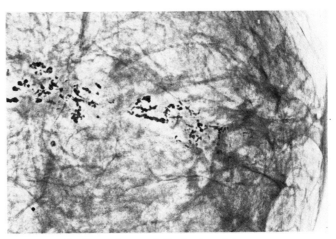

Fig. 82.19 The linear shape and distribution of these microcalcifications indicate ductal extension of this carcinoma from the irregular 2 cm tumour mass towards the nipple.

calcifications, as well as irregularity of their margins also raises the possibility of carcinoma.

Even when found over a wide area of the breast, calcifications which are grouped in clusters rather than diffusely distributed may indicate carcinoma, especially if there are no similar calcifications in the opposite breast.

Malignant intraductal calcifications in the retroareolar area, which may extend into the ducts of the nipple itself, may indicate Paget's carcinoma, an intraductal carcinoma which when it invades the epidermis of the nipple evokes the presence of Paget's cells: large cells with pale cytoplasm and irregular nuclei. These cells invade the epidermis. The patient's earliest symptom may be a burning or itching sensation in the nipple, followed by reddening, excoriation and finally erosion. These symptoms may lead some clinicians to the mistaken diagnosis of a benign dermatitis.

Differential diagnosis

When symmetrically distributed in both breasts, punctate microcalcifications indicate *benign adenosis* (See Fig. 82.5) and need not be biopsied.

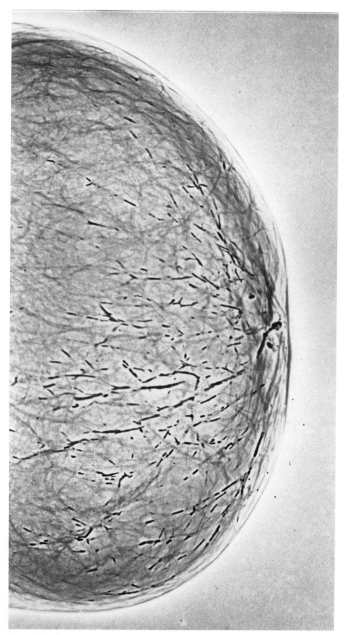

Fig. 82.20 Benign secretory calcifications. Typically, these are smoothly marginated, widely distributed, and bilateral.

Although linear in shape, *benign secretory calcifications* (Fig. 82.20) are clearly distinguishable from the linear type of malignant microcalcifications. Secretory calcifications also have a ductal distribution, but one which fans out along a series of smooth and orderly arcs, usually from the nipple to the upper outer quadrant. They are much wider and have an uneven width. Some are hollow cylinders; others have a solid core-like appearance. Many appear as round and solid or hollow circles when seen *en face*. They are frequently bilateral. Some result from calcified secretory debris within the lumen of the ducts. Others represent calcification of the duct wall itself. The retroareolar area on mammography may appear unremarkable or show dilated ducts. Most of these patients have a history of benign secretory disease: spontaneous nipple discharge — serous, blood-stained, or thick and pus-like.

Plasma cell mastitis (comedomastitis) is a complication of secretory disease. It results when the dilated, plugged ducts burst, releasing fatty secretory material into the breast causing a low grade inflammatory reaction accompanied histologically by plasma cells, leucocytes, giant cells and eosinophils. Fat necrosis may ensue with production of calcifications and parenchymal scarring (Fig. 82.21). The disease is frequently bilateral. Chronic episodes may produce retroareolar fibrosis which appears on the mammogram as a triangular area of increased density. Nipple retraction may be seen even without retroareolar fibrosis. In fact, most nipple retraction in older women is due to previous plasma cell mastitis.

The calcifications seen in *fat necrosis* may take many forms. Hollow spherical or oval calcifications are always benign and usually due to fat necrosis (Fig. 82.21). Coarse calcifications with no associated mass are always benign and are due to either a degenerated fibroadenoma or fat necrosis. Coarse calcifications within a mass usually indicate a partially degenerated fibroadenoma, much less often fat necrosis, and infrequently carcinoma. Microcalcifications occur in either malignant or benign breast disease such as fat necrosis. If the fat necrosis is due to a previous biopsy, the calcifications may be found beneath or along the incision site. Fat necrosis may also follow blunt trauma and is more common in large, fatty breasts.

Vascular calcifications run along the margins of arteriosclerotic vessels. They are seen as a series of dashes or as a solid line. Their appearance is usually typical, but a short segment of one or more calcifications in a single line can be mistaken for intraductal carcinoma. The chance of diagnostic error can be minimized if one looks for the presence of a vessel wall, making sure that it is not a duct, or for a parallel calcific line along the opposite wall of the vessel.

Idiopathic skin calcifications are punctate and/or ring-like calcifications of 1 to 2 mm size. When superimposed over breast tissue, they may be mistaken for benign adenosis when widely distributed, or for a possible malignancy when clustered. The correct diagnosis can be made by observing that some are ring-like or that others are imaged on profile

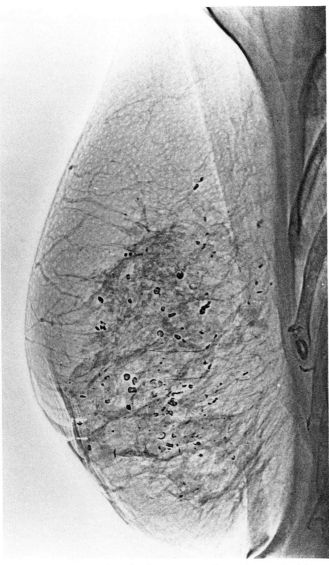

Fig. 82.21 In this patient, benign secretory disease has resulted in plasma cell mastitis causing fat necrosis with hollow spherical calcifications and nipple retraction. Similar calcifications may be associated with other causes of fat necrosis such as blunt trauma or surgery.

In cases where the calcifications are not definitely benign or malignant it is best to 'err on the side of conservatism' and advise biopsy, but the radiologist should also provide the surgeon with an estimate of the chance of malignancy so that a joint decision regarding biopsy can be made. This approach allows the radiologist to suggest a course of action, but avoids the possibility that he is either seen as causing excessive biopsies or missing a cancer found at a later time. Since breast biopsy is a relatively minor surgical procedure, this author does not like to follow the calcifications with serial mammography to observe any change. A stable appearance does not prove the existence of benign disease, since the malignancy may be in a phase of limited or no growth, or the calcifications may represent an indirect marker which does not reflect tumour growth.

MAMMOGRAPHY

Accuracy

Compared to other radiographic examinations, the accuracy of mammography is more highly dependent on technical quality and interpretive expertise. Many mistakes can be avoided through the practice of proper mammographic technique and the exercise of a reasonable degree of diagnostic skill [30]. The following factors can significantly influence mammographic accuracy, but can be largely controlled by the radiologist:

Technical quality deserves meticulous attention from the radiologist and the radiographic technologist. Equipment and technique for xeromammography and screen-film mammography will be discussed in subsequent sections of this chapter.

Clinical information is important for optimal mammographic interpretation and can be obtained from a questionnaire completed by the patient and/or technologist (Fig. 82.22). If the radiologist is not aware of the location of the suspicious lump or thickening on physical examination, he may overlook or fail to appreciate the significance of the corresponding mammographic abnormality. If the physical signs from a carcinoma are not by themselves sufficiently suspicious to merit biopsy, the mammographic report may then deter rather than encourage a necessary biopsy. If the area of clinical abnormality is not projected onto the mammographic field of the routine study, supplementary views e.g. rotated craniocaudal views, should be obtained.

The radiologist should also be aware of the patient's previous breast surgery and the location of any scars, because skin thickening, retraction and parenchymal distortion which result from biopsy may mimic carcinoma. In addition, removal of tissue during biopsy may suggest an asymmetrical increase in soft tissue density or calcifications in the opposite breast, which may then be mistaken for carcinoma.

in the skin. If necessary, tangential views can be taken to demonstrate that some are in the skin.

The term '*pseudocalcifications*' refers to metallic skin creams or powders, which when viewed *en face* simulate calcifications within the breast. These substances include zinc oxide cream, talcum powder, and aluminum containing deodorants. Often, the correct diagnosis can be made when these calcium-like densities are seen on the skin surface, particularly the medial or inframammary regions or along the creases of the axilla. At other times, it may be necessary to ask the patient if she has recently applied these materials to her skin and to repeat the mammogram after she has removed them.

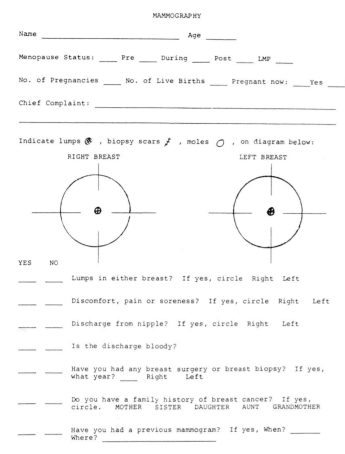

Fig. 82.22 Questionnaire for mammography patients.

A completed questionnaire should also include the location of any skin naevus, since it can simulate a mass within the breast.

History of nipple discharge can be a particularly helpful item of clinical information because intraductal papilloma and intraductal papillary carcinoma usually produce only subtle findings such as a slightly dilated retroareolar duct on routine mammography and may be apparent only on contrast ductography.

Comparison with previous mammography should always be made, since new findings, especially in post-menopausal women, may indicate carcinoma. On the other hand, absence of change from a previous study increases the possibility that a lesion is benign, though some slowly growing malignancies may show little or no change for as long as 1 to 2 years.

The tailored mammogram refers to any special projections taken to evaluate the patient's clinical signs and symptoms or a suspicious finding from the initial two view study. These projections will be discussed in the sections on xeromammography and screen-film mammography technique. The mammographer should review the patient's history and physical findings and then should check each study for both technical quality and the need for additional views before the patient leaves the radiology department.

Interpretive expertise requires experience and judgement. The mammographer must decide if the breast is normal or *definitely benign* — no further diagnostic work-up, only routine screening recommended; *indeterminate* — benign versus malignant, further diagnostic work-up — possible biopsy; or *probably malignant* — biopsy advised. Because the appearance of benign and malignant disease may overlap, mammography reports should often include diagnostic qualifications, i.e. 'probably benign but advise aspiration or biopsy for confirmation'.

Since mammographic signs of breast cancer are often subtle, requiring considerable observational skill, the radiologist should approach each study with caution and review it in a calm and deliberate manner. Hasty interpretation should never be undertaken. If the experienced mammographer has any doubts whether a lesion should be biopsied or not, it is best to decide in favour of biopsy because it is a simple and innocuous surgical procedure, which in many cases can be performed under local anaesthesia on an outpatient basis. Waiting until a lesion is more obviously cancer on follow-up mammography or physical examination carries the risk that the cancer may reach a less curable stage.

Mammography versus physical examination

The overall accuracy of mammography is considerably higher than that of physical examination. When women are screened by both modalities, 90 to 95% of cancers are seen on mammography, while only 50 to 60% are palpable on physical examination [31]. However, the relative accuracy of each study will depend on the following factors [32]:

Breast density exerts a significant influence. Mammography can detect 95 to 100% of cancers in fatty breasts, 90% of cancers in breasts of intermediate glandularity, and 80% of cancers in extremely glandular breasts. In these dense breasts, sensitivity rates of physical examination and mammography are similar, since the accuracy of one modality is defined in relation to the other.

Lesion depth below the skin surface also influences relative detection rates; deep lesions are more often nonpalpable.

Breast size is also significant. Clinical accuracy decreases with increasing breast size due to increased frequency of deep lesions in large breasts. Although mammography is more reliable than physical examination for large and intermediate breasts, it may in general be no more accurate than physical examination for small breasts. This may be related to tumour depth as well as the greater glandularity of small breasts.

Patient selection will also affect detection sensitivity of mammography, which will be lower among women referred for mammography because of a palpable mass than among women with no palpable masses who are referred for screening. This concept can be appreciated by means of the following. Assume that 100 cancers are detected on screening by mammography and physical examination, and of these 50 are found by physical examination and 90 are found by mammography. However, among the 50 cancers found by physical examination, 10 were missed by mammography. If only this skewed population of palpable cancers is considered, accuracy of physical examination is 100% (50/50) and that of mammography is 80% (40/50).

A negative mammogram should never deter the clinician from biopsy if the clinical findings are suspicious. When a mass or thickening is palpated and no corresponding mammographic abnormality is seen, the radiologist's report should state, 'it would be best to proceed on clinical grounds alone, since a small per cent of breast neoplasms may not be visible on mammography'.

Actually, the cancer yield for biopsies based on mammography is higher than that of physical examination. Among lesions biopsied on the basis of mammography, one of two to six cases is malignant, while among biopsies recommended by physical examination, one of five to nine patients is malignant. Although addition of mammography to physical examination will increase the total number of breast biopsies performed, the number of cancers detected will be increased by a higher percentage [31,33,34].

Indications for mammography

Mammography may be used as a *diagnostic* procedure to evaluate *signs and/or symptoms* of benign and malignant breast disease, such as pain, discharge, mass, skin and nipple abnormalities, or as a *screening* procedure to detect clinically unsuspected breast cancer.

Many clinicians do not appreciate the value of mammography in the preoperative work up of a mass which will be biopsied because it is clinically suspicious for carcinoma. While normal or benign mammographic findings should never deter the biopsy of a mass which is clinically convincing as carcinoma, there are other reasons for mammography in such cases. If the palpated mass is malignant, mammography may find a nonpalpable carcinoma in the same breast. Multicentric carcinoma should not be treated by local excision and radiation therapy; the mammographic demonstration of multicentricity will eliminate this treatment option. Mammography could also detect a nonpalpable carcinoma in the opposite breast. If the palpable mass is benign on biopsy, mammography would still be valuable to examine the breasts for possible nonpalpable carcinoma.

Mammography should also be part of the diagnostic *work up for metastatic carcinoma of unknown origin*.

Guidelines for *breast cancer screening* by mammography will be discussed in a subsequent section.

Biopsy method for nonpalpable lesions

The radiologist, by means of needle placement [35,36] can precisely localize a lesion at time of biopsy so that the surgeon need remove only the lesion and a small amount of surrounding tissue. Specimen radiography can then document the mammographic abnormality contained in the specimen. If needle placement were not performed, it might be necessary to remove an entire quadrant of the breast to insure that the lesion was contained in the biopsy specimen. Excessive postoperative deformity could result in patients with benign disease. Conversely, if the lesion were malignant, the pathologist would have to study an excessively large number of tissue sections in a quadrant biopsy, so that an accurate pathological diagnosis would be more difficult to achieve.

Lesion localization

The first step in localizing a nonpalpable lesion is to consider the breast as a grid with the nipple as origin. The *x* (horizontal) coordinate describes the medial or lateral distance of the lesion from the edge of the nipple. Its distance above or below the nipple determines the *y* (vertical) coordinate. These two coordinates are measured from the craniocaudal and lateral mammograms, respectively (Fig. 82.23), and together are transcribed as a single point on the patient's skin through which the needle is inserted (Fig. 82.24). To secure its placement, the needle is inserted to its full extent, even if its tip is beyond the lesion.

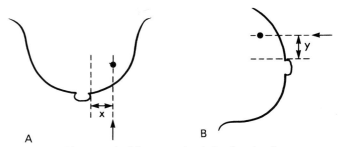

Fig. 82.23 Linear method for measuring lesion location from (A) craniocaudal and (B) lateral mammogram. Arrows indicate direction of needle insertion. (Reproduced with permission from Feig S A 1983 Radiol Clin North Am 21:155–172)

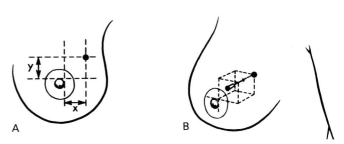

Fig. 82.24A & B Method of plotting point of needle insertion into the breast. View of patient's breast from (A) frontal and (B) oblique positions. Direction of needle insertion is shown in (B). (Reproduced with permission from Feig S A 1983 Radiol Clin North Am 21:155–172) [35]

Distances can be measured as either a straight line perpendicular to the nipple edge (linear method), or as a curved line along the skin surface (arc method Fig. 82.25). For most lesions, especially those where the overlying skin point is far from the nipple, the arc method is more accurate and allows the use of shorter needles.

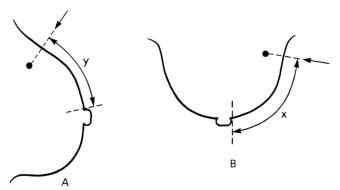

Fig. 82.25 Arc method for measuring lesion location from (A) lateral and (B) craniocaudal mammogram. Arrows indicate direction of needle insertion. (Reproduced with permission from Feig S A 1983 Radiol Clin North Am 21:155–172) [35]

For many cases, the linear and arc methods are used in combination: one method may be preferable for measuring on the horizontal axis. Another method may be better for measuring on the vertical axis.

The mammographic image will always be larger than the actual breast due to compression and the small degree of magnification inherent on 'nonmagnified' radiography of any three-dimensional object. Thus, if coordinates are directly transferred from the mammogram with no allowance for compression or magnification, the skin point will be peripheral to the true lesion location on both axes.

To facilitate the procedure, the patient is removed from the mammographic apparatus before measurements are plotted on the skin. Therefore, coordinates must be reduced. The exact fractional reduction depends on the mammographic unit, breast positioning and degree of compression. In the author's practice, both craniocaudal and lateral measurements are reduced by 25%.

A sheet of paper is placed against the mammogram perpendicular to the nipple edge for the linear method, or bent along the skin outline for the arc method. The vertical and horizontal distances are marked, measured with a ruler, and reduced. The paper is placed against the patient's breast and the measurements transferred.

If only "another hospital" mammographic study is available, it must be repeated on the mammographic unit where the needle localization is being performed, so that proper measurements can be made. This will document the appearance of the lesion on the imaging system. Subtle abnormalities may appear different or fail to appear on one imaging system or another.

Needle insertion

The point of insertion is marked on the patient's skin and the area is cleansed with alcohol. The localization marker needle should be the shortest that can reach the lesion from the skin. In most cases, a 0.5 inch or a 1.5 inch hypodermic needle will suffice. For these lengths, a 25-gauge needle is

preferable, as its small diameter is least traumatic to the patient. In some cases, lower gauge (wider diameter) needles are used, since they meet less resistance in denser tissues, and will not be extruded. At times, a 2.5 inch needle may be necessary for deep lesions. For this length needle, a 20-gauge calibre is best, since it will not bend when inserted deep in the breast. Insertion of the needle in the breast is relatively painless, therefore, local anaesthesia is seldom required. The needle is inserted to its full extent, even if its tip is beyond the lesion, so that its placement is secure. The needle is taped in place. Paper surgical tape is used as it can be removed without dislodging the needle, without trauma to the patient, and without leaving a residue on the skin. These qualities are important if the needle has to be repositioned in the radiology department and when the tape is removed in the operating room. The tape is transparent to X–rays.

Craniocaudal and lateral mammograms are repeated to determine the position of the needle with respect to the lesion. If it is more than 2 cm from the lesion on either mammographic view, a second needle is inserted while the first one is left in place as a positioning guide. The first needle is removed and the mammogram is repeated.

The procedure can usually be completed in 15 minutes. Preoperative medications are withheld until the procedure is completed so that the patient can cooperate. The patient is then taken to the operating room along with a set of mammograms that show the needle in place and the lesion circled (Fig. 82.26A & B).

If the lesion described by mammography contains calcifications, specimen radiography must be performed to ensure that they are contained in the biopsy specimen (Fig. 82.26C). This radiograph is taken at the time of surgery, preferably on a self-contained table top X–ray unit in the surgical pathology laboratory. While the patient is still on the operating room table, the surgeon is informed of the specimen X–ray results. If the calcifications are not all visible on the specimen radiograph, he is advised to excise additional tissue that is also radiographed.

Noncalcified lesions may be difficult to confirm on specimen radiography. The uneven tissue thickness and irregular shape of the specimen can obscure and/or mimic a soft tissue lesion. This problem is alleviated by the fact that most breast masses can be appreciated on gross surgical examination.

Alternative techniques

With the method described, the needle can be placed within 1 cm of the lesion on first insertion in 95% of cases. For this reason, the author has not used more elaborate localization equipment such as the *multiperforated plexiglass compression plate* [37,38]. This plate is placed over the breast for the mammogram and a needle is then inserted through the appropriate hole. It is advanced to a point at or beyond the expected lesion depth. With the needle in place, the plate is removed and rotated 90 degrees for another mammographic view. The needle may then be partially withdrawn to the proper depth.

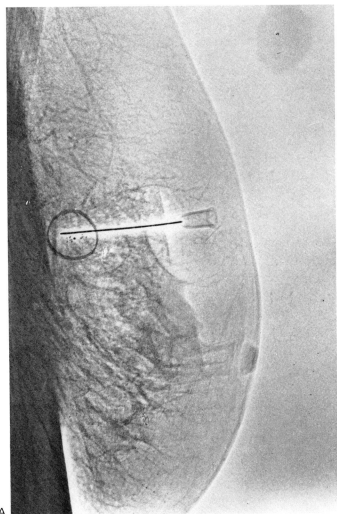

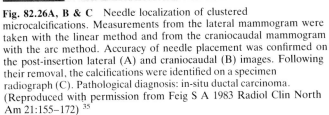

A

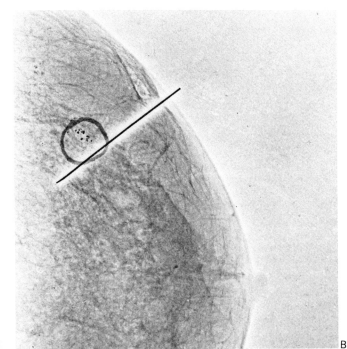

B

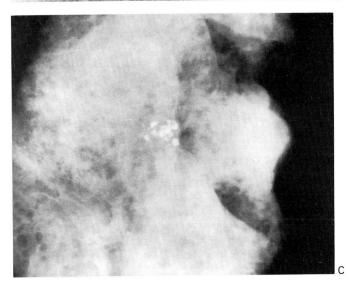

C

Fig. 82.26A, B & C Needle localization of clustered microcalcifications. Measurements from the lateral mammogram were taken with the linear method and from the craniocaudal mammogram with the arc method. Accuracy of needle placement was confirmed on the post-insertion lateral (A) and craniocaudal (B) images. Following their removal, the calcifications were identified on a specimen radiograph (C). Pathological diagnosis: in-situ ductal carcinoma. (Reproduced with permission from Feig S A 1983 Radiol Clin North Am 21:155–172) [35]

When the needle is securely taped in place, it does not dislodge. This has been a problem when other methods of securing the needle are used, and some investigators have advocated the use of a 25-gauge spring-hook wire because of its self-retaining feature [35–39]. This wire is contained within the lumen of a needle which is later withdrawn leaving the hook in place. However, the hook wire is traumatic to the patient. If a 25-gauge needle is used, the hookwire cannot be completely contained within the lumen. Since the hook protrudes beyond the needle tip, a small stab incision is necessary to introduce the needle and the protruding wire hook. An improperly placed guide wire cannot be easily removed or repositioned. Extraction can result in tissue damage. Containing the wire hook entirely within the needle

obviates these problems but requires the use of thicker (16–20 gauge) needles.

Technical requirements for mammography

The requirements for X-ray imaging of the breast are considerably different from those of other parts of the body. The glandular, fibrotic, and fatty tissues of the breast possess a relatively narrow range of radiographic density, yet the often subtle differences in soft tissue density both within and between these tissue components must be recorded as observable differences in radiographic contrast.

Also, the wide range of X–ray intensities transmitted by the thickest posterior and thinnest anterior portions of the breast must be portrayed on the same image without over– or underexposure.

Demonstration of small structures such as microcalcifications and trabeculae, often as small as 0.1 mm, requires a high degree of resolution to produce the sharpest possible image.

The posterior breast and axillary tail should be projected free of the overlapping structures of muscles and rib cage on which they rest.

Because the breast will move when the patient breathes, exposure time should be kept short to reduce motion unsharpness. Since mammography will often be performed as a screening procedure, it is important that dosage be maintained within acceptable limits.

In response to these problems, three methods of X–ray mammography have .been used [40–43].

Direct film mammography

This technique [44] employed a fine-grain double-emulsion industrial film to record optimal detail. It was performed without the screen-cassette combination used for most other radiographic procedures, which was felt to produce unacceptable geometric unsharpness and prevent close positioning near the chest wall. Instead, a lead-backed cardboard film holder was used. Direct film mammography was the only method available prior to 1971. Since it resulted in a relatively high X–ray dose (Table 82.1), it has now been supplanted by xeromammography and screen-film mammography.

Screen film mammography

Image receptors and image processing

In 1972, the Dupont company introduced the first low-dose screen-film system (Lo-dose I) for mammography, soon followed by Dupont Lo-dose II and Kodak Min-R (1975) [45,46]. These systems consisted of a single emulsion film held in intimate contact to a single intensifying screen. The screen converts X–ray energy into light energy, which then exposes the film so that considerable reduction in dosage is possible. Not only does the screen absorb more X–ray photons than would be absorbed by the film alone, but the effect of absorption is multiplied since each X–ray quantum produces hundreds of light photons.

The absorption of X–rays and their conversion into light occurs in the phosphor layer of the screen, which consists of phosphor crystals embedded in a plastic binder. Calcium tungstate is used in the Dupont screens and gadolinium oxysulphide (a rare earth) in the Kodak screens. Single emulsion rather than double emulsion film is used. Blurring occurs with films containing emulsion on both sides due to angled spreading of light from the screen phosphors.

Good screen-film contact is necessary to minimize blurring and is achieved when the screen-film combination is exposed in a plastic vacuum bag or specially designed mammographic cassette. The emulsion side of the film is placed against the screen. A polyethylene bag is preferable to a polyvinyl chloride bag, which absorbs and hardens the X–ray beam slightly more than the cassette cover does [47]. Once the screen and film are placed in the plastic bag, air is removed and an airtight seal is created by means of an electric pump. The screen-film combination is placed so that after exiting the breast, the X–ray beam first passes through the film, and then hits the screen.

The low dose mammography films are best developed in an automatic 90 or 120 second medical X–ray processor. Quality control of such factors as processing temperature and chemical replenishment is especially important because of the need for optimal image quality.

Comparison of screen-film systems

Since the introduction of the Dupont Lo-dose I system, other screen-film systems have produced images of comparable quality with further reduction in dose [48]. These include the Dupont Lo-dose II system (Lo-dose films and Lo-dose II screens), the Kodak Min-R system (Min-R film and Min-R screens) and Kodak Min-R screen-NMB system (Kodak nuclear medicine B-film and Min-R screens).

The mean breast dose from a two view study with any of these latter three systems is 0.1 to 0.3 rad, less than half the dose received from the Lo-dose I system (0.6 rad) (Table 82.1).

Table 82.1 Radiation dose of mammographic image receptors. (Reproduced with permission from Feig S A 1982 In: Bassett L W, Gold R H (eds) Mammography, thermography and ultrasound in breast cancer detection. Grune and Stratton, New York

Year introduced	Image receptor	Skin dose rads per exposure	Mean breast dose rads per 2-view exam	mid breast dose
Before 1971	Nonscreen industrial film	6.0–8.0	3.2	1.7
1971	Xeromammography	3.0–4.0	1.6	1.1
1972	DuPont Lo-Dose I screen-film system	1.0–1.3	0.6	0.3
1976	Reduced-dose xeromammography Positive mode	0.7–1.1	0.5–0.8	0.7
	Negative mode	0.5–0.8	0.3–0.5	0.5–0.6
1976	DuPont Lo-Dose II and Kodak Min-R screen-film systems	0.4–0.7	0.1–0.3	0.1

Each of these four systems is similar in terms of resolution. The three lowest dose systems, especially Min-R-NMB, exhibit slightly more noise than Lo-dose I. There is no significant difference in contrast between Lo-dose I and II, but Min-R has more contrast and Min-R-NMB even slightly more. Thus, the three lower dose systems would seem preferable to Lo-dose I since they accord marked reduction in dose with little or no loss of image quality. The choice among these three systems is largely a matter of personal preference.

Besides reduction in dose, another advantage of screen-film over industrial film is improvement in image quality. Although screen-film systems have lower resolution and greater noise than industrial film, these factors are more than offset by other imaging advantages. *Noise* refers to a visible image mottle resulting from random distribution of X–ray photons at low doses, especially at high contrast levels and with coarse grain film. The lower resolution of the screens and coarse grain film needed to reduce doses is countered by other resolution factors, such as decreased patient motion from shorter exposure, and decreased geometrical blurring since low-dose systems allow the use of X–ray units with smaller focal spots and longer focal spot-skin distances.

Since tube loading is reduced by the shorter exposure, lower kV settings can be used resulting in much higher film contrast. If such low kV settings were used with industrial film, tube overloading would occur when mAS was increased to maintain adequate exposure. The low dose screen-film systems also possess greater inherent contrast than industrial films. Despite the marked reduction in dose, screen-film methods may provide more diagnostic information than direct exposure mammograms [43].

Exposure factors

Molybdenum target X-ray units are preferred for screen-film mammography since their low energy photons can provide high subject contrast (Fig. 82.27). A 0.03 mm molybdenum filter will further soften the beam by suppressing photons with energies above 20 keV. Thus, screen-film mammography requires considerably less filtration than reduced dose xeromammography (Table 82.2). Tungsten target tubes and aluminum filtration result in a higher energy beam with decreased contrast and impaired detection of microcalcifications and other subtle signs of carcinoma [42].

Table 82.2 Equipment factors for xeromammography and screen-film mammography.

	Xeromammography	Screen-film
Peak kilovoltage	45–55	25–28
Filtration	2–3 mm Al	0.03 mm Mo
Target material	Tungsten	Molybdenum

Al = aluminium; Mo = molybdenum

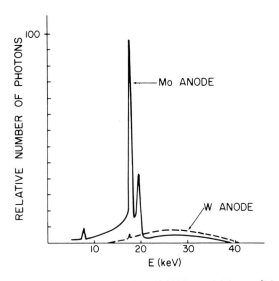

Fig. 82.27 X–ray spectra emitted at 40 kV by molybdenum [Mo] and tungsten [W] anodes. The molybdenum target produces a lower kV spectrum necessary for adequate contrast in screen/film mammography. The higher kV spectrum produced by a tungsten target is preferred for xeromammography since it allows a lower dose. In xeromammography, edge-enhancement compensates for the contrast lost at high kilovoltage. (Reproduced with permission from Haus A G, Doi K, Metz E G et al 1977 Radiology 125:83)

To achieve the highest contrast, most screen-film mammography should be performed in the 25 to 26 kV range. Extremely glandular breasts may require a harder beam of 27 to 28 kV. The mAS for an initial view of one breast can be estimated from the compressed thickness of the breast. This image is developed and checked for technique; the mAS for the remaining views can be modified accordingly. Automatic exposure control (phototiming) is not always helpful because of the relatively small area of the phototimer and the wide variation in positioning of the glandular tissue.

Positioning and compression

The standard screen-film mammographic examination consists of a craniocaudal view and an oblique view [47,49,50]. The oblique view includes more tissue in the posterior breast and the axillary tail than a contact lateral view. The oblique view is taken with the X–ray beam directed from supero-medial to inferolateral at an angle of approximately 45° (Fig. 82.28). Both breasts should be compressed at identical angles so that their images can be compared. Since the pectoralis muscle will be parallel to the plane of compression, the breast can be pulled away from the chest and onto the film. Conversely, compression for the contact lateral view 'fights' the direction of the pectoralis muscle so that the breast is less well compressed and incompletely displaced from the rib cage. With the patient standing, her arm is raised 90°, but kept as close to the breast as possible, since retracting or elevating the arm tightens the muscle. The

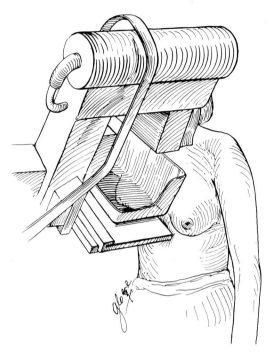

Fig. 82.28 Positioning for the oblique view. (Reproduced with permission from Bassett L W, Gold R H 1983 Radiology 149:585–587) [49]

axillary tail should be positioned onto the film by slightly rotating the breast (Fig. 82.29).

Visualization of the posterior breast on xeromammography does not require an oblique view; the standard chest wall lateral view is used instead. This view cannot produce technically satisfactory screen-film images because of the narrower latitude and lower kV employed in screen-film studies.

Because the recording latitude of screen-film mammography is less than that of xeromammography, the breast must be compressed to a more homogeneous thickness so that no portion will be overexposed or underexposed. Since screen-film mammography is performed at a lower kV, the degree of compression must also be greater to achieve adequate penetration. Vigorous compression should be applied parallel to the film surface to reduce the average breast to about 4 cm thickness. A rigid, flat compression device bent at a 90° angle posteriorly is needed. With a posteriorly sloped compression device, the base of the breast will be inadequately compressed and underexposed [47].

Dedicated mammography units

Low energy beam and compression

Prior to the introduction of a dedicated molybdenum target mammography unit with a breast compression device in 1969 [53], no X-ray unit specifically designed for mammography was commercially available in the US; only general radiographic tungsten tube machines were used, usually without the benefit of compression. Today, a dedicated mammography unit is necessary to provide the low energy X-ray beam and vigorous compression needed for proper screen-film technique. Dedicated units make it easier to perform a fast, efficient and high quality examination. Many such units are now available from numerous manufacturers.

This unit is not essential for xeromammography, as a higher energy beam and only moderate compression are employed. The study can be performed using an overhead tungsten tube with 2 to 3 mm added Al filtration and a Xerox compression device, placed on the X-ray table.

Benefits from compression include:

1. Reduced geometrical unsharpness — breast structures are closer to the image receptor.
2. Contrast improvement — scatter is reduced by decreased breast thickness.
3. Diminished motion unsharpness — the breast is immobilized so motion does not occur.
4. Reduction of X-ray dose — less entrance dose is needed; the mean glandular dose is reduced.
5. More uniform image density — underpenetration of thicker portions of the breast and overpenetration of thinner portions will be less likely.
6. Accentuation of normal versus abnormal tissue densities — normal breast tissue and cysts are easily compressible while carcinomas are more rigid.
7. Dispersion of tissue elements — tissue structures are spread apart so there is less superimposition.
8. Use of lower kV — results in increased contrast.

Focal spot size and focal spot-breast surface distance

Geometrical unsharpness is reduced via a small focal spot, a long focal spot-breast surface distance, and diminished object-image receptor distance. Most specialized mammography units use focal spots of 0.6 mm or less nominal size, smaller than those of most general purpose units. Focal spots of this size should be used in units with focal spot-breast surface distances of at least 50 cm. Smaller focal spots can tolerate shorter distances [42].

Grids

Visualization of glandular breasts and/or poorly compressible breasts may be impaired due to reduced contrast from scattered radiation. The amount of scattered radiation is proportional to breast thickness, and is more apparent in glandular breasts where contrast is lower. Mammographic grids [51,52] can increase image contrast by reducing the amount of scattered radiation reaching the image receptor. The grids used in other X-ray studies are not adaptable to mammography because of their excessive absorption of low kV radiation. Mammography grids must be constructed of materials such as carbon or extremely fine strips of aluminium, which have low X-ray absorption.

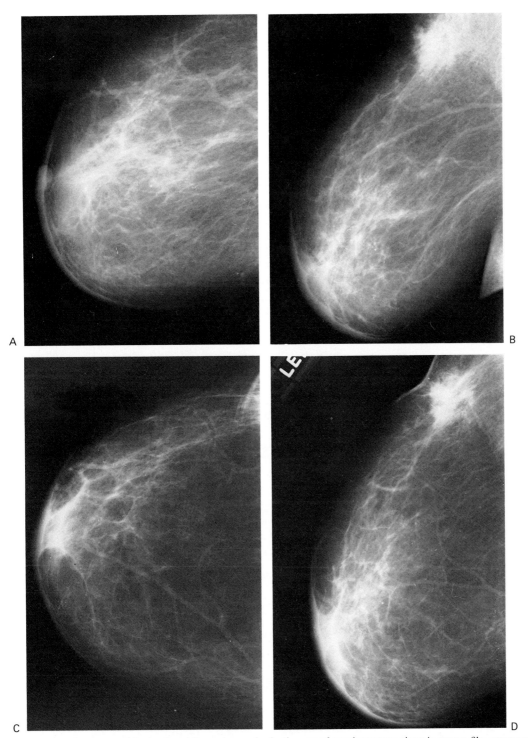

Fig. 82.29A–D Importance of proper positioning for oblique view and selective use of supplementary views in screen-film mammography. Poorly positioned oblique view (A) does not include posterior breast tissues since the breast was not pulled forward and the axillary tail was not rotated onto the film. Properly positioned oblique view (B) reveals a carcinoma in the axillary tail not visible on image (A). The standard craniocaudal view (C), though well positioned, demonstrates only the tip of the carcinoma. A laterally rotated craniocaudal view (D), was therefore obtained as a supplementary projection and demonstrates the carcinoma along with overlying skin thickening and retraction.

Most new mammography units contain moving grids, but older units can be adapted with either moving or stationary grids.

Grids are used primarily for screen-film mammography. They are needed less in xeromammography because of the edge enhancement effect and the higher kV employed. Microcalcifications and soft tissue abnormalities in glandular breasts are better seen on xeromammography than screen-film mammography. However, a grid can improve screen-film studies so that visualization of such findings is comparable to xeromammography.

For a given technique and screen-film system, grid studies require more than double the exposure to compensate for radiation absorbed by the grid. However, an increase of 4 to 5 kV and higher speed films e.g. Kodak Ortho M and Dupont MRF-31, may partly offset the increased exposure while retaining the improvement in image quality. Because of the improved image contrast resulting from the grid, the diminished latitude and increased mottle of these more sensitive films can be tolerated.

Disadvantages of a grid include a decrease in geometrical sharpness, since the breast is further from the film, and nonvisualization of the posterior 5 mm of breast due to grid frame and increased dose. Accordingly, grids should not be used routinely, but reserved for glandular breasts and poorly compressible breasts.

Other features

Specialised mammography units can *angle* the X-ray beam, allowing projections such as the oblique view and others which may be diagnostically helpful. By increasing the distance between the breast and the image receptor, *magnification views* [54] can be taken. These are useful in evaluating suspicious findings seen on the routine, nonmagnified images. *Coned down views* of suspicious areas increase contrast by reducing scatter. The use of *phototiming* has been discussed earlier in this chapter.

Xeromammography

Image receptors

Xeromammography [55] became commercially available for breast imaging in 1971. In xeroradiography, a selenium-coated aluminum plate is the counterpart of the X-ray film. Since selenium is a photoconductor, once an electrical charge is placed on the plate, the magnitude and distribution of the charge will remain unchanged unless the plate is discharged by light, heat, electricity or X-rays.

The xeroradiographic process begins before X-ray exposure, when the plate is charged in the Xerox conditioning unit. The plate now contains positive charges within the selenium layer and an equal number of negative charges (electrons) attracted to the selenium surface adjacent to the aluminum plate. A light-tight, electrically insulated cassette is then inserted into the conditioner to receive the charged plate. The cassette is then removed and positioned under the breast. X-rays passing through the breast selectively discharge the plate in inverse proportion to the radiographic density of the overlying tissue e.g. the discharge is greatest below fatty tissue and least below calcifications. A high-resolution latent image in the form of nonuniformly distributed electron charges is thus formed on the selenium-coated plate. (Fig. 82.30)

Image processing

After exposure, the cassette is inserted into the processing unit where charged blue toner particles are sprayed onto the selenium plate and then encapsulated into plastic-coated paper to form a permanent image.

Positive and negative mode

Xeroradiographic images may be developed in either a positive or a negative mode. The photoelectric charges placed on the selenium plate are identical in both. The differences in image appearance are due to the development process. In the positive mode, a positive-bias voltage is applied to the back of the plate, and the negatively charged blue toner particles are attracted toward the least-discharged regions which correspond to high radiographic densities, such as calcifications.

In the negative mode, a negative-bias voltage is applied, and the positively charged blue toner particles are attracted toward the most heavily discharged regions. These areas correspond to low radiographic densities, such as fatty tissue.

Due to its greater developing power, the negative mode requires 20 to 25% less X-ray exposure than the positive mode. Nevertheless, the positive mode is preferred by most xeromammographers. However, breasts containing silicone implants are better imaged in the negative mode to avoid 'toner-robbing' in the tissues adjacent to these dense objects.

Exposure factors

Entrance exposures for xeromammography have been reduced by increasing the aluminum filtration of the X-ray beam, thereby causing a preferential reduction in lower-energy radiation [56]. The 'softer' radition previously used contributed more to absorbed dose than to image detail. To compensate, the peak kV is raised from 35–45 to 45–55 kV. (If mAS rather than kV were increased, lengthened exposure times would create motion unsharpness.) Unlike screen-film mammography, xeromammography can be performed at a higher kV because the edge-enhancement effect offsets decreased image contrast. The decreased image contrast is partially restored by lowering the back-bias voltage of the processor. In large or dense breasts, the 'hardened' beam results in improved penetration. Aluminum filters thicker than 2.5 mm should not be used, as they produce a low-contrast image of suboptimal quality with little additional dose reduction.

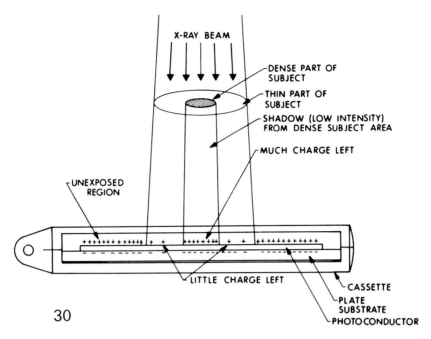

Fig. 82.30 Partially discharged xeroradiographic plate, enclosed within cassette, following X–ray exposure. Amount of regional discharge is inversely proportional to density of overlying tissue. (Reproduced with permission from Principles of the Xeroradiographic Process 1975 Xerox Corporation, California

Because dose reduction results from 'hardening' the X–ray beam, the reduction in absorbed dose is proportionately less than the reduction in skin dose. Doses from mammographic imaging systems are shown in Table 82.1. The mean breast dose is the best indicator of hypothetical carcinogenic risk. The mean breast dose from a two-view positive-mode xeromammographic examination is 0.5 to 0.8 rad, approximately twice that of screen-film mammography, 0.2 to 0.4 rad. The dose from a two-view negative mode examination is 0.3 to

0.5 rad, 1.5 times that of a screen-film study. The mean breast dose from either imaging system is well below 1.0 rad and is considered negligible in terms of carcinogenic risk.

Dedicated mammography units are not necessary for xeromammography if adequate compression and filtration are available on conventional radiographic equipment. The equipment requirements for xeromammography and screen-film mammography are listed in Table 82.2. To maintain dosage at acceptable limits, higher kV and greater beam

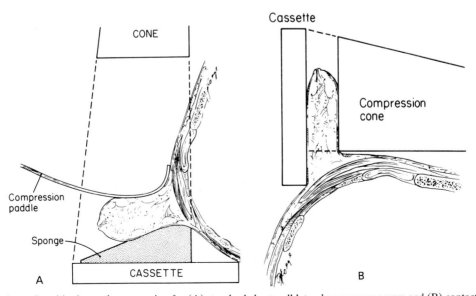

Fig. 82.31 Comparison of positioning and compression for (A) standard chest wall lateral xeromammogram and (B) contact lateral xeromammogram and lateral screen-film mammogram. Chest wall lateral xeromammogram includes more posterior breast tissue but employs less compression. (Reproduced with permission from Pagani J J, Bassett L W, Gold R H, et al 1980 A J R 135:141–146)

filtration are required for xeromammography. Because of edge-enhancement, the higher kV does not result in diminished image quality. Indeed, in dense breasts the 'harder' beam will yield better penetration. While a molybdenum target can produce high-quality xeromammograms, it produces higher doses than those obtained from a tungsten target.

Positioning and compression

The two standard projections for xeromammography are the craniocaudal and the chest wall mediolateral (lateral) views. Positioning for the craniocaudal view is identical to that used for screen-film mammography. Supplementary projections include rotated medial or lateral craniocaudal views to visualize the extreme medial or lateral portions of the breast and the contact mediolateral view for better resolution of lesions.

For the lateral view, the cassette must be separated from the lateral breast surface so as to partially overlie the adjacent rib cage. A radiolucent sponge is interposed between the breast and the cassette to support the breast and prevent skin folds (Fig. 82.31). A posteriorly sloped compression device is used. The contact mediolateral view is similar to that used with the screen-film technique. Here the cassette is placed in direct contact with the breast surface, without an intervening sponge. This projection provides greater resolution, but does not include the chest wall and the most posterior breast tissue (See Fig. 82.14). Because of its wider recording latitude and higher kV, less compression is required for xeromammography than for screen-film mammography.

Xeromammography versus screen-film mammography

Image characteristics

Xeromammograms possess two unique characteristics that improve visualization of breast pathology: wide recording latitude and edge-enhancement. The characteristic curves for xeromammography and screen-film mammography shown in Figure 82.32 illustrate that for equivalent exposure differences, density gradients for xeromammography are less than for screen-film. Because of this wide recording latitude, both the denser chest wall and the thinner peripheral portions of the breast are clearly visualized on a single xeromammogram.

By comparison, the narrower recording latitude (steeper characteristic curve) of screen-film combinations results in areas of overexposure or underexposure if the breast is not compressed to nearly uniform thickness. Thus the chest wall cannot be imaged in screen-film mammograms. The disadvantage of a wide recording latitude is that the overall difference in density between a mass and surrounding tissue (broad area contrast) is less in a xeromammogram than in a screen-film mammogram (Fig. 82.33).

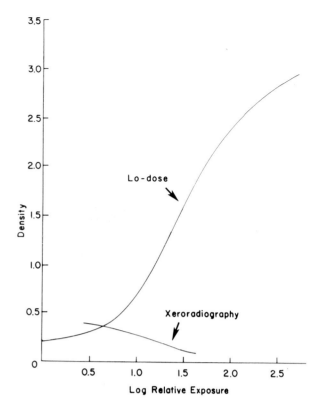

Fig. 82.32 Characteristic curves for DuPont Lo-Dose I screen-film system and xeroradiography. (Reproduced with permission from Haus A G 1983 In: Feig S A, McLelland R (eds) Breast carcinoma: current diagnosis and treatment. Masson, New York) [42]

Xeroradiographic edge-enhancement, on the other hand, accentuates the margins of breast masses, spiculations, and calcific particles (See Figs 82.7, 82.13 & 82.19) This phenomenon can be explained by lines of electrical force resulting from the interaction of charges on the Xerox plate with those applied in the development chamber. Although the charge pattern on the plate is not edge-enhanced, the toner-particle distribution during development results in edge-enhancement in the final image. As a result, an area of uniform greater density will have a higher concentration of toner particles at its border than at its centre. An area of lesser density will have a lower concentration of toner particles at its borders than at its centre (Fig. 82.34).

Image quality

Experiments on breast phantoms show that xeromammography can detect smaller abnormalities than screen-film mammography [55]. Although this advantage is tempered by the reduced dose screen-film technique, many radiologists assert that microcalcifications and spiculations are more readily discerned on xeromammograms because of edge-enhancement especially in dense breasts which are more easily penetrated at the higher kV. It is debatable whether xeromammography is better than screen-film mammography

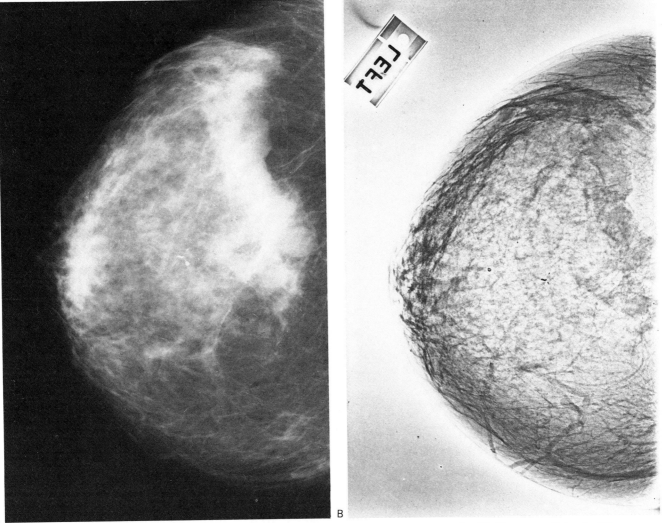

Fig. 82.33 Broad area contrast is greater in screen-film mammography (A) than in xeromammography (B). Hence overall density differences among soft tissue structures are better demonstrated with screen-film technique.

in fatty breasts, but it is generally agreed that xeromammography is preferred in glandular breasts. However, well-circumscribed masses may be less easily detected by xeromammography because of its relatively poor broad area contrast.

Imaging Projections

Visualization of the rib cage should not be attempted on screen-film mammography. Since the chest wall is curved and rigid, inclusion of the rib cage can only be accomplished by decreasing the extent of breast compression (Fig. 82.31). Therefore, the thick posterior tissues could not be sufficiently compressed for the lower kV technique used in screen-film mammography.

This projection can be used on xeromammography because:

1. The higher kV technique requires only moderate compression to obtain adequate penetration of denser structures.
2. The wider recording latitude requires the breast to be compressed to a lesser and inhomogeneous extent.
3. Increased resolution from edge-enhancement compensates for the geometrical unsharpness resulting from interposition of the sponge between the breast and the image receptor.

Nevertheless, it may not be necessary to include the rib cage in order to visualize the most posterior breast tissue. Some experts contend that the lateral oblique screen-film mammogram includes as much breast tissue as the chest wall lateral xeromammogram [47,57]. Unfortunately, there are no comparative studies to assess this issue. Positioning for the craniocaudal view is identical for both xeromammography and screen-film mammography.

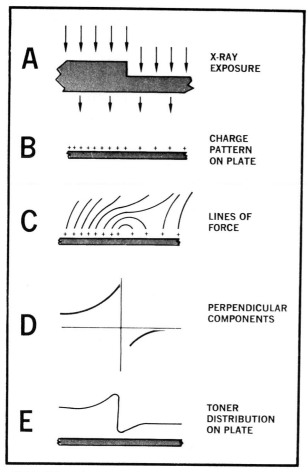

Fig. 82.34 Edge enhancement in xeroradiographic development. (Reproduced with permission, from Xerox Corporation 1974 Technical Application Bulletin 1: What is edge enhancement and how does it affect the mammographic image? Xerox Corporation, California)

Subjective assessment of the radiologist

Most radiologists believe that xeromammography is easier to interpret than screen-film mammography. Since the xeromammogram is viewed by reflected rather than transmitted light, there may be less eyestrain, especially when reading for long periods of time. Much of the viewbox glare encountered when reading screen-film studies can be reduced by covering the bare portions of the illuminated viewboxes with black cardboard.

Although xeromammography and screen-film mammography are more accurate than non-screen-film mammography, patient studies have not shown any difference in accuracy between these two newer methods [55,58]. It is likely that diagnostic accuracy largely depends on the radiologist's interpretive skills and the technical quality of the image.

Risk from mammography

High dose risk

An increased incidence of breast cancer has been observed in several groups of women exposed to high doses of radiation. These were Japanese survivors of atomic bombings at Hiroshima and Nagasaki [59]; Canadian [60] and American [61] sanatoria patients who received multiple chest fluoroscopies; American women treated with radiotherapy for post-partum mastitis (Fig. 82.35) [62]; Swedish women who received radiation therapy for a variety of benign breast conditions [63]; and radium dial workers who ingested radioactive material [64].

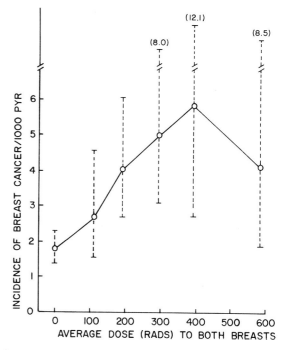

Fig. 82.35 Dose-response curve for American women treated with radiation therapy for postpartum mastitis. Because no women received doses below 100 rads, this study provides only indirect evidence of risk at low doses. (Reproduced with permission from Feig S A 1983 Radiol Clin North Am 21:173–192) [67]

Possible low dose risk

It is not clear whether very low doses of radiation such as those from current mammographic techniques induce breast cancer. Its existence has only been inferred from the excess breast cancer incidence seen in women exposed to high doses.

The estimated risk would depend on the shape of the dose response curve in the low dose region (Fig. 82.36). In a linear situation, a ten-fold reduction in exposure should lead to a ten-fold reduction in risk: risk per rad remains constant. In a curvilinear (quadratic) situation, the drop in cancer incidence would be considerably greater. The risk per rad at

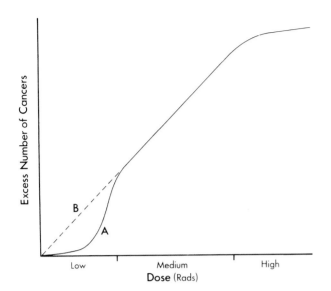

Fig. 82.36 Typical dose-response curve for radiation induced tumours among laboratory animals. At medium doses, there is a linear dose-response relationship so that risk per rad remains constant. At high doses, the curve flattens due to cell killing. At low doses, (below 50–100 rads) a quadratic dose-response relationship [A] is seen so that risk per rad is less than expected from a linear extrapolation [B] from medium doses. There is an obvious resemblance between human and animal curves at medium and high doses, but at low doses insufficient human data precludes comparison. (Reproduced with permission from Feig S A 1984 A J R, 143:469–476 [69]

low doses would be much less than that expected from a linear extrapolation. Most animal experiments involving a variety of radiation induced tumours, including breast cancer, show a curvilinear relationship at low doses.

Radiogenic breast cancers in humans do not appear until a minimum of 10 years following exposure. For younger women, the latent period is longer. The duration of carcinogenic effect is unknown, but it is at least 15 years and may persist for lifetime.

For the years following this latent period, a risk estimate of 7.5 excess breast cancers/million women/year/rad has been made from the Western women studied [65]. This estimate is a linear extrapolation from high doses due to lack of significant low dose data.

The risk estimate is even lower for older women. It has been estimated by the US National Cancer Institute that the risk for women over 30 years of age at time of exposure is 3.5 excess cancers/million women/year/rad [65]. Since this estimate is based on linear extrapolation from high dose data, it may be considered the upper limits of risk. However, it is likely that an ongoing study of Canadian sanatoria patients will reduce this estimate even further [66]. The reasons for decreased risk in older women are not entirely clear, possibly relating to parity, hormonal factors, or age-related changes in breast tissue.

Hypothetical risk from mammography

According to this estimate, if 2 million women above age 30 were each to receive a low dose mammogram (mean breast dose of 0.3 rad for a two view study), there would, after a latent period of 10 years, be one excess cancer/year in the population. Assuming a 50% breast cancer mortality rate, the hypothetical risk is 1 excess death/2 million women examined; equated with the following: 200 miles air travel, 30 miles car travel, smoking 1/2 of one cigarette, 3/4 minute of mountain climbing, and 10 minutes of being a man aged 60 [67].

The very small risk from mammography can be appreciated by comparison with the much larger magnitude of the natural breast cancer incidence: 800 cases/million women/year at age 40, 1800 cases/million women/year at age 50, and 2500 cases/million women/year at age 65 [67]. A substantial number of these cases could be detected at a curable stage if mammographic screening were performed.

Since radiation-induced and naturally-occurring breast cancers are identical pathologically, they can be distinguished only in a statistical sense. Because the risk from 1 rad is so small, a 20 year follow-up of 25 million exposed and 25 million nonexposed women from age 50 would be necessary to prove or disprove risk at this level [67]. However, it is possible to derive an indirect estimate of 3.5 excess breast cancers/million women/rad/year as the upper limits of such risk if existent.

In this regard, the BEIR III report (Biological Effects of Ionizing Radiation) [68] issued by the US National Academy of Sciences may be relevant. For all human cancers, the committee adopted a linear-quadratic model where risk is half that expected from the linear model. Estimates for the linear and quadratic models were taken as the upper and lower limits of risk, respectively. Because of insufficient data, the linear-quadratic model was not used for breast cancer risk. If it had been, the risk would be only half the previous estimate, 1.8 versus 3.5. If breast cancer were found to comply with the quadratic model used for some tumours, the risk could be only 1/100 that of the current estimate, 0.035 versus 3.5. Thus, the magnitude of possible risk from low dose mammography appears negligible, especially when compared to the substantial benefits which would result from early detection. [69]

BREAST CANCER SCREENING

Criteria for benefit

The role of mammographic screening in detecting unsuspected breast cancer in asymptomatic women is based on its ability to find the disease at an early nonpalpable stage. Breast cancer survival depends on two related factors: lesion size and lymph node status. Smaller lesions with no histological evidence of axillary metastasis have a better prognosis (Table 82.3). Mammography is currently the most effective means of detecting such lesions (Table 82.4). Thus it would appear that mammographic screening could greatly diminish

Table 82.3 Breast cancer survival according to pathological stage of disease and method of cancer detection.

Pathological stage of disease	Per cent survival		
	5 year	10 year	20 year
Minimal	98	95	93
Negative nodes	85	74	62
Positive nodes	55	39	23
Distant metastases	10	2	
Method of detection			
Screening by mammography and physical examination	93	*	*
Clinical detection in absence of screening	64	51	37

1. Per cent survival relative to normal life expectancy
2. Data compiled from SEER Report (NIH Publication No. 81–2330) 1981; Wanebo et al 1974 Cancer 33:349–357; Fraizer et al 1977 Am J Surg 133:697–701; Letton et al 1981 Cancer 48:404–406
3. Five and 10 year survival for minimal breast cancer as defined by Wanebo, 1974.
4. 20 year survival for minimal breast cancer as defined by Gallager 1971 Cancer 28:1505–1507
* Data not yet available due to insufficient follow up.

Table 82.4 Accuracy of mammography and physical examination in breast cancer screening according to stage of disease. (From Beahrs et al 1979 JNCI 62:640–709) (Detection rates for minimal carcinoma as defined by Beahrs.)

Stage of disease	Per cent detection	
	Mammography	Physical examination
Minimal carcinoma	97	33
Negative nodes	92	51
Positive nodes	93	77

the effects of a disease which now afflicts one of every 11 American women in her lifetime.

Since the risk of mammography is negligible, its use in screening should be beyond controversy. While a majority of investigators have endorsed mammographic screening for women over 50, some have questioned its efficacy in screening below this age. Their arguments could be summarized as follows: there is no proven benefit is screening younger women. Therefore, the risk, though insignificant, will exceed the benefit, which is zero.

Evidence of benefit

HIP study

A randomized trial was conducted by the Health Insurance Plan of New York. Sixty-two thousand women who volunteered for screening were divided into study and control populations of 31 000 women each. Women in the study group were offered screening by mammography and physical examination for 5 successive years (1963–1968). When compared to the control group, a 40% mortality reduction

was found among women above age 50 at time of detection. No such benefit was found among younger women. Reduced mortality for women screened above age 50 is still evident on 10 to 14 year follow up [70]. These results offer incontrovertible proof of benefit from screening.

The lack of decreased mortality among women screened below age 50 in the HIP study is the basis for the mammography controversy. It raises questions concerning the efficacy of screening these younger women. The most plausible explanation for the absence of decreased mortality in younger women seems to be that mammography as practiced in the HIP study was less effective in women below age 50. Among cancers detected among women above age 50, 30% were found on mammography alone. For cancers detected among women below age 50, only 20% were found by mammography alone (Fig. 82.37).

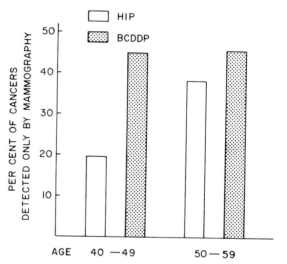

Fig. 82.37 Comparison of HIP and BCDDP screening studies. Per cent of cancers detected by mammography only according to patient age. (Reproduced with permission from Feig S A 1979 JAMA 242:2107–2109)

BCDDP study

In the more recent Breast Cancer Detection Demonstration Projects (BCDDP) (1973–1981) [31,71], sponsored by the American Cancer Society and the National Cancer Institute, the number of nonpalpable cancers detected among younger women has risen markedly. Among women below age 50, approximately 45% of cancers were found by mammography alone compared to 20% in the HIP study (Fig. 82.37). Cancer detection rates for women of all ages at the BCDDP centres were approximately twice as high as those from the HIP: 5.5 versus 2.8 cancers/thousand women on initial screening. There was also a remarkable shift in detection towards smaller lesions. Minimal carcinomas constituted 36% of all cancers at the BCDDP versus 8% in the HIP study. As seen in Table 82.4, mammography was largely responsible for the increased detection of minimal cancers. Although the HIP and BCDDP populations are not strictly comparable, these data indicate that mammography has become a more sensitive screening modality, especially in women below age 50.

Since a 40% mortality reduction was seen in HIP women over age 50, an equivalent or greater mortality reduction can be expected among women in the 40 to 50 year age range. The BCDDP study is not a randomized trial where mortality rates in control and study populations can be measured simultaneously. Rather, it suggests that the ability of mammography to detect early breast cancer in younger women will yield decreased mortality.

Benefit/risk comparison

Although incontrovertible proof of benefit depends upon the randomized clinical trials now underway in Sweden [72] and Canada [73], the expected benefit can be calculated from the BCDDP data and compared to the estimated risk from mammography as shown in Figure 82.38 [74]. These estimates of benefit/risk probably represent minimum value since the risk at low doses may be much less than assumed, especially for older women. Since the incidence of naturally occurring breast cancers increases with patient age, the benefit from screening is greater among older women. Benefit seems to exceed risk at age 40.

Benefit is greater among women with breast cancer risk factors such as family history, nulliparity, breast 'lumps', discharge, prior breast surgery, etc. Cancer detection rates on initial (prevalence) screening are approximately twice the natural breast cancer incidence due to the detection of prevalent cancers, which in the absence of screening would contribute to the incidence rate over the next several years. With subsequent annual screenings, detection rates approach the breast cancer incidence for the patient's age group.

The case for screening women above age 40 is so compelling that it is prudent to follow the recommended guidelines of the American Cancer Society and the American College of Radiology (Table 82.5).

Table 82.5 Screening recommendations for asymptomatic women[1].

Age	Breast self-examination	Physical examination by physician	Mammography
20–40	monthly	every 3 years	baseline study by age 40 [2]
40–50	monthly	annual	1–2 year intervals [3]
50–	monthly	annual	annual

1. Based on recommendations of Amercian Cancer Society (Ca — A Cancer J Clin 30:194–240, 1980; 33:255, 1983), and American College of Radiology (ACR Bulletin 38:6–7, 1983).
2. An earlier age for baseline study is preferable when there is a personal history of breast cancer or a history of premenopausal breast cancer in the patient's mother and/or sisters.
3. Intervals for screening women between age 40 and 50 determined by combined analysis of physical and mammographic findings and other risk factors, unless medically indicated sooner.

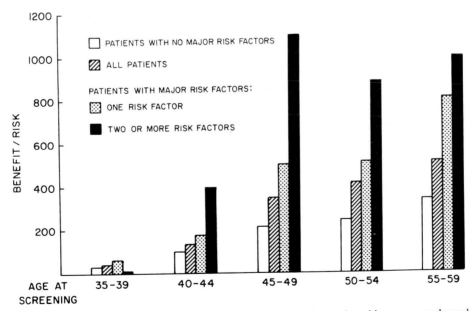

Fig. 82.38 Benefit/risk expressed as years of life expectancy gained/lost from first annual screening with mammography and physical examination at the BCDDP. Graph based on data from Seidman (1977) [74], modified to assume a mean breast dose of 0.17 rad and a risk estimate of 3.5 excess cancers/10^6 women/rad/year beginning 10 years post-exposure. (Reproduced with permission from Feig S A 1984 In: Feig S A, McLelland R (eds) Breast Carcinoma: current diagnosis and treatment Masson, New York pp 391–401)

THERMOGRAPHY

The increased metabolic rate of some benign and malignant breast conditions may produce a positive thermogram (Fig. 82.39). The major attraction of breast thermography has been that it does not involve ionizing radiation and thus has no known carcinogenic risk.

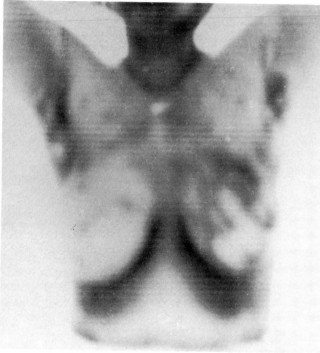

Fig. 82.39   Positive thermogram: excess vascularity in left breast.

Teletherography

This study is performed with a thermographic camera, which records infrared radiation emitted by the patient. Deeper structures are not imaged, but heat from within the breast is transferred by venous convection to the superficial veins.

In a normal thermogram, the venous pattern of each breast is similar, but need not be completely identical. An abnormal thermogram may be recognized as a significant increase in venous calibre, length, temperature, number or configuration, or as excess heat which does not conform to a venous pattern. No one pattern is specific for carcinoma. Any pattern may be associated with fibrocystic disease, fibroadenoma, breast abscess, trauma, fat necrosis, haematoma, or may occur in the absence of breast disease.

Initial studies indicated that teletherography could detect 75 to 85% of cancers, mostly large, clinically palpable lesions occurring in symptomatic patients [75,76]. Later, teletherography was employed in the BCDDP, and showed considerably lower detection rates since a greater proportion of these

cancers were small and nonpalpable. In this study, the cancer detection rate for thermography was only 40% vs 57% for physical examination and 91% for mammography. Moreover, for every true positive thermogram, there were 90 false positive thermograms [70].

Other thermography methods

Liquid crystal thermography utilizes cholesterol ester crystals contained in thin plastic sheets which are draped over the breasts. The colour of these crystals is altered by the temperature of the underlying breast producing the temperature map which can be viewed directly or photographed.

Computer assisted thermography involves computer analysis of temperature readings at standardized locations on each breast. The computer calculates a 'likelihood of malignancy' index which is independent of observer performance.

Graphic stress telethermography (GST) performs computer interpretation of breast skin temperature measurements pre- and post-vasoconstriction produced when the patient immerses her hands in ice water. This procedure is based on the premise that vessels supplying the tumour are less responsive than normal vessels to cold stress.

These newer thermographic methods have not been shown to be any more accurate than telethermography [77].

Limitations of thermography

Diagnostic evaluation

Thermography cannot be used to determine the aetiology of breast signs or symptoms, since carcinoma, cyst, abscess, and fibroadenoma can produce a positive thermogram. A negative thermogram does not reliably exclude the presence of carcinoma [76].

Thus, thermography should not be used to determine whether breast symptoms are due to benign or malignant disease, nor should it be used to determine whether palpable breast masses should be biopsied [76].

Screening

Thermography should not be used as a pre-screening examination to determine which patients should be further studied by mammography. If such procedure had been followed at the BCDDP, and mammography reserved for only women with positive thermograms, 80% of nonpalpable cancers would have been missed [70].

Determination of prognosis

Several studies suggest a tentative relationship between breast cancer survival and degree of thermographic positivity, possibly because faster growing, less differentiated, larger cancers result in more heat production than slower growing, less anaplastic ones. However, these studies are poorly documented and not corrected for known prognostic factors such as lesion size, lymph node involvement, and histological grade [77].

Prediction of breast cancer risk

It has been suggested that a positive thermogram may be a high risk indicator for breast cancer. These studies are unconfirmed and based on data that have not been corrected for known risk factors. At present, there is insufficient evidence to support the use of thermography for cancer risk prediction [77,78].

Thermography guidelines

The American College of Radiology policy statement on breast thermography [79] concludes that 'The addition of thermography to physical examination and mammography for diagnosis and screening provides little if any clinically meaningful information while substantially increasing the cost of medical care. Accordingly, thermography of the breast is a purely experimental procedure with no established clinical indications.'

BREAST ULTRASOUND

Ultrasound equipment

Palpable breast masses may be evaluated on *general purpose ultrasound equipment*, with the patient in an oblique supine position. In *contact scanning*, the transducer is hand held or mounted on a mechanical arm. It is placed directly over the mass after a coupling agent such as mineral oil or sonic gel is applied to the skin. The mass may be immobilized by one hand. In *water bath scanning*, the transducer is inside a water filled plastic bag, which is placed over the breast. This permits imaging the mass in the optimal focal length range. It also allows a more complete survey of the breast and provides breast compression. For optimal resolution, grey scale imaging and medium to high frequency transducers (5–10 MHz) should be used [80,81].

Visualization of the entire breast is most easily accomplished with *automated whole breast scanners*, since general purpose ultrasound units cannot generate rapid and reproducible thin section images through all portions of the breast. Even if such an examination were performed by a general purpose scanner, the time necessary for the ultra-sonographer to evaluate 150 hard copy images from each breast would be excessive.

These dedicated breast scanners record the entire study on disc or tape. It can then be rapidly viewed on a video monitor and transparent film images made from any portion. The patient is examined prone with her breast immersed in a water bath. The units contain from one to eight transducers of 2.5 to 3.5 MHz and are capable of 2 mm resolution. Spacing between scan planes is 1 to 5 mm [81].

Whole breast scanners may be a convenient method to evaluate nonpalpable lesions initially detected by mammography, but there is no evidence that they are more accurate than the cheaper general purpose scanners in this regard.

Diagnostic criteria

Normal breast

The topography of the breast on B-mode ultrasound relates to that seen on mammography. The skin appears as a highly reflective line below which is an anechoic zone of subcutaneous adipose tissue, at times traversed by the perpendicular linear reflections of Cooper's ligaments. The subcutaneous tissue zone may widen with age. In younger patients, fibroglandular tissue produces a cone shaped region of homogeneous high intensity echoes in the midportion of the breast. In older women, this region is smaller and shows spotty replacement by anechoic fatty tissue. Although the presence of fluid filled masses establishes the diagnosis of gross fibrocystic disease, it is otherwise difficult to differentiate fibrocystic disease from the highly echoic glandular breasts expected in the younger patient. The lactiferous ducts can be visualized as echo-free tubular structures radiating from the nipple. At times, on prone, whole breast scans performed with a single transducer scanner, there may be a wide, echo-free core extending from the nipple to the midportion of the breast. This phenomenon is believed to represent shadowing from nipple, lactiferous ducts, and fibroglandular tissue, and can be eliminated by compression at the time of scanning. At the back of the breast can be seen a thin curvilinear band of anechoic retromammary fat beneath which is the broader, highly echogenic band of the pectoralis muscle.

Breast masses

The ultrasonic appearance of commonly occurring breast masses is shown in Table 82.6.

Cyst

Fluid-filled cysts are free of internal echoes on low ultrasonic gain setting and remain so on high gain, as the sensitivity setting is increased. Their anterior and posterior margins are well defined. Cysts are usually round or oval, but multiple cysts and multiloculated cysts may appear lobulated or septated. Acoustic enhancement is seen behind the mass (Fig. 82.40).

Fibroadenoma

These masses have smooth, well defined anterior and

Table 82.6 Ultrasound diagnostic criteria for breast masses.

Mass	Criteria			
	Internal echoes	*Contour*	*Far wall echoes*	*Through transmission*
Cyst	absent	smooth	strong	increased
Fibroadenoma	uniform	smooth or slightly irregular	strong to weak	decreased
Carcinoma	nonuniform	irregular	weak or absent	decreased or absent

N.B. Criteria can reliably differentiate cystic from solid masses if sufficiently large, but often cannot distinguish benign from malignant solid masses.

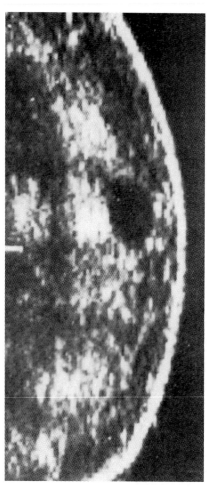

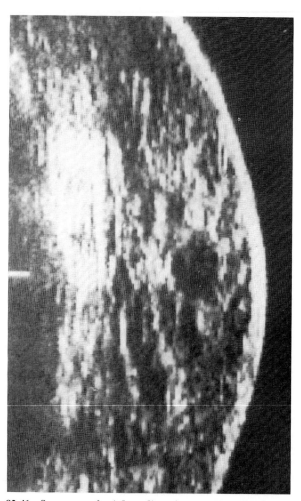

Fig. 82.40 Sonogram of a 2 cm cyst. Typical features include absence of internal echoes, smooth margins, and echo enhancement posteriorly. (Figs 82.40, 82.41 and 82.42 Reproduced with permission from Sickles E A, Filly R A, Callen P W 1983 In: Feig S A, McLelland R (eds) Breast carcinoma: Current diagnosis and treatment. Masson, New York pp 191–206) [81]

Fig. 82.41 Sonogram of a 1.5 cm fibroadenoma. Note low level internal echoes, nodular contour, and slightly increased posterior echoes.

posterior margins and are round, oval, or nodular. They contain weak, homogeneously distributed echoes. This moderate acoustic attenuation results in intermediate strength echoes behind the mass. Coarse calcifications within a fibroadenoma may be brightly reflective (Fig. 82.41).

Carcinoma

Breast cancer frequently has poorly defined anterior and posterior margins and an irregular or nodular contour. Internal echoes are usually faint and nonuniform. Because of marked acoustic attenuation through the mass, pronounced acoustic shadowing beyond the mass may be seen. In some cases, this may be the only ultrasonic evidence of the lesion. Architectural distortion without direct evidence of a mass has also been reported (Fig. 82.42) [82].

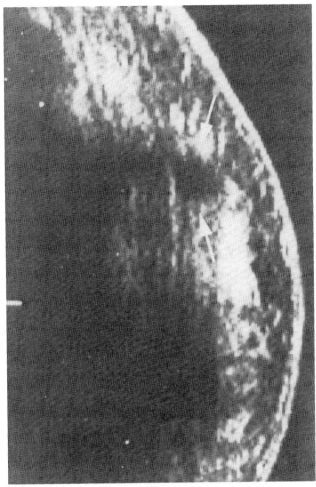

Fig. 82.42 Sonogram of a 1 cm infiltrating ductal carcinoma. Irregular contour and decreased through transmission are characteristic.

Other lesions

A *breast abscess* has irregular margins and may contain internal echoes. A *haematoma* is also irregular in shape. It is initially weakly echogenic, but manifests increasing echogenicity as it becomes organized.

Simple and compound scans

Both whole breast and general purpose scanners can be used to obtain single sector (simple) scans, which is the best means to demonstrate posterior sonic enhancement in fluid-filled masses and retrotumoural shadowing in solid masses. Only the multiple transducer whole breast scanners can produce compound images, which permit clear delineation of the lateral walls.

Accuracy

The ability of ultrasound to image a breast mass depends on the nature of the lesion and the surrounding tissue. Since cancers and fibroadenomas are weakly echogenic, they are better identified against the high level echoes of glandular breasts than against the low amplitude echoes of fatty breasts. Because cysts are free of internal echoes, they are more readily imaged than solid lesions.

Reports of high levels of accuracy of ultrasound in cancer detection approaching or equalling those of mammography are misleading for several reasons. Most of the cancers studied by sonography were large, obvious lesions, which do not challenge the sensitivity of the modality. The mammograms, collected from various hospitals and offices, were in many instances technically poor. Properly conducted studies indicate that even when sonography is interpreted with knowledge of the clinical and mammographic findings, it detects only a small proportion of nonpalpable cancers.

Smaller lesions are less well detected by ultrasound. In one study [83], ultrasound demonstrated 80% of cancers of 2 cm, 59% of cancers 1.0 to 1.9 cm, and 8% of cancers less than 1 cm (Table 82.7).

Once a mass has been visualized on sonography, a distinction of cystic versus solid can be realiably made if the lesion is of sufficient size. Since a cyst is better distinguished from surrounding tissue, it is easier to detect than a solid lesion. In another study, ultrasound correctly diagnosed 96% of cysts from 0.2 to 12.0 cm (average size 1.3 cm) [80]. However, it is not known if the diagnostic accuracy for cysts of 1 cm or less is the same as for larger ones.

Ultrasound frequently cannot distinguish benign from malignant solid masses. Some malignancies, especially ductal carcinoma of 2 cm or less, medullary carcinoma, and cystosarcoma phylloides appear as well-defined solid masses with weak internal echoes. They are difficult or impossible to distinguish from fibroadenoma.

Table 82.7 Accuracy of breast cancer detection: mammography vs. sonography.

Category	Per cent detection by		Total cancers
	Mammography	Sonography	
All cancers	97	58	64
Palpable cancers	98	73	41
Nonpalpable cancers	96	30	23
Cancers with negative axillary nodes	95	48	44
Cancers smaller than 1 cm	92	8	12
Cancers seen as micro-calcifications only on mammography	100	6	17

1. Sickles et al 1983 AJR 140:843–845 [83]
2. Sonography was performed and interpreted with knowledge of results from physical examination and mammography. 'Expanded' ultrasound diagnostic criteria were used i.e. all visualized masses not purely cystic were interpreted as potentially malignant.

Indications

Even though ultrasound can distinguish cystic from solid

masses with a higher degree of accuracy than either physical examination or mammography, it is not commonly used for palpable lesions, since needle aspiration is equally accurate, less expensive, and simpler, and can be performed in the the referring physician's office. Although aspiration is an invasive procedure, it is as innocuous as venepuncture and can be easily learned.

The major value of ultrasound is as a supplement to mammography in selected problem cases. These include evaluation of a nonpalpable mass or density which cannot be aspirated. Here, the establishment of its cystic nature can avert the need for biopsy. Ultrasound can also be used in the glandular breast to evaluate a questionably palpable mass if it is not seen on mammography. It should be stated that the lack of internal echoes in a mass of 1 to 2 cm or greater is a reliable indication of a cyst, but the accuracy of this sign among smaller masses is less well documented.

Ultrasound should not be used as a screening procedure, since it is unable to detect many nonpalpable breast cancers, especially those associated with negative axillary nodes and those seen on the basis of mammographic microcalcifications (Table 82.7). Although ultrasound may seem superficially attractive because it has not been implicated as a cause of breast cancer, the risk from low dose mammography is so slight that detection accuracy and not oncogenic risk should be the only consideration.

Some physicians have advocated ultrasound instead of mammography as the initial imaging procedure for evaluation of palpable breast masses. In this approach, mammography would be performed only if ultrasound showed no cyst. This practice could result in a serious clinical mistake. First, ultrasound might show a cyst, which could be mistaken for the palpated mass — an adjacent carcinoma not visualized on ultrasound. Second, a nonpalpable carcinoma in either breast could also be missed.

Mammography serves as a diagnostic procedure for the mass itself, and as a screening procedure for both breasts. Ultrasound is a diagnostic procedure only. The use of ultrasound to evaluate a palpable mass precludes the screening function of mammography. This distinction is especially important among women with breast lumps who are in a high risk group for breast cancer. Ultrasound does not have the requisite sensitivity to substitute for mammography in either diagnosis or screening. Accordingly, it should only be performed after a mammogram.

BREAST COMPUTERIZED TOMOGRAPHY

Because it is computer assisted, breast CT can discern even smaller differences in tissue radiodensity than mammography. These differences are enhanced by intravenous injection of iodinated contrast agent. Pre- and post-contrast injection scans are compared for changes in CT density ($\triangle$CT number) in the breast for specific points. Absolute

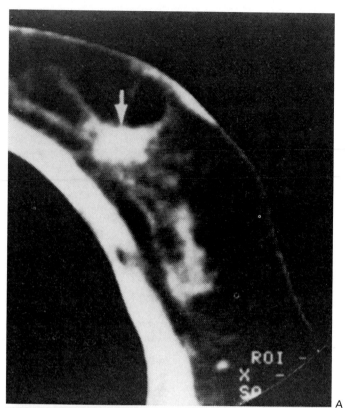

A

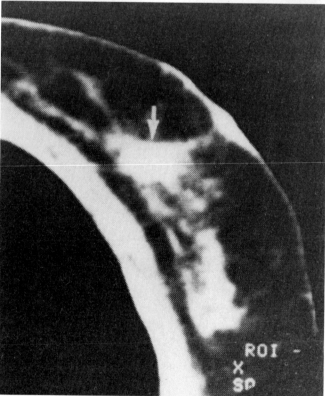

B

Fig. 82.43A & B Carcinoma demonstrated on CT mammography using a body scanner. An irregular spiculated mass with a $\triangle$CT value of 29 from (A) precontrast to (B) post-injection scan is seen. (Reproduced with permission from Chang C H J, Nesbit D E, Fisher D R 1982 AJR 138:553–558) [84]

density values as well as lesion shape and size are of lesser diagnostic importance (Fig. 82.43).

The ability of the $\triangle$CT number to differentiate benign from malignant breast disease has been the subject of several conflicting reports. One study [84] found that $\triangle$CT numbers of carcinoma and fibroadenoma tend to be higher than those of fibrocystic disease. It suggested that a $\triangle$CT number of 25 could serve as a useful cutoff point to obviate the need for biopsy nearly, since all carcinomas had a $\triangle$CT number of above 25. Two other studies [85,86] found significantly greater overlap in $\triangle$CT numbers, and suggested that CT should not be used to assess the need for biopsy.

Because of its sensitivity to small density differences, CT may detect some lesions in glandular breasts not visualized on mammography. However, its spatial resolution is considerably less than that of mammography. Carcinomas of less than 1 cm and microcalcifications cannot be commonly recognized, and may have an incorrectly low CT number due to partial volume effect. Also, breast CT is a lengthy and costly examination which requires intravenous contrast injection and higher radiation exposure than mammography with no concomitant improvement in diagnostic accuracy. For these reasons, it has not been widely accepted.

MAGNETIC RESONANCE IMAGING Nuclear magnetic resonance

Magnetic resonance imaging [87,88] is based on the application of an external magnetic field and a radiofrequency (RF) pulse to the tissue to be studied

Most currently available data on breast MRI has been obtained from *in vitro* analysis of breast tissue. Some studies have found significant difference in relaxation times of benign and malignant breast tissues, while others have described a considerable overlap.

Thus far, the number of MRI studies on *in vivo* breast tissue has been limited [89]. One study suggested that the configuration of abnormal areas on MRI scans may allow a distinction between benign and malignant processes. Cysts have very well defined borders. Like cysts, fibroadenomas are well defined on spin echo (SE) images, but on inversion recovery (IR) image, a calcified fibroadenoma has a heterogeneous appearance. Carcinoma has ill-defined, irregular margins (Fig. 82.44) [90].

It would seem that MRI may have difficulty in detecting small carcinomas visualized on mammography since, at present, the spatial resolution of MRI is significantly poorer. The examination is time consuming and costly. However, MRI carries no known risk to the patient and could conceivably provide information which is not obtainable from mammography e.g. improved imaging of dense breasts and detection of preneoplastic physiological abnormalities. Despite these potential advantages, the future of breast MRI remains unclear.

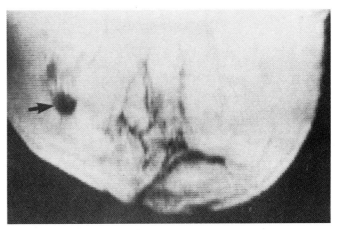

Fig. 82.44 Magnetic resonnance image obtained with a surface coil shows an irregular mass. Carcinoma was confirmed at biopsy. Reproduced with permission from El Yousef S J et al 1984 Radiology 150:761–766)[90]

TRANSILLUMINATION LIGHTSCANNING (Fig. 82.45)

There has been renewed interest in transillumination since it does not involve ionizing radiation and is therefore free of oncogenic risks. New modifications of this technique are now being evaluated. In place of the standard transilluminator, an infrared light source is now used since infrared is preferentially absorbed by the nitrogen rich compounds found in

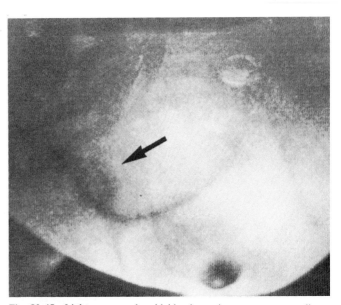

Fig. 82.45 Lightscan reveals a highly absorptive area corresponding to a 0.4 cm carcinoma found on biopsy. (Reproduced with permission from Bartram R J, Crow H C 1984 AJR 142:409–414)

rapidly growing cancer cells. Tumour vasculature may also contribute to infrared absorption since blood, especially haemoglobin, has a high nitrogen concentration. Although real-time viewing (diaphanoscopy) is still performed, the images are also recorded on infrared sensitive film (diaphanography) because the unaided human eye does not perceive infrared radiation.

On transillumination, carcinoma is darkest, fibroglandular tissue less dark, and fatty tissue which contains almost no nitrogen is lightest. Studies currently underway suggest that this method is considerably less sensitive than mammography for detecting deep lesions or small cancers [88,91].

BIBLIOGRAPHY

REFERENCES

1. Wolfe J N 1967 A study of breast parenchyma by mammography in the normal woman and those with benign and malignant disease. Radiology 89:201–205.
2. Haagensen C D 1971 Diseases of the breast. Saunders, Philadelphia pp 155–291
3. Barth V 1979 Atlas of diseases of the breast. Year Book, Chicago pp 53–56
4. Ingleby H, Gershon-Cohen J 1960 Comparative anatomy, pathology and roentgenology of the breast. University of Pennsylvania Press, Philadelphia: pp 121–288
5. Hoeffken W, Lanyi M 1977 Mammography. Saunders, Philadelphia pp 82–127
6. Gershon-Cohen J 1970 Atlas of mammography. Springer-Verlag, New York pp 39–126
7. Humphrey L J 1983 Fibrocystic disease and breast cancer. In: Feig S A, McLelland R (eds) Breast carcinoma: current diagnosis and treatment. Masson, New York pp 61–68
8. Kalisher L, McLelland R, Feig S A 1983 Mammographic patterns and breast cancer risk. In: Feig S A, McLelland R (eds) Breast carcinoma: current diagnosis and treatment. Masson, New York pp 77–88.
9. Wolfe J N, Albert S, Belle S, Salane M 1982 Breast parenchymal patterns: analysis of 332 incident breast carcinomas. Am J Roentgenol 138:113–118
10. Wellings S R, Wolfe J N 1978 Correlative studies of the histological and radiographic appearance of the breast parenchyma. Radiology 129:299–306
11. Egan R L, McSweeney M B 1979 Mammographic parenchymal patterns and risk of breask cancer. Radiology 133:65–70
12. Moskowitz M, Gartside P, Wirman J A, McLaughlin C 1980 Proliferative disorders of the breast as high risk factors for breast cancer in a self-selected screened population: pathologic markers. Radiology 134:289–291
13. Moskowitz M, Gartside P, McLaughlin C 1980 Mammographic patterns as markers for high-risk benign breast disease and incident cancers. Radiology 134:293–295
14. McDivitt R W, Stewart F W, Berg J W 1968 Tumors of the breast. Atlas of tumor pathology, second series, fascicle 2. Armed Forces Institute of Pathology, Washington D C
15. Young J L Jr, Percy C L, Asire A J (eds) 1981 Surveillance, epidemiology, and end results: incidence and mortality data, 1973–77. National Cancer Institute Monograph 57. NIH Publication No 81–2330. National Cancer Institute, Washington D C
16. Feig S A 1980 Biological determinants of radiation-induced human breast cancer. Crit Rev Diag Imaging 13:229–248
17. Gallager H S, Martin J E 1969 The study of mammary carcinoma by mammography and whole organ sectioning. Cancer 23:855–873
18. Feig S A, Shaber G S, Patchefsky A S et al 1978 Tubular carcinoma of the breast. Mammographic appearance and pathological correlation. Radiology 129:311–314
19. Millis R R 1979 Mammography In: Azzopardi J G (ed) Problems in breast pathology. Saunders, Philadelphia pp 437–460
20. Gold R H, Montgomery C K, Rambo O N 1973 Significance of margination of benign and malignant infiltrative mammary lesions: roentgenographic-pathological correlation. Am J Roentgenol 118:881–894
21. Sickles E A, Herzog K A 1980 Intramammary scar tissue: a mimic of the mammographic appearance of carcinoma. Am J Roentgenol 135:349–352
22. Bassett L W, Gold R H, Cove H C 1978 Mammographic spectrum of traumatic fat necrosis. The fallibility of 'pathognomonic' signs of carcinoma. Am J Roentgenol 130:119–122
23. Haagensen C D 1971 Traumatic fat necrosis of the breast. In: Diseases of the breast. Saunders, Philadelphia pp 202–211
24. Meyer J E, Kopans D B 1981 Stability of a mammographic mass, a false sense of security. Am J Roentgenol 137:595–598
25. Tabar L, Dean P B, Pentek Z 1983 Galactography: the diagnostic procedure of choice for nipple discharge. Radiology 149:31–38
26. Millis R R, Davis R, Stacey A J 1962 The detection and significance of calcifications in the breast: a radiological and pathological study. Br J Radiol 49:12–26
27. Murphy W A, DeSchryver-Kecskemeti K 1978 Isolated clustered microcalcifications in the breast: radiologic-pathologic correlation. Radiology 127:335–341
28. Sigfusson B F, Andersson I, Aspegren K, Janzon L, Linell F, Ljungberg O 1983 Clustered breast calcifications. Acta Radiol Diagn 24:273–281
29. Wolfe J N 1977 Xeroradiography. Breast calcifications. Thomas, Springfield
30. Kalisher L 1979 Factors influencing false negative rates in xeromammography. Radiology 133:297–301
31. Beahrs O H, Shapiro S, Smart C R 1979 Report of the working group to review the National Cancer Institute — American Cancer Society Breast Cancer Detection Demonstration Projects. JNCI 62:640–709
32. Feig S A, Shaber G S, Patchefsky A S et al 1977 Analysis of clinically occult and mammographically occult breast tumours. Am J Roentgenol 128:403–408
33. Dodd G D 1977 Present status of thermography, ultrasound and mammography in breast cancer detection. Cancer 39:2796–2805
34. DeLuca J T 1974 A statistical comparison of patients undergoing breast biopsy at a community hospital over a 16-year period. Radiology 112:315–318
35. Feig S A 1983 Localization of clinically occult breast lesions. Radiol Clin North Am 21:155–172
36. Hall F M, Frank H A 1979 Preoperative localization of nonpalpable breast lesions. Am J Roentgenol 132:101–105
37. Tabar L, Dean P B 1979 Interventional radiologic procedures in the investigation of lesions of the breast. Radiol Clin North Am 17:607–621
38. Goldberg R P, Hall F M, Simon M 1983 Preoperative localization of nonpalpable breast lesions using a wire marker and a perforated mammography grid. Radiology 146:833–835
39. Kopans D B, DeLuca S 1980 A modified needle — hookwire technique to simplify the preoperative localization of occult breast lesions. Radiology 134:781
40. Dance D R, Davis R 1983 Physics of mammography In: Parsons C A (ed) Diagnosis of breast disease. University Park Press, Baltimore pp 76–100.
41. Gajewski H 1977 Basic physical aspects of mammographic technique. In: Hoeffken W, Lanyi M (eds) Mammography. Saunders, Philadelphia pp 4–24
42. Haus A G 1983 Physical principles and radiation dose in mammography. In: Feig S A, McLelland R (eds) Breast carcinoma: current diagnosis and treatment. Masson, New York pp 99–114
43. Muntz E P, Wilkinson E, George F W 1980 Mammography at reduced doses: present performance and future possibilities. Am J Roentgenol 134:741–747

44. Egan R L 1960 Experience with mammography in a tumor institution. Evaluation of 1000 studies. Radiology 75:894–900

45. Wayrynen R E 1979 Fundamental aspects of mammographic receptors: film process. In: Logan W W, Muntz E P (eds) Reduced dose mammography. Masson, New York pp 521–528

46. Roth B, Hamilton J F Jr, Bunch P C 1979 Fundamental aspects of mammographic photoreceptors: screens. In: Logan W W, Muntz E P (eds) Reduced dose mammography. Masson, New York pp 529–536

47. Logan W W 1983 Screen/film mammography technique. In: Feig S A, McLelland R (eds) Breast carcinoma: current diagnosis and treatment Masson, New York pp 141–160

48. Sickles E A 1979 Controlled evaluations of image quality and diagnostic accuracy of low-dose mammography screen-film systems. In: Logan W W, Muntz E P (eds) Reduced dose mammography. Masson, New York pp 379–387

49. Bassett L W, Gold R H 1983 Breast radiography using the oblique projection. Radiology 149:585–587

50. Tabar L, Dean P B 1983 Screen/film mammography: quality control. In: Feig S A, McLelland R (eds) Breast carcinoma: current diagnosis and treatment. Masson, New York 161–168

51. Logan W W, Stanton L 1979 Grid versus magnification in clinical mammography. In: Logan W W, Muntz E P (eds) Reduced dose mammography. Masson, New York pp 265–279

52. McSweeney M B, Sprawls P, Egan R L 1983 Mammographic grids. In: Feig S A, McLelland R (eds) Breast carcinoma: current diagnosis and treatment. Masson, New York pp 169–176

53. Gros C M 1967 Methodologie. Symposium sur le sein. J Radiol Electrol 48:638–655

54. Sickles E A 1979 Microfocal spot magnification mammography using xeroradiographic and screen-film recording systems. Radiology 131:599–607

55. Feig S A 1982 Xeromammography. In: Bassett L W, Gold R H (eds) Mammography, thermography, and ultrasound in breast cancer detection. Grune and Stratton New York pp 73–86

56. Van De Riet W G, Wolfe J N 1977 Dose reduction in xeroradiography of the breast. Am J Roentgenol 128:821–823

57. Schmitt E L, Threatt B 1982 Tumor location and detectability in mammographic screening. Am J Roentgenol 139:761–765

58. Dodd G D 1981 Radiation detection and diagnosis of breast cancer. Cancer 47:1766–1769

59. Tokunaga M, Norman J E, Asano M, et al 1979 Malignant breast tumors among atomic bomb survivors, Hiroshima and Nagasaki, 1950–1974. JNCI 62:1347–1359

60. Myrden J A, Hiltz J E 1969 Breast cancer following multiple fluoroscopies during artificial pneumothorax treatment of pulmonary tuberculosis. Canad Med Assoc J 100:1032–1034

61. Boice J D, Monson R B 1977 Breast cancer following repeated fluoroscopic examinations of the chest. JNCI 59: 823–832

62. Shore R E, Hempelmann J H, Kowaluk E et al 1979 Breast neoplasms in women treated with x–rays for acute postpartum mastitis. JNCI 59:799–811

63. Baral E, Larrson L–E, Mattson B 1977 Breast cancer following irradiation of the breast. Cancer 40:2905–2910

64. Adams E E, Brues A M 1980 Breast cancer in female radium dial workers first employed before 1930. J Occupat Med 22:583–587

65. Upton A C, Beebe G W, Brown J M et al 1977 Report of the NCI Ad Hoc Working Group on the Risks Associated with Mammography in Mass Screening for the Detection of Breast Cancer. JNCI 59:481–493

66. Howe G R 1984 Epidemiology of radiogenic breast cancer. In: Boice J D Jr, Fraumeni J F Jr (eds) Radiation carcinogenesis: epidemiology and biological significance. Raven, New York pp 119–129

67. Feig S A 1983 Assessment of the hypothetical risk from mammography and evaluation of the potential benefit. Radiol Clin North Am 21:173–192

68. Committee on the Biological Effects of Ionizing Radiation 1980 The effect on populations of exposure to low levels of ionizing radiation. National Academy of Sciences — National Research Council, Washington D C

69. Feig S A 1984 Radiation risk for mammography: is it clinically significant? Am J Roentgenol 143:469–476

70. Shapiro S, Venet W, Strax P, Venet L, Roeser R 1982 Ten to fourteen year effect of screening on breast cancer mortality. JNCI 69:349–355

71. Baker L H 1982 Breast Cancer Detection Demonstration Project: five year summary report. Ca-A Cancer J Clin 32:194–225

72. Tabar L, Gad A, Akerlund E, Holmberg L 1983 Screening for breast cancer in Sweden. In: Feig S A, McLelland R (eds) Breast carcinoma: current diagnosis and treatment. Masson, New York pp 315–326

73. Miller A B, Howe G R, Wall C 1981 The National Study of Breast Cancer Screening. Clin Invest Med 4:227–258

74. Seidman H 1977 Screening for breast cancer in younger women, life expectancy gains and losses: an analysis according to risk indicator groups. Ca-A Cancer J Clin 27:66–87

75. Feig S A, Shaber G S, Schwartz G F et al 1977 Thermography, mammography and clinical examination in breast cancer screening: review of 16 000 studies. Radiology 122:123–127

76. Dodd G D 1983 Heat sensing devices and breast cancer detection. In: Feig S A, McLelland R (eds) Breast carcinoma: current diagnosis and treatment. Masson, New York pp 207–225

77. Sickles E A 1983 Breast thermography. In: Feig S A, McLelland R (eds) Breast carcinoma: current diagnosis and treatment. Masson, New York pp 227–231

78. Moskowitz M 1983 Screening for breast cancer: how effective are our tests? A critical review. Ca-A Cancer J Clin 33:26–39

79. American College of Radiology 1984 College policy reviews use of thermography. ACR Bull 40 (1):13

80. Fleischer A C, Muhletaler C A, Reynolds V H et al 1983 Palpable breast masses: evaluation by high frequency, hand held real-time sonography and xeromammography. Radiology 148:813–817

81. Sickles E A, Filly R A, Callen P W 1983 Breast ultrasonography. In: Feig S A, McLelland R (eds) Breast carcinoma: current diagnosis and treatment. Masson, New York pp 191–206

82. Kopans D B, Meyer J E, Steinbock R T 1982 Breast cancer: the appearance as delineated by whole breast water bath ultrasound scanning. J Clin Ultra 10:313–322

83. Sickles E A, Filly R A, Callen P W 1983 Breast cancer detection with sonography and mammography: comparison using state-of-the-art equipment. Am J Roentgenol 140:843–845

84. Chang C H J, Nesbit D E, Fisher D R 1982 Computed tomographic mammography using a conventional body scanner. Am J Roentgenol 138:553–558

85. Gisvold J J, Reese D F, Karsell P R 1979 Computed tomographic mammography (CTM). Am J Roentgenol 133:1143–1149

86. Muller J W T, van Waes P F G M, Koehler P R 1983 Computed tomography of breast lesions: comparison with x–ray mammography. J Comput Assist Tomogr 7:650–654

87. Partain C L, James A E, Rollo F D, Price P R 1983 Nuclear magnetic resonance (NMR) imaging. Saunders, Philadelphia

88. Sickles E A 1983 Breast C T scanning, heavy-ion mammography, N M R imaging, and diaphanography. In: Feig S A, McLelland R (eds) Breast carcinoma: current diagnosis and treatment. Masson, New York pp 233–250

89. Ross R J, Thompson J S, Kim K, Bailey R A 1982 Nuclear magnetic resonance imaging and evaluation of human breast tissue: preliminary clinical trials. Radiology 143:195–205

90. El Yousef S J, Duchesneau R H, Alfidi R J, Haagen J R, Bryan P J, LiPuma J P 1984 Magnetic resonance imaging of the breast. Radiology 150:761–766

91. Geslien G E, Fisher J R, DeLaney C 1985 Transillumination in breast cancer detection: screening failures and potential). Am J Roentgenol 144:619–622.

SUGGESTIONS FOR FURTHER READING

Azzopardi J G 1979 Problems in breast pathology. W. B. Saunders, London

Brünner S, Langfeldt B, Andersen P E (eds) 1984 Early detection of breast cancer. Springer-Verlag, Heidelberg

Feig S A, Kalisher L, Libshitz H I et al 1985 Breast disease. Self-evaluation syllabus. American College of Radiology, Chicago

Feig S A, McLelland R (eds) 1983 Breast carcinoma: current diagnosis and treatment. Masson, New York

Gallager H S, Leis H P, Snyderman R K, Urban J A (eds) 1978 The breast. Mosby, St Louis

Haagensen C D 1985 Diseases of the breast 3rd edn Saunders, Philadelphia

Hoeffken W, Lanyi M 1977 Mammography. Saunders, Philadelphia; Thieme, Stuttgart

Margolese R (ed) 1983 Breast cancer. Churchill Livingstone, Edinburgh

Martin J E 1982 Atlas of mammography. Williams and Wilkins, Baltimore

Netter F H 1954 Anatomy and pathology of the mammary gland, Section XIII, In: Reproductive system, Vol 2 of the Ciba Collection of Medical Illustrations. Summit, N J: Ciba Pharmaceutical Products Inc

Parsons C A (ed) 1983 Diagnosis of breast disease — imaging, clinical features and pathology. Chapman and Hall, London: University Park Press, Baltimore

Rothenberg L, Feig S A, Jans R et al 1985 Mammography: a user's guide NCRP report 72. Washington DC: National Council on Radiation Protection and Measurements

Tabar L Dean P B 1983 Teaching atlas of mammography. Thieme, New York

Witten D M 1969 The breast. In: Atlas of tumor radiology. Year Book, Chicago

Wolfe J N (ed) 1983 Mammography. The Radiological Clinics of North America Vol 21 No 1. Saunders, Philadelphia

Wolfe J N 1982 Xeroradiography of the breast, 2nd edn. Thomas, Springfield

9 The Central Nervous System

Editor: Ivan F. Moseley

Contents

83 The skull and brain: Methods of examination; diagnostic approach *J. Brismar, B. Lane, I. F. Moseley, J. Theron*
84 Cranial pathology (1) *J. Brismar, B. Lane, I. F. Moseley, J. Theron*
85 Cranial pathology (2) *J. Brismar, B. Lane, I. F. Moseley, J. Theron*
86 Cranial pathology (3) *J. Brismar, B. Lane, I. F. Moseley, J. Theron*
87 The spine: Methods of examination; diagnostic approach *V. L. McAllister, I. F. Moseley, J. Theron*
88 Spinal pathology *V. L. McAllister, I. F. Moseley, J. Theron*
89 Radionuclide scanning *John C. Harbert*

83 The skull and brain:
Methods of examination: diagnostic approach

J. Brismar, B. A. Lane, I. F. Moseley, J. Theron

Methods of examination

Plain radiography

Computerized tomography

Ultrasound

Vascular procedures
 Arteriography
  Anatomy of the cerebral arteries and veins
   The carotid system
   Anastomotic pathways
   The cerebral veins
   Vertebrobasilar arterial system
   Vertebrobasilar venous system
 Phlebography
 Sinography

Pneumography
 Anatomy
 Interpretation of air studies

The radiological diagnostic approach to clinical neurological problems

 Acute presentations

 Chronic presentations

METHODS OF EXAMINATION

Radiological techniques employed for the examination of the brain, skull and associated structures include the following:
 plain radiography (and tomography)
 computerized tomography
 nuclear magnetic resonance imaging
 radionuclide studies
 sonography
 vascular procedures:
  arteriography
  phlebography
  sinography
 pneumography
  pneumoencephalography
  ventriculography
 cisternography

Each of these will be considered in turn, together with the relevant radio-anatomy, with the exception of magnetic resonance imaging, which is discussed in Chapter 5 and techniques with radio-isotopes, which are dealt with in the section on nuclear medicine. Radio-isotope techniques have fallen into general disuse in clinical neuroradiology, because of the competition from computerized tomography, except as research techniques. In a final section, the diagnostic imaging approach to common clinical situations is discussed. Fuller details of pathological appearances are to be found in Chapters 84, 85 & 86.

Plain radiography

General considerations

Only skull radiographs of high technical quality are of clinical value, and this is more than ever true in the CT era. Scrupulous attention to positioning is essential. High definition films in grid cassettes (24–40 lines per cm) are preferred. Special compensating filters, which even out the contrast range over the radiodense skull base and less dense vault, are available. Tube kilovoltages of 50–90 kVp are employed, with a focal spot no larger than 0.6 mm, and a focus film

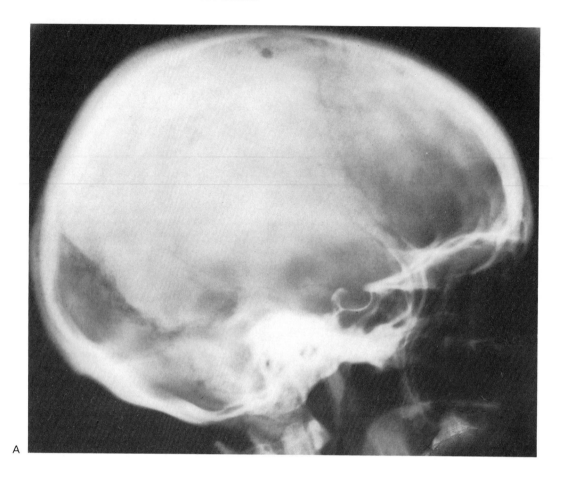

A

distance of 90 cm. Whenever possible, an isocentric dedicated skull unit should be available.

Recommendations in this chapter are based on those of the 1961 Commission on Neuroradiology of the World Federation of Neurology, with certain modifications suggested by Du Boulay [1]. Most isocentric systems use a customized system based on similar principles. The technique is based on the following lines and planes.

Lines [2]

1. *Anthropological base line.* This may be drawn from the lower margin of the orbit to the superior border of the external auditory meatus (EAM): Reid's or Frankfurt line; or from the outer canthus to the centre of the meatus (orbitomeatal OM line).

2. The *auricular line* is perpendicular to the above, passing vertically downwards through the EAM.

3. The *interpupillary line* passes through both ocular pupils, perpendicular to the median sagittal plane (see below).

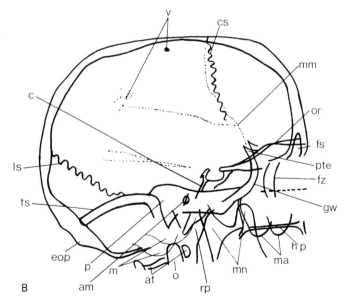

Fig. 83.1A & B   Lateral radiograph and diagram of the skull.

Planes

1. The *median sagittal plane* corresponds to the anatomical midline.

2. The *horizontal (Frankfurt) plane* contains both anthropological base lines; it is perpendicular to the median sagittal plane. A corresponding orbitomeatal plane contains both orbitomeatal lines.

3. The *frontal bi-auricular plane* lies perpendicular to both the preceding planes, through the centre of the EAM.

The standard skull series consists of four projections. In many cases, not all of these will be essential, while in others supplementary views will be added to or replace the conventional projections.

1. The lateral projection (Fig. 83.1)

The midsagittal plane is strictly parallel to the film. Du Boulay [1] recommends a centring point 2.5 cm anterior to the external auditory meatus and 1 cm above the orbitomeatal line, which has the merit of placing the sella turcica in the centre of the beam in most patients. On the resulting radiograph the anterior clinoid processes and the orbital roofs on the two sides should be superimposed.

The practice of placing the patient prone and rotating the head through 90° to obtain the lateral film using a vertical beam should be abandoned. Many skull radiographs are obtained in cases of head injury, when rotation of the neck may exacerbate an unsuspected upper cervical lesion; fluid levels will not be appreciated with a vertical beam. If the patient is placed supine, or sitting, using a horizontal beam, these potential disadvantages are avoided, and the more comfortable position makes for a straighter and improved film.

2. Posteroanterior (occipitofrontal) (Fig. 83.2)

The midsagittal plane is strictly perpendicular to the film, as is the orbitomeatal plane; in practice this is achieved by resting the nose and forehead on the film. The tube is angled 20° caudally, and the beam is centred on the nasion. A fronto-occipital (anteroposterior) projection should not be used unless the patient's condition presents no alternative, as it causes magnification and blurring of the important anterior structures.

The petrous ridges should be projected at or near the infraorbital margins. Many individuals have asymmetrical temporal fossae, and the best method of assessing rotation is to identify an anterior structure such as the base of the nasal septum and a more posterior structure such as the odontoid. If these are not in the same sagittal plane, the projection is not adequate.

3. Half-axial (Towne's) projection (Fig. 83.3)

The median sagittal plane is again strictly perpendicular to the film. Placing the occiput on the film, with the orbitomeatal or anthropological line perpendicular to it, combined with caudal tube angulation of 30°, gives an effective caudal angulation of 25–45° respectively. The beam is centred on the foramen magnum. Opinions differ on which degree of tilt is preferable; much depends on the configuration of the individual patient and the clinical problem.

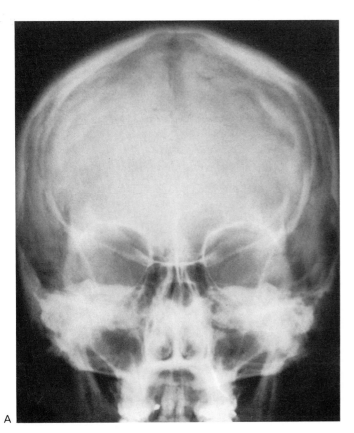

A

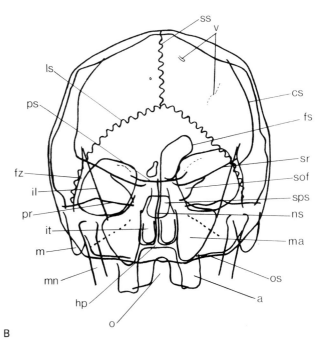

B

Fig. 83.2A & B Occipitofrontal radiograph and diagram of the skull.

Lateral rotation is assessed as described above. Care must be taken not to exclude the anterior temporal and facial regions from the film; they appear elongated, due to the distortion introduced by the tube/film angulation.

4. Submentovertical (basal) projection (Fig. 83.4)

With the patient supine, the head is fully extended such that the anthropological base line is parallel with the film; the median sagittal plane is perpendicular to it. The beam is centred along the biauricular line, between the angles of the mandible. A satisfactory radiograph is one in which there is no rotation and the angles of the mandible lie just anterior to the middle ear cavities. In order to achieve full extension of the neck, a thick pillow or bolster may be placed between the table and the patient's shoulders.

Other commonly used projections

Pituitary fossa

When the lateral projection is centred on the sella turcica, as described, 'coned views' are unnecessary. If, as occasionally occurs, the floor of the fossa is not visible on the frontal projection, inspection of the lateral film may indicate an alternative angulation which will bring the central ray parallel or tangential to the floor.

Optic canal

With a posteroanterior beam, the neck is extended so that the anthropological base line lies at 55° to the film; the head is then rotated to one side so that nose, malar eminence and supraorbital ridge make a 'three point landing' on the film. Centring is through the external auditory meatus further from the film, through the orbit being examined.

The optic canal should be seen *end on*, lying in the posteroinferior quadrant of the orbit. Since comparison between the two sides is helpful, both optic canals are usually examined and the two radiographs should correspond as closely as possible. Minor deviations from the ideal projections cause considerable distortion.

Jugular foramen

A position similar to that for the submentovertical projection is used, but the head is extended 20–30° less. The foramen is seen as a crescentic or bilobular translucency anterolateral to the cervical spine.

Anatomy [2]

The standard projections are shown in Figures 83.1 to 83.4 and the detailed radioanatomy of the pituitary fossa in Figure 83.5.

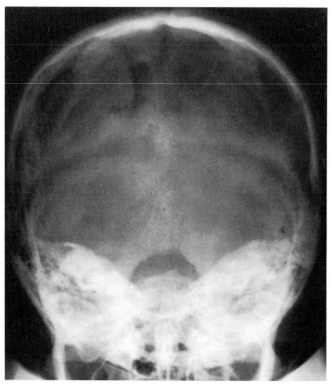

A

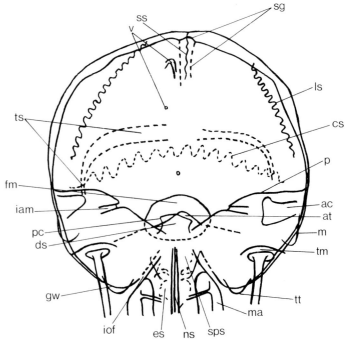

B

Fig. 83.3A & B   Half-axial (Towne's) radiograph and diagram of the skull.

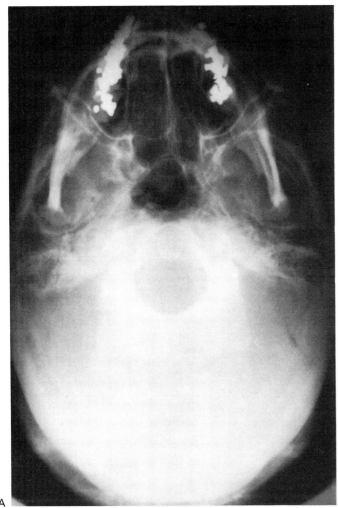

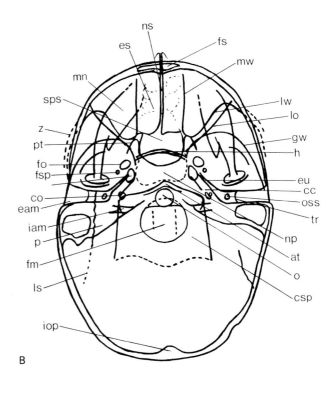

Fig. 83.4A & B Submentovertical radiograph and diagram of the skull. *Key for Figs 83.1–83.4* [a = alveolus; ac = air cells in petrous bone; am = external and internal auditory meatuses (superimposed on lateral projection); at = atlas; c = clivus; cc = carotid canal; co = cochlea; cs = coronal suture; csp = cervical spine; ds = dorsum sellae; eam = external auditory meatus; eop = external occipital protruberance; es = ethmoid sinus; eu = eustachian tube; fm = foramen magnum; fo = foramen ovale; fs = frontal sinus; fsp = foramen spinosum; fz = frontozygomatic synostosis; gw = greater wing of sphenoid bone; h = hyoid bone; hp = hard palate; iam = internal auditory meatus; il = innominate line; iof = inferior orbital fissure; iop = internal occipital protruberance; it = inferior turbinate; lo = lateral wall of orbit; ls = lambdoid suture; lw = lateral wall of maxillary antrum; m = mastoid process; ma = maxillary antrum; mm = groove for middle meningeal artery; mn = mandible; mw = medial walls of orbit and maxillary antrum (superimposed); np = nasopharynx; ns = nasal septum; o = odontoid; or = roof of orbit; os = occipital squame; oss = ossicles (auditory); p = petrous bone; pc = posterior clinoid process; pr = petrous ridge; ps = planum sphenoidale; pt = pterygoid plates; pte = pterion; rp = retropharyngeal soft tissue; sg = groove for superior sagittal sinus; sof = superior orbital fissure; sps = sphenoid sinus; sr = sphenoid ridge; ss = sagittal suture; tm = temporomandibular joint; tr = tympanic ring; ts = groove for transverse sinus; tt = temporal tubercle; v = venous markings; z = zygomatic arch]

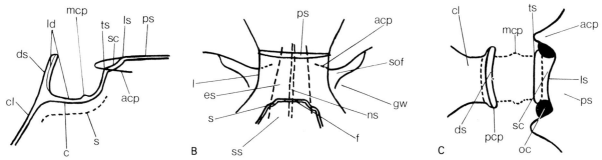

Fig. 83.5 Diagram of the sellar region. (A) lateral projection; (B) frontal projection; (C) from above [acp = anterior clinoid process; c = cortical bone lining sphenoid sinus; cl = clivus; ds = dorsum sellae; es = ethmoid sinus; f = floor of sella turcica; gw = greater wing of sphenoid; l = lamina papyracea; ld = lamina dura (cortical bone lining sella turcica); ls = limbus sphenoidale; mcp = middle clinoid process (inconstant); ns = nasal septum; oc = optic canal; pcp = posterior clinoid process; ps = planum sphenoidale; s = carotid sulcus; sc = sulcus chiasmaticus; sof = superior orbital fissure; ss = sphenoid sinus; ts = tuberculum sellae.].

For neuro-anatomical purposes, the basal portions of the cranial cavity are divided into three fossae: anterior, middle and posterior. The *anterior cranial fossa* is the space above the orbital roofs, anterior to the ridge formed by the lesser and greater wings of the sphenoid. It contains the frontal lobes and the olfactory bulbs and tracts.

The *middle cranial fossa* lies posteroinferior to the sphenoid ridge, on either side of the basisphenoid, and is bounded laterally by the squamous temporal bone and posteriorly by the petrous ridge. It contains the temporal lobe of the brain, and should not be confused with the temporal fossa, which is the extracranial space deep to the zygomatic arch.

The *posterior cranial fossa* comprises all the space below the tentorium or the central tentorial hiatus, and above the foramen magnum. It is bounded anteriorly by the clivus (basisphenoid and basiocciput) in the midline, anterolaterally by the posterior surface of the petrous bone, and elsewhere by the occipital bone. Superolaterally its extent is indicated on the skull radiographs by the groove for the transverse dural venous sinus, but in the midline the apex of the tentorium lies almost at the level of the pineal gland. Variations in the shape of the tentorium make plain film assessment of the size of the posterior cranial fossa unreliable. The fossa contains the brain stem, cerebellum, fourth ventricle, lower cranial nerves and the basilar artery.

The major compartments of the cranial cavity defined by the dural structures are shown diagrammatically in Figure 83.6.

Figure 83.7 shows two common plain film findings which should not be confused with significant pathology: calcification of portions of the dura and *normal* radiolucencies in the occipital bone.

The base of the skull contains a number of *foramina and canals*. The important data about them are summarized in Table 83.1.

Intracranial calcification

There are a number of causes of intracranial calcification that can be detected on plain radiography of the skull. These are listed in Table 83.2.

Fig. 83.6 The cranial fossae and dural reflections. The right side of the cranial vault has been removed, as have all the cranial contents apart from the dura mater. [acf = floor of the anterior cranial fossa (= orbital roof); acp = anterior clinoid process; cg = crista galli; cr = cribriform plate region; ds = dorsum sellae; f = falx cerebri; fe = free edge of the tentorium; h = tentorial hiatus; iss = inferior sagittal sinus; lst = lateral (transverse) sinus; mcf = middle cranial fossa; pr = petrous ridge; pt = pterion; s = cavernous sinus; sr = sphenoid ridge; ss = straight sinus; sss = superior sagittal sinus; t = tentorium; th = torcular Herophili (confluence of the dural venous sinuses].

Table 83.1 *The cranial foramina and canals*

Foramen/canal	Site	From	To
Optic canal	Basisphenoid	Orbital apex	Middle cranial fossa
Superior orbital fissure	Between wings of sphenoid	Orbital apex	Middle cranial fossa
Foramen rotundum	Greater wing of sphenoid	Middle cranial fossa	Pterygopalatine fossa
Pterygoid (vidian) canal	Body of sphenoid, lateral to f. rotundum	Foramen lacerum	Pterygopalatine fossa
Foramen ovale	Greater wing of sphenoid, posteriorly	Middle cranial fossa	Infratemporal fossa
Foramen spinosum	Greater wing of sphenoid, posterolateral to f. ovale	Middle cranial fossa	Infratemporal fossa
Carotid canal	Petrous temporal	Skull base	Middle cranial fossa, above f. lacerum
Internal auditory meatus	Petrous temporal	Posterior cranial fossa	
Jugular foramen	Between petrous temporal and basiocciput	Posterior cranial fossa	Extracranial jugular fossa
Foramen magnum	Basiocciput	Posterior cranial fossa	Cervical spinal canal
Hypoglossal (anterior condylar) canal	Occipital condyle	Foramen magnum	Medial to jugular fossa

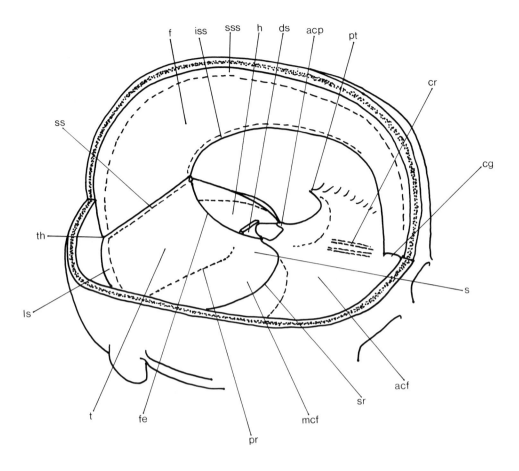

Fig. 83.6

Contents	Size	Best projection	Notes
Optic nerve and sheath; ophthalmic artery	6 mm diameter 8 mm long	Optic canal view	1 mm difference in size suspicious; keyhole and figure of eight variants
III, IV, V¹, VI; superior ophthalmic vein; middle meningeal artery branch	Very variable	Occipitofrontal	Thin greater wing may simulate erosion of lower border
V², artery of the foramen rotundum	3–4 mm diameter	Occipitofrontal	May be surrounded by extensive sphenoid sinus
Vidian nerve and artery	smaller than f. rotundum	Occipitofrontal	
V³, accessory meningeal artery; veins	5 × 9.5 mm	Submentovertical	Frequently poorly seen on one or both sides. May be confluent with f. spinosum
Middle meningeal artery	2.5–3 mm; rarely 5 mm	Submentovertical	May be double
Internal carotid artery and sympathetic plexus	6–9 mm diameter; 1.5 cm + in length	Submentovertical	Runs posteromedial to Eustachian tube; rarely passes through middle ear; absent in aplasia of internal carotid artery.
VII, VIII and dural sheath; internal auditory artery	5–6 mm in height	Perorbital	Height difference of 2 mm+ or difference in length of 2.5 mm+ suspicious
Pars nervosa: IX, inferior petrosal sinus; pars vascularis: X, XI, internal jugular vein and ascending pharyngeal and occipital artery branches	11 × 17 mm; right often larger	Under tilted submentovertical	Partes nervosa and vascularis may be separate
Medulla oblongata, meninges and ligaments; XI (spinal root); vertebral and spinal arteries and veins	30 × 35 mm	Lateral; submentovertical	Shape very variable
XII; branch of ascending pharyngeal artery	5 mm diameter	Reversed Stenvers'; Stockholm 'C'	

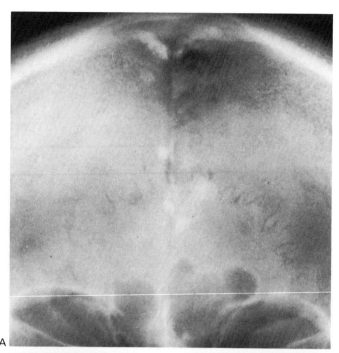

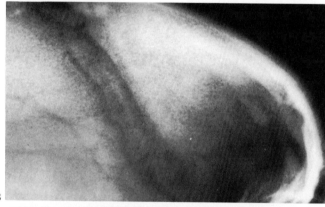

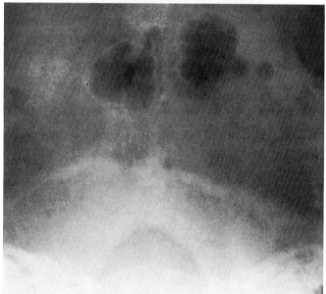

Fig. 83.7A, B & C   Common normal skull variants. (A) & (B) Dural ossification; (C): 'glial rests' in the occipital bone.

Table 83:2 Causes of intracranial calcification

Pineal gland

Habenular commisure

Choroid plexus (10% of normal persons)

Arachnoid granulations

Dura
    Falx cerebri (7% of normal individuals)
    Falx cerebelli
    Diaphragma sellae
    Dural plaques

Ligaments (petroclinoid and interclinoid)

Basal ganglia

Dentate nucleus

Carotid syphon (in elderly)

Lens (in elderly people)

Computerized tomography (CT)

A standard CT examination of the head consists of a series of tomographic sections 1 cm in thickness, at 1 cm intervals, from skull base to vertex. The orbitomeatal line is commonly used as the base line, but sections may be angled in either direction. Views with increased extension may be preferred for examination of the posterior fossa since if the chin is extended, the beam will not pass through the orbits, thereby reducing radiation dose to the eyes. Most adult heads can be covered in 10 to 20 sections.

Modifications of this protocol are employed in studies of localized areas such as the posterior cranial fossa, the cranio-cervical junction, the sella turcica, orbits, nasopharynx and petrous bone. In these contexts, the clinical features usually indicate precisely the area of interest. In general, the modifications consist of the use of thinner sections, with or without overlap, changes in the plane of section, computer reformation into other planes, magnification of small areas of interest, and the use of contrast media, usually intra-venous or intrathecal.

The *posterior cranial fossa* poses difficulties in CT imaging: the surrounding dense bony structures, the petrous pyramids and the occipital protuberances induce artefacts which obscure important detail; lesions tend to be relatively small when they cause symptoms, making their detection more difficult. The disease processes which occur in the cerebellum and brain stem are sufficiently different from those above the tentorium to render CT interpretation more problematic.

These inherent difficulties may be countered by using more sections, with overlap between them, thinner sections, or both. A common routine in cases of suspected posterior fossa mass lesion is to scan the posterior cranial fossa with 5 mm contiguous cuts, and to complete the examination of the supratentorial structures with 10 mm sections. Intravenous or intrathecal contrast medium is more frequently required for the establishment of normality in the posterior fossa than above the tentorium.

Studies of the *petrous bone* are carried out with a dense bone algorithm, if available, and many workers use only the coronal projection for this type of study, rather than the axial; the result more resembles conventional tomography of the petrous bone.

If standard CT studies show no evidence of an intracranial lesion when an VIII nerve tumour is suspected, the internal auditory meatus can be conveniently and expeditiously examined using a small volume of air (or oxygen) as the contrast medium [3]. Meatography can be carried out as an outpatient procedure and is very effective in excluding even very small neuromas. The patient lies in the lateral decubitus position with the suspect side uppermost. The head is elevated by the patient raising himself up on one elbow and 2 to 3 ml of air are injected via lumbar puncture. Thin sections are then obtained through the internal auditory meatus and cerebellopontine angle cistern. In the normal, the air enters the meatus (accompanied by a subjective 'pop'), but tumours obstruct the passage of air into the canal, and may project into the cistern.

The *craniocervical junction* is best studied with intrathecal contrast medium, since soft tissue detail at this level is unreliable even with advanced machines. Thin, closely spaced CT sections are obtained, which may be subjected to computer reformation into coronal, sagittal or other planes.

The *pituitary fossa*, being a relatively small structure in which microadenomas only a few millimetres in size may be sought, is best studied with contiguous fine (1.5 mm) CT sections. Reformation in coronal and sagittal planes is extremely helpful for assessment of the configuration of the diaphragma sellae, which is of importance. On most machines, artefacts interfere with direct coronal sections. Intravenous contrast medium is essential for clear definition of small tumours. Intrathecal contrast medium is not usually necessary if high quality computer reformations are available.

Contrast media for CT [4]

These are discussed in more detail elsewhere. In general neuroradiological practice, only intravenous and intrathecal water soluble contrast media are used, apart from air, as mentioned above, which is generally reserved for the very specific problem of small cerebellopontine angle tumours.

For *intravenous contrast enhancement*, any of the commercially available water soluble contrast medium solutions is acceptable. There are theoretical reasons for avoiding large doses of sodium salts, but in practice they do not seem of great importance. At least 35 to 40 g of iodine should be injected, by bolus or drip infusion; some authorities advocate twice this dose, but renal failure is a greater risk, and the diagnostic gain is very limited. Delayed studies at 30 minutes to 1 hour after injection have some theoretical advantages, but in practice are rarely necessary; most scans can be carried out immediately after injection of the contrast medium.

The question of when to or when not to use contrast medium for cranial CT cannot always be answered in a 'cookbook' fashion. Each case must be analyzed from the aspects of clinical presentation, previous diagnostic studies, renal and cardiac function, and allergic diathesis. In addition, a clear idea of the information required from the CT study will help in the decision. General rules can, however be formulated. Clinical suspicion of acute traumatic or other haemorrhagic lesions indicates a study without intravenous contrast medium, as does evaluation of hydrocephalus, chronic dementia and many congenital malformations. A history of allergy to contrast medium is a relative contraindication to its use, as are impaired renal function, multiple myeloma and sickle cell disease.

Indications for contrast medium administration hinge on the suspicion that an abnormality of the blood brain barrier (other than cerebral oedema) will be present, or that a hypervascular lesion is to be found. Most primary brain tumours, metastases and arteriovenous malformations are visible without the use of contrast medium; but the slightly increased detection rate and, the significantly increased accuracy of diagnosis make contrast scanning the method of choice in such cases. Infective or inflammatory processes, arteriovenous malformations, some aneurysms and a small proportion of extracerebral fluid collections may also benefit diagnostically from intravenous contrast medium.

A major category of patients referred for CT studies has not been mentioned: those with ischaemic lesions (stroke, cerebrovascular accident, transient ischaemic attack, etc.). It is arguable that most typical cases of acute stroke do not need CT examination. Moreover, the most cogent argument for CT in this context is to exclude a cerebral haemorrhage or haemorrhagic infarction, and for this no contrast medium is necessary. While it is true that cerebral infarcts usually exhibit contrast enhancement at some point in their evolution, it rarely aids in diagnosis, and has no known prognostic significance [5]. The preferred method of CT study of cases of acute stroke is therefore without intravenous contrast medium, and only if the images suggest an alternative diagnosis is contrast medium given.

Ideally, all patients should be studied in the first instance without intravenous contrast medium, and the decision as to whether to proceed is based on the clinical and CT findings in each case. This may be a counsel of perfection in the busy department, and in many centres patients who will need intravenous contrast medium are injected before the CT study begins.

Metrizamide, iopamidol and iohexol are the only currently available *intrathecal contrast agents*. The contrast medium is injected in isotonic solution, usually by lumbar puncture; 4 to 5 ml are usually adequate. The contrast medium is run up to the upper cervical region by slight head down tilt, with fluoroscopic control. The latter also detects extra-arachnoid injection. Complications and contraindications are discussed in Chapter 87.

The major indications for cranial CT with intrathecal contrast medium are:

1. Study of the cerebrospinal fluid circulation in suspected hydrocephalus
2. Examination of the craniocervical junction
3. Investigation of small extra axial tumours, e.g. acoustic neuroma

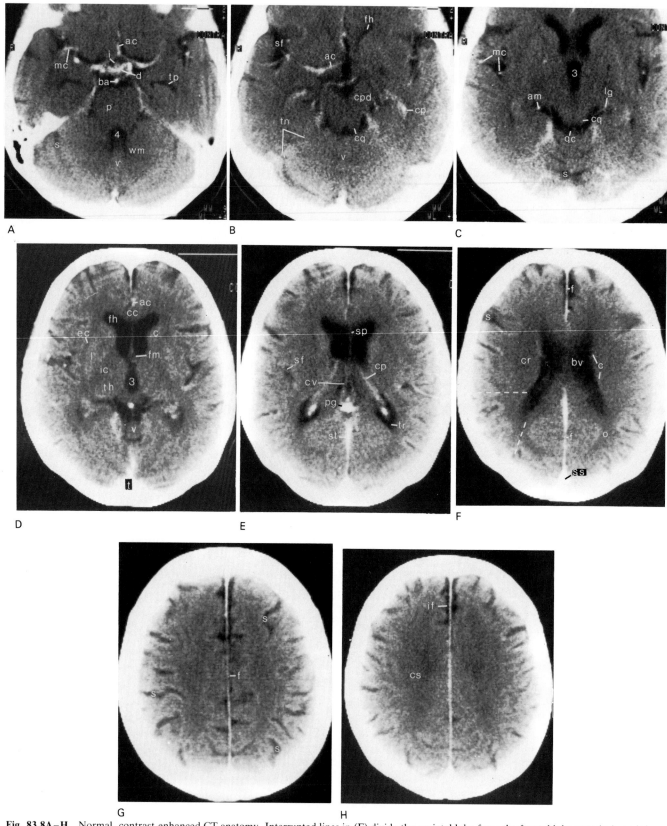

Fig. 83.8A–H Normal, contrast-enhanced CT anatomy. Interrupted lines in (F) divide the parietal lobe from the frontal lobe anteriorly and the occipital lobe posteriorly; note how small the parietal lobe is. [3,4 = third and fourth ventricles; ac = anterior cerebral artery; am = ambient cistern; ba = basilar artery; bv = body of the lateral ventricle; c = caudate nucleus; cc = corpus callosum (genu); cp = choroid plexus; cpd = cerebral peduncle; cq = corpora quadrigemina; cr = corona radiata; cs = centrum semiovale; cv = internal cerebral vein; d = dorsum sellae; ec = external capsule; f = falx cerebri; fh = frontal horn of lateral ventricle; fm = foramen of Monro; i = infundibulum; ic = internal capsule (posterior limb); if = interhemispheric fissure; l = lentiform nucleus; lg = lateral geniculate body; mc = middle cerebral artery and branches; o = white matter tracts, including optic radiations; p = pons; pg = pineal; qc = quadrigeminal cistern; s = sulcus; sf = Sylvian fissure; ss = superior sagittal sinus; st = straight sinus; t = torcular Herophili; th = thalamus; tn = tentorium; tp = temporal horn and tr = trigone of lateral ventricle; v = vermis; w = white matter of cerebellum].

4. Assessment of degree of communication of presumed cystic lesions and the subarachnoid space
5. Study of cerebrospinal fluid fistulae.

Exquisite detail of the posterior fossa, suprasellar and cisternal anatomy can also be obtained, which may be diagnostically significant.

Anatomy [6]

The normal brain CT study can of course be interpreted only with a working knowledge of classical and sectional anatomy. Numerous atlases are available, but day to day practice affords the opportunity to become familiar with the wealth of detail demonstrated on modern CT images. The accompanying Figure 83.8 shows a normal brain study. Normal structures which show contrast enhancement (because they do not have a blood-brain barrier) are indicated. Cisternal anatomy is displayed with intrathecal non-ionic, water-soluble media.

When viewing a CT examination, one should always seek and evaluate certain anatomical features [7]. The lateral ventricles should always be symmetrical but allowance must be made for the fact that in the majority of normal subjects the volumes of the left (dominant) cerebral hemisphere, and the ventricle within it, are greater than on the right side. The occipital horns of the lateral ventricles especially may be very unequal in size. Coaption of one frontal horn, also seen in normal individuals, may cause that side (usually the right) to appear smaller than its fellow. However, the midline structures, the septum pellucidum, fornices, third ventricle and pineal gland should not lie more than 1 to 2 mm from the midline. The insular cistern (Sylvian cistern, circular sulcus) is often slightly larger on the right than on the left. The other subarachnoid cisterns: suprasellar, pineal, quadrigeminal and ambient should, however be symmetrical.

Cerebral (and cerebellar) sulci are an index of the relative volumes of brain and cranial cavity, and give valuable information about mass effect on the hemispheres, from within or from without. Much has been written concerning the size

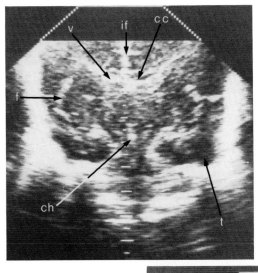

A

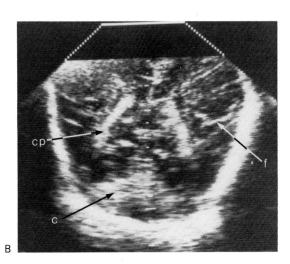

B

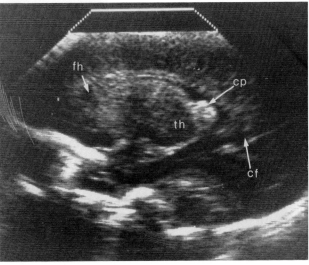

C

Fig. 83.9 Normal cranial ultrasound via the anterior fontanelle. (a) coronal, (b) coronal, posterior angulation and (c) para-sagittal images. Key: c = cerebellum; cc = corpus callosum; cf = calcarine fissure; ch = chiasmatic cistern; cp = choroid plexus; f = Sylvian fissure; fh = frontal horn of lateral ventricle; if = interhemispheric fissure; t = temporal lobe; th = thalamus; v = lateral ventricle.

of the sulci relative to the age of the patient, and normal indices have been proposed. In general, one learns from experience the normal range of size and distribution of the sulci, depending on the patient's age, the patient population with which one normally works, and the individual CT scanner. Asymmetrical enlargement or obliteration of sulci, however, is always abnormal.

In the posterior cranial fossa, the fourth ventricle is midline and symmetrical, and lies approximately half way along Twining's line, ie. between the tuberculum sellae and the torcular Herophili. The cerebellopontine angle cisterns should also be symmetrical.

After the ventricles, cisterns and sulci have been evaluated, the radiodensity of the cerebral substance should be analyzed. Normal deep white matter is well delineated from the overlying cortex and the basal ganglia, which appear more radiodense. The less dense cerebellar white matter can also be identified, as can the internal and external capsules. Among the basal ganglia, the head of the caudate nucleus is usually more radiodense than the lentiform nucleus and thalamus, especially in the elderly. Its body and tail are seen as a thin dense strip running along the superolateral margin of the lateral ventricle.

A small proportion of older individuals (from middle age onwards) exhibit asymptomatic bilateral calcification of the globus pallidus; unless there are associated clinical features, investigation of calcium metabolism is not indicated, as the finding is almost invariably without apparent significance.

Calcified structures which are normally visible include the pineal gland, the glomus of the choroid plexus, and not infrequently, portions of the falx cerebri or other reflections of the dura mater (tentorium, petroclinoid ligaments, etc). Pineal calcification is only remarkable if it is unusually extensive (more than 1 cm in diameter), or present before the age of 10 years, when it may indicate a pineal region tumour. Calcification in portions of the choroid plexus other than the glomus is often normal, but, when extensive, is suggestive of neurofibromatosis.

Ultrasound [8]

Cranial ultrasound has fallen into general disuse, except in one area in which it has recently burgeoned: examination of young children. Utilizing the anterior fontanelle as an acoustic 'window' into the infant brain, a wide range of intracranial anatomy and pathology can be displayed. The most widely used technique employs real-time sector scanning with a transducer frequency of 5 to 7 MHz. Real-time scanning, as opposed to static B-mode scanning, is highly desirable if pertinent details are not to be overlooked. High frequency is required because spatial resolution must be extremely high, given the tiny structures to be visualized in the neonatal brain. A sector scanner is much more useful than the linear array type, because of its relatively wide field of view compared to the size of the fontanelle.

A standard examination consists of a series of coronal and parasagittal sections, taken at the bedside or in the incu-

bator. Supplementary views through the posterior fontanelle may be obtained, as may transaxial scans. It should be noted that these planes of scanning are complementary to the planes usually obtained at CT, so that if both ultrasound and CT are used in the investigation of a difficult problem, the data from each are also complementary.

Fine anatomical detail can be displayed in the infant cranium by this technique (Fig. 83.9). The ventricular system, choroid plexus, many of the cisterns and sulci, the mesencephalon, including the aqueduct of Sylvius, and the pulsating arteries of the circle of Willis can be visualized routinely. The posterior cranial fossa is less well delineated, but the pons, fourth ventricle and cerebellum are usually seen.

Vascular procedures

Arteriography [9]

General principles and basic arteriographic techniques are described in Chapter 94. The present discussion is therefore concerned specifically with details of the approach to the cerebral vessels.

Arch aortography is used relatively little in neuroradiological practice, although it may be indicated for examination of suspected cases of the subclavian steal syndrome. Right and left anterior oblique projections are usually employed. *Digital subtraction angiography* is now preferred in many cases (Ch. 96).

The arteries supplying the brain can be approached in various ways:

1. *Carotid artery*
   direct puncture
   transfemoral catheterization
   transaxillary catheterization

2. *Vertebral artery*
   direct puncture (anterior or lateral approach)
   transfemoral catheterization
   transaxillary catheterization
   retrograde brachial artery injection
   subclavian artery injection

Choice of technique

Puncture of the carotid artery.

In many cases this is a relatively easy procedure, and requires the minimum of equipment. It offers a rapid means of visualizing one artery, especially in the elderly, in whom catheterization may be more difficult; all neuroradiologists should be familiar with the technique. It has the disadvantages that only one major vessel is available per puncture: selective catheterization of the internal and external carotid arteries may be possible, but is more difficult than by the transfemoral route; furthermore, the hands of the operator are near the X–ray beam. Specific complications include possible subintimal injection of contrast medium, which although radiographically spectacular is usually (but not always) without clinical sequelae, except that it renders the examination useless. Hemiplegia and death may (rarely) follow a major subintimal dissection. A false aneurysm may develop at the puncture site. The needle may pass directly through an atheromatous plaque, causing distal embolism. A rare complication is formation of an arteriovenous fistula between the carotid artery and adjacent veins when both are punctured. Formation of a large haematoma in the neck is not only unsightly and uncomfortable, but can compromise the airway, and, should it occur during the procedure, may result in displacement of the larynx anterior to the contra-lateral carotid artery, which cannot then be punctured. Direct puncture of the carotid and/or vertebral arteries is more disturbing to the patient than femoral catheterization, and many radiologists prefer general anaesthesia for direct puncture techniques.

If the common carotid artery has been ligated, direct puncture above the ligature may be the only feasible approach.

Femoral artery catheterization

This is currently the method of choice in most patients without severe aorto-iliac disease. Puncture of the femoral artery is easier than that of the carotid, less unpleasant for the patient and less hazardous; peripheral spasm or symptomatic thromboembolism are rare. Almost the entire vascular tree can be reached from the one site. In elderly or extremely atherosclerotic patients, however, catheterization of the cerebral vessels may be impossible. Even if they are eventually entered, prolongation of the procedure increases both patient discomfort and the risk of complications. Specific complications of catheterization of the neck vessels include peripheral embolism due to the guide wire damaging a friable atheromatous plaque in the carotid arteries, and spasm and dissection of the cervical vessels [10]. Femoral catheterization is virtually painless and local anaesthesia is preferred by many radiologists (see below).

Transaxillary artery catheterization

In most centres this is an ancillary method. It is slightly more difficult than using the femoral artery, and attended by a significantly increased risk of complications, including damage to the brachial plexus and formation of a pseudo-aneurysm in the axilla. Access to certain vessels is more difficult. The position of the patient's arm required for manipulation of the catheter can become very tiresome during extended procedures. For these reasons, many workers prefer carotid puncture as their 'second string' technique to the preferred primary method of femoral catheterization.

Retrograde brachial angiography

Retrograde brachial angiography, by unilateral or bilateral cannulation of the brachial artery in the antecubital fossa, is now little used. It is unpleasant for the patient, involving pressure injection into the brachial artery with a distal sphygmomanometer cuff inflated above arterial pressure, and often gives poor images, since retrograde filling is totally nonselective and dependent on variations in anatomy and collateral flow. Damage to the brachial artery with peripheral ischaemia is a possible complication.

Subclavian artery puncture

This has also fallen into disuse; it is similarly nonselective, and carries the risk of pneumothorax, but was previously used for vertebral arteriography.

Direct puncture of the vertebral artery

This has been abandoned almost universally. In addition to being unpleasant for the patient, it had a well recognized failure rate, due to extravasation or spasm (avoided by gentle injection, which often gave inferior images), or even to an absent or markedly hypoplastic vessel. Damage to the vessel itself (with possible formation of an arteriovenous fistula to the vertebral veins) or to the brachial plexus, is a recognized complication. A rare but potentially fatal complication is injection of contrast medium into the cervical subarachnoid space via a long cervical nerve root sheath.

Preparation of the patient

Informed consent is essential. Assessment of the peripheral pulses is followed by shaving and skin preparation of the relevant area(s).

In many European centres, general anaesthesia is preferred for angiography. In addition to the elimination of patient discomfort, it has the advantages that movement, which can be troublesome with direct magnification e.g. of the external carotid artery, does not occur. Moreover, hyperventilation of the paralyzed, intubated patient slows cerebral blood flow in normal vessels, but not in tumours or in some ischaemic regions, where autoregulation is defective. Conversely, general anaesthesia without hyperventilation is counterproductive. Ventilation is suspended during the angiographic series, to avoid movement. Disadvantages of general anaesthesia include its own complications, increased cost and duration of the procedure, and the concealment of adverse effects of angiography.

Apparatus

Assuming femoral catheterization to be the usually preferred method, a fluoroscopic table permitting rapid changeover to serial radiography is essential, preferably with facilities for lateral fluoroscopy; video may be helpful in difficult cases. Focal spot size for radiography should not exceed 0.3 mm; for direct magnification of two or three times, without loss of definition, a 0.1 to 0.2 mm focus is essential. A serial changer for 30 × 24 cm or 35 × 35 cm films, capable of at least three films/second should be available.

Choice of catheter shape and material is a question of personal preference and the case under examination. A selection of 5F tip catheters should be available, as should straight, tapered tip, curved and exchange guide wires.

Contrast medium for intracranial use should not exceed 280 mg iodine/ml; meglumine salts are preferable to sodium salts. Low osmolar media are theoretically preferable to conventional ionic monomers (see Ch. 7). A maximum safe dose of contrast medium has not been established; it is rarely a relevant consideration, except in small children. It should be remembered that much of the contrast medium given during a prolonged angiogram has been excreted by the time later injections are given.

Technique

The Seldinger method of catheterization, (described in Ch. 94) is used. The catheter is eventually introduced into the common, internal or external carotid artery, or into the vertebral artery, depending on the clinical problem. If proximal stenosis of the vertebral artery is suspected, an injection may be made into the subclavian artery, proximal to the origin of the vertebral artery, and an anteroposterior spot radiograph obtained. This often affords a better image of this region than an arch aortogram, with much less contrast medium, and a smaller catheter. Significant stenotic disease at the aortic origin of the other major vessels is rare, and not usually amenable to treatment. It may be necessary to exclude disease at the common carotid artery bifurcation before passing the catheter more distally. This should be documented radiographically; fluoroscopic inspection is seldom adequate.

The left vertebral artery is at least as large as the right in 80 per cent of cases and should therefore be used routinely as the approach route to the vertebrobasilar system. Should it appear to be absent, it probably arises from the arch of the aorta between the left common carotid and left subclavian arteries. If the left vertebral artery is very small, catheterization of the right side is preferred. When both vertebral arteries are small and one of them must be injected, it is frequently wise to withdraw the catheter into the aortic arch between injections, unless catheterization proved difficult initially and the vertebral may be difficult to re-enter.

Catheterization of the external carotid artery and its branches is facilitated by rotation of the head to the opposite side, but if the examination is likely to be protracted, lateral fluoroscopy is desirable. Once the catheter is beyond the arch of the aorta, a double flush technique — withdrawing into one syringe and flushing with another — should be used to decrease the risk of embolism.

Injection of contrast medium may be manual or mechanized; 6 to 8 ml of contrast medium are delivered in 1.5 to 2.0 seconds. Slower injection is used in the external carotid artery.

When general anaesthesia is employed, a series of two films per second for 2 seconds, then one film per second for five to seven films is often used for lateral series; the faster filming over the first 2 seconds can be omitted for the anteroposterior projection. A mask film, for subtraction purposes, can be exposed at the beginning of the series, at its end, or

both. Shorter series of films may be used when only the arterial phase is of interest (as in some series in patients with subarachnoid haemorrhage); a prolonged or more widely spaced series may be necessary for satisfactory demonstration of the venous sinuses.

For the vertebrobasilar system, a series of three films at one per second, followed by a pause of 3 to 4 seconds, then a further three films at one per second, is often adequate to display the arterial and venous phases.

For lateral carotid arteriography, the film is centred on the sella turcica, while for the anteroposterior series the petrous ridge is projected approximately over the roof of the orbit; this may be achieved by flexion of the neck, or angulation of the tube, and the angle may be changed depending on the shape of the individual patient, and the clinical problem. Further projections are described in the appropriate sections of Chapters 84, 85 & 86.

Three standard projections are employed for the vertebrobasilar system: lateral, half axial (Towne's) and anteroposterior, in which the petrous bone is superimposed on the lower border of the orbit.

Direct magnification (usually 2:1) series can be obtained to supplement standard projections, or if the clinical problem is restricted to a small area, this may be the only series required. The use of 35 × 35 cm films permits routine macroangiography. Photographic subtraction is frequently employed.

Digital subtraction angiography is described in Ch. 96 The indications for this and other radiological investigations are discussed at the end of this chapter.

Contraindications

There are very few absolute contraindications to cerebral angiography, but since the procedure is expensive, time consuming and not without risk, it should never be carried out if it is clear that the results will not influence management. A well documented history of allergic reactions to angiographic contrast medium administered intra-arterially is a relative contraindication. Patients with acute cerebral ischaemia may react poorly to angiography, and it should probably be avoided; conversely, treatment with anticoagulant drugs does not prohibit arteriography, providing the prothrombin level is within the normal therapeutic range. Surgical ligation of vessels may render angiography impossible.

Anatomy [11] of the cerebral arteries and veins

The skull, together with its contents and external coverings, is supplied by two carotid and two vertebral arteries.

The carotid system

The *right common carotid artery* is the first main branch of the *innominate* or *brachiocephalic artery*; the latter is often only a few centimetres long. The *left common carotid artery* is the second main branch of the aortic arch, after the innom-

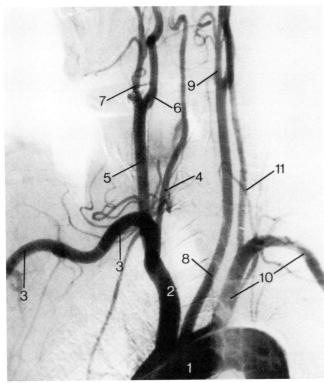

Fig. 83.10 Arch aortogram, left anterior oblique projection, arterial phase [1 = arch of aorta; 2 = innominate (brachiocephalic) artery; 3 = right subclavian artery; 4 = right vertebral artery; 5 = right common carotid artery; 6 = right internal carotid artery; 7 = right external carotid artery; 8 = left common carotid artery; 9 = left external carotid artery; 10 = left subclavian artery; 11 = left vertebral artery].

inate artery (Fig. 83.10). The two common carotid arteries run in a fascial plane, the carotid sheath, lateral to the vertebral column, dividing around the level of the fourth cervical vertebra into the *external* and *internal carotid arteries*. In the neck, the internal carotid artery lies posterior to the external, at first lateral, and then medial to it.

The internal carotid artery

The internal carotid artery usually gives no major branches before entering the skull, which it does at the base of the petrous bone. It then runs forwards, medially and slightly downwards in the bony carotid canal, posteromedial and parallel to the Eustachian tube, turning upwards above the foramen lacerum. Within the cranial cavity, it lies at first external to the dura mater, then within the cavernous sinus, before entering the subarachnoid space at the level of the anterior clinoid process. The tortuous portion formed by the cavernous and supraclinoid segments is the *carotid siphon*. Just beyond the siphon, the internal carotid artery terminates by dividing into the *anterior* and *middle cerebral arteries* (Fig. 83.11).

Principal branches of the internal carotid artery are:

1. The *meningohypophyseal artery* (which is small, but occasionally of diagnostic importance), which is given off within the cavernous sinus, and whose territory of supply is indicated by its name.
2. The *ophthalmic artery*, which is usually given off just after the internal carotid artery leaves the cavernous sinus, but whose origin is variable.

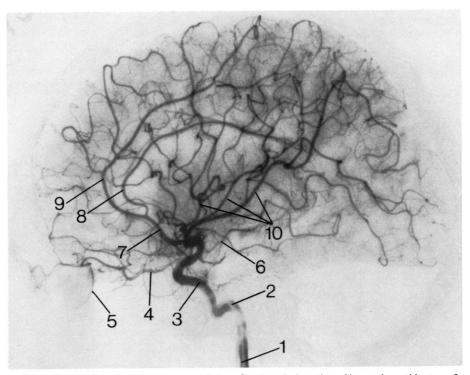

Fig. 83.11 Internal carotid arteriogram; lateral projection, arterial phase [1 = cervical portion of internal carotid artery; 2 = petrous portion; 3 = cavernous portion (siphon); 4 = ophthalmic artery; 5 = choroidal (ophthalmic) crescent; 6 = anterior choroidal artery; 7 = anterior cerebral artery; 8 = pericallosal artery; 9 = callosomarginal artery; 10 = middle cerebral artery branches].

3. The *posterior communicating artery*, which arises posteriorly from the distal portion of the carotid siphon, and links the internal carotid artery with the posterior cerebral artery; it is very variable in size and, when small, is inconstantly opacified by carotid injection.
4. The *anterior choroidal artery*, which arises from the posterior aspect of the carotid siphon just above the posterior communicating branch, to run posterosuperiorly and medially to the temporal horn of the lateral ventricle, and the surrounding structures.
5. The *anterior cerebral artery*.
6. The *middle cerebral artery*.

The *anterior cerebral artery* runs medially beneath the brain to the midline, where it is joined to its fellow of the opposite side by the *anterior communicating artery*. This first segment has one major branch, the *recurrent artery of Huebner*, so called because it arcs superolaterally to join the lenticulostriate arteries, which arise from the middle cerebral artery (vide infra). Variations occur: the first segment of the anterior cerebral artery may be hypoplastic on one side, in which case the distal segments are filled preferentially from the other side via the anterior communicating artery, or two separate segments can fuse in the midline to give rise to a single, large 'azygos' anterior cerebral artery distally, which supplies both cerebral hemispheres.

Distal to the anterior communicating artery, the anterior cerebral first turns upwards and then curves backwards on the upper surface of the corpus callosum. Its branching system is variable, but three main trunks are often identified: *frontopolar*, *callosomarginal* and *pericallosal*. The names of the first and last are self explanatory; the callosomarginal artery runs from the pericallosal up to the superior border of the hemisphere in the frontoparietal region. On the anteroposterior projection, these vessels lie near to the midline, then branch out laterally more distally. They supply the anterior two thirds of the medial surface of the cerebral hemisphere, turning over its superomedial angle to anastomose with branches from the middle cerebral artery.

The middle cerebral artery runs laterally and enters the Sylvian fissure, overlying the insula. Occasionally, an accessory middle cerebral artery arises from the distal internal carotid, or even from the proximal anterior cerebral artery. As it reaches the insula, the middle cerebral artery divides, typically into three main cortical branches, but before it does so it gives of a leash of fine vessels, the *medial* and *lateral lenticulostriate arteries*. These run a serpentine posterosuperior course, turning first medially, then laterally in a wider arc, before running medially again (Fig. 83.12); they supply the basal ganglia and capsular region.

The main divisions of the middle cerebral artery give *temporal branches*, which emerge from the Sylvian fissure over its inferior operculum, formed by the temporal lobe, to supply the latter. *Frontal* and *parietal branches* run up under the superior operculum, still on the insula, then turn downwards before turning up again to exit from the fissure. The characteristic loops formed by this upward and downward course generally lie with their superior curves in a straight line, the upper border of the 'Sylvian triangle'; its inferior

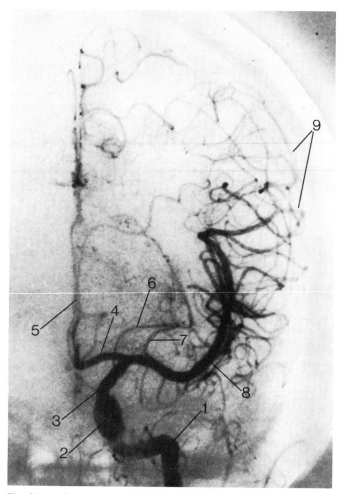

Fig. 83.12 Internal carotid arteriogram; anteroposterior projection, arterial phase [1 = petrous segment of internal carotid artery; 2 = cavernous portion; 3 = supraclinoid (subarchnoid) portion; 4 = anterior cerebral artery precommunicating segment, lying above the pituitary fossa; 5 = pericallosal and callosomarginal arteries, superimposed, lying in the midline; 6 = anterior choroidal artery; 7 = lenticulostriate artery; 8 = major divisions of the middle cerebral artery; 9 = cortical branches, which extend to the cranial vault].

border is formed by the temporal branches mentioned above. On an anteroposterior projection, these arteries are seen to pass first medially, then laterally before reaching the cranial vault; the most superomedial point of their course is referred to as the 'Sylvian point'.

Branching of the middle cerebral artery is variable, but *temporal*, *ascending frontoparietal*, *parietal*, *angular* and *posterior temporal* branches can usually be identified (Fig. 83.13). The deep territory of the middle cerebral artery, supplied by the lenticulostriate arteries, has already been described; the cortical branches supply most of the lateral surface of the cerebral hemisphere, excluding a narrow superomedial strip supplied by the anterior and posterior cerebral arteries. The middle cerebral artery also supplies a portion of the inferior surface of the temporal lobe, which may extend back to the occipital pole.

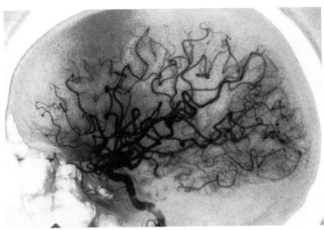

Fig. 83.13 Internal carotid angiogram, showing a common variant: hypoplasia of the anterior cerebral artery. Only the middle cerebral artery branches are filled; note how extensive they are.

External carotid artery [12]

The major branches of the *external carotid artery* are shown in Figures 83.14. They are best examined using the lateral projection. The first, anterior branch, directed inferiorly, is the *superior thyroid artery*; it may arise from the terminal common carotid artery. The *lingual* and *facial arteries* (Fig. 83.15) also arise anteriorly, sometimes from a common trunk, and run forwards, the former deep to and the latter lateral to the mandible. In addition to the structures from which they take their names, they also

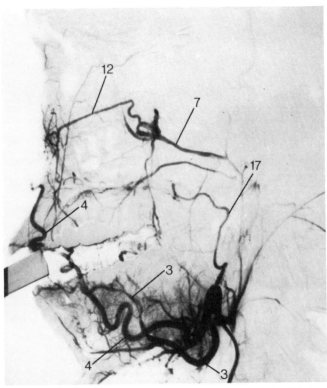

Fig. 83.15 Injection of a common linguofacial trunk; the infraorbital and internal maxillary arteries fill in a retrograde fashion.

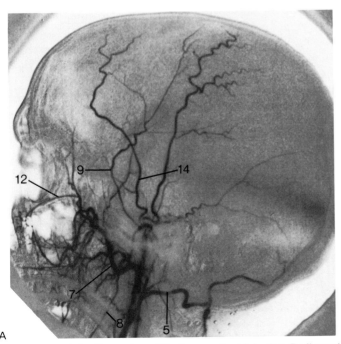

A

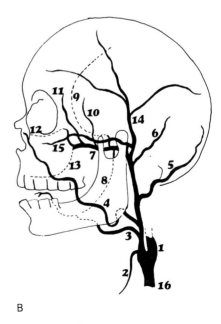

B

Fig. 83.14A & B External carotid artery proximal injection. Radiograph (A) and diagram (B) of principal branches. See Figure 83.19 for key.

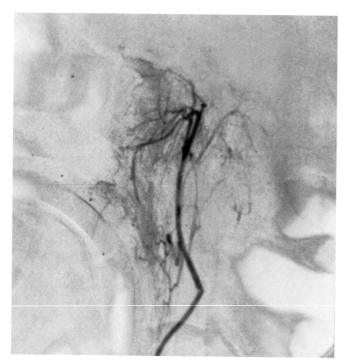

Fig. 83.16 Injection of the ascending pharyngeal artery.

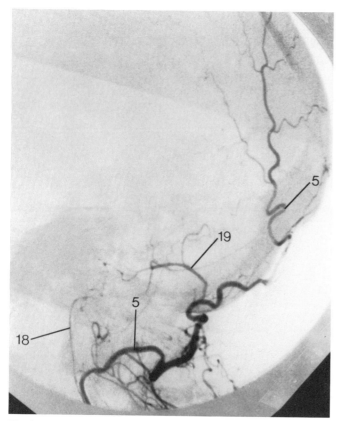

Fig. 83.17 Injection of the occipital artery; the ascending pharyngeal artery is filled by reflux. See Figure 83.19 for key.

supply the salivary glands. The *ascending pharyngeal artery* (Fig. 83.16) runs vertically upwards, often obscured on common carotid injections by the internal carotid artery, giving fine branches to the pharynx, the dura mater of the posterior cranial fossa and, in many individuals, the posterior lobe of the pituitary gland.

Posterior branches include the *occipital artery* (Fig. 83.17), through which the carotid system often communicates with the vertebrobasilar system; the artery supplies muscles, scalp and, via a petromastoid branch, the dura mater. The *posterior auricular artery* is often small.

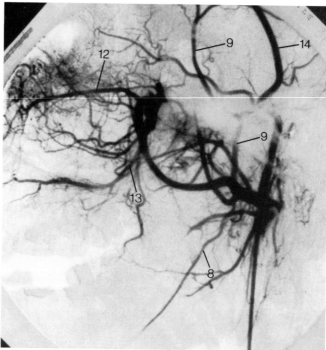

Fig. 83.18 Injection of the internal maxillary artery. See Figure 83.19 for key.

The terminal branches of the external carotid artery are the *internal maxillary* (Fig. 83.18) and *superficial temporal arteries*. The former turns forwards, deep to the mandibular condyle, giving *inferior dental, middle meningeal, deep temporal, accessory meningeal, sphenopalatine, infraorbital* and *descending palatine* branches. Of these, the middle meningeal artery (Fig. 83.19) is of greatest interest radiologically; it runs upwards, often appearing to cross the superficial temporal artery on the lateral film, through the foramen spinosum, where it makes an angular turn forwards to run in a smooth curve around the greater wing of the sphenoid and over the convexity, up to the midline. It also gives a posterior branch which runs backwards across the squamous temporal bone towards the lambda. Supplying the dura mater and the inner table of the cranium, it may also give off the ophthalmic artery; conversely, it can arise as a recurrent branch of the latter.

The superficial temporal artery is the main feeder to the scalp. It branches over the cranium, with a more tortuous

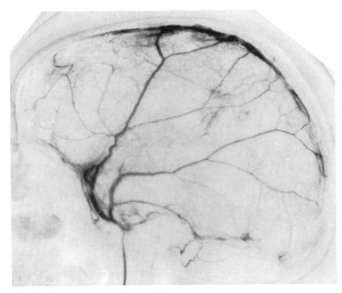

Fig. 83.19 Injection of the middle meningeal artery.
Key for Figs 83.14–83.19 [1 = internal carotid artery; 2 = superior thyroid artery; 3 = lingual artery; 4 = facial artery; 5 = occipital artery; 6 = posterior auricular artery; 7 = internal maxillary artery; 8 = inferior dental artery; 9 = middle meningeal artery; 10 = middle deep temporal artery; 11 = anterior deep temporal artery; 12 = infraorbital artery; 13 = descending (greater) palatine artery; 14 = superficial temporal artery; 15 = transverse facial artery; 16 = common carotid artery; 17 = ascending palatine artery; 18 = ascending pharyngeal artery; 19 = meningeal branch of occipital artery].

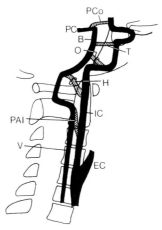

Fig. 83.20 Persistent caroticovertebral connections [B = basilar artery; EC = external carotid artery; H = hypoglossal artery; IC = internal carotid artery; 0 = otic artery; PAI = pro-atlantal intersegmental artery; PC = posterior cerebral artery; PCo = posterior communicating artery; T = trigeminal artery; V = vertebral artery].

Table 83.3 *Persistent caroticovertebral anastomoses*

Artery	Origin	Termination	Route
Pro-atlantal intersegmental	Cervical internal carotid artery	Vertebral artery	Via foramen magnum
Hypoglossal	Internal carotid artery	Vertebral artery	Via hypoglossal canal
Otic (exceptionally rare)	Petrous internal carotid artery	Basilar artery	Via internal auditory meatus
Trigeminal	Precavernous internal carotid artery	Basilar artery	Transdural

course than the middle meningeal artery. A major branch, the *transverse facial artery*, arises near its origin and runs forward parallel with the zygomatic arch.

Anastomotic pathways

The internal and external carotid systems have many actual or potential anastomotic connections, which are of importance in collateral vascularization and in interventional angiography. Principal anastomoses include:

facial artery
middle meningeal artery   } ophthalmic artery
superficial temporal artery

artery of foramen rotundum } internal carotid artery
vidian artery

Anastomotic pathways between external carotid and vertebrobasilar systems are also potentially significant:
occipital artery   } vertebral artery
ascending pharyngeal artery

The posterior communicating artery, which is very variable in size, connects the internal carotid artery to the vertebrobasilar system. When of large calibre, it is often referred to as a 'fetal' posterior communicating artery. Other developmental anastomoses can survive into adult life (Fig. 83.20 and Table 83.3). Of these, only the *trigeminal artery* is encountered with any frequency, but its incidence is still less than 1% of individuals. All of these anomalies are associated with an increased incidence of intracranial aneurysms [13].

The cerebral veins (Fig. 83.21)

The *cerebral veins* consist of two groups: the deep, *subependymal veins* and the *cortical veins*. The former are rather constant, while the latter are extremely variable. In the angiographic series, the cortical veins fill before the deep ones, and usually from frontal to occipital, but deviations from this pattern are not necessarily abnormal. *Medullary veins* run a straight course, perpendicular to the surface of the brain, between the deep and superficial groups; although they are always present, their radiological demonstration usually indicates hyperaemia.

The deep *septal vein*, courses directly posteriorly in the septum pellucidum, to join the *thalamostriate* vein as it runs anteromedially across the floor of the lateral ventricle; the two meet at the posterior lip of the foramen of Monro. This point, the *venous angle*, lies at a point midway between the external auditory meatus and the internal surface of the skull at the bregma on the lateral projection. From this

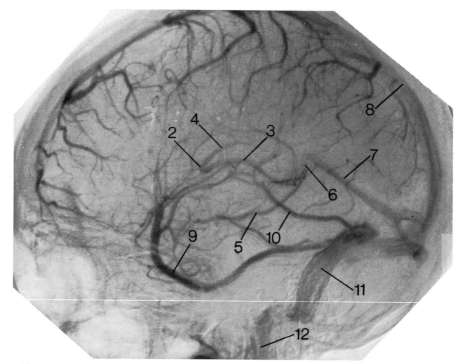

Fig. 83.21 Internal carotid arteriogram. Lateral projection, venous phase [1 = septal vein; 2 = venous angle indicating the foramen of Monro, formed by junction of 3 = internal cerebal vein and 4 = thalamostriate vein; 5 = basal vein (of Rosenthal); 6 = great vein of Galen; 7 = straight sinus; 8 = superior sagittal sinus; 9 = superficial middle cerebral vein; 10 = temporoparietal cortical vein (inferior anastomotic vein of Labbé); 11 = lateral sinus; 12 = internal jugular vein].

point, the *internal cerebral vein* runs posteriorly on the roof of the third ventricle, just to one side of the midline. All of the aforementioned veins are bilateral, as is the *basal vein (of Rosenthal)*, which arises in the region of the choroidal fissure, and arcs posterosuperiorly around the midbrain. The confluence of both internal cerebral and both basal veins gives rise to the *great vein of Galen*. This latter, despite its name, is only 1 to 2 cm long, lying in the midline, and showing a characteristic superior concavity as it lies in the quadrigeminal cistern. It discharges into the *straight sinus*, a dural venous sinus running down to the *torcular Herophili* in the junction of the falx cerebri and tentorium.

Because of their constant relationships to the ventricular system, the deep cerebral veins are very useful in the assessment of ventricular size and configuration. The position of the thalamostriate veins indicates the size of the cella media of the lateral ventricle on the anteroposterior projection, and is a much more sensitive indicator of ventricular size than the anterior cerebral arteries. Generally, the subependymal veins become visible at the point at which they reach the ventricle. An accurate impression of the shape and size of the lateral ventricles can therefore be gained from a study of the venous phase of the lateral angiographic projection.

In assessment of midline displacements, the deep veins should also be inspected. The anterior cerebral artery branches are the key to frontal displacements, but deeper, more posterior masses affect principally the deep veins.

Cortical veins divide into three main groups. The largest number drain upwards and medially to the *superior sagittal sinus*, which runs posteriorly in the midline, just below the

cranial vault, from just above the crista galli to the torcular Herophili where, being joined by the straight sinus, it bifurcates to drain into the *transverse* or *lateral sinus* on each side; the right is usually the larger. These dural sinuses run within the major dural septa: the superior sagittal sinus in the upper part of the falx cerebri and the *inferior sagittal sinus* in its lower border (running backwards to join with the great vein of Galen, discharging into the straight sinus), while the transverse sinuses run in the outer border of the tentorium itself.

Veins in the inferior frontoparietal and temporal region drain to the *superficial middle cerebral vein* and thence to the *sphenoparietal sinus*, while inferior parietal, posterior temporal and occipital veins drain directly to the transverse sinus. Large cortical veins running posterosuperiorly across the parietal lobe to the superior sagittal sinus and posteroinferiorly over the temporal lobe to the transverse sinus are the *superior and inferior anastomotic veins* (of Trolard and Labbé respectively); it is uncommon for both to be well developed.

Vertebrobasilar arterial system [14] (Figs 83.22 & 83.23)

The right and left vertebral arteries arise as the first branches of the corresponding subclavian arteries. Each vertebral artery then enters the foramen transversarium of the sixth cervical vertebra and runs directly upwards in the vertebral canal formed by these foramina before arcing laterally then medially around the arch of the atlas to pass through the

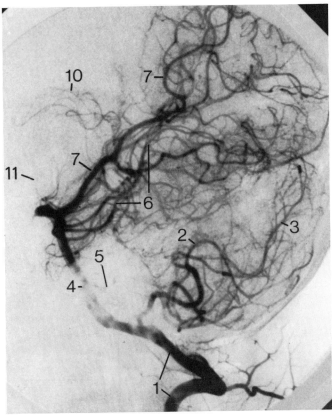

Fig. 83.22 Vertebral angiogram. Lateral projection, arterial phase
Key for Figs 83.22 & 83.23 [1 = vertebral artery; 2 = posterior inferior cerebellar artery; 3 = inferior vermian branch; 4 = basilar artery; 5 = anterior inferior cerebellar artery; 6 = superior cerebellar artery (duplicated on left); 7 = posterior cerebral arteries; 8 = posterior temporal branches; 9 = internal occipital and calcarine branches; 10 = posterior choroidal arteries; 11 = thalamoperforating arteries; 12 = filling of middle cerebral arterial branches via posterior communicating artery].

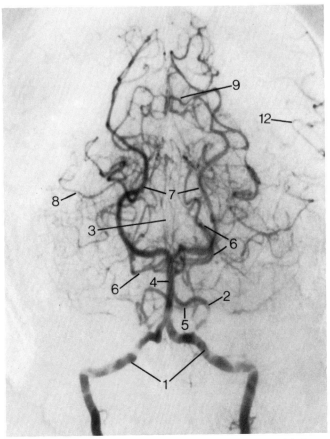

Fig. 83.23 Vertebral angiogram. Half-axial projection, arterial phase.

dura mater and enter the subarachnoid space at the level of the foramen magnum, subsequently fusing with its fellow behind the lower clivus and in front of the lower pons, to give rise to the midline *basilar artery*. The vertebral arteries give muscular branches, which frequently anastomose with those of the ascending pharyngeal and occipital arteries, and they commonly also furnish branches to the cervical spinal cord. One or other of the vertebral arteries commonly gives off the *posterior meningeal artery*, which passes upwards through the foramen magnum to run posteriorly in the midline over the dura mater of the occipital bone. Soon after entering the cranial cavity, each vertebral artery gives off a *posterior inferior cerebellar artery*, which runs around the medulla oblongata, to lie near its fellow in the midline behind it, before running posteriorly, over the cerebellar tonsil, where it lies close to the roof of the fourth ventricle, and continuing on the undersurface of the cerebellum, as the *inferior vermian artery*. The posterior inferior cerebellar artery also gives tonsillar and hemispheric branches.

The two vertebral arteries are commonly unequal in size: when this is the case, the left is usually the larger of the two; the right is, however, larger in about 20% of cases. When one of the two arteries is very small, it frequently supplies only the ipsilateral posterior inferior cerebellar artery territory. Partial duplication or 'fenestration' of the vertebral artery is a relatively rare anomaly, of no clinical significance.

The basilar artery runs upwards on the anterior surface of the pons, separating it from the clivus and giving off *anterior inferior cerebellar, superior cerebellar* and *posterior cerebral arteries* on both sides. Terminating just above the tip of the dorsum sellae, it generally shows a slight anterior convexity, and deviates from the midline in a curve away from the dominant vertebral artery; its form is sufficiently variable, especially in the elderly, to render assessment of lateral displacement difficult. It may also lie up to 1 cm from the clivus in the lateral projection.

The *anterior inferior cerebellar arteries* arise about 1 cm distal to the origin of the basilar artery, to run laterally on the pons and anteroinferior surface of the cerebellum; they loop in the cerebellopontine angle, and supply the surrounding structures. Their branches include the *internal auditory arteries*, to the structures in the internal auditory meatuses. The cerebellar branches anastomose with those of the posterior inferior cerebellar artery, and there is frequently an inverse relationship: if the posterior artery is small on one side, the corresponding anterior artery is larger, branching more extensively, and vice versa.

Right and left superior cerebellar arteries arise several millimetres below the posterior cerebral arteries which are the terminal branches of the basilar artery; they are below the tentorium. One or both are frequently duplicated, in which case the individual vessels are smaller. They pass around the brain stem to fan out over the superior surface of the cerebellar hemispheres, often with a very regular ladder-like pattern, while their main trunks run backwards over the superior vermis, giving a *precentral branch* which passes downwards between the roof of the fourth ventricle and the central lobule of the cerebellum.

A T shaped bifurcation of the terminal basilar artery gives rise to the *posterior cerebral arteries*. Running first laterally, and connecting with the posterior communicating arteries, these then turn posteriorly to encompass the brain stem, lying above the tentorium. There is a reciprocity in calibre of the precommunicating segments of the posterior cerebral arteries and the posterior communicating arteries: if the latter are large, and the main source of the posterior cerebral blood flow is from the carotid arteries (sometimes referred to as the 'fetal' arrangement), the first segments of the posterior cerebral arteries may be very small. The appearances are commonly asymmetrical.

These two vessels, the proximal posterior cerebral and posterior communicating arteries, give off fine *thalamoperforating arteries*, which pass posterosuperiorly into the interpeduncular fossa to enter the posterior perforated substance; in the lateral projection, they are characteristically serpentine. A *medial posterior choroidal artery* also arises from the proximal posterior cerebral artery and passes round the midbrain, then superolaterally, describing a curve over the pulvinar of the thalamus, to reach the third ventricle. Two or more *lateral posterior choroidal arteries* arise from the posterior cerebral artery alongside the midbrain.

Although the distal cortical branching system of the posterior cerebral arteries is complex, it can be divided into two main groups: the *posterior temporal arteries*, which supply a considerable portion of the inferior surface of the temporal lobe (anastomosing with the middle cerebral artery branches) and the branches of the *internal occipital artery*, among which the *parieto-occipital* and the more inferior *calcarine arteries* supply the posterior one third of the medial surface of the cerebrum, including the visual cortex, forming anastomoses with the anterior cerebral artery anterosuperiorly and with the middle cerebral artery around the occipital pole.

Vertebrobasilar venous system (Figs 83.24 & 83.25)

Posterior mesencephalic veins run around the upper midbrain, overlying the basal veins on the lateral projection, and being continuous with smaller *circumpeduncular* veins anteriorly. In the half-axial projection, these veins outline the mesencephalon (Fig. 83.25). Posteriorly, the posterior mesencephalic veins run up to the great vein of Galen, as does the *precentral cerebellar vein*, which lies in the midline on the anterior surface of the cerebellum, posterior to the superior medullary velum, the superior part of the roof of the fourth ventricle. Its most anterior point therefore indicates the front of the cerebellum on the lateral projection, and should lie half way between the tuberculum sellae and

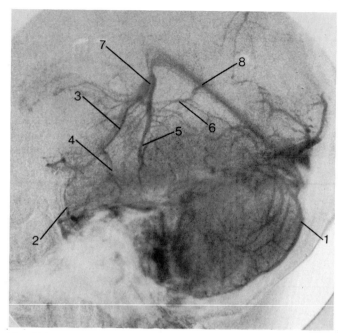

Fig. 83.24 Vertebral angiogram. Lateral projection, venous phase.

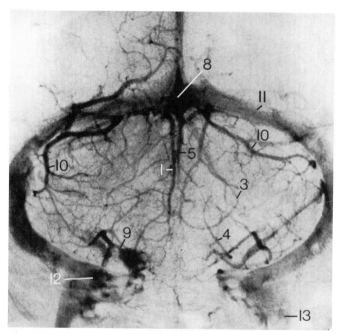

Fig. 83.25 Vertebral angiogram, half-axial projection; venous phase. *Key for Figs 83.24 & 83.25* [1 = inferior vermian vein; 2 = anterior pontomesencephalic vein; 3 = posterior mesencephalic vein; 4 = lateral mesencephalic vein; 5 = precentral cerebellar vein; 6 = superior vermian vein; 7 = great vein of Galen; 8 = straight sinus; 9 = petrosal vein; 10 = cerebellar hemispheric veins; 11 = transverse sinus; 12 = sigmoid sinus; 13 = internal jugular vein]. Note the normal asymmetry of the posterior fossa.

the torcular Herophili. *Superior and inferior vermian veins*, outlining the cerebellum above and below, typically drain to the great vein of Galen and the straight sinus respectively, but are variable (Fig. 83.24).

The *anterior pontomesencephalic vein* runs down the anterior surface of the pons and medulla, closely related to the basilar artery. It is frequently continuous with the circumpeduncular veins above, and commonly drains to the *petrosal vein*. This latter is relatively large, and closely related to the internal auditory meatus, and in turn drains to the *superior petrosal sinus*. The petrosal vein and its tributaries are normally seen clearly on the half-axial projection, often connected to the posterior mesencephalic vein by the *lateral mesencephalic vein* which, although running down the brain stem, appears on the same projection to have a medial convexity. The *vein of the lateral recess of the fourth ventricle*, often also a tributary of the petrosal vein, is small, inconstant and frequently not identified with certainty, especially when displaced.

Phlebography [15]

The orbital veins and the basal sinuses of the skull lack valves, and may thus be opacified via an anterior approach (orbital phlebography) or a posterior approach (inferior petrosal sinography). [16]. The technique of orbital phlebography is simple, although even in trained hands it has a small failure rate. Moreover, no serious complications have been described in cases in which prolonged jugular compression has been avoided.

The configuration of the inferior petrosal sinus precludes the posterior approach in almost 10% of individuals. Complications, although rarely significant, are also more frequent with this technique. The anterior approach is superior for depiction of the intraorbital veins and the cavernous sinuses, while the posterior approach is essentially used for the evaluation of problems in the jugular foramen region, or as a supplementary technique for demonstration of the posterior extent of a venous occlusion demonstrated by orbital phlebography. The indications for the latter are discussed in more detail in the chapter on orbital disease.

Either technique can be used on outpatients. No special preparation is required, although a mild sedative (such as diazepam) may be given before the examination. General anaesthesia is usually required in children.

The patient is placed on the X–ray table in the supine position, with the head extended and dependent. A tourniquet is placed around the head just above the eyes and the forehead is inspected and palpated for veins. A frontal vein will usually be found, running in the midline or close to it. A medium size conventional intravenous cannula with a coaxial catheter is advanced, with gentle suction, as far down towards the bridge of the nose as possible. After removal of the tourniquet, the position of the catheter and the venous anatomy is checked on a single film (or fluoroscopically), following slow injection of 5 to 10 ml contrast medium. To direct the flow of contrast medium into the orbits, the tourniquet is reapplied, this time just cranial to the tip of the catheter, and the angular veins are occluded manually (by the patient), or with another tourniquet. A complete examination of the orbits may include radiographs in anteroposterior, semiaxial (10 to 40° craniad angulation) basal, and straight (and/or oblique) lateral projections. Because of

radiation dose and contrast medium dose, not all of these views are routinely obtained. The basal view is usually sufficient for evaluation of the cavernous sinus and adjacent structures. For each projection, three to five films are exposed at 1 to 2 second intervals; 8 to 10 ml contrast medium are injected rapidly, commencing immediately after the first exposure. If a venous anomaly is being sought, a more extended series may be required.

For examination of the jugular bulb, injection into the internal jugular vein is adequate, but for a study of the cavernous sinus by the posterior route, injection into the inferior petrosal sinus may be required. Satisfactory opacification may not be obtained without simultaneous bilateral injections.

The jugular vein may be catheterized from the femoral vein, or punctured percutaneously. For the latter procedure, the patient lies supine, prepared as for percutaneous puncture of the carotid artery. While the patient strains to dilate the jugular veins, blind puncture is performed immediately lateral to the common carotid artery, and the needle or cannula slowly withdrawn during continuous aspiration until venous blood flows. A catheter is then introduced using the Seldinger technique. Catheterization of the inferior petrosal sinus is then attempted.

Anatomy of the veins [17–19]

The *facial veins* are connected via the orbital veins to the cavernous sinuses and the basal venous sinuses of the skull. The major intraorbital vein, the *superior ophthalmic vein* (Figs. 83.26 & 83.27), is formed behind the trochlea of the superior oblique muscle by the junction of tributaries from

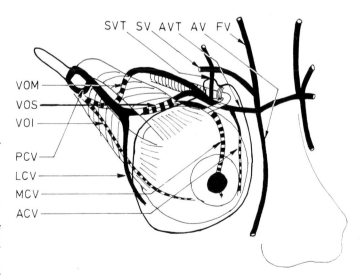

Fig. 83.26 Diagram of the right orbit, to show the veins. Tributaries [SVT, AVT] from the supraorbital [SV] and frontal [FV] veins join behind the trochlea to form the superior ophthalmic vein [VOS], which crosses laterally below the superior rectus muscle, then runs posteriorly, to leave the orbit via the superior orbital fissure. During its course it gives off medial [MCV] and lateral [LCV] collateral veins, which pass on either side of the muscle cone. Inferior [VOI] and middle [VOM] ophthalmic veins, anterior [ACV] and posterior [PCV] collateral veins and the angular vein [AV] are also shown.

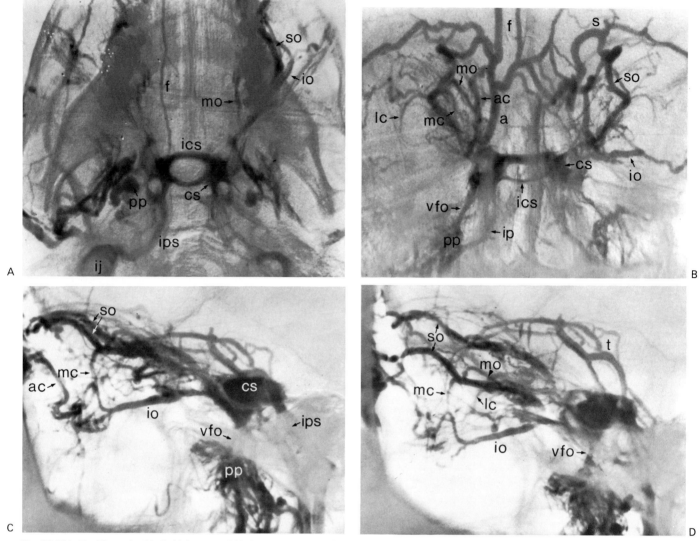

Fig. 83.27A–D   Normal orbital phlebogram. (A) Anteroposterior; (B) submentovertical; (C) true and (D) oblique lateral projections
[a = angular vein; ac, lc, mc = anterior, lateral and medial collateral veins; cs = cavernous sinus; f = frontal vein; ics = intercavernous sinus;
ij = internal jugular vein; io, mo, so = inferior, middle and superior ophthalmic veins; ips = inferior petrosal sinus; pp = pterygoid plexus;
t = temporal veins (extracranial); s = supraorbital vein; vfo = vein of the foramen ovale].

the *angular and supraorbital veins*. It crosses laterally below the superior rectus, and follows its lateral border back to the superior orbital fissures, through which it passses to empty into the cavernous sinus. The vein normally appears narrowed as it passes through the fissure. The superior ophthalmic vein is connected to *inferior orbital veins* by the *collateral* or *absidal veins* on either side of the muscle cone.

The *cavernous sinuses* are located on either side of the sella turcica, extending from the superior orbital fissure to the petrous apex. They are connected to each other by the *anterior* and *posterior intercavernous sinuses* and through the *basilar venous plexus*, which lies on the clivus. Anteriorly, the sinus has connections with the superior ophthalmic vein and the *sphenoparietal sinus*, running along the sphenoid ridge, and posterosuperiorly with the *superior petrosal sinus*. It drains laterally through the foramen ovale to the *pterygoid plexus*, and posteriorly, via the *inferior petrosal sinus*, to the *internal jugular vein*.

Sinography

Occasionally, when the integrity of the dural venous sinuses is of surgical importance, sinography, direct injection of contrast medium into the sinus via a surgical exposure, is carried out. With improvements in angiographic techniques, including digital subtraction angiography, which shows the veins to great advantage, this procedure has become a rarity.

Pneumography [20]

The introduction of CT has markedly reduced the indications for both *pneumoencephalography* and *ventriculography*, and when CT of high quality is universally available, it is highly probable that none will remain. The spatial resolution of CT is still inferior to that of pneumography, however, and thin septa and discrete nervous structures may be impossible to demonstrate by CT. Pneumoencephalography and ventriculography also give some information, albeit unphysiological, on the patency of the cerebrospinal fluid pathways, and on communications between the subarachnoid space and presumed cystic lesions.

Pneumoencephalography causes very significant discomfort to the patient and should therefore be performed only on very good clinical grounds, and when facilities are sufficient for an optimal examination. A complete pneumographic study is rarely indicated in the CT era: the examination is usually directed at answering specific questions which remain in spite of, or are posed by CT.

In some neurosurgical centres, ventricular drains are liberally inserted for preoperative management of patients with a possible posterior fossa space occupying lesion, or aqueduct stenosis. Ventriculography can then be performed on less stringent indications. It may be carried out with gas, oily or water soluble contrast medium. Water soluble media, because of surfaction, penetrate narrow spaces more easily than air or oil, and in contrast to oil are eliminated rapidly from the subarachnoid space. Oily media have therefore fallen into disuse.

Equipment [21]

Many varieties of sophisticated pneumoencephalographic devices have been developed, equipped with somersaulting chairs permitting an isocentric study, and with tomographic facilities enabling sections to be made with all possible combinations of beam orientation and head positioning. These purpose designed equipments greatly simplify pneumoencephalography, and provide an optimal examination. However, the small number of pneumographic studies currently performed argues against the purchase of such machines. Minimum requirements are as follows: horizontal beam tomographic facilities (preferably non-linear), and a chair suitable to support an anaesthetized patient. A somersaulting chair is desirable but not essential, and fluoroscopic facilities greatly reduce the length of the examination, and make less likely complications such as prolonged studies in patients with cerebellar tonsillar herniation, or large extra-arachnoid injections.

Gas ventriculography requires the same equipment as pneumoencephalography, but *positive contrast ventriculography* can be carried out on a normal skull unit.

Positive contrast cisternography necessitates a tilting table, and lateral fluoroscopy is extremely useful, and makes the examination safer.

Preparation of the patient

If the patient is very cooperative, pneumoencephalography or ventriculography can be carried out under local anaesthesia, but general anaesthesia is preferred and is used routinely in children. Even with local anaesthesia, the patient must fast before the study, since vomiting is not uncommon. Atropine and a sedative drug such as a barbiturate are commonly used for premedication; an anti-emetic can usefully be added.

Ventriculography with water soluble or other contrast medium requires appropriate anaesthesia for the burr hole and any other preceding surgical procedure; the radiological study itself causes minimal discomfort to the patient.

For water soluble cisternography, the patient must be fully cooperative or examined under general anaesthesia, since rapid, unplanned changes in position can be disastrous as regards the radiographic results, and hazardous for the patient. Barbiturates may be given as premedication to reduce the risk of seizures, but since they take 48 to 72 hours to be effective, this is not always feasible.

Techniques

Pneumoencephalography

The patient is placed in the chair with the upper part of the neck well flexed so that the orbitomeatal plane is angled at least 10° downwards in the sitting position. Lumbar puncture is then performed at L2/3 or below. A fine (e.g. 22 SWG) needle is used, to minimize postencephalographic headache; withdrawal of spinal fluid for analysis is kept to a minimum for the same reason.

A small amount of air (5 to 10 ml) is then injected, with fluoroscopic observation of the craniocervical junction to detect any cerebellar tonsillar herniation at as early a stage as possible. If fluoroscopy is not available, a spot film is taken after 5 ml of gas have been injected, and no further injections made until this has been inspected. If downward herniation of the tonsils blocks the passage of air (Fig. 83.28), the examination is usually terminated, unless prompt

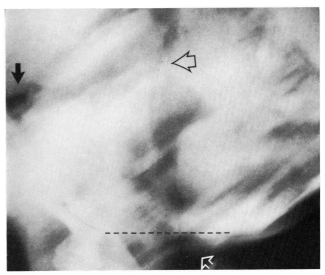

Fig. 83.28 Tonsillar herniation. The cerebellar tonsils [lower arrow] project through the foramen magnum, indicated by the dotted line. Air does not enter the aqueduct, which is displaced posteriorly [open arrow]. The floor of the third ventricle is pushed downwards [arrow]. The examination was terminated forthwith.

neurosurgical assistance is at hand. If no block is encountered, a further 10 to 15 ml of gas are injected slowly. Normally, the air fills the cisterna magna, and then, following its entrance into the fourth and third ventricles, can be seen bubbling up into the lateral ventricles. Occasionally an 'incompetent' cisterna magna permits the air to escape upwards over the cerebellum. This should not be mistaken for a subdural injection of air. In the subdural space, the air is seen as sharply defined slits of low density beneath the tentorium, which do not outline the normal contours of the brain.

Three films are then exposed: one posteroanterior film, with the beam parallel to the floor of the anterior fossa, a lateral projection, centred on the sella turcica or posterior cranial fossa, and a midline lateral tomogram, centered in the same way (Fig. 83.29). The chin of the patient is then extended, and another 10 cm³ of gas are injected, to fill the basal cisterns. After positioning the patient as before, three further films are exposed: a posteroanterior, as previously, another with the beam parallel to the clivus, and a lateral projection or tomogram (Fig. 83.30). The radiologist then has to decide whether the examination of the posterior fossa is complete (before the patient is moved to another position), or, as is frequently the case, further films are required. If the cerebellopontine angle is suspect, axial tomography, with the beam parallel to the clivus, is performed.

The patient is then rotated backwards to the supine position, which usually improves filling of the supratentorial ventricular system, and films are again exposed in the three standard projections. If the suprasellar region is of special interest and filling of the third ventricle is suboptimal, the supine patient can be tilted further backwards and the head extended to the 'hanging head' position. Horizontal and vertical beam tomography is often then performed, preferably with complex motion (Fig. 83.31).

The full pneumoencephalographic examination then continues with forward rotation of the patient to the prone or brow down position, and films are exposed as before to demonstrate the posterior portions of the ventricles. In practice, this part of the examination is rarely helpful, and can usually be omitted.

The patient is then subjected to a full 180° forward somersault, to fill both temporal horns. This may be accomplished manually if no somersaulting chair is available. Three or four films are then exposed (Fig. 83.32): a transorbital anteroposterior, another anteroposterior view with the beam parallel with the clivus, and a straight lateral projection; a slightly oblique lateral view will throw one horn above the other.

Ventriculography

Gas ventriculography. Cerebrospinal fluid is exchanged with gas (usually room air), via a ventricular cannula introduced through a burr hole, until 15 to 30 ml. of gas have been injected. In small children, a needle may be passed through the open fontanelle. The total volume of gas will depend on the size of the ventricles and the clinical problem.

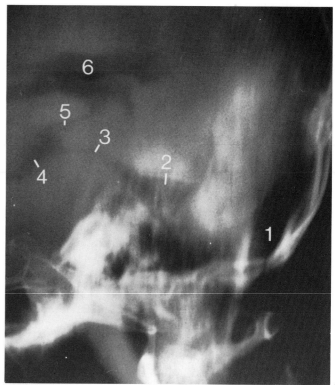

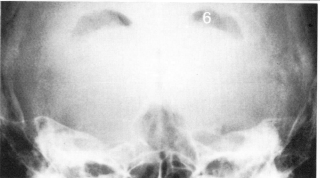

Fig. 83.29A & B Normal pneumoencephalogram, early filling phase. (A) Midline lateral tomogram; (B) posteroanterior projection [1 = cisterna magna; 2 = fourth ventricle; 3 = aqueduct of Sylvius; 4 = third ventricle; 5 = suprapineal recess of third ventricle; 6 = trigone and posterior body of lateral ventricle].

The patient may then be positioned as described above for pneumoencephalography, but ventriculography is usually required when the third ventricle, aqueduct or fourth ventricle are in question. The patient is then subjected to a slow backward somersault, to the brow down position, where appropriate films are exposed. Tomography is frequently required. Small children are easily examined without a somersaulting chair, being supported and rotated by the radiologist or an assistant.

Ventriculography with water soluble contrast medium [22]. The surgeon introduces a ventricular catheter so that its tip lies in a frontal horn, near the foramen of Monro. The patient is then sat erect, with the neck flexed and a small quantity

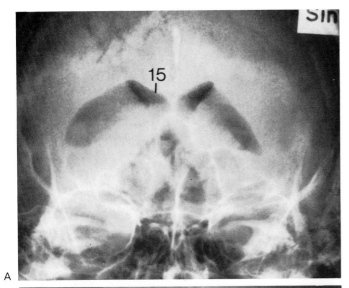

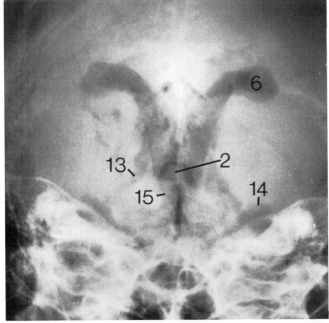

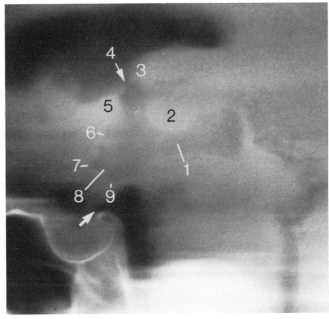

Fig. 83.31 Normal pneumoencephalogram. Midline lateral tomogram in supine (brow up) position [1 = body of third ventricle; 2 = massa intermedia; 3 = paraphysis; 4 = foramen of Monro; 5 = anterior commissure; 6 = lamina terminalis; 7 = optic recess; 8 = optic chiasm; 9 = infundibular recess; lower arrow = Liliequist's membrane].

of contrast medium (3 to 5 ml) is injected slowly, after which the head is tilted to the uninjected side and slowly raised so that the contrast medium, being heavier than cerebrospinal fluid, slowly passes down through the foramen of Monro to the third ventricle. Fluoroscopic control greatly increases the reliability of the manipulation, but is not essential. Appropriate films are then exposed in sitting and usually also supine positions. Tomography may be required but is often superfluous. The procedure is fast and simple, and causes little discomfort to the patient.

Cisternography with positive contrast media [23]. This examination is used to examine specifically the cerebellopontine angle. Iophendylate (2 to 3 ml) or a larger quantity of metrizamide, iopamidol or iohexol is injected by lumbar or cervical puncture. The use of water-soluble media entails tomography. The patient is placed in the prone position with the side of the head of interest downwards and the head turned at 45° to the trunk, so that the posterior surface of the petrous bone of the suspect side is parallel to the table top. The contrast medium is then manipulated into the cerebellopontine angle

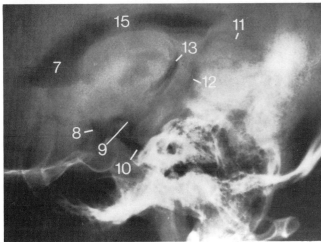

Fig. 83.30A, B & C Pneumoencephalogram, sitting position after filling of the basal cisterns. (A & B) Posteroanterior projections parallel to the floor of the anterior fossa and the clivus respectively. (C) lateral projection [1–6: as Fig. 83.29; 7 = frontal horn of lateral ventricle; 8 = chiasmatic cistern; 9 = interpeduncular fossa; 10 = pontine cistern; 11 = superior cerebellar cistern; 12 = quadrigeminal cistern; 13 = ambient cistern; 14 = cerebellopontine angle cistern; 15 = cella media of lateral ventricle].

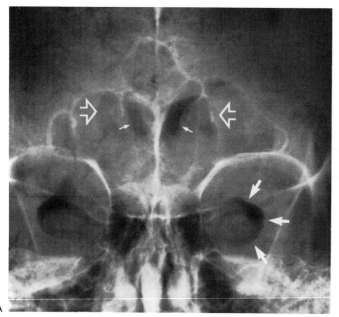

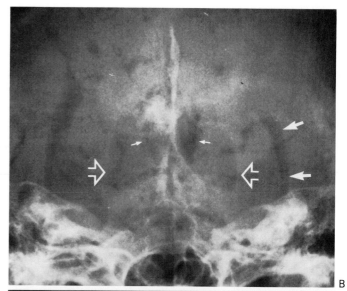

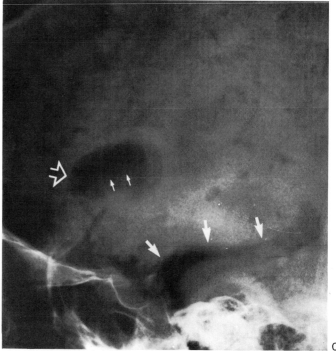

Fig. 83.32A, B & C   Pneumoencephalogram, following somersault. Brow up position perorbital (A), anteroposterior (B) and lateral projections (C). [Closed arrows = temporal horns; open arrows = tips of frontal horns; small arrows = heads of caudate nuclei].

by lowering the head, and horizontal cross table and vertical projections are obtained, to demonstrate the contrast medium in the internal auditory meatus. Alternatively, a small quantity of air can be injected to show the upper of the two meatuses; tomography is required [24]. All these techniques are little used since the development of CT gas meatography.

Complications

Pneumoencephalography. Pallor, nausea and vomiting frequently occur during the injection phase. Transient syncope is not uncommon; the examination can usually be continued, but the necessity to lower the head may prejudice the radiographic results.

Slight pyrexia is common on the following day; an increase in the cell content of the spinal fluid, mainly polymorphonuclear cells, is noted almost immediately following the procedure.

Headache is also common, and may last for several days. Some patients are prostrated after the study, and require bed rest, without elevation of the head, for some days.

Serious complications are rare. The most feared is herniation of brain through the foramen magnum (coning), under the falx cerebri or through the tentorial hiatus, due to altered pressure relationships in the subarachnoid space following tapping of the spinal fluid and gas injection. Patients with papilloedema or known brain distortions should not be submitted to pneumoencephalography.

Ventriculography. The major complication is infection; strict sterility must be observed during manipulation of the ventricular catheter. Passage of the catheter or cannula can cause intracerebral or subdural haemorrhage.

The risks and treatment of complications of water soluble contrast media are dealt with in Chapter 7.

Anatomy [15]

It is assumed that the reader is acquainted with the anatomy and nomenclature of the ventricles and subarachnoid space compartments, which are illustrated in Figures 83.29–83.32, and described in detail in textbooks of neuroanatomy. Some of the more important variants will however be discussed, along with diagnostic criteria.

Lateral ventricles

Differences in gas filling of the two lateral ventricles, which are the rule rather than the exception, may, in frontal projections suggest depression of the roof of one lateral ventricle, leading to an erroneous impression of a tumour close to the midline above the ventricle, the only sign of which may be such a depression. In the lateral view, both lateral ventricles should be smoothly outlined and symmetrical.

The floor of the anterior horn of the lateral ventricle may show a marked impression at the junction of the head of the caudate nucleus and the corpus callosum. The roof of the ventricle may show pronounced ridging caused by radiating fibre tracts. The choroid plexus is seen as a rounded filling defect, usually about 1 cm in diameter, but sometimes much larger.

The lateral ventricles are separated by the septum pellucidum, a thin membrane which is occasionally defective, and may be absent. The septum is in fact a double membrane, which commonly encloses a fluid-filled slit-like space, the cavum of the septum pellucidum, which can communicate with the lateral or third ventricles. The cavum may continue posteriorly as a cavum vergae, bordered superiorly by the body of the corpus callosum, posteriorly by the posterior column of the fornix and inferiorly by the hippocampal commissure.

The occipital horns are subject to extreme individual variations. On one side the horn may extend to within a centimetre of the occipital bone, it may be absent on the other. The shape is also very variable and rarely of diagnostic utility.

The temporal horns normally appear symmetrical. From the trigones they form a smooth gentle curve downwards and laterally to the junction of the anterior and middle thirds, where they curve medially and downwards like the bowl of a spoon.

The maximum transverse diameter of the frontal horns divided by the internal transverse diameter of the cranial cavity (Evans's encephalographic ratio) is the most commonly used index of ventricular size. The normal upper limit is 0.29 [26].

The third ventricle

This cavity (Fig. 83.31) is slit-like, its width increasing with age, and ranging from 2 to 10 mm in normal subjects. The massa intermedia is present in most cases; it is a non-neural adhesion between the thalamus on the two sides of the ventricle and should not be confused with an intraventricular mass.

The third ventricle has two recesses directed downwards and anteriorly: the *optic recess*, directed towards the cranial end of the optic canals, and behind it the *infundibular recess*, directed at the sella turcica. These recesses normally appear sharply pointed at ventriculography with water soluble contrast medium, but present a more rounded appearance at pneumoencephalography. The optic chiasm lies between them. Distortion of the recesses is an important observation in cases of suprasellar mass lesion.

The posteriorly situated *suprapineal recess* is subject to greater variation: it may measure 1–2 mm or be as much as 30 mm in length. The *pineal recess*, below the suprapineal recess and lying between the habenular and posterior commissures, is a small dimple.

The posterior commissure and the anterior commissure, (which forms the anterior margin of the foramen of Monro) are important landmarks in ventriculograms used to plan stereotactic surgery on the basal ganglia.

The aqueduct (of Sylvius)

This channel (Fig. 83.29) is usually seen best on the first filling films of the pneumoencephalogram; tomography is often necessary for clear delineation. It describes a gentle curve, most pronounced in its upper third, connecting the third and fourth ventricles. The minimum diameter is usually 1–2 mm.

The fourth ventricle

This cavity (Fig. 83.29) connects the ventricular system with the extracerebral subarachnoid space via the foramina of Luschka, which constitute the orifices of the lateral recesses of the ventricle, and the foramen of Magendie, the main outlet, which opens in the midline, where it is continuous with the vallecula. While the lateral recesses are directed laterally, forwards and downwards, two posterosuperior recesses project posterolaterally and appear on anteroposterior films as two ear-like extensions on either side of the body of the ventricle. The fourth ventricle is normally very symmetrical, and minor asymmetries usually indicate pathology.

On the lateral projection, the normal position of the fourth ventricle may be estimated by reference to Twining's line [27], which connects the tuberculum sellae and the internal occipital protuberance. The midpoint of this line lies within the fourth ventricle, near its floor.

The subarachnoid cisterns

Visualization of the subarachnoid cisterns was mandatory before the CT era for the pneumoencephalographic assessment of possible masses in the posterior fossa or suprasellar regions. Such information is still required in cases where doubt persists in these areas and may also be required to establish whether a tumour is extra-axial and potentially removable, or whether it lies within the brain.

The basal cisterns (Fig. 83.30): the cisterna magna, pontine cistern, interpeduncular and chiasmatic cisterns are connected to the cortical subarachnoid space via the ambient cisterns, passing up on each side around the brain stem to the quadrigeminal cistern, then around the splenium of the corpus callosum to the interhemispheric fissure; the Sylvian cisterns, and the cistern of the lamina terminalis, which extends upwards around the genu of the corpus callosum.

The pontine cistern is best visualized in lateral midline tomograms; it is normally 5 to 10 mm in anteroposterior dimension. Anteroposterior tomograms, with the central ray parallel with the clivus, are best for the cerebellopontine angle and ambient cisterns.

The chiasmatic cistern requires complex motion tomography for optimal demonstration. As encephalography is nowadays usually performed to exclude small lesions in this region, access to such facilities is very desirable.

There is normally free communication between the subarachnoid cisterns, which are no more than arbitrary divisions of a continuous space. However, within the interpeduncular cistern, the membrane of Liliequist (Fig 83.31), between the third nerves often causes a temporary arrest of gas flow; this is a normal finding, and should not be misinterpreted as a sign of basal arachnoiditis.

Interpretation of air studies

When a pneumoencephalogram or ventriculogram is being analyzed, the following are assessed.

1. The ventricular system

  (a) Enlargement
    — generalized, as in communicating hydrocephalus or global cerebral atrophy
    — involving one lateral ventricle only, due to focal atrophy or obstruction at the foramen of Monro
    — asymmetrical, in combination with dislocation (and probably also herniation), as caused by a tumour
    — localized, due to local cerebral atrophy
  (b) Dislocation
    — of the midline structures
    — of various portions of the system
  (c) Deformity
  (d) Filling defects

2. The subarachnoid cisterns

  (a) Enlargement, or compression, due to a mass
  (b) Obliteration or obstruction
  (c) Filling defects

3. The cortical subarachnoid space

  (a) Enlargement of sulci, generalized or focal, due to atrophy; this is notoriously difficult to assess, but it is generally accepted that sulci wider than 5 mm are suspect, and those wider than 10 mm definitely pathological.
  (b) Obliteration or non-visualization of sulci.

THE RADIOLOGICAL DIAGNOSTIC APPROACH TO CLINICAL NEUROLOGICAL PROBLEMS

Although the brain and cranial nerves are not amenable to inspection, palpation and auscultation, the mode of clinical presentation and abnormal physical signs often give a clear idea of the site and probable nature of a lesion. Neuroradiological investigation has two roles: first, the identification of an abnormality in terms of site, size and, if possible, nature; and second, provision of the information necessary for surgical intervention, if indicated. These two roles frequently overlap, but it is often the case that the classical invasive diagnostic techniques are now employed to facilitate surgery rather than to establish a diagnosis. Differential diagnosis is less commonly a serious consideration in neuroradiology than in other branches of radiology.

Neurological presentations can for convenience be divided into acute and chronic. In either case, a history of head injury is of prime diagnostic significance.

Acute presentations

I. With a known or suspected head injury

Skull radiographs should probably be obtained in any patient who presents to hospital having lost consciousness as the result of a presumed head injury. The demonstration of a skull fracture greatly increases the probability of an intracranial lesion and in many centres indicates admission and overnight observation. If the patient is uncooperative or has other injuries which require prior treatment, the skull films can often be delayed until a convenient time. Only good quality radiographs are useful, and the radiographer should not be asked to struggle with a restless, perhaps violent patient.

Radiographs of the cervical spine are desirable in any patient with a moderately severe head injury, and all patients admitted unconscious should have at least a frontal *chest film*. *Cranial CT* is indicated when the patient arrives comatose or with a deteriorating conscious level, or develops focal physical signs. A history of a penetrating injury, or signs of an intracranial mass or of a lesion requiring surgery (such as a depressed fracture) on plain films may also indicate a CT study, not necessarily as a emergency.

Ultrasound is a poor substitute for CT, except in small children.

Invasive investigations such as *angiography* may be required if CT is unavailable or if its findings are equivocal. Many surgeons prefer emergency exploration if clinical signs and other evidence point to a rapidly expanding intracranial haematoma.

II. Acute headache, with or without physical signs, i.e. suspected subarachnoid haemorrhage.

Skull radiographs are desirable if there is any possibility of trauma; the number of projections may be limited.

CT should be carried out in the early stages (but not as an emergency); it may obviate lumbar puncture, exclude other diagnoses, and serve as a baseline for subsequent developments.

Angiography is mandatory when subarachnoid haemorrhage not due to trauma is proven, *provided that the patient would be fit for operation*. In cases with a very suggestive history of subarachnoid haemorrhage, in which cerebral angiography reveals no cause for haemorrhage, *myelography* should precede possible *spinal angiography*, as the latter is virtually never positive if the myelogram is normal.

III. Acute onset of neurological deficit, without head injury

This will usually indicate a vascular cause, but the onset of some demyelinating diseases, infections or metabolic disturbances may also be relatively rapid.

1. Loss of consciousness or coma, without focal signs

Skull radiographs may provide a useful clue, particularly if trauma cannot be excluded.

Cranial CT is strongly indicated. If it is positive, further investigation will depend on the CT findings. If it shows no abnormality in the acute stage, brain stem or massive cerebral infarction or possibly encephalitis are possibilities when metabolic and other causes have been excluded. Repeat CT studies will probably clarify the situation.

Angiography has virtually no part to play, unless CT shows evidence of haemorrhage; even then, it can be deferred unless emergency surgery is contemplated.

2. Cranial nerve palsies

In this and the following categories, a distinction must be made between transient and established defects. Investigation of the former is directed at detection of a treatable lesion, preventatively; when the deficit is established, such investigations may not only be of little practical significance, but may contribute to long-term morbidity.

Comprehensive *skull radiographs* are not usually contributory in cases of acute cranial nerve lesions, but a lateral projection at least should be obtained in every case, since underlying lesions such as pituitary tumours or mucoceles of the paranasal sinuses may manifest themselves acutely, and can be readily detected. Changes of raised intracranial pressure may be the clue to the aetiology of visual obscurations or sixth nerve palsies. Acute lesions of the lower cranial nerves are relatively uncommon, and are usually not amenable to radiological detection. Clinically typical Bell's (facial) palsy does not call for petrous bone examination (*chest radiography* to exclude sarcoidosis is more relevant) and acute vertigo is very rarely due to otherwise silent ear disease which may be detectable on plain films.

CT is also of limited value, except in the detection of underlying lesions, including those causing raised intracranial pressure, or the demonstration of associated abnormalities such as multiple cerebral infarcts. Nevertheless, it is indicated for these reasons.

Angiography is indicated in many cases: amaurosis fugax, and acute ocular motor palsies which can be the result of aneurysms are obvious examples. Digital subtraction angiography of the cervical arteries is the technique of choice.

3. Acute cerebral hemisyndromes

Hemiplegia or sensory disturbance, hemianopia, dysphasia or parietal lobe dysfunction.

Skull radiographs are rarely contributory, but a lateral projection should be obtained as it may give an aetiological clue. Radiographic views of the ears and sinuses may be obtained if an abscess is suspected, but can usually be deferred.

CT is the fundamental investigation when the cerebral deficit is established. If normal in the acute stage, an infarct is by far the most likely cause, although encephalitis and acute demyelination cannot be excluded; repeat studies will usually make the diagnosis evident. If a haemorrhage is shown on CT, *angiography* will often be requested before surgery; it can be limited in extent, at least in the acute stage. The policy of the referring surgeon will determine whether angiography or other investigations are carried out when CT demonstrates other pathology: primary or metastatic tumours, abscess, or even infarction. Angiography is not indicated if changes at CT are thought to represent meningitis, encephalitis, demyelination, etc., unless cortical or dural venous thrombosis is considered, in which case a digital subtraction study is probably superior.

With *transient cerebral deficits*, almost always due to ischaemia, *CT* is characteristically normal, but serves to exclude an alternative diagnosis. *Angiography* of the cervical and intracranial arteries, which can be of the *digital intravenous type*, is the prime investigation for transient ischaemic attacks and the various forms of stroke in evolution, and may be regarded as an emergency. *Noninvasive imaging techniques* of the carotid arteries, including *ultrasound* and *isotope studies* are usually reserved for low suspicion cases; very few vascular surgeons will operate on the basis of the resulting images.

Although reconstruction or transluminal dilatation of the origin of the vertebral arteries is on the increase, the diagnosis of embolic occlusion of a posterior cerebral artery is usually made on clinical and CT grounds; angiography is not generally performed.

The indications for *cerebral angiography* in fixed cerebral deficit are debatable, depending on the strength of the belief of the vascular surgeon in the beneficial effects of endarterectomy and arterial anastomotic procedures. Lack of well documented follow up series and comparison with untreated controls has contributed to this subject remaining controversial.

4. Acute brain stem deficit

Skull radiography can be limited to a lateral projection, to detect signs of raised intracranial pressure, and may be omitted.

CT in ischaemic disease of the brain stem is generally contributory only in excluding other pathology such as pineal region or brain stem tumours with acute decompensation, haemorrhage or large aneurysms.

Angiography is rarely contributory in a positive sense unless an aneurysm is shown, and if the patient's condition would permit surgery.

5. Acute cerebellar disturbance

This is usually due to haemorrhage or infarction. *Skull radiographs* are generally noncontributory, while *CT* may also be unrewarding in cases of infarction. *Angiography* may be carried out before evacuation of a haematoma, to exclude an underlying arteriovenous malformation.

Chronic presentations

I. Headache, facial or occipital pain

A full set of *skull radiographs* should be obtained; supplementary views of the paranasal sinuses, temporomandibular joints, teeth, petrous bones or cervical spine may be indicated by the clinical features. To proceed to more sophisticated studies before these have been obtained is a misuse of resources. The vast majority of typical cases of migraine, migrainous neuralgia, tic doloureux and occipital neuralgia will show no abnormality, and extensive radiological investigation is rarely required.

CT is also generally unhelpful; careful clinical selection of cases with atypical or suggestive features (or plain film abnormalities) is required to prevent CT services being swamped with totally unnecessary examinations. When CT is normal, there is rarely any indication for further radiological investigation, except in a small proportion of patients in whom clinical findings suggest an intracranial vascular anomaly. Abnormal CT will determine the sequence of further studies, if required.

II. Progressive or recurrent neurological disturbances

1. Cranial nerves

(a) Optic nerve and optic chiasm. Unilateral visual impairment is assumed in the absence of systemic disease to be due to compression of the optic nerve, until proved otherwise. *Skull radiographs* are a rapid way of excluding a number of causes; optic canal views may be helpful. *Tomography* is of limited value if CT is available.

CT of the orbits and parasellar region is usually required; studies with intrathecal water soluble contrast medium may be indicated for delineating the intracranial portion of the optic nerve.

Carotid angiography, orbital phlebography and even *pneumoencephalography* may be required (in that order) for the elucidation of difficult problems.

Papilloedema is investigated by *skull films*, which may show evidence of raised intracranial pressure when all other radiological investigations are normal, and may indicate the cause of the papilloedema. *CT* is of prime importance; if it is normal, lumbar puncture can be performed, while any abnormality will determine the sequence of subsequent investigations.

Lesions of the optic chiasm are usually compressive. *Skull radiographs* are very valuable; they enable a diagnosis of the nature of very many compressive lesions. *Tomography* may be helpful in elucidating an area of calcification or hyperostosis, but has no part to play in diagnosis of pituitary tumours large enough to compress the optic chiasm.

CT is also valuable in confirming the plain film diagnosis and showing the extent and internal composition of a compressive lesion prior to surgery. If high quality reformation of coronal and sagittal images is not available, water soluble CT *cisternography* is probably the best adjunct for demonstration of the topography of parasellar masses.

Many surgeons require *cerebral angiography* before operating on pituitary adenomas, while a few prefer *orbital phlebography* if the trans-sphenoidal approach is to be employed; many of the surgeons using the latter route also require preoperative *tomograms* of the sphenoid sinus.

Preoperative *pneumoencephalography* is carried out in very few, relatively conservative institutions.

(b) Upper cranial nerves (III to VI). Lesions arising between the brain stem origins of these nerves and their egress from the skull are frequently elusive, requiring the combination of several imaging modalities.

Skull radiographs may be extremely helpful; *tomography* is sometimes an asset.

CT should include the orbital region, since intraorbital lesions may simulate disorders of the ocular motor nerves. Water soluble *cisternography* may be helpful.

Angiography is frequently required to supplement these techniques and is essential if aneurysm is considered a likely cause.

(c) Lower cranial nerve and bulbar problems. Most patients with tinnitus and/or vertigo have no macrostructural abnormality; radiological investigation is usually restricted to *skull radiographs*, and views of the petrous bones. *CT* is performed in selected cases, when the clinical or plain radiographic features indicate a structural lesion.

If an acoustic neuroma with intracranial extension is strongly suspected and *CT* is inconclusive, the study is repeated with *intrathecal water soluble contrast medium*, but if the lesion is thought to be intracanalicular, *CT air meatography* is preferred.

Lower cranial nerve lesions possibly due to neoplastic involvement of the skull base require careful *plain radiographs and tomograms*; *CT* is very helpful. *Angiography* is frequently required for diagnosis and/or treatment.

When the lower brain stem is involved, water soluble *CT cisternography* or *pneumoencephalography* may be most informative. *Myelography* is probably the best study for cerebellar tonsillar ectopia.

2. Cerebral disorders

Hemisyndromes, hemianopia, epilepsy, dementia, involuntary movements.

Basic radiological investigation includes a *lateral skull radiograph*, with further views if indicated by clinical localizing factors (e.g. a lump on the head) or plain film findings, a *chest radiograph*, and *CT*.

If CT shows no abnormality, or merely generalized atrophic or involutional changes, other radiological investigations are rarely required. Many abnormal findings, e.g. congenital anomalies, hemiatrophy, most white matter disorders, evidence of old trauma or infarction, etc. may be of diagnostic significance in their clinical context but similarly merit no further radiology.

When CT shows a 'surgical' lesion such as a tumour, abscess or chronic subdural haematoma, further radiological studies will depend almost entirely on the plan of treatment and the preferences of those who will carry it out. Various combinations of *radionuclide scans, angiograms* and even *ventriculography* may be requested. It is to be anticipated that dissemination of improvements of CT technology and surgical familiarity with them will render most of these additional conventional techniques unnecessary.

Angiography will continue to be mandatory for vascular anomalies.

In the investigation of hydrocephalus without obvious obstructive cause, *water soluble CT cisternography* is now the preferred technique; *ventriculography* is sometimes desirable.

III. Developmental problems

1. Abnormal size and/or growth of head

Skull radiographs may be very informative; at least a lateral film should be obtained. *CT* is, however, usually the definitive study and will indicate the need for further investigation or treatment. In *young children, ultrasound* is probably preferable.

2. Retarded development, reading difficulties, etc

Only rarely is radiological investigation of value, and even less commonly does it reveal a treatable lesion. The prime function of *CT* in most cases would appear to be reassurance of parents and paediatricians; the extent to which its use for this purpose is justified, is an ethical problem.

3. Evident malformations and developmental anomalies

Radiological investigation of such conditions, while it may provide spectacular textbook examples, is justifiable only when the nature or extent of the malformation is not clear, or when treatment of the underlying condition or its complications is considered.

IV. Endocrine disturbances

These are commonly manifestations of lesions of the hypothalamic pituitary axis. They may arise not only from hyperfunction or hyperplasia but also, less commonly from compressive or neoplastic lesions such as craniopharyngioma, glioma, pineal region tumour etc.

It is evident that *skull radiographs* and *CT* are the fundamental modes of radiological investigation. Small pituitary adenomas without neurological manifestations are diagnosed on clinical and biochemical grounds. Extensive exposure of affected patients to ionizing radiations is rarely justified; it can be argued that if patients are to be treated surgically, the only role of radiology is to exclude a macroadenoma, which can be done simply by means of a lateral skull radiograph and CT. The extent to which repeated high dose CT of the pituitary region in patients being treated medically (with bromocryptine) is justified for other than research purposes is also debatable.

When surgery is planned, radiological investigations will be determined by the wishes of the surgeon, but once again it should be noted that, in the case of tumours within a small pituitary gland, radiological localization of the adenoma has very little effect on the surgical exploration.

Radiology provides little help in the diagnosis of *acromegaly*, which is clinical and biochemical, and is of limited value in follow up. Its main role is to confirm the presence of a pituitary adenoma and provide the data necessary for its treatment.

V. Cerebrospinal fluid rhinorrhoea or otorrhoea; recurrent meningitis

When one or other of these symptoms follows a known head injury, the causative breach in the dura mater and/or skull base may be very difficult to identify precisely enough to enable surgical repair. Fluid can escape from one nostril, for example, as a result of a dural defect on the same side, the other side, in an anterior or posterior location, or even as the result of a fracture of the petrous bone.

High quality *plain radiographs of the skull* are therefore required, and will frequently be supplemented by *views of the sinuses or petrous bone; tomography* is often necessary.

CT is sometimes useful, but, as with plain films, is often unrewarding. *CT cisternography* with water soluble contrast medium is probably the technique of choice, although it also, is fallible.

A number of more sophisticated techniques are employed in different centres, combining contrast media or isotopes with plain films and conventional tomography; their multiplicity reflects their unreliability.

BIBLIOGRAPHY

REFERENCES

1. Du Boulay G H 1980 Principles of X-ray diagnosis of the skull. Butterworth, London
2. Newton T H, Potts G 1971 Radiology of the skull and brain, Vol I (Books 1 and 2): The skull. Mosby, St Louis
3. Sortland O 1979 Computed tomography combined with gas cisternography for the diagnosis of expanding lesions in the cerebellopontine angle. Neuroradiology 18: 19–22.
4. Moseley I F 1977 The use of contrast media as an adjunct to C T scanning. In: Kühler W J (ed) Computer assisted tomography. Excerpta Medica, Amsterdam pp 26–45
5. Pullicino P, Kendall B E 1980 Contrast enhancement in ischaemic lesions. I. Relationship to prognosis. Neuroradiology 19:235–239; II Effect on prognosis. Neuroradiology 19:241–243
6. Salamon G, Huang Y P 1980 Computed tomography of the brain. Springer, Berlin
7. Valentine A R, Pullicino P, Bannan E 1980 A practical introduction to cranial CT. Heinemann, London
8. Haber K, Wachter R D, Christenson P C et al 1980 Ultrasonic evaluation of intracranial pathology in infants: a new technique. Radiology 134:173–178
9. Osborn A G 1980 Introduction to cerebral angiography. Harper and Row, Hagerston
10. Mani R et al 1978 Complications of catheter cerebral angiography. Am J Roentgenol 131:861–874
11. Newton T H, Potts G 1974 Radiology of the skull and brain, Vol 2 (Books 1–4): Angiography. Mosby, St Louis
12. Djindjian R, Merland J J 1978 Super-selective arteriography of the external carotid artery. Springer, Berlin
13. Lie T A 1968 Congenital anomalies of the carotid artery. Excerpta Medica, Amsterdam
14. Huang Y P, Wolf B S 1970 Differential diagnosis of fourth ventricle tumours from brain stem tumours in angiography. Neuroradiology 1:4–9
15. Brismar J 1974 Orbital phlebography I Technique. Acta Radiol 15:369–382.
16. Hanafee W, Rosen L M, Weidner W, Wilson G H 1965 Venography of the cavernous sinus, orbital veins and basal venous plexus. Radiology 84:751–753
17. Brismar J 1974 Orbital phlebography II Anatomy of superior ophthalmic vein and its tributaries. Acta Radiol 15:481–495
18. Brismar J 1974 Orbital phlebography III Topography of intraorbital veins. Acta Radiol 15:577–594
19. Brismar J 1975 Orbital phlebography IV The cavernous sinuses and adjacent venous sinuses of the skull base. Acta Radiol 16:1–16
20. Robertson E G 1967 Pneumoencephalography. Thomas, Springfield
21. Ruggiero G 1974 Radiological exploration of the ventricles and subarachnoid space. Springer, Berlin
22. Cronqvist S 1977 Ventriculography with metrizamide. Acta Radiol Suppl 355:237–246
23. Baker H L 1963 Myelographic examination of the posterior fossa with positive contrast medium. Radiology 81:791–801
24. Isherwood I 1972 Air meatography. Clin Radiol 23:65–77
25. Di Chiro 1971 An atlas of detailed normal pneumoencephalographic anatomy. Thomas, Springfield
26. Evans W A 1942 An encephalographic ratio for estimating the size of the cerebral ventricles; further experience with serial observations. Am J Dis Child 64:820–830
27. Twining E W 1939 Radiology of the third and fourth ventricles II. Br J Radiol 12:569–598

SUGGESTIONS FOR FURTHER READING

Burrows E H, Leeds N E 1981 Neuroradiology. Churchill Livingstone, Edinburgh

Caillé J, Salamon G 1980 Computerized tomography. Springer, Berlin

Davidoff L M, Dyke C G 1951 The normal pneumoencephalogram. Lea and Febiger, Philadelphia

Du Boulay G H (ed) 1984 A textbook of X-ray diagnosis by British authors: Neuroradiology. Lewis, London

Felix R, Kazner E, Wegener O H 1981 Contrast media in computed tomography. Excerpta Medica, Amsterdam

Fischgold H, ed 1971–6 Traité de Radiodiagnostic. Tomes 13, 14: Neuroradiologie. Masson, Paris

Gonzalez C F, Grossman C B, Palacios E 1976 Computed brain and orbital tomography. Wiley, New York

Harwood-Nash D C, Fitz C R 1976 Neuroradiology in infants and children. Mosby, St Louis

Leighton R S 1971 Neuroradiologic anatomy. A stereoscopic atlas. Williams and Wilkins, Baltimore

Newton T H, Potts G 1978 Radiology of the skull and brain, Vol 2: Angiography. Volume 4: ventricles and cisterns. Mosby, St Louis

Peterson H O, Kieffer S A 1972 Introduction to neuroradiology. Harper and Row, Hagerston

Raimondi A J 1972 Pediatric neuroradiology. Saunders, Philadelphia

Ramsey R G 1981 Neuroradiology, with computed tomography. Saunders, Philadelphia

Salamon G, Huang Y P 1976 Radiologic anatomy of the brain. Springer, Berlin

Taveras J M, Morello F 1979 Normal neuroradiology. Year Book Medical Publishers, Chicago

Wilson M 1963 The anatomic foundation of neuroradiology of the brain. Little Brown, Boston

Intracranial tumours
    The skull in raised intracranial pressure

  Cerebral tumours
    Glioma
    Colloid cyst
    Pineal region tumours
    Medulloblastoma
    Haemangioblastoma
    Choroid plexus papilloma

  Metastases to the brain
    Effects of radiation therapy
    Angiography

  Pituitary tumours
    Other pituitary tumours
    Computerized tomography
    Angiography
    Empty sella

  Other tumours in the sellar region
    Craniopharyngioma
    Optic chiasm glioma

  Meningioma
    Plain film manifestations
    Computerized tomography
    Angiography

  Other intracranial tumours
    Pearly tumours
    Chordoma
    Glomus tumours

INTRACRANIAL TUMOURS

Many different tumours can arise in relation to the bony skull, its external investing layers, the meninges, or almost any component of the central nervous system (Fig. 84.1). Some of these tumours will produce more or less specific changes on plain skull radiographs, but the majority of intracranial masses will be manifest simply as raised intracranial pressure. The alterations produced are therefore discussed here, but it should be remembered that most of them are quite nonspecific; reference should also be made to this section when such problems as hydrocephalus are under consideration.

The skull in raised intracranial pressure [1]

Changes to be found in plain radiographs depend on the age of the patient, the duration of the elevation of intracranial pressure and, in some cases, its cause. They affect the cranial vault, the sutures and the sella turcica.

Children

In *infants*, raised pressure is usually manifest as enlargement of the cranium, the bones of which are thin. In the first few months of life, apparent defects in the bones of the vault, craniolacunae, may be present although convolutional markings are not prominent. The sutures are wider than normal and show excessive interdigitations. Erosion of the lamina dura of the dorsum sellae may be present, but is generally less marked than the other changes. Some evidence of the cause of the increased pressure may be present (see below).

In *older children*, acutely raised pressure causes suture diastasis (Fig. 84.2); it can occur within a few days, but is less common after 10 years of age. Erosion of the lamina dura of the sella turcica develops more slowly, and is generally not seen within 1 month. It is first manifest as fluffiness or fine discontinuity of the cortex lining the posteroinferior angle of the sella at the base of the dorsum, and may progress to massive demineralization of the skull base. Erosion first

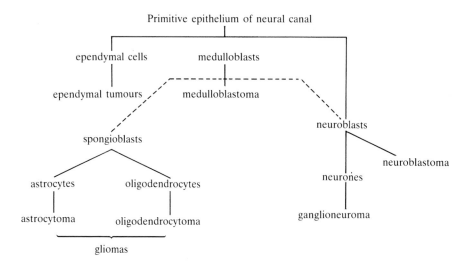

Primitive epithelium of neural canal

ependymal cells   medulloblasts

ependymal tumours   medulloblastoma

spongioblasts   neuroblasts

astrocytes   oligodendrocytes   neuroblastoma

astrocytoma   oligodendrocytoma   neurones

gliomas   ganglioneuroma

Fig. 84.1 Neuroectodermal tumours (after Treip [3])

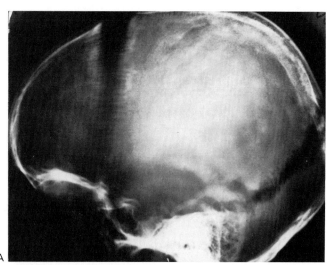

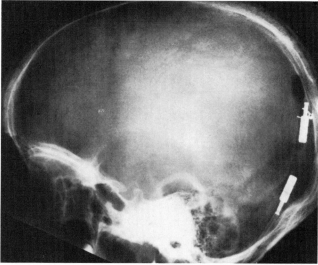

Fig. 84.2 Raised intracranial pressure in a child with a pineal tumour. (A) At time of presentation: the sutures are splayed, with exaggerated interdigitations; convolutional markings are mildly increased; the vault is thin. The sella turcica is slightly enlarged and the lamina dura is defective. (B) Some months later after shunting: the skull is virtually normal.

occurs where the cortex overlies soft, cancellous bone; that portion of the lamina dura abutting the cortex within the sphenoid sinus is more resistant. Erosive changes are seen in only about one third of patients with raised intracranial pressure, but can be a valuable observation in patients with no clinical signs.

Chronically raised pressure produces marked changes in the cranial vault, which becomes expanded (Fig. 84.3). The anterior cranial fossa frequently shows the greatest expansion, with depression of the orbital plates and, on the lateral projection, a rounded appearance. The occipital bones may be markedly ballooned when a posterior fossa mass or cystic lesion is responsible (as in the Dandy-Walker syndrome). Conversely, the posterior fossa may appear small, although it is usually of normal size, when the supratentorial compart-

ment alone is greatly expanded. The bone of the vault is thin, with exaggerated convolutional markings ('digital impression'), giving a 'beaten copper' appearance (Fig. 84.4). Convolutional markings are normally present in children, especially on those parts of the vault which bear the weight of the brain, but they decrease in prominence before puberty. Widespread frontoparietal or vertex impressions are usually pathological, but caution is required in diagnosing raised intracranial pressure on the basis of this sign alone. If the elevation of pressure has been intermittent, the vault may become thicker than normal, showing a characteristic laminated appearance.

The sutures and occasionally the fontanelles, are prominent with excessive interdigitation. Erosion of the sella turcica and skull base may be advanced. When the third

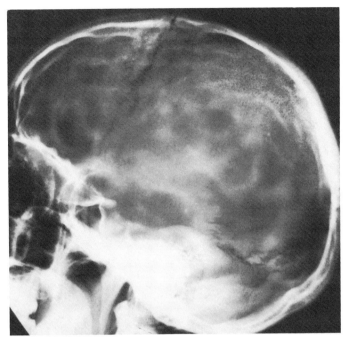

Fig. 84.3 Chronic raised intracranial pressure in an older child, due to aqueduct stenosis. The cranial cavity is large, particularly the anterior cranial fossa, which is abnormally rounded, while the posterior fossa is of normal size. The vault is thin, and convolutional markings are increased. All the sutures are slightly diastatic. The orbital plates are depressed. The sella shows a 'J' configuration: truncated, thin dorsum, shallow pituitary fossa, prominent sulcus chiasmaticus and large anterior clinoid processes, indicating enlargement of the anterior end of the third ventricle.

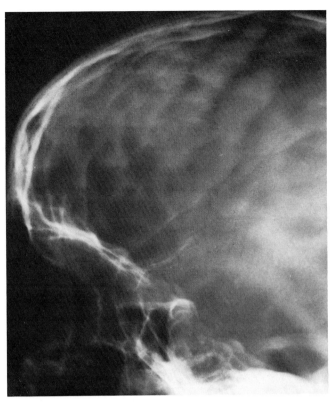

Fig. 84.4 Craniopharyngioma, causing longstanding increase of intracranial pressure in a young adult. Evidence of generalized increased in pressure: exaggeration of convolutional markings and widening of coronal suture. Truncation of the dorsum sellae and enlargement of the pituitary fossa, which contains calcified material.

ventricle is particularly enlarged, sellar erosion may take a characteristic form: the dorsum is short, thin and anteflexed, while the sulcus chiasmaticus is deep, causing the pituitary fossa, which is in fact small, to appear enlarged; the anterior clinoid processes are large and square (Fig. 84.3). This 'J' configuration is the result of direct pressure of the third ventricle and should not be confused with the normal appearance of a deep sulcus chiasmaticus in young children, nor with the excavation of the presellar region produced by gliomas of the optic chiasm. Marked erosion of the sella, especially the dorsum, with less marked changes in the skull vault in children, is suggestive of craniopharyngioma; when suprasellar calcification is also present, the picture is virtually pathognomonic (Fig. 84.4).

Adults

In adults, changes in the cranial vault are seen only when a large mass itself erodes bone, or when the elevation of pressure dates from childhood. Thus, the major change occurring in the vault is enlargement of the foramina for emissary veins, particularly in the occipital bone, and of the areas of bone thinning due to Pacchionian granulations. It is said that emissary foramina more than 2 mm in diameter are pathological, but as an isolated sign this is unreliable.

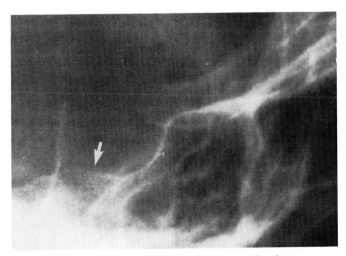

Fig. 84.5 Erosion of the lamina dura of the dorsum sellae due to raised intracranial pressure. Skull, lateral projection: the cortex is eroded where it overlies cancellous bone (posterior to the arrow).

The skull base is usually affected to a much greater degree. The earliest changes consist of erosion of the lamina dura at the base of the dorsum sellae, as in children. Du Boulay [1] categorized sellar changes as follows.

Category 1: destruction of the lamina dura only; this is not seen in communicating hydrocephalus (Fig. 84.5).

Category 2: truncation of the dorsum sellae (and posterior clinoid processes). When present as a solitary abnormality, it generally indicates a suprasellar mass or a dilated third ventricle; when the lamina dura is also defective, an intracranial mass lesion is likely.

Category 3: marked deossification of the skull base, including the sella, planum sphenoidale and the floor of the anterior cranial fossa, which may be bulged downwards (Fig. 84.6). The base view shows marked thinning of bone, the basal foramina being enlarged and poorly defined. These changes occur in chronic, severe elevation of pressure, with downward transtentorial herniation, often due to a frontal mass lesion.

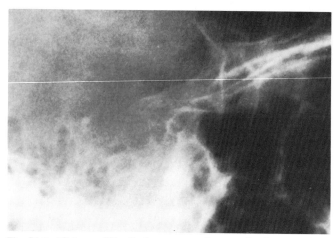

Fig. 84.6 'Category III' sella due to severe, longstanding increase of intracranial pressure. The lamina dura is absent, and the whole skull base, particularly the floor of the anterior cranial fossa, is markedly deossified.

Category 4: increase in the depth of the sella turcica, sometimes accompanied by less marked expansion in other planes, without cortical erosion. This is the typical picture of an empty sella, which, although usually of no clinical significance, is a frequent accompaniment to chronically raised pressure, as in benign intracranial hypertension. The description of these appearances by Bonneville and Dietemann [2] is exemplary:

. . . above a poorly aerated sphenoid . . . a double floor of the sella, with two parallel lines corresponding to the floor and occasionally also to the dorsum sellae and the anterior wall; the lower line . . . is very well defined and thick, but the upper one is blurred. On the frontal projection the floor shows a symmetrical downward convexity. . . .

Generalized enlargement of the sella turcica can also occur as the result of raised intracranial pressure, giving a 'ballooned' appearance similar to that caused by a pituitary tumour. The combination of ballooning and erosion of the lamina dura, however, is strongly suggestive of raised pressure.

When increased pressure is relieved, the cranial vault often thickens; sutures may close prematurely. The sella turcica reossifies and if deformed, may remodel.

Cerebral tumours (Table 84.1)

Brain tumours are found in approximately 2% of autopsies [3]; 75% are primary, and about one half are gliomas. Cerebral gliomas are often graded by the proportion of cells showing mitotic figures, Kernohan grades 1 to 4, Grade 1 being the least malignant. Grades 3 and 4, classed together as glioblastoma multiforme, constitute about 50% of gliomas, and are more common in males. At least 50% of the remaining gliomas are astrocytomas. Ependymomas arise in relationship to the cerebral ventricles, especially the fourth ventricle; the term 'subependymoma' refers simply to a subependymal astrocytoma, while microglioma is a synonym for cerebral lymphoma.

Table 84.1 *Incidence of intracranial tumours*

Primary		
Glioma		45%
Glioblastoma multiforme	25	
Astrocytoma	9	
Ependymoma	3*	
Medulloblastoma	3*	
Oligodendroglioma	2	
Other	3	
Meningioma		14%
Pituitary adenoma		11%
Acoustic neuroma		7%
Craniopharyngioma		3%
Pineal tumours		
Dermoid/epidermoid		each 1%
Colloid cyst		or less
Choroid plexus papilloma		
		80%
Secondary		20%

* predominantly in children

Glioma

On plain films, cerebral gliomas are manifest as raised intracranial pressure, as discussed above. Calcified structures such as the pineal and choroid plexus may be displaced.

Glioma is the commonest cause of pathological intracerebral calcification on plain films, taking the form of amorphous blobs, streaks and nodules, usually rather faint, and most common in patients with a long history. Ring shadows are very rare, but band or track like calcification is typical of oligodendrogliomas. The latter type of tumour is rare, however, so that calcification usually denotes an astrocytoma (Fig. 84.7).

Rarely, slow growing gliomas will erode and expand the overlying cranium.

Computerized tomography [4]

Astrocytoma

The 'benign' or Grade 1 astrocytoma may cause very subtle CT abnormalities; indeed, many of these indolent lesions are difficult for the pathologist to identify with the brain in front of him. Such tumours are characterized by increased cellu-

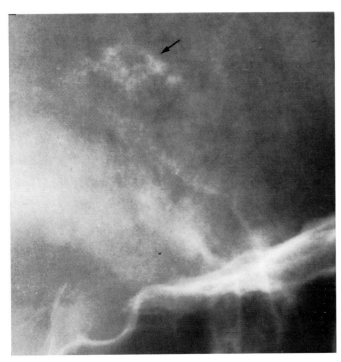

Fig. 84.7 Cerebral glioma: amorphous tumour calcification and erosion of the lamina dura of the dorsum sellae.

larity or gliosis, manifest on CT as ill defined increased or decreased density; oedema is usually absent and there is never necrosis or increased vascularity. The blood brain barrier is at most minimally affected, so that intravenous contrast medium causes no enhancement. Mass effect is often subtle: slight asymmetry of a cistern or minimal impression on a ventricle.

Moreover, no other standard imaging modality (except possibly nuclear magnetic resonance or positron emission tomography) can show these lesions, so that indefinite CT findings may be the only evidence for a slow growing tumour producing occasional seizures or vague neurological deficit. These patients are generally followed with serial CT studies until a well defined lesion appears.

Calcification is not infrequently detected in astrocytomas (and oligodendrogliomas); it is inhomogeneous, punctate, linear or patchy. The presence of calcification generally correlates with a slow progression, but very malignant tumours may also show foci of calcium. Similar patterns of calcification may also be seen in some cases of arteriovenous malformation.

Astrocytomas are more common in the deeper white matter than in the cortex. A relatively common location is in the anterior part of the corpus callosum, where the tumour may become very large before it is detected, the frontal lobes being relatively 'silent' neurologically. The tumour compresses the frontal horns and extends across the midline. Tumours of this type are not resectable and have a poor prognosis (Fig. 84.8).

Malignant glioma

This type of tumour, more anaplastic than the Grade 1

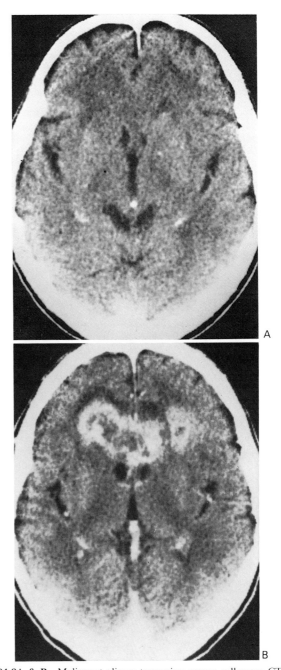

Fig. 84.8A & B Malignant glioma traversing corpus callosum; CT. (A) The frontal white matter is of abnormally low density, and the frontal horns are compressed. (B) After intravenous contrast medium, irregular enhancement gives a classic 'butterfly' appearance. The thick, irregular tumour margins, central area of reduced enhancement suggesting necrosis, and perilesional oedema are all highly suggestive of a malignant glioma.

lesion, is characterized on CT by areas of mixed high and low density, mass effect and surrounding oedema. Cyst formation, or small zones of necrosis within the tumour are common. A very round focus of low density surrounded by obviously compressed parenchyma is strongly suggestive of a cyst; layering of denser material in its dependent part is, however the only unequivocal indication. Its recognition is of clinical significance, since cyst drainage may be the only beneficial procedure available to the neurosurgeon.

A reliable predictor of malignancy in an intrinsic tumour is contrast enhancement. A defective blood brain barrier generally indicates an anaplastic tumour, a malignant glioma of at least Grade 2. In this category of malignant glioma (including astrocytomas, oligodendrogliomas, ependymomas and mixed types), contrast enhancement may be diffuse, nodular, or peripheral (Fig. 84.9).

Oedema around malignant gliomas is of the 'vasogenic' type, largely confined to the white matter. It is probable that oedema contributes significantly to the symptomatology of many of these tumours, and response of clinical state and CT oedema to systemic steroid therapy may be striking.

Glioblastoma multiforme

This most anaplastic member of the glioma series (with histology so undifferentiated that the cell of origin is often unidentifiable) is unfortunately also the most common; prognosis is uniformly poor.

CT appearances are typical: marked mass effect, moderate oedema, contrast enhancement, usually peripheral and often ragged. Haemorrhage completes the picture; calcification is not rare. Solitary, necrotic metastases and rare malignant tumours can, however produce similar appearances, as can radionecrosis, which should always be considered when tumours apparently recur after treatment.

Oligodendroglioma

This type of glioma has two striking tendencies: a predilection for the frontal lobes, and calcification. In other respects, its CT features are those of gliomas in general (Fig. 84.10).

Brain stem glioma [5]

These tumours, commonly seen in childhood, tend to be diffusely infiltrative, very anaplastic, and most are glioblastomas. Despite this, they differ markedly from supratentorial glioblastomas in that they do not characteristically show marked contrast enhancement; cyst formation, calcification and haemorrhage are also not conspicuous.

The earliest CT sign of these tumours is enlargement of the brain stem, manifest as subtle alterations in the configuration of the pontine or ambient cisterns and the fourth ventricle. The latter may be displaced posteriorly to a minor degree. These changes later become more marked. In the early stages, pneumoencephalography can be more sensitive than CT, particularly if the scanner is not of the highest quality (Fig. 84.11).

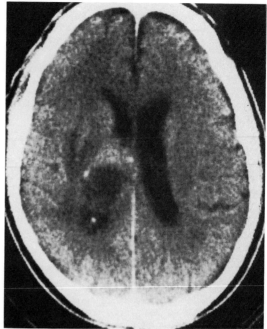

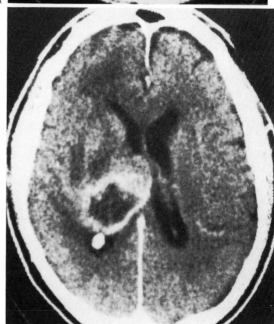

Fig. 84.9A & B Malignant glioma; CT (A) In the right thalamus, a low density zone is surrounded by increased density, particularly anteriorly, within which are at least two flecks of calcification. Oedema spreads along the white matter tracts of the internal and external capsules. The body of the right lateral ventricle is obliterated. (B) After intravenous contrast medium: the margins of the lesion enhance markedly, and are thick and irregular. Biopsy revealed a highly malignant mixed astrocytoma/ependymoma. Note that the presence of calcification does not necessarily imply benignity.

Most gliomas in the brain stem have CT numbers equal to or less than those of normal brain, and are usually rather homogeneous. Hyperdense or cystic tumours are less common; focal calcification should suggest the possibility of another lesion such as a vascular malformation. Contrast enhancement is present in more than half of cases, but is often not striking.

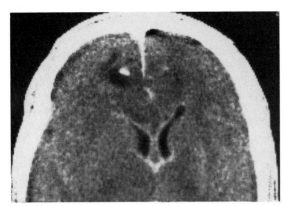

Fig. 84.10 Oligodendroglioma; CT. A right frontal calcific focus is surrounded by a low density zone, with moderate mass effect, indicating that the tumour is more extensive than it appears at first sight.

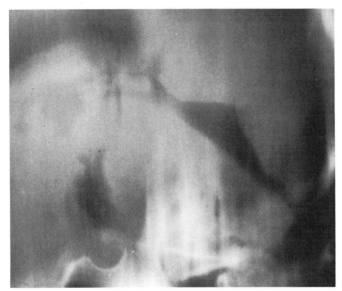

Fig. 84.11 Brain stem glioma; pneumoencephalography, midline lateral tomograms in sitting position, (child aged 8 years). The pons is too bulky, and the fourth ventricle is flattened posteriorly.

An exophytic type of brain stem glioma grows out as a circumscribed mass into the cisterns around the brain stem, or into the fourth ventricle, simulating an extra-axial lesion. Intrathecal contrast medium can be extremely valuable in the correct indentification of the site of origin, which is of considerable importance as regards management.

Cerebellar astrocytoma [6]

This relatively benign childhood tumour has a good long term prognosis. It is seen most often on CT as a low density lesion, round or ovoid, in one of the cerebellar hemispheres, or less commonly in the vermis. The usual clinical presentation is with raised intracranial pressure, and most of these tumours show CT evidence of hydrocephalus; the fourth ventricle is grossly distorted, displaced to the opposite side or obliterated. Less commonly it will appear hugely dilated when the tumour lies below it, and can mimic a large tumour cyst.

The contents of the cystic tumour show CT density ranging from that of cerebrospinal fluid to that of brain tissue, the latter indicating a high protein content. A tumour nodule in the wall may be shown as a focus of contrast enhancement (Fig. 84.12), but a ring pattern is more frequent. Differential diagnosis of thin walled cysts in the posterior fossa is extensive, so that identification of a tumour capsule is of some value. Haemangioblastoma can show identical appearances, while in adults cystic or necrotic metastases are more common. Ventriculography is sometimes used for differentiation of brain stem and cerebellar masses (Fig. 84.13).

Ependymoma [7]

This variety of glioma generally arises in the posterior fossa in children, and within the cerebrum in adults; its nature may be suggested on CT by its para- or intraventricular site (Fig. 84.14). The tumour, which is spontaneously denser at CT than surrounding brain, may be calcified, and shows marked contrast enhancement. Differentiation from medulloblastoma may be difficult (although the latter very rarely calcifies).

If the tumour grows predominantly within the fourth ventricle, it will be seen as an intraventricular mass, the ventricle enlarging to accomodate it. A characteristic feature is downward extension into the cisterna magna, or into the cerebellopontine angle, via the foramina of Luschka. Ependymomas show a high recurrence rate after surgery and radiotherapy, at the site of the original tumour, within the ventricular system, and throughout the cranial and spinal subarachnoid space.

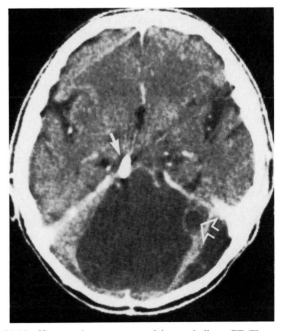

Fig. 84.12 Huge cystic astrocytoma of the cerebellum; CT. The slowly growing tumour has enlarged the posterior cranial fossa. The cystic component is of water density; a daughter cyst is present on the left [open arrow]. Small remnants of cerebellar tissue only remain. [White arrow = shunt tube]. (Figs. 84.12, 84.19, 84.20, 84.22, 84.27, 84.28, 84.38, 84.39 and 84.42 by courtesy of Dr W Marshall, Stanford University, California)

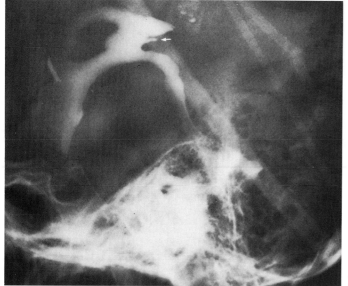

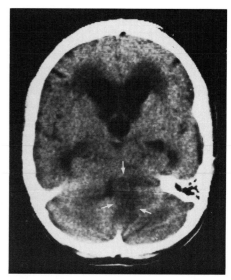

Fig. 84.14 Ependymoma of the fourth ventricle in a child; CT. The tumour [small arrows], which is of decreased density, expands the fourth ventricle and burrows into the left cerebellar hemisphere. There is obstructive hydrocephalus, with marked interstitial oedema around the frontal horns.

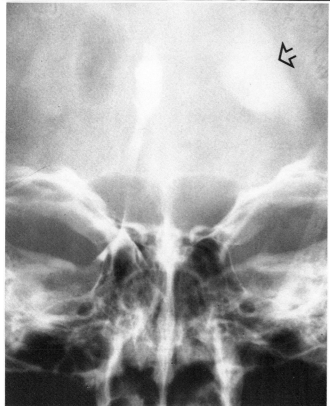

Fig. 84.13A & B　Left cerebellar astrocytoma; metrizamide ventriculogram. (A) Lateral and (B) anteroposterior projections, brow up: the fourth ventricle is dislocated anteriorly and to the right. Note excellent demonstration of massa intermedia and pineal recess [arrow]. There is contrast medium in the left occipital horn [open arrow].

Colloid cyst [8,9]

The cell of origin of colloid cysts is unclear, but it is thought that they may arise from ependymal rests, and are therefore considered here. Their characteristic site is at the paraphysis,

the posterior lip of the foramina of Monro; their enlargement gives rise to biventricular hydrocephalus. The anterior end of the third ventricle may, however also be enlarged, so that the skull radiographs may show a truncated dorsum sellae.

This typical location is evident at CT, when the tumour is seen just behind the columns of the fornix, lying between dilated lateral ventricles, while the third ventricle is slit-like or deformed (Fig. 84.15). When the classical site is combined with a remarkably rounded form of the cyst and intrinsically high radiographic density, unchanged after intravenous contrast medium, the diagnosis is virtually certain, and most cases are now operated on the basis of CT findings alone. Some cases will show unilateral hydrocephalus and if the offending tumour is small, air encephalography may be very helpful (Fig. 84.16). Since the differential diagnosis may be thought to include aneurysm (although both contrast enhancement and calcification are very rare in colloid cysts), angiography may be carried out. It reveals signs of hydrocephalus and a typical elevation and separation of the anterior portions of the internal cerebral veins, which are draped over the cyst.

Pineal region tumours

Tumours which grow in the region of the pineal (loosely called 'pinealomas') tend to cause obstructive hydrocephalus early in their development when the tumour itself is relatively small, because of their proximity to the aqueduct of Sylvius and the posterior third ventricle (Fig. 84.17). They are more common in children. The plain film findings include the signs of raised intracranial pressure discussed above, and, in a small proportion of cases, excessive calcification (more than 1 cm in diameter) in the region of the pineal (Fig. 84.18).

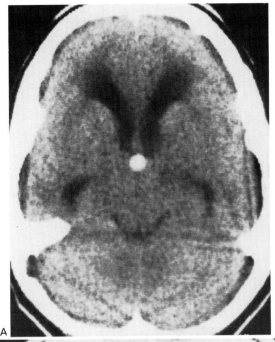

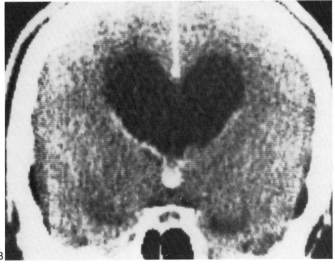

Fig. 84.15A & B Colloid cyst; CT. (A) A dense, rounded mass, 1 cm in diameter, lies in the position of the foramina of Monro, causing marked hydrocephalus of the lateral ventricles only; the third ventricle is collapsed. A coronal section after intravenous contrast medium (B) shows no pathological enhancement, and demonstrates that the mass lies largely within the third ventricle. Subependymal veins outline the dilated ventricles. (Courtesy of Dr J Price, Oakland, California)

At the time of clinical presentation, the CT findings include dilatation of the lateral ventricles and the anterior portion of the third ventricle, and a mass commonly up to 2 cm in diameter, engulfing or displacing the calcified pineal [10]. (Fig. 84.19) The quadrigeminal cistern is distorted or obliterated; if this sign is not recognized, a small isodense lesion may be overlooked. Differential diagnosis from benign aqueduct stenosis hinges on the normality of the posterior third ventricle and quadrigeminal cistern in that latter condition.

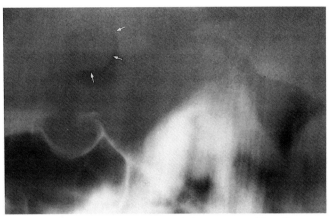

Fig. 84.16 Colloid cyst. Pneumoencephalogram, erect filling film, demonstrates a rounded filling defect projecting into the upper part of the third ventricle, from the foramen of Monro [arrows], and blocking the passage of air.

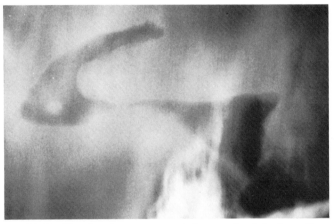

Fig. 84.17 'Pinealoma'; pneumoencephalogram. A relatively small mass in the region of the pineal narrows the aqueduct. The suprapineal recess is a large one.

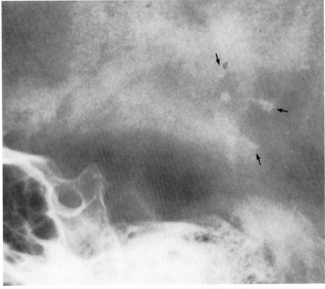

Fig. 84.18 Teratoma of the pineal region; skull lateral projection. Extensive spotty calcification [arrows] over an area larger than the normal pineal, in a boy of 12 years.

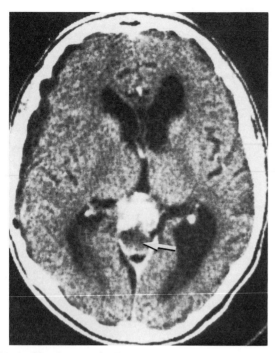

Fig. 84.19 Pineal tumour (malignant astrocytoma); CT. A large, contrast enhancing tumour occupies the quadrigeminal cistern and bulges into the posterior end of the third ventricle, causing obstructive hydrocephalus. Part of the tumour is probably cystic [arrow]. A subdural effusion underlies a right temporal craniotomy.

Injection of contrast medium is mandatory, and the majority of pineal tumours will show enhancement (the only invariable exception being the pure lipoma).

A minority of patients with pineal region tumours will not have hydrocephalus, but will present with Parinaud's syndrome (paresis of upward gaze) due to compression of the tectal plate. Diabetes insipidus, cranial nerve palsies or long tract signs may also be encountered.

There is no consensus in the CT literature on useful specificity of CT findings for the various histological types of tumour found in this region. Some differentiating features may however be helpful.

Germinomas, (the most common type) are virtually never calcified, but may surround normal pineal calcification. They tend to be uniformly hyperdense on precontrast CT studies, and enhance markedly and homogeneously after intravenous contrast medium. They are generally rounded and well defined, but more aggressive, infiltrative types do occur.

A hallmark of the germinoma is subependymal spread along the third and lateral ventricles, subtle on precontrast CT scans, but clearly enhancing in a smooth or nodular fashion. An uncommon but classical finding is a second enhancing mass in the suprasellar region [11]; the pineal mass may be much smaller than the suprasellar tumour, and either may exist in isolation. Pineal lesions should be sought in all cases of suprasellar tumour of unclear aetiology (and are also associated with retinoblastomas).

The *embryonal cell carcinoma* and the *teratoma*, related to the germinoma, are often similar at CT, but may show calcification, which is not a feature of germinoma. Teeth may be found in teratomas. The margins of these tumours are more often irregular, indicating their invasive nature. If fat is present within the tumour, a teratoma is most likely.

True *pinealomas* and *pineoblastomas* are much less common than germ cell tumours. Their CT appearances overlap with those of the germinoma/teratoma group, although lipomatous elements are not observed. Extensive calcification is quite characteristic, especially in young children, and points to a pineal rather than glial origin. The occasional *glioma* arising adjacent to the pineal can in many respects mimic pineal tumours, being CT isodense or hyperdense with respect to the surrounding brain, with contrast enhancement and occasional calcification. A helpful differential clue is initial low density, not often seen with germ cell or pineal tumours.

Lipomas offer few problems in CT identification, being uniformly fatty in CT density, extremely well marginated, without calcification or contrast enhancement. *Epidermoids* are rather similar, but closer to cerebro-spinal fluid CT density.

Medulloblastoma

This is the commonest intracranial tumour in childhood, but may be encountered throughout life. It arises in the region of the roof of the fourth ventricle (the superior medullary velum) and causes hydrocephalus. It very commonly recurs after surgery, to infiltrate and spread throughout the subcharachnoid space. Presentation is frequently with raised intracranial pressure; plain film findings are nonspecific.

The tumour appears on CT as a solid lesion, slightly denser than the cerebellum, and surrounded by a low density 'halo' [12]. It is usually midline, growing into the fourth ventricle from behind, but frequently extends into the cerebellar hemispheres, and up into the brain stem. The almost universal lack of calcification is a differentiating feature from the considerably rarer ependymoma. Patchy or homogeneous contrast enhancement occurs in the large majority of medulloblastomas (Fig. 84.20).

A subtype of medulloblastoma, with a better prognosis, classified as '*desmoplastic* or *cerebellar sarcoma*, is found in adults and older children. It is frequently more eccentric in location, and may extend into the cerebellopontine angle, mimicking an acoustic neuroma.

Postoperative scans in cases of medulloblastoma are of considerable importance. Subarachnoid seeding is difficult to detect; a frequent manifestation is progressive hydrocephalus. CT may also reveal diffuse enhancement of the cisterns and sulci. The entire head should always be examined.

Haemangioblastoma

This tumour also typically arises in the cerebellum, although supratentorial lesions are reported. The tumours may be multiple and form part of the von Hippel-Lindau syndrome.

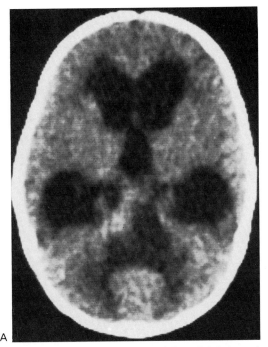
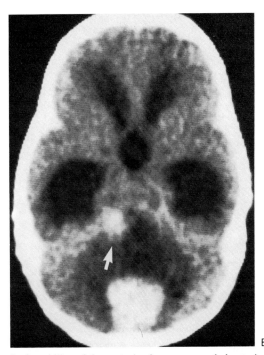

Fig. 84.20A & B Medulloblastoma; CT. (A) A slightly hyperdense mass is present in the midline of the posterior fossa, surrounded anteriorly and laterally by extensive oedema. The fourth ventricle cannot be seen, and there is gross obstructive hydrocephalus. (B) After intravenous contrast medium: the tumour shows homogeneous enhancement, and another lesion is revealed to the right of the brain stem [arrow].

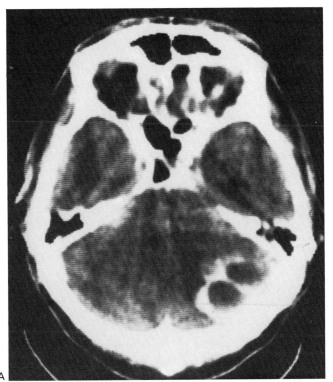
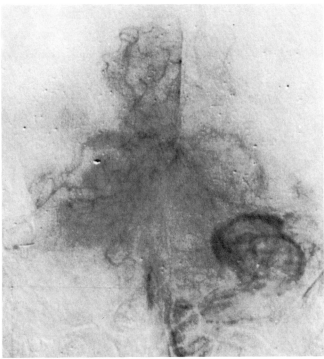

Fig. 84.21A & B Cerebellar haemangioblastoma. (A) CT, after intravenous contrast medium: a double ring of contrast enhancement surrounding low density cysts is seen in the left cerebellar hemisphere. (B) Vertebral angiogram, half axial projection, capillary phase, showing a vascular tumour whose form corresponds exactly to that seen in (A).

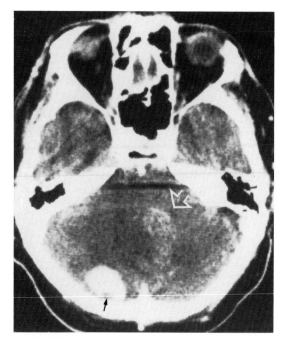

Fig. 84.22 Cerebellar haemangioblastoma; CT. A contrast enhancing tumour peripherally in the right cerebellar hemisphere is associated with extensive oedema; the fourth ventricle [open arrow] is almost obliterated. A very small lucent area within the tumour [arrow] corresponded to a small cyst found at surgery.

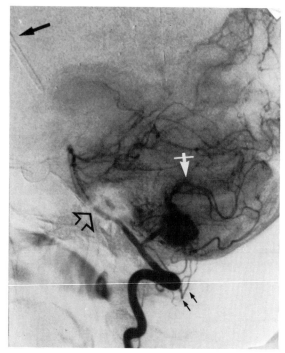

Fig. 84.23 Cerebellar haemangioblastoma; vertebral angiogram, lateral projection. Typical dense tumour nodule in the cerebellar tonsil, displacing the supratonsillar segment of the posterior inferior cerebellar artery upwards [white arrow], the basilar artery forwards [open arrow] and the arteries around the cerebellar tonsils down through the foramen magnum [small arrows]. [Upper arrow = shunt tube].

Plain film findings are those of raised intracranial pressure.

The most typical CT feature is a low density cyst, generally very well defined, with attenuation values only slightly higher than those of cerebrospinal fluid. The lesions are occasionally multiple.

Contrast enhancement classically produces intense increase in CT density of the margin of the cyst (Fig. 84.21 & 84.22), but the vascular component, in the form of a mural nodule, may be very small, and overlooked at CT. Occasionally a small nodule is present, unaccompanied by a cyst and less commonly a large solid tumour may have no cystic component.

Differential diagnosis of the CT appearances includes cerebellar astrocytoma or metastases, or extra-axial tumours such as meningioma.

Angiography is almost always performed if the diagnosis is suspected preoperatively. Unilateral vertebral arteriography usually suffices. It reveals one or more very vascular nodules (Fig. 84.23), supplied by cerebellar arteries, with rapidly draining veins. The vascular nodule may appear to have an avascular centre, or can be so intense that it mimics an arteriovenous malformation. A large avascular mass in association with the vascular nodule usually indicates a cyst. It is not uncommon for angiography to show the presence of multiple small tumours in individuals thought on CT findings to have a single lesion [13].

Choroid plexus papilloma

Papilloma of the choroid plexus is a rare tumour occurring

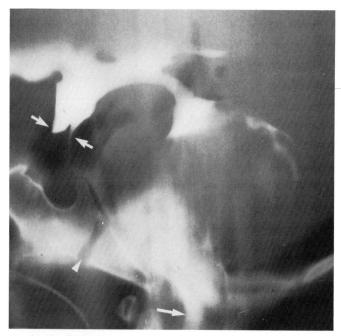

Fig. 84.24 Choroid plexus papilloma of the fourth ventricle; metrizamide ventriculogram, sitting position, midline lateral tomogram. The large, irregular tumour is outlined by contrast medium, within the fourth ventricle. Despite the presence of hydrocephalus, the contrast medium has reached the subarachnoid space [lower arrow]. Note truncated, widened aqueduct; also excellent demonstration of optic and infundibular recesses [arrows]. The spheno-occipital synchondrosis [arrowhead] is unfused.

in children and young adults, arising in the fourth or lateral ventricles (Fig. 84.24). The tumour does not usually invade the surrounding tissues, and remains mobile; malignant change is rare, although seeding may occur via the cerebrospinal fluid. It does however cause hydrocephalus due to increased production of cerebrospinal fluid, and plain films may therefore show evidence of raised intracranial pressure. Calcification is rare.

CT shows a well defined lesion of increased density, usually situated in the atrium of the lateral ventricle, which is dilated. Intravenous contrast medium causes marked increase in density. Angiography characteristically shows a hypervascular mass supplied predominantly by choroidal arteries, the anterior choroidal, and the choroidal branches of the posterior cerebral artery. The mobility of the tumour has proved a problem in pneumographic diagnosis, since it flops into the dependent part of the dilated ventricle, where it is concealed by ventricular fluid; lateral decubitus films with the affected side uppermost can avoid the need for injection of larger quantities of air.

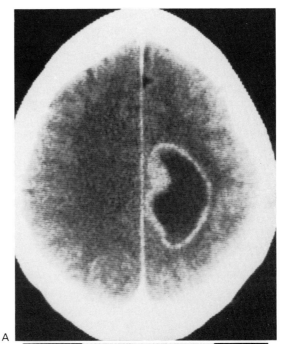

A

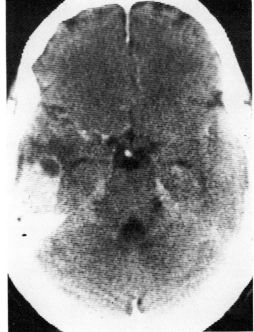

B

Metastases to the brain

Secondary tumours are the most commonly encountered in clinical practice, and in the average CT experience in a general hospital outside neurosurgical centres. Plain films may be extremely helpful if they demonstrate other evidence of metastatic disease especially in the patient with a solitary cerebral lesion. Since metastases often produce symptoms over a short period, signs of raised intracranial pressure are characteristically lacking.

The most useful observation as regards CT diagnosis of metastases is their multiplicity (Fig. 84.25): multiple masses are metastatic tumours until proven otherwise, or unless the history indicates another cause, such as multiple abscesses in a patient with known endocarditis. A history of prior malignant disease on the other hand is very suggestive, and practically very useful, because most of the CT patterns shown by metastases are relatively nonspecific.

There is a tendency for metastases to seed peripherally in the cerebral substance, especially at the grey/white matter junction. This sign is helpful when present, but secondary deposits can, of course, be found in the midbrain, basal ganglia or corpus callosum. Peripheral lesions can lie so near the skull that they are difficult to identify.

Metastases are characterized by surrounding white matter oedema, often out of proportion to the size of the tumour itself. This type of oedema responds promptly but transiently to systemic steroid therapy.

Almost all metastases demonstrate marked contrast enhancement because of blood brain barrier deficiency. It is strongly advised to give intravenous contrast medium in any CT search for metastatic disease as a mass which shows no contrast enhancement is unlikely to be a metastasis.

Fig. 84.25A & B Metastases; CT following intravenous contrast medium. The higher section (A) shows a very large, deep. frontoparietal mass with an enhancing rim, which is thin and well defined laterally, but thick and irregular on the medial side. The centre of the lesion is of uniformly low density, which often indicates that it is fluid, or necrotic. Oedema is limited. The correct diagnosis is indicated by the presence of a second lesion in the right temporal lobe (B), which is mainly solid, and has more obvious oedema around it.

The histology of the primary tumour has limited influence upon the CT appearances of cerebral secondary deposits. Squamous cell carcinomas, usually bronchogenic, tend to outgrow their blood supply and become necrotic; a low attenuation, 'cystic' central portion is then seen, surrounded by an enhancing rim (Fig. 84.25). The latter may be thick and shaggy, but is not uncommonly thin and regular.

Deposits of breast carcinoma may also cavitate but are more frequently solid; they can be very numerous. Most metastases from breast and lung (the most common sites) are similar in density to normal brain on precontrast CT scans, but some types of tumour are spontaneously dense, due to their dense cellularity, the presence of haemorrhage or, rarely calcification. The most characteristic and frequently encountered is *malignant melanoma* [14]. This tumour, which in some series is the third most common cerebral metastasis, shows well defined increased density in over 90% of cases due primarily to haemorrhage, but in some instances related to intense cellularity and/or the presence of melanin. This increased density is usually uniform. Other haemorrhagic metastases described are from alimentary tract and breast carcinomas, choriocarcinoma, hypernephroma and sarcomas. Focal calcification within a secondary deposit at CT is rare, but has been observed in bone tumours. and in breast and colonic carcinomas; it may follow irradiation.

Meningeal invasion is also characteristic of melanoma, manifest as focal increased density within a part of the subarachnoid space, with strong enhancement following intravenous contrast medium. Increased meningeal enhancement is a classical but rather uncommon finding in carcinomatous meningitis.

Other multiple brain lesions, including abscess, infarction, haematoma, aneurysm, meningioma, neuroma and lymphoma enter into the radiographic differential diagnosis. Clinical features may be of paramount importance in indicating the correct choice. The solitary metastasis presents an even greater CT dilemma; it should not be forgotten that even in specialized centres, metastasis is the commonest cerebellar tumour. The major differential choice above and below the tentorium, is primary malignant tumour. However, when in doubt, biopsy is always indicated: a patient should never be allowed to deteriorate or succumb to a benign lesion in the mistaken assumption that it is metastatic.

Angiography may be helpful in differential diagnosis. In addition to the expected mass displacement, it often shows increased capillary density in the tumour, and a dense blush with malignant vessels is common, as are early filling veins. Frank malignant circulation is not rare. Multiple haemangioblastomas represent a source of misdiagnosis.

Cerebral lymphoma (*microglioma*) [15] may be part of disseminated disease, but many patients present with cerebral lesions. These resemble metastases in being denser than normal brain, well defined, with surrounding oedema and in generally showing dense, homogeneous enhancement with intravenous contrast medium. A typical feature is a deep paraventricular location, and the tumour may grow around the ependyma lining the ventricle. Tumour circulation is not a prominent angiographic feature.

Effects of radiation therapy [16]

Although treatment for malignant disease is generally based on radical excision, this is rarely possible in cases of cerebral

tumour, and postoperative irradiation is commonly used. Deleterious effects of such treatment may be evident radiologically.

Radionecrosis of the skull (Fig. 84.26) is now seen rarely; it is manifest as patchy bone lysis. Sclerosis is uncommon (as in cranial osteomyelitis), probably because of the excellent blood supply from scalp and dural vessels.

Occlusion of small vessels within the brain leads to cerebral infarction, atrophy and, occasionally, calcification (Fig. 84.27). In the acute stage, however, radionecrosis may be manifest at CT as reduced or mixed density, swelling and

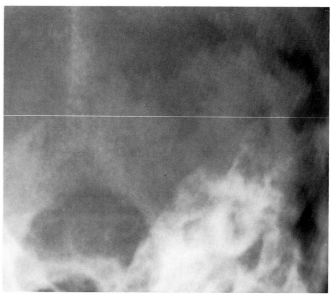

Fig. 84.26 Radionecrosis following treatment of a posterior fossa tumour. Skull, half axial projection: irregular deossification of the left side of the occipital bone.

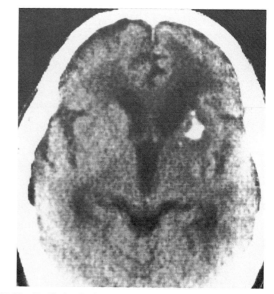

Fig. 84.27 Radiation leukoencephalopathy; CT. The frontal white matter of the left frontal lobe is of abnormally low radio-density, and there is calcification in the basal ganglia. Atrophic dilatation of the adjacent ventricle indicates demyelination rather than oedema or recurrent tumour.

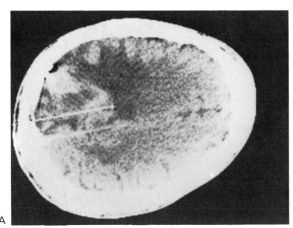

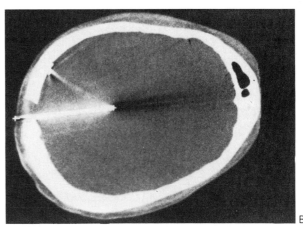

Fig. 84.28 Radiation necrosis, with CT guided biopsy; CT with intravenous contrast medium shows a large, irregular, enhancing lesion in the right parietal lobe, with surrounding oedematous white matter (A). A smaller mass is present on the left. To exclude recurrent glioma, needle biopsy was performed through an occipital burr hole (B) Histological examination revealed radiation necrosis with no evidence of recurrent tumour.

pathological enhancement, exactly simulating a recurrent malignant tumour. No CT features permit reliable differentiation, and biopsy may be necessary for decisions as to further management (Fig. 84.28); decompressive excision of a necrotic mass is sometimes required.

The combination of radiation and methotrexate, particularly when the latter is given intrathecally, can cause the rapid development of *disseminated necrotizing leukoencephalopathy*, manifest on CT as low density of white matter, with the appearance of calcification within a period of weeks; the latter may be dense enough to be visible on plain films.

Angiography in suspected intra-axial brain tumours

Historically, angiography became the classical means of investigating possible cases of brain tumour, after pneumography, and it remained so until recently. The role has now been assigned to computerized tomography, but in centres in which CT is not available, or where neurosurgeons are reluctant to change old habits, angiography is still widely used. Its task has changed however: refinement of preoperative diagnosis, mapping of major blood vessels and, in some cases, preoperative embolization are now the indications.

The extent of angiographic investigation will be determined by a combination of clinical and radiographic factors. If it is clear that a circumscribed intra- or extra-axial mass is present, full scale carotid and vertebral angiography is not required, but lesions in certain situations, e.g. near the falx cerebri or tentorium, around the pineal or the midline portion of the skull base, may necessitate bilateral internal and selective external carotid injections, as well as study of the posterior fossa. For this reason, femoral catheterization is the preferred method.

Angiographic abnormalities [17] include abnormal vessels within or at the margins of the tumour, and secondary effects on blood vessels, near and remote. In practice, the latter are more common, and are considered first. What follows is not a detailed discussion, but this can be found in any of the

Table 84.2 *Angiography of intracranial tumours (modified from Wickbom* [17]*).*

Type	Increased vascularity	Tumour vessels	Blush	Venous filling	Meningeal supply
Intra-axial					
Glioma (1 2)	rare	(+)	(+)	normal	v. rare
Glioblastoma	increased (50%)	+ +	+	early	rare
Metastases	increased (50%)	+ + +	+ +	early	(+)
Lymphoma	normal	(+)	rare	normal	rare
Haemangioblastoma	+ +	+ + to + + +	+ +	rapid	(+)
Intra-ventricular					
Plexus papilloma	increased	+	+	early	no
Meningioma	increased	+	+ to + +	early	no
Colloid cyst	no	no	no	normal	no
Extra-axial					
Meningioma	increased (75%)	+ (angioblastic)	+ +	early/normal	typical
Neuromas	normal/increased	(+)	(+)	can be early	+
Pituitary adenoma	can be increased	no	(+)	normal	from ICA
Craniopharyngioma	normal	no	no	normal	no
Chemodectoma	+ + +	+ + +	+ +	rapid	+ +
Chordoma	normal/increased	+ to + +	+ to + +	early	+

older standard texts — see Suggestions for Further Reading.

Mass lesions of any kind displace both arteries and veins. Many tumours are relatively avascular, and angiographically manifest essentially as *displacements* (Table 84.2); this is particularly true of gliomas. When assessing displacements, the vessels should be thought of not as isolated conduits, but as outlining the adjacent neural structures. Displacements which characterize specific types of tumour are indicated in the appropriate sections.

Displaced vessels indicate:

1. The *position* of the tumour: arteries and veins are stretched around the lesion (Fig. 84.29 & 30). Shift of midline structures is often present.

2. The *site* of the tumour relative to the neuraxis. A superficial lesion within the brain will compress vessels against the cranial vault or falx cerebri, whereas one outside the brain will separate them from these structures. Lesions within the temporal lobe will elevate the middle cerebral arteries which remain draped over the expanded lobe.

3. The *location* of the tumour *relative to the ventricular system*. Masses within the supratentorial ventricles separate the periventricular, subependymal or deep cerebral veins, while lesions within the fourth ventricle part the posterior inferior cerebellar arteries. Brain stem lesions push the vessels around the fourth ventricle (posterior inferior

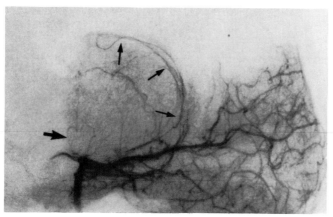

Fig. 84.29 Thalamic tumour; vertebral angiogram, lateral projection. The posterolateral choroidal artery [arrows] is greatly stretched as it runs up and over the thalamus. The normal tortuosity of the thalamoperforating arteries [arrow] is lost. Apparent hypervascularity of the thalamus is a normal finding.

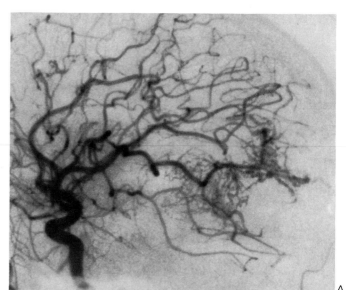

A

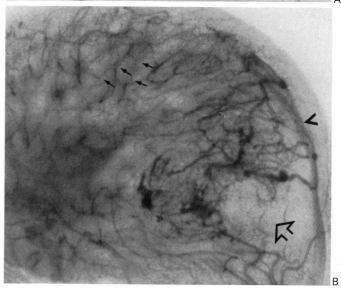

B

Fig. 84.31A & B Malignant glioma; carotid angiogram, lateral projection. (A) Arterial phase: upward and anterior displacement of the middle cerebral artery branches. Tumour vessels are evident posteriorly. (B) Capillary phase: the extent of pathological circulation is better seen, with widespread arteriovenous shunting and early filling of the posterior portion of the superior sagittal sinus [arrowhead]. Note absence of normal capillary blush in the tumour [open arrow], possibly due to cyst formation, and crowding together of convolutions more anteriorly [small arrows].

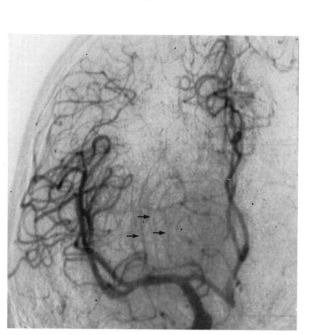

Fig. 84.30 Deeply seated glioma, centred on the caudate nucleus; carotid angiogram, anteroposterior projection. The lenticulostriate arteries [arrows] are straightened and displaced medially, but midline displacement is minimal. As with the haematoma shown in Figure 85.27 (p 1756), there is no direct evidence of the nature of the lesion.

cerebellar arteries and precentral veins) backwards, whereas cerebellar masses push them forwards.

4. *Herniations.* (a) Across the midline. Above the tentorium, anteriorly: anterior cerebral artery, and posteriorly: internal cerebral veins. Below the tentorium: circummesencephalic vessels and posterior inferior cerebellar arteries. (b) Through the tentorial hiatus: medial displacement of the anterior choroidal artery and inferior displacement of the proximal posterior cerebral artery. (c) Through the foramen magnum: tonsillohemispheric branches of the posterior inferior cerebellar artery originating below the foramen magnum.

Increased vascularity in tumours is of two types: increased number of normal vessels (or an accentuated capillary blush), and actual tumour vessels which are irregular and tortuous, sometimes bearing microaneurysms (Fig. 84.31). Arteriovenous shunting and early venous drainage may occur. *Increased density of vessels* can be seen with most types of tumour, but is particularly marked in meningiomas. *Tumour vessels* are typical of glioblastoma (and very rare in 'benign' gliomas) and metastases, but may be seen with other malignant tumours (such as chordoma) and in haemangioblastomas and angioblastic meningiomas.

The vessels feeding a tumour are usually but not invariably a clue to its site of origin (cerebral tumours being fed by cerebral vessels (Fig. 84.32), extracerebral tumours by meningeal vessels). However, meningiomas not infrequently acquire pial supply, while dural supply to gliomas and, particularly, metastases is well documented.

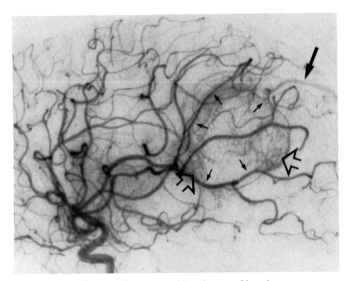

Fig. 84.32 Malignant glioma; carotid angiogram. Vessels are stretched around the tumour [small arrows] and the Sylvian vessels are displaced forwards. Pathological (tumour) vessels are seen within the tumour [open arrows] and there is early filling of a cortical vein [large arrow].

Pituitary tumours

From the viewpoint of the radiologist, pituitary tumours fall into two major groups: those producing endocrine abnormalities which often draw attention to themselves when rather small; and those producing neurological abnormalities, which are characteristically much larger at presentation.

These tumours may be classified according to their plain film appearances:

1. *Microadenomas* (Fig. 84.33)

These are by definition less than 10 mm in diameter, lying within the substance of the pituitary gland. They cause localized thinning and expansion of the floor of the pituitary fossa, usually unilateral, which may be anterior or posterior. Many can be detected on standard lateral and occipitofrontal projections, but in some cases tomography is performed. Recent work has suggested a rather poor correlation between abnormalities shown on sellar tomography and localization of the tumour.

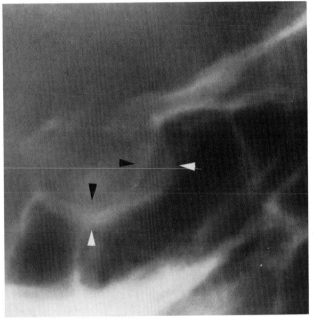

Fig. 84.33 Small pituitary tumour enlarging central portion of sella turcica. Lateral projection: black and white arrowheads indicate inner and outer components respectively of 'double floor'.

2. *Enclosed*

These tumours, more than 10 mm in diameter, 'balloon' the pituitary fossa, which becomes rounded and expanded in all directions, but they remain enclosed by the dura matter. The floor of the fossa is frequently asymmetrical, the occipitofrontal projection showing that one side is deeper than the other, while on the lateral view two parallel lines are seen, one upper representing the less affected side (and sometimes

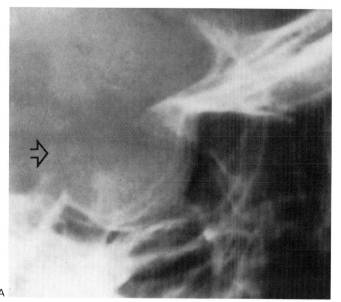

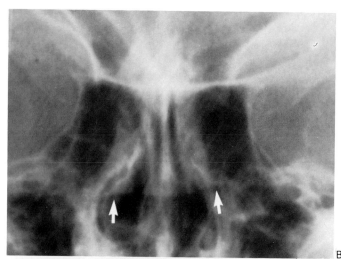

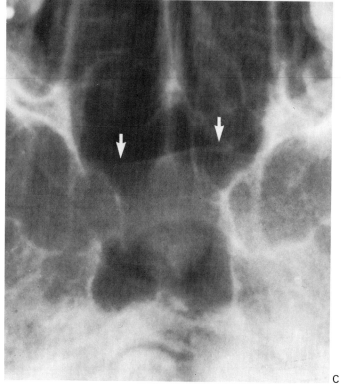

Fig. 84.34A, B & C Large pituitary adenoma. (A) Lateral, (B) occipitofrontal and (C) submentovertical plain films. The sella turcica is enlarged in all planes; the dorsum is very attenuated (open arrow). The floor is lower on the right but extends further forward on the left [arrows in B, C], explaining the multiple 'floors' seen in (A).

virtually normal) and the lower, describing a larger arc beneath it, indicates the true size of the tumour. Similar appearances may be seen on the basal projection.

3. Locally invasive (Fig. 84.34)

This type of tumour (usually a nonsecretory chromophobe adenoma) causes more extensive erosion of the basi-sphenoid. Destruction of bone is, however relatively uncommon; an enlarged sella with absent cortical margins is more suggestive of raised intracranial pressure.

4. Diffusely invasive

This less common variety invades the floor of the pituitary fossa, the sphenoid sinus and the dorsum sellae. The supero-medial border of the superior orbital fissure on one or both sides may be involved, and undercutting of the anterior clinoid processes (erosion of the inferior surface, giving an elongated, pointed appearance) may be seen. Very advanced tumours can even cause a mass in the nasopharynx.

Calcification occurs in less than 5% of pituitary adenomas; it may be granular or nodular. When curvilinear calcification is present, apparently in a suprasellar extension of the tumour, it may represent a flake of bone carried upwards. Other diagnoses such as giant aneurysm or craniopharyngioma should also be considered in this context.

Eosinophil (*growth hormone-producing*) *tumours* have frequently caused less marked enlargement of the pituitary fossa than nonsecretory tumours by the time of diagnosis. As part of the generalized acromegalic changes, the sella sometimes appears rather chunky, square or angular. Other

manifestations of acromegaly on the skull radiographs are: thickening of the vault, especially at muscle attachments, but with a normal bone texture; enlargement of air cells and paranasal sinuses, particularly frontally, with prominence of the supraorbital ridge; increase in the mandibular angle, prognathism and widely spaced teeth; hypertrophy of the soft tissues (Fig. 84.35).

Basophil (ACTH-producing tumours) are rarely large at the time of presentation.

Demonstration of the degree of sphenoid sinus pneumatization and the disposition of longitudinal septa within the sinus may be important in the assessment of patients for trans-sphenoidal surgery. Pneumatization may be sellar, extending back to the floor of the sella (in 86%), presellar, extending only as far as the tuberculum sellae (in 11%), or

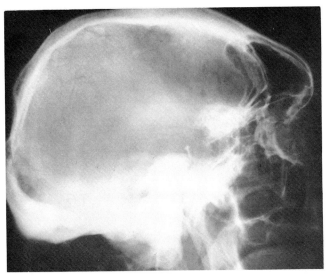

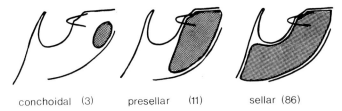

conchoidal (3)   presellar (11)   sellar (86)

Fig. 84.36 Variations in pneumatization of the sphenoid sinus (relative incidence given in %).

Fig. 84.35 Acromegaly; skull, lateral projection. The vault is large and thick, with overgrowth of the paranasal sinuses, particularly the frontal. The facial skeleton, especially the mandible, is hypertrophic. The pituitary fossa is only mildly enlarged.

conchoidal — rudimentary (in 3%), (Fig. 84.36). Surgery is usually contraindicated in the third group and in patients with active inflammatory disease of the sinuses. Tomograms may be required for adequate assessment.

Following surgery or, more rarely, spontaneous involution of a pituitary tumour, an enlarged sella turcica may reossify and show remodelling towards a more normal size and shape.

Other pituitary tumours

Craniopharyngioma can arise almost entirely within the pituitary fossa; the diagnosis is suggested by the presence of calcification. *Glioma* and *choristoma* rarely occur in the neurohypophysis, which is the site of election for the much commoner metastasis. Irregular expansion of the sella turcica with bone destruction may be seen. Mucocele of the sphenoid sinus can mimic sellar expansion (Fig. 84.37).

Computerized tomography [18]

Microadenomas

These tumours may be visualized on CT only with a high resolution apparatus, and with careful attention to detail. Contiguous sections 1.5 mm in height are obtained in the axial plane, with computer reformation into coronal and sagittal planes. Direct coronal sections may be of higher quality. Scanning is carried out only after intravenous contrast medium.

The adenoma appears as a relatively low density area within the denser gland (Fig. 84.38). Contrast enhancement of the tumour itself is rare. Additional signs of the presence

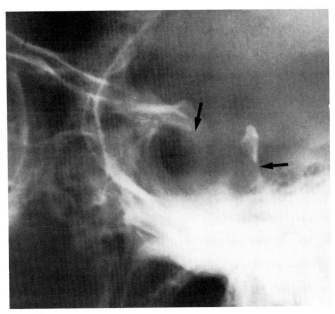

Fig. 84.37 Mucocele of the sphenoid sinus, causing optic nerve compression. Skull, lateral projection: the floor of the sella turcica is eroded, simulating a pituitary adenoma, but remnants of the floor and anterior wall [arrows] suggest that the sella is not, in fact, enlarged. The sphenoid sinus is opaque.

of a microadenoma are: focal erosion of the floor of the pituitary fossa, upward convexity of the superior surface of the gland and deviation of the infundibulum.

CT studies can be carried out during bromocriptine therapy to document disappearance or shrinkage of the tumour.

Larger adenomas

The typical pituitary 'macroadenoma' has CT features which allow confident diagnosis in the majority of cases. The characteristic CT finding is soft tissue within an enlarged pituitary fossa. In contradistinction to microadenomas, its density is most often greater than that of brain. Most pituitary adenomas enhance strongly with intravenous contrast medium, usually uniformly, indicating a solid tumour. Low density areas within the tumour may represent cysts, while peripheral rim enhancement, or absence of enhancement

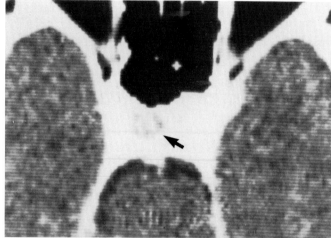

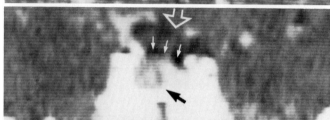

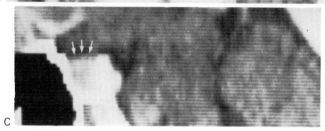

Fig. 84.38A & B   Pituitary microadenoma (prolactinoma); CT. (A) Axial section through pituitary fossa. (B) coronal and (C) sagittal reformations. After intravenous contrast medium, the tumour [black arrows] is less dense than the normal gland. The superior surface of the gland is bulged upwards [small arrows] and the infundibulum [open arrow] is displaced.

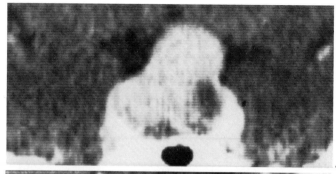

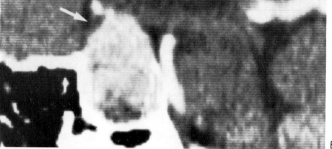

Fig. 84.39A & B   Pituitary adenoma. (A) Coronal and (B) sagittal images, after intravenous contrast medium. A lobulated tumour has considerably enlarged the sella turcica. Low density, unenhancing regions within it are compatible with cyst formation or necrosis. Substantial suprasellar extension of the tumour encroaches on the region of the optic chiasm [arrow] and anterior third ventricle; the patient presented with visual disturbance.

suggest a necrotic lesion (Fig. 84.39). If the entire sellar contents are of low density, a search should be made for the infundibulum within the low density area, since an empty sella (see below) is more likely.

The extent of the tumour is best assessed on contrast enhanced images. The adjacent cavernous sinuses can also be better seen for assessment of lateral extension of the tumour. Suprasellar extension is present if the tumour reaches above the clinoid processes. In the case of very large tumours, the mass fills the suprasellar cisterns and can invade the frontal or temporal lobes or hypothalamus; hydrocephalus is rare.

Calcification is uncommon, and often suggests an alternative diagnosis such as aneurysm or craniopharyngioma.

When high resolution CT is not available, plain film studies (usually with tomography) and/or CT following intrathecal injection of water soluble contrast medium can be employed to give an accurate impression of possible suprasellar extension of the tumour.

Angiography

Many surgeons require angiography before operating on pituitary tumours, particularly if the subfrontal approach is employed. In addition to demonstrating the disposition of the major vessels, the study also serves to exclude the presence of a suprasellar aneurysm either mimicking a tumour or as an additional, incidental lesion.

Bilateral injections of the internal carotid arteries are performed, often using direct magnification. The lateral projection is centred on the pituitary fossa, while the anteroposterior projection is performed with the chin raised, so that the petrous bone overlies the lower border of the orbit, allowing precise estimation of lateral displacement of the carotid siphons and elevation of the first segment of the anterior cerebral arteries. The lateral projection also demonstrates 'opening' or 'closing' of the siphon, indicating the relative site of lateral extension: above the siphon, between its limbs, or below it. Small hypophyseal vessels are often seen arising from the siphon to supply the tumour, and occasionally a well defined tumour blush indicates the shape of the lesion. The internal carotid arteries commonly appear irregular in calibre adjacent to the tumour, but this does not usually imply that they are encased by it.

If the mass is very large and posteriorly placed, vertebral angiography may also be requested. It shows posterior displacement of the termination of the basilar artery and stretching of the thalamoperforating arteries.

In the absence of high quality computerized tomography, *pneumoencephalography* is still performed for the assessment of pituitary adenomas (Fig. 84.40). In addition to demonstration of the mass lesion, it may provide valuable information as to the position of the anterior end of the third ventricle. Dislocation of the anterior recesses is an important observation. Suprasellar extension of the mass may be obscured by gas in the surrounding cisterns, even at linear tomography. Lateral tomography of the third ventricle in such cases usually shows clearly upward displacement and spreading apart of the chiasmatic and infundibular recesses, indicating the position of the tumour relative to the optic chiasm. *Orbital venography* is also performed in some centres (Fig. 84.41).

Empty sella

CT studies have made it abundantly clear that an empty sella, i.e. a pituitary fossa largely filled with cerebrospinal fluid, is very common and in the large majority of cases is unassociated with clinical deficit, either endocrine or neurological. It should not be regarded as abnormal unless other

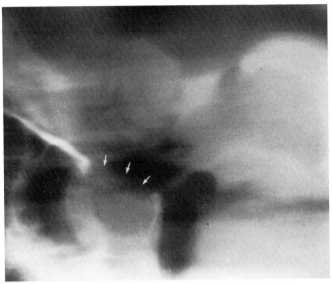

Fig. 84.40 Pituitary adenoma. Pneumoencephalogram, brow up position, midline lateral linear tomograms: extension of the tumour is largely downwards into the sphenoid sinus; a small suprasellar extension [arrows] does not reach the chiasm or third ventricle (cf. Fig. 84.39)

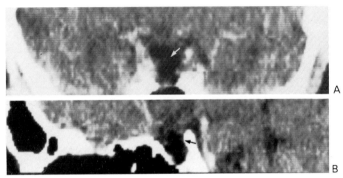

Fig. 84.42A & B Empty sella; CT coronal and sagittal reformation. The contents of the sella are of water density. The infundibulum can just be discerned posteriorly [arrows].

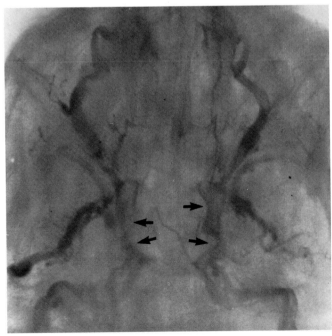

Fig. 84.41 Pituitary adenoma; orbital phlebogram, submentovertical projection. The cavernous sinuses are compressed from the medial aspect and dislocated laterally by the tumour.

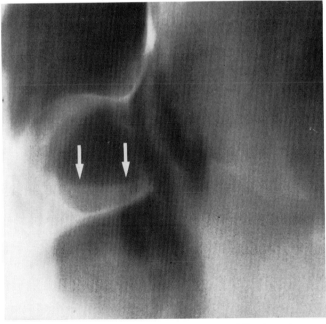

Fig. 84.43 Empty sella; pneumoencephalogram, midline lateral tomogram in brow up position. Arrows indicate a fluid level within the 'empty' sella; there is very little residual pituitary tissue, but the patient had no endocrine abnormality. The anterior end of the third ventricle lies just above the dorsum sellae. Note the characteristic deep shape of the sella turcica.

factors suggest that this is the case. Problems arise when an enlarged pituitary fossa is detected on plain films, although the finding of typical CT features in an asymptomatic patient should probably not prompt further investigation.

CT reveals a sella turcica of normal size, or slightly enlarged (Fig. 84.42). High resolution studies usually show the infundibulum as a small spot of soft tissue density extending down posteriorly to the bottom of the sella, thereby excluding a low density tumour.

In those cases in which the infundibulum cannot be shown, intrathecal contrast medium — water soluble or gaseous — can be used to confirm the diagnosis. If air is combined with conventional tomography (Fig. 84.43) it may be necessary to shake the head to induce the fluid within the sella to run out.

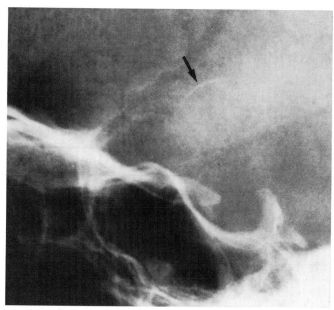

Fig. 84.44 Craniopharyngioma; skull, lateral projection. Curvilinear calcification in the dome of the tumour [arrow]. Enlargement and flattening of the sella turcica.

Other tumours in the sellar region

These include craniopharyngioma, meningioma, optic chiasm glioma, hypothalamic glioma, germinoma and metastasis. Chordoma can also arise in the sellar region.

Craniopharyngioma [19]

This tumour arises in displaced remnants of hypophyseal duct in the capsule of the pituitary and infundibulum, between the sella turcica and the floor of the third ventricle. It is a relatively common tumour in childhood, but can be seen at any age. Characteristically cystic, it produces three types of change on plain skull radiographs:

1. *Calcification.* Craniopharyngioma is the commonest cause of midline suprasellar calcification; it is present in about 85% of children and 50% of adults with the disease. It can be nodular, commonly composed of specks about 2 mm in diameter, lying in the basal part of the tumour, sometimes extending into the pituitary fossa; when this is the case, the extent of calcification gives no idea of the size of the tumour. Alternatively, it may be curvilinear, lying in the capsule, often near the vertex of the lesion, in which case it does indicate the extent of the tumour. The calcification is usually symmetrical about the midline and is best seen in the lateral projection (Fig. 84.44).

2. *Bone erosion.* Typically, this takes the form of truncation of the dorsum sellae, and is more common in adults. The sella turcica may simply be ballooned, as by a pituitary adenoma. Extensive destruction, usually symmetrical, of the planum sphenoidale, orbital roofs and anterior clinoid processes, with enlargement of the superior orbital fissures, is rare.

3. *Signs of raised intracranial pressure.* These are much more frequent in children.

The CT profile of craniopharyngioma: *suprasellar location, cyst formation, calcification and peripheral contrast enhancement*, is characteristic.

The tumour is often rather large especially in children who present with hydrocephalus due to obstruction of the foramina of Monro; most are over 2 cm in diameter. They tend to be lobulated and extend more posteriorly than pituitary adenomas (Fig. 84.45).

Calcification is visible by CT in almost all childhood craniopharyngiomas, and in up to 75% of adult tumours. The basal portion may be very densely calcified, and impossible to remove at surgery; calcification in the wall of the upper, cystic portion is also typical.

Cysts may be small and multiple or very large. The density of the fluid within them encompasses the range from slightly less than that of cerebrospinal fluid to that of calcium, the latter attributed to high protein content. An isodense cyst can easily be overlooked at CT. Contrast enhancement is observed in many craniopharyngiomas but is often not striking, and its absence does not exclude the diagnosis. The enhancing components are the solid portions and the rim of cysts, but not calcified tissues or the cyst contents.

Exceptional presentations are difficult to diagnose by any imaging technique. There may be no calcification or identifiable cyst, and the tumour can be located apparently within the third ventricle, in the posterior fossa or within the thalamus. Calcified teratomas, cystic meningioma, partially thrombosed aneurysms and hypothalamic glioma must be considered.

The role of invasive investigations is the same in cases of craniopharyngioma as in pituitary adenoma i.e. preoperative assessment (Fig. 84.46).

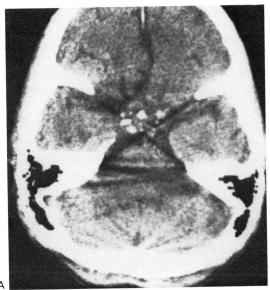
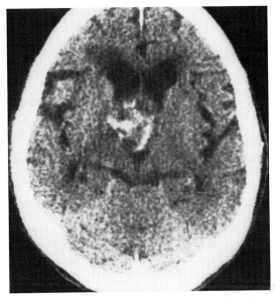

Fig. 84.45A & B   Craniopharyngioma; CT (A) before and (B) after intravenous contrast medium. A partly calcified, but also partly cystic mass displaces the midbrain posteriorly and causes hydrocephalus, by obstructing the foramina of Monro. The cyst fluid is denser than CSF. There is inhomogeneous contrast enhancement of the superior portion of the tumour.

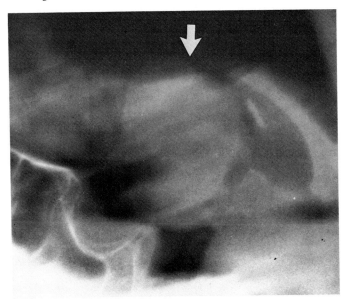

Fig. 84.46   Craniopharyngioma; pneumoencephalogram, midline tomogram in supine, 'hanging head' position. Huge craniopharyngioma, causing marked dislocation of the anteroinferior portion of the third ventricle, obstructing the foramina of Monro [arrow] and causing hydrocephalus. Note the posterosuperior orientation of the tumour.

Optic chiasm glioma [20]

These relatively benign astrocytic tumours constitute 7% of all childhood gliomas, with a peak incidence between 2 and 9 years of age, greatest at 4 years.

The characteristic feature on the lateral skull film is erosion of the sulcus chiasmaticus and anterior portion of the sella turcica, with undercutting of the planum sphenoidale, giving an 'omega' or 'cottage loaf' sella (Fig. 84.47), which should not be confused with the 'J' sella, nor with the normally prominent sulcus chiasmaticus of young children. Erosion occurs slowly, the cortex being preserved, and is only obvious in advanced cases.

Views of the optic canals may show enlargement on one or both sides, as evidence of extension into the optic nerves. The canals are fully developed by 3 years of age, with a diameter of 3.5 to 5.5 mm. A change in shape from oval (the greatest diameter being vertical) to round is the earliest sign; a difference in diameter of 2 mm, or an absolute measurement of more than 7 mm is usually pathological (but does not

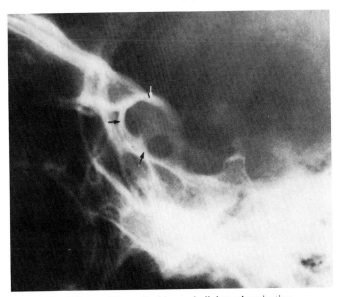

Fig. 84.47   Glioma of the optic chiasm; skull, lateral projection. Undercutting of the planum sphenoidale, with enlargement of the optic canals [arrows]; the dorsum sellae is truncated, but is thick and pushed backwards. This 'omega' or 'cottage loaf' sella should not be confused with the 'J' sella of hydrocephalus (Fig. 84.3).

necessarily indicate a glioma). Enlargement may be bilateral in cases of optic chiasm glioma. When it is marked, the optic canals become visible on the occipitofrontal projection, lying medially at the orbital apex. The bony cortex is preserved.

In later phases, changes of raised intracranial pressure are seen. The incidence of optic gliomas is increased in neurofibromatosis and skull films may show other evidence of that disease (Ch. 86).

At CT, the chiasmal glioma infiltrates and enlarges the chiasm in a diffuse manner, without major change in its radiographic density; large lesions may contain low attenuation cysts. Some lesions calcify, especially after radiotherapy. Contrast enhancement is very variable, being more striking in the larger, more malignant types.

The clue to the presence of isodense tumours is effacement of the chiasmatic cistern; coronal or sagittal images may be very helpful. Other causes of expansion of the chiasm: inflammatory or metastatic, demyelinating or vascular, are excessively rare.

Extension into the optic nerves, tracts and hypothalamus should be carefully sought, as this may influence surgical management. Conversely, the region of the chiasm should be carefully inspected in children with optic nerve gliomas. Some authors believe that pneumoencephalography is a more accurate way of assessing the intracranial optic nerves; CT with intrathecal water soluble contrast medium is probably equally effective. In cases in which the diagnosis rests between an extra-axial lesion and a chiasmal or hypothalamic glioma, pneumoencephalography can render surgical exploration unnecessary (Fig. 84.48).

Hydrocephalus is a common complication in advanced cases; sometimes the cause is not clear until after ventricular drainage, when the CT study is repeated.

Angiography plays little or no part in the diagnosis or presurgical assessment of chiasm gliomas. They are occasionally hypervascular, however.

Meningioma

Meningiomas represent 10 to 15% of primary intracranial neoplasms; they are thus less common than either gliomas or metastases. They arise from rests of arachnoid cells in relation to the dura mater, and are therefore found at the site of arachnoid villi, along venous sinuses, especially the superior sagittal, lateral, transverse and petrosal. Common sites also include the pterion, the sphenoid wings, around the cavernous sinus, the tentorium and on the floor of the anterior cranial fossa. The sheath of the optic nerve can also be a primary site, as may the choroid plexus. Although histologically 'benign', these tumours can be life threatening; malignant change is commonest in the hypervascular 'angioblastic' variety and in tumours involving the skull base.

Plain film manifestations [1]

Hyperostosis is the commonest abnormality, being present in 90% of basal tumours (Fig. 84.49). Thickening and increased density of the bone usually involves the inner and middle table; the latter may be effaced. The outer table can also be affected with a bony, spiculated or soft tissue mass outside the skull. The site of hyperostosis generally indicates the centre of attachment of the tumour to the meninges, but its extent is not proportional to the size of the tumour. *Ossification* may occur in the falx cerebri, tentorium or dural ligaments, but is also seen in normal subjects; in meningiomas, it may be extensive and unilateral.

Alteration of bone texture, giving a spotty appearance (Fig. 84.50), is very common, and may be seen at some distance from the tumour, especially with basal lesions. Very occasionally, the tumour arises within the cranial vault, expanding the diploic space. Frank lytic lesions of the vault or base are not rare.

Pressure changes are more common around the skull base with enlargement of a superior orbital fissure, erosion of the petrous apex, orbital walls, etc.

Blistering or expansion of the sphenoid sinus, with elevation of its roof, which may nevertheless be thickened, is extremely suggestive of a planum sphenoidale menin-

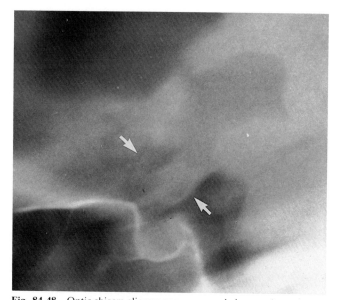

Fig. 84.48 Optic chiasm glioma; pneumoencephalogram, brow up position, midline tomogram. Mass in the region of the chiasm, outlined above and below by air [arrows] ,but blending with the floor of the third ventricle posteriorly (cf. Fig. 84.55).

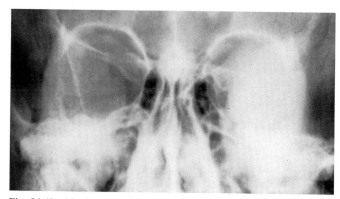

Fig. 84.49 Meningioma of sphenoid wing; skull, occipitofrontal projection. Marked thickening and increased density of the greater wing of the sphenoid on the left.

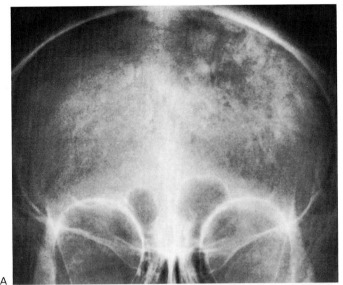

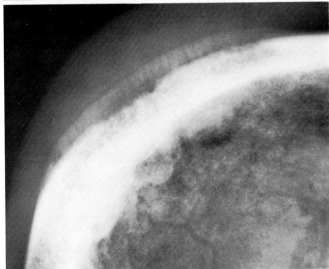

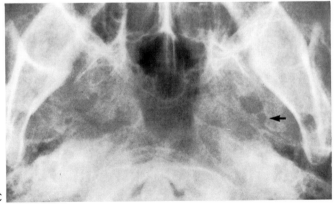

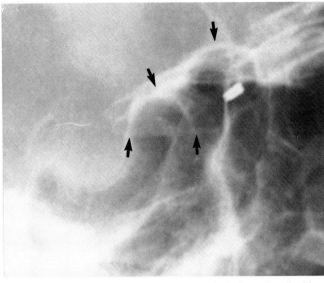

Fig. 84.51 Meningioma; skull, lateral. 'Blistering' of anterior clinoid process [arrows] in relation to a meningioma. Note sellar erosion (due to raised intracranial pressure) and surgical clips.

gioma; it is present in more than half of such lesions (Fig. 84.51).

Enlarged arterial and venous grooves reflect dilatation of meningeal arteries supplying the tumour, and of draining veins. The foramen spinosum may also be enlarged on the side of the lesion; as an isolated observation, asymmetry is rarely important (Fig. 84.50).

Calcification is visible on plain skull films in about 15% of meningiomas, as faint nodules, isolated or conglomerate or, less commonly, a faint homogeneous density (Fig. 84.52).

Nonspecific changes of raised intracranial pressure are often present. Soft tissue masses may be evident, either overlying a vault lesion, within the paranasal sinuses or, rarely, extending into the nasopharynx.

Fig. 84.50A, B & C Frontal meningioma; skull.
(A) Occipitofrontal projection shows irregular thickening and lysis, with abnormal texture, of left frontal bone. (B) Soft tissue lateral film showing extracranial new bone formation and soft tissue swelling. (C) Submentovertical projection: enlargement of left foramen spinosum [arrow].

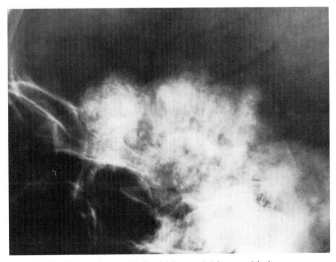

Fig. 84.52 Meningioma of left middle cranial fossa, with dense calcification.

Computerized tomography [21]

Meningiomas are often sufficiently characteristic in their CT appearances to be diagnosed with confidence. A number of asymptomatic meningiomas are also detected in this way.

A reliable CT feature is the uniform intrinsic raised density of the lesion, which ranges from just above brain density to very high, almost bony. The high density is homogeneous, or accompanied by flecks of calcification (Fig. 84.53).

These tumours are generally very well circumscribed, noninfiltrative, and often round, ovoid or lobulated. The characteristic sites have been detailed above.

A second, almost invariable CT finding is intense, uniform contrast enhancement, which is due to the intrinsic vascularity of the tumours and to the lack of a blood brain barrier (Fig. 84.54).

The presence or absence of oedema is of no diagnostic consequence in cases of meningioma: they may cause extensive white matter oedema, or show none. Usually, a meningioma discovered incidentally will have no associated oedema, while the acutely symptomatic one has considerable oedema, but all combinations are possible and the obser-

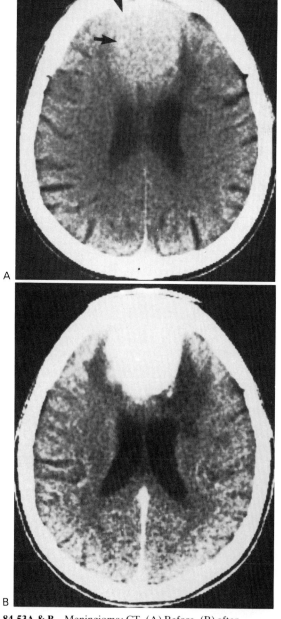

Fig. 84.53A & B Meningioma; CT. (A) Before, (B) after intravenous contrast medium: a large, rounded lesion, denser than the surrounding brain, lies in the midline anteriorly. It has small foci of calcification within it [arrows]. There is oedema in the frontal lobes, and the ventricles are displaced posteriorly. After contrast medium, there is typical, marked, homogeneous enhancement. The tumour arises in relation to the anterior part of the falx cerebri.

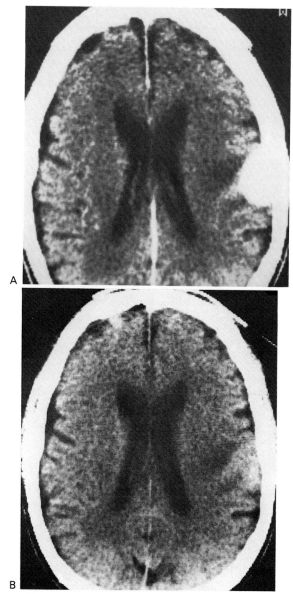

Fig. 84.54 Meningioma, low convexity; CT after intravenous contrast medium. The tumour appears to have a base against the bone, laterally, indicating its extra-axial location.

vation of oedema does not help in the differentiation of meningioma from malignant brain tumours.

Parasagittal meningiomas and tumours of the convexity and tuberculum sellae have characteristic dural attachments, which may be shown by CT. Thin CT sections, or special projections such as coronal sections can be obtained. If no proximity to a dural surface can be shown, the likelihood of a lesion being a meningioma is reduced. This does not apply in the case of the rare intraventricular meningioma, which for some reason is almost always found at the trigone of the left lateral ventricle. It may be heavily calcified, and the ventricle may be enlarged to accomodate it, but true hydrocephalus (as is seen with choroid plexus papilloma) is not found [22].

Meningiomas in the parasellar region may cause more diagnostic difficulty by CT that those in other locations, not only because of the larger variety of lesions which occur in that site, but also because the adjacent skull base renders their detection more difficult. Contrast enhancement is typical of many parasellar lesions: adenomas, aneurysms, chiasmatic gliomas, etc.; bony sclerosis or blistering favours the diagnosis of meningioma. A sella turcica of normal size and shape is usually present in cases of meningioma. If CT or pneumoencephalography show a lesion extending forwards along the planum sphenoidale, meningioma is a prime consideration (Fig. 84.55).

Cystic or necrotic meningiomas have been demonstrated by CT, preferentially located in the parasagittal region. The low density nonenhancing cystic component may be a very small part of the tumour, or leave only a narrow rim of enhancement. These areas contain fluid, necrotic tumour or even fat. They have no prognostic significance but can lead to misdiagnosis as a malignant tumour. Angiography may be helpful in establishing the correct diagnosis.

Cerebellopontine angle meningiomas can mimic acoustic neuromas, but are usually hyperdense on the unenhanced CT images, unlike the latter. Some workers emphasize the flatter shape of the meningioma, plastered on the posterior surface of the petrous bone, in contrast to the more rounded neuroma. Bone sclerosis is in favour of meningioma, while enlargement of the internal auditory meatus is much more common in cases of neuroma.

Tentorial meningiomas can arise on either the upper or lower surface of the tentorium, a distinction of some importance to the neurosurgeon. Coronal CT images will generally clarify the situation.

Angiography

Opinions differ greatly as to the role of angiography in cases of meningioma demonstrated by CT: some neurosurgeons regard it as mandatory, while others deem it unnecessary in the large majority of cases. When it is carried out, it often involves selective internal and external carotid angiography on one or both sides, sometimes with vertebral artery injections in addition.

The cardinal angiographic findings are supply to the tumour from meningeal vessels, and a dense, persistent, homogeneous blush, although the latter is frequently absent in basal lesions (Fig. 84.56). Meningeal supply is particularly common from the middle meningeal artery, but supply is frequently from several vessels (Fig. 84.57), and parasitization of cortical arteries is not rare. The blush can be very irregular, particularly in the 'angioblastic' variety, and difficult to distinguish from a malignant tumour.

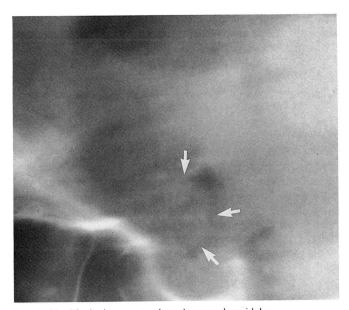

Fig. 84.55 Meningioma centred on planum sphenoidale; pneumoencephalogram, brow up position, midline tomogram. The lesion is 'capped' by air [arrows] and is therefore extra-axial (cf. Fig. 84.48). Note the typical extension forwards along the planum.

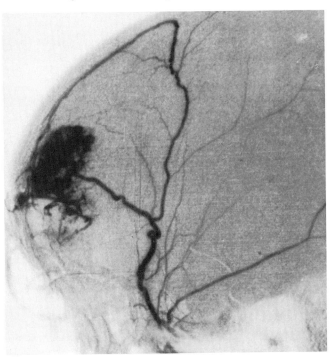

Fig. 84.56 Frontal, parasagittal meningioma; injection of internal maxillary artery. The hypertrophied anterior division of the middle meningeal artery supplies the tumour; one branch runs up to the falx before turning forwards to the tumour.

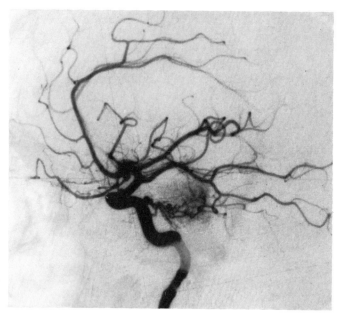

Fig. 84.57 Meningioma of the tentorium; internal carotid arteriogram, lateral projection. Meningohypophyseal vessels emerge from the carotid siphon to supply the tumour, which elevates the posterior communicating artery. Such meningeal vessels are frequently visible only when enlarged.

Cerebral vessels are displaced away from the skull, falx cerebri or tentorium, indicating the extra-axial location of the tumour (Fig. 84.58). Venous drainage is often early. Veins or major dural sinuses adjacent to the tumour may be compressed, and the radiologist is often asked to determine whether a parasagittal tumour has invaded or obliterated the superior sagittal sinus, observations which modify the surgical approach. Suitable angiographic techniques are discussed in Chapter 83.

If preoperative embolization (Fig. 84.59) is not a consideration, it is probable that adequate presurgical data can be obtained by means of digital subtraction intravenous angiographic studies.

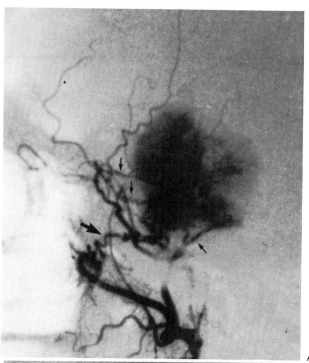

A

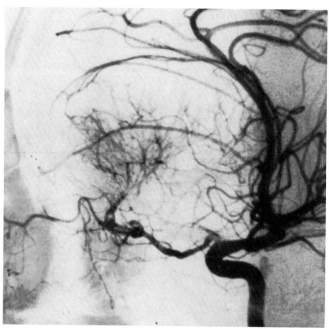

Fig. 84.58 Subfrontal meningioma; internal carotid arteriogram, arterial phase. The tumour, which receives its blood supply from the meningeal branches of the ophthalmic artery, elevates the vessels on the lower surface of the frontal lobes, indicating its extra-axial location.

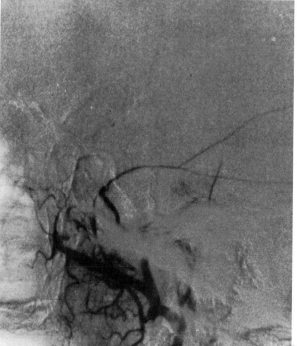

B

Fig. 84.59A & B Pterional meningioma. (A) External carotid arteriogram: a typical tumour blush arises from branches of the middle meningeal [arrows] and internal maxillary [large arrow] arteries. (B) after preoperative embolization.

Other intracranial tumours

Other tumours which characteristerically develop within the skull, but outside the brain include neuromas of the cranial nerves (especially the acoustic nerve), dermoids and epidermoids (pearly tumours) and chordoma.

Acoustic neuroma [23]

'Neuromas' develop from the neurilemmal or Schwann cell elements of the cranial nerves, and are sometimes referred to as neurilemmomas or Schwannomas, but the term 'neuroma' is established by usage. While these tumours can arise from any cranial nerve, the VIII (acoustic) nerve is by far the most common site, followed by V and IX. Only tumours arising from VIII will be considered here.

Neuromas can develop almost entirely inside the internal auditory meatus, or extend into the cranial cavity. Small tumours are capable of producing symptoms such as tinnitus and partial hearing loss, and give abnormal audiometric tests and evoked responses. Extensive radiological investigation of patients in whom these tests have not been performed is not indicated.

Most lesions large enough to cause clinical symptoms and signs enlarge the internal auditory canal. Abnormalities of the petrous bone are described further in Chapter 86. It should be noted that meningiomas in the cerebellopontine angle, brain stem glioma and, rarely, such conditions as vertebral artery ectasia or raised intracranial pressure can also enlarge the meatus. When CT is available, conventional tomography is rarely indicated.

Most medium size and large acoustic neuromas, projecting more than 5–10 mm into the cerebellopontine angle, can be identified on standard CT with intravenous contrast medium. Many of the smaller tumours will not be identifiable on CT without contrast medium, because they are of the same density as the surrounding brain. Artefacts from the petrous bone may also obscure the cerebellopontine angle, but if the cistern is well seen, it may be noted to be widened on the affected side.

Acoustic nerve tumours enhance strongly in most cases, most often homogeneously or peripherally; they are usually round or ovoid, with a flattened border along the petrous bone.

Additional CT signs are present with very large lesions. Not only is the cerebellopontine angle cistern widened or distorted, but the brain stem is rotated and asymmetrical. The fourth ventricle is distorted and displaced, and hydrocephalus may be present particularly in the elderly.

If the CT examination is apparently negative, an intracanalicular tumour is not excluded. Air meatography (Ch. 83) is then carried out. It is positive when air fails to fill all or part of the internal auditory canal. This is suggestive of acoustic neuroma, particularly if the canal is large, but false positive studies are reported with very small canals or with arachnoid adhesions. The study is unequivocally positive when, in addition to not filling the canal, the air outlines

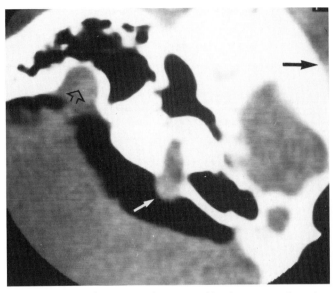

Fig. 84.60 Acoustic neuroma, demonstrated by air meatography and CT. Patient in left lateral decubitus postion [black arrow points anteriorly]. The tumour emerges from the internal auditory meatus [white arrow] and is surrounded by air in the cerebellopontine angle. Open arrow: sigmoid sinus.

a small rounded mass protruding from the meatus (Fig. 84.60).

If CT is unavailable, *pneumoencephalography* is a sensitive means of demonstrating acoustic tumours, which appear as a filling defect in the cerebellopontine angle cistern; tomography in the half axial projection, with the patient erect, is the most graphic technique. The other changes described above: widening of the ipsilateral cistern and rotation of the fourth ventricle, are noted with large tumours. The extra-axial location of the tumour is clearly displayed (Fig. 84.61).

Angiography plays little part in diagnosis, but is often carried out preoperatively [24]. It is usually limited to vertebral angiography, although carotid supply to large tumours is not uncommon. The angiographic signs are those of a mass in the

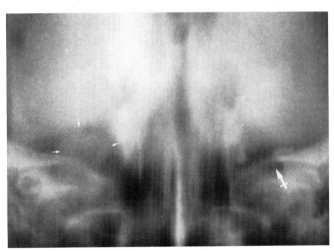

Fig. 84.61 Acoustic neuroma; pneumoencephalogram, tomography in sitting position, half axial projection. Small right sided neuroma [small arrows]; the internal auditory meatus is enlarged — compare with normal side [crossed arrow].

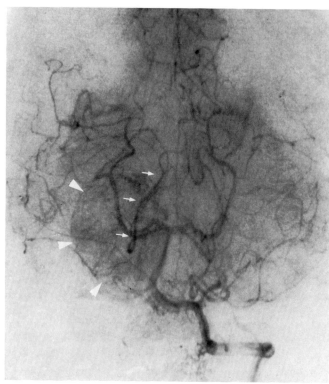

Fig. 84.62 Acoustic neuroma; vertebral angiogram, half axial projection, late arterial phase. Deformity of the superior cerebellar artery [arrows] indicating indentation of the brain stem by the large, slightly hypervascular tumour [arrowheads].

cerebellopontine angle: backward and usually downward stretching of the anterior inferior cerebellar artery, and elevation and underfilling of the petrosal vein. With larger tumours there is elevation of the superior cerebellar artery (Fig. 84.62) and contralateral displacement of the posterior inferior cerebellar artery; massive tumours displace the basilar artery. Large tumours often show a capillary blush, and variable hypervascularity with contributions from the cerebellar arteries, the meningohypophyseal branches of the internal carotid artery, and the meningeal vessels arising from the branches of the external carotid artery, viz. ascending pharyngeal, occipital and middle meningeal (Fig. 84.63). The observation of a hypervascular tumour should not lead to misdiagnosis of a meningioma if other features point to a neuroma.

Pearly tumours (dermoid and epidermoid) [25]

These developmental tumours can arise at almost any site in relation to the neuraxis, depending on the stage of ontogenesis at which faulty development occurred. Thus, they can be found within the cerebral substance or ventricular cavities, in the subarachnoid space, extradurally, in the cranium or even external to it.

Given these possibilities, the radiological manifestations are very varied. Intracranial lesions can produce raised intracranial pressure (see section on pineal tumours, p. 1712) or focal expansion of the cranial cavity. Erosion of bone, at the petrous apex, for example, may be very marked. Lesions arising within bone have characteristic sites: at the outer angle of the eye, in the midline, and in the cranial vault, above the ear. They produce expansion of the vault with loss of bone density and texture, with well defined scalloped margins (Fig. 84.64).

The keratin, cholesterol and fat within the lesions give them a characteristic low density on CT [25], but this is miti-

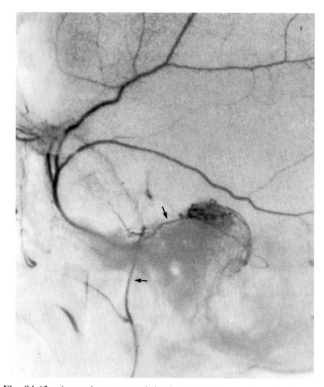

Fig. 84.63 Acoustic neuroma; injection of middle meningeal artery, lateral projection. A posterior branch gives considerable supply to the left sided tumour.

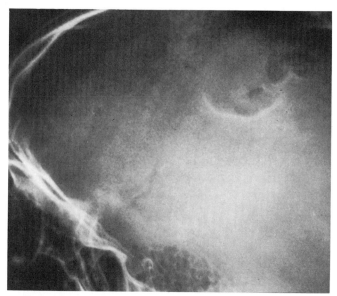

Fig. 84.64 Epidermoid of cranial vault; skull lateral projection. Well defined, scalloped expansion of middle table, with sclerotic margin, in typical location.

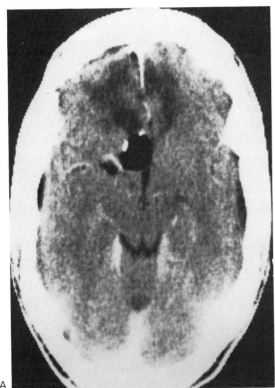

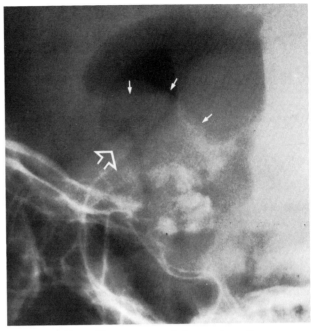

Fig. 84.66 Epidermoid; pneumoencephalogram, lateral brow-up projection. An unusual, partly calcified mass of juxtasellar location indents the frontal horn of the lateral ventricle [arrows]; the opposite frontal horn is normal [open arrow].

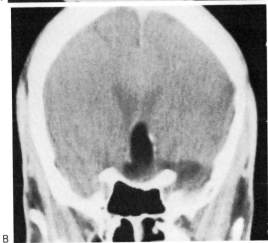

Fig. 84.65A & B Suprasellar dermoid; CT. Three characteristic features: midline location, calcification and fat, are shown. Low density lesions in the frontal lobes are postoperative. The coronal section (B) shows scalloping of the planum sphenoidale.

gated by their tendency to grow in a frond-like fashion throughout the subarachnoid space, so that the result is a lesion very similar in density to the surrounding cerebrospinal fluid (Fig. 84.65). Calcification and contrast enhancement are both rare. A fat-fluid level within the subarachnoid space or a ventricle, is highly suggestive of rupture of one of these tumours.

In suspicious cases without clear cut CT findings, intrathecal water soluble contrast medium should be used to outline the tumour. Air encephalography reveals a typical picture of an irregular mass, with air in its interstices (Fig. 84.66).

Angiography shows an avascular mass.

Chordoma [26]

The primitive notochord is the site of origin of this tumour; in about one third of cases the lesion arises in the region of the clivus, most of the remainder being in the sacral area.

Calcification, visible on plain films, is seen in the majority of cases: it can be of almost any type (Fig. 84.67). *Bone destruction* of the clivus, dorsum sellae, basisphenoid, petrous bones or upper cervical vertebrae is equally common; the combination of the two is virtually pathognomonic. *Soft tissue masses* in the nasopharynx or sphenoid sinus complete the picture (Fig. 84.68). The lesions are usually, but by no means always, midline.

CT shows a dense, calcified mass, and the associated bone destruction. Contrast enhancement on CT is of variable degree, but can be very marked. Neither of these features is specific, and the nature of the tumour is usually suggested by the midline position.

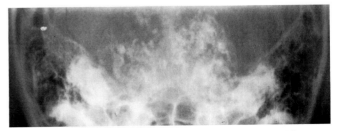

Fig. 84.67 Densely calcified chordoma in the posterior cranial fossa.

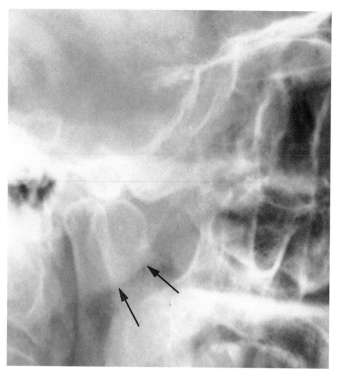

Fig. 84.68 Chordoma. Extensive destruction of skull base and upper cervical spine; large retropharyngeal mass [arrows].

Angiographic appearances are also very variable, from an avascular mass to a grossly hypervascular lesion taking supply from all adjacent vessels.

Glomus tumours

Glomus tumours in general are considered elsewhere. The glomus jugulare tumour arises in the region of the jugular bulb at the level of the jugular foramen and may cause marked enlargement, often rather irregularly marginated, of the latter foramen (Fig. 84.69). CT shows a soft tissue mass,

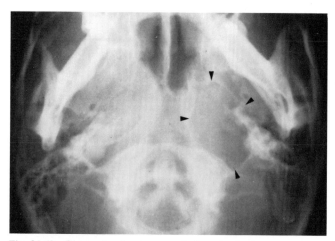

Fig. 84.69 Glomus jugulare tumour; skull, undertilted submentovertical projection. Gross enlargement of left jugular foramen [arrowheads].

with a variable extension through the jugular foramen, up into the posterior cranial fossa and down into the neck. Contrast enhancement on CT is often rather disappointing, given the very vascular nature of these tumours.

Angiography is the essential preoperative investigation. The tumours are extremely vascular, supplied largely from the occipital, posterior auricular, ascending pharyngeal and internal maxillary branches of the external carotid artery (Fig. 84.70). However, the internal carotid and vertebral arteries not infrequently contribute. *Jugular venography* plays no part in diagnosis, but may show extensive invasion or even occlusion of the vein at the base of the skull; tumour may be present within the lumen of the vessel. Preoperative embolization is frequently undertaken.

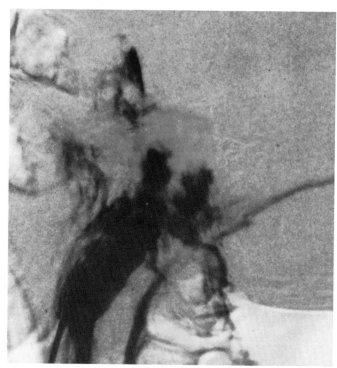

Fig. 84.70 Glomus jugulare tumour; external carotid arteriogram, lateral projections. The hypervascular tumour is supplied by the ascending pharyngeal artery.

BIBILOGRAPHY

REFERENCES

1. Du Boulay G H 1980 Principles of Xray diagnosis of the skull. Butterworth, London
2. Bonneville J F, Dietemann J L 1981 Radiology of the sella turcica. Springer, Berlin
3. Treip C S 1978 Colour atlas of neuropathology. Wolfe, London
4. Butler A R, Horii S C, Kricheff II, Shannon M B, Budzilovich G N 1978 Computed tomography in astrocytomas. Radiology 129:433–39
5. Bilaniuk L T, Zimmerman R A, Littman P et al. Computed tomography of brain stem gliomas in children. Radiology 1980; 134:89–95

6. Weisberg L A 1982 Computed tomographic findings in cerebellar astrocytoma. Comput Radiol 6:137–44

7. Swartz J R, Zimmerman R A, Bilaniuk L T 1982 Computed tomography of intracranial ependymomas. Radiology 143:97–101

8. Sage M R, McAllister V L, Kendall B E, Bull J W D, Moseley I F 1975 Radiology in the diagnosis of colloid cysts of the third ventricle. Br J Radiol 48:708–23

9. Isherwood I, Pullan B R, Rutherford R A, Strang F A 1977 Electron density and atomic number determination by computed tomography. Br J Radiol 50:613–19

10. Zimmerman R A, Bilaniuk L T, Wood J A, Bruce D A, Schut L 1980 Computed tomography of pineal, parapineal and histologically related tumours. Radiology 137:669–77

11. Takeuchi J, Handa H, Otsuka S, Takebe Y 1979 Neuroradiological aspects of suprasellar germinoma. Neuroradiology 17:153–59

12. Enzmann D R, Norman D, Levin V, Wilson C, Newton T H 1978 Computed tomography in the follow up of medulloblastomas and ependymomas. Radiology 128:57–63

13. Seeger J F, Burke D P, Knake J E, Gabrielsen T O 1981 Computed tomographic and angiographic evaluation of hemangioblastomas. Radiology 138:65–73

14. Enzmann D R, Kramer R, Norman D, Pollock J 1978 Malignant melanoma metastatic to the nervous system. Radiology 127:177–80

15. Spillane J A, Kendall B E, Moseley I F 1982 Cerebral lymphoma. J Neurol Neurosurg Psychiatry 45:198–208

16. Mikhael M A 1978 Radiation necrosis of the brain: correlations between computed tomography, pathology and dose distribution. J Comput Assist Tomogr 2:71–80

17. Wickbom I 1974 Tumor circulation. In: Newton T H, Potts D G (eds) Radiology of the skull and brain. Vol 2 Angiography Book 4 Specific disease processes. Mosby, St Louis pp 2257–85

18. Banna M, Baker H L, Houser O W 1980 Pituitary and parapituitary tumours on computed tomography. Br J Radiol 53:1123–43

19. Banna M 1976 Craniopharyngioma: based on 160 cases. Br J Radiol 49:206–23

20. Oxenhandler D C, Sayers M P 1978 The dilemma of childhood optic gliomas. J Neurosurg 48:34–47

21. Vassilouthis J, Ambrose J 1979 Computerized tomography scanning appearances of intracranial meningiomas. J Neurosurg 50:320–27

22. Mani R L, Hedgcock M W, Mass S I, Gilmor R L, Enzmann D R, Eisenberg R L 1978 Radiographic diagnosis of meningioma of the lateral ventricle. J Neurosurg 49:249–55

23. Dubois P, Drayer B P, Bank W O, Deeb Z L, Rosenbaum A E 1977 An evaluation of current diagnostic radiologic modalities in the investigation of acoustic neurilemmomas. Radiology 126:173–79

24. Numaguchi Y, Kishikawa T, Ikeda J et al 1980 Angiographic diagnosis of acoustic neuromas and meningiomas in the cerebellopontine angle. A reappraisal. Neuroradiology 19:73–80

25. Mikhael M A, Mattar A G 1978 Intracranial pearly tumors. J Comput Assist Tomogr 2:421–29

26. Kendall B E, Lee B C P 1977 Cranial chordomas. Br J Radiol 50:687–98

SUGGESTIONS FOR FURTHER READING

Di Chiro G 1967 An atlas of pathologic pneumoencephalographic anatomy. Thomas, Springfield, Ill

Du Boulay G H, Moseley I F (eds) 1977 First European seminar on computerised axial tomography in clinical practice. Springer, Berlin

Krayenbühl H A Yaşargil M G 1978 Cerebral angiography. Butterworth, London

Lee K F, Lin S R 1979 Neuroradiology of sellar and juxtasellar lesions. Thomas, Springfield, Ill

Russell D S, Rubinstein L J 1977 Pathology of tumours of the nervous system, 4th edn. Arnold, London

85 Cranial pathology (2)

J. Brismar, B. Lane, I. F. Moseley and J. Theron

Intracranial infections
    Brain abscess
    Subdural empyema
    Tuberculosis
    Encephalitides
    Meningitis
    Parasitic infections

Degenerative disorders

Demyelinating disorders
    Multiple sclerosis

Subarachnoid haemorrhage
    Intracranial arteriovenous malformations
    Spontaneous cerebral haemorrhage

Cerebral ischaemia
    Contrast enhancement
    Angiography
    Vertebrobasilar insufficiency
    Intracranial abnormalities
    Arteritis

INTRACRANIAL INFECTIONS [1]

Intracranial infections take the following forms:

Abscess: a focal, encapsulated infection of the neuraxis.

Empyema: an abscess forming in an enclosed space or potential space, sub- or extradural.

Granuloma: a focal, more or less encapsulated, inflammatory lesion, without pus formation.

Encephalitis: direct infection of the brain, usually rather diffuse.

Meningitis: infection of the meninges, which may be suppurative or granulomatous.

Osteomyelitis of the skull may also occur; infective lesions of the paranasal sinuses are discussed elsewhere.

Brain abscess

Direct evidence of a brain abscess on skull radiographs is rare; gas within the abscess, or a fluid level, may very occasionally be seen (Fig. 85.1). More common findings are displacement of the pineal or choroid plexuses due to mass effect.

Cerebral abscesses are most often streptococcal, the result of extension from adjacent structures (in about 50%) or of haematogenous dissemination. The value of skull radiographs thus lies in the demonstration of the causative lesion: an infected paranasal sinus or middle ear cavity, a fracture or foreign body or, more rarely, osteomyelitis or an extracranial or periorbital soft tissue mass. A chest film — for detection of a cardiac lesion or pulmonary abscess — is mandatory.

If CT is not available, opaque material may be injected into the abscess cavity during surgical aspiration (Fig. 85.1). On subsequent films the cavity should become progressively smaller; a concave border may suggest a second loculus. Leakage of the contrast medium (and pus) into the ventricles is a grave complication.

A cerebral abscess has a stereotyped appearance on the postinjection CT study: a 'ring' or 'doughnut' lesion with surrounding oedema, often extensive (Fig. 85.2). The ring represents the spherical wall or capsule of the abscess, the

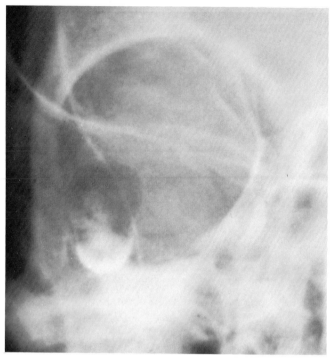

Fig. 85.1 Air and barium in an otogenic abscess within the temporal lobe, following aspiration. Occipitofrontal projection showing nonpneumatized petrous bone.

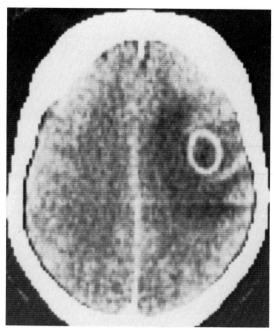

Fig. 85.2 Cerebral abcess; CT. A uniform contrast enhanced ring surrounds a nonenhancing cavity. Extensive oedema is confined to the white matter.

contrast enhancement being the result of breakdown of the blood brain barrier, as well as hypervascularity of granulation tissue. The nonenhancing centre is pus or nonviable debris, while the associated oedema is of the white matter 'vasogenic' type. Before intravenous contrast medium, abscesses do not generally contain high density material, although the capsule may be appreciated as a ring of less decreased attenuation; this is a valuable differentiating feature from cerebral tumours, which may be partly dense.

The CT pattern is by no means specific for a pyogenic abscess; it can be mimicked closely by such diverse lesions as metastatic tumour, glioblastoma, or even an infarct or resolving haematoma. Moreover, the enhanced ring pattern occurs only at a certain stage in the evolution of the abscess i.e. after a capsule is formed; an abscess at an earlier stage is indistinguishable from a more diffuse cerebritis, although pus may be present. The ring shape is also modified by the location and site or origin of the abscess. The margin alongside a ventricle may be less well developed than the remainder, or the wall of the abscess may abut bone, taking a less typical shape. The wall may be so thick that the abscess cavity cannot be identified, or several loculi may be present.

Nevertheless, when a ring lesion is seen with a clinical history suggesting infection, the diagnosis should always be borne in mind, because early treatment is more likely to be effective. CT has been responsible for a marked improvement in the morbidity and mortality of cerebral abscess.

The site of brain abscesses is dependent upon their mode or origin: an infected frontal sinus will result in abscess formation in the adjacent frontal pole or beneath it, while mastoiditis will give rise to a temporal or cerebellar lesion. Blood-borne infection can arise anywhere in the brain, but has a predilection for the territory of the middle cerebral arteries, particularly the frontoparietal region. Abscesses are frequently subcortical or periventricular.

There is a tendency for cerebral abscesses to be multicystic or loculated; instead of a solitary ring, CT discloses a number of contiguous, partly circular portions. Multiple abscesses indicate an embolic origin, often related to cardiac disease and bacterial endocarditis. Metastatic neoplasms can simulate this pattern, however.

Gas may rarely be detected within a cerebral abscess, usually indicating communication with an air-containing space such as a frontal sinus, but the presence of gas-forming organisms is a possibility, particularly when the lesion is deeply placed.

CT-controlled stereotaxic aspiration of the cavity is sometimes the optimal diagnostic and therapeutic manoeuvre. Instillation of radio-opaque substances is not recommended when CT is available for follow up. It was believed at one time that persistent contrast enhancement of the capsule of an abscess indicated that infection was still active, but it is now clear that this is not the case.

Cerebral abscesses due to *fungal infections* are seen most typically in patients with deficient immunity; Nocardia and Aspergillus are the commonest causative organisms. The lesions are radiologically similar to pyogenic abscesses (Fig. 85.3), but tend to be smaller, and show more homogeneous contrast enhancement. They are often multiple.

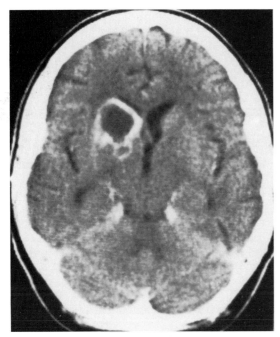

Fig. 85.3 Fungal abscess in a patient with suppressed immune responses. CT: a very small second loculus is seen posterior to the abscess in the right caudate nucleus, following intravenous contrast medium. Oedema is minimal. A malignant tumour might produce very similar appearances.

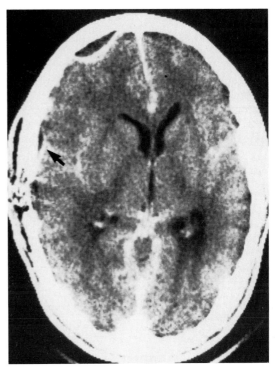

Fig. 85.4 Extradural empyema, secondary to frontal sinusitis; CT with intravenous contrast medium. A small, low density collection lies anterior to the right frontal pole; the high density rim represents the dura mater. A smaller lesion [arrow] lies anterior to a temporal burr hole. Considerable mass effect is in part due to cerebral oedema.

Subdural empyema

Subdural suppuration is generally the result of local extension from sinus or mastoid infection; extradural empyema also occurs, but is less common. The CT features are of a cresentic collection over the cerebral convexity, or widening of the interhemispheric fissure. The CT density of the collection is usually higher than that of cerebrospinal fluid, but lower than that of blood. Its infected nature is revealed by marked peripheral enhancement with intravenous contrast medium (Fig. 85.4); empyemas also tend to be loculated, multiple or complex.

Angiography is seldom indicated in cases of intracranial abscess, unless the diagnosis is in doubt. A cerebral abscess appears most commonly as an avascular mass; increased circulation in the capsule, although classical, is seen in a minority of cases. *Subdural empyema* is manifest as separation of the superficial cerebral arteries and veins from the cranial vault, or, in the case of interhemispheric lesions, separation of the vessels on the medial surfaces of the hemispheres. Cortical venous thrombosis may be evident.

Tuberculosis [2]

Mycobacterial infection rarely causes cranial osteomyelitis, manifest as slowly progressive, poorly defined erosion of the vault, or, less commonly, the base. There are no specific features.

Tuberculous meningitis used to be a common complication of miliary tuberculosis, but like central nervous system granulomas is now seen predominantly in adults. It produces a chronic granulomatous reaction in the basal cisterns, over the cerebellum and tracking along the major arteries, with a consequent arteritis. Tuberculomas occur in the brain, especially the cerebellum, and in the spinal cord.

Acute tuberculous meningitis produces no change in the skull radiographs, unless hydrocephalus supervenes, when signs of raised intracranial pressure may appear. Later, following treatment, small flakes of calcification appear, predominantly in the basal cisterns (Fig. 85.5), but sometimes along the course of the major arteries. Obstructive arteritis can result in the development of collateral channels, with enlargement of vascular grooves. If infection occurs early in life, the vault remains small, thickened and featureless.

Tuberculomas are often rather indolent, and may present with the picture of raised intracranial pressure, especially when situated in the cerebellum. Calcification dense enough to be visible on plain skull films is rare in Western countries; many patients in whom densely calcified 'brain stones' are labelled as tuberculomas have no clinical evidence of the disease.

Chronic granulomatous meningitis, as typified by tuberculosis, is manifest at CT as obliteration of the basal cisterns,

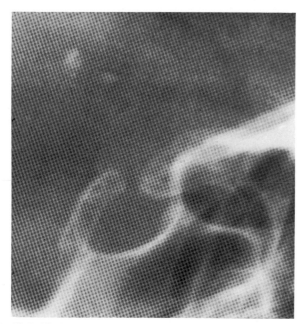

Fig. 85.5 Flecks of calcification above the sella turcica, resulting from tuberculous meningitis.

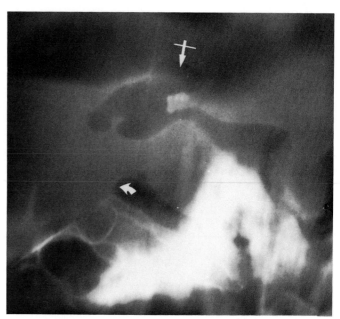

Fig. 85.6 Hydrocephalus secondary to basal meningitis. Midline lateral tomogram, pneumoencephalogram: obstruction to the flow of gas at the level of the membrane of Liliequist [lower arrow]. The fourth ventricle, aqueduct and third ventricle are widened, while the suprapineal recess [crossed arrow] is dilated.

which are filled to a variable extent with material isodense with brain, showing marked enhancement with intravenous contrast medium [3]. In advanced cases, there is visible enhancement of much of the brain surface. Obstruction to flow of cerebrospinal fluid in the basal cisterns or at the exit foramina of the fourth ventricle results in hydrocephalus (Fig. 85.6).

Other causes of this radiological picture are subarachnoid haemorrhage, in the subacute stage, carcinomatous meningitis or noninfective diseases such as sarcoidosis [4]. *Fungal infections* may produce an identical pattern: coccidioidomycosis, torulosis, blastomycosis and nocardia should be considered.

Tuberculomas are seen at CT as rounded lesions, often isodense with brain, or slightly denser. There may be little or no surrounding oedema, so that a tuberculoma may be overlooked without intravenous contrast medium. The lesions tend to be smaller than pyogenic abscesses and enhance strongly with intravenous contrast medium, revealing a rounded, thick walled or solid mass. Often multiple, they may show a variety of appearances in any one case. They tend to lie superficially in the brain, often adjacent to the Sylvian fissure; brain stem and cerebellum are other favoured sites. Chronic lesions may calcify, but, as noted above, this is not a striking feature [5].

CT demonstration of miliary tuberculous lesions (numerous small, round, enhancing dot lesions) is rare.

Intracranial lesions similar to tuberculomas may be seen in *sarcoidosis*; chest radiographs are therefore mandatory. *Metastases* must also be excluded; they generally cause more widespread white matter oedema.

In tuberculosis, as in most types of chronic meningitis, angiography shows arteritic changes in the intracranial vessels,

particularly the basal arteries, progressing in some cases to a 'moyamoya' picture. Venous occlusions may also be present. Hydrocephalus is often noted.

When a granuloma is present, arteritic changes may be focal. Other characteristic patterns are of an avascular mass, or one with slight, poorly defined hypervascularity.

Encephalitides

Encephalitis, whatever the infective agent, produces cerebral oedema of vasogenic (white matter) type. The most commonly observed abnormality at CT is therefore focal or more generalized low attentuation in white matter. There is breakdown of the blood brain barrier, but contrast enhancement is often not striking; it commonly affects the overlying cortex.

Specific causes of encephalitis may show variations from the basic pattern. *Acute disseminated encephalitis* results in large areas of white matter oedema, with considerable mass effect, involving one cerebral hemisphere, or both; the brain stem and cerebellum are often affected.

An identical picture is seen with *acute haemorrhagic leukoencephalopathy*: despite its name, its CT features are of oedema, not blood density, because the haemorrhage is petechial. Contrast enhancement is usually absent or faint.

Herpes simplex encephalitis takes two forms, the first in young children, the second in older children and adults. In the former, the infection in the brain is overwhelming, and usually rapidly fatal. Early CT findings (within the first few days after the onset of symptoms) are of diffuse, severe oedema with brain swelling obliterating the ventricles and cisterns. The severe oedema leads to necrosis, and the end result is of multicystic encephalomalacia, with the cerebrum appearing of CSF density. If the infant survives in a vegetative state, follow up CT may show prominent calcification in the remaining cortical ribbon.

The adult form is quite different, although the prognosis is also frequently grave. Its predilection for focal, often unilateral involvement of the frontal and anterior temporal region gives rise to a characteristic CT pattern [6]. A low density lesion is the first manifestation, often with some mass effect, located usually in the temporal pole or at the fronto-temporal junction. Over a few days, the lesion enlarges, and swells, sometimes irreversibly. A not uncommon feature at this stage is focal haemorrhage at the heart of the lesion. Contrast enhancement is occasionally marked. The end result is severe cerebral atrophy.

Angiography, although now rarely carried out, reveals characteristic abnormalities in herpetic encephalitis: evidence of a mass, usually temporal, with shift of the midline structures, although the latter may be absent within the first week after the onset of symptoms [7]. In the capillary phase, persistent filling of peripheral arteries, with areas of blush or hypervascularity (usually venous) and early filling of veins are seen. Multiple lesions are commonly present. Other types of encephalitis rarely show temporal swelling, and the other abnormalities are both less common and less marked.

Subacute sclerosing panencephalitis, due to measles virus, has, in addition to low density lesions of the white matter, a characteristic CT feature: cerebral atrophy; however, this is because most cases are studied long after the active phase of demyelination. Some of the lesions are indistinguishable from infarcts, and the diagnosis is made from clinical and E.E.G. features rather than radiologically.

Progressive multifocal leukoencephalopathy, also due to viral infection, is seen at CT as one or more focal areas of white matter oedema, with mass effect and variable contrast enhancement.

Meningitis

Chronic, granulomatous meningitides have been discussed above. It is well established that uncomplicated acute pyogenic meningitis is very rarely detected at CT; this is not entirely surprising, because there are no structural changes in the cerebrum.

There is little reason, therefore to recommend CT in uncomplicated meningitis, but refractory or difficult cases may benefit from the study, since CT can demonstrate significant sequelae such as abscess, empyema, hydrocephalus or venous thrombosis.

Parasitic infestations

Toxoplasma gondii infection in the brain of a host depends on the latter's reaction to it, which is often modified by immunosuppression. A ring pattern of enhancement, with surrounding oedema, similar to that seen in pyogenic

abscess, indicates some degree of host response; pathologically, an abscess capsule is found.

Conversely, a single or multifocal, poorly defined low density lesion, deeply situated and often subtle, indicates deficient host defences, and has a very poor prognosis (Fig. 85.7).

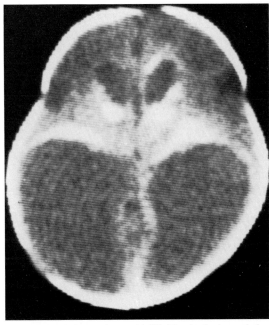

Fig. 85.7 Congenital toxoplasmosis; CT. Massive hydrocephalus involves particularly the posterior portions of the lateral ventricles. The ependyma is densely calcified, while low density in the frontal lobes indicates extensive parenchymal damage. Other congenital infections, notably cytomegalic inclusion disease, can result in a similar CT pattern.

Cysticercosis also presents an array of CT findings [8], because of its varied neuropathological features. Solitary or multiple areas of calcification, in the parenchyma of the brain but without surrounding oedema, are typical of inactive cysticerci, representing dead larvae. These small, round calcifications may be seen on plain films (Fig. 85.8) or CT; the latter is much more sensitive.

Viable larvae may cause focal low density lesions on CT, due to cyst formation or to oedema. Contrast enhancement may occur, with a ring configuration in more advanced cases. Less commonly, parenchymal cysts are spontaneously dense.

Meningobasal cysticercosis has a triad of CT features: obstructive hydrocephalus, extra-axial cystic lesions of low density, and contrast enhancement of the basal cisterns. Hydrocephalus is caused by cysts and inflammatory reaction in the basal meninges; the lesions, if large enough, can appear as grapelike clusters of low density, especially in the posterior cranial fossa.

Intraventricular cysticerci are usually of cerebrospinal fluid density, and, being thin walled, tend to escape detection. The diagnosis should be suspected if there is unexplained hydrocephalus in a patient from an endemic area. Water

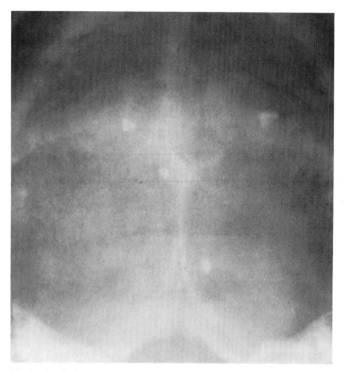

Fig. 85.8 Calcified intracerebral cysticerci in a patient with epilepsy.

soluble contrast medium instilled via a ventricular drain may be necessary to confirm the diagnosis. It will outline the cyst, which appears as a low density filling defect; it may be evident that it is mobile.

Hydatid cysts appear on CT as large cystic lesions of water density [9]. They virtually never calcify in the brain, and there is only rarely any perilesional contrast enhancement. Expansion of the cranial cavity on the side of the lesion, indicating the long course of the infestation, is common. Ventricular deformity and mass effect are considerable. The cysts are most commonly parenchymal, but extradural and orbital lesions are also encountered.

DEGENERATIVE DISORDERS

Many of the degenerative disorders which affect the brain are of unknown aetiology: a number are familial. Atrophy of the brain substance — loss of neural tissue — is a common feature. Atrophy is manifest on CT or pneumoencephalography as diminished brain volume. However, although volume loss and atrophy are often synonymous, other mechanisms may be responsible for a reduction in the expected volume of the brain.

Fluid shifts from the brain, for example, can cause a pseudoatrophic state which mimics atrophy; this has been documented in patients treated with systemic steroids [10] and with osmotic diuretics. It is also seen in cases of anorexia nervosa, in which case pseudoatrophy is presumed to be secondary to protein starvation; CT appearances return to normal with adequate nutrition. Some chronic alcoholics also show apparent atrophy. In all of these conditions, the changes are reversible, while in true atrophy, they are not.

Failure of normal development of the brain, agenesis or hypoplasia, may resemble atrophy, but with different prognostic implications. A variety of conditions may cause focal or even diffuse hypoplasia of the developing brain, but because of the plasticity of the growing tissue, the neurological consequences may be minimal.

The most important distinction is that of cerebral atrophy from hydrocephalus, since the latter may be amenable to treatment; the features which distinguish the two are discussed in Chapter 86.

Diffuse cerebral atrophy appears on CT or pneumoencephalography as increased volume of cerebrospinal fluid, reflecting loss of neural tissue volume. Assessment of the size of the sulci, fissures and cisterns is a matter of experience, and mental comparison of the study in question with those of normal patients of a similar age group examined in the same way, e.g. with the same type of CT scanner. Tables of normal measurements are to be found in the literature, but in practice no measurement is necessary, because subtle changes are unimportant, and gross findings are obvious and unequivocal. It should be remembered that most causes of atrophy are not treatable, and that the correlation between 'atrophy' shown radiologically and decreased higher cerebral functions is poor: nothing is to be gained by labelling brains as atrophic unless the changes are gross.

In general, the atrophic or involutional process which is a normal function of ageing, affects the brain diffusely [11]. The frontal sulci often appear largest at CT, because the brain tends to settle posteriorly in the supine position. The Sylvian fissures also become prominent with atrophy: the left is often the larger. The interhemispheric fissure becomes wider. The basal cisterns also enlarge, and if there is cerebellar atrophy, the superior vermian, pontine and cerebellopontine angle cisterns become prominent.

As the subarachnoid space reflects atrophy from without, so the ventricles are the index of deep atrophy: both are usually involved. Diffuse atrophic dilatation affects the frontal horns to the greatest degree. They become smoothly rounded, as do the bodies of the ventricles. Temporal horn enlargement is not such a prominent feature, and when marked, is more suggestive of hydrocephalus. The third ventricle enlarges from side to side, becoming rather rectangular on axial CT sections; the foramina of Monro are often clearly identifiable.

In cerebellar or pontocerebellar atrophy, the fourth ventricle appears on CT as a smoothly rounded lozenge rather than the normal slit-like 'boomerang'; this change is accompanied by enlargement of posterior fossa cisterns and cerebellar sulci [12].

The changes described can be focal: old trauma, infection, infarction or haemorrhage, surgical intervention, demyelination and certain specific degenerative disorders can result in focal destruction or shrinkage of the brain.

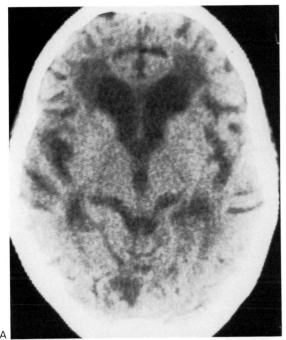

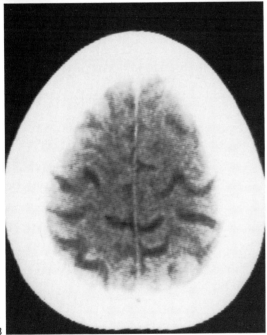

Fig. 85.9 Cerebral atrophy, with subcortical arteriosclerotic encephalopathy (Binswanger's disease); CT. Typical atrophic features: enlargement of cerebral and cerebellar sulci and fissures, ventricles and cisterns, are seen. In addition, there are probably old areas of infarction, in both occipital lobes. The white matter around the ventricles is of abnormally low density, compatible with diffuse arteriosclerotic encephalopathy.

Huntington's chorea affects predominantly the heads of the caudate nuclei, which become atrophic. The characteristic CT or pneumoencephalographic pattern is therefore one of very rounded frontal horns [13]. Unfortunately, this is a late finding, not entirely specific, and of no value in early diagnosis.

Olivopontocerebellar degeneration and other atrophic brain stem or cerebellar disease (such as the hereditary ataxias) show a shrunken midbrain and pons surrounded by capacious cisterns, while the supratentorial structures are normal.

Wilson's disease (hepatolenticular degeneration) affects the brain stem and the basal ganglia; the latter show low density lesions in about half of cases [14].

Cerebellar atrophy involving especially the vermis is occasionally seen in *chronic alcoholics*; atrophy of the cerebellum is also seen in some epileptic patients on long term phenytoin therapy, and may be associated with thickening of the cranial vault.

A number of elderly patients with dementia show areas (sometimes very extensive) of low density in the cerebral white matter, often most marked around the frontal horns. It has been shown [15] that this is the radiological correlate of subcortical arteriosclerotic encephalopathy (Binswanger's disease) (Fig. 85.9), a chronic and only partially reversible disease caused by atheroma of the medullary arteries. It is more common in hypertensives. There is some correlation between the degree and extent of CT changes and clinical deficit.

It is possible that this condition represents the erstwhile elusive state of 'multi-infarct dementia'.

DEMYELINATING DISORDERS

The *congenital leukodystrophies* have as a common CT characteristic, abnormally low density of the cerebral white matter in a more or less symmetrical bilateral pattern; the internal capsule is often relatively spared [16]. The most striking changes are seen in *spongy degeneration, Alexander's disease* (in both of which the brain is also abnormally large) and *globoid cell leukodystrophy*. More patchy white matter demyelination is the rule in *metachromatic leukodystrophy, mitochondrial cytopathy* (in which basal ganglia calcification is also seen) [17], and in *adrenoleukodystrophy*, in which the occipital lobes are first affected. Clear cut contrast enhancement near the periphery of the lesions is common in the last named disorder, and has been described in Alexander's disease.

The *gangliosidoses* have variable CT manifestations. As with the leukodystrophies, the late result of these inherited diseases is cerebral atrophy, at times severe. The CT study may be quite normal in the early stages, but if demyelination is prominent, as in some cases of *Tay-Sachs disease*, the appearances may be those of a leukodystrophy.

Abnormal white matter may also be seen in the *mucopolysaccharidoses*, as may arachnoid cysts and/or hydrocephalus.

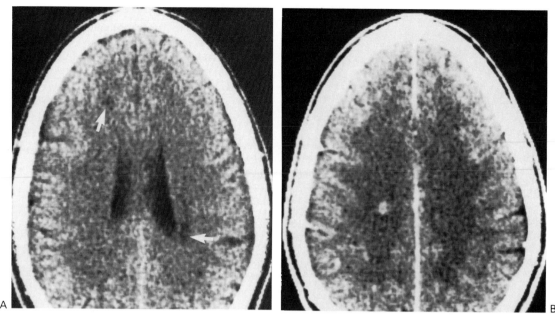

Fig. 85.10A & B   Multiple sclerosis; CT. Before intravenous contrast medium (A): two (and possibly more) low density plaques are seen, in typical paraventricular sites — frontal lobe and adjacent to the trigone. After contrast medium (B), another, enhancing lesion is evident in the right centrum semiovale.

Multiple sclerosis [18]

This disease, which is of unknown aetiology, but which closely resembles some of the slow virus infections, is very common in temperate climates, especially in Western Europe. It is characterized by neurological deficits which are separated in time and space; some patients are only mildly affected, with more or less complete recovery, but many are crippled by a succession of lesions involving the brain, spinal cord and optic nerves.

CT findings in an acute phase are of one or more 'plaques' of reduced density, classically around the trigones of the lateral ventricles or in the white matter of the frontal lobes, which show variable contrast enhancement [19] (Fig. 85.10). These plaques may resolve completely, or persist as foci of low attenuation, without contrast enhancement. Cerebral, cerebellar and brain stem atrophy are common in chronic cases.

Certain viral infections, such as progressive multifocal leukoencephalopathy and subacute sclerosing panencephalitis also show evidence of demyelination of the cerebral white matter, with a variable degree of subsequent atrophy.

Nuclear magnetic resonance is a more sensitive modality than radiological CT for demonstrating demyelination foci in multiple sclerosis and similar conditions (Ch. 5).

SUBARACHNOID HAEMORRHAGE

Skull radiographs in patients with subarachnoid haemorrhage are frequently normal, but may reveal evidence of one or other of the common causes: trauma, intracranial aneurysm, arteriovenous malformation, or, more rarely, other lesions such as cerebral tumours.

Trauma is the most common cause of subarachnoid haemorrhage. An adequate history is often lacking, and although such abnormalities as vault fractures may be a secondary result of loss of consciousness, they should orientate investigation towards a traumatic aetiology.

Aneurysms, which account for about 75% of nontraumatic subarachnoid haemorrhage, are not generally evident on plain skull films, but are occasionally manifest by calcification (curvilinear or plaque) or bone erosion (Fig. 85.11). The latter is most common around the sella turcica; enlargement of the superior orbital fissure and truncation of an anterior clinoid process are typical (Fig. 85.12). Enlargement of the pituitary fossa is a feature of giant aneurysms, as is erosion of one side of the basisphenoid, so that the lateral film may appear almost normal.

At CT, increased density of the subarachnoid spaces is the hallmark of subarachnoid haemorrhage [20]. Detection rate for subarachnoid blood should approach 90% if the scan is carried out within a week of bleeding. As in all types of haemorrhage, the haemoglobin content is the major determinant of detectability: a few red cells in the cerebrospinal

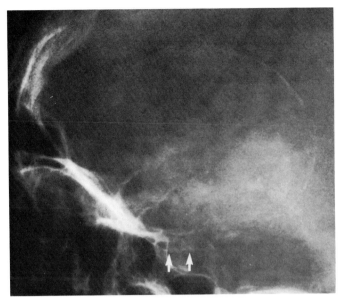

Fig. 85.11 Giant aneurysm; plain skull films lateral. A fine rim of calcification outlines the huge terminal carotid aneurysm. There the also calcification in the carotid siphon [arrows].

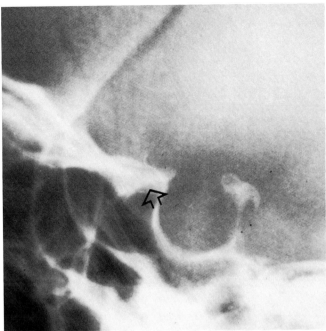

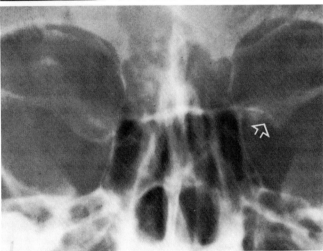

Fig. 85.12 Amputation of the anterior clinoid process from its inferolateral aspect [arrows]. Erosion of this type may be caused by an intracavernous aneurysm, a pituitary adenoma, or a meningioma.

fluid will not be detectable, but once the haematocrit of the cerebrospinal fluid reaches only a few percent, the increased density is evident.

Most aneurysms are located on or close to the circle of Willis (Table 85.1), and the blood is therefore seen around the suprasellar cisterns. If bleeding is profuse, the entire cistern becomes white on CT, and the carotid arteries, optic chiasm, and pituitary stalk appear as negative filling defects.

Table 85.1 Location of aneurysms giving rise to subarachnoid haemorrhage

Site	%
Anterior communicating artery	30
Posterior communicating artery	25
Middle cerebral artery	21
Terminal carotid artery	13
Basilar and posterior inferior cerebellar arteries	3

There is no barrier to the flow of blood in the subarachnoid space, and with a lot of bleeding the entire intracranial subarachnoid space may be opacified, with reflux or breakthrough into the ventricular system. An intracerebral haematoma may also be present. However, the blood tends to clot around the site of aneurysmal rupture, and forms a valuable clue to its location (Fig. 85.13).

Aneurysms of the *posterior communicating artery*, because of their location within the suprasellar cistern, tend to cause the most opacity of that region on rupturing. In many cases, laterality will be evident. The most dense subarachnoid blood is seen with these aneurysms, and with those at the termination of the basilar artery. Posterior communicating artery aneurysms infrequently rupture into the brain substance, a feature which distinguishes them from the ante-

rior communicating and middle cerebral artery aneurysms, with which intraparenchymal haematomas are more common. On the other hand, they may become very large before they rupture, especially in elderly females, and may then be visible on CT.

The aneurysm of the *anterior communicating artery* is strategically located to give rather stereotyped CT findings. Lying in the relatively confined cistern of the lamina terminalis, it tends to bleed upwards into that space and into the septum pellucidum, or into the third or lateral ventricles. A clot in the septum pellucidum, possibly extending into one or other frontal lobe, is virtually diagnostic of this type of aneurysm.

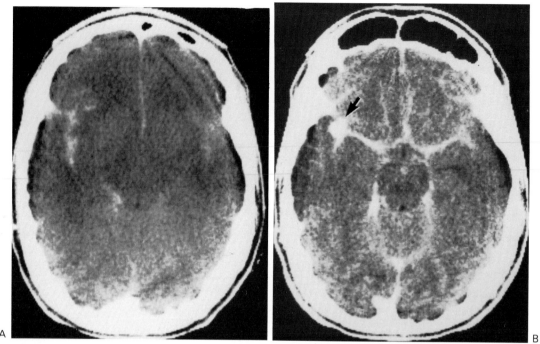

Fig. 85.13A & B   Subarachnoid haemorrhage from a right middle cerebral artery aneurysm. CT: (A) high density blood is seen throughout the subarachnoid space, but is most abundant in the right Sylvian fissure. (B) After intravenous contrast medium, at a lower level, the aneurysm is seen clearly [arrow]. Marked enhancement surrounding the basal cisterns is also typical of acute subarachnoid haemorrhage.

Middle cerebral artery aneurysms are found almost exclusively at the major branching point of that vessel into the temporal and Sylvian branches. Bleeding usually occurs adjacent to the anterior temporal lobe. Features which suggest the diagnosis at CT are a clot within the temporal lobe associated with blood in the Sylvian fissure, which may track into the suprasellar cistern or into the convexity sulci (Fig. 85.13).

Aneurysms of the *basilar artery* are usually located at its termination, where it branches into the posterior cerebral and superior cerebellar arteries. They are frequently 'giant' aneurysms, which present with mass effect, but when they rupture blood is found in the suprasellar cistern, usually not lateralized. Parenchymal clot from such aneurysms is usually located in the pons or midbrain, or higher up in the thalamus and basal ganglia, and is frequently associated with a grim prognosis.

The other classical site on the posterior circulation is at the origin of one or other *posterior inferior cerebellar artery*. Haemorrhage often occurs upwards into the fourth ventricle, thence to spread throughout the ventricular system, and downwards into the spinal subarachnoid space.

The terminal bifurcation of the *internal carotid artery* is a relatively common site for aneurysms giving rise to subarachnoid haemorrhage, after which come the origins of the *ophthalmic* and *anterior choroidal arteries* and the division of the *anterior cerebral artery* into pericallosal and callosomarginal arteries. The same general rules apply; intracerebral clot identifies the site of rupture, and visible subarachnoid blood tends to lateralise the aneurysm, although

exceptions occur. CT may be especially helpful in the case of multiple aneurysms, when angiography does not indicate which has bled; if angiography reveals no cause for haemorrhage, positive focal CT findings will indicate any region which perhaps needs further scrutiny.

CT studies performed after subarachnoid haemorrhage disclose a number of associated findings. Ischaemic lesions and hydrocephalus are the most important.

Ischaemic infarction is, unfortunately, well recognized in cases of subarachnoid haemorrhage, and is probably due to intense vasospasm, with or without thrombosis. Much of the morbidity of subarachnoid haemorrhage is due to ischaemia, which is difficult to prevent or to treat. Infarcts in this context do not present different appearances from typical ischaemic lesions; they are almost always nonhaemorrhagic. Reversible ischaemia is also manifest as a focal area of low density, which subsequently resolves; differentiation of infarction and ischaemia is impossible in the early stages.

Hydrocephalus following subarachnoid haemorrhage is of the communicating type (Ch. 86). The inflammatory effects of the subarachnoid blood block the flow of cerebrospinal fluid at the tentorial hiatus, over the cerebral convexities or at the Pacchionian granulations. The rapidity of onset of hydrocephalus is striking: it is not rare to find it on a CT study a few hours after subarachnoid haemorrhage. It frequently evolves over several days, as seen on serial CT. Most patients recover or succumb regardless of the hydrocephalus, however, because it tends to be self limiting. If progressive, it may necessitate ventricular shunting procedures.

An unruptured berry aneurysm, if small, will almost always be asymptomatic, and will not be studied by CT. It may well be overlooked, or be detected as an incidental finding at CT. Such aneurysms appear as tiny dense 'dots' on the course of a major vessel, often the middle cerebral artery, which enhance with intravenous contrast medium (Fig. 85.13). Calcification is rare. Angiography may be required to confirm the nature of the aneurysm.

The so-called *'giant' aneurysm* on the other hand, manifests itself clinically by mass effect on adjacent structures. It grows slowly over many years without leaking, and may reach a diameter of several centimetres. Internal thrombosis is common, leading to a thick walled, organized aneurysm with a relatively small lumen and a calcific wall. The base of the brain is the favoured site, the aneurysms arising from the distal internal carotid, middle cerebral or basilar arteries.

Virtually all of these large aneurysms will be evident at CT. They are seen as round or ovoid areas of raised density, often calcified in part, but frequently homogeneous; less often they are isodense or only subtly hyperdense if there is no thrombus within them. Following intravenous contrast medium, they show total enhancement or, when thrombus is present, partial enhancement. Confusingly, the enhancement may be mainly peripheral. Differential diagnosis is from parasellar meningioma, craniopharyngioma or pituitary tumour.

Many giant aneurysms have no obvious mass effect, because they have slowly burrowed into the brain, rather than displacing it. It is not rare for them to appear intra-axial at CT.

In certain individuals, cerebral atherosclerosis takes the form of aneurysmal tortuosity and elongation of the arteries, especially the basilar, internal carotid and middle cerebral. Such ectatic vessels are demonstrable by CT, especially with intravenous contrast medium. They appear as serpentine, tubular shadows; the basilar artery may project up into the floor of the third ventricle, mimicking an intraventricular mass, or simulate a mass in the cerebellopontine angle.

Mycotic and *traumatic* aneurysms must also be considered. Mycotic aneurysms arise from septic or malignant emboli. They tend to be more peripheral than the usual type of aneurysm, often on the branches of the middle cerebral artery. A common presentation is with intracerebral haemorrhage, usually with a parenchymal clot, shown by CT. While nonspecific, such a finding in a patient with known septicaemia or bacterial endocarditis is highly suggestive of a mycotic aneurysm.

Traumatic aneurysms are usually overlooked at CT, being obscured by concomitant haemorrhage; they are diagnosed by angiography.

Angiography in subarachnoid haemorrhage and intracranial aneurysms [21]

Angiography is essential for diagnosis and treatment of the large majority of intracranial aneurysms and other lesions giving rise to subarachnoid haemorrhage. When the latter is confirmed by lumbar puncture or CT, bilateral carotid angiography and uni- or bilateral vertebral angiography is indicated. The timing of the angiogram varies from centre to centre, but the study is usually obtained as soon as the general condition of the patient permits, so that surgery, which is directed at excluding the aneurysm from the circulation, can be carried out before further, possibly fatal, bleeding occurs.

An acceptable study may be obtained by bilateral carotid artery puncture and retrograde brachial angiography, but much the most satisfactory approach is transfemoral catheterization of both internal carotid and at least one vertebral artery at a single session. The carotid portion of the study

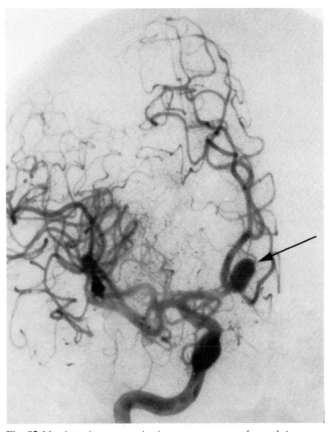

Fig. 85.14 Anterior communicating artery aneurysm [arrow] shown on internal carotid angiography. The oblique position (anteroposterior projection, head turned away from the injected side) clearly demonstrates its relationship to surrounding vessels.

requires not only lateral and anteroposterior series, but also oblique projections (Fig. 85.14) in order to unravel looping arteries, which may simulate an aneurysm. When it is thought that an aneurysm has been detected, further views, depending on the individual anatomy, may be required to confirm the diagnosis and to facilitate the surgical approach by demonstrating the neck of the aneurysm and its relationship to the surrounding arteries. These additional oblique series can be reduced: one film per second for 3 seconds is adequate.

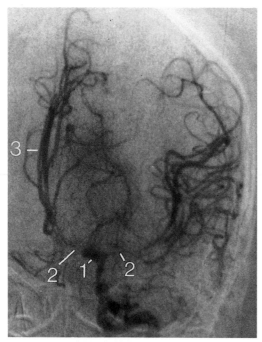

Fig. 85.15 Supraclinoid internal carotid artery aneurysm [1], with spasm of the adjacent middle and anterior cerebral arteries [2]. The anterior cerebral artery [3] is displaced to the right by a haematoma.

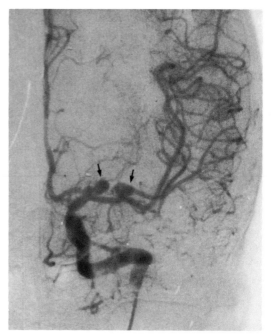

Fig. 85.16 Multiple aneurysms. Left carotid arteriogram shows terminal carotid and middle cerebral bifurcation aneurysms. A further two aneurysms were present on the right.

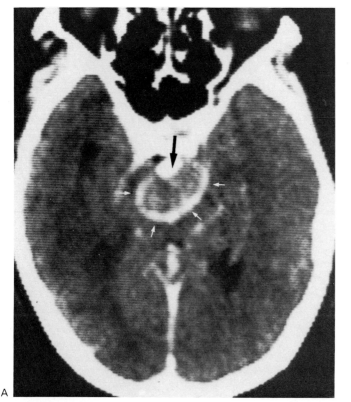

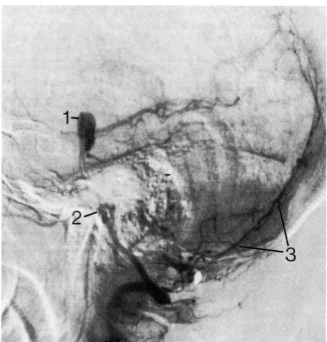

Fig. 85.17A & B Aneurysm at the termination of the basilar artery. (A) CT, with intravenous contrast medium, showing enhancement of the wall [small arrows] and lumen [arrow] of the aneurysm, with thrombus between them. (B) Vertebral angiogram: only the nonthrombosed portion is shown, and the aneurysm appears deceptively small [1]. There is severe spasm of the basilar artery [2]; note prominent posterior meningeal artery [3].

An aneurysm appears as an additional bleb somewhere along the course of an artery, almost always at a branch point; contrast medium may remain in it when the arteries have already cleared. Adjacent vessels often appear narrowed and/or irregular, indicating spasm (Fig. 85.15); they may also be displaced, due to a focal clot.

Angiography demonstrates multiple aneurysms in about 20% of cases (Fig. 85.16). Since there are often no clinical localizing features, the decision as to which has bled may be made on CT and angiographic evidence. The largest, or the most irregular, multilocular aneurysm is usually incriminated; focal spasm or evidence of a haematoma also point to the offending aneurysm. An aneurysm at the anterior communicating artery is also more likely to have bled than one elsewhere, but the only absolute evidence of rupture of an aneurysm is extravasation of contrast medium during angiography; it is also an absolute indication to terminate the study forthwith.

Large aneurysms are often partially thrombosed, in which case only the patent portion of the lumen is demonstrated angiographically (Fig. 85.17). Disparity in size between the sac shown at angiography and a mass demonstrated by CT may suggest this possibility.

Angiography shows no cause for subarachnoid haemorrhage in about 10% of cases.

Some surgeons require *postoperative angiography*. *Peroperative angiography* is less commonly employed because images of adequate quality are difficult to obtain. Postoperative films should show the surgical clip obliterating the entire neck of the aneurysm without occluding any adjacent vessels. Extensive spasm may, however be present, as may evidence of cerebral swelling or even a subdural collection.

Mycotic aneurysms, as stated above, are usually distally placed; they are often small and multiple. Similar lesions may be seen following penetrating injuries or rarely, as a manifestation of metastatic tumour.

Aneurysms arising from the internal carotid artery within the cavernous sinus pose different problems (Fig. 85.18). They do not give rise to subarachnoid haemorrhage, but compress the nerves within the sinus (III to VI nerves). A direct surgical approach is usually impossible, but occlusive balloon catheters have revolutionized their treatment.

Intracranial arteriovenous malformations

Arteriovenous malformations ('angiomas') account for 10% of cases of subarachnoid haemorrhage. They may also present with headache, epilepsy or progressive neurological deficit. They are usually classified according to the vessels involved as *arteriovenous fistulae* with direct shunting, *angiomas* with a bed of abnormal capillaries, *cavernous* or *capillary* angiomas, and *venous* angiomas. Clinically, the cerebral arteriovenous malformation is the most significant.

Changes due to enlargement of the feeding arteries are the commonest plain film manifestations: thus, the internal carotid artery causes increased diameter of the carotid canal, best seen on the base view, enlargement of the carotid sulcus and undercutting of the anterior clinoid process; the groove for the vertebral artery on the upper surface of the atlas is deepened, so that the posterior arch is very thin. When a malformation has a dural blood supply, the foramen spinosum may be enlarged, and meningeal vascular grooves become deeper, more tortuous and more numerous (Fig. 85.19). Venous grooves, including those of the dural venous sinuses, may also enlarge, as may the jugular foramen and superior orbital fissure. All these changes can be progressive if the lesion is untreated.

Venous calcification occurs in about 20% of cerebral arteriovenous malformations. Typically faint and spotty, it may be curvilinear; dense calcification is rare.

The cranial vault overlying an arteriovenous malformation may be eroded or, if the underlying brain is atrophic, reflect that atrophy. The overlying soft tissues are rarely thickened.

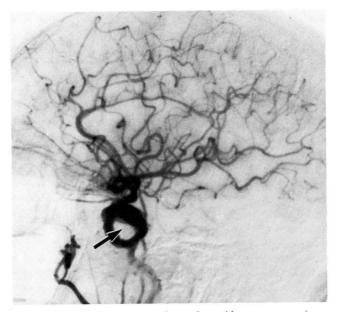

Fig. 85.18 Large intracavernous internal carotid aneurysm, causing proptosis; mural thrombus is evident as a filling defect (arrow) in the aneurysm; treated by balloon catheter.

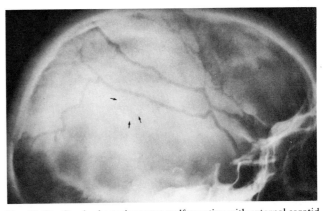

Fig. 85.19 Cerebral arteriovenous malformation with external carotid component. Grooves for both middle meningeal arteries are enlarged. Arrows indicate faint flecks of calcification. The sella turcica is deep, and probably empty.

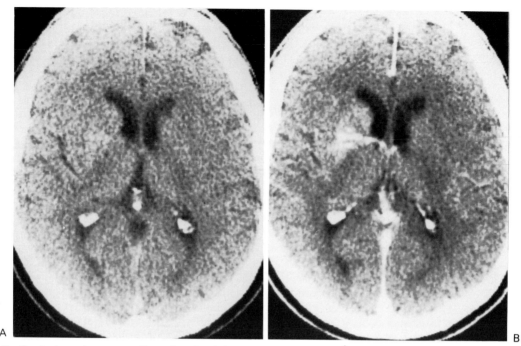

Fig. 85.20A & B   Cerebral arteriovenous malformation; CT. (A) subtle increase in density is discernible in the right lentiform nucleus. (B) After intravenous contrast medium, the lesion shows considerable enhancement. Serpiginous structures within the lesion are continuous with an enlarged thalamostriate vein.

Changes of raised intracranial pressure (Ch. 84) can result from hydrocephalus, obstructive or communicating, or increased venous pressure; only rarely does the malformation act as a mass lesion. Pineal or other displacements may, however, be present if haemorrhage has occurred.

With good quality CT studies, very few intracranial arteriovenous malformations will pass undetected, because their pathological features give them a well defined radiographic appearance [22]. CT findings include: haemorrhage, calcification, low density areas representing ischaemia, draining veins and feeding arteries, and secondary atrophy or hydrocephalus. Arteriovenous malformations likely to be overlooked on a good quality study are therefore those in which these features are lacking, many of which will be clinically insignificant. The major exception is the dural malformation or fistula, which can nevertheless produce profound symptoms; angiography is required for the detection of many of these lesions.

The most common CT abnormality in a cerebral arteriovenous malformation is a focus of increased density, caused by calcification or haemosiderosis. There is often also low density, due to ischaemia, atrophy or focal encephalomalacia; oedema is rare, as is mass effect. When the latter is present, it is attributable to the bulk of draining veins or to recent haemorrhage.

Enhancement following intravenous contrast medium is of two types: a diffuse 'blush' within the lesion, due to a deficient blood brain barrier, and opacification of feeding arteries and especially draining veins, as serpentine, tubular or rounded structures (Fig. 85.20). The latter feature is virtually pathognomonic for an arteriovenous malformation, but when it is absent, the lesion may closely resemble a primary brain tumour of low or intermediate malignancy. Biopsy may be necessary to make this distinction, particularly because a malformation with very slow flow (cavernous type) or one which is substantially thrombosed may show no clear abnormality on angiography. These so-called 'cryptic' malformations are, paradoxically, more reliably detected by CT than by angiography.

Venous angiomas are usually small, appearing at CT as a circumscribed area of abnormal contrast enhancement, sometimes denser than surrounding brain before injection [23]. Their clinical significance is unclear.

Malformations may be encountered anywhere in the cerebral substance, but the classical site for cerebral arteriovenous malformations is in the posterior half of the cerebral hemisphere, extending from the lateral ventricle to the cortex. Less often they are encountered in the cerebellum; lesions in the brain stem are excessively rare.

Angiography

Arteriography is essential for detailed diagnosis and preoperative assessment. Because feeding vessels regularly arise from more than one of the major arterial axes, it is customary to inject both internal carotid and at least one of the vertebral arteries. Rapid sequence serial angiography (up to six per second) may be necessary to sort out feeding vessels if shunting is very rapid.

The following features are studied:

1. The *vessels* involved, both their type and site of origin.

Generally there is an abnormal connection between arteries and veins, without any intervening tissue, as may be seen in very vascular tumours (Fig. 85.21), but as noted above, malformations may involve solely arteries, capillaries or veins (Fig. 85.22).

2. The exact *disposition* of the feeding arteries and the draining veins; this information is essential for surgery.

3. The *extent* of the lesion and its *relationship* to the adjacent nervous structures, both of which may affect its operability (Fig. 85.23).

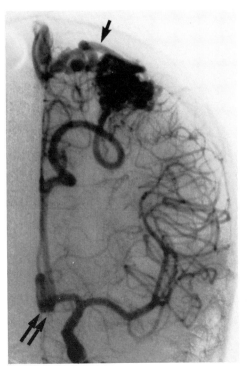

Fig. 85.21 Cerebral arteriovenous malformation, fed by a dilated callosomarginal branch of the anterior cerebral artery. Internal carotid arteriogram, anteroposterior projection in arterial phase. There is rapid venous drainage towards the superior sagittal sinus [arrows]. Note how vascular loops can simulate aneurysms [double arrows].

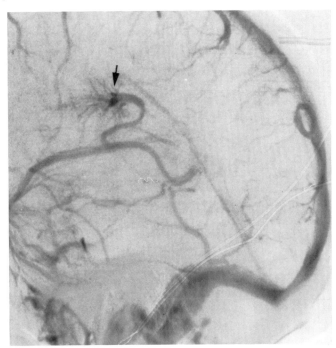

Fig. 85.22 Venous 'angioma' [arrow] draining into a large thalamostriate vein. Internal carotid arteriogram, lateral projection, venous phase.

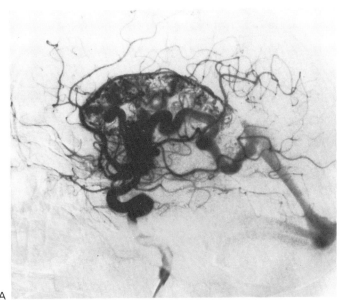

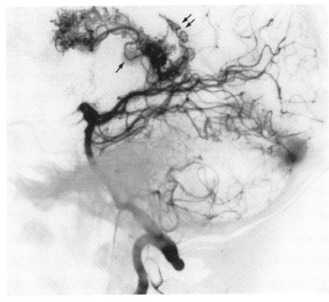

A

B

Fig. 85.23A & B Arteriovenous malformation in the corpus callosum. (A) Internal carotid injection, showing supply from the pericallosal artery and rapid drainage via a markedly dilated deep vein and the straight sinus. (B) Vertebral artery injection: a posterior component is supplied by the medial posterior choroidal [arrow] and posterior pericallosal [double arrow] arteries. Note the small calibre of the remaining cerebral arteries.

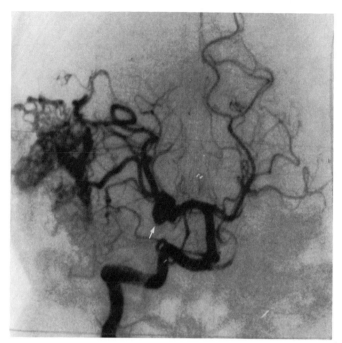

Fig. 85.24 Cerebral arteriovenous malformation with associated aneurysm. Vertebral angiogram, half axial projection. A posterior temporal malformation is fed by branches of the posterior cerebral artery, one of which bears an aneurysm [arrow].

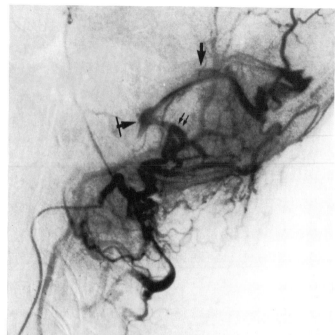

A

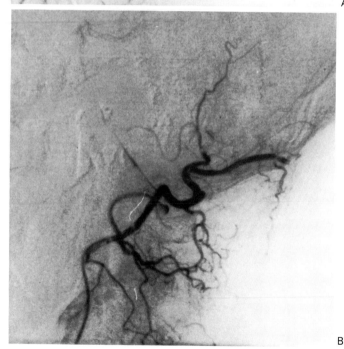

B

Fig. 85.25A & B Dural arteriovenous fistula. (A) Superselective injection of the occipital artery (lateral projection), the meningeal branch of which [double arrow] shunts directly [crossed arrow] into the lateral sinus (arrow). (B) Following embolization.

4. *Associated anomalies*, notably aneurysms on the feeding arteries (Fig. 85.24).

5. The *feasibility of nonsurgical treatment*, in the form of embolization of contributions from the external carotid artery, or even direct embolization of an intracerebral lesion.

Extracerebral malformations are supplied essentially by the external carotid artery branches, but may also receive supply from the internal carotid or vertebral arteries. Many lie on the dura mater.

Although *dural arteriovenous fistulae* are relatively rare vascular anomalies, they are being revealed with increasing frequency as the technical quality of angiography improves. Abnormal connections between the meningeal arteries and the veins of the dura mater are frequently situated near the lateral, superior sagittal or cavernous sinuses (Fig. 85.25); they often come to light, particularly in menopausal women, as the cause of a subjective bruit, which can be confirmed by auscultation. They may also cause subarachnoid haemorrhage if they drain to cerebral veins.

These lesions are easily overlooked at CT but the skull radiographs, showing hypertrophied vascular channels, may indicate the diagnosis.

Angiographic exploration requires selective catheterization of the external carotid arteries, preferably with superselective injection of their branches [24]. The internal carotid and vertebral systems should also be injected.

Since treatment is by surgery and/or embolization, radiological investigation should take account of the following:

1. The *relative contributions of the arteries which cannot be obliterated*, i.e. the internal carotid and vertebral arteries.

These may increase if the external carotid branches are embolized.

2. Possible *anastomoses* between these vessels and the external carotid artery, through which emboli may pass to reach the eye or brain.

3. The *risks* of overly effective embolization — cutaneous ulceration, cranial nerve palsies, etc.

4. The *calibre* of arteriovenous connections, especially when drainage is to cerebral veins, which may become blocked should emboli pass through the fistula.

The treatment of fistulae in the region of the cavernous sinus is discussed elsewhere.

Spontaneous cerebral haemorrhage

In patients presenting with an acute neurological syndrome, or 'stroke', which is thought to be due to haemorrhage rather than ischaemia, skull radiographs are usually obtained, although their contribution is minor. As in subarachnoid haemorrhage, they may show evidence of trauma, of a known cause of intracerebral bleeding (arteriovenous malformation, etc.), or rarely, of a tumour.

CT is the most accurate diagnostic method [25]. Detection of intracranial haemorrhage depends upon the scanner's ability to distinguish the high radiographic density of blood from the density of surrounding structures; this is possible because of the high protein content of clotted blood.

Depending on the initial haemoglobin content of the extravasated blood, its dilution by extracellular fluid, and the size of the clot relative to the thickness of the CT section, blood within the brain has a density which varies from isodensity with brain to almost 100 Hounsfield units. This range is, of course not specific for blood: calcified and highly protein-aceous materal can fall within the same range. Nevertheless, the combination of the clinical presentation and the CT features is usually highly suggestive of the diagnosis. Contrast enhancement of tumours can also render them of the same density as clotted blood, and for this reason, CT is always performed without intravenous contrast medium when haemorrhage is suspected. If doubt persists, a post-injection scan resolves most problems, because many tumours or other dense lesions show additional contrast enhancement, while blood clot does not.

When blood leaks into the ventricles, as it frequently does in cases of intracerebral haemorrhage, the appearances may vary from small amounts of liquid blood in the occipital horns (the most dependent part) to a dense cast of the whole ventricular system. There is often associated ventricular dilatation (Fig. 85.26).

Hypertension is a potent cause of spontaneous intracerebral haemorrhage, particularly in older individuals. Small Charcot-Bouchard aneurysms of the lenticulostriate arteries are the probable cause. This explains why the territory of these arteries, the basal ganglia, is the most frequent site for hypertensive haemorrhage. Spontaneous haemorrhage can however, occur anywhere in the cerebrum, cerebellum or brain stem.

A fresh intracerebral clot is usually round or ovoid, dense and homogeneous; its size may vary from a few millimetres to the greater part of a cerebral hemisphere. Prognosis is directly related to size, for any given situation. There is usually no oedema around the fresh clot, but a fine rim of low density represents clot retraction. Contrast medium

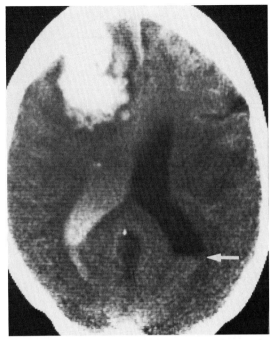

Fig. 85.26 Intracerebral haemorrhage, in a patient with systemic lupus erythematosus and thrombocytopenia. A right frontal haematoma is characteristically irregular in outline, but well defined and relatively homogeneous; a surrounding zone of clot retraction appears of lower density. Mass effect is much less than with a tumour of comparable size. There is also blood in the right lateral ventricle, and a blood fluid level is seen on the left [arrow].

injection is unrevealing and is not in general indicated. Mass effect is often surprisingly small, but herniation of brain is a frequent cause of death in large lesions.

Over the course of several days, an untreated haematoma becomes of lesser density, from the periphery towards the centre, and therefore appears smaller. In this phase, oedema may be seen in the surrounding white matter, and intravenous contrast medium may produce a halo of enhancement; this latter observation does not indicate an underlying lesion.

The end result of cerebral haemorrhage is a focal low density lesion, usually well defined, and of cerebrospinal fluid density; focal atrophy may also be present.

Angiography

In an elderly or hypertensive patient, the combination of clinical and CT features is so stereotyped that angiography, which very rarely reveals an underlying vascular anomaly, is infrequently performed. It is sometimes carried out if either clinical or radiographic features are atypical, or to locate the lesion relative to major vessels if surgery is to be performed.

Intracerebral haemorrhage cannot be demonstrated directly by angiography; vascular displacements may however be evident, compatible with the presence of a clot. Its cause may be revealed.

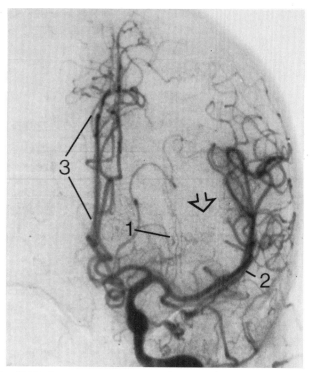

Fig. 85.27 Spontaneous intracerebral haematoma. Left carotid angiogram, anteroposterior projection, arterial phase: there is a mass in the region of the external capsule [open arrow], shown by medial displacement of the lenticulostriate arteries [1], and lateral displacement of the middle cerebral artery [2]. There is a 'square' shift of the anterior cerebral artery [3]. Note that no cause for haemorrhage is shown, and that the presence of a haematoma is merely inferred from clinical data and vascular displacements.

Selective injection of only the vessels supplying the appropriate territory is adequate, unless an aneurysm or vascular malformation is disclosed. A haematoma is manifest as an avascular mass, stretching adjacent vessels. Before the advent of CT, attention was paid to the position of the lenticulostriate arteries on the anteroposterior projection: lateral displacement, indicating a deeply placed clot, was generally regarded as unfavourable for surgical exploration, as opposed to medial displacement, indicating a more superficial lesion (Fig. 85.27).

The causative lesion may be revealed: aneurysm, arteriovenous malformation, tumour, etc. Demonstration of Charcot-Bouchard aneurysms by means of high quality magnification angiography is of no therapeutic significance.

Ultrasonography

In *infants*, *ultrasonography* is the technique of choice for the demonstration of intracranial haemorrhage. Haemorrhage is, indeed the commonest pathological finding with this technique.

The sonographic appearance of a small *germinal matrix haemorrhage* is that of a focus of high echogenicity, adjacent to the frontal horn of the lateral ventricle, in the region of the head of the caudate nucleus. Even very small haematomas deform the wall of the ventricle, a feature best appreciated in coronal images.

With larger subependymal haemorrhages, the echogenic area is more extensive and involves the surrounding parenchyma. Acutely, the haematoma is homogeneous, but within a few days its centre gradually becomes less echogenic, and a ring or circle echo is then obtained. Eventually, a porencephalic cyst with no internal echoes, results.

Intraventricular blood, which often accompanies haemorrhage into the germinal matrix, also appears echogenic, but its location depends on gravity, so that the clot may be found only in the dependent portion of the ventricles. It may vary in extent from a pin-point echo to an entire lateral ventricle. In the infant, it often adheres to the choroid plexus, which then loses its smooth contour and appears irregular or lumpy. Fluid levels are rare.

Ultrasonic demonstration of *subarachnoid haemorrhage* is considerably less satisfactory, but this is rarely a problem in practice, since isolated subarachnoid haemorrhage is relatively rare in this group of patients.

CEREBRAL ISCHAEMIA

Ischaemic episodes may be due to interruption of flow by occlusion of vessels, by thrombosis or embolism, or transient diminution in cardiac output. Vascular disease causing cerebral ischaemia is the province of the neuroradiologist.

Ischaemic episodes may be classified as follows:

1. *Transient ischaemic attacks* (*TIA*): all symptoms and signs resolve within 24 hours. Transient ischaemic visual loss, *amaurosis fugax*, is included in this category.
2. *Reversible ischaemic neurological deficit* (*RIND*): the duration of symptoms and/or signs is longer, but resolution is complete.
3. *Stuttering lesions*, in which an ischaemic deficit is repeated, and frequently becomes definitive.
4. *Stroke in evolution*: neurological deficit is progressive.
5. *Completed stroke*: a definitive neurological deficit is established; return of function, if it occurs, is often slow and only partial.

Radiological investigation is directed at confirming the diagnosis, excluding other causes of the symptoms, and detecting lesions such as carotid stenosis before they produce a completed stroke.

Skull radiographs are generally noncontributory. Carotid siphon or bifurcation calcification may be revealed, but correlates poorly with symptomatology. Plain films are of more value when they suggest an alternative diagnosis, such as an arteriovenous malformation or tumour which can simulate embolic transient ischaemic attacks.

Ischaemic cerebral infarction is shown most frequently with CT as a focal area of low attenuation within the cerebral substance. The appearances are, however, variable, depending on time course and severity of tissue damage, location within the brain, and other poorly understood modifying factors [26].

In true transient ischaemic attacks, CT generally reveals no pertinent abnormality.

CT demonstration of low density may be possible in ischaemic lesions as early as 2 hours following the onset, but as a general rule, infarcts are rarely demonstrable before 12 hours. After 1 or 2 days, about 90% of all hemispheric infarcts will be visible. The initial low density has been shown to be due to tissue anoxia, with intracellular (cytotoxic) oedema; the increased water content of the cerebral tissue lowers the CT numbers, and causes mass effect, effacement of sulci, cisternal compression and ventricular displacement. This oedema affects both white and grey matter; in some cases minimal mass effect alone will precede altered density. Cytotoxic oedema does not affect the blood brain barrier, so that contrast enhancement is rarely visible in the first 12 hours.

Vasogenic oedema however then supervenes: the vascular endothelium becomes permeable and fluid leaks into the extracellular space; this process can be very marked with mass effect accounting for the clinical deterioration seen in many patients with large infarcts a few days after the initial ictus. Contrast enhancement also occurs.

The configuration of the low density lesions of cerebral infarction is a function of the vascular territory which has been compromised. The majority of clinically apparent infarcts involve the *middle cerebral artery* territory (Fig. 85.28); they may be cortical, in the temporal, posterior frontal or parietal lobes, or proximal, in the basal ganglia. The typical finding is either a wedge shaped superficial lesion, with well defined borders, affecting both grey and white matter, or a smaller, rounded, deeply placed lesion.

The *posterior cerebral artery* territory is a common site of ischaemia (Fig. 85.29): all or part of the occipital lobe is involved, frequently with a wedge configuration. A homonymous visual field defect is the clinical correlate.

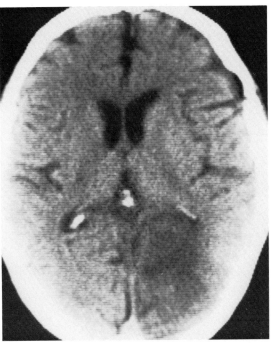

Fig. 85.29 Acute ischaemic infarction in the territory of the posterior cerebral artery. CT: the infarcted tissue is of reduced density. Mass effect is manifest as effacement of sulci and of the interhemispheric fissure on the left; the occipital horn and trigone are also compressed.

Anterior cerebral artery infarcts are rare, reflecting the small likelihood of embolism into the anterior cerebral artery and the generally excellent collateral flow from the other side via the anterior communicating artery. The medial portions of the frontal and parietal lobes are affected.

Small infarcts in the basal ganglia ('lacunar infarcts' or 'lacunes') are common, especially in hypertensives [27]. Often multiple and bilateral, they are of low density, and are often not seen well until the acute stage has passed. The internal capsule, lentiform nucleus and thalamus are the favoured sites (Fig. 85.30).

Cerebellar infarcts are often manifest acutely because of their mass effect, leading rapidly to brain stem compression and/or hydrocephalus. Their CT appearance is similar to that of supratentorial infarcts, but they are more commonly haemorrhagic. Urgent surgical decompression may be indicated.

Brain stem infarcts are difficult to demonstrate by CT; they are generally small, since large lesions are usually incompatible with survival, and occur in a region in which artefacts often degrade the CT images. Some individuals with massive infarcts do survive, however. If the underlying lesion

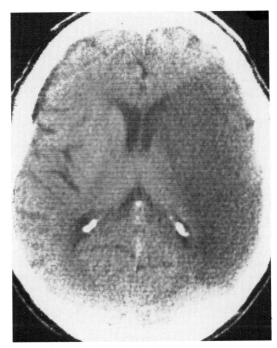

Fig. 85.28 Acute ischaemic infarction in the left middle cerebral artery territory. CT: the lesion is of reduced density, approximately wedge shaped, well defined and homogeneous. Both white and grey matter are affected, but the thalamus is spared. Diffuse mass effect is evident as effacement of sulci (as compared with the other side), and mild compression of the frontal horn. This pattern of infarction is often associated with acute occlusion of the internal carotid artery.

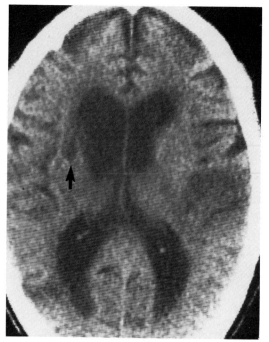

Fig. 85.30 Lacunar infarct; CT. There is a cleft-like lucency in the right lentiform nucleus, with considerable atrophic dilatation of the adjacent frontal horn, indicating that the lesion is not recent.

is occlusion of the basilar artery, the cerebellum and occipital lobes may also be affected.

Global cerebral hypoperfusion may lead to cellular damage in the most distal part of the vascular bed, the 'watershed' areas between major cerebral arterial territories. The CT correlate is linear or wedge shaped low density in the zones between the anterior and middle and/or middle and posterior cerebral artery territories. A broad line of low density may parallel the falx cerebri from front to back. Anoxia of the brain, as opposed to hypoperfusion, may cause infarcts in sensitive regions, such as the basal ganglia on both sides (which can show cavitation after carbon monoxide poisoning, for example), or may be manifest as widespread low density of the cerebral white matter.

Contrast enhancement of cerebral infarcts

It seems likely that the large majority of infarcts will show contrast enhancement if examined at some stage from 24 hours to 2 months after the onset of symptoms[28]. However, there is some evidence that administration of intravenous contrast medium to patients with acute defects in the blood brain barrier is deleterious in the long run, and it should probably be avoided. Since the main purpose of CT in suspected infarction is to exclude another lesion, such as a haemorrhage, and since the pattern of enhancement has not been shown reliably to indicate prognosis, the further information to be gained does not outweigh the possible risk. If the diagnosis is in doubt, the possible contribution of

contrast medium injection in the individual case should be assessed.

The pattern of contrast enhancement is extremely variable: marginal, central, patchy, dense, cortical and other patterns are all described. Even ring enhancement can occur; when present, it is usually at the periphery of the area of low density, in contrast to tumours, abscesses, etc., in which oedema characteristically surrounds the lesion.

Haemorrhagic infarction (Fig. 85.31). It is probable that any infarct, whatever its cause or location, may become frankly haemorrhagic. Standard teaching is that haemorrhagic infarcts are embolic in origin, the embolus first causing ischaemia in a region which then becomes suffused with blood when the embolus breaks up. However, since it is now believed that the majority of infarcts are embolic, this explanation is not helpful. A well founded association of haemorrhagic infarction is with venous occlusion.

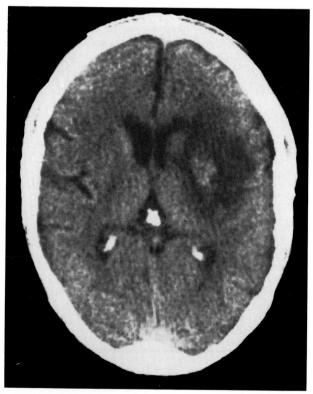

Fig. 85.31 Haemorrhagic infarct. A low density region surrounds an area of blood density, indicating secondary haemorrhage, and contra-indicating anticoagulants.

Venous infarction may be caused by spontaneous dural sinus or cortical vein thrombosis; it occurs with trauma, infection and from tumour invasion. CT shows cerebral swelling with small ventricles, and diffuse low density in the cerebral white matter, which may be haemorrhagic[29]. Intravenous contrast medium often produces striking cortical enhancement; filling defects within the dural sinuses may be detected. Rarely, the sinuses and cortical veins will be dense from contained thrombus before injection (Fig. 85.32).

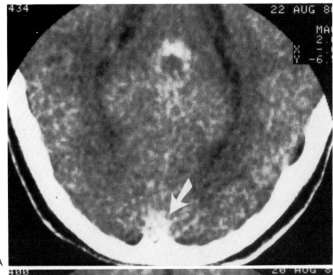

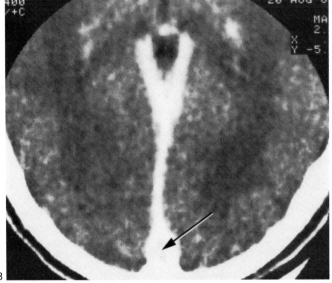

Fig. 85.32A & B Sagittal sinus thrombosis; CT. (A) Without contrast medium: the contents of the sagittal sinus are of high density [arrow]. (B) After intravenous contrast medium, there is abnormal enhancement of the straight and superior sagittal sinuses, which become denser than their contents [long arrow]: the 'delta sign'.

It is of practical value to divide haemorrhagic lesions into *petechial haemorrhage*, *haemorrhagic infarction* and *haematoma*, using CT data. In *petechial haemorrhage*, the lesion resembles a simple infarct, but shows areas of vaguely increased density within it. Subtle punctate foci of blood leakage may be visible. Clear cut *haemorrhagic infarction* is diagnosed when CT shows more or less homogeneous density close to that of blood, within a typical infarct. The configuration of the lesion, if it is typical of an infarct in the middle cerebral artery territory for example, may suggest that a dense area which would otherwise be labelled a haematoma is in fact the end result of infarction. A *haematoma* is a circumscribed homogeneous collection of blood density with mass effect. It will be evident that a number of cases are borderline.

The practical significance of the demonstration of blood in a patient with an acute 'stroke' is that it countermands the administration of anticoagulants. It also has prognostic significance, patients with haemorrhagic infarction tending to fare worse as a group, than those with uncomplicated infarcts. A haemorrhagic cerebellar lesion will occasionally necessitate prompt removal, because of its mass effect, be it an infarct or haematoma.

Haemorrhagic infarcts often show very marked enhancement with intravenous contrast medium, in keeping with the more severe breakdown of the blood brain barrier. Use of contrast medium is, however, contraindicated.

The late effects of infarction

Infarction causes tissue necrosis and volume loss. Within weeks of the insult, the lesion becomes well defined, and of progressively diminishing density, until that of water is approached. This process is accompanied by shrinkage of the brain, shown by enlargement of the adjacent ventricle and subarachnoid space. A cortical lesion may appear simply as a region of enlarged sulci. Resolution to normal is rare.

Angiography in cerebral ischaemic disease

Demonstration of the intracranial effects of cerebrovascular disease is of limited value; the role of angiography is the discovery of surgically treatable lesions. Surgical procedures currently performed are carotid endarterectomy and grafting, and external to internal carotid anastomoses. Other operations: vertebral endarterectomy, anastomoses to the vertebrobasilar system, etc., are not performed in a large number of centres. Endoarterial procedures such as transluminal dilatation of the vertebral artery are still in an experimental stage.

Angiography may show lesions at the level of the aorta and the origins of the main vessels, in the cervical portions of those vessels, or within the head.

Arch angiography is used to show lesions of the proximal portions of the great vessels; since these are rarely of surgical significance, aortography is of questionable value, except in the diagnosis of the *subclavian steal syndrome*. In this condition, a proximal stenosis of the subclavian artery reduces pressure distally to the extent that collateral flow occurs through the carotid arteries, then, in a retrograde fashion, down the vertebral artery, to perfuse the distal territory of the subclavian artery. Delayed films may be necessary to show the retrograde opacification of the vertebral artery (Fig. 85.33).

In the *cervical carotid arteries*, atheromatous lesions occur predominantly around the bifurcation into external and internal carotid arteries. Angiography shows atheromatous plaques as smooth or irregular constrictions of the vessels, typically involving the origin of the internal carotid artery (Fig. 85.34). Demonstration of some plaques requires at least two projections: a true lateral and an anteroposterior oblique with the head turned away from the side under

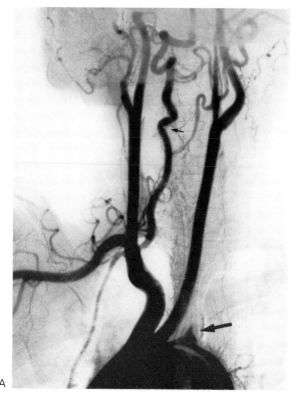

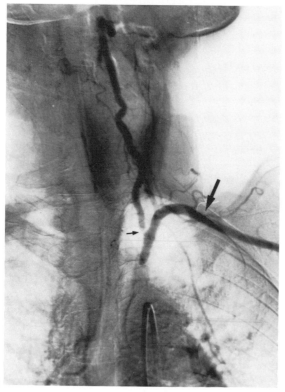

Fig. 85.33A & B Subclavian steal; arch aortogram. (A) Left anterior oblique projection, arterial phase: proximal occlusion of the left subclavian artery [arrow]. Note irregularity and tortuosity of right vertebral artery, related to degenerative changes in the cervical vertebrae [small arrow]. (B) Right anterior oblique projection, late phase: the distal segment of the left subclavian artery (arrow) fills via retrograde flow in the left vertebral artery, despite this vessel being stenotic at its origin [small arrow].

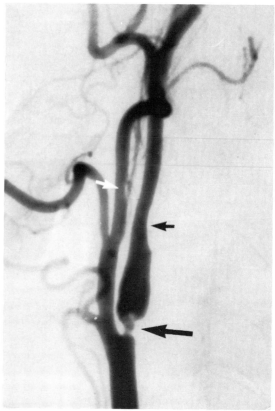

Fig. 85.34 Irregular, high grade, artheromatous stenosis at the origin of the internal carotid artery [large arrow]. Shallow atheromatous plaques are seen on the internal [black arrow] and external [white arrow] carotid arteries.

investigation are the most commonly used (Fig. 85.35). Dense contrast medium may obscure some lesions, and some workers 'trickle' small amounts of contrast medium along the inferior wall of the vessel (the patient being supine) in order to display small irregularities. Many centres expose a single film only in each projection, centred on the bifurcation.

Atheromatous ulcers are thought to be particularly likely to give rise to distal embolization. They are seen as small, irregular outpouchings of the lumen, similar to ulcer craters on barium studies (Fig. 85.35). It may, however, be impossible to distinguish between an ulcer crater and a normal segment of vessel between two raised plaques. Rarely, loose or attached *thrombus* is seen within the artery, commonly distal to an irregular portion of the wall, surrounded by contrast medium.

Atheromatous irregularity should be differentiated from *spasm* due to the presence of a needle or catheter (inconstant, and most severe at the tip of the provoking agent); from *fibromuscular dysplasia* [30] (extensive, regular, concentric corrugation of the vessel, frequently bilateral) (Fig. 85.36) and from *dissection* [31] — spontaneous or iatrogenic (extensive narrowing, with some irregularity and slow flow, often extending up to the level of the ophthalmic artery).

The *internal carotid artery* may also be occluded; it usually comes to an end within 1 cm of its origin (Fig. 85.37). Since

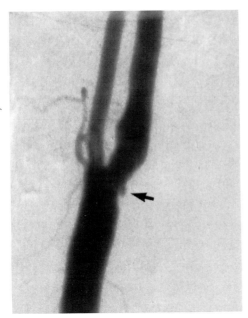

Fig. 85.35 Ulceration of an atheromatous plaque. Injection of common carotid artery. There is moderate, concentric narrowing of the internal carotid artery just distal to its origin. An oblique projection shows a probable ulcer [arrow].

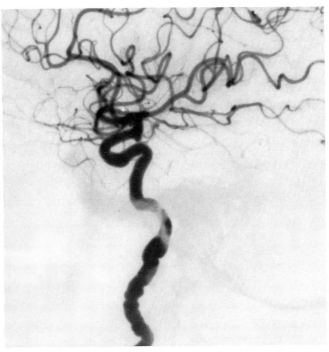

Fig. 85.36 Fibromuscular dysplasia; internal carotid arteriogram, lateral projection. The cervical portion of the artery shows regular, concentric corrugations; appearances were similar on the other side.

total occlusion generally countermands surgical reconstruction, whereas subtotal obstruction is a strong indication for endarterectomy, their distinction is most important. A tapering artery may fill very slowly due to distal obstruction, and this should not be confused with a thrombotic occlusion [32].

Consideration of surgery necessitates a number of data:

1. The *state of the vessels distal to the carotid bifurcation*; in particular, the possible presence of a stenotic lesion at the level of the carotid siphon.

2. The *flow pattern* distal to a thrombosis or severe stenosis, which occurs:

   a. From the contralateral carotid system, via the anterior communicating artery. Should the opposite carotid artery also be stenotic, it will usually be treated. But it may be found to be occluded; asymptomatic carotid occlusion is not rare, and may be discovered only when a cerebrovascular accident draws attention to its patent fellow.

   b. From the branches of the ipsilateral external carotid artery, principally the internal maxillary, which, via its terminal branches, anastomoses with the ophthalmic artery, filling it, and the intracranial internal carotid artery by reflux (Fig. 85.38). Pial anastomoses between meningeal and cerebral arteries may also arise. If these external carotid pathways are widely patent, surgery may be unnecessary.

   c. From the vertebrobasilar system, via the posterior communicating artery (Fig. 85.39).

It is thus clear that angiographic assessment of cerebral ischaemia requires a radiologist who is not only adept, since

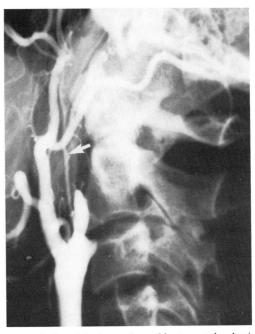

Fig. 85.37 Occlusion of the internal carotid artery at the classical site, just beyond its origin; the stump is irregular. The ascending pharyngeal artery [arrow] should not be confused with a very narrow internal carotid artery.

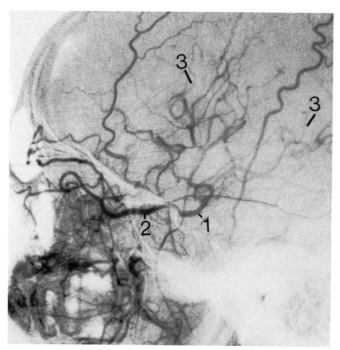

Fig. 85.38 Occlusion of the internal carotid artery in the neck. Common carotid injection, lateral projection, late arterial phase: collateral flow through the facial artery fills the dilated ophthalmic artery [2] in a retrograde fashion, thence the irregular, narrowed internal carotid siphon [1], and branches of the middle cerebral artery [3].

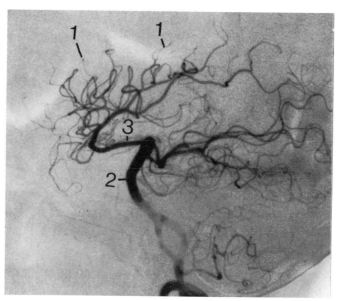

Fig. 85.39 Occlusion of the internal carotid artery in the neck. Vertebral artery injection, lateral projection, arterial phase: there is filling of cortical branches of the middle cerebral artery [1] from the basilar artery [2], via a wide posterior communicating artery [3].

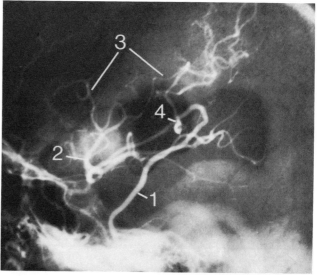

Fig. 85.40 External carotid artery injection following surgical anastomosis between the superficial temporal [1] and middle cerebral [2] arteries, for carotid occlusion, with good opacification of the cortical branches [3]. [4 = site of anastomosis — note craniectomy].

manipulation of catheters is more difficult in tortuous, atheromatous vessels, but also understands the type of pathology he may encounter, and the information the surgeon will want. The patients are often in poor condition, and the risk of complications is high. Digital intravenous angiography is changing the diagnostic approach to the investigation of these patients, greatly reducing the number of intra-arterial injections. A digital study of the neck vessels should always include images of the carotid siphons, since no diligent vascular surgeon will operate on the vessels in the neck without knowledge of their run-off.

Postoperative angiography may be required to assess an endarterectomy or a superficial temporal-to-middle cerebral anastomosis (Fig. 85.40). It can usefully be carried out by the digital method. In the case of the anastomosis, it should be appreciated that rather unsatisfactory immediate postoperative appearances often improve as flow patterns change [33].

Vertebrobasilar insufficiency

This syndrome is difficult to diagnose with confidence, since the clinical picture is often misleading, and the radiological verification frequently unsatisfactory. Angiography may show proximal disease of the subclavian artery, including a steal phenomenon, stenotic lesions of the vertebral artery or vascular occlusions. Vertebral artery stenosis is especially common just distal to the origin of the vessel: it is often circumferential and associated with tortuosity, preventing catheterization of the artery. Radiographic documentation requires arch angiography or preferably, injection into the proximal subclavian artery; a single film in the arterial phase will suffice. Tortuosity and/or narrowing of the cervical portions of the vertebral arteries is frequent in the elderly, and associated with degenerative disease in the cervical spine. The changes may be exaggerated by rotation of the head to either side; the angiographer may be asked to inject the arteries with right and left rotation of the head in patients with positional symptoms, but the procedure is rarely informative.

Complete occlusion of one vertebral artery may be revealed. However, the vertebral artery may be tiny or absent on one side in normal individuals, and the left vertebral artery may arise from the aortic arch; furthermore, technical factors may impair filling of the vertebral artery, so that apparently complete occlusion unaccompanied by evidence of collateral flow should be regarded with suspicion. Occlusion of the basilar artery, usually a grave event, is more common. The intracranial branches may show atheroma, manifest as irregularity and angularity. Arterial ectasia, i.e. increase in length and diameter, often accompanied by marked irregularity of outline, is relatively more common in the vertebrobasilar system than in the carotid arteries.

Intracranial abnormalities in ischaemia

A number of intracranial abnormalities may be seen following ischaemic attacks [34]. Occlusion of major vessels, particularly the middle cerebral or posterior cerebral arteries (Figs. 85.41 & 85.42), with a variable degree of collateral filling of their distal territories (Fig. 85.43), is relatively rare. Localized occlusions of cortical branches (Fig. 85.44), manifest as interruption, defects, or stasis of contrast medium, are more frequent. Emboli can be seen as rounded filling defects within the arteries (Fig. 85.45); they generally arise from atheromatous lesions in the cervical arteries, or in the heart. Occasionally they are septic, and can lead to formation of a mycotic aneurysm.

Cerebral swelling may be present in the acute stage, especially after about 1 week, and may suggest falsely the presence of a tumour or haematoma; the former may be further mimicked by hypervascularity within or around the infarcted area, prominence of medullary veins, or early venous drainage.

Angiography frequently reveals no abnormality. When this is the case, particular attention should be given to the venous phase of the angiogram, since cortical or dural sinus venous

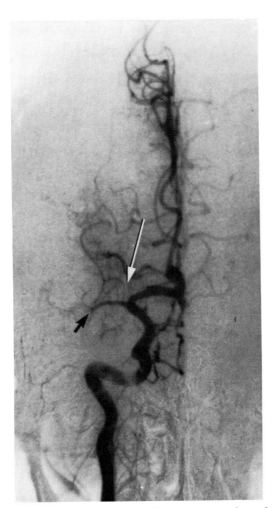

Fig. 85.41 Occlusion of the right middle cerebral artery [arrow], just distal to the origin of the lenticulostriate arteries [long arrow].

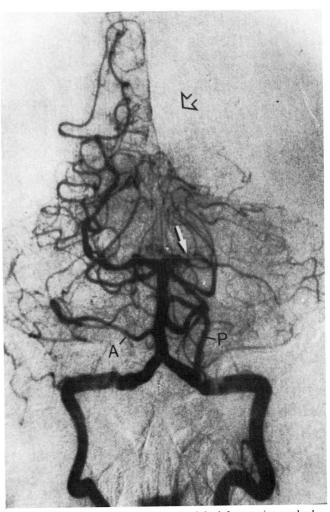

Fig. 85.42 Occlusion of the main trunk of the left posterior cerebral artery [arrow]; vertebral angiogram, anteroposterior projection. Vessels are absent in the region of the left occipital cortex [open arrow]. Note normal disparity in size of the vertebral arteries, the left being the larger; also large right anterior [A] and left posterior [P] inferior cerebellar arteries.

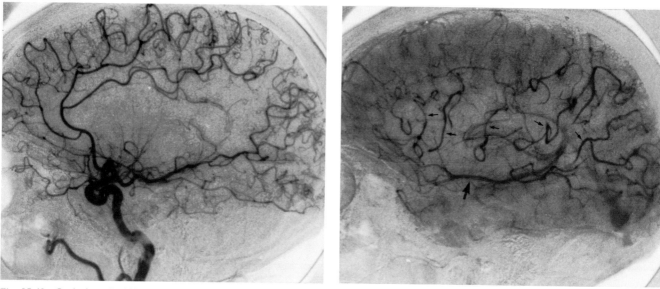

Fig. 85.43 Occlusion of middle cerebral artery (common carotid injection, lateral projection, arterial (A) and early venous (B) phases). In (A), the cortical branches of the middle cerebral artery are not seen; note normal extent of the anterior and middle cerebral arterial territories. (B) Subsequent filling of cortical branches via retrograde flow from anterior and posterior cerebral arteries (small arrows). Lower arrow: prompt filling of basal vein.

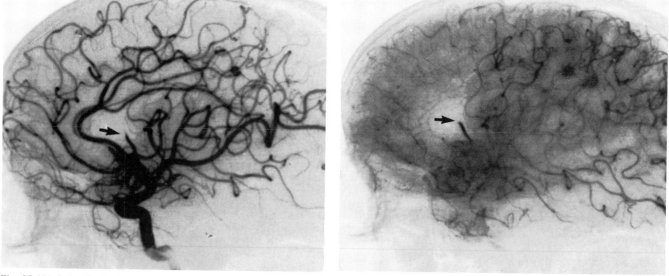

Fig. 85.44A & B Occlusion of a cortical branch of the middle cerebral artery; internal carotid angiogram, lateral projection. (A) Arterial phase: a cortical artery is interrupted [arrow], and in the capillary phase (B) it is surrounded by a zone of decreased capillary blush; contrast medium is stagnant within it [arrow]. Similar films two months later were normal.

thrombosis can produce a clinical picture similar to that of arterial occlusion.

Venous thrombosis may occur in association with intracranial infection, as a complication of vascular anomalies or of pregnancy, or without evident cause. Thrombosis of cortical veins is difficult to recognize unless it is extensive, because of variations in the number and pattern of these vessels. A prolonged angiographic series may be required to exclude or confirm the possibility.

Demonstration of thrombosis (or neoplastic invasion) of the superior sagittal sinus is best obtained by digital subtraction angiography. If this is not available, an extended internal carotid series in the anteroposterior oblique position (to separate the anterior and posterior portions of the sinus) is preferred. Compression of the contralateral carotid artery during injection reduces influx of unopacified blood to the sinus. Subtraction is often required, and it may be necessary to inject both carotid arteries before the diagnosis can be

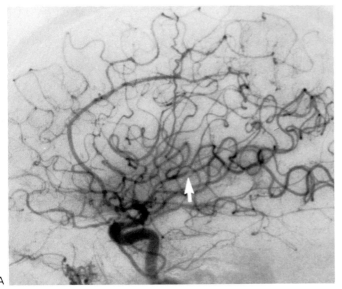
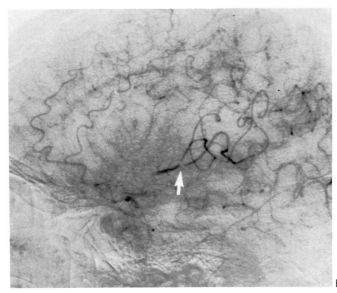

A   B

Fig. 85.45A & B   Embolus in a cortical artery [arrow]. Common carotid injection, (A) arterial phase: a filling defect is seen at a bifurcation. (B) Flow is slowed beyond and just proximal to the embolus.

established. Direct injection (sinography) is nowadays rarely employed.

Anatomical variations in the drainage to the lateral sinuses often render their demonstration problematic. Most of the blood from the superior sagittal sinus frequently drains to the right side, regardless of which artery has been injected, and opacification is often patchy, due to inflow from tentorial and posterior fossa veins. Once again, a prolonged series is sometimes required.

With obstruction of the dural sinuses there is often evidence of diverted flow, in the form of tortuous cerebral veins bridging gaps in the sinuses, or draining anteriorly or inferiorly (Fig. 85.46).

The venous phase of the arteriogram can also be used to study the cavernous sinuses and the veins of the skull base. Retrograde phlebography often gives superior results.

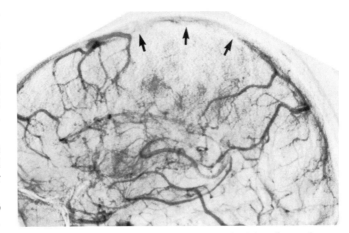

Fig. 85.46   Partial occlusion of the superior sagittal sinus [arrows], with poor filling of adjacent cortical veins.

Arteritis [35]

Inflammatory changes in the intracranial arteries can accompany a large number of systemic diseases:
1. Infective: bacterial, mycobacterial, fungal, syphilitic, rickettsial or viral.
2. Necrotizing: polyarteritis nodosa, rheumatic fever, giant cell arteritis.
3. Collagen diseases (especially systemic lupus).
4. Toxic (ergot, amphetamine) or radiation damage.
5. Idiopathic, e.g. Takayasu disease.

The intracranial vessels may show stenoses, thromboses, or a beaded appearance; a combination of these abnormalities is highly suggestive of an inflammatory aetiology, but none of them is specific (Fig. 85.47). Collateral flow may be evident. Some of the diseases causing arteritis affect primarily the large, basal arteries (tuberculosis, systemic lupus) while others, such as polyarteritis, affect vessels which are too small to be visualized angiographically, so that a normal angiogram may accompany profound clinical deficit. In giant cell (temporal) arteritis, the diagnosis is suggested by an obliterated superficial temporal artery.

Fibromuscular dysplasia [30] presents a typical symmetrically corrugated appearance in the upper part of one or both of the cervical internal carotid arteries, almost always ceasing at the skull base, but similar changes have been described in the intracranial vessels. There is an increased incidence of intracranial 'berry' type aneurysm; arteritides may also be accompanied by aneurysm formation.

Moyamoya [36] is a term strictly reserved for an occlusive disease of unknown aetiology, although the literal meaning of the Japanese is 'puff of smoke', which describes the radio-

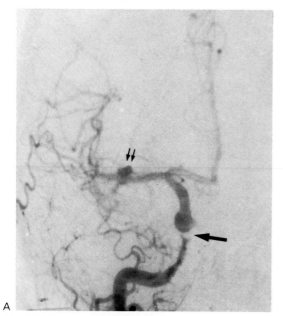

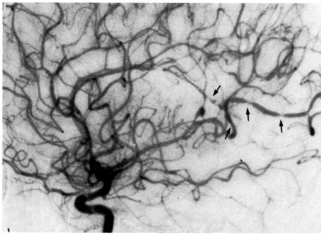

Fig. 85.47A & B   Arteritis, caused by septic emboli of cardiac
origin. (A) Common carotid arteriogram anteroposterior
projection. Filling defects are seen [arrows], many vessels are
irregular and underfilled and the middle cerebral artery bears a
mycotic aneurysm (double arrows). (B) Beaded appearance of cortical
arteries [arrows] lateral projection.

logical appearance of the collateral vessels. The arteries
involved are the terminal internal carotid and proximal
anterior and middle cerebral arteries, which show a
progressive stenosis, and eventually become occluded.
Collateral flow occurs via hypertrophied lenticulostriate
arteries, and many other collateral pathways (from the
external carotid and vertebrobasilar system) also open up to
supply the cortical branches, some of which may also be
involved in the arteritic process. The collateral vessels may
show aneurysm formation. Many of the aforementioned
causes of arteritis can produce a similar picture.

The condition was originally described in Japan; both children and adults are affected. Presentation is with cerebral
ischaemia, or haemorrhage: subarachnoid, intracerebral or
subdural, from the collateral vessels. The disease in children
seems to be self limiting.

CT is frequently normal, but areas of low density in the
basal ganglia have been reported, as have classical infarcts.
Evidence of haemorrhage may be seen when the patients
present acutely.

The Tolosa Hunt syndrome

Arteritis is also a part of the syndrome of painful ophthalmoplegia caused by an inflammatory lesion of the cavernous
sinus region. The aetiology is generally obscure, but fungal
infection is incriminated in some cases. Response to systemic
steroid therapy is dramatic, and is one of the major diagnostic features. Other lesions in the vicinity, such as aneurysm or meningioma can mimic this syndrome. Angiography
shows irregular constriction of the intracavernous portion of
the internal carotid artery, sometimes with pseudoaneurysm
formation. Often, however, the only unequivocal abnormality is obstruction of the superior ophthalmic vein at its
entry into the cavernous sinus, and lack of opacification of
the ipsilateral cavernous sinus at orbital phlebography.

BIBLIOGRAPHY

REFERENCES

1. Claveria L E, Du Boulay G H, Moseley I F Intracranial infections:
    investigation by computerized axial tomography. Neuroradiology
    12:59–71
2. Rovira M, Romero F, Torrent O, Ibarra B 1980 Study of tuber-
    culous meningitis by computed tomography. Neuroradiology
    19:137–41
3. Enzmann D R, Norman D, Mani J, Newton T H 1976 Computed
    tomography of granulomatous basal meningitis. Radiology 120:341–44
4. Kendall B E, Tatler G L V 1978 Radiological findings in neurosar-
    coidosis. Br J Radiol 51:81–92
5. Bhargava S, Tandon P N 1980 Intracranial tuberculomas: a CT
    study. Br J Radiol 53:935–45
6. Davis J M, Davis K R, Kleinman G M, Kirchner H S, Taveras J M
    1978 Computed tomography of herpes simplex encephalitis with
    clinicopathological correlation. Radiology 129:409–17
7. Pexman J H W 1974 The angiographic and brain scan features of
    acute herpes simplex encephalitis. Br J Radiol 47:179–84
8. Carbajal J R, Palacios E, Azar Kia B, Churchill R 1977 Radiology
    of cysticercosis of the central nervous system including computed
    tomography. Radiology 125:127–31
9. Özgen T, Erbengi A, Bertan V, Sağlam S, Gürçay O, Pirnar T 1979
    The use of computerized tomography in the diagnosis of cerebral
    hydatid cysts. J Neurosurg 50:339–42
10. Lagenstein I, Willig R P Kühne D 1978 Cranial computed tomog-
    raphy (CCT) findings in children treated with ACTH and dexa-
    methasone. Neuropädiatrie 10:370–84
11. Hughes C P, Gado M 1981 CT and aging of the brain. Radiology
    138:391–96
12. Allen J H, Martin J T, McLain L W 1979 Computed tomography
    in cerebellar atrophic processes. Radiology 130:379–82
13. Terrence C F, Delaney J F, Alberts M C 1977 Computed tomo-
    graphy for Huntington's disease. Neuroradiology 13:173–75

14. Merland J J, Chiras J, Melki J P, Cassan J L 1978 Etude tomographiques dans la maladie de Wilson. Neuroradiology 16:269–70

15. Goto K, Ishii N, Fukusawa H 1981 Diffuse white matter disease in the geriatric population. Radiology 141:687–95

16. Kendall B E, Kingsley D P E 1980 The diagnostic and prognostic significance of CT in neurodegenerative, metabolic and leucodystrophic diseases in childhood. In: Wackenheim A, Du Boulay G H (eds) Choices and characteristics in CT. Kugler, Amsterdam pp 65–80

17. Seigel R S, Seeger J F, Gabrielsen T O, Allen R J 1979 Computed tomography in oculocraniosomatic disease. Radiology 130:159–64

18. Delouvrier J J, Tritschler J L, Desbleds M T, Cambier J, Nahum H 1980 Computerized tomography in multiple sclerosis. In: Wackenheim A, Du Boulay G H (eds) Choices and characteristics in CT. Kugler Amsterdam pp 81–91

19. Radue E W, Kendall B E 1978 Iodine and xenon enhancement of computed tomography (CT) in multiple sclerosis (MS). Neuroradiology 15:153–58

20. Kendall B E, Lee B C P, Claveria L E 1976 Computerized tomography and angiography in subarachnoid haemorrhage. Br J Radiol 49:483–501

21. Moseley I F 1981 Aneurysms of the cerebral arteries. Br J Hosp Med 26:612–18

22. Kendall B E, Claveria L E 1976 The use of computed axial tomography (CAT) for the diagnosis and management of intracranial angiomas. Neuroradiology 12:141–60

23. Michels L G, Bentson J R, Winter J 1977 Computed tomography of cerebral venous angiomas. J Comput Assist Tomogr 1:149–54

24. Djindjian R, Merland J J 1978 Super-selective arteriography of the external carotid artery. Springer, Berlin

25. Kendall B E, Radue E W 1978 Computed tomography in spontaneous intracerebral haematoma. Br J Radiol 51:563–73

26. Alcala H, Gado M, Torack R M 1978 The effect of size, histologic elements and water content on the visualization of cerebral infarcts. Arch Neurol 35:1–7

27. Nelson R F, Pullicino P, Kendall B E, Marshall J 1980 Computed tomography in patients presenting with lacunar syndromes. Stroke 11:256–61

28. Caillé J M, Guibert Tranier F, Bidabé A M, Billerey J, Piton J 1980 Enhancement of cerebral infarcts with CT. Comput Tomogr 4:73–77

29. Kingsley D P E, Kendall B E, Moseley I F 1978 Superior sagittal sinus thrombosis: an evaluation of the changes demonstrated on computed tomography. J Neurol Neurosurg Psychiatry 41:1065–68

30. Osborn A G, Anderson R E 1977 Angiographic spectrum of cervical and intracranial fibromuscular dysplasia. Stroke 8:617–26

31. O'Dwyer J A, Moscow N, Trevor R, Ehrenfeld W K, Newton T H 1980 Spontaneous dissection of the carotid artery. Radiology 137:379–85

32. Macpherson P 1978 Pseudo-occlusion of the internal carotid artery. Br J Radiol 51:5–10

33. Latchaw R E, Ausman J I, Lee M C 1978 Superficial temporal-middle cerebral artery bypass. A detailed analysis of multiple pre- and postoperative angiograms in 40 consecutive patients. J Neurosurg 51:455–65

34. Bradac G B, Oberson R 1980 CT and angiography in cases with occlusive disease of supratentorial cerebral vessels. Neuroradiology 19:193–200

35. Sole Llenas J, Pons Tortella E 1978 Cerebral angiitis. Neuroradiology 15:1–11

36. Takeuchi S, Kobayashi K, Tsuchida T, Imamura H, Tanaka R, Ito J 1982 Computed tomography in moyamoya disease. J Comput Assist Tomogr 6:24–32

SUGGESTIONS FOR FURTHER READING

Du Boulay G H 1965 Some observations on the natural history of intracranial aneurysms. Br J Radiol 38: 721–757

Kendall B E 1979 Symmetrical white matter low attenuation in children. Xtract 7: 3–14

Locksley H B 1966 Report on the co-operative study of aneurysms and subarachnoid hemorrhage. J Neurosurg 25, 219–39: 321–68

Meyer J S, Shaw T 1982 Diagnosis and management of stroke and TIAs. Addison Wesley, London

Patten J 1977 Neurological differential diagnosis. Harold Starke, London

Probst F P 1979 The prosencephalies, Morphology, neuroradiological appearances and differential diagnosis. Springer Berlin

Zülch K J 1981 Cerebrovascular pathology and pathogenesis as a basis of neuroradiological diagnosis. In: Dietheim L, Wende S (eds.) **Encyclopedia of medical radiology, Vol. XIV, 1A. Springer, Berlin.** pp 1–192

86 Cranial pathology (3)

J. Brismar, B. Lane, I. F. Moseley and J. Theron

Cranial, facial and cerebral malformations
  Midline defects
    Holoprosencephaly
    Septo-optic dysplasia
    Corpus callosum defects
    Hydranencephaly
    Dandy-Walker syndrome
    Chiari malformation
    Arachnoid cysts
    Ependymal cysts
  Developmental anomalies of the skull
    Cranial sutures
    Skull base and foramen magnum area

The phakomatoses
    Neurofibromatosis
    Sturge-Weber syndrome
    Tuberous sclerosis
    Von Hippel-Lindau disease

Trauma to the skull and brain
    Fractures
    Intracranial haemorrhage
    Intracerebral and subarachnoid haemorrhage
    Other findings
    Late effects
    Arteriovenous fistulae

Bone pathology
    Fibrous dysplasia
    Paget's diseases
    Tumours of the skull
    Calcification of basal ganglia

Disturbances of cerebrospinal fluid circulation
    Aqueduct stenosis
    Communicating hydrocephalus
    External hydrocephalus
    Neonatal ultrasound
    Ventricular shunting procedures

CRANIAL, FACIAL AND CEREBRAL MALFORMATIONS

The range of congenital anomalies involving the skull and neuraxis is enormous, with many variations on a large number of basic patterns, and the majority are, unfortunately, untreatable [1]. Only common or therapeutically significant lesions will be considered here.

Midline defects

Because of the embryological mechanisms by which the neuraxis and its coverings develop, many defects involve midline structures.

Cranium bifidum occultum, without herniation of brain or meninges, is rare as an isolated entity. Most common in the frontal region, but sometimes extending to involve the parietal bones, it is manifest as a variable midline separation of the bones of the cranial vault, without evidence of raised intracranial pressure.

Meningoceles, in which there is also herniation of meninges through the defect, and *encephaloceles*, which contain brain, are rare: less than 50/100 000 live births, of which 15% are associated with spina bifida. The occipital region is the most common site (75%), the remainder being parietal (10%), frontal (5%) or basal (15%) (Fig. 86.1). Occipital and parietal lesions are manifest clinically, the diagnosis usually being evident. Plain film changes are limited to a well defined midline defect of variable size, with an overlying soft tissue mass. When the latter is very large, it may be evident that the cranial cavity is correspondingly reduced in size. With the use of CT, the soft tissue component of the malformation may be visualized, in addition to the bone defect. If surgery is considered, angiography may be required to show any herniation of major cerebral vessels into the sac.

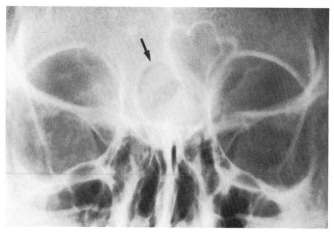

Fig. 86.1 Frontonasal encephalocele; occipitofrontal projection. The orbits are abnormally separated (hypertelorism) and the cribriform plate is bowed downwards; a small bone defect [arrow] is seen above it.

Basal *encephaloceles* usually involve the sphenoid/ethmoid or fronto/nasal regions. Their recognition is important because they may present as pharyngeal, nasal or intraorbital masses, provoking biopsy. Plain films show a well defined midline defect, of variable size, sometimes small enough to require tomography, in the bones of the base, hypertelorism, and occasionally a mass in the paranasal sinuses. At CT, the lesions are of soft tissue density; they are best studied by a thin section technique, with computer reformations to outline their size and extent, if surgical repair is planned. True coronal sections may be extremely helpful. The bony defect may be very small in relation to the herniated sac, which may appear to originate in the sinuses or nose: the differential diagnosis then includes mucocele. Arteriography may be required before surgery, since major branches can loop into the encephalocele.

Evaluation of the underlying brain is also important, because in the case of large malformations, the state of the cerebral tissue may influence the decision to proceed with surgery.

Related midline anomalies are holoprosencephaly, septo-optic dysplasia, and defects of the septum pellucidum and corpus callosum.

Holoprosencephaly

This is a severe craniofacial defect, classified as follows:

1. *Alobar*: the most advanced form, with no development of cerebral lobes or fissures, massive facial anomalies, and in extremes cases a single, central eye: *cyclopia*.

2. *Semilobar*: lobes are present, but there is no inter-hemispheric fissure.

3. *Lobar*: lobes and fissures are developed, but other anomalies, such as frontal midline continuity, olfactory tract agenesis and corpus callosum defects are seen [2].

Plain film findings range from bizarre craniofacial malformations, (including a single orbit and absence of the bones surrounding the nasal cavity) to cleft palate and hypotelorism (shallow 'half moon' orbits, orientated superomedially). The alobar type appears at CT as a single large ventricle, which is mis-shapen to a variable degree. Normal brain structure may be entirely lacking; if cerebral tissue is present, it is usually more recognizable posteriorly than anteriorly. Even in the lobar type, the frontal lobes may be fused with the frontal horns in continuity. These anomalies can be confirmed by pneumoencephalography, but with the availability of CT this is rarely required.

A characteristic feature of holoprosencephaly is absence of the falx cerebri; this is an important distinguishing feature from similar conditions such as hydranencephaly (see below).

Septo-optic dysplasia (De Morsier's disease) [3]

This consists of hypoplasia of the anterior optic pathways (optic nerves and chiasm) and the hypothalamus. The full clinical picture is of a child with poor vision, retarded development, because of hormonal deficiency, and hypoplastic optic discs, but the extent of involvement is variable. Plain films may show small optic canals. CT is more helpful, showing hypoplastic optic nerves, a large chiasmatic cistern (the chiasm itself being difficult to recognize), and rather 'squared off' frontal horns, the septum pellucidum being absent. The same features may be recognized on air studies. There is no treatment.

Corpus callosum defects

Corpus callosum defects are not generally detectable on plain films unless a *lipoma* is present (Fig. 86.2). This congenital tumour may manifest itself simply as a more radiolucent area in the region of the genu of the corpus callosum. It is more

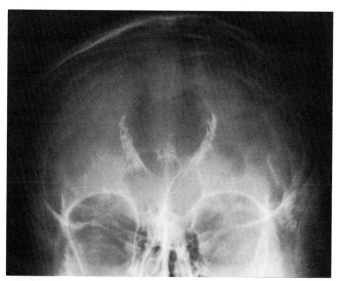

Fig. 86.2 Lipoma of the corpus callosum. Occipitofrontal plain film showing characteristic flakes of calcification surrounding a radiolucent area in the midline.

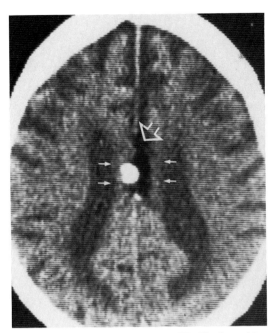

Fig. 86.3 Lipoma of the corpus callosum; CT. The frontal horns and bodies of the lateral ventricles are abnormally separated [small arrows], and the third ventricle projects up between them. An area whose density is less than that of CSF represents the lipoma [open arrow]; it is partially calcified.

Hydranencephaly

This is another developmental anomaly with characteristic CT or pneumographic appearances [6]. Plain films usually show a small cranial vault, without convolutional markings, but without the anomalies seen in holoprosencephaly. On CT, the vault is seen to be filled with water. The only recognizable brain tissue is small nubbins at the base of the skull, representing hypoplastic basal ganglia, and occasionally a rim of frontal lobe is present; the posterior cranial fossa structures appear relatively normal. The fluid within the cranium extends to the periphery, with no overlying cerebral tissue, which distinguishes this condition from gross hydrocephalus. Should doubt remain, angiography, showing absence or extreme hypoplasia of the anterior and middle cerebral artery branches, will distinguish hydranencephaly from either extreme hydrocephalus, in which the vessels are present but very stretched, and from huge chronic subdural collections, in which the cortical arteries will be compressed and displaced towards the midline.

It should be noted that manipulation of CT window level settings can give cerebrospinal fluid the visual appearance of brain density; it is possible to mistake hydranencephaly for massive brain swelling with compressed ventricles if this is not appreciated. In hydranencephaly the falx may be intact but it is invariably absent in holoprosencephaly.

readily recognized, however, when typical, bilaterally symmetrical, slightly irregular crescents of calcification, seen most clearly on the frontal projection, lying to either side of the midline, are present. This picture is pathognomonic, but atypical cases also occur [4].

CT or air studies in cases of *agenesis of the corpus callosum* show the lateral ventricles to be separated by a high third ventricle, so that their medial borders do not approximate; this is the cardinal sign [5]. As in other midline anomalies, coronal images may be most useful in assessing the abnormalities. When only part of the corpus callosum is deficient, it is always the most posterior portion. The occipital horns of the lateral ventricles are commonly enlarged.

The CT appearance of *lipoma* of the corpus callosum is unmistakable: a rounded mass of fatty density, with typical negative CT numbers, lies within the anterior part of the corpus callosum, which is usually extensively deformed; calcification in the lateral margins of the mass is characteristic (Fig. 86.3).

Angiography shows that the anterior cerebral arteries do not have their characteristic course, particularly on the lateral projection. They appear to 'wander'. In cases of lipoma, the arteries pass upwards through the tumour; this is one reason why resection of these lesions is not attempted.

Minor *defects in the septum pellucidum* are occasionally detected at CT, and have little or no clinical significance. The most common is *cavum of the septum pellucidum*: the septum is seen as two fine, parallel leaves, and the lateral ventricles may appear a little wider than usual. Cava of this type, as well as *cavum of the velum interpositum* and *cavum vergae*, both seen at the posterior end of the third ventricle, are much more common in small infants.

The Dandy-Walker syndrome [7]

Like so many other developmental aberrations, this condition exhibits a spectrum of morphological and clinical expression. It consists of malformation of the cerebellum, with hypoplasia of the vermis, and atresia of the outlet foramina of the fourth ventricle. This combination leads to enormous dilatation of the fourth ventricle and expansion of the posterior cranial fossa, sometimes with hydrocephalus of the supratentorial ventricles. Corpus callosum defects, described above, are occasionally associated with this syndrome.

Skull radiographs show expansion of the posterior fossa in about half of cases; this may reach a marked degree (Fig. 86.4). As well as thinning and ballooning of the occipital bones, the enlargement may be recognized by upward displacement of the groove for the lateral dural sinus, indicating elevation of the attachment of the tentorium.

Both skull films and CT may show only minor abnormalities in in mild forms of the syndrome. At CT, a fourth ventricle enlarged posteriorly, at the expense of the cerebellar vermis, and apparently continuous with a large cisterna magna may be the clue to the diagnosis; absence of the vermis is the hallmark (Fig. 86.5). In advanced cases, the posterior fossa is seen to be grossly expanded and apparently filled by a large cyst of cerebrospinal fluid density, which no longer retains the form of the fourth ventricle. Once again, the dysplastic appearance of the cerebellum is the key observation. Hydrocephalus involving the lateral and third ventricles is usually but not invariably present.

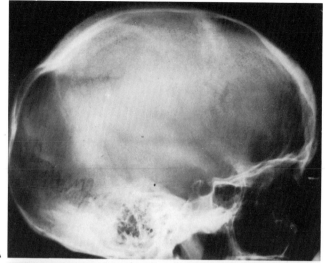

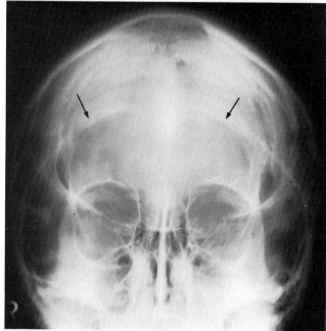

Fig. 86.4A & B   Dandy-Walker syndrome. The posterior fossa is grossly enlarged. The grooves for the transverse sinuses [arrows] indicate the abnormally high position of the tentorium.

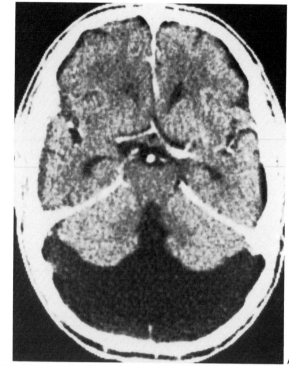

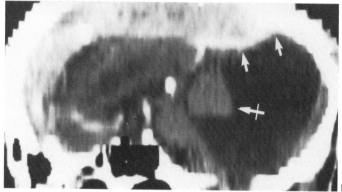

Fig. 86.5A & B   Dandy-Walker syndrome; CT. Axial sections (A) show a large CSF containing space in the posterior fossa, which is greatly enlarged. The cerebellar hemispheres are hypoplastic, the vermis is absent, and the fourth ventricle opens into the huge cyst. A sagittal reformation (B) shows the markedly elevated straight sinus and torcular Herophili [arrows]; a small nubbin of tissue represents the superior vermis [crossed arrow]. (Figs. 86.5, 86.9 & 86.17 reproduced by courtesy of Dr W. Marshall, Stanford University)

Both a *large cisterna magna* and an *arachnoid cyst* may superficially resemble a Dandy-Walker malformation, but in these conditions, some portion of the vermis lies posterior to the fourth ventricle. A fourth ventricle dilated because of a tumour at its base usually retains its normal form and relationship to the cerebellar vermis. Even a huge cisterna magna is not associated with hydrocephalus, and may be seen to extend around the cerebellar hemisphere, in continuity with the superior cerebellar cistern. Conversely, arachnoid cysts, unless incidental findings, usually present with symptoms of raised intracranial pressure, and therefore show ventricular dilatation.

The Chiari malformation

This is discussed in some detail in Chapter 88 and only the intracranial manifestations will be discussed here.

Chiari Type I malformation consists of herniation of the cerebellar tonsils, which normally lie above the line joining anterior and posterior margins, through the foramen magnum, where they lie in the upper cervical spinal canal, behind or on either side of the cervicomedullary junction (Fig. 86.6).

In the *Chiari Type II* malformation, the medulla and an elongated fourth ventricle are also herniated, and there is general downward migration of the posterior fossa contents.

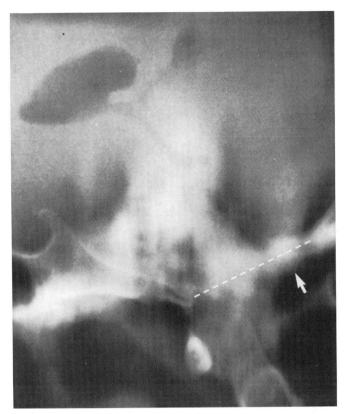

Fig. 86.6 Chiari I malformation; pneumoencephalogram. A midline lateral tomogram demonstrates dislocation of elongated cerebellar tonsils [arrow] through the foramen magnum, the level of which is indicated by the dotted line.

Type I is frequently associated with bony anomalies around the foramen magnum or in the upper cervical spine Chapter 88. The skull is otherwise normal. CT is often unrewarding if performed without intrathecal contrast medium, although high quality coronal images through the foramen magnum may document the tonsillar herniation. Mild hydrocephalus may be present, and the cisterna magna is small or invisible. However, with intrathecal contrast medium, the abnormally low position of the cerebellar tonsils becomes evident.

Type II presents a spectrum of plain film and CT findings, but their expression in the individual case is very variable [8]. *Lacunar skull* 'lückenschädel' is present in a number of cases from birth. The foramen magnum may be enlarged.

CT reveals dilatation of the lateral ventricles; the septum pellucidum is frequently deficient, and if absent, gives the appearance of a single ventricle. The third ventricle is very attenuated, due to fusion of the thalami, by an enlarged massa intermedia. Its suprapineal recess is larger than normal, as is the quadrigeminal cistern.

A characteristic malformation of the midbrain appears on CT as a prominent posterior 'beaking'. The surrounding mesencephalic cisterns are compressed in a 'tight' posterior fossa. The volume of the latter is small, and the petrous bones show a typical posterior scalloping. The fourth ventricle is low in position, and very small or even invisible.

The *sine qua non* of the syndrome is downward herniation of the brain stem and cerebellar tonsils, which is usually more marked than in Type I, but not necessarily more easily demonstrated without intrathecal contrast medium.

Type II is relatively uncommon as an isolated entity, and is frequently associated with spinal dysraphism.

Arachnoid cysts

These are collections of cerebrospinal fluid whose degree of communication with the subarachnoid space is variable. They are often incidental findings, but may present as mass lesions, epilepsy, etc. Classical sites are in the regions of the anterior middle cranial fossa and Sylvian cistern, above the sella turcica (Fig. 86.7), in the quadrigeminal cistern, and in the posterior cranial fossa. Temporal lesions often expand the cranial vault, and cause focal thinning of bone (Fig. 86.8).

At CT, the lesions are characteristically of water density [9]. Thinning and or bulging of the overlying bone may be evident. The shape of middle cranial fossa cysts often has a typical angularity (Fig. 86.9); the same may be seen in posterior fossa lesions as they fill the fissures and crevices of the brain. The wall of the cyst does not enhance with intravenous contrast medium, although calcification is occasionally seen. Focal atrophy or hypoplasia of adjacent brain is often striking, particularly with middle fossa lesions: the temporal

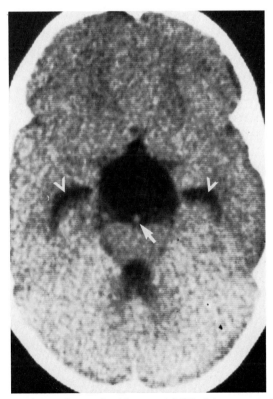

Fig. 86.7 Suprasellar arachnoid cyst; axial CT. A large mass of CSF density occupies the chiasmatic and interpeduncular cisterns, displacing the pons and basilar artery [arrow] posteriorly, and the uncus of the temporal lobes laterally. Moderate dilatation of the temporal horns [arrowheads], due to obstruction of the anterior third ventricle and foramina of Monro.

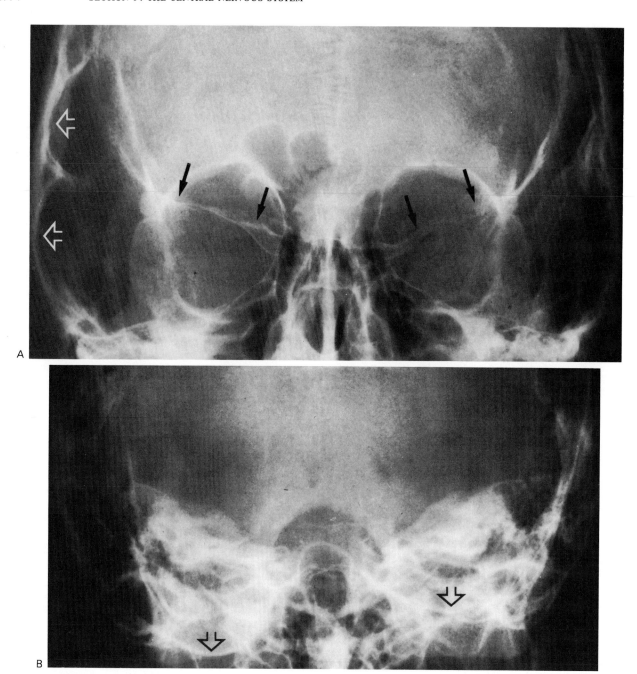

Fig. 86.8 Arachnoid cyst in the middle cranial fossa. Plain skull films: (A) occipitofrontal, (B) half axial. The middle cranial fossa is expanded on the right [arrows in B], with elevation of the sphenoid ridge [arrows in A] and the right side of the planum sphenoidale. The vault is extensively scalloped on the right [open arrows in A].

lobe appears shrunken, and the temporal horn of the lateral ventricle is dilated. Mass effect may be apparent, but surrounding oedema is absent. There is a well recognized but unexplained association between arachnoid cysts, especially those in the middle fossa, and ipsi- or even contralateral subdural haematomas. Moreover, many lesions previously referred to as 'chronic juvenile subdural haematoma' were probably arachnoid cysts.

Pneumoencephalography is rather unrewarding in cases of arachnoid cyst, since if the communication between the lesion and the subarachnoid space does not allow ingress of air, the cystic nature of the lesion may not be evident

(Fig. 86.10). Distinction of a suprasellar lesion from a tumour such as a craniopharyngioma is then impossible; direct needling of the cyst may be attempted. CT with intrathecal contrast medium is more satisfactory: the cyst frequently does not communicate freely, and will therefore be outlined by the contrast medium, but delayed scans often show progressive increase in density of the cyst fluid.

Ependymal cysts

These lesions may be intra- or paraventricular. The former

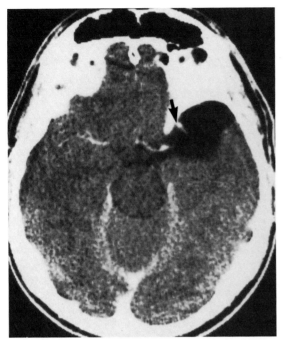

Fig. 86.9 Arachnoid cyst in middle cranial fossa. CT: a zone of CSF density occupies the left middle cranial fossa, displacing the temporal lobe and middle cerebral artery [arrow]; the middle fossa is expanded.

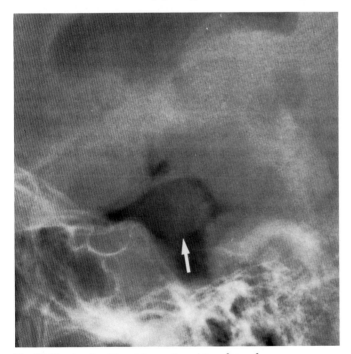

Fig. 86.10 Arachnoid cyst in pontine cistern [arrow]; pneumoencephalography does not indicate the cystic nature of the lesion.

are challenging at CT, since, being thin walled and of water density, they occupy the ventricle, or even fill it completely, without visible borders. The lateral ventricle is the site of predilection, so that the picture resembles unilateral hydrocephalus. If the diagnosis should be suspected, intrathecal or intraventricular contrast medium will indicate the nature of the lesion.

Paraventricular ependymal cysts resemble cystic brain tumours, but without a discernible cyst wall. *Hydatid cyst* is another diagnostic possibility.

Developmental anomalies of the skull

Craniolacunia (lacunar skull, lückenschädel) is a dysplasia of the skull vault; cartilage bones are affected. Often associated with midline or other anomalies, it is generally seen in patients with a very poor prognosis for survival or normal development.

Radiologically, craniolacunia is manifest as bilateral clusters of oval areas in which the vault is extremely thin, separated by thicker bone strands. Some areas may be normal. The appearances should not be confused with increased convolutional markings due to raised intracranial pressure, in which the intervening strands are less prominent, and the degree of bone thinning is usually not so marked.

These appearances are present at birth, but resolve before 6 months of age.

Abnormalities of the cranial sutures

The coronal, sagittal and lambdoid sutures, unlike the other sutures, do not close early in life, and are not completely fused until adulthood. A *metopic suture*, in the midline between the frontal bones, persists into adult life in about 10% of individuals; it should not be mistaken for a fracture.

Premature fusion of the sutures (craniosynostosis) [10] can result in increased intracranial pressure or cranial deformity. A classification is as follows:

1. *Primary.* This is the most common variety, and is probably the result of defective development of the skull base. It is five times as common in males as in females. The resulting deformity (Fig. 86.11) depends on which sutures are affected:

coronal and/or lambdoid
(a) bilaterally: brachycephaly (short head)
(b) unilaterally: plagiocephaly (lopsided head)
  sagittal: scaphocephaly, dolichocephaly (long head)
  all: oxycephaly, acrocephaly, turricephaly (pointed head).

2. *Secondary*, i.e., as an essential component of a complex malformative syndrome, e.g. Apert's syndrome, Crouzon's disease, etc.

3. In association with other diseases: metabolic (rickets); bone dysplasias (achondroplasia); microcephaly; haematological disorders (sickle cell disease, thalassaemia major); following ventricular shunting for hydrocephalus.

The radiological features include premature closure of all or part of the involved suture line(s), lack of the normal interdigitations at the borders of the sutures, and heaping up of bone along the margins. Deformity of the cranium may be minimal or gross, as may changes of raised intracranial pressure (Fig. 86.11).

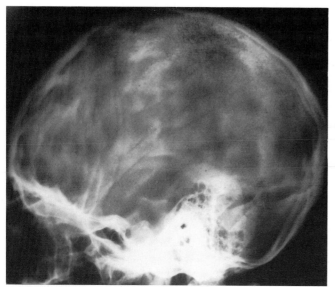

Fig. 86.11 Premature fusion of the cranial sutures. Note 'turret' deformity of the vault, which is abnormally small compared to the facial skeleton, and exaggerated convolutional markings.

Widening of the sutures occurs most commonly in raised intracranial pressure, which may have a large number of causes (Ch. 84). It is also seen with extradural metastases of neuroblastoma, in which case the adjacent bone is often clearly eroded.

Defective ossification in a number of conditions (e.g. cleidocranial dysostosis, osteogenesis imperfecta) results in very wide sutures, with Wormian bones. It is usually evident that the patient has a generalized bone disorder.

Congenital anomalies of the skull base and foramen magnum area [11]

Basilar invagination

This is a term reserved for conditions in which the margins of the foramen magnum are invaginated. The aetiology is usually developmental, but similar changes may complicate rickets, Paget's disease or other conditions in which the bone is softened. The condition should not be confused with platybasia (see below).

The following lines may be used for the assessment of basilar invagination (Fig. 86.12).

1. *Chamberlain's line*: drawn on the true lateral projection of the craniocervical junction from the posterior end of the hard palate to the posterior lip of the foramen magnum. Not more than 2 mm of the odontoid process should lie above the line.

2. *MacGregor's line*: as above, but the lowest point of the occipital squama being the posterior landmark, as the margin of the foramen magnum may not be identifiable. This line, is, however vitiated if the head is tilted to one side. Not more than one half of the odontoid should project above MacGregor's line.

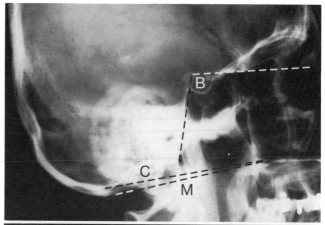

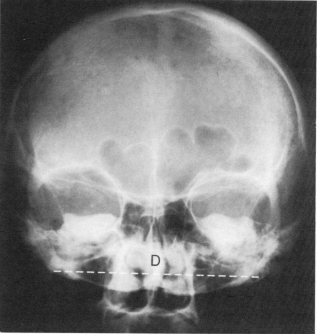

Fig. 86.12A & B Lateral and occipitofrontal skull radiographs, showing Chamberlain's line [C], MacGregor's modification [M], Boogaard's angle [B] and the digastric line [D]. The reference points are described in the text.

3. *The digastric line*: drawn on the occipitofrontal projection, between the right and left digastric notches. Basilar invagination is present when the atlanto-occipital joints are not below this line.

Basilar invagination is, however, not the only condition in which the odontoid is unduly high with respect to these lines; an abnormally short clivus and/or occipitalization of the atlas can give similar appearances.

In *platybasia* there is an increase in the basal angle, which lies between lines drawn from the nasofrontal junction and from the anterior lip of the foramen magnum to a point at or near the tuberculum sellae. The normal range is 120° to 140°. When the angle exceeds 140°, the base of the skull is abnormally flat. Chamberlain and MacGregor's lines do not apply in this context.

Occipitalization of the atlas

In this anomaly, the atlas is fused to the skull base. It is present to a variable extent in almost 1% of the population; in its mildest degree, the distance between the posterior arch of the atlas and the occipital bone is reduced and does not change with flexion or extension. In 'assimilation' of the atlas, fusion is complete, and no separate components of the atlas can be identified. The normal relationship of the atlas and axis is, however preserved, so that the odontoid lies in an abnormally high position.

The significance of this anomaly lies in its association with the *Chiari malformation* (see Ch. 88). Logue [12] noted occipitalization in 17% of patients with Chiari malformations, of which one quarter were assimilated. Basilar invagination was present in 10%.

Occipital vertebra

This anomaly is discussed in Chapter 87.

THE PHAKOMATOSES

The term phakomatoses refers to a group of neuroectodermal disorders, which include neurofibromatosis, the Sturge-Weber syndrome, tuberous sclerosis, and von Hippel Lindau disease; ataxia-telangiectasia and naevus of Ota and Ito are rare members of the group.

Neurofibromatosis (von Recklinghausen's disease) [13]

This is the commonest of the group; it is inherited as an autosomal dominant, but males are affected twice as often as females. About 90% of affected individuals have the typical skin changes, but in the remainder the affection is mainly central. Many neoplasms show an increased incidence, especially acoustic neuroma and optic glioma. There are associations with other phakomatoses and with fibrous dysplasia (Ch. 74).

Skull radiographs

The most characteristic lesion is *aplasia of the sphenoid wings*, particularly the greater wing, giving rise to to a 'bare' orbit on the affected side (Fig. 86.13). This appearance is virtually pathognomonic and does not warrant further investigation. CT shows the absent bone, allowing the temporal lobe to prolapse forwards into the orbit, displacing its contents forwards and explaining the typical symptom of pulsatile exophthalmos.

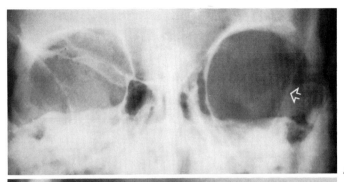
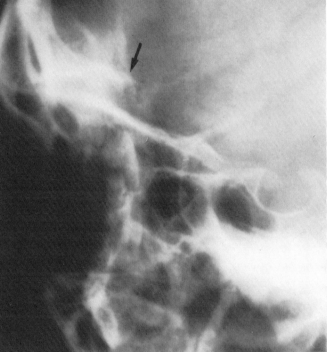

Fig. 86.13 Neurofibromatosis; dysplasia of the sphenoid bone on the left. (A) Occipitofrontal projection: the left orbit is enlarged, with elevation of the left side of the planum sphenoidale. The sphenoid ridge and superior orbital fissure are absent [open arrow = innominate line which, unrelated to the orbit, is normal.] (B) Lateral projection: the orbital roof is truncated [arrow]. These appearances are classical and warrant no further investigation.

Enlargement of the eye, or of the orbit, without a bony defect, may occur, as may enlargement of the optic canal. The latter may however be the result of an associated optic nerve glioma or nerve sheath meningioma extending into the canal. Asymmetry of the cranial vault and/or facial bones can reflect unilateral hypertrophy or contralateral hemiatrophy; both occur in neurofibromatosis. The vault may also show patchy increase in bone density, and osseous defects at the lambdoid suture are reported.

Skull films may also show evidence of tumours: acoustic neuroma (virtually pathognomonic of neurofibromatosis when bilateral). (Fig. 86.14), optic nerve or chiasm glioma, meningioma, etc.. The abnormalities are not specific to neurofibromatosis. Neuromas arising from other cranial nerves may also enlarge the basal foramina; a plexiform

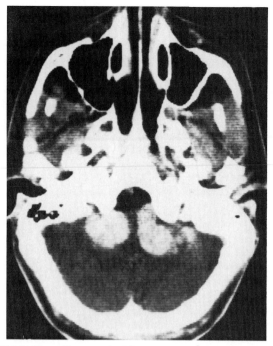

Fig. 86.14 Neurofibromatosis; bilateral cerebellopontine angle tumours. In this case, there are multiple, contiguous neuromas involving many cranial nerves, but multiple meningiomas may also occur in this condition. (Figs 86.14, 86.24, 86.25 & 86.31 reproduced by courtesy of Dr M. Brant-Zawadski, University of California, San Francisco)

neuroma can arise in any superficial site, but characteristically enlarges the orbit, causing increased density, due to hypertrophied soft tissues and/or bone sclerosis. Faint soft tissue shadows representing the cutaneous neurofibromas appear rounded and often rather poorly defined.

Extensive calcification in the choroid plexuses is characteristic but uncommon.

CT confirms the abnormalities shown on plain films. It may also show evidence of focal or generalized cerebral atrophy, or of ventricular enlargement.

Angiography is usually carried out in this condition for associated neoplasms; the appearances are similar to those seen in similar tumours in patients without neurofibromatosis and are described elsewhere.

The sphenoid dysplasia so typical of neurofibromatosis causes anomalies of the course of the ophthalmic arteries and veins, and the cavernous sinus may also be anomalous. *Vascular dysplasia*, with segments of dilatation and stenosis, is found in this disease, as in many of the phakomatoses. Some patients show actual occlusion of vessels, including the internal carotid artery.

The Sturge-Weber syndrome [13]

This condition is frequently stated to consist of the combination of a cerebral arteriovenous malformation and a cutaneous angioma in the distribution of the trigeminal nerve (encephalotrigeminal angiomatosis). Neither of these statements is correct: the intracranial lesion is a leptomeningeal

angiodysplasia, with atrophy and calcification of the underlying cerebrum, while the cutaneous naevus flammeus or port wine stain does not correspond to the territory of the 5th nerve; as a general rule, only naevi extending above the palpebral fissure are associated with intracranial abnormalities. They are usually, but not invariably on the same side as the cerebral lesion.

Up to 50% of patients with this syndrome, who usually present with intractable epilepsy accompanied by lateralizing signs, show calcification on plain radiographs, classically in parallel linear streaks corresponding to the convolutions of the atrophic parieto-occipital cortex (Fig. 86.15). The cerebral lesion is rarely bilateral. Evidence of focal cerebral shrinkage — separation of the calcified cortex from the cranial vault — and of cranial hemiatrophy is frequently present.

The most characteristic CT feature is the calcification, which has the appearance of a thin, atrophic, cortical ribbon. One or two gyri or the larger part of an entire hemisphere may be affected. The calcification is more frequently visible on CT than on plain films, and appears within a few months of birth. The affected hemisphere is classically small and atrophic, but may be paradoxically enlarged.

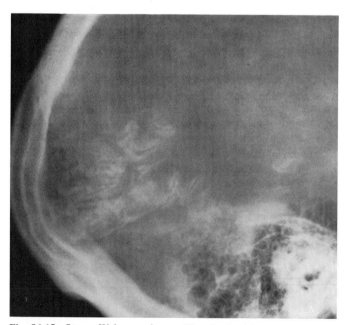

Fig. 86.15 Sturge Weber syndrome. 'Tramline' calcification of the occipital cortex, with evidence of hemiatrophy.

The angiodysplasia is not visible on CT, but collateral venous drainage through deep medullary and subependymal veins, secondary to occlusion of cortical veins, may be observed after intravenous contrast medium.

Angiography is not generally indicated, but may be carried out if hemispherectomy is being considered because of intractable epilepsy. It often shows little or no abnormality, but close inspection reveals dysplastic cortical and meningeal vessels in the affected region. The collateral veins referred to above may be evident. Arterial occlusions are also reported.

Tuberous sclerosis [14] (adenoma sebaceum, epiloia, Bourneville's disease)

This disease, inherited as an autosomal dominant, causes epilepsy and, in about 50% of cases, mental deficiency. 'Tubers' (glial nodules) form in the cerebrum, especially around the ventricles, and less commonly in the cerebellum. Giant cell astrocytic tumours supervene in about 10% of affected individuals, characteristically around the foramen of Monro, where they cause obstructive hydrocephalus.

At least half of patients with this condition show calcification on plain films, but it is rarely visible before the age of 1 or 2 years. Small, rounded calcific foci lie deeply, corresponding to their subependymal position; they are multiple in 75% and bilateral in 50% of cases. Calcification may rarely present in the choroid of the eye. Poorly defined areas of sclerosis in the skull vault, affecting the middle table in the frontparietal region, are said to occur in up to 50% of cases, but in some series are much less common.

When tumours develop, signs of intracranial pressure occur (Fig. 86.16).

The condition is well suited to early CT diagnosis, which may be of importance as regards genetic counselling (Fig. 86.17). The tubers show as dense nodules along the edges of the ventricles, into which they may project. When calcified, they appear to be stable and inactive. It is not certain whether uncalcified tubers, which may become more apparent with intravenous contrast medium, continue to grow.

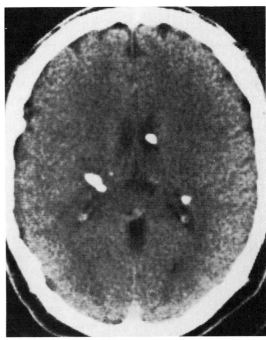

Fig. 86.17 Tuberous sclerosis in father and son. CT of the father discloses typical small calcified tubers along the borders of the lateral ventricles; the cerebrum appears otherwise normal. (The son had one large, calcified tuber at the right foramen of Monro, with mild obstructive hydrocephalus of the ipsilateral ventricle. A cortical lesion was present in the left temporo-occipital region.)

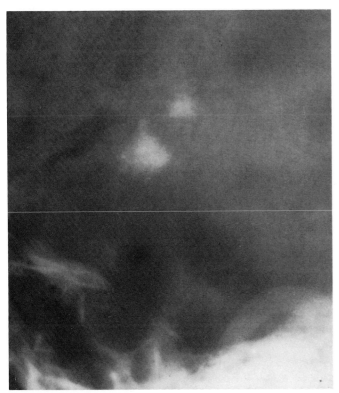

Fig. 86.16 Tuberous sclerosis, with tumour around foramina of Monro, containing dense plaques of calcification. The lamina dura of the sella turcica is deficient, and the dorsum is truncated.

Giant cell tumours are seen around the foramina of Monro in a small proportion of cases. They frequently cause hydrocephalus involving the lateral ventricles only, and may show homogeneous contrast enhancement.

Other CT findings include low density areas within the cerebrum, due to demyelination, and rarer cortical dysplastic lesions. Bone sclerosis may be evident.

Cerebral angiography shows no specific abnormalities [14]. When tumours are present, displacement of the subependymal veins may indicate a mass at the foramen of Monro, with hydrocephalus. A slight, diffuse increase in capillary vascularity is sometimes observed in giant cell tumours.

The classical abnormality at pneumoencephalography is 'candle grease guttering' — nodular irregularity of the walls of the ventricles, but in practice this is seen only occasionally, in advanced cases.

Von Hippel-Lindau disease [15]

This complex, autosomal dominant angiodysplasia consists of the association of retinal capillary angioblastomas with multiple haemangioblastomas of the brain (especially the cerebellum) and spinal cord. Malignant tumours may arise in other organs, particularly the kidney. Haemangioblastomas secrete erythroblastic factors and may be associated with a raised haematocrit.

Radiological features of haemangioblastoma are discussed in Chapter 84.

TRAUMA TO THE SKULL AND BRAIN

The indications for the various diagnostic modalities are discussed in Chapter 83. The present discussion is concerned with pathological appearances.

Fractures of the skull

Fractures of the skull vault are characteristically linear, although they may be irregular (Fig. 86.18). When acute, they are typically well defined, particularly when the injured

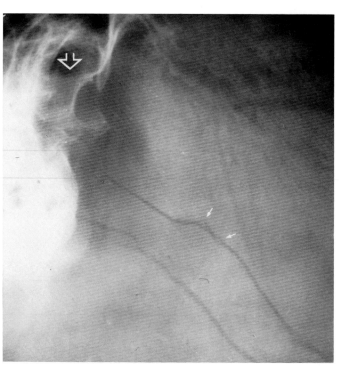

Fig. 86.19 Bilateral vault fracture, with fluid level in sphenoid sinus [open arrow]. Two fracture lines are seen; the more anterior is better defined and is therefore on the side nearer the film. Apparent islands of bone within [small arrows] are typical of an acute fracture. (Brow-up.)

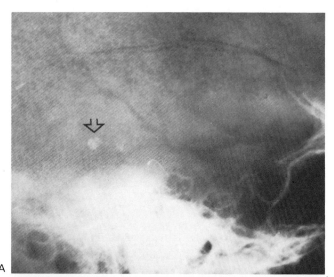

A

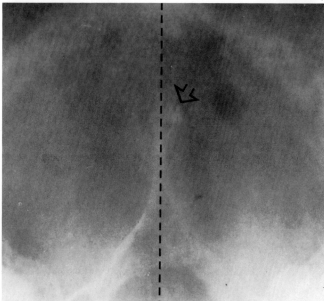

B

Fig. 86.18 Horizontal fracture through frontal and parietal bones, seen on lateral projection (A). The fracture is narrower and better defined than the prominent vascular markings. The pineal is displaced downwards (A) and laterally (B), by a large subdural haematoma [dotted line = midline; open arrow = pineal].

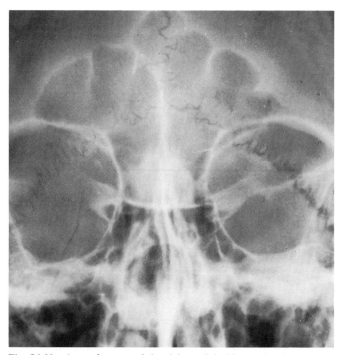

Fig. 86.20 Acute fracture of the right occipital bone; the fracture apparently traverses the orbit and the petrous bone; it therefore lies posteriorly. There is diastasis of the left lambdoid suture.

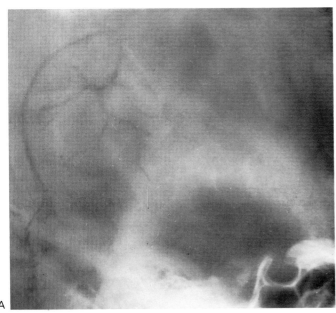

A

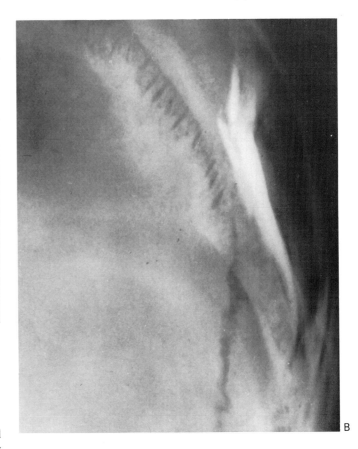

B

Fig. 86.21A & B Stellate depressed fracture produced by a direct blow. Lateral (A) and half axial (B) projections; the latter shows the typical appearance of a dense flake deep to the skull vault.

side is against the film, and are seen as fine lines of decreased density. Slight obliquity of the margins to the central ray may cause the fracture to appear double in places (Fig. 86.19). Fractures, which sometimes branch, must be distinguished from vascular markings, particularly the groove in the squamous temporal bone caused by the deep temporal artery. Fractures are usually straighter, more translucent, and do not have corticated margins. Particular attention should be paid to whether a linear fracture passes through a sinus or air cell, since this effectively converts a simple fracture into a compound one.

More severe fractures may be associated with suture diastasis, particularly in young people; one or more of the sutures (frequently the lambdoid) appears wider than its fellows, with more prominent interdigitations (Fig. 86.20). A tangential view sometimes reveals slight elevation of the bone on one side of the diastasis. This should not be confused with bathrocephaly, a normal variant in which the occipital bone projects beyond the parietal bone at the lambda. A diastatic suture may remain permanently widened, but in younger children premature fusion can result.

A fragment of bone can be depressed, usually by a direct blow. One border of the fragment appears dense where it overlaps the adjacent bone, and a projection at right angles shows a dense bony flake lying beneath the cranial vault (Fig. 86.21). This observation has important therapeutic consequences, and the possibility should not be overlooked.

Fractures of the skull base, manifest clinically as bleeding or leakage of cerebrospinal fluid from one or more orifices, are often difficult to demonstrate radiologically, to the extent that a submentovertical projection is frequently omitted in cases of acute trauma. However, secondary manifestations,

such as opacity or fluid levels in paranasal sinuses or middle ear cavities should be sought (Fig. 86.22).

The demonstration of simple fractures of the vault is of little practical significance, although there is a considerably increased incidence of intracranial complications in patients with fractures. However, the other types of fracture described here are of great clinical importance, since compound fractures have attendant risks of infection, cerebrospinal fluid fistulae, etc.

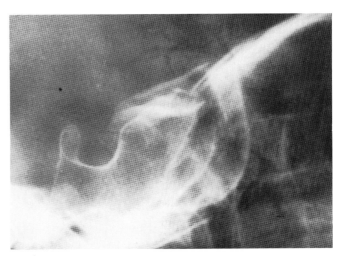

Fig. 86.22 Fracture through the anterior part of the planum sphenoidale seen in lateral projection, in a child with c.s.f. rhinorrhoea; all the paranasal sinuses were opaque.

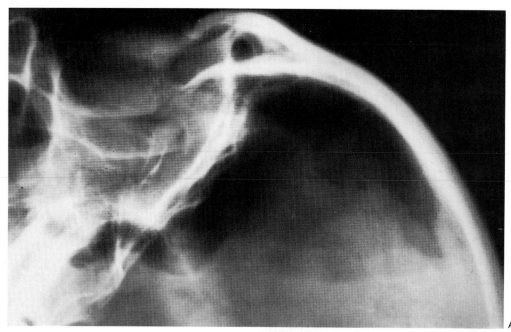

In acute trauma, the skull radiographs should also be examined for the presence of foreign bodies, displacement of the calcified pineal gland (see Fig. 86.18) or choroid plexuses, and associated injuries to the upper cervical spine and facial skeleton.

CT plays little or no part in the assessment of simple skull fractures, although some basal fractures are best demonstrated by this technique. Depressed fractures present no difficulties with CT, as long as the 'bone window' setting is used in every case [16]. With a standard 'brain window' a fragment of bone just deep to the vault may be obscured by blood, or even by partial volume effects. In children, depression can be of the 'ping pong ball' type, but in older individuals the depressed fragments are always completely detached from the skull. Penetrating trauma such as that caused by high velocity missiles can drive bone and metallic fragments deep into the brain; their location by CT can be very helpful to the exploring surgeon.

Occasionally, plain films will show air within the cranium in the absence of a known penetrating injury. When it appears sharply defined, lying superficially, adjacent to the midline or in the expected position of the tentorium, the air is usually subdural; it may be very extensive (Fig. 86.23). If the air is diffuse, in bubbles, or outlining any part of the brain, it is subarachnoid, in which case the meninges have been torn. Intraventricular air will rarely be seen.

Such aeroceles are readily appreciated at CT; it may be evident that subdural or extradural air is under tension, displacing the brain. In very severe injuries, air can be seen within the damaged brain itself.

Growing fractures (leptomeningeal cysts) usually occur with severe head injuries sustained in early life. The dura mater underlying a linear fracture is torn, often with damage to the underlying brain. Exposure of the remodelling bone

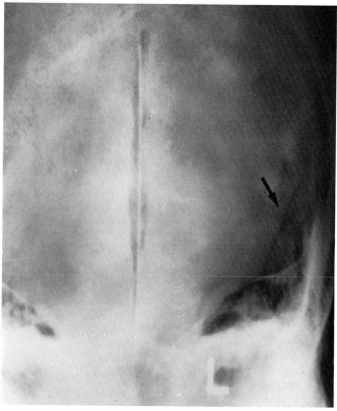

Fig. 86.23 Intracranial air following fracture [arrow]. Lateral (A) and half axial (B) projections in brow up position. Air outlines the falx cerebri but not the cerebrum itself, and is therefore subdural.

to the direct pulsation of the cerebrospinal fluid results in progressive widening of the fracture over weeks, or more commonly months. The edges of the fracture become everted, with predominant erosion of the inner table. The process may become arrested, with simple widening of the original fracture line, or the formation of a bubble-like expansion covered by a fine rim of bone. However, it often progresses to result in a large, rather poorly defined bone defect, with irregular margins and extensive thinning and/or sclerosis of the surrounding bone; a large extracranial soft tissue mass is usually evident, and is the cause of the patient's referral to hospital.

CT is very satisfactory for the investigation of growing fractures, but pneumoencephalography can be used if CT is unavailable. The brain substance is seen to herniate through the wide skull defect. A prominent porencephalic cyst or focal dilatation of the lateral ventricle usually underlies the fracture and may communicate with an extracranial fluid collection [17].

Traumatic intracranial haemorrhage [18]

The aim of radiological investigation is to identify those patients with an intracranial haemorrhage requiring surgery; they represent less than 1% of patients with significant head injury.

Trauma can cause bleeding into the scalp, between the cranial vault and the dura mater (extradural), between the dura and arachnoid mater (subdural), into the subarachnoid space, the brain or the ventricular system.

Extracranial haematomas

Extracranial swelling is the rule rather than the exception in significant head injury. Swollen soft tissues may be the clue to the site of an underlying fracture and should not be mistaken for bone sclerosis. Periorbital swelling causes a marked difference in density between the two orbits on the frontal skull films.

Cephalhaematoma is an extracranial haematoma in neonates, typically following a traumatic delivery, often with forceps. The lesion frequently calcifies; within a very short time, a rim of calcium is seen parallel to the cranial vault; resorption is also rapid. A chronic calcified extracranial haematoma is much less common, being seen chiefly in older patients subject to repeated head injuries, such as recidivist alcoholics and epileptics. Irregular calcification lies within a soft tissue density swelling. The underlying vault may be thinned or thickened.

All of these lesions are evident at CT. An orbital haematoma can also be detected, as a mass of greater than brain density within the orbit. It can be diffuse, or, more commonly, subperiosteal, lying typically along the lateral wall of the orbit, displacing the globe and optic nerve medially.

Extra- and subdural haematomas

In cases of *extradural* haematoma, usually due to arterial bleeding from the middle meningeal artery, plain skull films frequently show a fracture, crossing the groove of that vessel in the temporoparietal region. Contralateral displacement of the pineal may be evident.

Subdural haemorrhage is usually associated with damage to the brain, and arises mainly from rupture of veins in the subdural space. However, vault fractures are usually present in cases of acute subdural haematoma. Subacute subdural collections, presenting 7 to 10 days after injury, are less commonly accompanied by fractures. Signs of an intracranial mass are also seen, but displacement of pineal or choroid plexuses may be absent if the lesions are bilateral.

Haemorrhage is one of the most readily identifiable features in a CT study without intravenous contrast medium. The highly proteinaceous blood components cause high radiographic density, distinguishing clot from adjacent brain, and proportionate to the haematocrit. Even acute haemorrhage appears dense, but clot retraction, which starts immediately, intensifies the density even more. After a few days, the density of the clot begins to decrease, and, depending on local conditions and the haematocrit, will pass through a period when it is the same density as that of brain. After 2 or more weeks, the clot is less dense than brain.

The *acute extradural haematoma* is a relatively stereotyped lesion (Fig. 86.24). Because of the adherence of the dura mater to the skull, the haematoma assumes an ellipsoid shape and is seen on CT sections as a biconvex lentiform high

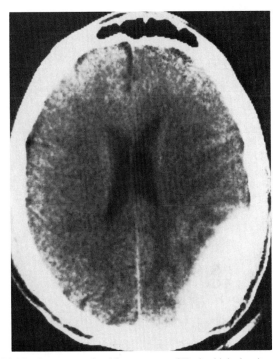

Fig. 86.24 Acute extradural haematoma. CT: the high density collection is focal and biconvex (cf. Fig. 86.25). Buckling of the subjacent white matter (medial displacement of the corticomedullary junction) is a reliable indication that the mass is extra-axial.

density area immediately underlying the vault. The temporal and parietal convexity is the most common site, the lesions being easily detected on axial sections. More troublesome are frontal, posterior fossa and vertical extradural haematomas: coronal images may be required. Even then, small extradural collections may be overlooked, especially if they are adjacent to contused or haemorrhagic brain. Wide window images may help distinguish the relatively denser extracerebral clot from the brain.

Chronic extradural haematomas are rarely discovered; their form is unchanged, but they are usually less dense than the adjacent brain. The margin of the collection may show marked enhancement with intravenous contrast medium; very occasionally it is calcified.

Acute subdural haematomas are also dense and peripherally situated, but usually differ from extradural collections in being more or less crescentic, i.e., having a concavoconvex lens form (Fig. 86.25). This is because the blood within them is under less pressure, but is less restricted in extent. Very extensive subdural haemorrhage may spread over an entire cerebral convexity. Their high mortality in the aged is due in large part to the associated swelling, contusion or laceration of the underlying hemisphere; it is often apparent at CT that midline displacement is greater than would be accounted for by the mass effect of the haematoma alone. Dilatation of the contralateral ventricle is a bad prognostic sign.

A variant is the *interhemispheric subdural haematoma*, which spreads along the falx cerebri, sometimes on both sides. If the collection extends onto the tentorium, a characteristic 'comma' shape is seen on the axial sections.

Coronal images may be very helpful in distinguishing supra- and infratentorial bleeding. Very low posterior cranial fossa sub- or extradural collections (which can be life-threatening) may be overlooked. The presence of hydrocephalus in cases of acute head injury should therefore prompt a thorough examination of the posterior fossa.

If an acute subdural haematoma is not drained surgically, it may disappear spontaneously, or evolve into a subacute or even a chronic lesion.

The density of the blood in a *subacute subdural haematoma* slowly reduces. As a rule of thumb, it is denser than the underlying brain for about 1 week, and less dense after about 3 weeks. There is thus an interim period of about 2 weeks when it may be 'isodense' with brain [19]. Indirect signs as to its presence may then be crucial: midline shift, with contralateral ventricular enlargement, compression of the ipsilateral ventricle, medial displacement of the junction between the white and grey matter ('buckling'), and effacement of cerebral sulci. Intravenous contrast medium, by opacifying the vessels on the cerebral cortex, may remove any doubts about the extracerebral location of the lesion (Fig. 86.26). Some of these signs will be absent if there are bilateral subdural collections; the frontal horns may then lie closer together than normal, with a 'rabbit's ear' configuration.

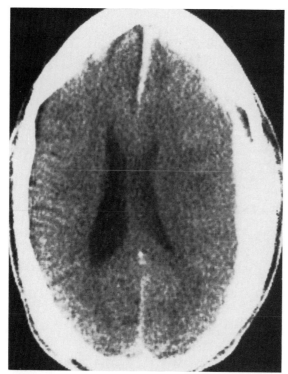

Fig. 86.25 Acute subdural haematoma; CT. A high density crescent of fresh blood spreads over most of the convexity. Anteriorly, it has tracked into the interhemispheric fissure, along the falx; this feature distinguishes it from an extradural lesion. The midline structures are displaced to the right, the sulci are effaced on the left, and there is ipsilateral extracranial soft tissue swelling.

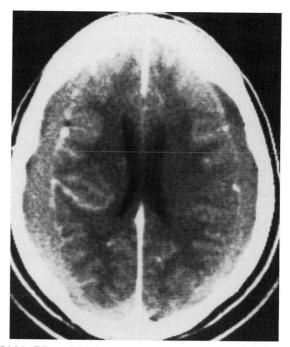

Fig. 86.26 Bilateral 'isodense' subdural haematomas. Crescentic extracerebral collections are in part isodense with the underlying brain, but are denser posteriorly, due to dependent layering of cellular debris. There is buckling of the white matter on both sides, and the lateral ventricles are distorted, but not displaced. After intravenous contrast medium, opacification of the cortical vessels delineates the extracerebral lesions.

Not all isodense subdural haematomas are subacute: a very anaemic patient may show an isodense acute lesion. Conversely, because of continued leakage of venous blood into the collection, a chronic lesion may also be isodense.

A chronic extracerebral collection may be manifest on plain radiographs in several ways, depending on the age at which the causative trauma occurred and its effects on the underlying brain.

In children, chronic bilateral effusions may simply cause enlargement of the cranium, which will, however, frequently show focal expansion, often unilateral, and involving predominantly the middle cranial fossa. If the injury has occurred early in life, and interfered with brain growth, the cranial vault may be thick, with an abnormal lack of convolutional impressions and hypertrophy of the air cells and sinuses; one side is frequently more severely affected. Calcification, in the form of streaks or plaques, resembling pleural calcification but often parallel to the cranial vault, is occasionally seen in the capsule of the haematoma (Fig. 86.27). Other signs of old trauma: fractures, burr holes, etc., are commonly present.

In adults, the skull is frequently normal, or shows signs of raised intracranial pressure (Ch. 84); the pineal or choroid plexuses may be displaced.

At CT, the density of chronic subdural collections is low, i.e. less than that of brain substance, and approaching that of cerebrospinal fluid (Fig. 86.28). Their form is usually biconvex, in contrast to that of the acute subdural bleed. The inner membrane of the collection usually shows contrast enhancement. Fluid/fluid levels between denser blood

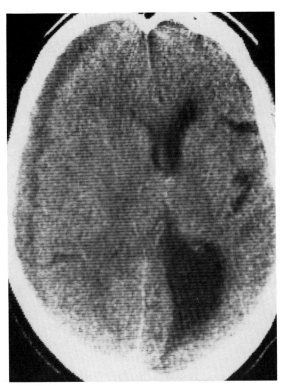

Fig. 86.28 Subacute subdural haematoma; CT. The lesion is less dense than brain but denser than CSF; it is denser posteriorly. Displacement of midline structures is greater than would be expected from the size of the lesion, suggesting extensive swelling of the underlying hemisphere. The contralateral ventricle is dilated.

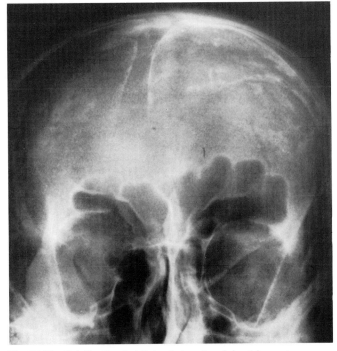

Fig. 86.27 Calcification in bilateral chronic subdural haematomas. The relatively small cranial vault and extensive paranasal sinuses, evidence of atrophy of the underlying brain, indicate trauma early in life.

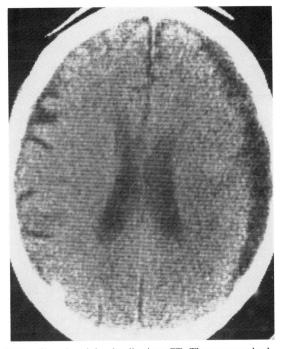

Fig. 86.29 Chronic subdural collection; CT. The extracerebral collection is of CSF density; underlying sulci are effaced.

constituents in the more dependent portion and serous fluid above may be seen, particularly if repeated haemorrhage has occurred; they are, not, however, specific for chronic lesions (Fig. 86.29).

Angiography in extracerebral haemorrhage

When CT is available, angiography is carried out only rarely for the investigation of suspected extra- or subdural haemorrhage.

In *acute extradural bleeding*, the cardinal sign is displacement of the cortical arteries and veins inwards from the cranial vault, often indicating a concave deformity to the brain, as described above (Fig. 86.30). The anteroposterior projection, showing a mass underlying the vault, is the most useful, but anteroposterior oblique series are sometimes required by surgeons to document the extent and relative size of the haematoma. Midline displacement and medial displacement of the anterior choroidal artery indicating herniation of the uncus into the tentorial hiatus are often present. If a dural venous sinus or the middle meningeal artery is also displaced inwards from the vault, the extradural

location of the lesion is proven. Careful examination of the angiographic series sometimes reveals other abnormalities of the middle meningeal artery: occlusion, extravasation, arteriovenous shunting; they are of academic interest only.

The *acute subdural haematoma* may have appearances very similar to those of the extradural lesion, but more classically is seen as a diffuse, crescentic separation of the cortical vessels from the vault. As noted above, however, chronic lesions tend to assume a biconvex shape.

In any extracerebral collection, the absence of commensurate midline displacement should suggest the possibility of a contralateral lesion; traumatic lesions are frequently multiple.

Traumatic intracerebral and subarachnoid haemorrhage

In suspected traumatic haemorrhage, the skull radiographs should be examined carefully for evidence of injury, while remembering that head injury may be the result rather than the cause of a cerebrovascular accident.

Traumatic intracerebral bleeding is usually divided into *haematoma* and *haemorrhagic contusion*, although the distinction is not always easy, even with CT. In general, a focal, well defined, oval or rounded dense area in the brain represents a clot, which may be amenable to surgical drainage. A fluid level within it makes the diagnosis surer still. An ill defined, patchy, slightly dense area within a zone

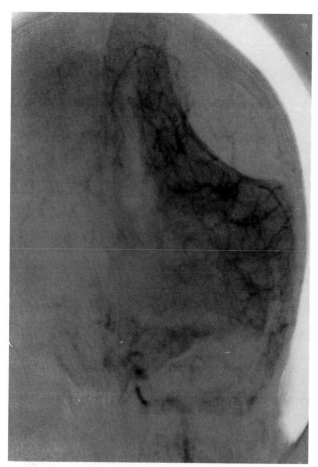

Fig. 86.30 Acute extradural haematoma; carotid angiogram, anteroposterior projection. Both arteries and veins show a focal separation from the vault, indicating a biconvex extracerebral lesion; the midline structures are displaced away from the haematoma. Similar appearances may be seen with a chronic subdural collection.

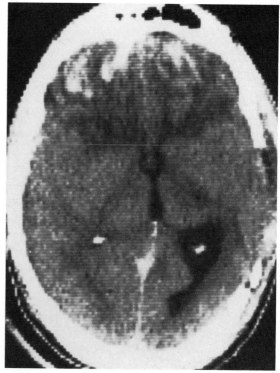

Fig. 86.31 Haemorrhagic contusion; CT. Both frontal lobes show inhomogeneous density due to a mixture of haemorrhage and oedema, with considerable mass effect, effacing the frontal horns. There has been a left temporal decompressive craniectomy.

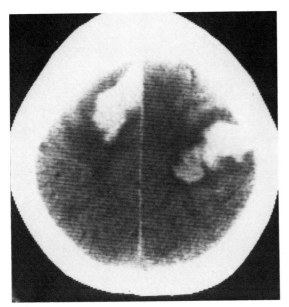

Fig. 86.32 Multiple high density acute intracerebral haematomas following head injury. Low density surrounding the lesions is due to clot retraction, not oedema.

of low density implies an area of petechial haemorrhage, oedema and damaged brain, without a circumscribed clot (Fig. 86.31).

The commonest sites of traumatic cerebral haemorrhage are the frontal, temporal and occipital poles. The bleeding is often subcortical. Contrecoup injuries — a haemorrhage on the side opposite a skull fracture — are classical.

Traumatic intracerebral lesions are frequently multiple, unlike spontaneous haemorrhage (Fig. 86.32).

Subarachnoid haemorrhage is frequent following severe head injury. It is commonly diffuse, and may contribute to nonvisualization of the basal cisterns. The CT appearances are described more fully elsewhere (Ch. 85). As a solitary abnormality it is easily overlooked, but is of some importance, particularly in children, indicating that a severe injury has occurred.

Other findings in acute trauma

Cerebral swelling is difficult to assess by CT, unless it is focal and accompanied by low density in the swollen brain[20]. *Shearing injuries* in white matter — particularly the corpus callosum — have a poor prognosis but may be accompanied by subtle CT abnormalities.

A low density area may represent shearing, simple oedema, whose consequences are less significant, or contusion. The latter may subsequently develop frank haemorrhage within it — 'delayed intracerebral haemorrhage'. Identification of these different lesions in the acute stage is often impossible.

Diffuse cerebral swelling without alteration in density is especially common in children. The prognosis is good; even slit like ventricles do not necessarily indicate raised intra-

cranial pressure[21]. However, the older the patient and the more persistent the swelling, the poorer the outcome.

Infarction can result from massive brain herniations, transtentorial or subfalcine, involving the territories of the posterior and anterior cerebral arteries respectively.

Cerebral angiography is rather unhelpful in the distinction of cerebral haemorrhage, contusion and simple swelling, all of which are manifest as avascular intra-axial mass lesions. If the swelling is in the posterior cranial fossa, hydrocephalus may be evident as stretching of the subependymal veins. Other findings, such as a shallow extracerebral collection or vasospasm secondary to subarachnoid haemorrhage, are sometimes present.

Vasospasm can be sufficiently severe as to cause poor peripheral filling, and is indeed another cause of infarction in acute head injury.

Vascular occlusion can also result from direct trauma in the neck or at the skull base: extensive irregular narrowing indicates traumatic dissection. An aneurysm can subsequently form at the site of injury. Penetrating wounds can cause similar appearances. Direct trauma to an intracranial vessel can give rise to a traumatic aneurysm, typically situated on a peripheral vessel, not necessarily at a bifurcation, and without the 'neck' of a 'berry' aneurysm. An intracerebral haematoma is frequently evident (Fig. 86.33).

When intracranial pressure is very high, contrast medium injected into any of the main neck vessels does not enter the head. The usual picture is of a static column of contrast medium in a narrowed vessel, from catheter tip to carotid siphon. The grave prognostic significance of such an 'agonal'

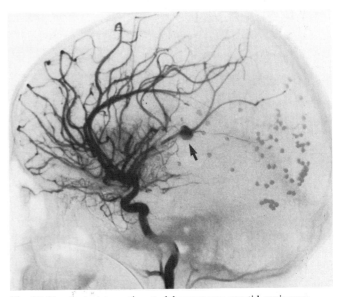

Fig. 86.33 Acute traumatic arterial aneurysm; carotid angiogram, lateral projection. Metallic fragments are seen posteriorly; the vessels around them are stretched and narrowed, and a rounded collection of contrast medium, representing the aneurysm is seen, unrelated to an arterial bifurcation [arrow].

angiogram will be appreciated; it has in the past been accepted as evidence of brain death. The CT correlate is that normal intracranial contrast enhancement does not occur. It is evident that the angiographic picture should not be confused with similar patterns produced by arterial dissection, embolic occlusion just beyond the ophthalmic artery, severe catheter-induced spasm or subintimal injection.

The late effects of head injury

Possible late effects of trauma on the skull have been mentioned above: suture diastasis, growing fracture, chronic subdural haematoma, etc.

The end results of intraparenchymal contusion or haematoma are focal atrophy, or, in more advanced cases, softening and cyst formation — *encephalomalacia*. Focal shrinkage of the brain occurs in the usual nonspecific way: enlargement of the sulci, adjacent cisterns and underlying ventricle (Fig. 86.34). Cystic areas, usually rather smaller than the original area of clot or contusion, are a striking feature of many CT studies following trauma. Extensive bifrontal atrophy, with low density lesions in the frontal white matter, is common after severe injuries.

Traumatic hemiatrophy may affect the brain and the overlying skull. It occurs as the result of injury early in life, and is frequently due to associated vascular damage rather than to direct trauma. Growth of the cranium during childhood is stimulated by brain growth, so that impaired cerebral development is reflected by a small cranium. Post-traumatic

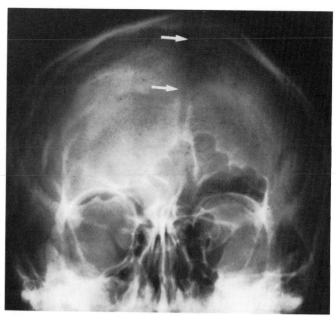

Fig. 86.35 Cranial hemiatrophy. The left hemicranium is smaller than the right (arrows indicate the groove for the superior sagittal sinus); the left petrous bone is elevated, and the paranasal sinuses are more extensive on the affected side. These changes are secondary to impaired growth of the underlying cerebral hemisphere.

atrophy is usually unilateral, affecting only the anterior and middle cranial fossae, which are smaller than their fellows, with a thicker vault, reduced convolutional markings and hypertrophy of the ipsilateral air cells and paranasal sinuses, particularly the frontal sinus. The calcified pineal may appear displaced towards the affected side, but it will often be evident that it lies in the midline plane as defined by the groove for the superior sagittal sinus (Fig. 86.35).

These plain film features are also seen at CT or pneumoencephalography, which show the affected hemisphere to be small; focal cortical atrophy is less common. [22] At angiography, the internal carotid artery on the atrophic side is usually small, but patent, and its branches are attenuated to a variable extent. Ipsilateral shifting of the venous sinuses is evident, as is enlargement of the lateral ventricle.

Post-traumatic *cerebrospinal fluid leakage* from the ear (otorrhoea) or nose (rhinorrhoea) is evidence of a basal fracture in communication with the subarachnoid space. (Leakage without preceding trauma may be due to congenital anomalies of the ear, tumoral erosion or raised intracranial pressure.) The mode of external leakage is, however, a poor guide to the site of the fistula: fluid may enter the ear but leave the nose, via the Eustachian tube.

Whatever the aetiology, the significance of cerebrospinal fluid leakage is the presence of pathway for infection from the exterior to the subarachnoid space: it must be repaired.

Plain films may give valuable evidence, showing for example a fracture passing through the middle ear. Tomography is frequently necessary: fractures frequently involve the ethmoid region, but are often difficult to identify with certainty. Opacity of, or a fluid level within the middle ear

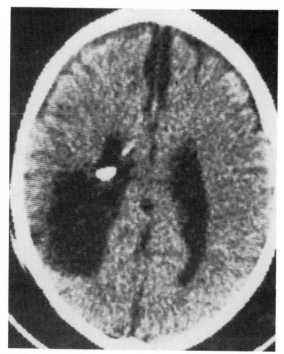

Fig. 86.34 Porencephalic cyst; CT. A CSF-containing cyst communicates with the ventricular system. Such cysts can exert mass effect.

cavity or one of the air sinuses are valuable clues. Very occasionally, intracranial air bubbles may be seen.

With thin section CT, small fractures or bone defects can usually be identified. Intrathecal water soluble contrast medium can be used to demonstrate the site of leakage. The patient is placed prone in the scanner after injection of the contrast medium. Serial CT studies should demonstrate dense contrast medium in the sphenoid or ethmoid sinuses, then in the nasal cavity. While not uniformly successful, this is probably the optimal approach [23]. Oil or air injection followed by conventional tomography is less uniformly successful, and radio-isotopic methods lack the desirable spatial resolution.

Any radiological investigation for cerebrospinal fluid oto- or rhinorrhoea must be carried out at a time when the patient is actively leaking fluid.

Traumatic arteriovenous fistulae

Arteriovenous fistulae can arise in relation to any fracture, if an artery and the adjacent veins are ruptured. Common sites in the head and neck include: the temporoparietal region (middle meningeal artery) in relation to the transverse sinus (involving dural arteries, including the middle meningeal and occipital), in the neck (internal carotid or vertebral arteries), the scalp (usually superficial temporal artery), and above all, in the region of the *cavernous sinus*, where the internal carotid artery actually lies within a venous sinus.

Such fistulae produce plain film abnormalities. Those in relation to the skull vault frequently cause hypertrophy of

the feeding arteries and/or draining veins, with enlargement of, for example, the foramen spinosum and meningeal vascular grooves; an extracranial soft tissue mass may be present. *Traumatic caroticocavernous fistulae* may result in enlargement of the carotid canal, and of the carotid sulcus. Drainage is usually to the superior ophthalmic vein, among others, and longstanding lesions often cause enlargement of the superior orbital fissure on one or both sides.

Arteriovenous fistulae are studied by angiography, but the initial clinical diagnosis can be supported by CT findings of a highly vascular lesion. In the commonest type — the caroticocavernous fistula, the proptosis accompanying the lesion may be evident, but, since some of these fistulae are most pronounced under the influence of gravity, proptosis may be optimally demonstrated in the prone position. The most prominent abnormality is often the hugely dilated superior ophthalmic vein, resembling a worm in the upper part of the orbit, and showing marked contrast enhancement. Muscle swelling is an inconstant feature.

Investigation, and indeed treatment, of these lesions is arteriographic [24]. The large majority of traumatic carotico-cavernous fistulae are direct communications between the intracavernous carotid artery and the sinus. Drainage is via the superior and inferior ophthalmic veins and inferior petrosal sinus. Almost all the contrast medium injected into the carotid artery may leave via the fistula (Fig. 86.36), and not uncommonly contrast medium will cross intercavernous connections, draining to both sides. Bilateral internal and external carotid angiography is required for full assessment, since a number of post-traumatic fistulae are supplied by the external carotid artery alone. Localization of the exact site of the fistula is often difficult because the abnormal orifice is obscured by the contrast medium flooding around it; injection with ipsilateral carotid compression, or vertebral angiography with retrograde filling of the fistula can be useful.

Fistulae on the cranial vault are usually supplied exclusively by branches of the external carotid artery. Extensive superselective angiography is required, as a single lesion may be fed by several vessels from one or both sides.

Treatment is currently by means of detachable balloons in the case of large, direct arteriovenous connections and by particulate emboli in the the more widespread dural lesions.

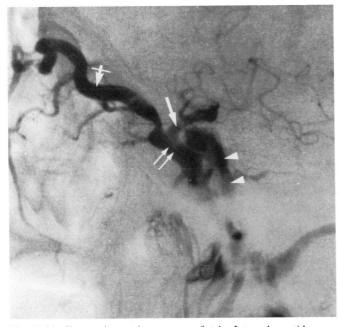

Fig. 86.36 Traumatic caroticocavernous fistula. Internal carotid arteriogram, lateral projection, midarterial phase: most of the blood from the carotid siphon [arrow] has entered the cavernous sinus [double arrows], whence it drains via the superior ophathalmic vein [crossed arrow] and the inferior petrosal sinus [arrowheads]. Distal filling of the intracranial vessels is greatly reduced.

BONE PATHOLOGY

Fibrous dysplasia [25]

The systemic manifestations of this condition are discussed in Chapter 74.

In the skull, fibrous dysplasia takes two main forms. The *sclerotic form* is the commoner of the two, especially in the polyostotic form of the disease; it affects the base and/or facial bones, which are expanded and dense, sometimes showing the classical 'ground glass', i.e. featureless pattern (Fig. 86.37). This variety is the commonest form of 'leontiasis

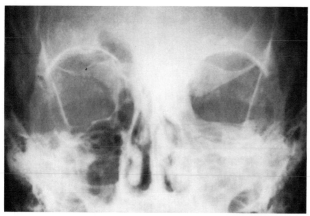

Fig. 86.37 Fibrous dysplasia of the skull base. Dense 'ground glass' appearance, with loss of the normal bone texture, extending from the nasion to the clivus, into the sphenoid wings on both sides, and the left maxilla.

ossea'. Meningioma represents the important differential diagnosis. In the latter, sclerosis is usually more marked than expansion of bone, and extension from the basisphenoid or sphenoid wings into the facial bones is much less common. Prominent vascular grooves are more common in meningioma, but may be present in fibrous dysplasia. Lower density areas within the sclerotic bone, representing cysts, are strongly in favour of fibrous dysplasia. If *malignant transformation* occurs, ragged bone destruction is seen.

The *cystic form* of fibrous dysplasia, often an incidental finding, affects the vault, expanding the outer table and producing a 'blistered' appearance (Fig. 86.38). Here, the

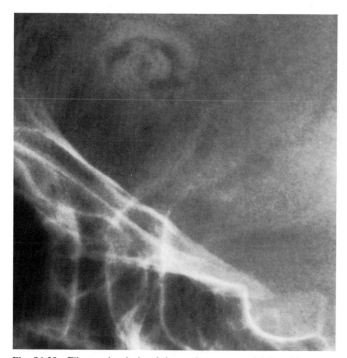

Fig. 86.38 Fibrous dysplasia of the vault: an arcuate 'blister' is surrounded by bone of abnormal texture.

differential diagnosis is from epidermoid, the borders of which are finer and better defined, whilst the translucent area is more homogeneous.

CT shows the same features as plain films; angiography is rarely, if ever required.

Paget's disease [26]

This condition, of unknown aetiology, but possibly an infection, is rare before middle age. It affects males more frequently than females; familial and strong geographical variations in incidence are also noted. The skull is involved in about two thirds of cases presenting clinically.

In the vault, a pure sclerotic form may be encountered, but a mixture of sclerosis and lysis is much more common. Unless the condition is discovered incidentally, the radiological changes are frequently advanced by the time of diagnosis. The earliest change is a spotty 'cotton wool pledget' increase in density of the bone, which becomes thicker and irregular in texture. Generalized thickening of the vault may, however, be the first manifestation. The middle and outer tables are most affected. When the disease is focal, it can resemble the sclerotic variety of fibrous dysplasia, but the increased density is more patchy than in the latter and the trabeculae are coarsened rather than effaced. Vascular grooves may be prominent and the foramina spinosa can enlarge.

Osteoporosis circumscripta is a form of Paget's disease which may progress to the more advanced form. The vault is demineralized, from the base upwards (Fig. 86.39), most frequently in the occipital region; the abnormal bone often has a clearly defined border. This form is frequently found in association with skeletal Paget's disease.

Complications of Paget's disease of the skull include:

—Basilar invagination (Fig. 86.40), due to softening of the bone; this occurs in about one third of cases, producing a 'Tam O'Shanter' deformity in the advanced stage
—Narrowing of basal foramina, producing cranial nerve palsies, especially deafness and occasionally medullary or spinal cord compression;
—Malignant tumours; these arise in about 1% of cases (Fig. 86.41). Osteosarcoma is the commonest variety; this tumour very rarely affects the skull in patients without Paget's disease. The tumour is generally manifest as an irregular area of lysis within a previously dense area. A soft tissue mass may be visible but new bone formation is uncommon. Benign giant cell tumour, a well recognized complication, is much rarer than osteosarcoma, but radiologically indistinguishable.

CT of the skull in Paget's disease shows a thickened vault, which appears irregular in outline, due to the irregular sclerosis. Basilar invagination may be recognized if the entire clivus is seen on one normally angled section, or if the ring of bone around the foramen magnum appears to lie in the centre of the posterior fossa.

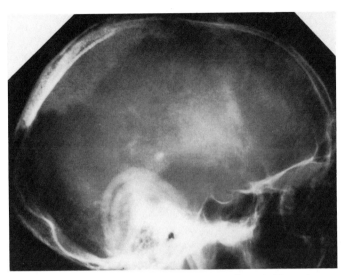

Fig. 86.39 Osteoporosis circumscripta (Paget's disease). Extensive loss of bone density affects the lower part of the cranial vault; the margin between abnormal and normal bone is sharp.

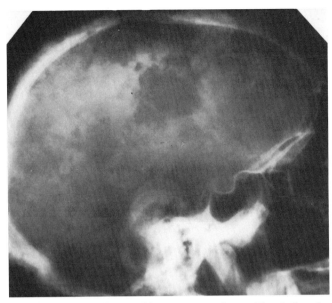

Fig. 86.41 Paget's disease with sarcomatous change. The skull vault shows irregularity of texture and slight thickening, evidence of Paget's disease. An irregular area of bone destruction is seen near the vertex. Biopsy confirmed sarcomatous degeneration.

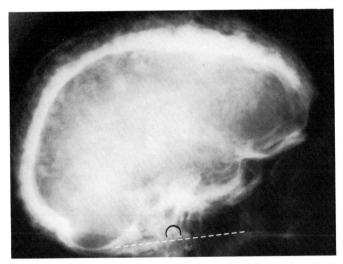

Fig. 86.40 Advanced Paget's disease, with basilar invagination. Skull lateral projection: gross thickening and alteration of bone texture affects the entire skull. Basilar invagination is manifest as extension of the odontoid (outlined in black) above Chamberlain's line (dotted line).

External carotid angiography shows hypertrophied vessels supplying the vault from the middle meningeal and superficial temporal arteries.

Tumours of the skull

Primary tumours of all kinds can occur in the skull vault, but most are exceedingly rare.

Haemangioma of the cranial vault sometimes presents as a lump on the head or focal tenderness. It is typified by a well circumscribed area of punctate or stellate rarefaction without

expansion. Prominent vascular grooves may also be present in the vicinity of the lesion (Fig. 86.42), and external carotid angiography sometimes shows a tumour blush. The tumour is not progressive and treatment is not generally required.

Osteomas of the vault are benign condensations of cortical bone which may project either external to the skull (exostosis) (Fig. 86.43) or towards the cranial cavity (enostosis). Treatment is not usually required, unless the bony mass is large. Differential diagnosis includes fibrous dysplasia and meningioma. Osteomas are generally more circumscribed, and do not show abnormal bone texture.

Malignant tumours of the skull are generally secondary; sarcomas are very rare. Local invasion from superficial tumours, such as basal cell carcinoma or from nasopharyngeal tumours may occur. Metastases are common in disseminated malignancy; their characteristics are similar to those found in other sites: irregular lysis and/or sclerosis of bone, and multiplicity (Fig. 86.44).

Calcification of the basal ganglia

Calcification of the basal ganglia may be noted on plain radiographs and is frequently observed in normal, older individuals (Fig. 86.45). Other causes include hypoparathyroidism and pseudohypoparathyroidism, and mitochondrial cytopathy, but many cases are idiopathic and affected individuals shown no evidence of disturbed calcium metabolism; some cases are familial (Fahr's syndrome).

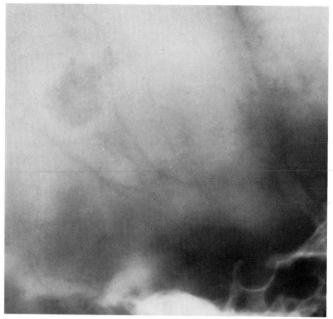

Fig. 86.42 Haemangioma of skull vault. A typical rounded area of punctate loss of bone density is seen in the parietal bone; prominent vascular grooves run to and from the lesion.

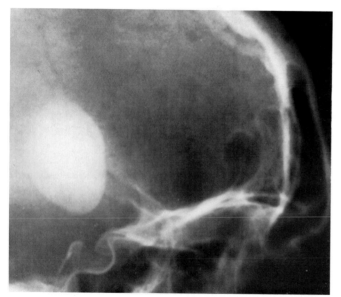

Fig. 86.43 Osteoma of the skull vault. Skull, lateral projection. The extracranial nature of the lesion is suggested by its very well defined border. The tangential view clearly showed only the outer table to be affected. This appearance should not be confused with hyperostosis due to a meningioma.

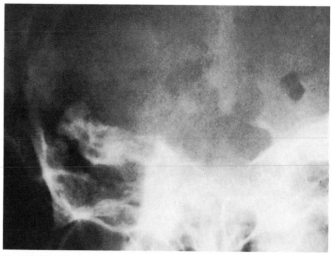

Fig. 86.44 Metastasis producing irregular erosion of right occipital and petrous bones

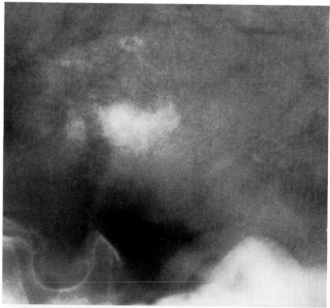

A

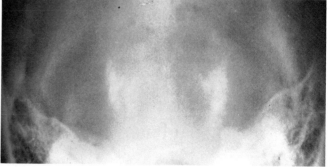

B

Fig. 86.45 Bilaterally symmetrical asymptomatic basal ganglion calcification (A) lateral, (B) half-axial projections: the calcification is typically fluffy and centred on the caudate nuclei.

DISTURBANCES OF CEREBROSPINAL FLUID CIRCULATION

Cerebrospinal fluid is produced essentially within the ventricles by the choroid plexuses, and absorbed at the arachnoid villi. Reduced absorption results in hydrocephalus — 'water on the brain'. The American neurosurgeon Walter Dandy noted that dyes introduced into the ventricles reached the subarachnoid space in some patients with what he therefore termed 'communicating' hydrocephalus, but not in others, with 'noncommunicating' or obstructive hydrocephalus.

Causes of obstructive hydrocephalus are dealt with in sections on congenital anomalies, infections, tumours, etc. However, the commonest cause in young children who present with enlargement of the head is stenosis of the aqueduct [27].

Aqueduct stenosis

This is a condition of unknown, possibly multifactorial aetiology. It is not clear whether the majority of cases are due to primary atresia of the aqueduct of Sylvius, and it has even been suggested that occlusion of the narrow channel is secondary to collapse of its walls as a result and not a cause, of hydrocephalus. Although the majority of cases are discovered in early life, initial presentation in adulthood is not rare.

The skull shows changes of raised intracranial pressure (Fig. 84.3), typically of chronic type, with a 'J' sella. CT reveals marked enlargement of the lateral and third ventricles; the latter may be so marked as to suggest a suprasellar arachnoid cyst, but in aqueduct stenosis the transverse diameter of the ventricle rarely exceeds 3 cm. Interstitial oedema is often lacking. The fourth ventricle is normal in size. Differential diagnosis therefore includes a mass lesion in the midbrain, and it is important to exclude impression on the posterior part of the third ventricle, which in aqueduct stenosis appears ballooned and convex.

If there is doubt about the diagnosis pneumography, ventriculography, or a combination of the two may be required (Fig. 86.46).

Communicating hydrocephalus

In communicating hydrocephalus, the barrier to absorption of cerebrospinal fluid lies distal to the exit foramina of the fourth ventricle: at the tentorium, within the basal cisterns or over the cerebral convexity. Intracranial pressure may be raised or apparently normal: 'normal pressure hydrocephalus'. The major causes of communicating hydrocephalus are trauma, subarachnoid haemorrhage and infection, but in a number of cases the causative factor is not identified.

Plain skull films may show no abnormality or changes of raised intracranial pressure (Ch. 84); there may be evidence of the underlying lesion. At CT or pneumography

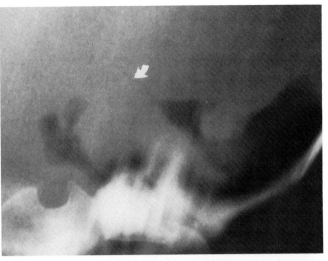

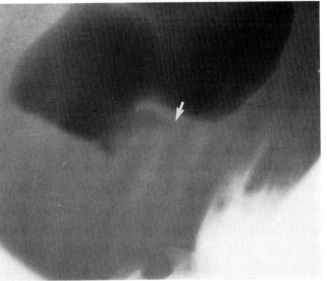

Fig. 86.46 Aqueduct stenosis in a young child.
(A) pneumoencephalogram, lateral midline tomogram in sitting position: tapering and occlusion (arrow) of the aqueduct. The fourth ventricle is small, but the basal cisterns are capacious.
(B) ventriculogram, midline tomogram in brow down position confirms complete occlusion (arrow) and demonstrates gross dilatation of the lateral and third ventricles.

(Figs. 86.47 & 86.48), the hallmark of communicating hydrocephalus is ventricular dilatation, usually marked and generalized. In young children the occipital horns are often most enlarged, but in adults the frontal and temporal horns show the greatest enlargement. Interstitial oedema may be present. The basal cisterns and fissures are sometimes prominent, but the cerebral sulci are characteristically not enlarged.

The major diagnostic consideration is cerebral atrophy; the differentiation is important since patients with communicating hydrocephalus may show a dramatic response to ventricular shunting procedures. If CT features do not enable distinction of atrophy from hydrocephalus, water-soluble cisternography can be employed. The results, which are exactly analogous to those of radionuclide cisternography,

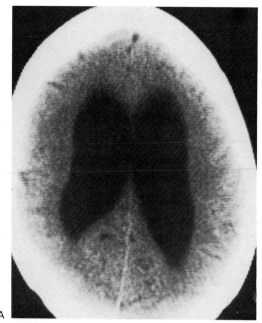

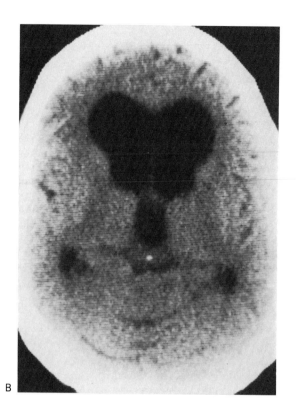

Fig. 86.47A & B Communicating hydrocephalus, CT. Enlargement of the lateral, third and (to a lesser extent) fourth ventricles. The features which indicate the diagnosis, rather than that of atrophy are: absence of enlarged sulci, fissures and cisterns; acute angle between frontal horns; large, rounded third ventricle, and prominence of the temporal horns.

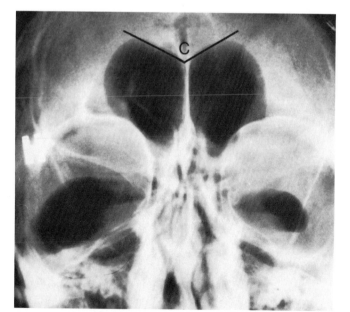

Fig. 86.48 Communicating hydrocephalus (same patient as Fig. 86.47), pneumoencephalogram, anteroposterior brow up projection. The ventricles, particularly the temporal horns, are enlarged and abnormally rounded, but no air is seen over the convexity. The callosal angle [C] is not acute in this case.

are indicated in Table 86.1, which summarizes the differential diagnostic features of hydrocephalus and atrophy [28].

External hydrocephalus [29]

A small number of young children with enlarged heads are found to have wide subarachnoid spaces over the cerebral hemispheres, paradoxically suggesting cerebral atrophy. The sulci and fissures are wide, a feature which aids in the differentiation from bilateral chronic subdural effusions. There is occasionally a history of preceding infection or trauma.

This condition is thought to represent an 'external' hydrocephalus, in which failure of the normal absorption of cerebrospinal fluid results in increased volume of the subarachnoid space; it is generally benign, and often self limiting.

Neonatal ultrasound (Fig. 86.49) (Ch. 103)

Ventricular dilatation is a common observation on cranial ultrasound studies in premature infants. It is usually attributable to intracranial haemorrhage, with subsequent blockage of the ventricular outflow or of the tentorial and convexity pathways. Fortunately, hydrocephalus requiring shunting procedures in exceptional; mild, transitory ventricular dilatation is the rule. Such infants can be followed by ultrasound, firstly at two or three day intervals, then weekly until stabilization.

Table 86.1 *Communicating hydrocephalus and atrophy: radiological and other investigations.*

Test	Communicating hydrocephalus	Atrophy
Skull radiographs	Usually normal; sometimes raised pressure	Normal
CT	All ventricles enlarged (4th may be normal)	Temporal horns and 4th ventricle not large; dilatation may be focal
	sulci not enlarged (but fissures may be) interstitial oedema may be present	sulci enlarged; may be focal white matter generally may be low density
Pneumography	Ventricles large no visualisation of sulci callosal angle less than 120° ventricles larger next day	ventricular enlargement not so marked sulci large angle more than 120° usually no change in size
CT/radionuclide cisternography	Ventricular reflux marked, persistent delay in passage over convexity increased periventricular hypodensity	ventricular reflux absent or minimal rapid absorption at vertex
Cerebral blood flow	Reduced frontally frontal flow increases after shunt	variable; may be globally or focally reduced no change
Lumbar infusion test	Pressure rises	no effect
Intracranial pressure monitoring	Plateau waves	normal

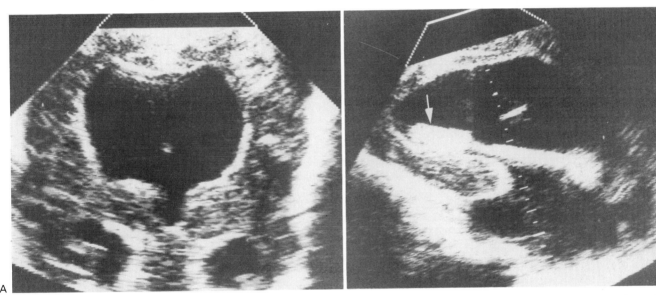

A   B

Fig. 86.49 Hydrocephalus, presumed due to aqueduct stenosis. (A) Coronal sonogram: the frontal horns of the greatly enlarged lateral ventricles merge with the third ventricle. A remnant of the septum pellucidum forms an echogenic dot in the centre of the image. Inferiorly, dilated temporal horns are visible. (B) Parasagittal image through left lateral ventricle, after placement of a ventriculoperitoneal shunt, which is seen running from right to left. Its tip [arrow] is larger than the rest because of terminal flanges; it is correctly sited in the frontal horn, although the ventricles remain dilated. A small echogenic remnant of the septum pellucidum is again seen just above the catheter.

Other forms of hydrocephalus are also easily diagnosed by ultrasound, including those associated with aqueduct stenosis, Dandy Walker syndrome, Chiari malformation, etc. The majority of infants studied by ultrasound need no other type of intracranial imaging. It is, however standard practice to use CT in cases of complex malformation.

Results of ventricular shunting procedures

CT is often employed to follow the size of the ventricles following shunting procedures for communicating or obstruc-

tive hydrocephalus. A satisfactory result is indicated by disappearance of interstitial oedema and reversion of ventricular size towards normal.

Complications which may be detected by CT include:
1. Malfunction of the shunt, with failure of the hydrocephalus to resolve. This may be because of discontinuity in the shunt tubing, which is better assessed by plain films.
2. Incorrect placement of the intraventricular catheter.
3. Intraventricular, intracerebral or extracerebral haemorrhage. Subdural effusions, which are of low density from the outset, are not uncommon.
4. Infection: ventriculitis, abscess or subdural empyema.

BIBLIOGRAPHY

REFERENCES

1. Kendall B E, Kingsley D 1978 The value of computerized axial tomography (CAT) in cranio-cerebral malformations. Br J Radiol 51:171–90
2. Osaka K, Matsumoto S 1978 Holoprosencephaly in neurosurgical practice. J Neurosurg 48:787–803
3. O'Dwyer J A, Newton T H, Hoyt W F 1980 Radiologic features of septo-optic dysplasia: de Morsier syndrome. AJNR 1:443–50
4. Wallace D 1976 Lipoma of the corpus callosum. J Neurol Neurosurg Psychiatry 39:1179–85
5. Byrd S E, Harwood Nash D C, Fitz C R 1978 Absence of the corpus callosum: computed tomographic evaluation in infants and children. J Can Assoc Radiol 29:108–12
6. Dublin A B, French B N 1980 Diagnostic image evaluation of hydranencephaly and pictorially similar entities, with emphasis on computed tomography. Radiology 137:81–92
7. Carmel P W, Lobo Antunes J, Hilal S K, Gold A P 1977 Dandy-Walker syndrome: clinicopathological features and re-evaluation of modes of treatment. Surg Neurol 8:132–38
8. Naidich T P, Pudlowski R M, Naidich J B, Gornish M, Rodriguez F J 1980 Computed tomographic signs of the Chiari II malformation. Radiology 134:65–72, 391–98 and 657–64
9. Anderson F M, Segall H D, Caton W L 1979 Use of computerized tomography scanning in supratentorial arachnoid cysts. J Neurosurg 50:533–38
10. Duggan C A, Keever E B, Gay B B 1970 Secondary craniosynostosis. Am J Roentgenol 109:277–93
11. Wackenheim A 1974 Roentgen diagnosis of the craniovertebral region. Springer, Berlin
12. Logue V 1971 Syringomyelia: a radiodiagnostic and radiotherapeutic saga. Clin Radiol 22:2–16
13. André J M 1974 Les angiodysplasies systematisées. L'Expansion Scientifique, Paris
14. Lee B C P, Gawler J 1978 Tuberous sclerosis: comparison of computerized tomography and conventional neuroradiology. Radiology 127:403–08
15. Fill W L, Lamiell J M, Polk N O 1979 The radiographic manifestations of von Hippel-Lindau disease. Radiology 133:289–95
16. Moseley I F, Zilkha E 1976 The role of computerized axial tomography (EMI scanning) in the diagnosis and management of cranio-cerebral trauma. J Neuroradiol 3:277–96
17. Kingsley D, Till K, Hoare R 1978 Growing fractures of the skull. J Neurol Neurosurg Psychiatry 41:312–18
18. Merino de Villasante J, Taveras J M 1976 Computerized tomography (CT) in acute head trauma. Am J Roentgenol 126:765–78
19. Naidich T P, Moran C J, Pudlowski R M, Naidich J B 1979 CT diagnosis of isodense subdural hematoma. In: Thompson R A, Green J R (eds) Advances in neurology Vol 22. Raven Press, New York pp 73–105
20. Bruce D A, Alavi A, Bilaniuk L, Dolinskas C, Obrist W, Uzzell B 1981 Diffuse cerebral swelling following head injuries in children: the syndrome of 'malignant brain edema'. J Neurosurg 54:170–78
21. Roberson F C, Kishore P R S, Miller J D, Lipper M H, Becker D P 1979 The value of serial computerized tomography in the management of severe head injury. Surg Neurol 12:161–67
22. Danziger A, Price H I 1980 CT findings with cerebral hemiatrophy. Neuroradiology 19:269–71
23. Manelfe C, Cellerier P, Sobel D, Prevost C, Bonafé A 1982 Cerebrospinal fluid rhinorrhea: evaluation with metrizamide cisternography, Am J Roentgenol 138:471–76
24. Peeters F L M, Kröger R 1979 Dural and direct cavernous sinus fistulas. Am J Roentgenol 132:599–606
25. Liakos G M, Walker C B, Carruth J A S. Ocular complications of craniofacial fibrous dysplasia. Br J Ophthalmol 1979; 63:611–16
26. Du Boulay G H 1980 Principles of X-ray diagnosis of the skull. Butterworth, London
27. Kingsley D, Kendall B E 1978 The value of computed tomography in the evaluation of the enlarged head. Neuroradiology 15:59–71
28. Huckman M S 1981 Normal pressure hydrocephalus: evaluation of diagnostic and prognostic tests. AJNR 2:385–395
29. Kendall B E, Holland I M 1981 Benign communicating hydrocephalus in children. Neuroradiology 21:93–96

SUGGESTIONS FOR FURTHER READING

See Chapter 84

87

The spine
Methods of examination: diagnostic approach

V. L. McAllister, I. F. Moseley and J. Theron

Methods of examination
  Plain radiography
  Anatomy
  Computerized tomography
  Myelography
    Endomyelography
  Angiography
    Arteriography
    Phlebography
  Discography
  Epidurography
  Ultrasound
  Magnetic resonance imaging

Radiological diagnostic approach to common problems
  Acute presentations
  Chronic presentations

METHODS OF EXAMINATION

Many imaging techniques are available for the investigation of diseases of the spine and its contents (Table 87.1). Plain radiography and myelography are by far the most widely used in neurological practice, although CT is rapidly becoming of great clinical use. Where possible, information required for diagnosis and treatment should be obtained from noninvasive techniques before proceeding to invasive procedures such as myelography or CT with intrathecal contrast media. The decision to resort to these potentially hazardous techniques should always be a matter of consultation between clinician and radiologist, and the techniques employed should be tailored to the individual case.

Nuclear medicine studies, which are often orientated towards the demonstration of neoplastic or inflammatory disease of the spinal column in patients known to have systemic disease, are considered in Chapters 2, 79.

Table 87.1 *Diagnostic imaging of spinal pathology (Modified from Park [1]).*

Noninvasive	Invasive
Plain radiography (chest, spine, skeletal survey)	Myelography
Tomography	Epidurography
Isotope bone scans	Computerized metrizamide myelogram
Ultrasound	Vascular studies
CT	Spinal angiography Epidural venography Digital vascular radiology
Magnetic resonance imaging	Provocation radiology Discography Facet joint arthrography Interventional radiology Chymopapein injection Embolization Aspiration needle biopsy

Plain radiography of the spine[1] in neuroradiology

The vertebral column may be divided into six regions for radiographic purposes; the extent of the radiological examination in each patient will be determined by localizing features of the clinical picture. The standard projections are as follows:

1. Atlanto-occipital region

Anteroposterior: supine or seated position, with the baseline of the skull (see Ch. 83) extended 10° relative to the beam, which is centred on the mouth.

Lateral: with the baseline parallel to a line across the centre of the casette, centring 2.5 cm below and behind the external meatus. In radiography of the atlanto-occipital and cervical regions, as of the skull, a true lateral, without rotation of the head, is mandatory.

In practice, tomography in both planes is much more satisfactory for examination of this region; autotomography, with gentle side to side rotation of the head, may suffice for the lateral projection. The posterior end of the hard palate should be included in this view.

2. Cervical spine

Anteroposterior: supine or seated, with the baseline extended 20°, centring (a) through the mouth, which is held open, for the upper vertebrae or (b) at the sternal notch, perpendicular to the film, for the lower vertebrae. The jaw may be moved gently during the exposure, to produce an autotomogram. To show the posterior intervertebral joints and lateral masses, 30° caudal angulation may be employed.

Lateral: erect, neck extended, shoulders forcibly depressed, particularly in obese individuals (weights may be held in the hands), centred 2.5 cm behind the angle of the mandible.

Oblique: anteroposterior, neck and head rotated 45°, with chin depressed, centring at midcervical level, with 15° cephalad tube angulation. To show the lower neural foramina clearly, it is often necessary to rotate the shoulder as well as the neck, to avoid foreshortening the foramina. Note that the foramina displayed *en face* are those *away from which* the head is rotated, i.e. furthest from the film (c.f. lumbar spine). To avoid confusion, each oblique projection should show both right and left side markers.

3. Thoracocervical

Anteroposterior: centring point: the sternal notch. This projection is not often required, but is a useful supplement to (4) below.

Lateral: a 'swimmer's' or Twining's view is obtained; the arm adjacent to the film is elevated above the head, while the other remains down by the side. The beam is centred above the shoulder further from the film, to the opposite axilla, with 15° cephalad tube angulation. Tomography is often preferable.

4. Thoracic

Anteroposterior: centring point: midway between cricoid and xiphoid cartilages, i.e. about 2.5 cm below the sternal angle. The film should show the entire thoracic portion of the vertebral column.

Lateral: the beam is centred on the sixth thoracic vertebra, i.e. through the axilla. If there is a scoliosis, the convexity is placed nearer the film, so that the divergent rays are more nearly parallel to the disc spaces. The patient may breathe gently during the exposure, blurring out the rib cage.

5. Lumbar

Anteroposterior: flexion of the hips and knees will reduce the lumbar lordosis. Centring for all lumbar projections is at the lower costal margin.

Lateral: the beam is centred 10 cm anterior to the third lumbar spinous process. Convexity of any scoliosis is nearer the film.

Anteroposterior obliques: 30°–45° of obliquity will serve to show *en face* the pedicles and neural foramina *towards which* the trunk is rotated (i.e. nearest the film).

6. Lumbosacral

The lowest disc space is often best assessed separately from the remainder of the lumbar spine.

Anteroposterior: supine, with 20°–30° cephalad angulation of the tube, centring in the midline, between the anterior superior iliac spines.

Lateral: centring point is 10 cm anterior to the spinous process of the fifth lumbar vertebra.

Anatomy

Certain common anomalies are mentioned here; most are without clinical significance in the large majority of cases.

Spina bifida of the atlas and/or the first sacral segment is common; the atlas may also be bifid anteriorly. The midline defect is easily identified on the anteroposterior projection in the lumbar region. In the cervical spine it is manifest as absence of the cortical line on the anterior surface of the spinous process, as seen on the lateral projection, and can be verified by oblique projections, or by a half axial projection of the skull, when the posterior arch of the atlas is seen through the foramen magnum.

Intervertebral fusions are most often encountered in the cervical region. One level only is usually involved, C2/3 being the commonest. When fusion is extensive, mobility of the neck is reduced, and the neck is short (the Klippel-Feil syndrome), but the majority of cases show no neurological abnormality, unless there is an associated Arnold-Chiari malformation.

Transitional vertebrae may be encountered:
1. At the atlanto-occipital articulation. Assimilation of the

atlas is considered elsewhere. The converse tendency, the formation of extra bone elements between the skull base and the first cervical vertebra, is referred to as 'manifestation of an occipital vertebra'. It is not usually significant.

2. At the thoracocervical junction. The seventh cervical vertebra may show long, pointed transverse processes, or bear ribs; both may be present, in which case the former are more likely to be associated with a nerve entrapment syndrome. Oblique or lordotic projections may be necessary for good demonstration.

3. At the thoracolumbar junction. A vertebra bearing vestigial ribs may be found to represent the twelfth thoracic or the first lumbar vertebra.

4. At the lumbosacral junction. The last lumbar vertebra may be more or less completely fused with the sacrum (sacralization), or the first sacral segment may not be fused with the body of the sacrum (lumbarization). Some workers believe that asymmetrical fusion may predispose to back strain. The abnormal segmentation is not usually significant, but may lead to confusion in patients with root compression syndromes, when the level is wrongly identified clinically or radiologically.

An individual with one of these anomalies will frequently show another anomaly.

Computerized tomography of the spine[2]

Although most modern scanners provide good images of the vertebral column, demonstration of the intraspinal structures is a rigorous test of any machine. Movement, poor natural contrast and the small size of the lesions sought are major problems. CT is therefore often combined with water soluble myelography.

Spinal CT is carried out in the supine position, with the spinal column as perpendicular to the plane of section as possible. The neck should be moderately flexed, so as to reduce the normal lordosis; the beam will then be more nearly parallel to the disc spaces. However, artefacts from dental fillings may then obscure the upper part of the cervical spine, so that some neck extension may be necessary. Gantry tilt can assist in overcoming this problem, but the result is often a compromise. Artefacts are often severe around the shoulder girdle; when CT of this region is essential, it may be necessary to carry out trial scans with the arms up alongside the head or down by the trunk to assess which gives the better results. Gantry tilt is often useful in the lower lumbar region, but on many machines is inadequate for an axial scan of the last disc space. Flexion of hips and knees, supported by a pillow, may bring the plane of the disc space within the range of the machine, and is often more comfortable for the patient.

The straight, supine position may be intolerable for patients with for example, metastatic disease of the spine, and adequate analgesia must be ensured; examination of the spine is often a lengthy procedure. Otherwise, no preparation is necessary.

A digital CT radiograph of the region to be studied ('scanogram', 'scout film'), while not mandatory is extremely useful for selection of the levels to be scanned, and for retrospective localization of abnormalities. Examination of the intervertebral discs is virtually impossible without this facility. A number of methods of external identification of scan levels have been described, but are now essentially obsolete.

Assuming that the scan times are short enough, the patient is instructed not only to remain still, but also not to breathe, and, for the cervical region, not to swallow; this is a potent source of artefact.

The thickness of the CT sections will depend on the capacities of the machine, and the clinical problem. For suspected disc disease, 5 mm thick sections through the disc space, 5 mm above and 5 mm below will usually provide diagnostic information. The number of sections and the number of levels examined will be dictated by the clinical picture and the CT findings. If coronal and sagittal reformations are to be carried out, thinner sections may be preferred. High resolution or bone algorithm programmes can be employed.

Contrast media may be administered for spinal scans. These studies which are not uniquely concerned with the vertebral column itself are generally carried out only after intravenous iodinated contrast medium, which increases the contrast between the epidural tissues and spinal cord on the one hand and the cerebrospinal fluid on the other. Patients with suspected intraspinal vascular lesions (malformations or tumours), in whom abnormal contrast enhancement is sought, are exceptions to this practice.

Spinal CT often follows myelography, and if this is foreseen, a water soluble contrast medium is used. Any patient, who may undergo subsequent CT, should not be examined with oil contrast medium, as this causes artefacts. CT can follow myelography by several hours, and indeed may be more informative when the aqueous contrast medium is more diluted. In the search for a syrinx or a cystic lesion with a narrow communication with the subarachnoid space, delayed scans may be mandatory. CT alone may be carried out with a smaller dose of contrast medium than is needed for conventional myelography, but information from the two modalities is often complementary. CT may also follow endomyelography.

Inhaled stable xenon gas has also been recommended as a contrast agent: being liposoluble, it is concentrated in the white matter of the spinal cord. It is, however, expensive and in the concentrations desirable for CT imaging has an anaesthetic effect. Its use is therefore limited.

Combination of intravenous or inhaled contrast media with intrathecal water soluble medium is counterproductive, as contrast differences are thereby reduced.

CT anatomy (Fig. 87.1)

The vertebral column

The atlas (the first cervical vertebra) is defined by the absence of a body; the odontoid peg of the axis occupies its expected position. CT sections often pass obliquely through the craniocervical junction, so that the anterior margin of the foramen magnum (the lower end of the clivus) appears on the same section as the posterior arch of the atlas, or vice versa. This may be important in assessing tonsillar herni-

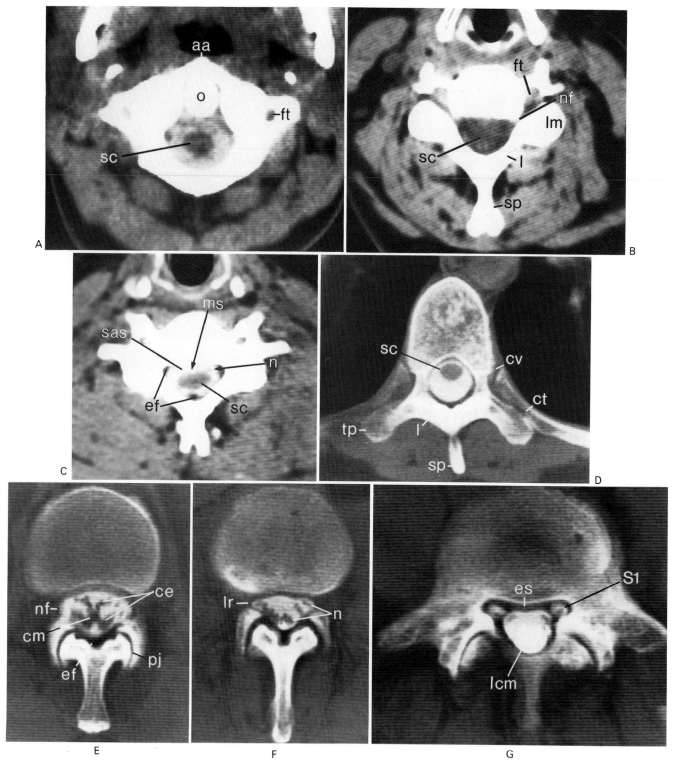

Fig. 87.1 CT of normal spine; sections at: (A) C1/2; (B & C) Mid-cervical; (D) mid-thoracic; (E) T12/L1; (F) L3; and (G) L5/S1 levels. All but (B) with intrathecal metrizamide. Note the poor visualization of the spinal cord in (B), and its typical size, shape and position in (C) and (D)

aa = anterior arch of atlas; ce = cauda equina; cm = conus medullaris; ct = costotransverse joint; cv = costovertebral joint; ef = epidural fat; es = wide extradural space (containing veins anteriorly at L5/S1; ft = foramen transversarium; l = lamina; lcm = layering of contrast medium, which is denser posteriorly (patient supine); lm = lateral mass; lr = lateral recess of spinal canal; ms = median anterior sulcus of spinal cord; n = nerve roots; nf = neural foramen; o = odontoid; pj = posterior intervertebral joint; sas = subarachnoid space; sc = spinal cord; sp = spinous process; S1 = first sacral nerve root in dural sheath; tp = transverse process.

ation. The lateral masses of C2 to C6 show rounded defects, the foramina transversaria, through which run the vertebral arteries. A vertical cleft in the spinous processes of the cervical vertebrae is a normal finding, in no way related to spina bifida. The cervical spinal canal is widest at C1, where it is approximately circular in cross section, but it rapidly funnels down to become triangular, the flattened base lying anteriorly. The lateral recesses are often the most anterior portions of the canal on the CT sections.

In the thoracic region the vertebral bodies are more massive, often appearing elongated in the anteroposterior plane because the normal kyphosis causes them to be oblique to the plane of section. The spinal canal is relatively small, and more circular in cross section. Identification of segments at the thoracocervical and thoracolumbar junctions is simplified by recognition of the ribs.

The lumbar vertebrae more closely resemble the cervical vertebrae in overall form, having a rounded body and a triangular spinal canal. In contrast with those of the cervical spine, however, the posterior intervertebral joints lie perpendicular to the plane of section. Their articular surfaces and adjacent osteophytes can therefore be accurately assessed, as can their position relative to the pedicles and lateral recesses, of great importance in evaluation of spinal stenosis.

Throughout the spine, thin sections which pass exclusively through the vertebral body show a normal cortical and trabecular pattern, while sections through the discs show a less dense, amorphous and smoothly rounded structure, with a concave posterior border, except at the lumbosacral level, where the disc is convex. CT sections which are oblique to the disc spaces in any plane will show a variable mixture of these appearances, which should not be misinterpreted as disc calcification or vertebral erosion.

The contents of the spinal canal

Most CT scanners show the spinal cord clearly only in the cervical region, and then only in its upper half. Throughout the remainder of the spine, the theca may be visible, outlined by epidural fat, which is most abundant posteriorly, giving the appearance of a 'pseudocord'. The cervical spinal cord appears rounded or elliptical, with its greater diameter transversely, surrounded by the lower density of the cerebrospinal fluid.

When CT is carried out after intrathecal injection of water soluble contrast medium, the cord is clearly outlined, and in the cervical region the anterior median sulcus can often be identified. The thoracolumbar cord is more circular in cross section, and whereas the cervical cord lies in the centre of the subarachnoid space, this portion of the cord lies more anteriorly. Since the lower end of the spinal cord normally lies at about L1 or 2, there is no central spinal cord filling defect below this level in the normal.

Nerve roots cannot usually be identified within the theca at any level without contrast medium, although images suggestive of the cauda equina have been published. The dorsal root ganglia and some nerve roots can, however be shown as blobs of soft tissue density lying in the intervertebral foramina in the lumbar region and within the sacrum, and occasionally higher up. With intrathecal contrast

medium, the sheaths around these nerve roots may be filled. Demonstration of intrathecal roots above the cauda equina remains difficult; the lumbar and sacral roots can, however, be seen surrounding the lower end of the spinal cord and spreading out in a typical cruciate pattern below it. They should normally be separate, in the absence of arachnoid adhesions, and lie posteriorly in the lower lumbar canal.

The dura mater as such is not visible at CT, but its position can be inferred from the low density epidural fat around it.

Prominent epidural veins may be seen, especially anteriorly at the L5/S1 level; they should not be mistaken for a bulging disc.

The ligamentum flavum is identified as a V shaped soft tissue structure lining the posterior aspect of the spinal canal, and extending into the lateral recesses. It is most evident in the lumbar region.

Myelography

The technical aspects of myelography are mainly the type of contrast medium to be used, the site of its injection into the subarachnoid space and special details of its manipulation. These will vary according to the clinical and anatomical problems presented by each patient.

Types of contrast medium

An ideal contrast medium for opacification of the cerebrospinal fluid should possess:

1. Optimal radio opacity for demonstration of the spinal cord, nerve roots and nerve root sheaths
2. Complete reabsorbability from the subarachnoid space
3. Thorough miscibility with the cerebrospinal fluid.
4. No inflammatory or toxic effects on either the nervous system or the meninges [3].

If it were to be truly ideal, it would also be administered orally or perhaps intravenously.

Three main types of contrast medium are currently in use:

1. Nonionic water soluble: metrizamide, iopamidol, iohexol
2. Oily: iophendylate (Myodil, Pantopaque), and lipiodol derivatives (Duroliopaque)
3. Gaseous: air, oxygen, carbon dioxide.

Water soluble contrast media

This type of contrast medium is the most recently developed, and is increasingly supplanting other types. The most widely used at present is *metrizamide* (*Amipaque* (and its derivatives); a nonionic compound introduced in 1972, which is derived from metrizoic acid and glucosamine (2[3-acetimido 2,4,6-triiodo 5-(n-methyl acetimido) benzamido] 2-deoxy-D-glucose) (Fig. 87.2). Its chief advantage over the earlier water soluble contrast media (Conray, Dimer X) is that it does not dissociate into positive and negative ions in aqueous solution, and therefore yields solutions with considerably lower osmolarity, and more importantly, with lower toxicity to the nervous system. It is dispensed as a freeze dried powder, which can be used in any desired concentration by dissolving it in a specially supplied bicarbonate buffer solution. Although this has the advantage that the concentration can be varied (a table of dilutions is supplied by the manufacturers), it must be made up at the time of the study, as the solution is not stable. A solution with 180 mg iodine/ml is isotonic with cerebrospinal fluid.

The low neurotoxicity of metrizamide allows its use throughout the subarachnoid space. Its moderate radio-opacity and its ability to permeate narrow spaces result in excellent visualization of the spinal cord, cauda equina and nerve root sheaths. It is, however, expensive, and much more demanding in terms of radiological manipulation and of radiography than iodized oil.

About 85% of metrizamide injected into the subarachnoid space is excreted within 24 hours through the kidneys. Metrizamide is absorbed into the blood stream through the arachnoid villi in both the spinal and cranial subarachnoid spaces. Most of the contrast medium is absorbed from the spinal theca [4]. Maintaining the patient erect, therefore, after myelography, encourages spinal absorption and reduces the amount of contrast medium reaching the head.

There has as yet been no proven case of arachnoiditis (inflammation of the leptomeninges) following the use of metrizamide in humans. Arachnoiditis has been provoked in animal experiments, but with doses which far exceed those used in clinical practice [5]. Metrizamide has a slight but well documented epileptogenic effect and is therefore contra-indicated in patients with a history of epilepsy and in those taking drugs which lower the seizure threshold: e.g. tricyclic antidepressants, phenothiazines, monoamine oxidase inhibitors and central nervous system stimulants. The increased risk of seizures is not, however, an absolute contraindication, but patients having predisposing factors should have any offending drug withdrawn at least 48 hours before the examination. Premedication with antiepileptic agents is often not practicable, as they may take 48 hours or more to reach therapeutic plasma levels. If fits or spasms should occur, intravenous diazepam is the treatment drug of choice.

Detailed and authoritative accounts of the indications, technique and interpretation of metrizamide myelography are to be found in Acta Radiologica, Supplements 335 (1973) and 355 (1977).

Iopamidol (Niopam) is a more recent nonionic water soluble contrast medium. A derivative of 2,4,6 tri-iodo benzioc acid, substituted with hydrophillic polyalcohols (Fig. 87.2), it is similar to metrizamide as regards side effects and quality of examination, but has the advantage that it is stable in solution, and is therefore provided ready for injection. It is also considerably less expensive and causes less headache so will probably replace metrizamide.

Iohexol is another nonionic contrast medium suitable for myelography; its structure is shown in Figure 87.2. Its chemical and pharmacological properties are similar to those of metrizamide and iopamidol, but is probably the least epileptogenic after intracranial spill. Like iopamidol, it is stable in solution, supplied ready for injection and is about the same price as iopamidol.

Metrizamide will almost certainly be replaced by iohexol and iopamidol. An even newer product (a non-ionic

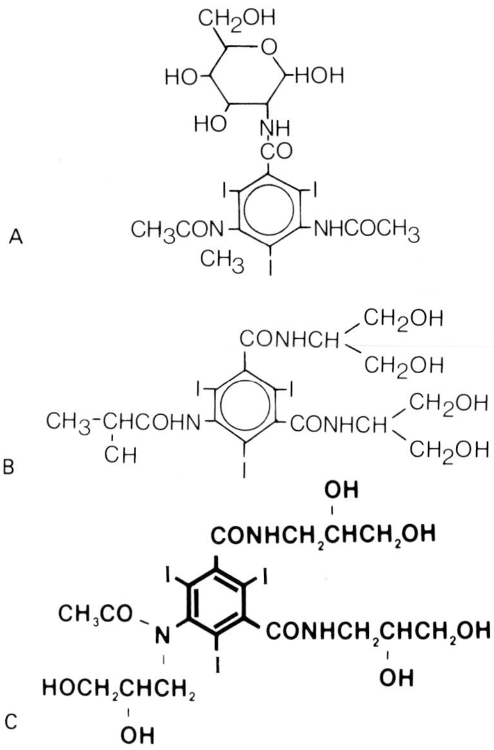

Fig. 87.2   Structure of (A) metrizamide; (B) iopamidol; (C) iohexol.

dimer-Iotrol) may well become the myelographic agent of choice.

Oily contrast media

The entire cerebrospinal fluid compartment from the sacral sac to the ventricles can be examined with iophendylate. Re-screening of the difficult or doubtful diagnostic case, or of patients who have meanwhile undergone surgery, is possible if the contrast medium has not been removed. The marked opacity of the oil may obscure anatomical detail, and its high surface tension results in poor penetration into the nerve root sheaths. The tendency to form oil globules increases difficulties in interpretation.

Oil contrast media have been shown to induce an inflammatory reaction in the meninges, which is exacerbated by subarachnoid blood [6]. The contrast medium is absorbed very slowly from the subarachnoid space, and in many centres it has been considered necessary to remove it on completion of the examination because of the fear of producing arachnoiditis. However, removal of the oil is often a painful procedure, usually incomplete, which may provoke haemorrhage and may require a second lumbar puncture.

Retained oil also has the disadvantage of interfering with CT or angiographic studies of the spine.

Gaseous contrast media

Air is usually used. It has low radiographic contrast, and its use as a myelographic agent requires meticulous radiographic technique, almost always involving tomography, to obtain good results. This tends to lengthen the procedure; it also increases radiation dose and requires relatively sophisticated equipment. The exchange of a large volume of cerebrospinal fluid with air causes the patient considerable discomfort, even with general anaesthesia, which is often employed. For detailed consideration of the technique and interpretation of air myelography the reader is referred to the review by James and Lassman [7].

This technique has been largely rendered obsolete by nonionic water soluble contrast media, but is still carried out in some centres for the investigation of spinal dysraphism and syringomyelia. It is *less* reliable for the demonstration of disc protusions (unless they are central), arteriovenous malformations, arachnoid cysts and arachnoiditis.

Choice of contrast medium

The introduction of nonionic water soluble media has greatly clarified this problem. They are now generally regarded as the best available contrast media in terms of both diagnostic effectiveness and freedom from significant side effects and there are now relatively few indications for either oil or gas myelography. Iohexol and iopamidol are currently the aqueous media of choice.

Oil is still used in some centres for certain patients with cervical problems, others whose clinical picture gives no clear spinal level, or difficult patients in whom delays or difficulties in obtaining radiographs may be problematic because of dilution of the contrast medium. Some workers have doubts about the use of water soluble contrast media in circumstances where delayed filming may be required, such as spinal or sacral cysts [8]. The use of CT as an adjunct to water soluble myelography can be an acceptable alternative to delayed films.

Puncture site

Contrast medium is generally introduced by lumbar puncture, cisternal puncture or a lateral puncture at C1/2. Other levels are occasionally used.

Lumbar puncture

Many neuroradiologists prefer to carry out lumbar puncture with the patient sitting and the back well flexed so that the vertebral spinous processes and laminae are separated to the maximum extent. This position also ensures that the spine is straight (something which is very difficult in the lateral decubitus position, which many believe should only be used when absolutely necessary) and facilitates a midline puncture. Other workers prefer the prone position, flexing the lumbar spine by a pillow under the abdomen. This position removes the necessity for moving the patient before commencing the myelogram proper, and is thus useful for uncooperative patients or those with whom oral communication is limited. A line joining the iliac crests passes through the fourth lumbar vertebra, and injection of the intervertebral space immediately above this landmark may be carried out with safety.

A 20 or 22 gauge needle is used; local anaesthetic should be used by less experienced operators. The site of puncture should be away from expected pathology and is usually therefore at L2/3 or 3/4, since these levels are both below the normal termination of the spinal cord and above most lumbar disc lesions. The needle is advanced, slightly cranially, in the midline, a few millimetres at a time, until the dural 'pop' is obtained, and cerebrospinal fluid flows. It is then advanced further so that the entire bevel lies within the subarachnoid space. Fluoroscopic control of contrast medium injection is highly desirable, to avoid extra-arachnoid injection, and to titrate the amount of contrast medium injected to the capacity of the spinal canal.

Contrast medium injected into the *subdural* space tends to move slowly. On the anteroposterior projection it often presents angular margins, and appears dense, since it does not mix with CSF. A prone lateral radiograph will show the dorsal or ventral position of the contrast medium as compared with any in the subarachnoid space (Fig. 87.3). Contrast medium does not move freely in the *extradural* space. It coats the periphery of the dura mater and runs out along the nerve roots, beyond the intervertebral foramina (Fig. 87.4). Water soluble media have the advantage over oil that extra-arachnoid contrast medium is quickly absorbed and repeat injection at another level is usually possible. The lateral projection is often the best for appreciation of the fact that the contrast medium is not in the subarachnoid space.

Occasionally, the contrast medium will be seen to enter the epidural veins during the injection, and disappear rapidly from the spinal canal.

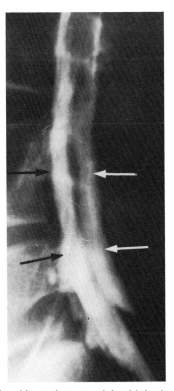

Fig. 87.3 Metrizamide myelogram; subdural injection of contrast medium posteriorly [white arrows]. Contrast medium in the subarachnoid space anteriorly [black arrows] is in close contact with the discs and vertebral bodies.

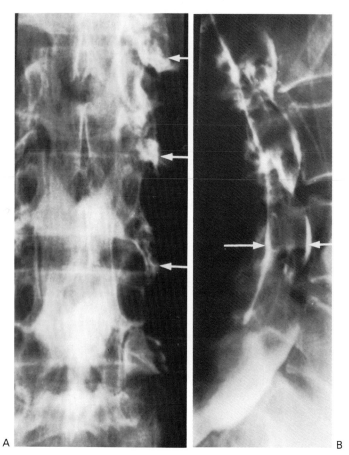

Fig. 87.4 Oil (Myodil) myelogram; epidural injection. (A) AP projection shows contrast medium along the nerve roots, beyond the intervertebral foramina [arrows]. (B) Lateral projection; contrast medium outlines the theca from without [arrows].

Failure to enter the subarachnoid space (a 'dry tap') is usually the result of faulty technique, but may also occur in cases of obliteration of the spinal canal (by a tumour, an abscess or a major disc prolapse) or a very restricted subarachnoid space, in arachnoiditis or severe canal stenosis.

Ideally, myelography should not be attempted within a week of a previous lumbar puncture since there is a danger of contrast medium being injected into a pool of cerebrospinal fluid in the subdural space. Oil should not be injected if the cerebrospinal fluid is bloody, except in an emergency; this does not apply to water soluble media.

Lateral cervical puncture [9]

The patient is placed prone and under careful lateral fluoroscopic control, the space between the posterior arches of the first and second cervical vertebrae is identified. A 22 gauge needle is inserted two thirds of the way back in that interspace. The technique is otherwise as for lumbar puncture, except that the needle is not usually advanced once fluid is obtained.

Cisternal puncture

This technique is used less now that water soluble contrast media are in use, but the neuroradiologist should be familiar with the method.

The puncture is carried out with the patient in the lateral decubitus position, the neck well flexed and supported so that it is parallel with the table top. Local anaesthetic is injected in the midline midway between the external occipital protuberance and the spinous process of C2. A cisternal needle is then inserted, and directed at the glabella. As it is advanced slowly through the atlanto-occipital membrane and dura mater, the resistance suddenly falls. Cisternal needles are calibrated in centimetres, and a flow of cerebrospinal fluid, indicating that the needle has entered the cisterna magna, usually occurs at a depth of 5 to 6 cm. The main risk of this technique is damage to the posterior inferior cerebellar artery, but this is very rare.

Lateral cervical or cisternal puncture may be indicated in the following situations:

1. Patients with severe lumbar canal stenosis or other diseases in whom lumbar puncture has failed
2. Patients with suspected lumbar infection, cutaneous or epidural;
3. Patients in whom it is desirable to demonstrate the superior limit of an obstructive lesion when this is considered necessary for surgical management;
4. Patients with suspected lumbar dysraphism, with a low cord. However, if a water soluble medium is introduced by the cervical route, there is often excessive dilution of the contrast medium by the time it reaches the lower end of the canal. Most workers have therefore adopted lumbar injection, and very few complications have as yet been described [10].

Cervical or cisternal injection is contraindicated:

1. in patients with a suspected lesion at the foramen magnum level, such as meningioma or tonsillar ectopia, or those in whom the upper cervical cord may be very expanded;
2. in patients with cervical spondylosis or other lesions which may be causing an obstruction at a high level, although below the injection site. It may not be possible to inject an adequate amount of contrast medium to show the pathology clearly without running the risk of its mainly entering the head;
3. in patients who are suspected of having an obstructive lesion over several segments. Although cervical injection may turn out to be necessary eventually, lumbar puncture should generally be the first approach.

Technical considerations

Most patients are examined initially in the prone position, ideally on a tilting table (90°–90°), with a suitable harness, which should support the top of the shoulders so as to avoid any damage to the brachial plexus. A cradle to rotate the patient around his long axis and the capacity to carry out tomography on the same table are useful but not essential. The contrast medium is moved up and down the spinal canal by means of gravity (even the water soluble media are heavier than spinal fluid) and spot radiographs are taken as required, usually as anteroposterior and lateral or oblique pairs.

Water soluble media have the very significant disadvantage that they may mix very rapidly with the spinal fluid, becoming dilute and giving poor contrast. Within a few seconds of injection into a very capacious theca, it may be impossible to obtain diagnostic images. It is advisable therefore that the examination be directed initially at the specific level indicated by the clinical features or by findings on preliminary plain films of the spine. Control films of each region to be examined will obviate unsatisfactory exposures. The aqueous medium should never be moved to another part of the spinal canal, or the patient moved to a new position, e.g. supine, until the radiographs of the region being examined have been inspected.

The full extent of any lesion encountered should be defined as accurately as possible so that the extent of surgical exposure or radiotherapy field may be planned. This may represent a problem when an apparently complete block is found. Some workers recommend the technique of injecting air by cervical puncture to demonstrate simultaneously the upper and lower borders of a lesion on one film, one outlined by air and the other by positive contrast. If a block is suspected at the outset, the lumbar needle should be left in place, and the patient placed immediately in the head down position. Further injection of the aqueous contrast medium often causes the contrast medium to pass the level of apparent obstruction and enables demonstration of the upper border of the lesion. It may cause transient discomfort to the patient, but this is often preferable to a second puncture. The latter may be necessary if this manoeuvre fails. If the block is low down in the spinal canal, some workers prefer to inject a small quantity of iodized oil by cervical puncture, thereby avoiding possible dilution.

Marker films

The level of a surgical lesion should be marked on the skin by the radiologist at the time of myelography. This will avoid possible inaccuracies in counting spinous processes; it is most important in the middle portion of the spine where external landmarks are lacking. Anteroposterior and lateral films are obtained with a radio-opaque marker at the site of the lesion. The latter should be in the centre of the field to minimize errors due to parallax. The films should not be tightly coned, but should include identifiable landmarks, such as the first or last ribs. A fairly deep scratch is made at the appropriate level, but lateral to the spine so that the operative site is not involved should it become infected. Occasionally, the surgeon will request a rib marker: the shaft of a fine hypodermic needle is embedded in the posteromedial portion of the appropriate rib and broken off flush with the skin.

Endomyelography [11,12]

Endomyelography is the intentional introduction of contrast medium into the spinal cord itself, almost always when the cord is believed to contain a cyst or fluid collection. Its purpose is to confirm the presence of the fluid filled space,

determine its extent, show any mural nodules of tumour and, in some cases, to decompress it. The procedure is contra-indicated if myelography suggests the presence of a hyper-vascular lesion.

Endomyelography is usually carried out under general anaesthesia, to minimize movement, with the patient prone. A spinal needle is inserted in the midline at the point at which the spinal cord is most expanded, and the canal gently traversed from back to front. Paramedian needling may be carried out if no fluid is encountered; an adjacent level may be explored, but excessive passages of the needle are avoided. When fluid is obtained, it is aspirated for diagnostic purposes, and contrast medium (usually water soluble) injected. Should the fluid be bloody, the procedure is terminated.

Complications of myelography

These may be due to the spinal puncture or to the contrast medium itself.

Lumbar puncture

Headache following simple lumbar puncture occurs in between 10 and 35% of patients [13]. It is generally accepted that the headache arises from traction on blood vessels crossing the subarachnoid space, due to loss of fluid through the needle hole in the meninges. The incidence and severity of headache are reduced if a small gauge needle is used. [14]

Infection at the site of the puncture, or meningitis, are very rare if adequate sterile technique is employed. Iatrogenic intraspinal epidermoid has been described, due to implantation of cutaneous tissue at the time of lumbar puncture. It is extremely rare, usually occurring in patients who have undergone numerous lumbar punctures for e.g. tuberculous meningitis; pain and severe spinal rigidity are typical clinical features.

Inadvertent puncture of a lumbar tumour or cyst may occur. Injection is characteristically very painful and the contrast medium may appear to be subdural.

Cisternal and cervical puncture

Damage to the neuraxis should not occur if the procedure is performed with due care. The possibility of haemorrhage has already been mentioned.

Direct effects of the contrast medium

Water-soluble media (Metrizamide, Iopamidol, Iohexol).

Adverse reactions have been classified into three broad groups: hyperexcitation states, radicular effects and meningeal reactions [15]. Allergic or cardiovascular reactions occur very infrequently.

Hyperexcitation states. Focal or generalized epileptic seizures may occur. In the clinical trials of metrizamide which included almost 10 000 cases, seizures occurred in 25 patients (an incidence of 0.25%). Epilepsy was much more frequent in cervical myelography: incidence 0.8%. Fits usually occur as a result of faulty technique:

1. Excessive dose
2. Uncontrolled intracranial diffusion;
3. Use of metrizamide in patients with a lowered threshold due to epilepsy or certain drugs.

They are usually short lived and respond rapidly to intravenous diazepam.

Psycho-organic disturbances such as confusion, hallucinations, mental depression and stupor have been reported after metrizamide in a few patients, but minor psychic symptoms are probably experienced by most.

Iohexol and iopamidol produce much less psycho-organic disturbance as well as less epilepsy.

Focal neurological disturbances, including dysphasia and other cortical signs, cranial nerve palsies, etc., are rare, and often associated with faulty technique.

Radicular effects. These include aggravation or recurrence of the patient's pain and the development of lower limb paraesthesiae. They usually occur during the first 24 hours after injection.

Meningeal reactions. Headache, nausea and vomiting are the most frequent side effects of myelography. They are usually mild to moderate in severity, last at most 48 hours, and respond to simple medications. They may occasionally be severe and persist for days; headaches tend to be more frequent and persistent in female patients and in those who are not well hydrated [16].

These side effects can be minimized by careful attention to detail:

1. Use of a small (22) gauge needle
2. Removal of as little spinal fluid as necessary
3. Good hydration of the patient before and after the procedure
4. Sitting the patient upright following the procedure, for six hours, to encourage maximal absorption of the contrast medium from the spinal theca
5. Ensuring that the contrast medium is not run higher in the spinal canal than is essential for diagnostic purposes.

2. Iophendylate (oil)

Transitory spinal or root pain and low grade pyrexia are not uncommon. The possibility of arachnoiditis has prompted removal of the contrast medium at the end of the procedure, especially in the United States. Arachnoiditis is diagnosed if any of the following radiological signs are present on subsequent myelography [17]:

1. Impaired filling of the lumbar nerve root sheaths (Fig. 87.5)
2. Loss of the normal striated pattern of the cauda equina
3. Narrowing, shortening or irregularity of the caudal subarachnoid space
4. Abnormally thickened nerve roots.

Adhesive arachnoiditis may also follow water-soluble myelography with Conray and Dimer X (Fig. 87.5).

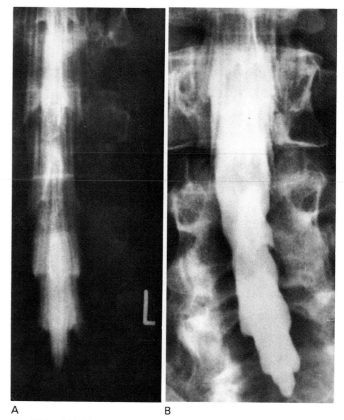

A   B

Fig. 87.5 (A) Dimer X myelogram with normal demonstration of the roots of the cauda equina and their sheaths. (B) Repeat study with metrizamide 7 months later, with changes of arachnoiditis: poor filling of the nerve root sheaths, poor definition of the cauda equina, no nerve roots visible in lower cul-de-sac, abnormal outline of subarachnoid space.

It should be emphasized, however, that no close correlation has been established between symptoms, radiological appearances and surgical findings, in patients with these radiological signs. The presence of arachnoiditis seriously reduces the diagnostic value of a subsequent myelogram. There is evidence that adhesive arachnoiditis may increase the acute neurotoxicity of subsequent water soluble contrast media by impairing absorption from the spinal theca [18].

Pulmonary oil embolism is a rare complication which may follow venous intravasation of the contrast medium (Fig. 87.6).

Anatomy

Normal anatomical features are best appreciated from a careful study of radiographs. Important anatomical features fundamental to myelographic interpretation will, however, be described.

Lumbar region

There are significant variations in the shape, size and level of termination of the lumbar subarachnoid space. In the anteroposterior projection, the contrast medium normally occupies 30 to 80% of the distance between the pedicles. It usually terminates at the first or second sacral level, but a

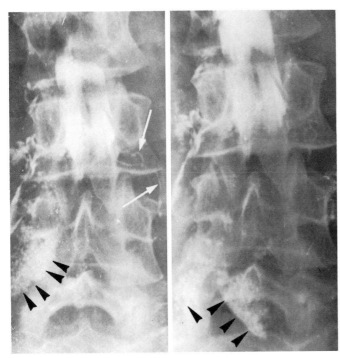

Fig. 87.6 Myodil myelogram with venous intravasation. Contrast medium is seen in the vertebral venous plexus [white arrows] and in the iliac veins [arrowheads]. There were no pulmonary complications.

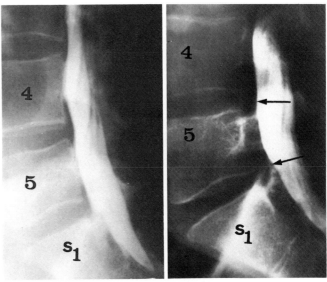

Fig. 87.7   Fig. 87.8

Fig. 87.7 Normal metrizamide myelogram; lumbar region, lateral projection. The anterior surface of the contrast medium column has a smooth convexity, in close contact with the vertebrae and disc spaces. The caudal sac tapers and terminates in a (rounded or) pointed extension at about S2.

Fig. 87.8 As Fig. 87.7. In this case, there is prominent separation of the contrast medium from the L4/5 and L5/S1 disc spaces. A central disc protrusion can be missed in the presence of this normal variant.

short dural sac may end at or above the lumbosacral disc space. In the lateral projection, the anterior margin of the contrast medium is smooth, slightly convex or flat, and closely applied to the posterior aspects of the discs and vertebral bodies (Fig. 87.7). In some cases however there may be a considerable gap between the contrast medium and the intervertebral disc at the lumbosacral level (Fig. 87.8), due to a wide epidural space; this may conceal a disc lesion at this level.

Each of the paired nerve roots, as it approaches its point of exit from the subarachnoid space, lies against the lateral aspect of the theca. The dura and arachnoid mater form a sheath which surrounds each root to the level of the intervertebral foramen. These sheaths are normally symmetrical and closely related to the pedicles (Fig. 87.9); they are well outlined when water soluble contrast medium is used, and the root is seen as a fine linear translucency within each sheath. Oil does not fill the sheaths to the same degree. The root sheaths appear as triangular outpouchings on the lateral border of the contrast medium (Fig. 87.10).

The importance of obliques and/or lateral decubitus projections for the demonstration of the root sheaths is emphasized (Fig. 87.11).

The first sacral root sheath emerges from the theca at or just above the fifth lumbar (L5/S1) disc, and the fifth lumbar root at or just above the L4/5 disc, while the higher roots emerge below the respective discs [19]. The L5 root will therefore be compressed by a disc lesion at L4/5 and the S1 root by a lesion at L5/S1. The first sacral root is readily identified by its typical course down to the first sacral foramen (Fig. 87.12). The lumbar roots sweep around the pedicles of the corresponding vertebrae and so can be easily identified.

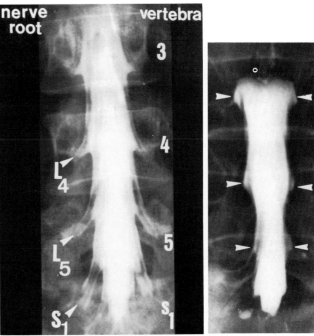

Fig. 87.9   Fig. 87.10

Fig. 87.9 Normal metrizamide myelogram, AP projection of lumbar region. Vertebral levels are identified on the patient's left and nerve root sheaths on the right. The L4 and L5 roots make a characteristic sweep around their respective pedicles. Note the symmetry of the roots and their sheaths.

Fig. 87.10 Normal oil myelogram. The nerve root sheaths are shown as blunted triangular outpouchings [arrows] and the roots are not as clearly demonstrated as in Fig. 87.9.

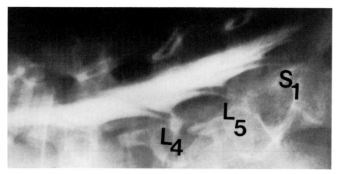

Fig. 87.11 Normal metrizamide myelogram, oblique lateral decubitus view, giving excellent demonstration of roots and root sheaths.

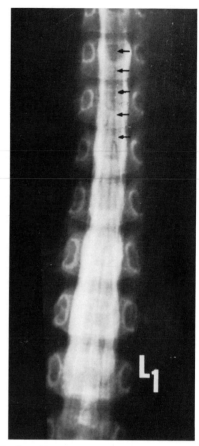

Fig. 87.13 Metrizamide myelogram showing the spinal cord terminating in the conus medullaris at the lower border of L1. The anterior spinal artery [arrows] is clearly visible.

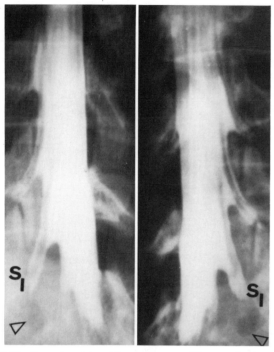

Fig. 87.12 Normal metrizamide myelogram, oblique projections. Note the characteristic course of the S1 nerve roots running down towards the first sacral foramina [arrows].

In the adult, the lumbar enlargement of the spinal cord is clearly outlined with water soluble contrast medium, ending in the conus medullaris at the L1/2 level (Fig. 87.13). The filum terminale may be identifiable as a narrow midline band extending down from the conus to the caudal end of the subarachnoid space, to fuse eventually with the periosteum of the first coccygeal segment. The lower spinal cord and the filum are best shown in the supine position. In the newborn the conus may lie as low as the L5 vertebral body, but it lies at the normal adult level (L1 or L2) by two months of age. The lumbar enlargement is often rather bulbous in young children, and the anterior spinal artery may appear rather tortuous.

Thoracic region

The anteroposterior projection shows the contrast medium as two radio-opaque columns on either side of a central radiolucency representing the spinal cord (Fig. 87.13). The contrast medium extends close to the medial borders of the pedicles. The subarachnoid space is narrower and the nerve root sheaths much shorter and less distinct than in the lumbar region. In the lateral projection, the spinal cord is clearly defined by water soluble medium (Fig. 87.14) since, unlike oil, or even gas, it outlines the subarachnoid space both anterior and posterior to the cord. The cord approximates to the anterior margin of the spinal canal.

The thoracocervical region is often difficult to demonstrate in the lateral projection, particularly with water soluble media, in patients who are obese or have broad shoulders. Well penetrated lateral films taken with the patient's arms in the Twining or swimmer's position are the best compromise (Fig. 87.15).

Irregularities of the contrast medium column are common, particularly when oil is used, and should not be confused with arachnoiditis or vessels. A defect is likely to be significant only if it produces obstruction to flow and is constant on serial films. The thoracic kyphosis forms an upward convexity when the patient is prone, and the contrast medium tends to break up over it. Fluoroscopy in the supine position is therefore preferred for this region.

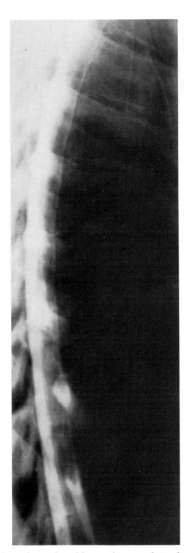

Fig. 87.14 Normal metrizamide myelogram, lateral projection of thoracic region. The spinal cord is clearly outlined front and back by contrast medium.

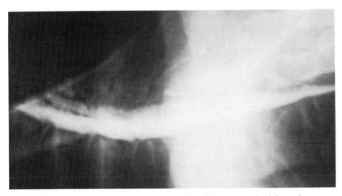

Fig. 87.15 Normal oil myelogram at the thoracocervical junction (swimmer's position).

Cervical region

The normal appearances with water soluble contrast media and iophendylate are illustrated in Figures 87.16 and 87.17. The cervical spinal cord shows a fusiform shape on the frontal projection, the cervical enlargement being widest at C5/6. The transverse diameter of the cord should be 50 to 75% of the diameter of the subarachnoid space [20]. A ratio greater than 80% suggests a widened cord, and less than 50% cord atrophy, but these figures are very variable. Values for the lateral projection are also available [21]. In the anteroposterior prone position, a prominent odontoid peg may produce a central oval defect in the contrast medium column (Fig. 87.17), which should not be mistaken for pathology.

Anteroposterior and oblique projections clearly demonstrate the nerve root sheaths, which are directed laterally, almost perpendicular to the theca in the upper cervical region, and progressively more obliquely downwards below this. Normal vessels on the surface of the cord are seen clearly with water soluble contrast medium.

On the lateral projection, the anterior surface of the contrast medium presents a shallow concavity extending from the lower margin of the odontoid peg to the anterior margin of the foramen magnum, due to the transverse ligament (Fig. 87.18). In the prone position water soluble contrast medium fills the entire subarachnoid space, so that the spinal cord is well outlined. The region of the foramen magnum, however, is not clearly demonstrated on prone fluoroscopy, and the supine position is nearly always necessary to show the position of the cerebellar tonsils, which normally lie above

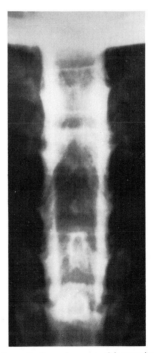

Fig. 87.16 Normal cervical myelogram with metrizamide, AP prone projection. The spinal cord appears as a central translucency. The emerging nerve roots are well seen; they run obliquely and laterally to enter the triangular nerve root sheaths, which are directed almost at right angles to the contrast medium column. The linear shadows of the ventral [upper] and dorsal [lower] nerve roots can be identified in the neural foramina.

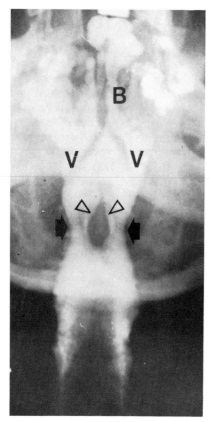

Fig. 87.17 Normal oil myelogram. The spinal cord apparently becomes narrower as it extends upwards. Note narrowing of the contrast medium column as it passes over the odontoid peg and transverse ligaments. The oval filling defect [open arrows] is also caused by the odontoid. Vertebral [V] and basilar [B] arteries are identifiable.

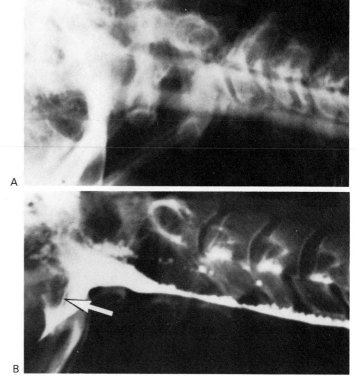

Fig. 87.19 Normal myelograms at the craniocervical junction, lateral projection in supine position. (A) Metrizamide; (B) oil. The spinal cord is less well seen in (B), but the cerebellar tonsils are more clearly outlined [arrow].

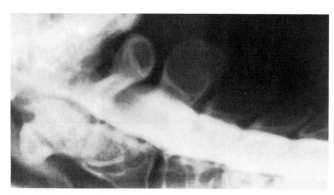

Fig. 87.18 Normal metrizamide myelogram, prone lateral projection. With a more penetrated exposure the spinal cord is clearly outlined.

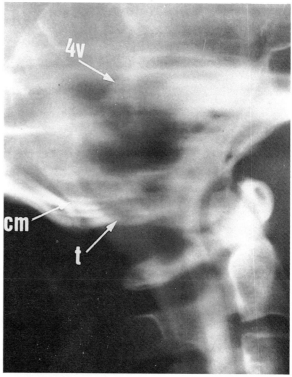

Fig. 87.20 Metrizamide myelogram: tomography of posterior fossa and foramen magnum [t = cerebellar tonsil; cm = cisterna magna; 4v = fourth ventricle].

a line joining the anterior and posterior margins of the foramen magnum (Fig. 87.19). Tomography has proved extremely valuable for visualization of the craniovertebral junction and posterior fossa (Fig. 87.20).

Interpretation of the myelogram

A systematic approach to the study of the myelogram is advocated, which, depending on the clinical problem, should include assessment of the following features:

1. Partial or complete obstruction to the flow of contrast medium
2. The site of any deforming structure: extradural, intradural—extramedullary or intramedullary (see Ch. 88).
3. The size of the spinal canal
4. The size and shape of the spinal cord, and the level of its termination
5. Filling and symmetry of the nerve root sheaths, presence and normal size of intrathecal nerves
6. Irregular shadows due to vessels, scarring, etc.
7. Position of the cerebellar tonsils
8. Abnormal extension of contrast medium beyond the spinal canal
9. The effects of flexing and extending the spine.

It must however be emphasized that not all variations or changes seen on myelography are significant; they must always be interpreted in the light of clinical features. It is not unusual to see large lumbar disc lesions in patients without a history of back pain when myelography is performed for cervical problems.

Spinal angiography

Arteriography [22]

This technique consists of identification and injection of arteries supplying the spinal cord, meninges and vertebral column. The radiological anatomy of these vessels is variable and it is often necessary to inject numerous intercostal and lumbar arteries on both sides.

The procedure is generally carried out under general anaesthesia, as injection of the appropriate vessels with conventional media may be painful; the examination is often prolonged. In patients with suspected arteriovenous malformations or intramedullary tumours, dexamethasone in full dosage (4 mg qds) is commenced 24 hours prior to the procedure. Bladder catheterization prior to arteriography is frequently helpful, as sphincter function may be impaired. The use of low osmolar, less neurotoxic contrast media e.g. iohexol, iopamidol or ioxaglate (Hexabrix) is strongly recommended.

A 7F viscerofemoral catheter is introduced via femoral artery puncture, unless the lesion is thought to be confined to the cervical region, in which case a 5F catheter may be used. If the femoral arteries are inaccessible (because of fixed flexion deformities at the hips), the axillary artery can be catheterized. Slow, gentle injections of 2–3 ml of angio-

graphic contrast medium are made into the intercostal and lumbar arteries on each side, using an anteroposterior series of a subtraction mask followed by three films at one every 2 seconds; opacification of the corresponding hemivertebra indicates a satisfactory injection. Ventilation is suspended during each series. When a vascular lesion is encountered, more rapid and/or prolonged series, or different projections can be obtained. If a number of injections are made into a single artery feeding the spinal cord, it is advisable to use a low osmolar medium such as metrizamide, iopamidol, iohexol or ioxaglate (Hexabrix), in a concentration giving 280 mg I/ml.

Selective injections of both vertebral arteries (near their origins) and of the deep cervical arteries may be required for examination of the cervical region. Theoretically, the cervical vessels can be opacified by subclavian injections, but in practice the results are often suboptimal. Study of the lumbar region occasionally involves injection of the sacral branches of the internal iliac arteries. It cannot be overemphasized that spinal angiography is a skillful and demanding procedure and that to embark on a search for a spinal arteriovenous malformation, for example, without appreciating that it may involve injection of all cervical, intercostal and lumbosacral vessels before a lesion can be excluded, is unjustifiable.

Indications for spinal arteriography include suspected angiomatous malformations or vascular tumours of the spinal cord, meninges or vertebral column; it may follow negative cerebral angiography in the investigation of subarachnoid haemorrhage. Therapeutic embolization may be carried out. Some neurosurgeons require demonstration of the origins of vessels feeding the spinal cord e.g. artery of Adamkiewicz before any surgery which might compromise them (scoliosis correction; costotransversectomy for thoracic disc protrusion, etc.).

Contraindications: since angiography is a costly, time consuming procedure with a slight but definite morbidity, no patient should be submitted to it if no action will be taken as a result of the findings. Patients considered unfit for surgery should not have spinal angiography. A positive myelogram should always precede the search for a spinal cord tumour or arteriovenous malformation.

Complications include minor deterioration in cord symptoms, relatively common but usually transient; permanent cord damage is rare if the examination is carefully performed.

Anatomy

The spinal cord is supplied via three main longitudinal arterial axes, the midline anterior spinal artery, and two posterolateral spinal arteries. In the cervical region, these arteries arise from the vertebral and deep cervical arteries, themselves branches of the subclavian arteries, while lower down they arise from intercostal or lumbar arteries (Fig. 87.21). At each vertebral level, a radicular artery runs alongside the nerve root, and some of these (the radiculomedullary arteries) continue to the spinal cord and join either the anterior or posterior spinal arteries (Fig. 87.22).

One major radiculomedullary artery (the arteria

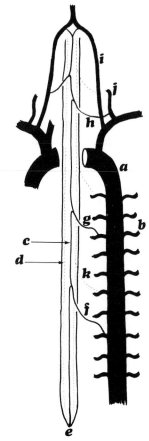

Fig. 87.21 The spinal arteries and their feeding vessels [a = aorta; b = intercostal artery; c = anterior spinal artery; d = posterolateral spinal artery; e = anastomosis at conus medullaris; f = arteria radicularis magna (of Adamkiewicz); g = thoracic and h = cervical radiculomedullary arteries; i = vertebral artery; j = deep cervical artery].

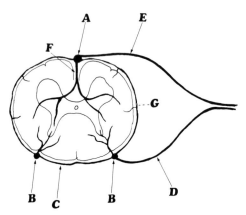

Fig. 87.22 Blood supply of the spinal cord [A = anterior spinal artery; B = posterolateral spinal arteries; C = posterior anastomotic artery; D = posterior and E = anterior radiculomedullary arteries; F = sulcocommissural arteries; G = lateral anastomotic artery].

radicularis magna of Adamkiewicz) is found in the thoracolumbar region; its level of origin is variable, but it is usually on the left side, between T8 and L1/2. Another radiculomedullary artery arises in the upper thoracic region. The level of origin of the posterior radiculo-medullary arteries is similarly variable. Occasion-ally, a single intercostal artery will give rise to both anterior and posterior radiculomedullary branches (Fig. 87.23). In the cervical region, anterior radiculomedullary arteries arise at every vertebral level, but they are very variable in size and importance (Fig. 87.24).

The anterior spinal artery is by far the most important of the axes, because it supplies the major portion of the cord substance, including the motor cells of the anterior horns. It gives off tiny sulcocommissural arteries which run into the cord; they are not visible at angiography unless pathologically enlarged.

Arteries supplying the vertebral column also arise at each vertebral level; their study involves catheterization of the same vessels as arteriography of the spinal cord (Fig. 87.25).

Phlebography [23]

This technique consists of opacification of the veins which run longitudinally in the epidural space, especially anteriorly, which are remarkably constant in distribution (Fig. 87.26). Because of their intimate relation to the intervertebral discs and neural foramina, they are a sensitive indicator of disc disease. Phlebography is most commonly carried out in the lumbar region; in some centres cervical phlebography is also performed.

Lumbosacral phlebography can be carried out in several ways:

1. bilateral cannulation of the femoral veins,
2. selective catheterization of the lateral sacral or ascending lumbar veins (Fig. 87.27)
3. direct injection into a lumbar spinous process; this method has been almost entirely superceded, although it has the theoretical advantage that it can be carried out at any level.

Using catheterization or direct injection into both femoral veins, the examination is carried out under local anaesthesia, and can be an outpatient procedure. An essential part of all methods is really effective abdominal compression, obliter-ating the inferior vena cava and forcing the contrast medium into the intraspinal veins. Depending on the method employed, about 30 to 40 ml of angiographic contrast medium is injected rapidly during a Valsalva manoeuvre, and films are obtained every 2 seconds over 10 seconds. One anteroposterior projection is usually sufficient, but oblique or lateral series may complement it in doubtful cases. Subtraction is virtually always required. Extravasation is uncommon and usually without major sequelae.

The femoral catheter approach is also used for cervical phlebography, with selective catheterization of the vertebral veins (Fig. 87.28).

The prime indication for phlebography, either cervical or

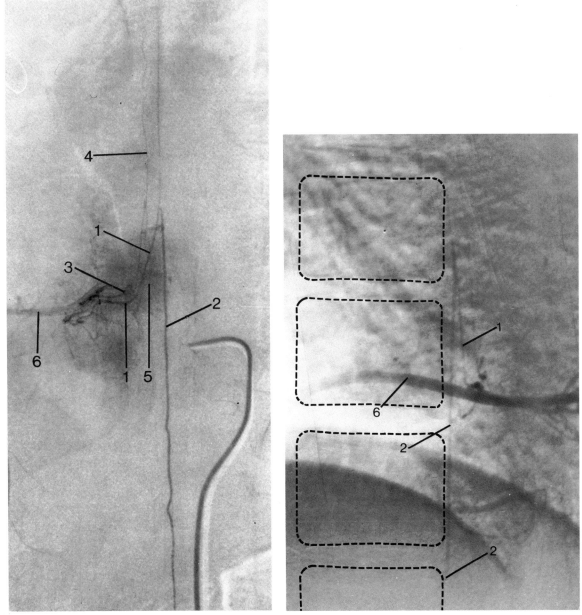

Fig. 87.23 Injection of arteria radicularis magna. (A) AP projection; (B) lateral projection [1 = arteria radicularis magna; 2 = anterior spinal artery; 3 = posterior radiculomedullary artery; 4 = posterior spinal artery; 5 = blush of hemivertebra at level injected; 6 = intercostal artery].

lumbar, is investigation of disc lesions and spondylosis, usually after an equivocal myelogram, or a normal study in patients with very suggestive clinical findings. Occasionally it may be used in the investigation of infiltrative processes of the epidural space. Its role in the assessment of large paraspinal masses has been largely taken over by CT. Phlebography is of very little value following intraspinal surgery, since the epidural veins are often damaged at operation, or involved in subsequent scar tissue.

Discography

Injection of contrast medium into the nucleus pulposus of the cervical or lumbar intervertebral discs is used more frequently in orthopaedic practice, for investigation of neck or arm pain or lumbago, than in neuroradiology. In some centres it is currently enjoying a vogue as an adjunct to chemolysis of the discs.

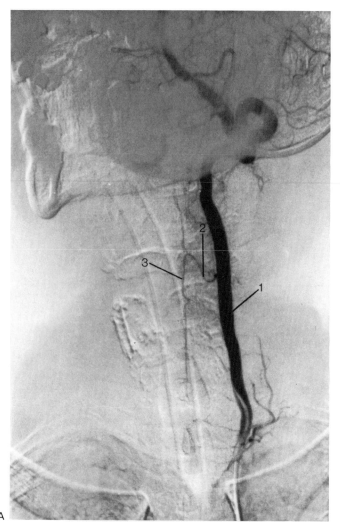

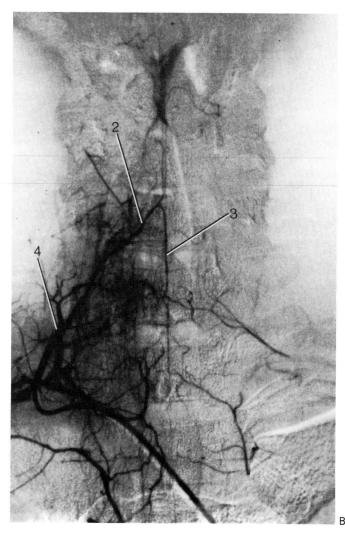

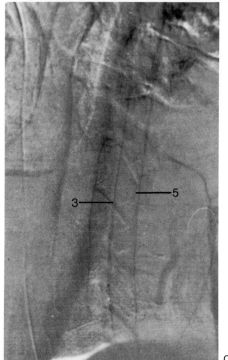

Fig. 87.24 Anterior spinal artery in cervical region, fed (A) from vertebral artery [1], (B) from deep cervical artery [4], via radiculomedullary arteries [2]. (C) lateral projection. Opacification of anterior [3] and posterior [5] spinal arteries.

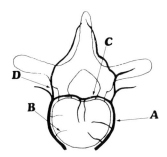

Fig. 87.25   Blood supply of the vertebral bodies.

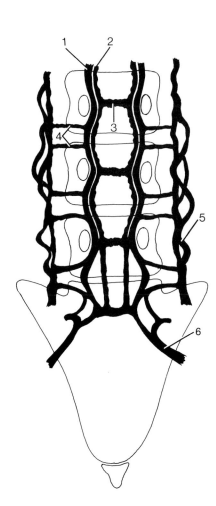

Fig. 87.26   Diagram of the epidural veins [1 = lateral epidural vein;
2 = medial epidural vein; 3 = retrocorporeal anastomotic vein;
4 = superior and inferior veins of intevertebral foramen;
5 = ascending lumbar vein; 6 = lateral sacral vein].

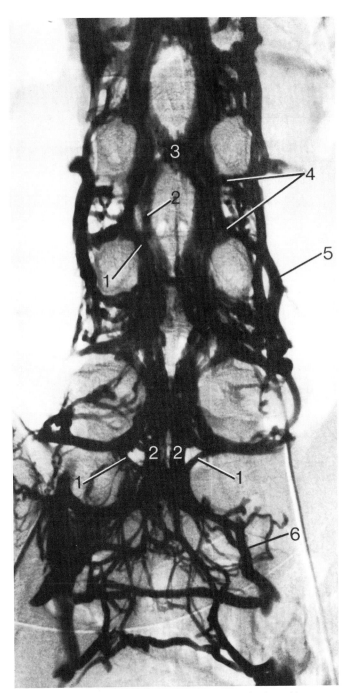

Fig. 87.27   Normal lumbar epidural veins, AP projection with
injection of right lateral sacral and left ascending lumbar veins
[arrow]. Key as in Fig. 87.26. Note the normal separation of the
medial and lateral epidural veins at L5/S1; above this, the more
tortuous medial vein is scarcely distinguishible from the lateral vein.
Poor filling at S1 on the left is the result of injection at a higher level
on that side.

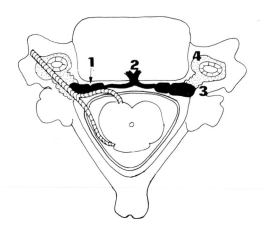

A

Fig. 87.28 A & B Cervical epidural veins: (A) Cross-section, (B) Frontal view [1 = medial and lateral epidural veins. Note relationship to lateral recess of spinal canal; 2 = basivertebral vein, draining to retrocorporeal anastomotic vein; 3 = venous plexus of the intervertebral foramen; 4 = vertebral venous plexus, surrounding the vertebral artery.

Epidurography [24]

Opacification of the epidural space with contrast medium occasionally occurs during attempted myelography. When it is carried out intentionally, the technique is referred to as epidurography. Water soluble nonionic contrast medium is used, and the technique has the advantage that no foreign substance is introduced into the cerebrospinal fluid.

The procedure can be carried out in the same way as a lumbar puncture, but instead of advancing the needle until spinal fluid is obtained, the resistance to injection of air is tested repeatedly. A 'pop' is generally felt when the posterior intraspinal ligaments are breached, and resistance is then markedly reduced. After aspiration to ensure that neither blood nor spinal fluid can be obtained, the contrast medium can be injected directly, under fluoroscopic control or, if a larger needle is used, a fine catheter may be passed into the epidural space. An alternative method of injection is the sacral approach, the needle being introduced into the sacral canal from below. The risk of entering the subdural or subarachnoid space is thereby reduced. The contrast medium spreads easily throughout the epidural space, in an irregular manner. When opacification appears optimal, the needle or catheter is withdrawn and anteroposterior, lateral and oblique projection radiographs are obtained.

The density of opacification of the epidural space is variable, but a dense line of contrast medium is generally seen delineating the posterior surface of the vertebral bodies and intervertebral discs, as well as tracking out along the dural nerve root sheaths (see Fig. 87.4). It is evident that this technique is reserved effectively for investigation of lumbar and lumbosacral disc and nerve root problems.

Contraindications include the possibility of an extradural tumour or abscess at the level of puncture. Among the possible complications are inadvertent injection into the subar-

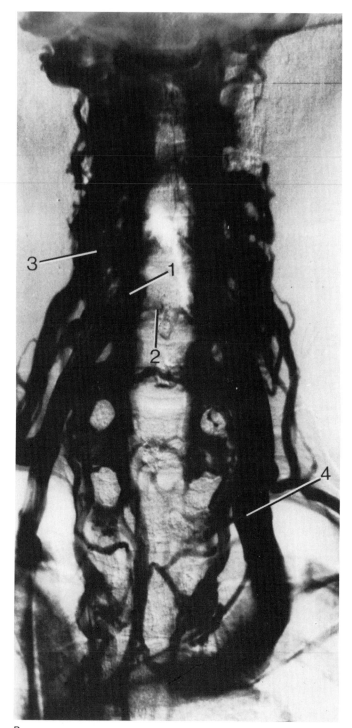

B

achnoid or subdural space, or an epidural vein, and the excitation of an epidural inflammatory reaction. In general, however, this investigation is well tolerated by the patient. Its relative lack of popularity as a prime imaging modality would appear to stem more from difficulties in interpretation and lack of demonstration of any intrathecal abnormalities.

Ultrasound [25]

Sonography has been recommended for measurement of the internal dimensions of the spinal canal in suspected cases of canal stenosis. The value and accuracy of the measurements are, however debated, and there is little doubt that plain films, complemented by CT if necessary, with myelography should surgery be contemplated, have not been supplanted by ultrasound.

Magnetic resonance imaging

Although this technique has, at present, little to offer in terms of investigation of bone disease, it is a remarkably effective way of showing the intervertebral disc and nucleus pulposus. Early images have also suggested that it may eventually be of considerable interest in the assessment of the spinal cord, which can be distinguished throughout its length, and imaged in transverse and longitudinal planes. Images suggesting demonstration of the grey and white matter have been published. There is thus considerable potential for investigation of both extra- and intramedullary spinal lesions.

THE RADIOLOGICAL DIAGNOSTIC APPROACH TO COMMON CLINICAL SPINAL PROBLEMS

Clinical problems may be divided into acute and chronic presentations.

Acute presentations

1. Back pain
2. Root syndromes
3. Spinal cord lesions

Acute back pain

Acute back pain, and many cases of acute extremity pain of presumed spinal origin are not generally investigated radiologically; rest and conservative treatment are tried first. Plain radiographs may, however, be indicated in cases of pain following significant trauma, and in patients with a known tendency to develop spinal lesions e.g., metastatic disease, steroid therapy, etc.

Acute root syndromes

Acute lower motor neurone weakness of one arm is uncommonly due to spinal disease in the absence of trauma. Nerve root avulsion is generally not investigated radiologically in the acute stage, but may subsequently require a combination of plain films, myelography and CT, as described in Chapter 88.

Lumbosacral disc protusion may present with sciatic nerve root compression which is predominantly motor, giving an acute foot drop. Depending on the severity of the clinical picture and the aggressive attitude of the surgeon, conservative treatment may be preferred, but if there is evidence of a major disc herniation with limb weakness and impairment of sphincter function, plain films and myelography may be required urgently.

Acute lesions of the spinal cord

Acute traumatic lesions of the spinal cord are often definitive and permanent. Careful clinical assessment in the early stages may, however, indicate a partial lesion with potential for some recovery. Plain films, CT and myelography may then be indicated, depending on the aggressiveness of the surgical approach.

An acute non-traumatic lesion of the spinal cord is assumed to be compressive, and amenable to surgery until proven otherwise and is a medical emergency, since the degree of recovery is directly related to the speed of diagnosis and treatment. A chest film is mandatory, since many cases are neoplastic or infective. Plain radiographs of the area indicated by the level of cord damage, or of the whole spine if a clear level is lacking, are obtained, followed by water soluble myelography by the lumbar route, with placement of a marker. CT may be a useful adjunct. The plain films often show changes indicating the level of spinal involvement, serving to orientate the myelographer, and may suggest the diagnosis. They will also help in the decision as to whether cervical injection of contrast medium is indicated, or, if they show extremely extensive disease, whether investigation and treatment are in fact justified.

If it is clearly established that the patient has demyelinating disease, the referring neurologist may choose not to carry out myelography: there is evidence that patients with multiple sclerosis deteriorate after oil myelography, although this may not be the case with water soluble contrast medium.

Spinal angiography is not indicated unless the plain film or myelographic findings indicate the presence of a highly vascular lesion. If a very vascular tumour or an arteriovenous malformation is suspected, there is probably nothing to be lost in delaying angiography until the acute stage has passed.

Chronic presentations

1. Pain
2. Root compression syndromes
3. Cord lesions

Chronic pain

(a) Chronic spinal pain should be investigated in the first instance by plain radiographs; although CT is proving increasingly useful in this context, it does not give the rapid, cheap overall picture which plain films afford. The decision to proceed to discography or myelography in the absence of diagnostic plain film changes is a clinical one. Many spinal arteriovenous malformations cause pain, and it may be their only symptom; water soluble myelography should nevertheless precede angiography, even in suspected cases as it is simpler and less hazardous.

(b) In sciatica, plain films and CT are fundamental investigations. However, in most centres, myelography is almost invariably carried out before spinal exploration, although advances in CT (and possibly MRI) may result in a number of patients being operated upon on the basis of noninvasive tests alone. Spinal phlebography is, in most departments, an ancillary investigation, reserved for cases in which either the clinical picture or the myelographic findings are equivocal. There is every reason to suppose that with more reliance on CT, the use of phlebography will decrease.

(c) When pain in the arm or shoulder is thought to be of spinal origin, plain films of the cervical spine are mandatory. They may show evidence of degenerative disease, cervical ribs, or more rarely, evidence of a neoplasm or of infection. The large majority of patients with cervical spondylosis are treated conservatively, although myelography may be required to make the therapeutic decisions. Alone or combined with CT, it should always precede surgery. Some surgeons still carry out cervical discography, but this is provocative diagnostic technique rather than an imaging procedure.

Root compression syndromes

These are generally investigated in the same way as chronic pain. Plain radiographs of the elbow, wrist, thoracic inlet or pelvis etc., may be required for the differentiation of distal from proximal nerve entrapment.

Chronic lesions of the spinal cord

Three main groups may be identified: extramedullary compressive lesions; intramedullary space occupying lesions (tumours and syringomyelia in the large majority) and inflammatory or vascular disease.

(a) Chronic compressive lesions are often cervical, spondylosis and cervical disc disease forming the major portion. They are investigated by plain films, which may be supplemented by tomography (for intraspinal calcification or craniovertebral junction anomalies associated with instability). CT may be helpful. Cases being considered for surgery will be investigated by myelography.

(b) Intrinsic space—occupying lesions of the spinal cord are rarely evidenced by plain films, but the detection of craniocervical anomalies will orientate the diagnosis towards syringomyelia. CT may confirm that diagnosis, or show an intraspinal fat containing tumour. Water soluble myelography is the definitive procedure, including views of the craniocervical junction, and followed by CT if a syrinx is suggested. Cord puncture may be required in difficult cases.

(c) If inflammatory or demyelinating disease is suspected, CT of the brain may provide valuable evidence of associated lesions, but myelography is indicated if there is any doubt as to the cause of the spinal problem. If it is negative, it is extremely unlikely that angiography will be revealing; even demonstration of anterior spinal artery occlusion is unreliable (and of academic interest only). This caveat also applies to the investigation of subarachnoid haemorrhage in which cerebral angiography has unearthed no cause, even when back pain has been prominent: water soluble myelography is easier and safer than spinal angiography.

Finally, it should be mentioned that some patients with spinal tumours may present with symptoms or signs suggesting intracranial lesions, and CT may show hydrocephalus or be normal[26]. The spinal fluid protein is often markedly elevated. Spinal investigations as indicated above for intramedullary or intradural extramedullary lesions are indicated.

BIBLIOGRAPHY

REFERENCES

1. Park W M 1980 Radiological investigation of the intervertebral disc. In: Jayson M V (ed) The lumbar spine and back pain, 2nd edn. Pitman Medical, London.
2. Post M J D 1980 Radiographic evaluation of the spine. Masson, New York
3. Shapiro R 1975 Myelography. 3rd edn. Medical Year Book Publishers, Chicago
4. Colman K, Wiik I, Salvesen S 1979 Absorption of a nonionic contrast agent from cerebrospinal fluid to blood. Neuroradiology 18: 227-233
5. Haughton V M, Ko K C, Larsen S J et al 1977 Experimental production of arachnoiditis with water soluble contrast media. Radiology 123:681-685
6. Howland W I, Parry JL 1966 Pantopaque arachnoiditis. Acta Radiol 5:1032
7. James MCC, Lassman L P 1981 Spina Bifida Occulta. Academic Press, London
8. Vonofakos D, Grau H, Stendel W 1981 Multiple spinal arachnoid cysts. The role of oily contrast medium. Surg Neurol 15:125-127
9. Lamb J T 1979 Cervical myelography by lateral C1/C2 puncture. In: Grainger R G, Lamb J T (ed) Myelographic techniques with metrizamide. Nyegaard (UK), Birmingham. pp 59-73
10. McAllister V L 1977 Myelography with metrizamide in occult spinal dysraphism. Acta Radiol (Suppl) 355:200-210 (see also papers by Fitz et al, Hugosson et al)
11. Kendall B, Symon L 1973 Cyst puncture and endomyelography in cystic tumours of the spinal cord Br J Radiol 46:198-209
12. Quencer R M 1980 Needle aspiration of intramedullary and intradural extramedullary masses of the spinal cord. Radiology 134: 115-126
13. Tourtelotte W W et al 1964 Post lumbar puncture headaches. Thomas, Springfield, Illinois
14. Harris L M, Harmel M H 1953 The comparative incidence of post lumbar puncture headache following spinal anesthesia administered through 20 and 24 gauge needles. Anesthesiology 14:390-397
15. Irstam L 1973 Side effects of water soluble contrast media in lumbar myelography. Acta Radiol 14:467-656
16. Eldevik O P, Haughton V M 1978 The effect of hydration on the acute and chronic complications of aqueous myelography. Radiology 129:713-714

17. Johnson A J, Burrows E H 1978 Thecal deformity after lumbar myelography with iophendylate (Myodil) and meglumine iothalamate (Conray 280). Br. J Radiol 51:196–202

18. Eldevik O P, Haughton V M 1978 Risk factors in complications of aqueous myelography (1), Radiology 128:415–416

19. Begg A C, Faulkener M A, McGeorge M 1946 Myelography in lumbar intervertebral disc lesions: a correlation with operative findings. Br J Surg 34:141–157

20. Di Chiro G, Fischer R L 1964 Contrast radiography of the spinal cord. Arch Neurol 11:125–143

21. Boltshauser E, Hoare R D 1976 Radiographic measurement of the normal spinal cord in childhood. Neuroradiology 10:235–237

22. Doppman J L, Di Chiro G, Ommaya A K 1969 Selective arteriography of the spinal cord. Green, St Louis

23. Théron J, Moret J 1979 Spinal phlebography. Springer, Berlin

24. Hattam H P 1980 Metrizamide lumbar epidurography with Seldinger technique through the sacral notch and selective nerve root injection. Neuroradiology 19:19–25

25. Porter R W, Wicks M, Ottewell D 1978 Measurement of the spinal canal by diagnostic ultrasound. J Bone Joint Surg (B) 60: 481–484

26. Ridsdale L, Moseley I F 1978 Thoracolumbar tumours presenting features of raised intracranial pressure. J Neurol Neurosurg Psychiatry 41:737–745

SUGGESTIONS FOR FURTHER READING

Crock H V, Yoshizawa H 1977 The blood supply of the vertebral column and spinal cord in man. Springer, Berlin

Du Boulay G H (ed) 1984 A textbook of X-ray diagnosis by British Authors. Neuroradiology. Lewis, London

Grainger R G 1984 The spinal canal. Techniques. In: Whitehouse G H and Worthington B S (eds). Techniques in diagnostic radiology. Blackwell, Oxford pp 263–284

Taveras J M. Morello F 1979 Normal neuroradiology. Year Book Medical Publishers, Chicago

Vakili H 1967 The spinal cord. Intercontinental Medical Book Corporation, New York

88 Spinal pathology

V. L. McAllister, I. F. Moseley and J. Theron

Congenital and developmental lesions
    Anterior sacral meningocele
    Lateral thoracic meningocele
    Occult spinal dysraphism
    Spinal cysts
    Sacral cysts
    Arnold-Chiari malformation
    Syringomyelia

Back pain and sciatica
  Disc protrusion and prolapse
    Stenosis of the lumbar spinal canal
    Functional myelography
    Postoperative myelography
    Spondylolisthesis

Degenerative disease in the cervical spine

Spinal cord compression
    Plain radiographs
    Myelography
    Extradural lesions
    Intradural extramedullary lesions
    Intramedullary lesions
    Inflammatory lesions

Trauma

Vascular lesions

CONGENITAL AND DEVELOPMENTAL LESIONS

Spina bifida in its mildest form (spina bifida occulta) consists simply of a failure of fusion of the neural arches, usually at the C1 or L5 and/or S1 levels. The abnormality is nearly always asymptomatic, and is usually an incidental radiographic finding.

In more advanced cases, there may be herniation of the spinal meninges (*meningocele*) or of the spinal cord itself (*myelomeningocele*). Gross spina bifida, with failure of fusion of the spinal cord, is termed *rachischisis*. Myelography is usually unnecessary in severely affected individuals.

CT will clearly demonstrate bony defects, and show whether there is protrusion of spinal contents through the defect (Fig. 88.1). However, it is often not possible to distinguish between spinal fluid collections within a meningocele and neural herniation in a more complex abnormality without intrathecal contrast medium. It may be necessary to position the patient appropriately for the contrast medium to enter the herniated sac, for instance head raised, supine for a lumbosacral lesion; this may present problems in introducing the patient into the scanner.

In the following sections consideration will be given to only those lesions which are potentially amenable to surgery and therefore may require radiological investigation.

Anterior sacral meningocele

In this anomaly there is a bony defect in the anterior surface of the sacrum, through which the meninges herniate, producing a soft tissue mass in the pelvis. Symptoms are those of a pelvic mass, exerting pressure on the bladder or rectum. Plain films may be diagnostic, showing a 'scimitar sacrum', but the diagnosis is confirmed at myelography when the contrast medium is seen to enter the meningocele (Fig. 88.2), clearly distinguishing it from a tumour invading the sacrum. Delayed films using oil contrast medium (or delayed CT studies with water soluble contrast) may be required to demonstrate that the contrast medium does enter the menin-

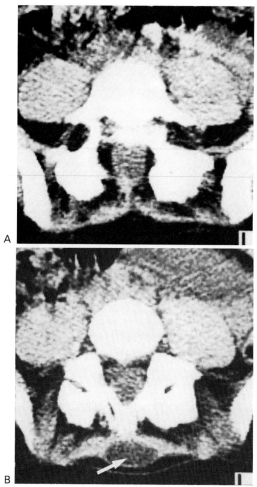

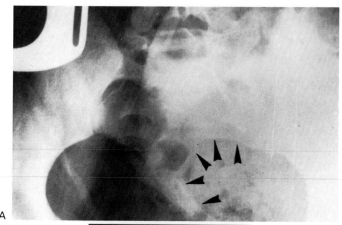

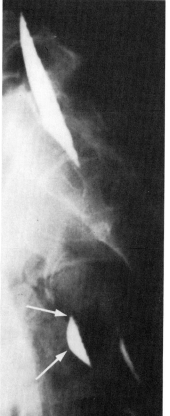

Fig. 88.1A & B Lumbosacral meningocele. CT shows spina bifida, the theca protuding through the bony defect (A). At a slightly higher level, a fluid collection of CSF density, the meningocele, lies in the soft tissues (arrow in B).

gocele if its communication with the subarachnoid space is very small.

CT has proved extremely valuable in the investigation of sacral lesions [1,2]. Detection of bony anomalies is easier than by means of plain films or conventional tomography. Confirmation of the nature of sacral lesions extending into the soft tissues of the pelvis, such as a meningocele, may require the bladder and/or rectum to be outlined by contrast medium.

Fig. 88.2A & B Anterior sacral meningocele. Plain radiographs (A) show the typical bony defect [arrowheads] in the sacrum (scimitar sacrum). Delayed film after oil injection (B) reveals the meningocele [arrows].

Lateral thoracic meningocele

A lateral thoracic meningocele is a protrusion of the arachnoid and dura mater through an enlarged intervertebral foramen into the paravertebral gutter, producing a soft tissue mass visible on plain films of the chest. It is usually discovered as an incidental paramediastinal shadow. The condition is associated with neurofibromatosis in 70% of cases.

Plain radiographs may show enlargement of the intervertebral foramen, increase in interpedicular distance, scalloping of the vertebra and/or separation and erosion of adjacent ribs. Differentiation from other paravertebral masses such as neurofibroma, bronchial neoplasm, neurenteric cyst, etc. may require myelography to fill the sac of the meningocele, but diagnosis may be possible by CT. Treatment is not usually required when the diagnosis is established.

Occult spinal dysraphism

This term covers a spectrum of anomalies of the spine and

spinal cord including an abnormally low, tethered spinal cord, traction bands, diastematomyelia, congenital tumours such as lipoma or dermoid and dermal sinus.

The usual presentations are abnormalities of the lower limbs, including inequality of foot and leg size, muscle wasting and talipes (the orthopaedic syndrome) or disturbances of bladder function (the urological syndrome). Abnormalities of the skin over the lesion, such as naevus, hairy patch or lumbosacral lipoma are frequent.

Plain radiographs invariably show dysraphic bony abnormalities more extensive than a simple lamina defect in L5 or S1. These anomalies can be confirmed by CT, which also demonstrates the abnormal shape of the spinal canal at the affected level. A bony spur traversing the canal in the sagittal plane is pathognomonic of diastematomyelia [4] with a split cord (Fig. 88.3), but if the dividing septum is fibrous or absent, splitting of the cord may not be detectable without intrathecal water soluble contrast, when the extent of the abnormality can be assessed accurately (Fig. 88.4) [3]. A low termination of the spinal cord is then also clearly shown, but is virtually impossible to identify without intrathecal contrast medium. Lipomas, on the other hand, are readily detectable, since their fat content renders them of strikingly lower density on CT than cerebrospinal fluid, they may be intra- and/or extraspinal (Fig. 88.5).

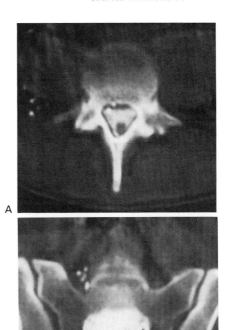

Fig. 88.5A & B   Low termination of the cord, with lipoma. CT with intrathecal metrizamide (A) at L4: the spinal cord is clearly visible as a filling defect, characteristically lying posteriorly; normally, only nerve roots should be seen at this level. The lower end of the cord cannot be distinguished from a thickened filum terminale. (B) The sacral canal is very wide, with spina bifida; an intrathecal mass of fat density is outlined as a filling defect.

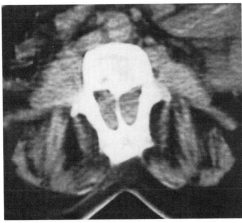

Fig. 88.3   Diastematomyelia with bony septum completely dividing the spinal canal; the patient also had cerebellar ectopia and a sacral meningocele

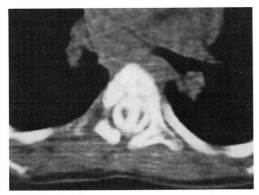

Fig. 88.4   Diastematomyelia without bony septum, demonstrated by CT with intrathecal metrizamide. Note spina bifida and abnormal shape of spinal canal extending from T2/3 to T5. The shape of the cord is abnormal above the level of the split.

Myelography is best carried out using water soluble contrast medium introduced by lumbar puncture; the reader is referred to publications by Fitz et al [3], and by Resjö et al [4] and James and Lassman [5] for a detailed account of techniques and interpretation. The myelogram will demonstrate a low placed conus medullaris, that is, lying below the third lumbar vertebra (Fig. 88.6), frequently associated with thickening of the filum terminale, which is greater than 3 mm in diameter. The low spinal cord is tethered posteriorly, a fact which may be demonstrated in the prone position. Traction bands appear at myelography as small, constant translucencies. Diastematomyelia, which may or may not be associated with a midline septum of bone, cartilage or fibrous tissue, is clearly seen as a midline streak or pool of contrast medium parallel with the long axis of the cord. A septum appears as a constant midline filling defect within this pool. In the presence of a septum the dura mater is divided into two halves; the extent of this division can be assessed (Fig. 88.7). Water soluble contrast medium, unlike oil, can demonstrate diastematomyelia without a septum (Fig. 88.8). Tethering bands are frequently present in cases of diastematomyelia without a septum.

Intrathecal masses (lipoma or dermoid cyst) may be present (Fig. 88.9). In cases of congenital dermal sinus, myelography is carried out early to assess whether the sinus communicates with the subarachnoid space or is associated

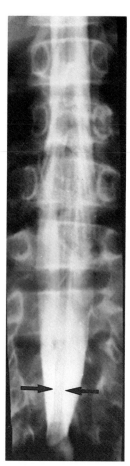

Fig. 88.6 Occult spinal dysraphism. Metrizamide myelogram: the conus medullaris is low, at the level of the L4 vertebral body. There is marked thickening of the filum terminale (arrows).

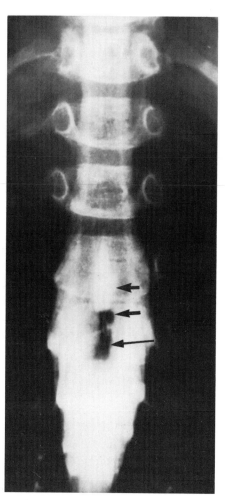

Fig. 88.7 Metrizamide myelogram showing diastematomyelia with a bony septum. The septum [arrow] is clearly demonstrated, as are the division of the theca above it and the low, split cord.

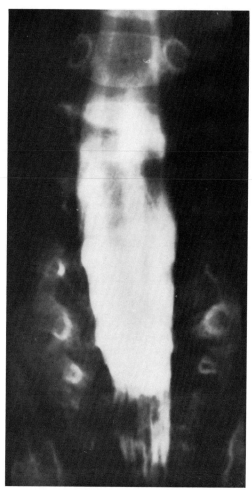

Fig. 88.8 Metrizamide myelogram: diastematomyelia without a septum.

with an intrathecal dermoid cyst. Congenital scoliosis is commonly associated with dysraphic lesions, and myelography should be carried out in such cases to exclude these lesions prior to spinal traction or fusion, especially if the plain films show congenital anomalies, or if there are skin lesions or positive neurological signs.

Spinal cysts

These are not infrequently an incidental finding at myelography and only rarely produce spinal cord or root compression. They may be classified according to their anatomical site as extradural or intradural, or as to whether the contrast medium enters the cyst at myelography: communicating or noncommunicating. Extradural spinal cysts arise as a result of arachnoid herniation through a small defect in the dura mater, and they enlarge due to a stop-valve effect of intermittent obstruction at the orifice. Most cases present in the second and third decades; there is a male predominance. The

majority occur in the thoracic region. Plain film abnormalities, including pedicular erosion and widening of the interpedicular distance are common. The diagnosis is established at myelography[6]. The majority of these lesions are located posteriorly, so that prone fluoroscopy often reveals merely a nonspecific lesion of extradural type. It is only with the patient supine that contrast medium may enter the cyst and define its extent (Fig. 88.10).

Intradural cysts are also most commonly posteriorly situated, and found in the thoracic region. Plain films are usually normal, in contradistinction to those in cases of extradural cyst.

CT without intrathecal contrast medium is of very little use in cases of intraspinal cyst, although the bony abnormalities may be demonstrated in the extradural type. With water soluble contrast medium however, the cyst may be shown as a rounded intraspinal mass, sometimes displacing or compressing the spinal cord. The intra- or extradural location of the lesion may not be evident, but poor or partial filling is more suggestive of the latter (Fig. 88.11).

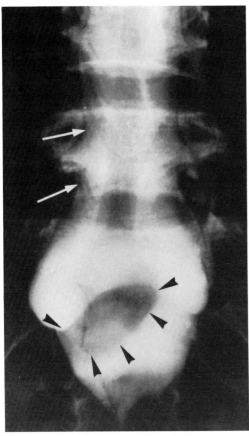

Fig. 88.9 Metrizamide myelogram showing the conus medullaris at the level of S1, with a rounded filling defect [arrowheads] due to an intrathecal lipoma. Note the upward course of the nerve roots from their abnormally low origin [white arrows].

Sacral cysts

Large arachnoid cysts communicating with the subarachnoid space may be found in the sacral canal (occult intrasacral meningocele) [7]. They often produce erosion and expansion of the canal, best demonstrated on the lateral projection. CT is valuable in excluding a tumour. The diagnosis is confirmed at myelography, contrast medium entering the cyst. However, delayed films or CT may be required to demonstrate this when there is merely a narrow connection with the subarachnoid space (Fig. 88.12) [8].

Small perineural ('Tarlov') cysts may occur around the sacral roots, most commonly the second and third; they are frequently multiple (Fig. 88.13). It is not clear what role, if any, they play in the production of sciatic pain [9]. They are usually asymptomatic.

The Arnold-Chiari malformation

This term should be used only in those situations in which there is a variable downward displacement of the brain stem and the lower portions of the cerebellum, the tonsils and inferior vermis, so that the elongated fourth ventricle may

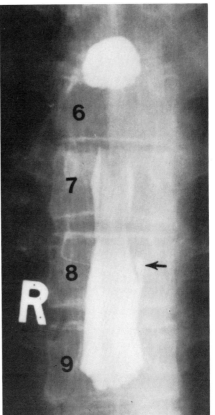

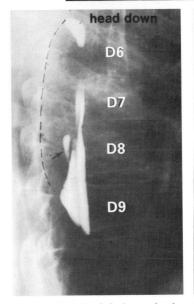

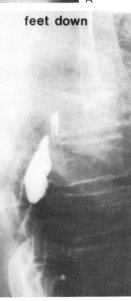

Fig. 88.10A & B Spinal extradural cyst; oil myelogram. (A) Supine AP projection: extradural type obstruction at the D6/7 level, with some contrast medium in the cyst above it. The arrow indicates a communication between the cyst and the subarachnoid space. (B) Lateral projection showing the full extent of the cyst in head and feet down positions.

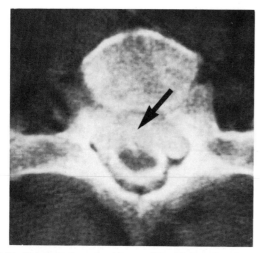

Fig. 88.11 Intraspinal arachnoid cyst. CT with intrathecal metrizamide, showing the cyst anterior to the main part of the theca [arrow], displacing it backwards and expanding the spinal canal. The contrast medium is less dense within the cyst, suggesting a limited connection between the two.

extend through the foramen magnum. The condition is frequently associated with spina bifida and meningocele. The term Chiari (type 1) malformation applies to patients in whom only the cerebellar tonsils project below the foramen magnum. This condition may, as the result of compression of nervous pathways at the foramen magnum, produce a number of diverse clinical syndromes including cranial nerve involvement, cerebellar dysfunction and, in slightly less than 50% of cases, is associated with syringomyelia.

Myelography is preferred to pneumoencephalography for demonstration of the Chiari malformation, and demonstrates the ectopic cerebellar tonsils, as a characteristic rounded or elongated posterior filling defect below the foramen magnum on the lateral projection, with the patient in the supine position. An anteroposterior projection will show them as bilateral filling defects on either side of the spinal cord (Fig. 88.14). It should be noted that, even with water soluble contrast medium, the tonsils may not be outlined in the prone position. The cisterna magna is characteristically small. These abnormalities can be confirmed by CT following myelography (Fig. 88.15).

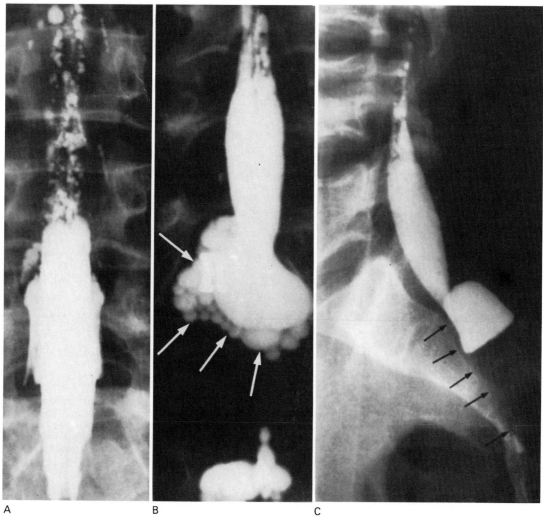

A   B   C

Fig. 88.12A, B & C Oil (Iophendylate) myelogram in a patient with a large sacral cyst (occult intrasacral meningocele). (A) Initially there is no gross abnormality. (B) 24 hour film shows contrast medium in a large cyst [white arrow], of which the lateral view (C) shows the upper margin. Note an eroded and expanded sacral canal [black arrows].

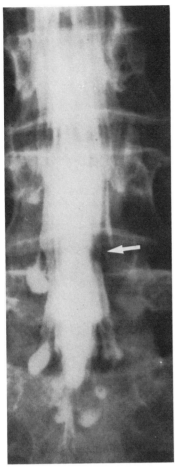

Fig. 88.13 Multiple small perineural (Tarlov) cysts. The left L5 nerve root sheath is obliterated by a disc lesion [arrow].

Syringomyelia

This term is used to describe those conditions in which there is a cavity within the spinal cord whose lining is composed mainly of glial tissue. It must be regarded as a syndrome which may be caused by a number of distinct pathological processes [10].

Cases may be classified as (1) communicating syringomyelia, due to a dilatation of the central canal of the spinal cord, which is associated in the large majority of cases with a Chiari malformation and (2) noncommunicating syringomyelia without primary involvement of the central canal, which may be the result of trauma, infection or a tumour.

Preliminary plain films of the spine should include good views of the craniocervical junction. Atlanto-occipital fusion is the most common primary bony anomaly in cases of Chiari malformation and syringomyelia, but other suggestive findings are manifestations of an occipital vertebra, spina bifida or abnormalities of segmentation, e.g. intervertebral fusions. The spinal canal may be enlarged, with flattening or concavity of the medial surfaces of the pedicles, the posterior surfaces of the vertebral bodies and the bases of the spinous processes. Such expansive changes are usually present only in advanced cases.

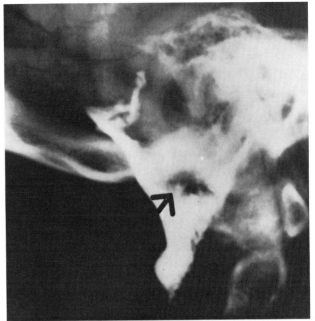

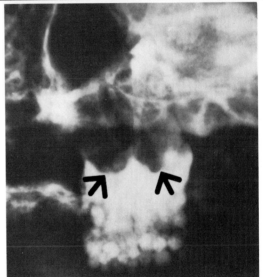

Fig. 88.14A & B Oil myelogram showing the cerebellar tonsils [arrows] in the Chiari Type 1 malformation. The low lying tonsils are seen in lateral (A) and AP oblique (B) projections.

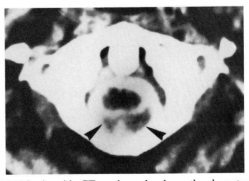

Fig. 88.15 Metrizamide CT myelography shows the characteristic filling defects of the cerebellar tonsils [arrows] posterior to the cord in a section just below the foramen magnum, passing through the odontoid and the atlas.

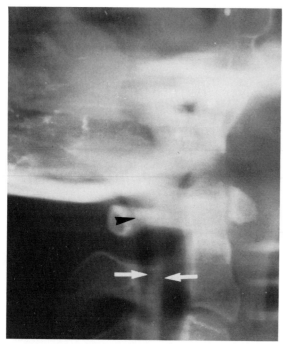

Fig. 88.16 Syringomyelia with a Chiari Type 1 malformation. Air myelography shows a collapsed upper cervical spinal cord [arrows] and low cerebellar tonsils [arrowhead].

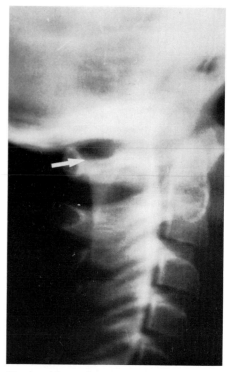

Fig. 88.18 Metrizamide myelogram showing an expanded cord (syringomyelia) and low cerebellar tonsils [arrow].

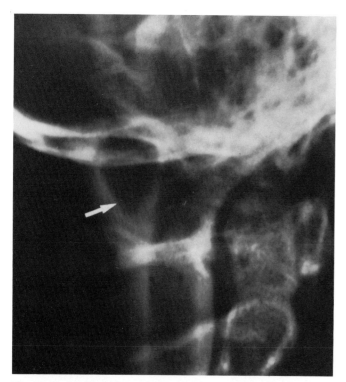

Fig. 88.17 Metrizamide myelogram showing tonsillar herniation [arrow]; the spinal cord is normal in size.

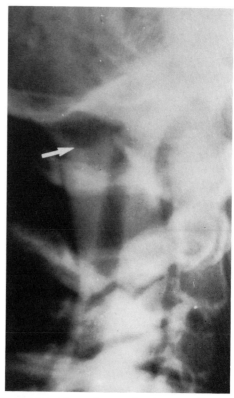

Fig. 88.19 Metrizamide myelogram showing a small, collapsed cord and ectopic cerebellar tonsils [arrow]. Note the expanded spinal canal.

CT may demonstrate a syrinx in the cervical spinal cord [11] and confirm the presence of a Chiari malformation, but is fallible in both respects without intrathecal contrast medium. It may however demonstrate evidence of hydrocephalus, a not uncommon association, and may exclude a tumour or cyst in the posterior cranial fossa, both of which have been described in association with syringomyelia [12].

Air myelography was at one time widely used to show the classic collapse of the spinal cord in the head up position (Fig. 88.16) when head down films showed it to be expanded, but is now rarely used. Myelography can be carried out with oil or water soluble contrast medium. Although the latter may give inferior demonstration of tonsillar ectopia, it shows the shape and size of the cord to more advantage, and may be combined with CT [13].

At water soluble myelography the spinal cord may appear normal in size, expanded or collapsed (Figs 88.17–88.19). Changes in cord size similar to those seen with air may be observed. Some degree of tonsillar ectopia is seen in as many as 90% of cases.

CT following myelography will confirm the presence of tonsillar herniation (Fig. 88.20). Delayed scans will also, in the majority of cases, show contrast medium within the intramedullary cavity (Fig. 88.20). This may occur early, in which case the contrast medium probably enters the syrinx via the fourth ventricle, through a patent central canal, or possibly through a defect in the cord itself. More frequently, filling is seen only on delayed examinations (at 6 to 24 hours), and there is strong evidence for transneural passage of metrizamide [14], possibly through enlarged Virchow-Robin spaces, as postulated by Ball and Dyan [15].

In up to 20% of cases a significant degree of arachnoiditis around the foramen magnum is found at surgery. Patients with this condition derive little benefit from foramen magnum decompression (the treatment of choice in cases with tonsillar ectopia), but may be treated by shunting procedures on the syrinx itself. A finding suggestive of arachnoiditis is that in the head down position, contrast medium fails to fill the cisterna magna, but instead flows forwards into the pontine cistern.

Post traumatic syringomyelia is discussed on page 1851.

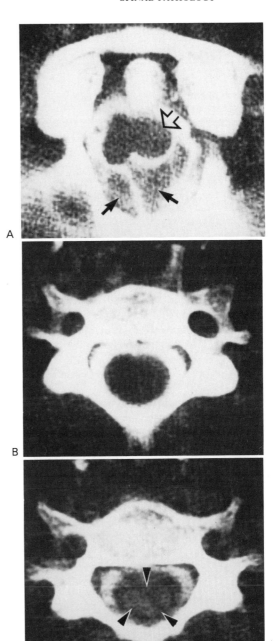

Fig. 88.20A, B & C Chiari Type 1 malformation and syringomyelia. Metrizamide CT myelography. (A) Just below the foramen magnum: the ectopic tonsils [arrows] and the distorted medulla oblongata [open arrow] are outlined. A section at C3 (B) shows the spinal cord to be expanded, while a similar section 6 hours later (C) reveals dilute metrizamide within a large syrinx [arrowheads].

BACK PAIN AND SCIATICA: DEGENERATIVE SPINAL DISEASE

Over 90% of cases of acute back pain need only symptomatic treatment, and only less than 10% have symptoms or signs of nerve root lesions [16]. Neuroradiological investigation is required only in those patients with persistent back and leg pain unresponsive to conservative treatment, and in patients with abnormal neurology.

Plain film evidence of degenerative disease is seen so commonly after the age of 50 years as to be considered within the normal range. Conversely, the plain films often show no significant abnormality in the presence of an acute lumbar disc protrusion. In spite of the lack of specific radiological changes of surgically significant degenerative disease, plain radiography of the lumbar spine should be carried out routinely prior to myelography. It may demonstrate:

1. Abnormalities of segmentation of the vertebral bodies, such as lumbarization of the first sacral segment or sacralization of the fifth lumbar vertebra, which will be of relevance to the surgeon in choosing the correct level for operation;
2. Evidence of lumbar canal stenosis;
3. Unexpected abnormalities such as tumour, infection, Paget's disease, haemangioma of bone, etc.; but such findings occur in only 2 or 3% of cases.

CT is being used in some centres as the prime imaging modality in the investigation of possible disc disease. High quality CT images show posterior or posterolateral bulging of the disc material, whose density is intermediate between that of bone and the epidural tissues. The normal posterior

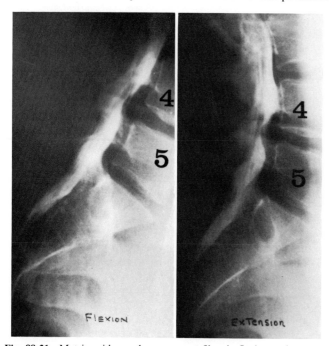

Fig. 88.21 Metrizamide myelogram; erect films in flexion and extension. A typical anterior impression due to a bulging annulus (disc protrusion) seen in extension, is greatly reduced on flexion.

concavity of the discs above L5/S1 is lost. Extruded material is occasionally calcified, although this is more common in the thoracic region. Displacement of the theca or of the nerve roots is sometimes evident, particularly when these are filled with intrathecal contrast medium following myelography See Fig. 88.23

In most centres, myelography is carried out as a routine prior to surgery for disc disease, for the following reasons:

1. It provides accurate confirmation and localization of the level of a disc protrusion, so that the surgeon's operative exposure can be limited. Clinical localization is adequate in only about half of the patients.
2. It assists the surgeon in choosing the type of surgical procedure, ranging from fenestration for small, lateral lesions, to extensive laminectomy for multiple, large, central disc protrusions.
3. It shows the presence and extent of lumbar canal stenosis, which may necessitate even more extensive decompression.
4. It may demonstrate unexpected pathology, such as a tumour of the lower spinal cord, arachnoid cyst, etc., which may not be appreciated on CT without intrathecal contrast medium, and may be coexistent with degenerative disease in older individuals.

Disc protrusion and prolapse

A tear in the annulus fibrosus of an intervertebral disc may allow protrusion of disc material into the space between the annulus and the intact posterior longitudinal ligament. A bulging disc produces a characteristic impression on the contrast medium column at myelography, and is referred to as a *disc protrusion*.

Disc material may however breach the longitudinal ligament, giving rise to a *disc herniation*. The anterior impression on the contrast medium associated with disc protrusion tends to disappear on flexion, due to stretching of the posterior longitudinal ligament (Fig. 88.21). If the impression persists on flexion and exceeds 3 mm from the adjacent bone on the lateral projection, disc herniation is usually confirmed at operation [17].

Myelographic appearances in disc lesions will depend on the size of the lesion, whether the ligament has been breached and its central, centrolateral or lateral position.

Central disc protrusions produce an anterior deformity of the contrast medium at the level of the disc space. This may diminish or disappear on flexion, while with central herniation, the deformity persists. Large central lesions cause focal decreased density of the contrast medium on the antero-posterior projection, and evidence of nerve root compression, often bilateral (Fig. 88.22). A massive central herniation can produce a complete block to the passage of contrast medium, especially in patients with canal stenosis. Such a block may be overcome in some patients by flexion of the back in the erect position.

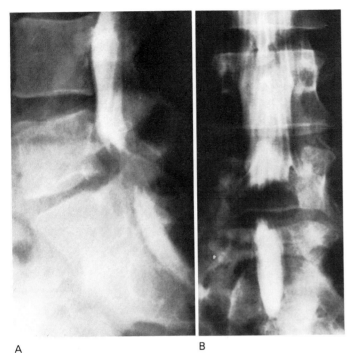

A
B

Fig. 88.22A & B Metrizamide myelogram. A large, central disc protrusion produces a very prominent anterior impression (A) and bilateral nerve root compression (B).

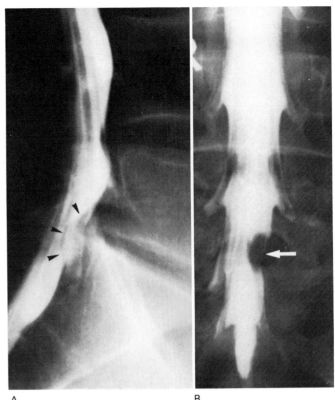

A
B

Fig. 88.24A & B Metrizamide myelogram; centrolateral L5/S1 disc herniation producing a typical double contour appearance on the lateral projection (A) [arrow heads]. The AP projection (B) shows a typical filling defect laterally, with impaired filling of the S1 nerve root sheath [arrow].

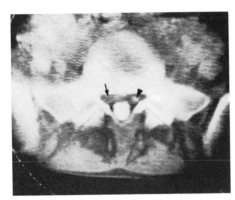

Fig. 88.23 Lumbosacral disc protrusion. CT following metrizamide myelography shows an anterolateral soft tissue mass within the spinal canal [arrow], deforming the theca. A contrast medium filled nerve root sheath (S1) is present in the same position on the other side [arrowhead].

Centrolateral disc herniation causes a variable anterior deformity of the contrast medium column, often giving a double contoured appearance. There is usually a typical filling defect on the lateral aspect of the column on the anteroposterior films, with evidence of underfilling, displacement or deformity of the nerve root sheaths (Fig. 88.23 & 88.24). Nerve roots may been seen to be displaced and thickened or swollen.

Laterally situated disc lesions may produce impaired filling, displacement, distortion or amputation of the nerve root sheath (Fig. 88.25) and this may be the main or only myelographic finding, particularly in patients with sciatica. A very laterally placed lesion may cause no abnormalities on the

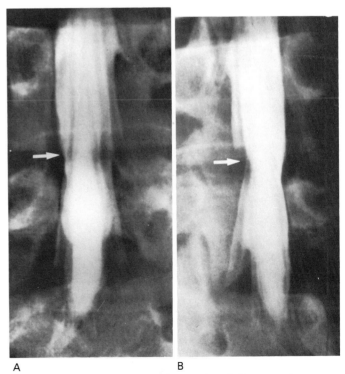

A
B

Fig. 88.25A & B Iopamidol myelogram; lateral disc protrusion at L4/5, with impaired filling of the L5 nerve root sheath (A), confirmed on an oblique projection (B) [arrow].

myelogram, particularly in individuals with short dural nerve root sheaths.

Lumbar phlebography is particularly suitable for detection of lateral disc protrusions which produce minimal or equivocal changes on myelography, lesions in the lateral recesses of the spinal canal and the neural foramina [18]. At the lumbosacral disc space the anterior epidural space is often very deep in normal individuals, particularly the more obese, and the veins, being more closely applied to the disc and the neural structures than the contrast medium filled theca, are a more sensitive index of disc lesions. CT may prove superior to either (as may magnetic resonance imaging), but for the present phlebography retains a place in the assessment of difficult cases.

Disc protrusion is manifest on phlebography as focal nonfilling of the epidural veins (Fig. 88.26), or as displacement or amputation of veins; occasionally, collateral filling of veins not normally opacified may be seen. Phlebo-

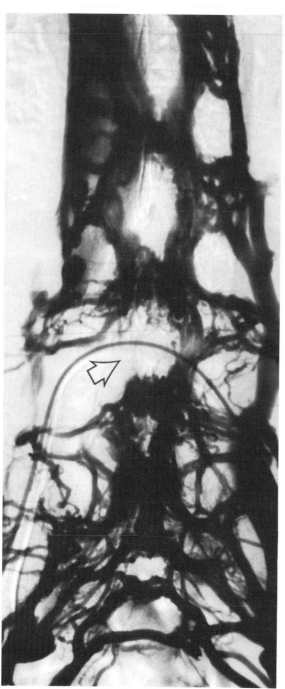

Fig. 88.26 Lumbar epidural phlebogram; injection of both lateral sacral veins (note catheters crossing just above arrow). Lateral disc protrusion: interruption of medial and lateral veins on the right side at L4/5.

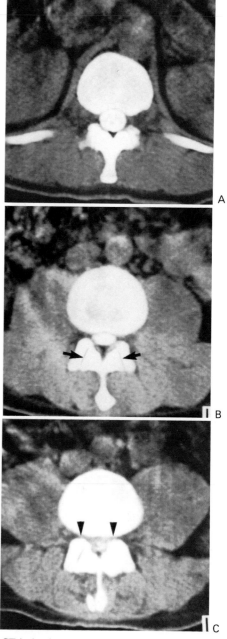

Fig. 88.27 CT in lumbar canal stenosis. On myelography, no contrast medium was visible below L3. (A) at L1 the theca is relatively normal, while at L3 (B) it is flattened from behind and at L4 (C) virtually no contrast medium is seen. Note the medial position of the bulky posterior intervertebral joints [arrows], and narrowing of the lateral recesses of the spinal canal [arrowheads]; there is no evidence of disc disease.

graphy is less helpful in the investigation of lumbago; it may, however, indicate at which levels discography may usefully be performed.

Stenosis of the lumbar spinal canal

This takes two forms: *congenital*, in which the anteroposterior diameter of the canal is reduced, the pedicles being both short and bulky, and the posterior intervertebral joints lie closer to the midline than normal; and *acquired*, in which degenerative changes around the posterior joints and buckling of the ligamentum flavum due to generalized loss of disc space height have the same effect: reduction in cross sectional dimensions of the canal. These features may be evident on plain films but CT is the ideal method of assessment of the dimensions of the spinal canal in the axial plane, especially of the lateral recesses of the canal, in which nerve roots may become trapped (Fig. 88.27).

Lumbar puncture may be very difficult and/or painful in this condition, and when injection of contrast medium commences, there may be doubt as to whether the contrast medium is really in the subarachnoid space. Fluoroscopy and spot films should be taken before an attempt to reposition the needle is made. The myelographic abnormalities which may be shown include the following:

1. Partial or complete obstruction to the flow of contrast medium, usually opposite the disc spaces (Fig. 88.28). The lateral projection will show if the compression is mainly anterior, due to disc disease, or posterior, due to osteophytes and ligamentous corrugation. The value of functional myelography in this context is described below.
2. The anteroposterior projections show waisting of the contrast medium column; if several levels are involved the column gives the appearance of multiple 'hourglass' constrictions at the level of the discs.
3. The nerve roots appear crowded together, and are often swollen, to give the 'bundle of twigs' appearance where the theca is constricted. This may be compounded by the presence of tortuous roots or prominent veins adjacent to obstructions.
4. The usual quantity of contrast medium often fills the canal into the lower or midthoracic region; if filling is controlled by fluoroscopy the volume injected can be reduced accordingly.

In canal stenosis, phlebography can show a range of abnormalities. In congenital constitutional narrowing, the epidural veins are crowded together (Fig. 88.29), but the epidural space is preserved. This crowding is not seen in stenosis involving only the lateral recess. Extensive narrowing of the epidural space may occur, with failure to fill the veins over a number of segments (Fig. 88.30). This may be seen in congenital or degenerative types, when the stenosis is severe.

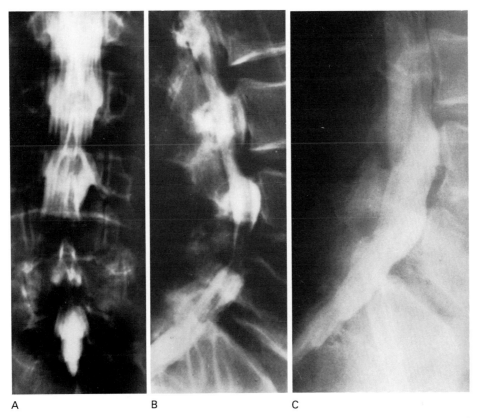

A   B   C

Fig. 88.28A, B & C Metrizamide myelogram in lumbar canal stenosis. (A) AP projection showing typical waisted constriction, most marked at L4/5 and L5/S1 disc levels. (B) A lateral projection shows narrow AP diameter of the spinal canal, from L2 to L5. (C) Following extensive laminectomy, the lumbar theca is of normal size.

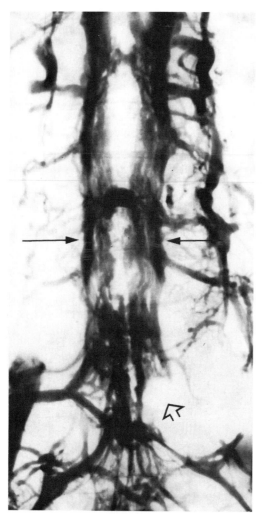

Fig. 88.29 Epidural phlebogram: lumbar canal stenosis. The right and left longitudinal veins lie closer together than normal [arrows], because of the reduced transverse diameter of the spinal canal. A lateral disc protrusion obliterates the lateral vein and the veins in the intervertebral foramen at L5/S1 on the left [open arrow].

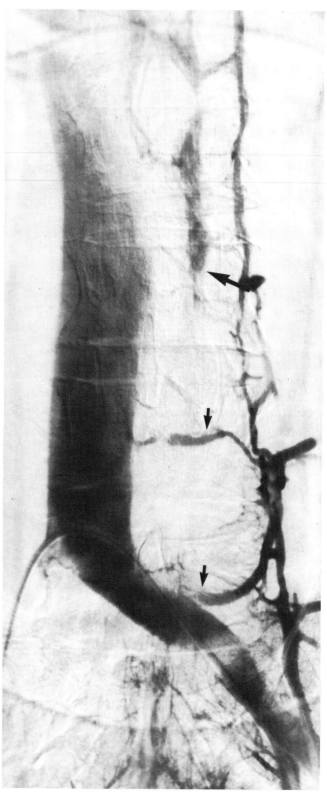

Fig. 88.30 Epidural phlebogram: severe spinal stenosis. Injection of the left lateral sacral and ascending lumbar veins produces very little opacification of the intraspinal veins below L2; the veins appear narrowed or occluded as they pass through the intervertebral foramina [arrows]. Epidural veins fill from L3 upwards [large arrow].

Functional myelography

Using water soluble contrast medium, it is possible to carry out flexion and extension studies in the erect or standing positions. This procedure more clearly demonstrates the anteroposterior diameter of the lumbar spinal canal; in the prone position, there is often layering of the contrast medium, which therefore fails to indicate the size of the canal. Flexion and extension films also give information as to what occurs during normal activities rather than the static myelographic data usually obtained.

Dynamic pathogenetic mechanisms can be demonstrated, such as constriction of the canal due to corrugation of the ligamentum flavum in extension (Fig. 88.31). The distinction between disc protrusion and disc herniation is made more

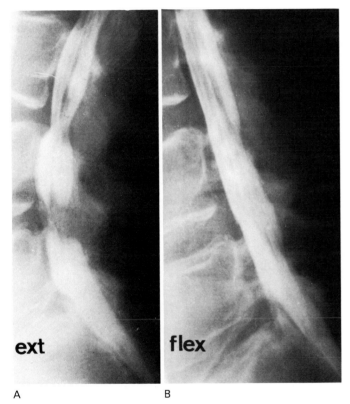

Fig. 88.31A & B Metrizamide myelogram, flexion and extension views. A localized area of canal stenosis seen in extension (A) is due to corrugation of the ligamentum flavum. It disappears when the spine is flexed (B).

easily on dynamic studies, as mentioned above. An apparently complete block at myelography in patients with canal stenosis is often relieved on erect flexion films, permitting examination of the lower lumbar segments (Fig. 88.32). Post-myelographic CT may assist in this respect, by showing opacification of the lower theca with contrast medium too dilute to appear on conventional films (see Fig. 88.27). A true anteroposterior diameter of the lumbar theca of 15 mm is considered the lower limit of normal; a diameter of less than 10 mm is encountered only in patients with severe symptoms [19].

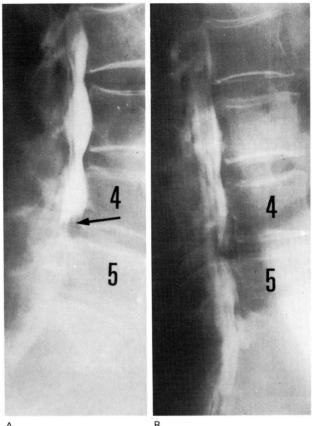

Fig. 88.32A & B L4/5 disc protrusion producing a virtually complete obstruction (A) [arrow]; the obstruction is relieved in flexion (B, erect film).

The accuracy of myelography in degenerative disease of the lumbar spine

Water-soluble myelography has a reported accuracy of 94 to 96% for the demonstration of surgically confirmed lumbar disc lesions [20,21].

Errors are most likely to occur at the lumbosacral level, and are usually related to (1) prominent anterior separation of the contrast medium from the L5/S1 disc space due to a deep epidural space at this level (which may be more than 1 cm in obese individuals) and (2) a high termination of the lumbar theca, above the last disc space, making examination of this level impossible.

A disc lesion situated extremely laterally, in the region of the intervertebral foramen, can also escape detection.

Postoperative myelography

Myelography following spinal operations may present considerable diagnostic problems when patients present with recurrent symptoms. It is frequently impossible to differentiate between myelographic changes due to a recurrent disc lesion and those due to postoperative scarring.

Myelography may show the following abnormalities:
1. Signs suggestive of a recurrent disc lesion at the operated

level. The only reliable sign is demonstration of an anterior impression on the contrast medium opposite the relevant disc space. Underfilling of the nerve root sheaths and deformity of the contrast medium column are seen frequently after myelography and surgery, and are not reliable indicators of a recurrent or residual disc protrusion.

2. A disc lesion at a new level. This should not prove unduly difficult to recognize, with the proviso that thecal scarring may cause obliteration of nerve roots at levels without disc protrusions. Occasionally it will be evident from the level of the laminectomy and/or any surgical clips in the vicinity that the original operation was not at the supposed level.

3. Inflammatory postoperative change (epiduritis and/or arachnoiditis). This will be suggested by marked irregularity, narrowing and shortening or the matting together or thickening of the nerve roots and loculation of the subarachnoid space. If a complete block is encountered, it may be very difficult to distinguish between a disc lesion and arachnoiditis. Absence of other signs of inflammation will make the former more likely, as will an indication that the obstruction is anterior; however, an extruded fragment of disc material may lie posteriorly, or even, rarely, intradurally. Moderate changes of inflammation usually bear no relationship to the patient's symptoms.

4. Previously unsuspected stenosis of the lumbar canal.

Spondylolisthesis

In this condition there are bilateral defects in the pars inter-articularis (spondylolysis) of one neural arch. commonly the fourth or fifth lumbar vertebra, permitting forward slip of the vertebral body, pedicles and superior articular processes on the next lower vertebral body. The remainder of the detached neural arch usually remains in place. Spondylolisthesis may also occur without spondylolysis, as a consequence of degenerative processes affecting the articular facets in such a way as to change their angulation and allow forward displacement of one segment on another. Fibrosis and bony overgrowth frequently occur around the bony defects or degenerative joints, contributing to narrowing of the spinal canal, particularly the lateral recesses, where the nerve roots may be trapped.

The diagnosis is made on plain radiographs, which demonstrate the bony defects on lateral and oblique projections (Ch. 87) and permit assessment of the degree of forward displacement. Myelography may be indicated if surgery is considered. The lateral projection usually shows posterior angulation of the contrast medium away from the body of the upper vertebra, with a step deformity at the affected level as the column again approximates the anterior border of the spinal canal at the next vertebra below. (Fig. 88.33).

In more severe degrees of spondylolisthesis, myelography shows more advanced deformity, with a partial or complete obstruction of the theca, due to anterior compression from the forward displacement of the vertebral body and posterior compression by the vertebral neural arch. Hypertrophy of the arch and thickening of the ligamentum flavum further accentuate these changes.

Spondylolisthesis may predispose to disc herniation, usually at the affected level, but also at other levels, probably

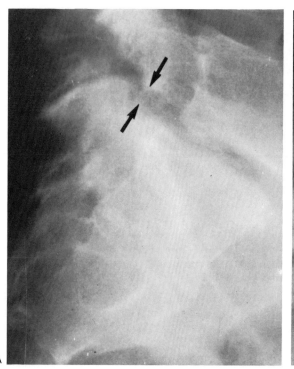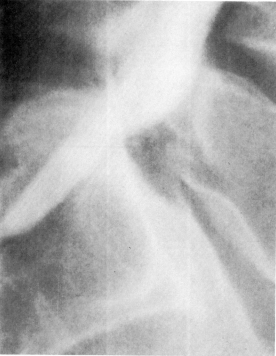

Fig. 88.33A & B   Spondylolisthesis at L5/S1. (A) Plain film showing forward slip of L5 on S1, with a prominent defect in the pars interarticularis [arrows]. (B) metrizamide myelogram: there is a marked step deformity at the affected level.

due to the disordered mechanics in the region. Disc protrusion at the level of the forward slip may be very difficult to assess myelographically.

DEGENERATIVE DISEASE IN THE CERVICAL SPINE: RADICULOPATHY AND MYELOPATHY.

The term cervical spondylosis refers to degenerative changes in the discs and posterior intervertebral joints, usually idiopathic, but sometimes the sequel to trauma, or associated with abnormal mechanical strains, as in patients with congenital intervertebral fusions, where the adjacent joints are often affected in relatively early life. Clinically, it gives rise to two entities, which may be combined: radiculopathy and myelopathy.

Cervical spondylotic *radiculopathy* is due to a lateral disc rupture or to lateral osteophytic encroachment on the neural foramina from the margins of the neurocentral joints. Compression of one root is the commonest neurological presentation.

Less frequently, the spinal canal may be narrowed from front to back by disc bulges, osteophytic bars along the disc margins, or posteriorly, by a corrugated ligamentum flavum, compressing the cord, and giving rise to a paraparesis of variable severity. This is spondylotic *myelopathy*. Ischaemia of the spinal cord may play an important part in its production. Patients with a congenitally narrow anteroposterior diameter of the canal are much more prone to develop these complications since there is less capacity for reduction of the area of the spinal canal.

There is often no clear clinical correlation between the findings on plain radiographs and the patient's signs and symptoms in cervical spondylosis. Marked degenerative changes are often seen in asymptomatic elderly patients, while soft, acute disc protrusions may occur without any plain film abnormality. Assessment of the size of the spinal canal is important; congenital canal stenosis is considered to be present if the anteroposterior diameter from the posterior margin of the vertebral bodies to the bases of the spinous processes is less than 13 mm at the C5 level. In such cases, the laminae appear on the lateral projection to be very foreshortened, so that the space between the pedicle and the spinous process seen in the normal lateral view is absent. It may be evident that the canal is further narrowed by posterior osteophytes projecting into the canal from the disc margins, in which case measurement from the posterior border of the osteophyte to the spinous process will indicate the space available for the spinal cord. It should be remembered that the cervical spinal cord is almost 1 cm in anteroposterior diameter. Oblique projections may show osteophytic encroachment on the intervertebral foramina or, rarely, enlargement due to a neurofibroma. Flexion and extension films in the lateral projection may show evidence of instability, which can of itself cause pain, and contributes to canal stenosis.

Plain films may also reveal other abnormalities such as cervical ribs, metastatic disease, rheumatoid arthritis or metabolic bone disease.

CT can be used, without contrast medium, to demonstrate narrowing of the spinal canal or lateral recess by disc material or osteophyte. Disc herniations in the cervical region are not infrequently calcified (Fig. 88.34).

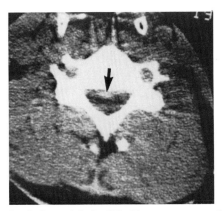

Fig. 88.34 Cervical spondylosis. CT without contrast medium shows a soft tissue disc protrusion at C3/4 [arrow].

Myelographic abnormalities in cervical spondylosis include the following:

1. In patients presenting with radiculopathy:

   (a) obliteration of one or more nerve root sheaths (Fig. 88.35) corresponding to the level(s) incriminated clinically. The most frequently involved roots are C5, C6 and C7. Asymptomatic nerve root sheath defects are commonly present. When multiple defects are seen, the largest is usually the clinically significant one. The cervical nerves emerge *above* the appropriately numbered vertebra (as opposed to the lumbar region).

   (b) anterior indentation of the contrast medium at the same level(s) by disc or osteophyte.

2. In patients with myelopathy:

   (a) evidence of complete or partial obstruction to flow of the contrast medium, most marked in extension, and commonly at C5/6 or C6/7, which may be substantially relieved by flexion of the neck (Fig. 88.36). It should be remembered that, whether myelography is carried out by lumbar or cervical puncture, the head and neck are usually placed in an exaggerated extended position, so that the apparent block may be unphysiological.

   (b) indentation of the contrast medium anteriorly due to ossified or cartilaginous bars at the disc margins, disc protrusions or subluxation, or posteriorly due to corrugation of the ligamentum flavum. The latter appears as a series of posterior 'thumbprints'.

   (c) evidence of canal stenosis, with generalized reduction in size of the subarachnoid space (Fig. 88.37).

3. In either group of patients, myelography may reveal unexpected pathology such as a tumour, syrinx or Chiari malformation.

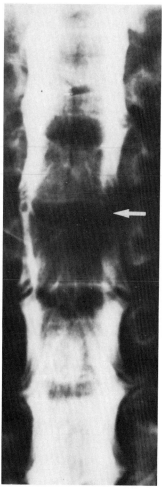

Fig. 88.35 Metrizamide myelogram in a patient with a left sided cervical radiculopathy, showing obliteration of the left C5 nerve root sheath [arrow].

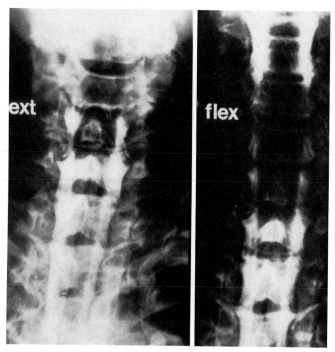

Fig. 88.36 Cervical myelogram: a complete obstruction to flow of the contrast medium in extension, at C4/5, relieved on flexion. There was a prominent anterior impression due to disc protrusion at the affected level, together with focal canal stenosis.

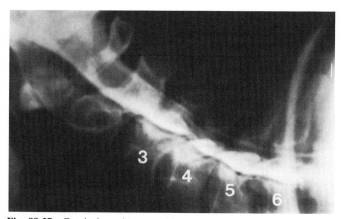

Fig. 88.37 Cervical myelogram with metrizamide showing canal stenosis extending from C3 to C6.

The findings at myelography will determine the operative approach. It is therefore important that the radiologist assess the degree of spinal cord compression in patients with myelopathy. The presence of degenerative changes does not mean that they are responsible for cord compression. The latter can be said to be present when the cord can be seen to be indented or deformed by osteophyte or disc protrusion, when it appears focally widened on the anteroposterior projection, or when there is obstruction to the passage of contrast medium.

According to the interpretation of the myelogram, the surgeon may opt for:

1. An anterior surgical approach, consisting of removal of disc material from the front, decompression of the cord and nerve roots and fusion of the vertebral bodies with a dowel of bone (the Cloward operation). This is not usually performed if multiple discs are involved, or if there is severe, extensive canal stenosis.

2. A posterior surgical approach, laminectomy, which is usually reserved for patients with canal stenosis or spondylotic myelopathy due to extensive degenerative disease. This approach is also used for intraspinal lesions.

3. Facetectomy, removal of material from around the neural foramen in cases of focal nerve root compression.

4. A combination of the above.

As in the lumbar region, epidural phlebography may provide additional information in troublesome cases, particularly in laterally placed lesions, and in the region of the intervertebral foramen, where the veins and nerve roots are closely related (Fig. 88.38).

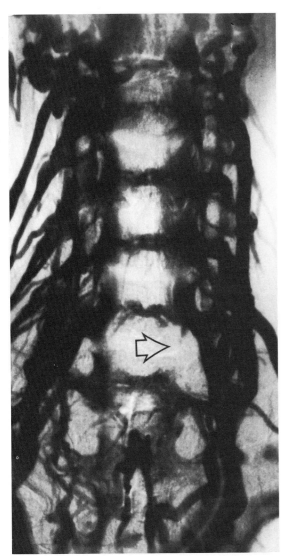

Fig. 88.38 Cervical epidural phlebogram. Complete occlusion of epidural veins at C6/7 on the left due to a lateral disc protrusion [arrow]. Less marked compression of the veins is present at other levels (e.g. C5/6 to C7/T1 on the right).

Table 88.1 Anatomical location of spinal lesions

Extradural

Benign
Disc prolapse
Haematoma
Abscess
Neurofibroma
Osteochondroma
Dermoid/epidermoid
Vertebral body tumours
   haemangioma
   osteoclastoma
   aneurysmal bone cyst
Paget's disease

Malignant
Metastases
Lymphoma
Myeloma
Sarcoma
Chordoma

Intradural/extramedullary
Neurofibroma
Meningioma
Dermoid/epidermoid   }
Lipoma   } also intramedullary
Ependymoma   }
Metastases in CSF
   medulloblastoma
   ependymoma
   melanoma
   carcinoma

Intramedullary
Tumours
   ependymoma
   astrocytoma
   glioblastoma
   developmental tumours
   haemangioblastoma
Syringomyelia
Myelitis
Abscess/granuloma
Haematomyelia

SPINAL CORD COMPRESSION

Mechanical compression of the spinal cord requires expeditious diagnosis, elucidation and treatment if irreversible damage is to be prevented. Clinical diagnosis is made difficult by two factors. First, the condition may be mimicked by a number of neurological diseases having spastic paraplegia as a dominant part of the clinical picture (Table 88.1). Second, due to the diversity of causes of cord compression in a variety of diseases, patients frequently present in nonneurological units, so that the diagnosis is not evident without a high index of clinical suspicion.

Patients with compression of the spinal cord may deteriorate following myelography, so that neurosurgical assistance should be at hand; if it is not, myelography is contraindicated.

Plain radiographs

Careful examination of plain films of the spine and chest should always precede myelography, as metastatic and infective bone lesions account for the majority of acute or subacute cases. Demonstration of disseminated metastatic lesions may influence the decision as to whether myelography should be carried out, or as to whether surgical decompression or radiotherapy should be the first line of treatment.

Primary neoplasms of bone are rare causes of spinal cord compression. Their radiological appearances are described in Chapters 69 & 70.

Plain film findings of bone lysis, collapse with or without pathological fracture, or sclerosis, accompanied by a paravertebral shadow will suggest metastatic disease, while collapse of an intervertebral disc space will orientate the diagnosis towards infection. In either case, the chest radiograph may provide valuable supplementary evidence.

Expansion of the bony spinal canal may be focal or generalized, and occurs with both intra- and extramedullary lesions, although it is more common with the former. A neurofibroma may enlarge both the spinal canal and an intervertebral foramen. Calcification within the canal can occur with meningioma or with intramedullary glioma, but is more frequent with thoracic disc protrusion, or in the condition of ossification of the posterior longitudinal ligament. Changes of cervical spondylosis may be present, but, since they are ubiquitous in the elderly, can be misleading.

Myelography

Myelography is the fundamental examination. When clinical features or plain film findings suggest a lesion at a single level, water-soluble myelography, using 12 ml of 200 to 250 ml I/100 ml solution (metrizamide or iopamidol), injected via lumbar puncture, is the method of choice. Some workers still use iodized oil in patients whose clinical level of involvement is uncertain or in whom involvement of several levels is expected, since these groups of patients may require detailed myelography of the entire spine, which in the absence of a major obstruction, may be difficult with water soluble contrast medium.

At myelography, particular attention is paid to defining the location of the lesion. Tumours and other space-occupying lesions can be classified according to their relationship to the dura mater and spinal cord into three groups:

1. *Extradural* lesions, which arise outside the spinal canal, from the vertebrae, the intervertebral discs or the epidural tissues. These form the large majority.
2. *Intradural, extramedullary* lesions, which lie within the subarachnoid space around the spinal cord and usually arise from nerve roots or the meninges.
3. *Intramedullary* lesions, arising within the spinal cord itself.

Extradural lesions

The value of plain films has already been mentioned. Plain CT (i.e., without intrathecal contrast medium) is of value only in showing associated changes: bone disease in inflammatory lesions (Fig. 88.39), primary or metastatic tumours (Fig. 88.40), paraspinal masses (Fig. 88.41), etc. Calcification within the spinal canal may be seen in tumours, or more commonly in disc protrusion. Unless the level of compression is evident clinically, or bone changes are equivocal, there is little to be gained from CT preceding myelography, and the delay in proceeding to myelography and surgery is scarcely justified.

CT may, however, usefully complement myelography with water soluble contrast medium: it may define the extent of an obstructive lesion if only a small amount of contrast medium, undetectable on plain radiography, has passed it. It can also aid in the differentiation of extradural, extra- and intramedullary masses.

At myelography, extradural lesions characteristically displace the contrast medium filled subarachnoid space away from the bony margins of the spinal canal. In the antero-posterior projection, the contrast medium normally comes

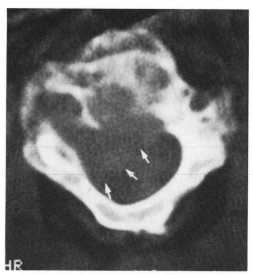

Fig. 88.39 Aneurysmal bone cyst. CT shows expansion and lysis of the body and lateral mass of a cervical vertebra. There is intraspinal tumour [arrows].

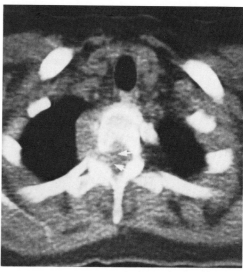

Fig. 88.40 Metastasis to an upper thoracic vertebra. CT: the right pedicle is absent, and a paraspinal mass is present. Intraspinal extension [arrows] is poorly defined.

into close opposition with the medial margins of the pedicles. When an extradural mass is present, there is a gap between the contrast medium and the pedicle, while in the lateral projection the contrast medium may appear displaced forwards, away from the posterior elements, or posteriorly, away from the vertebral bodies or intervertebral discs (Fig. 88.42).

Metastatic extradural lesions often cause a complete obstruction to the flow of contrast medium, particularly in the thoracic region, where the spinal canal is narrow. The upper edge of such an obstruction may show a horizontal serrated appearance, often likened to a bundle of twigs, or there may be a circumferential constriction of the column of contrast medium (Fig. 88.43). In the majority of cases there is evidence of bony disease at the same level, or of an adjacent vertebra.

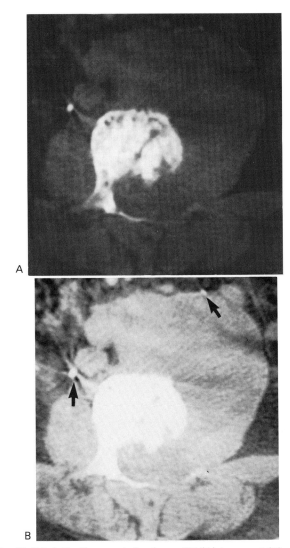

A

B

Fig. 88.41A & B Recurrent chordoma. CT (A) bone and (B) soft tissue windows. Extensive bone destruction is associated with a massive soft tissue paraspinal tumour; CT shows both to advantage. Arrows indicate the contrast medium filled ureters.

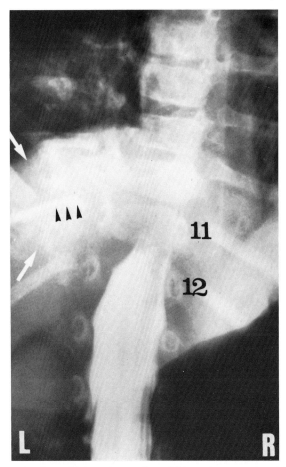

Fig. 88.42 Iopamidol myelogram in a child aged ten months with spinal cord compression due to neuroblastoma. AP projection: complete block at the level of T11 with a predominantly left sided extradural lesion displacing the theca and its contents to the right. Note mottled paravertebral calcification [arrows], and erosion and thinning of the left 11th rib [arrowheads].

Lymphomas often produce myelographic appearances indistinguishible from those of metastases. The bones, however, often appear normal, and the extradural lesion is more classically an incomplete obstruction extending over a number of segments.

Spontaneous epidural haematoma (or, less commonly subdural haematoma, which is myelographically very similar) is occasionally encountered in middle aged or elderly patients. There may be a history of mild trauma or straining, of hypertension, or of a coagulation defect. At myelography, the findings are usually of an incomplete block of extradural type, extending over a long segment. These appearances are not however specific, and the diagnosis is made on the clinical features such as acute onset of cord compression and local spinal pain. An epidural abscess can produce very similar myelographic appearances.

Symptomatic protrusion of thoracic intervertebral discs is uncommon (about 1% of the number of lumbar disc lesions), and usually presents as progressive compression of the spinal cord. Plain films may be very suggestive: calcified intraspinal material can be demonstrated in about 70% of cases, making the diagnosis virtually certain, especially if it can be seen to extend from the disc into the spinal canal (Fig. 88.44) [22]. Calcification within the disc is quite common in the senile, degenerate thoracic spine and is of no significance in this context. The myelographic features are typical (Fig. 88.45).

As noted above, spinal cord compression by benign primary tumours of the vertebral column (aneurysmal bone cyst, osteoblastoma) is uncommon. Haemangioma of bone is a rather common incidental finding, with the characteristic plain film findings of a honeycomb or vertically striated bone (Fig. 88.46). The range of plain film abnormalities is much larger however, and these lesions can cause compression of the spinal cord or nerve roots even when the bone does not appear particularly expanded [23]. When symptomatic, they are investigated by myelography and/or CT, and by angiography. The contribution of the latter is manifold:

1. It may confirm the diagnosis when the affected vertebra does not have the classical appearance. With injection of the relevant intercostal or spinal artery or arteries, pools of contrast medium are seen within the bone, giving a vascular pattern which is much more irregular and persistent than the normally homogeneous blush.

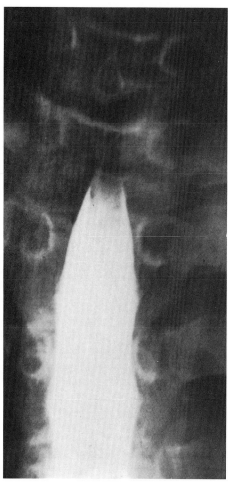

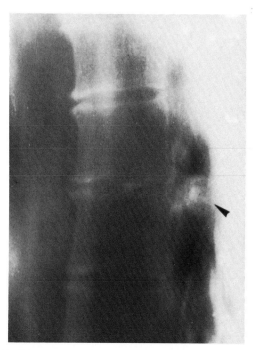

Fig. 88.44 Tomogram of thoracic disc protrusion, with calcified disc material in the spinal canal [arrowhead].

Fig. 88.43 Metrizamide myelogram: complete block at T2 due to an extradural secondary deposit, with circumferential constriction of the contrast medium column.

2. The extent of the malformation, both within the vertebra and in the surrounding soft tissues, can be assessed (Fig. 88.47). An arteriovenous malformation of the spinal cord is a rare but well documented association.
3. The radiculomedullary arteries in the region of the lesion can be identified preoperatively, so that the surgeon is forewarned of the potential dangers of interfering with them.
4. The arteries feeding the haemangioma can also be identified; they can then be ligated at operation, or embolized, should the disposition of the radiculomedullary arteries permit. Embolization can be carried out preoperatively (Fig. 88.47), or, in cases where the mode of presentation is with pain rather than cord compression, it can be a definitive therapeutic procedure.

It should be noted that the demonstration of a hypervascular vertebral lesion does not prove the diagnosis of haemangioma; aneurysmal bone cyst, osteoblastoma or some metastases can also appear very vascular.

Ossification of the posterior longitudinal ligament is a relatively rare form of extradural lesion which may cause cord compression, particularly in the cervical and upper thoracic region. It is of unknown aetiology, and appears to

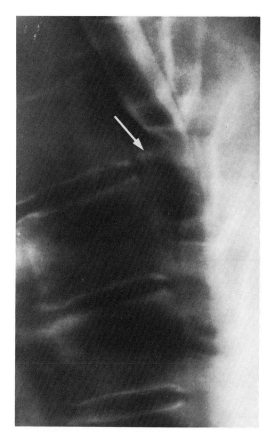

Fig. 88.45 Thoracic disc protrusion. Metrizamide myelogram shows backward displacement of the theca and spinal cord, centred on a disc space. Calcified disc material lies anteriorly in the canal [arrow].

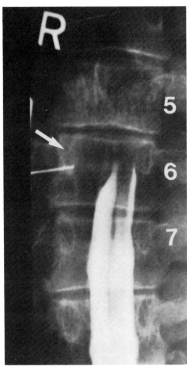

Fig. 88.46 Haemangioma of the T5 vertebral body, with the typical honeycomb appearance. The right pedicle of T6 also appears indistinct [arrow]. Myelography shows a complete obstruction of extradural type at this level, the contrast medium outlined theca being displaced to the left.

be more common in the Japanese. Plain films show a dense line of calcification just behind the vertebral bodies on the lateral projection, which CT shows to be narrowing the spinal canal. At myelography there is smooth anterior extradural compression, extending over several segments.

Thickening of the pachymeninges (the dura mater) may be the result of infection (e.g. syphilis), metabolic disease (Fig. 88.48) or idiopathic (Charcot's disease). CT of good quality may indicate the diagnosis by showing more or less concentric constriction of the subarachnoid space; myelography shows the constriction to be extensive and sometimes rather irregular.

Intradural extramedullary compressive lesions

This group is made up almost entirely of meningiomas and neurofibromas which are benign, potentially curable tumours.

CT is of little assistance unless water soluble myelography has been unsatisfactory due to dispersion or partial blockage of the contrast medium, when the further information gained about the site and extent of the lesion can salvage the examination (Fig. 88.49). If a large tumour has an extradural component which projects beyond the spinal canal, this can be demonstrated by CT (Fig. 88.50).

Both common types of extramedullary, intradural tumour are ovoid or spherical in shape, and lie within the subarachnoid space, producing a clearly defined, intradural type

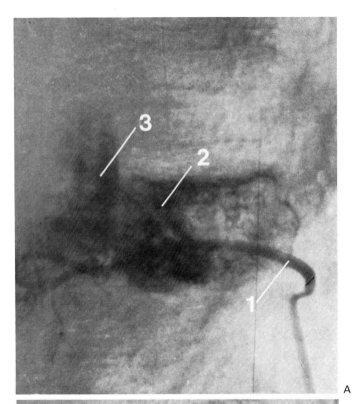

A

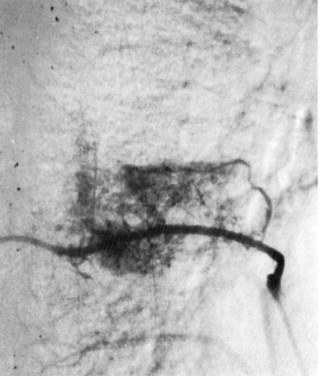

B

Fig. 88.47A & B Haemangioma of bone. (A) Injection of intercostal artery [1], lateral projection, showing grossly abnormal vascularity in the bone [2], extending into the spinal canal [3]. (B) After preoperative embolization, the hypervascularity is marked reduced, particularly within the spinal canal.

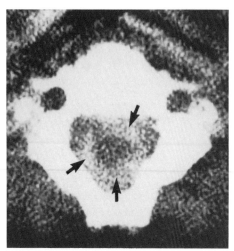

Fig. 88.48 Mucopolysaccharidosis V (Scheie's disease). CT with intravenous contrast medium showing grossly thickened meninges [arrows] surrounding the cervical spinal cord.

filling defect at myelography. The myelogram shows widening of the contrast medium outlined subarachnoid space on the side of the tumour, the contrast medium usually surrounding or directly outlining at least part of the margin of the lesion, producing a characteristic 'capping' appearance (Fig. 88.51). The spinal cord is displaced away from the tumour, to one side or in the sagittal plane, depending on whether the tumour lies predominantly laterally, anteriorly or posteriorly. The dura mater is *not* displaced away from the bodies or pedicles of the vertebrae and the contrast medium remains closely applied to these structures (Fig. 88.52), in contrast to lesions of extradural type. Obstruction to flow of the contrast medium is often incomplete, and, if the contrast medium has been introduced by lumbar puncture, the upper pole of the lesion can often be demonstrated by contrast medium which has found its way past the tumour; water soluble contrast medium is particularly advantageous in this respect. If this does not occur, and injection of further contrast medium via the lumbar needle does not encourage flow past the obstruction, it may be necessary to inject further contrast medium by cervical puncture.

Myelographic distinction between meningioma and neurofibroma is often not possible. Meningiomas in the spinal canal are much commoner in middle aged females than in males or at other ages, and the large majority are found in the thoracic region. They rarely produce bone erosion, and although histologically they may show calcification, this is rarely apparent radiographically. Meningioma is also the commonest intradural lesion at the level of the foramen magnum (although it should not be confused with an ectopic cerebellar tonsil). They commonly lie anteriorly.

Neurofibromas occur at any site in the spine and more commonly produce bone erosion. They show no sex predominance. The cerebrospinal fluid protein level is frequently markedly elevated. In neurofibromatosis, a large number of discrete lesions may be shown (Fig. 88.53). Angiography often shows them to be hypervascular, if the feeding vessel can be found (Fig. 88.54). The relationship of the tumour to surrounding vessels can be shown (Fig. 88.55); preoperative

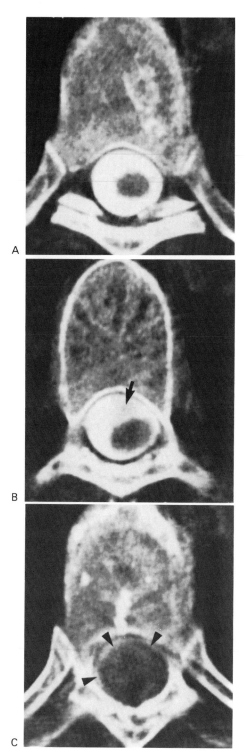

Fig. 88.49A, B & C Intrathecal, extramedullary tumour (meningioma). CT following metrizamide myelography shows the spinal cord to be displaced laterally above the level of the tumour (A). The upper pole of the tumour is a half shadow within the contrast medium (B) [arrow]. The body of the tumour is surrounded by a thin rim of contrast medium (C) [arrowheads], confirming its intradural position.

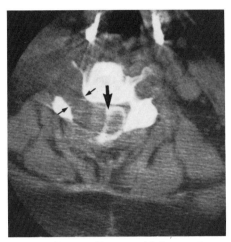

Fig. 88.50 'Dumb-bell' neurofibroma, with intra and extraspinal components. CT following metrizamide myelography: the contrast medium filled theca [arrow] is displaced away from the tumour, which widens the intervertebral foramen [small arrows]. The extraspinal component is not well defined, but the normal soft tissue pattern, present on the other side, is lost.

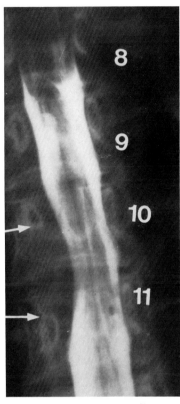

Fig. 88.52 Intradural, extramedullary neurofibroma at T8/9 and extradural neurofibroma at T10/11. Note erosion of the pedicles and increased distance between them in relation to the lower lesion [arrows].

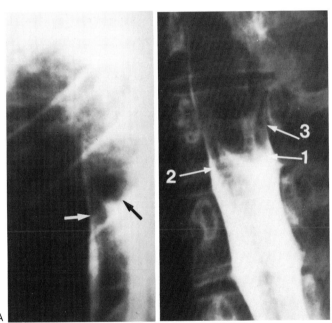

A   B

Fig. 88.51A & B Intradural extramedullary tumour (neurofibroma); metrizamide myelogram. In the AP projection, note characteristic features: the lower pole of the tumour [1] outlined by contrast medium; displacement of the spinal cord [2] away from the side of the tumour, while contrast medium remains in close contact with the pedicles [3].

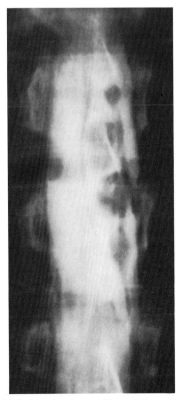

Fig. 88.53 Multiple intradural neurofibromas in a patient with neurofibromatosis.

embolization may be feasible, depending on the origins and configurations of the radiculomedullary arteries.

Developmental tumours such as *dermoids* and *lipomas* may have intradural extramedullary components, although they are essentially intramedullary tumours. Some *ependymomas* of the spinal cord have exophytic nodules which may be virtually indistinguishable from tumours lying alongside the cord, and when ependymomas arise from the filum terminale, below the termination of the cord, they are indistinguishable from extramedullary tumours. Further discussion of these lesions will be found in the next section.

Metatastatic neoplasms rarely show diffuse intradural spread; central nervous system tumours, especially medulloblastoma, ependymoma and melanoma are by far the most common to show intradural spread, but systemic neoplasms may metastasize in this way. Myelography shows multiple irregular filling defects (Fig. 88.56) and/or thickened nerve roots, due to infiltration by tumour. Differential diagnosis is from multiple neurofibromas and severe arachnoiditis.

Intramedullary lesions

Intrinsic lesions of the spinal cord consist essentially of tumours of the glioma series: ependymomas and astrocytomas, of which the former is by far the commoner. Syringomyelia is the prime differential diagnosis.

Plain films are rather unhelpful in the majority of cases. Abnormalities include expansion of the spinal canal, manifest as flattening of the medial surface of the pedicles, flattening or scalloping of the posterior surface of the vertebral bodies, etc., which may be diffuse or focal. The latter is more common with ependymomas, but is evident in only 10 to 15 per cent of intramedullary tumours. Congenital anomalies of the cervical spine, such as occipitalization of the atlas, spina bifida or intervertebral fusions, should orientate the diagnosis towards syringomyelia. Spina bifida may however accompany a tumour of developmental origin, such as a lipoma.

CT is of little value in the differentiation of neoplastic and other causes of swelling of the spinal cord, with the exception of developmental or post-traumatic syringomyelia (p.1851). Studies without intrathecal contrast medium may show densities significantly lower than those of cerebrospinal fluid, indicating the presence of fat, and suggesting a tumour of developmental origin, i.e. lipoma or dermoid (Fig. 88.57). Clear cut demonstration of either obvious cysts or marked heterogeneity within the cord, indicating malignant tumours, is relatively rare.

Intrathecal water soluble contrast medium outlines an expanded spinal cord, but tends to obscure detail within it (Fig. 88.58). Permeation of contrast medium into a cystic tumour is described, but is much less common than in syringomyelia. CT sections through the region of the foramen magnum, to assess tonsillar ectopia, are mandatory should doubt persist.

Myelography demonstrates a more or less fusiform expansion of the spinal cord, lying within the contrast medium filled subarachnoid space, in both anteroposterior and lateral

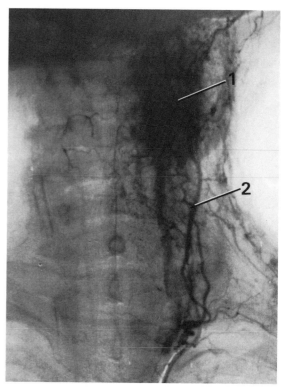

Fig. 88.54 Hypervascular neurofibroma [1] supplied by the ascending cervical artery [2].

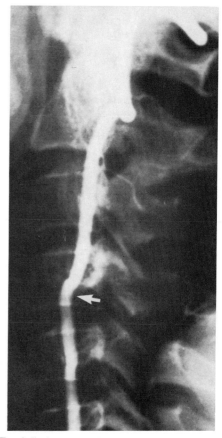

Fig. 88.55 Focal displacement of the vertebral artery [arrow] by the extraspinal component of a neurofibroma.

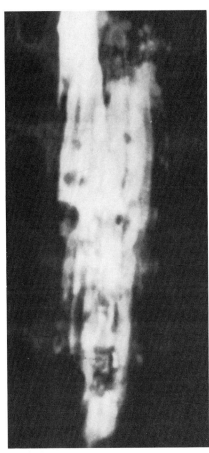

Fig. 88.56 Oil myelogram showing multiple irregular, nodular filling defects due to diffuse intradural spread of secondary deposits from an intracranial tumour. Note the similarity to neurofibromas (Fig. 88.53).

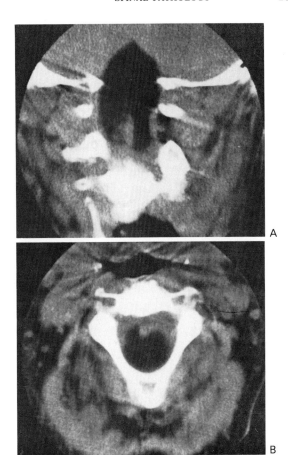

Fig. 88.57A & B Intramedullary lipoma; coronal and axial CT sections showing a mass of fat density extending from an enlarged upper cervical canal, up through the foramen magnum. Although the nature of the tumour is evident, its intramedullary location is not certain from this study.

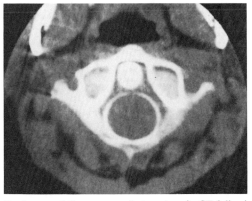

Fig. 88.58 Intramedullary tumour (astrocytoma). CT following metrizamide myelography shows contrast medium surrounding an expanded spinal cord at C1.

projections (Fig. 88.59). Cord expansion usually occurs over several segments, and there is rarely a complete obstruction to the flow of contrast medium. The subarachnoid space around the expanded cord is correspondingly narrowed, but retains its normal close proximity to pedicles and vertebral bodies.

It is essential that an intramedullary lesion not be confused with an anterior or posteriorly placed extradural lesion, such as a cervical disc protrusion, in which the cord can be splayed out over the lesion, with an increase in its transverse diameter. Such confusion can be of extreme therapeutic significance; it is therefore emphasized that the presence of apparent cord expansion must always be confirmed on both frontal and lateral projections.

As noted above, only extradural and intradural tumours can be distinguished below the level of the conus medullaris. A neurofibroma which grows to a large size in the lumbar region may be indistinguishible from a large ependymoma of the lower end of the spinal cord or the filum terminale (Fig. 88.60). Both of these, sometimes referred to as 'giant tumours of the cauda equina', can cause extensive bone erosion and expansion of the spinal canal.

Ependymomas at any level may show a fungating extramedullary appearing component, enlarging in the subarachnoid space and mimicking an intradural, extramedullary tumour.

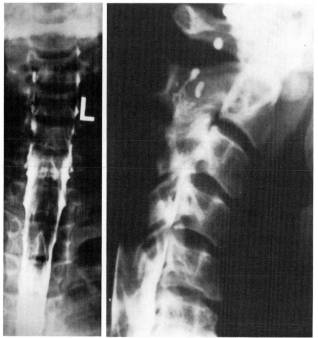

Fig. 88.59 Oil myelogram showing extensive cervical astrocytoma. AP (A) and lateral (B) projections both show expansion of the spinal cord, confirming the intramedullary location of the lesion.

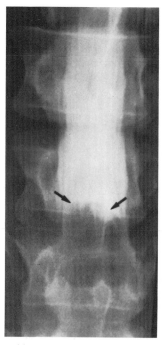

Fig. 88.60 Metrizamide myelogram. An ependymoma of the filum terminale causing a complete obstruction to the flow of contrast medium at the upper border of L1 [arrows]. This patient presented with backache and bilateral sciatica; the importance of including the lower end of the spinal cord in the examination of such patients is emphasised.

The differentiation between syringomyelia and an intrinsic tumour of the spinal cord may be problematic. Myelographic features which indicate the former include:

1. The presence of tonsillar ectopia,
2. Evidence of changes in size of the spinal cord with posture,
3. CT demonstration of entry of intrathecal contrast medium into the syrinx.

Conversely, a tumour would be suggested by:

1. Focal expansion of the cord,
2. Irregularity of outline, which may in part be due to dilated vessels on the surface of the tumour,
3. The absence of tonsillar ectopia or other congenital anomalies.

Angiography has little to offer in the differential diagnosis between syrinx and tumour, unless the lesion is a haemangioblastoma. Ependymomas and astrocytomas infrequently show a tumour blush, although with any intramedullary tumour, the spinal cord arteries may be larger than normal. Any cause of expansion of the cord will separate the anterior and posterolateral spinal arteries.

Another diagnostic difficulty is swelling of the cord in patients who have been irradiated for malignant disease. Radiation myelitis, with swelling, is unfortunately much commoner than intramedullary metastases.

Inflammatory lesions

Spinal inflammatory disease may arise either by direct extension of a local lesion, such as vertebral osteomyelitis, or as a blood borne metastatic infection, from a distant focus, such as an infected skin lesion. Offending organisms may be pyogenic, especially in haematogenous disease, or tuberculous, most commonly due to direct spread.

The epidural space is frequently involved, by virtue of its rich venous network. The diagnosis of pyogenic epidural abscess is essentially clinical, suggested by rapid onset of severe back pain and tenderness, followed rapidly by evidence of spinal cord or cauda equina compression. There may be evidence of an infective focus elsewhere. Plain films will frequently be normal, but may show vertebral or disc space changes suggestive of osteomyelitis.

Inflammatory lesions of the vertebral column can also be demonstrated by CT, as irregular rarefaction of the bone, at a stage when plain films are not clearly abnormal. Extension into the paravertebral soft tissues is also shown more effectively than by plain films, especially in the cervical and lumbosacral regions (Fig. 88.61). These appearances are however not specific, and differentiation of infection from a tumour such as a metastasis is rarely possible, unless the study shows incidental abnormalities (hepatic metastases, renal tuberculosis) which indicate the diagnosis. Intraspinal extension of infection is very difficult to assess without intrathecal contrast medium, but CT can sometimes be a useful adjunct to myelography.

Urgent myelography is indicated in cases of suspected intraspinal abscess, which is usually seen as a posterior

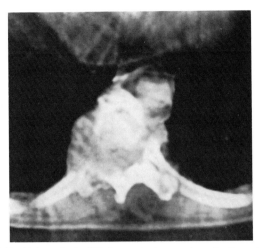

Fig. 88.61 Tuberculosis. CT demonstrates erosion of a thoracic vertebra and the adjacent rib. A soft tissue mass extends on both sides of the spine; intraspinal extension, which is of greater therapeutic importance, is less clearly seen. Note the similarity to malignant disease (Fig. 88.40).

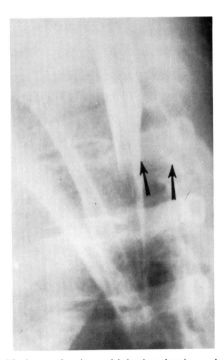

Fig. 88.62 Myelogram by cisternal injection showing a classical epidural abscess, with a tapering, posteriorly situated extradural type lesion [arrows].

extradural lesion, most frequently encountered in the lower thoracic region (Fig. 88.62). The abscess may cause the theca to taper over several segments. Spinal puncture should ideally be well away from the suspected site of the lesion to avoid the possibility of introducing infection into the subarachnoid space.

In extradural abscesses of tuberculous origin, the clinical picture is less dramatic and myelography shows a more focal partial or complete block of extradural type. Plain film abnormalities such as disc collapse, bone erosion and a paraspinal mass are common.

Chronic nonspecific extradural granuloma is a rare condition whose myelographic and operative characteristics are similar to those of a malignant tumour; the diagnosis can only be made histologically.

Myelographic evidence of spinal cord enlargement has been described in association with acute transverse myelitis due to demyelination and necrotizing myelitis, and in the Guillain-Barré syndrome. Large vessels may even be seen on the surface of the cord, so that differentiation from a tumour is difficult. Repeat myelography, showing a decrease in the size of the cord, may indicate the correct diagnosis. A 'contracting cord' has been described in multiple sclerosis [24]. As there is at least a suggestion that patients with this latter disease are more likely to have adverse reactions to myelography, it should probably be avoided if that diagnosis is established.

The very rare intramedullary abscess or granuloma may produce radiological changes indistinguishible from those of an intramedullary tumour; clinical features may be helpful. Inflammatory lesions may be due to schistosomiasis, cysticercosis, hydatid disease, cryptococcus, blastomycosis, coccidioidomycosis and other fungi, or to granulomas such as syphilis or sarcoidosis. The myelographic features are usually nonspecific, and diagnosis rests on other parameters.

TRAUMA

In the large majority of cases of acute spinal trauma where an acute paraplegia has developed, the patient is treated conservatively, to allow the spinal cord maximum potential for recovery. If loss of spinal cord function is complete at 24 hours it is almost certainly irreversible [25], and most radiological procedures are therefore not indicated.

Plain film findings are discussed elsewhere (Ch. 68). Damage to the vertebral column can be detected by CT, although there is little evidence that it contributes substantially to patient management. The presence and nature of fractures of the vertebral bodies and neural arches can be assessed, often more satisfactorily by CT than by plain films or conventional tomograms. Bone fragments within the spinal canal can be identified by CT. Subluxation or dislocation of the posterior intervertebral joints can be assessed, but anterior or posterior displacement is more graphically shown by plain films.

Acute disc protrusion can be demonstrated by CT, and this may be of therapeutic significance, especially in patients with incomplete transection of the cord. Foreign bodies which are not opaque to conventional radiography can also be recognized by CT.

Contrast resolution is often insufficient for demonstration of intramedullary haemorrhage (haematomyelia), but extensive, recent lesions can be detected as circumscribed areas of increased density in the expected position of the cord. Subarachnoid haemorrhage, in which the dense blood outlines the spinal cord in the same way as intrathecal

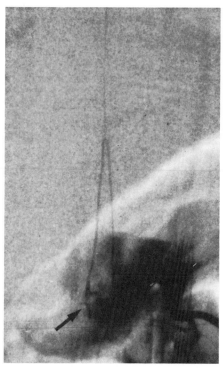

Fig. 88.63 Interruption of the anterior spinal artery [arrow] in a patient who was permanently paraplegic after spinal trauma.

contrast medium, is more easily recognised by CT. Extensive paraspinal or retroperitoneal haemorrhage may be present.

The most common indication for myelography is partial or progressive deterioration of spinal cord function in a patient with normal plain films. It is best carried out by a lateral C1/2 puncture with the patient supine, using water soluble contrast medium. Movement at the fracture site is thereby minimized [26]. The contrast medium outlines the whole spinal canal and allows detection of any encroachment on it from bony fragments, disc herniation, subluxation or haematoma. Water soluble media, unlike oil contrast media, have the advantage that they can safely be used when blood is present in the subarachnoid space, without fear of acute arachnoiditis.

Spinal angiography has been used in the assessment of acute spinal trauma, but there are doubts as to its utility. It can show lesions of the extraspinal vessels or occlusion of the radiculomedullary or spinal arteries (Fig. 88.63). This is a bad prognostic sign, but the converse does not apply; normal or dilated vessels may be seen on the surface of the cord for some time after trauma, without indicating good perfusion and a favourable prognosis (Fig. 88.64). Separated spinal arteries may indicate a swollen cord, due to haematomyelia or contusion.

Brachial plexus injury is most commonly caused by road traffic (particularly motorcycle) or industrial accidents, or by

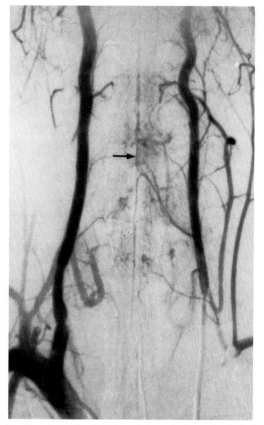

Fig. 88.64 Excellent opacification of the spinal vessels, including the anterior spinal artery [arrow] in a patient who was nevertheless permanently tetraplegic after injury to the cervical spinal cord.

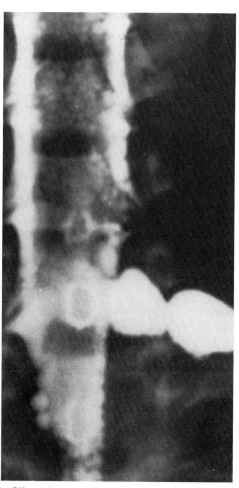

Fig. 88.65 Oil myelogram following brachial plexus injury, showing a typical post-traumatic meningocele.

falls. The roots most frequently detached from the spinal cord are C5 and C6 if the arm is adducted, and C7 to T1 if the arm is abducted at the time of injury.

Trauma results in a tear of the dural and arachnoid covering of the nerve roots, producing a cerebrospinal fluid containing traumatic meningocele, which may be outlined at myelography (Fig. 88.65). Such a meningocele may, however, be present without avulsion of the associated roots [27]. When the roots are avulsed, the normal linear radiolucencies representing the roots are lost (Fig. 88.66). Demonstration of normal roots and root sheaths excludes intrathecal rupture of the nerve fibres and will encourage exploration of the brachial plexus, where a sectioned or injured nerve may be repaired.

The residua of spinal fractures are easily detected by CT. In brachial plexus avulsion, intraspinal abnormalities are not usually evident without intrathecal contrast medium, but a post-traumatic meningocele is seen as a rounded, well circumscribed area of spinal fluid density, extending through a enlarged neural foramen into the paraspinal tissues. With intrathecal contrast medium and CT, loculi unfilled at myelography may be revealed. The spinal cord is often displaced by the intraspinal component of the meningocele, and may be atrophic (Fig. 88.67). Rupture of lumbar nerve roots produces similar appearances, but is much less common.

A small but significant number of patients who are paraplegic following spinal cord injury develop a progressive syndrome of ascending pain and loss of function in one or

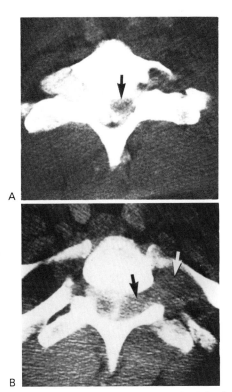

Fig. 88.67A & B Post-traumatic meningocele. CT following metrizamide myelography. (A) The meningocele, full of contrast medium, extends out through an enlarged intervertebral foramen; it displaces the spinal cord [arrow]. (B) At a lower level, an unopacified loculus is revealed [arrows].

both upper limbs [28]. This is due to an intramedullary cavity extending cephalad from the site of trauma, and is usually treated by a syringoperitoneal shunt at the level of the maximum expansion of the cord.

A post-traumatic syrinx of this kind is sometimes visible on CT, as a central lucent area within the cord shadow, but demonstration is not reliable. Bony abnormalities are usually evident at the level of the original injury. It is sometimes possible to show contrast medium within the cord a short time after intrathecal injection, possibly indicating a tear in the substance of the cord. CT may then be of value in demonstrating the extent of the cavity. The myelographic appearances are those of a diffusely swollen cord, with changes of arachnoiditis near the site of injury. As there is often a complete block to contrast medium at the damaged level, the study is carried out by cervical puncture. Endo-myelographic studies have confirmed that the widest part of the syrinx is usually just above the fracture site.

VASCULAR LESIONS

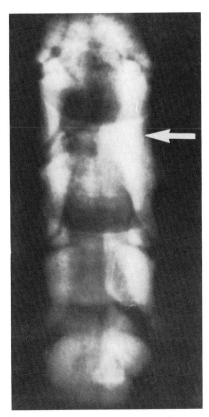

Fig. 88.66 Oil myelogram following brachial plexus injury, showing evidence of nerve root avulsion: absence of the normal linear filling defects due to the nerve rootlets [arrow].

There are two main types of vascular lesion involving the spine: arteriovenous malformations and vascular tumours

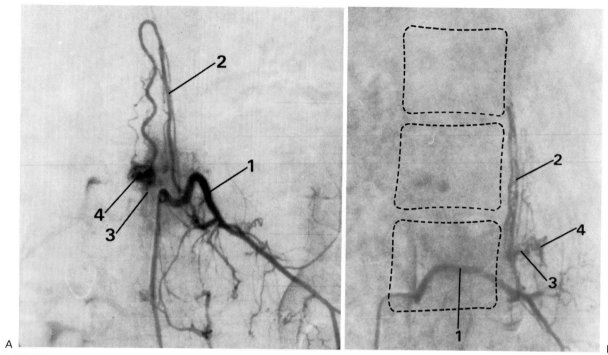

Fig. 88.68A & B   Intramedullary arteriovenous malformation. (A) AP and (B) lateral projections. [1 = intercostal artery; 2 = dilated arteria radicularis magna; 3 = enlarged sulcocommisural arteries feeding malformation (4)].

(haemangioblastoma, or more rarely haemangiopericytoma), which have been the subject of extensive reviews [29].

Spinal arteriovenous malformations (angiomas) appear to fall into two groups, which are distinct as regards their anatomical, haemodynamic and clinical features [30].

1. **Arteriovenous malformations** of the **spinal cord**. This type is commoner in children and young people and more frequently found in the cervical and upper thoracic region than the dural type described below. Subarachnoid haemorrhage is a common presentation.
2. **Arteriovenous malformations** situated in or on the **spinal dura mater**, but draining into the veins of the spinal cord. These lesions, which present in middle age and are commoner in males, are presumed to cause chronic, progressive neurological disturbances by interference with the venous drainage of the cord. The lower thoracic and upper lumbar region is the preferential site.

Plain films are almost always normal, although a rare association with a segmental angiomatosis involving vertebral and/or soft tissue angiomas is recorded.

CT may show irregular, spotty contrast enhancement representing the enlarged draining veins within the spinal canal; in the intramedullary type, this may involve the spinal cord. The contrast enhancement may be marked but is not constant; a spinal arteriovenous malformation cannot be excluded by this technique.

Spinal angiography is essential for confirmation of the diagnosis, presurgical identification of the feeding vessels and the radiculomedullary arteries; therapeutic embolization is also possible. Precise knowledge of the site, blood supply

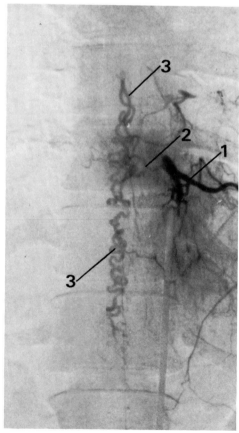

Fig. 88.69   Dural arteriovenous malformation of the spine. [1 = intercostal artery; 2 = site of malformation in intervertebral foramen, i.e. lateral to the spinal cord; 3 = draining veins on cord].

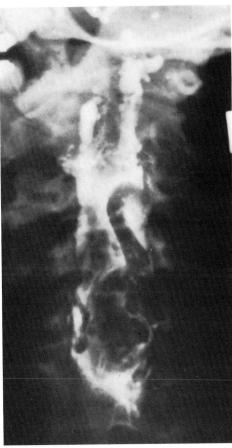

Fig. 88.70 Myelogram showing cervical arteriovenous malformation, with multiple serpiginous filling defects representing hugely dilated draining veins.

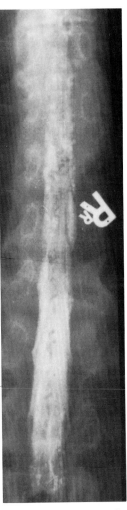

Fig. 88.71 Myelogram showing tortuous vessels on the spinal cord secondary to a dural arteriovenous malformation.

and venous drainage of the lesion is essential for surgical management. Some intramedullary malformations, previously considered inoperable, are now excised via a midline longitudinal cordotomy.

Angiography demonstrates the site of the abnormal arteriovenous communications relative to the spinal cord, showing the contribution of the anterior or posterior radiculomedullary arteries. In some cases, dilated sulcocommissural arteries can be demonstrated, by means of tomography or the lateral projection, confirming the intramedullary location of the lesion (Fig. 88.68). It should be noted that the vessels seen at myelography or CT usually represent the draining veins, and do not give a clear indication of the level of the feeding arteries. Multiple feeding vessels are commonly present in intramedullary malformations, but are rare in the dural type.

Dural malformations are seen at angiography, lying lateral to the presumed position of the spinal cord, often in the neural foramen, as a small knot of vessels, from which dilated veins course into the spinal canal, to lie on the anterior and posterior surfaces of the cord (Fig. 88.69).

Myelography typically shows serpiginous linear filling defects (Figs. 88.70 & 88.71). The spinal cord is usually not expanded. Similar myelographic appearances of tortuous filling defects may, however be found in association with

severe lumbar canal stenosis, vascular tumours or any condition causing obstruction of the subarachnoid space, and may be mimicked by redundant or hypertrophied nerve roots or arachnoiditis.

The exact site and size of the malformation cannot usually be predicted from the myelographic appearances, and spinal angiography is essential if surgery is considered. Fluoroscopy with the patient in the supine position is essential, as the majority of the draining veins lie on the posterior surface of the cord. A water soluble contrast medium should always be used if the diagnosis is suspected: it outlines the cord clearly and, once reabsorbed, it does not interfere with subsequent angiography (unlike iodized oil). Failure to demonstrate abnormal vessels on a myelogram of good quality virtually excludes the diagnosis of arteriovenous malformation.

Complications of arteriovenous malformations which may be shown at myelography include:

1. Subarachnoid haemorrhage, with irregular intradural filling defects representing clot, and subsequent arachnoiditis;
2. An epidural haematoma (rare);
3. Spinal cord swelling, due to haematomyelia;

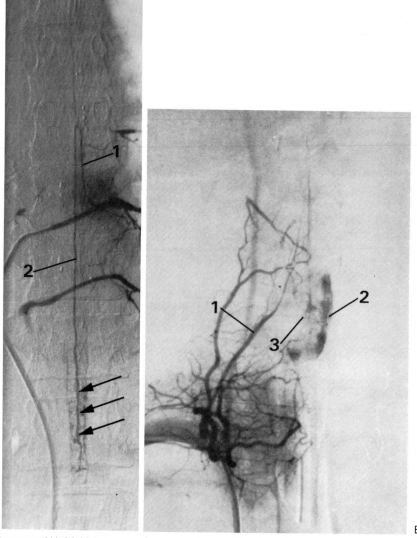

Fig. 88.72A & B Haemangioblastomas. (A) Multiple tumours [arrows] in the von Hippel-Lindau syndrome. [1 = radiculomedullary artery; 2 = dilated anterior spinal artery supplying vascular tumours in the lower extremity of the spinal cord]. (B) Large cervical tumour [1 = hypertrophied branch of ascending cervical artery; 2 = tumour blush; 3 = unopacified portion of the tumour, supplied by other vessels or representing an avascular cyst].

4. Spinal cord or nerve root compression
5. Infection and atrophy of the cord, as a result of chronic ischaemia.

There are recognized associations of spinal arteriovenous malformations with other neural or extraneural vascular anomalies such as vertebral or cutaneous angioma, haemangioblastoma and dysplastic nervous system lesions: spina bifida, syringomyelia.

Haemangioblastomas are intramedullary vascular tumours which may cause extensive cord swelling and expansion of the spinal canal. They may rarely be extramedullary or even extradural. If a large tumour nodule is present, CT may show definite pathological enhancement with intravenous contrast medium; small tumours are very likely to be overlooked however. Intramedullary cysts may be evident on unenhanced CT, while studies with intrathecal contrast medium often show rather widespread expansion of the spinal cord and bony canal, even when angiography subsequently demonstrates a relatively small tumour.

Myelography in cases of haemangioblastoma shows serpiginous filling defects on the surface of an expanded spinal cord. This picture indicates spinal angiography, which is essential for exact location of the lesion, since the cord expansion is much more extensive than the tumour. It shows a well defined tumour blush, without the dilated arteries and draining veins which are a feature of spinal arteriovenous malformations (Fig. 88.72).

BIBLIOGRAPHY

REFERENCES

1. Luken M G, Michelsen W J, Whelan M A, Andrews D L 1981 The diagnosis of sacral lesions. Surg Neurol 15:377–83
2. Haberbeck Modesto M A, Servadei F, Greitz T, Steiner L 1981 Computed tomography for sacral and intracorporeal meningocoeles. Neuroradiology 21:155–58
3. Fitz C R, Harwood Nash D C, Barry J F, Byrd S F, 1977 Pediatric myelography with metrizamide. Acta Radiol Suppl 355:182–93
4. Resjö I M, Harwood Nash D C, Fitz C R, Chuang S 1978 Computed tomographic metrizamide myelography (CTMM) in spinal dysraphism in infants and children. J Comput Assist Tomogr 2:549–58.
5. James M C C, Lassman L P 1981 Spina bifida occulta. Academic Press; London.
6. Raja I A, Hankinson J. Congenital spinal arachnoid cysts 1970 J Neurol Neurosurg Psychiat 33:105–10
7. Gelmers H J, Go K G 1977 Intrasacral meningocoele. Acta Neurochir 39:115–19
8. Grivegnee A, Delince P, Ectors P 1981 Comparative aspects of occult intrasacral meningocoele with conventional X-ray, myelography and CT. Neuroradiology 22:33–37
9. Tarlov I M 1953 Sacral nerve root cysts. Thomas; Springfield
10. Logue V 1971 Syringomyelia: a radiodiagnostic and radiotherapeutic saga. Clin Radiol 22:2–16
11. Bonafé A, Ethier R, Melançon D, Bélanger G, Peters T 1980 High resolution CT in syringomyelia. J Comput Assist Tomogr 4:42–47
12. Poser C M 1956 The relationship between syringomyelia and neoplasm. Thomas, Springfield 1956.
13. McAllister V L 1979 Metrizamide myelography combined with CT scanning in the diagnosis of syringomyelia and the associated Chiari malformation. In: Grainger R G, Lamb J T, (eds) Myelographic techniques with metrizamide. Nyegaard, Birmingham.
14. Aubin M L, Vignaud J, Jardin C, Bar D 1981 Computed tomography in 75 cases of syringomyelia. AJNR 2:199–204
15. Ball M J, Dayan A D 1972 Pathogenesis of syringomyelia. Lancet ii:779–80
16. Dillan J B, Fry J, Kalton E 1966 Acute back syndrome: a study from general practice. Br Med J ii:82
17. Pilling J R 1979 Water soluble radiculography in the erect position. Clin Radiol 30:665–70
18. Théron J, Moret J 1978 Spinal phlebography. Springer, Berlin
19. Sortland O, Magnaes B, Hauge T 1977 Functional myelography with metrizamide in the diagnosis of lumbar canal stenosis. Acta Radiol (suppl) 355:42–54
20. Cook P L, Wise K 1979 The correlation of surgical and radiculographic findings in lumbar disc herniations. Clin Radiol 30:671–82
21. Occleshaw J V 1979 Metrizamide myelography in the lumbar region. In: Grainger R G, Lamb J T (eds) Myelographic techniques with metrizamide. Nyegaard, Birmingham 37–51
22. McAllister V L, Sage M R 1976 The radiology of thoracic disc protrusions. Clin Radiol 27:291–99
23. McAllister V L, Kendall B E, Bull J W D 1975 Symptomatic vertebral haemangiomas. Brain 98:71–80
24. Haughton V M, Ho K C, Boedecker R A 1979 The contracting cord sign of multiple sclerosis. Neuroradiology 17:207–209
25. Braakman R, Penning L 1971 Injuries to the cervical spine. Excerpta Medica, Amsterdam
26. Pay N T, George A E, Benjamin M V, Bergeron T, Lin J P, Kricheff I I 1977 Positive and negative contrast radiography in spinal trauma. Radiology 123:103–111
27. Heon M 1965 Myelogram a questionable aid in diagnosis and prognosis in avulsion of brachial plexus components by traction injuries. Conn Med 29:260
28. Barnett H J M, Jousse A A 1973 Syringomyelia as a late sequel to traumatic paraplegia and quadriplegia: clinical features. In: Barnett H J M, Foster J B, Hudgson P (eds) Syringomyelia. Saunders, Philadelphia
29. Pia H W, Djindjian R 1978 Spinal angiomas; advances in diagnosis and therapy. Springer, Berlin
30. Kendall B E, Logue V 1977 Spinal epidural angiomatous malformations draining into intrathecal veins. Neuroradiology 13:181–89

SUGGESTIONS FOR FURTHER READING

Djindjian R 1970 Angiography of the spinal cord. Masson, Paris
Epstein B S 1976 The spine. Lea and Febiger, Philadelphia
Grainger R G, Lamb J T (eds) Myelographic techniques with metrizamide. Nyegaard, Birmingham.
Jirout J 1969 Pneumomyelography. Thomas, Springfield
Newton T H, Potts D G 1983 Modern neuroradiology, Vol 1: CT of the spine. Clavadel Press, San Francisco
Fischgold H (ed) 1971 Traité de radiodiagnostic. Tome 15. Masson, Paris
Sackett J F, Strother C M 1979 New techniques in myelography. Harper and Row, Hagerston

89 Radionuclide scanning

John C. Harbert

Brain scanning
  Radiopharmaceuticals
  Blood-brain barrier
  Nondiffusable tracers
  Diffusable tracers
  Scan interpretation
  Radionuclide cerebral angiogram

Tumours
  Gliomas
  Meningiomas
  Metastases
  Pituitary tumours
  Cerebellopontine tumours
  Comparison with CT

Inflammatory, cystic and demyelinating lesions

Trauma and lesions of the skull
  Contusions
  Subdural haematoma
  Carotid-carvernous fistulae

Cerebral vascular lesions
  Cerebral infarction
  Hypoperfusion syndromes
  Haemorrhage
  Vascular anomalies
  Comparison with CT scanning

Radionuclide cisternography
  CSF physiology
  Techniques
  Hydrocephalus
  Normal pressure hydrocephalus versus cerebral
    atrophy
  Paediatric cisternography
  Computerised tomography versus radionuclide
    cisternography
  Shunt patency studies
  CSF rhinorrhoea
  Radionuclide ventriculography

BRAIN SCANNING

The role of radionuclide brain scanning has changed appreciably with the remarkable developments in computed tomography (CT). No doubt further changes will result from the current development of magnetic resonance imaging and digital radiography. While the contribution of brain scanning to neurological diagnosis has declined, there remain numerous indications beyond the problem patients who are uncooperative, allergic to iodine or have surgical clips that make CT difficult. These indications include:

1. Detection and localization of primary and recurrent brain tumours.
2. Detection and localization of cerebral infarction, inflammation and intracranial haemorrhage.
3. Diagnosis and followup of congenital structural and vascular malformations.

We will attempt to indicate, wherever known, the relationships between brain scanning, CT and other neurodiagnostic modalities.

Radiopharmaceuticals

Table 89.1 lists the most common brain scanning agents currently used. All of these are nonspecific in that they localize in a wide variety of structural lesions in and around the brain. The mechanism of concentration within a brain lesion varies with the type of molecule and the lesion. In most cases there is probably little binding to identifiable elements within the lesion, but rather a differential rate of concentration occurs whereby transfer of the tracer into the lesion exceeds its clearance. This results in a transiently elevated concentration that permits the lesion's detection against a background of normal brain from which the tracer is excluded. The precise mechanisms of transfer and clearance are poorly understood.

The blood-brain barrier

The brain vasculature effectively excludes most substances that are not highly lipid soluble or not used directly in brain

Table 89.1 Principal non-diffusable brain scanning radiopharmaceuticals

Agent	$T_{\frac{1}{2}}$ physical	Principal gamma emission	Usual adult dose	Usual scan interval	Radiation dose		
					Whole body Gy or Sv	Critical organ mGy/MBq	rad/mCi
	hours	keV	MBq (mCi)	hours			
^{99m}Tc-pertechnetate	6 hours	140	550–750 (15–20)	1–3	0.01	2.7×10^{-5}	(0.1) (colon)
^{99m}Tc-DTPA*	6 hours	140	550–750 (15–20)	2–3	0.01	1.3×10^{-4}	(0.5) (bladder)
^{99m}Tc-glucoheptonate	6 hours	140	550–750 (15–20)	2–3	0.01	1.3×10^{-4}	(0.5) (bladder)
^{113m}In-DTPA	1.7 hours	392	400–550 (10–15)	1–3	0.1	1.6×10^{-4}	(0.6) (bladder)

* diethylenetriaminepentaacetic acid

cellular metabolism. This barrier is both anatomical and metabolic in nature. The capillaries of the brain are lined with endothelial cells which have tight intercellular junctions and a continuous basement membrane that inhibit transfer of most molecules [1,2].

The close approximation of astrocyte foot processes to the capillary basement membrane and groups of glial cells surrounding the capillaries constitute further physical barriers by excluding passive diffusion, pore filtration and cellular pinocytosis.

Certain anatomical and pathophysiological changes occur in brain lesions that permit localizations or abnormal transport of nondiffusible radiopharmaceuticals, and these changes account for 'positive' brain scans. It is simplistic and erroneous to ascribe positive brain scans solely to 'altered blood-brain barrier' (BBB) [3]. Bakay [3] has listed several mechanisms that account for localization of tracer substances in brain tumours, many of which apply equally to other brain lesions:

1. Increased vascularity
2. Abnormal vascular permeability
3. Pinocytosis
4. Enlarged extracellular space and reactive oedema
5. Cellular metabolism.

The uptake of a radiopharmaceutical in a given lesion results from several different processes, which explains why brain lesions accumulate molecules of widely varying size, ionic charge and chemical characteristics.

Blood-brain barrier (nondiffusible) tracers

These tend to be hydrophilic, ionized, protein bound or of large molecular size. All of these characteristics promote vascular retention and prevent crossing the intact blood-brain barrier. All of the tracers listed in Table 89.1 fall into this category.

Technetium-99 labelled chelates, particularly ^{99m}Tc-DTPA and glucoheptonate have largely supplanted ^{99m}Tc-pertechnetate as the most commonly used brain imaging radiopharmaceuticals because their higher rates of renal clearance result in reduced blood background and higher lesion-to-

brain ratios. This is especially important in lesions with low tracer uptake such as well differentiated gliomas, recent infarcts and lesions adjacent to vascular structures such as basal tumours, craniopharyngiomas and cerebellar tumours. The optimum scan interval for ^{99m}Tc-DTPA is longer (180 minutes) than ^{99m}Tc-glucoheptonate (90 minutes) but the radiation absorbed dose to the kidneys is four times higher with glucoheptonate [4].

^{113m}In-DTPA is primarily used in regions far from centres of commercial radionuclide production. The ^{113}Sn-^{113m}In generator needs to be replaced only a few times a year and provides a convenient source of short-lived radionuclide, the chemistry of which is well understood.

Diffusible tracers

Greatly renewed interest has developed for tracers capable of crossing the intact blood-brain barrier either by passive diffusion or active transport. Scanning with diffusible tracers offers the potential of mapping regions of altered blood flow and metabolism. The concomitant development of emission computed tomographic (ECT) scanners promises to yield greater information from these studies.

Diffusible tracers tend to be neutral, lipophilic substances that are almost completely cleared from the blood in a single pass through the brain. This requires low plasma protein binding and an octonol/water partition coefficient greater than about 0.5 [5]. The first of such tracers was ^{123}I-iodoantipyrine [6]. While this tracer is initially distributed according to regional cerebral blood flow (rCBF), it recirculates and is soon distributed according to brain volume.

A much more interesting and potentially useful tracer is ^{123}I-iodoamphetamine (IMP). The first-pass extraction efficiency is high, the washout is slow and the blood-brain ratios are high. Furthermore, the scanning properties of ^{123}I ($T_{\frac{1}{2}}$ = 13 hours, 150 keV photon) are favourable. Kuhl et al [7] have demonstrated well-resolved tomographic brain images using single photon emission computed tomography (SPECT) and good quantitative correlations with cerebral blood flow measurements.

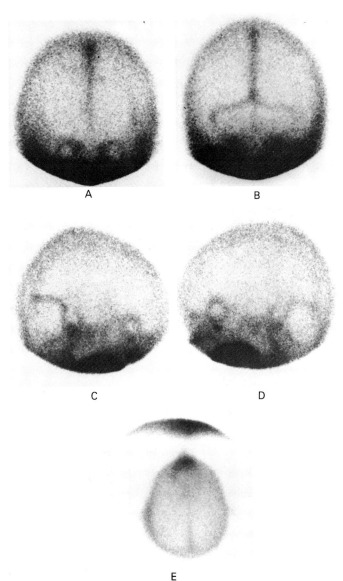

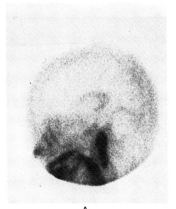

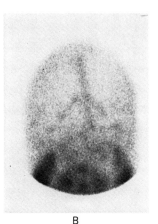

Fig. 89.2A & B Choroid plexus visualized with ^{99m}Tc-pertechnetate (without perchlorate blocking) (A) Left lateral. (B) Posterior slightly rotated to the left. Choroid plexus and salivary gland uptake

Fig. 89.1A–E Normal ^{99m}Tc-DTPA brain scans. (A) Anterior. (B) Posterior. (C) Left lateral. (D) Right lateral. (E) Vertex.

Scan interpretation

Figure 89.1 shows the five normal static brain scan views using ^{99m}Tc-DTPA. The vertex is usually obtained only to delineate superiorly located lesions or to compare periventricular lesions with CT. Normal cerebrum and cerebellum exclude non-diffusable tracers, while the cranial and vascular structures contain relatively high activity. Several variations may be seen:

Asymmetric transverse sinus is a frequent variation. The right transverse sinus is usually more prominent than the left. Enlargement of the left transverse sinus (30% of scans) is frequently associated with enlargement of the midline *occipital* sinus [8]. This must not be mistaken for a midline vermis tumour.

A *thick skull* (cranial hyperostosis) may give the appearance of symmetrical widening of the marginal rim of activity. In the lateral view, a thick skull may appear as two parallel bands of activity running the length of the superior longitudinal sinus. The skull radiograph usually confirms the true nature of this variation.

Choroid plexus. Pertechnetate is secreted by the choroid plexus (Fig. 89.2), salivary glands and nasal mucosa as well as the thyroid and stomach. Choroid plexus uptake is blocked by administering 500 mg potassium perchlorate or 10 drops of Lugol's iodine solution. Visualization of lateral ventricles after blocking doses, or whenever a chelate tracer is used has pathological significance. Among the causes are: ventriculitis, choroid plexus papilloma and ependymal metastases.

DTPA is not concentrated by the choroid plexus in significant amounts.

Malposition of the head is a common and serious cause of variation, particularly in the lateral view. If the forehead is tilted away from the detector, the anterior landmarks are blurred and the posterior rim of activity may appear as a double line of activity. If the occiput is tilted away from the detector, the transverse sinus is blurred. Head rotation increases the apparent thickness of activity on the side closer to the detector — a phenomenon that could be confused with a subdural haematoma (Figs. 89.2B & 89.10A). The usual clue to the presence of rotation is that the irregularity is seen in only one view or the sagittal sinus is not in the midline. Repeat views resolve this problem.

Brain scans performed soon after the administration of *intra-arterial contrast agents* must be interpreted with caution because they may cause transient alteration in the BBB and increased extracerebral capillary permeability, particularly if only one carotid artery has been injected [9].

Various drugs, especially chemotherapeutic agents, may produce unexpected changes in the brain scan appearance [10].

Radionuclide cerebral angiogram[11,12]

The radionuclide cerebral angiogram, or 'dynamic flow study' is usually performed in the anterior position, but

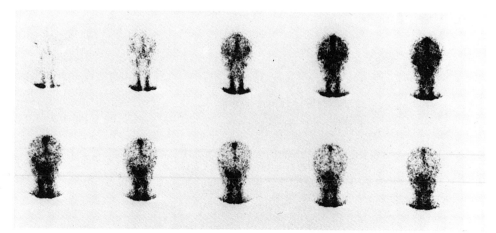

Fig. 89.3 Normal radionuclide cerebral angiogram. Each frame is 2 seconds in duration. Study begins in upper left frame.

posterior, lateral or vertex positions may provide better definition if the probable site of lesion is known before the examination. Images are collected at 2 to 3 second intervals by a multi-imaging device or computer. Figure 89.3 demonstrates a normal dynamic study in the anterior view. Three phases can be recognized. During the *arterial phase*, a five-pointed star pattern is formed by the two carotid arteries, the two middle cerebral arteries, and the combined anterior cerebral arteries. During the *capillary phase*, activity within the hemispheres becomes uniformly distributed. This is followed by a *venous phase* during which activity in the venous sinuses prevails. The radionuclide angiogram should form an integral part of the brain scan because it increases both the sensitivity and specificity of the test. It is of particular value in evaluating (1) arteriovenous malformations that may not be evident in the static images, (2) cerebral infarctions that may not become positive for 7 to 14 days following CVA, (3) subdural and epidural haematomas, and (4) cerebral death where internal carotid flow is absent.

TUMOURS

With current radiopharmaceutical imaging techniques, tumours of 1 cm or greater can usually be visualized. Smaller tumours are detected if associated haemorrhage or reactive oedema occurs.

Tables 89.2 and 89.3 indicate the frequency of the different intracranial tumours encountered in radionuclide scanning in adults and children.

Gliomas

Glial cell tumours are the most common tumours in both children and adults. They comprise a variety of cell types and

Table 89.2 Incidence and results of radionuclide imaging in 2551 adult brain tumours.
Modified from Schall and Quinn [11].

Type	Incidence %	% True positive
Gliomas	40–45	
glioblastoma	13–17	93
astrocytoma	7–9	73
oligodendroglioma	6–8	93
medulloblastoma	4–5	63
ependymoma	4–5	72
miscellaneous	6–7	
Meningioma	15–18	93
Metastasis	10–12	84
Pituitary adenoma	10–12	72
Craniopharyngioma	3–4	35
Acoustic neurinoma	6–7	66
Other	13–17	62
		Mean 84

Table 89.3 Incidence and results of radionuclide imaging in 422 brain tumours in children.
Modified from Conway [12].

Type	Incidence %	% True positive
Gliomas	81	
glioblastoma	7	100
astrocytoma	30	86
oligodendroglioma	0.5	100
medulloblastoma	18	63
ependymoma	7	69
brain stem glioma	13.5	38
miscellaneous	5	80
Meningioma	2	100
Metastasis	2.5	90
Pituitary adenoma	7	38
Others	7.5	
pinealoma	1	75
papilloma	0.8	100
sarcoma	3	100
miscellaneous	2.7	
	Total 100	Mean 73

RADIONUCLIDE SCANNING 1861

malignant potential. *Glioblastomas* are characterized by extensive neovascularization, mitosis and necrosis. They are the most aggressive of the glial tumours and confer a poor 5-year survival. The brain scan appearance is highly variable, probably due to their mosaicism. The distribution of activity is often irregular, often crosses arterial supplies and occasionally extends into the opposite hemisphere ('butterfly glioma'). Gliomas tend to outgrow their vascular supply, which results in central necrosis and causes the 'doughnut' sign, a rim of increased activity surrounding a colder centre (Fig. 89.4). This doughnut appearance is found in several

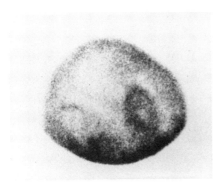

Fig. 89.4 Glioblastoma multiforme. Doughnut sign in right lateral view.

other conditions, including abscesses, subdural haematomas and skull lesions. The radionuclide angiogram often demonstrates increased vascularity.

Cystic astrocytomas are the most common brain tumour of childhood and generally arise in the cerebellum. The combination of a positive brain scan and the characteristic CT findings of cystic lesion with eccentric plaque is usually diagnostic. Well differentiated astrocytomas, grades 1 and 2, may be associated with negative brain scans because they produce little blood-brain alteration.

Oligodendrogliomas are usually small, discrete and located within the cerebral hemispheres (Fig. 89.5).

Ependymomas and medulloblastomas usually arise in the posterior fossa, particularly in the fourth ventricle which they

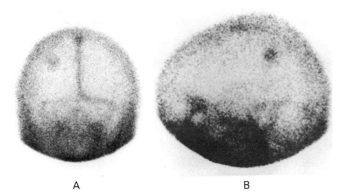

Fig. 89.5A & B Solitary left parietal oligodendroglioma. (A) Posterior. The larger right transverse sinus is a normal variation. (B) Left lateral.

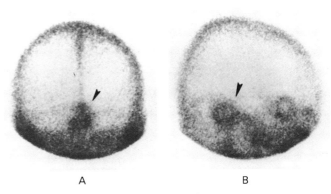

Fig. 89.6A & B Fourth ventricular ependymoma presents as a midline lesion in the anterior portion of the posterior fossa [arrows]. (A) Posterior. (B) Right lateral.

may obstruct, causing hydrocephalus. These tumours usually appear as a midline posterior fossa lesion (Fig. 89.6), and are rare in adults but account for 20% of tumours in children.

Meningiomas

Meningiomas are most often located parasagittally (27%). along the sphenoid wings (17%), on the convexity surfaces (17%), the floor of the anterior or posterior fossa (25%) and the falx (7%) [13]. They are often quite vascular and cause a blush on the radionuclide cerebral angiogram (Fig. 89.7), although the absence of this sign by no means rules out a meningioma. They may be associated with regional hyperostosis, are generally enhanced with contrast on CT, and are seen angiographically to derive their blood supply from branches of both the internal and external carotid arteries. The brain scan is positive in more than 90% of meningiomas, the accuracy varying according to location and vascularity. The most difficult to detect are small plaque-like meningiomas situated close to normal vascular structures.

Metastases

Brain metastases most frequently develop from carcinomas of lung, breast, kidney and from melanomas. They are often multiple (Fig. 89.8), but when solitary are indistinguishable from primary brain tumours. Most patients with metastases large enough to image by brain scanning have neurological symptoms. In asymptomatic patients, the brain scan is not a productive screening test.

Brain metastases are usually supratentorial and subcortical. When they occur in the cerebellum, they are usually peripheral, seldom in the midline.

Pituitary tumours

Pituitary adenomas and craniopharyngiomas are generally small, and the normally high activity at the base of the brain

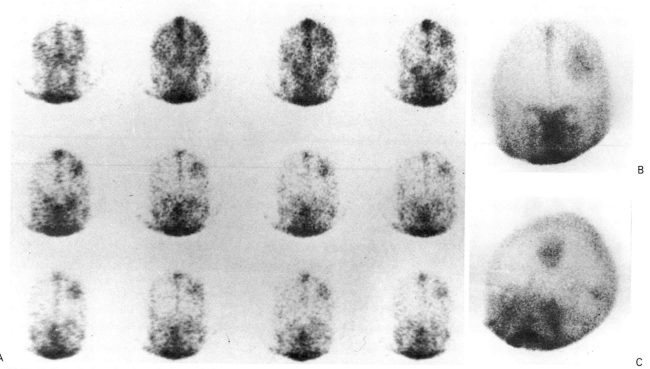

Fig. 89.7A, B & C Left parietal meningioma. (A) Posterior view Radionuclide cerebral angiogram showing progressive increase in activity. (B) Anterior. (C) Left lateral.

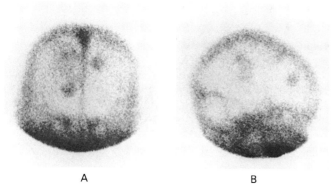

Fig. 89.8 Multiple metastases; (A) anterior view. (B) Lateral

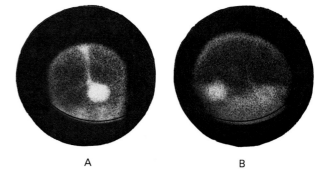

Fig. 89.9A & B Cerebellopontine angle tumour (^{99m}Tc-DTPA). (A) Posterior. (B) Right lateral.

makes them difficult to detect. CT scanning is much more successful than radiopharmaceutical scanning.

Cerebellopontine angle tumours

These may be demonstrable by brain scanning when they exceed 1.5 cm in size (Fig. 89.9).

Comparison with CT

CT has an overall sensitivity of 93 to 98%, and about 90%

specificity for detecting intracranial tumours [14,15]. Brain radiopharmaceutical scanning has a sensitivity of 75 to 93% and considerably lower specificity [14,15,16,17]. CT is clearly the first diagnostic procedure of choice when an intracranial mass lesion is suspected. Brain isotope scanning is useful when:

1. CT is negative but the clinical suspicion of tumour is high.
2. Technical problems prevent optimum CT images, e.g., excessive movement, surgical clips, iodine sensitivity.
3. There is uncertainty whether a lesion represents tumour or another lesion, e.g., cerebral infarcts.

It is too early to evaluate the impact of ECT scanning on brain tumour diagnosis. Lesions located near bone and vascular structures are more apparent, but early comparative studies, using first-generation ECT scanners and conventional tracers have shown little advantage over conventional scanning [18].

INFLAMMATORY, CYSTIC AND DEMYELINATING LESIONS

The brain isotope scan is useful in the differential diagnosis of meningoencephalitis by excluding the presence of a focal purulent collection that signals the need for surgical intervention. Brain scanning is highly sensitive for detecting abscesses. Four independent series have reported 100% accuracy in localizing abscesses [18,19,20,21]. A 'doughnut' sign (Fig. 89.4) is seen when a significant volume of nonvascular purulent material is surrounded by oedema and neovascularity. In serial brain scans, regression of lesion size is considerably slower than regression of clinical symptoms.

The scintigraphic characteristics of granulomas are similar to those of abscesses, although generally without a central photon-deficient region. Positive brain scans are also found in various focal inflammatory diseases such as Herpes simplex, sarcoidosis and tuberculosis. A positive brain scan in these diseases appears to signify a localized process of especially intense reaction.

Encephalitis and meningitis commonly produce diffusely increased activity over the convexities or throughout both hemispheres. These patterns may be mistaken for bilateral subdural haematomas, although the clinical picture seldom causes confusion.

Cystic lesions have a variety of causes (trauma, infections, haemorrhage) and may be congenital or acquired. While brain cysts are common, those that produce symptoms are rare. An example is cystic hygroma which occurs after intracranial trauma or haemorrhage. Radionuclide brain scanning has little role in the diagnosis of cystic lesions of the brain because CT is more accurate.

Focal brain scan lesions have been reported in some demyelinating diseases including multiple sclerosis [22], Schilder's disease [23] and adrenoleukodystrophy [24].

TRAUMA AND LESIONS OF THE SKULL

Head trauma may produce both intracranial and extracranial lesions and thus a variety of abnormal brain scan patterns. Care must be exercised when interpreting these studies because without tomographic projections it is difficult to distinguish between superficial, bony and intracerebral lesions. Skull fractures, skull metastases and craniotomy lesions are generally evident radiologically, and superficial soft tissue lesions (e.g. lacerations and haematomas) are clinically apparent.

Lesions that cause increased tracer uptake, either focal or generalized include:
1. **Extracranial lesions**
   scalp contusion, laceration, and haematoma
   surgical incision
   subgaleal haematoma
   dermal neoplasm
2. **Skull lesions**
   craniotomy and burr holes
   fibrous dysplasia
   Paget's disease
   hyperostosis frontalis
   sickle cell disease
   neoplasms, especially skull metastases
   granulomata
   osteomyelitis
3. **Intracranial lesions**
   subdural haematoma
   epidural haematoma
   cerebral contusion
   meningitis
   subarachnoid cyst
   leptomeningeal cyst
   Sturge-Weber disease
   neoplasm

Cerebral contusions

While frequently positive on radionuclide brain scanning, often they cannot be distinguished from associated superficial trauma.

Subdural haematomas

These result from rupture of veins that bridge the cerebral hemispheres and veins that insert into the dural sinuses, which remain fixed at the time of injury. These haemorrhages do not generally become apparent on static brain scans earlier than 7 to 10 days after the injury, at which time oedema, new vessel formation, and other factors create a peripheral crescentic or lenticular lesion with increased uptake that may persist for several months (Fig. 89.10).

The sensitivity of brain scanning for chronic subdural haematomas is about 80% [25]. Using dynamic as well as early and late (3 to 4 hour) static images, Razzak et al [26] reported 92% sensitivity without regard to the age of the lesion. In the same series, only 52% of subdural haematomas were detected by CT as a secondary ventricular shift. Haematomas that elude detection by CT are usually bilateral isodense collections that produce no ventricular shift, or small (less than 45 ml) unilateral, isodense lesions.

Carotid-cavernous fistula

The radionuclide angiogram is useful both to identify the lesion and to assess the results of therapy.

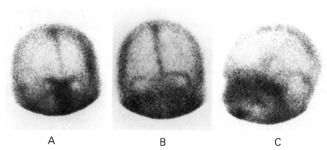

Fig. 89.10A, B & C Subdural haematoma (⁹⁹ᵐTc-DTPA).
Radionuclide cerebral angiogram showed diminished left peripheral
perfusion, (Anterior view). Static images (A) anterior, (B) posterior &
(C) lateral demonstrate increased activity along the left convexity.

CEREBRAL VASCULAR LESIONS

Cerebral vascular accidents (CVA), also called 'strokes', are
the third most common cause of death in the industrialized
world.

Cerebral infarction

Cerebral infarctions are classified as ischaemic or haemorrhagic, a distinction important to treatment and prognosis.
Thrombosis generally leads to ischaemic infarction. Less
frequently, infarction results from emboli arising from
carotid atheroma or from thrombi on the walls and valves of
the heart. Emboli more often give rise to haemorrhagic
infarction.

Infarctions may result from a failure of cerebral blood flow
due to a fall in blood pressure, a change in calibre of the
arterial lumen, altered vascular permeability, increased
blood viscosity and hypoxia. As cardiopulmonary resuscitat-
ive measures have improved, these hypoperfusion syndromes
and ischaemic cerebral infarctions have increased.

The anatomical basis for the scintigraphic patterns found
in cerebral infarction is shown in Figure 89.11. It is useful
to compare this figure with examples of infarcts presented
in Figures 89.12 to 89.15. The scan pattern of ischaemic
infarction evolves slowly. In the first week after the onset
of symptoms only 21 to 27% of the static scans are
positive [27]. In the second week, 24 to 71% become
positive, owing to neovascularization. In the third week,
over 75% become positive, falling to 50 to 70% in the
fourth week and progressively diminishing thereafter.

Occlusion of the anterior cerebral artery, often due to
embolism, causes infarction of the frontal lobe and the
paramedian convolutions of the frontal and parietal lobes
above the corpus callosum (Fig. 89.12).

Infarction in the distribution of the posterior cerebral
artery involves the medial occipital lobe, parts of the
temporal lobe, and thalamus. Occlusions of the occipital
branches of the posterior cerebral artery produce
parasagittal lesions (Fig. 89.13A). Occlusions of the
temporal branches produce lesions located along the
tentorium (Fig. 89.13B) while combinations of the two may
produce a so called 'hockey stick' lesion [27]. Occlusions of

REGIONAL CORTICAL DISTRIBUTION OF THE CEREBRAL ARTERIES

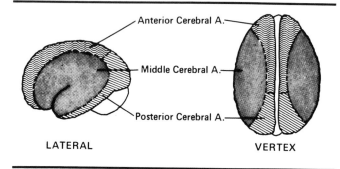

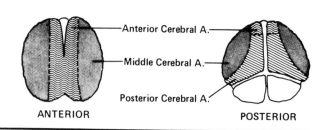

Fig. 89.11 Distribution of cerebral artery perfusion.

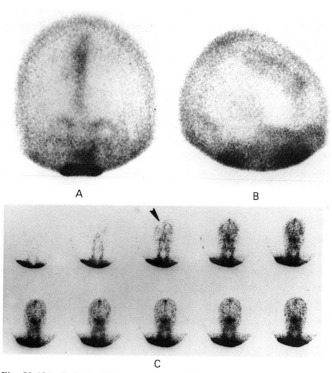

Fig. 89.12A, B & C Right anterior cerebral infarction. (A) Anterior.
(B) Right lateral showing increased uptake. (C) Radionuclide
angiogram demonstrating diminished right anterior cerebral flow in
early arterial phase [arrow].

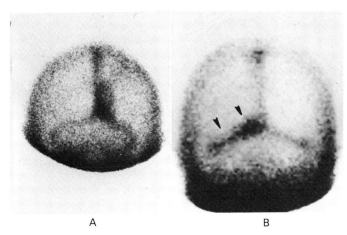

Fig. 89.13A & B Posterior cerebral artery infarction. (A) Posterior view showing involvement of occipital and thalamic branches of the right posterior cerebral artery. (B) Infarction of the left temporal branches.

the posterior cerebellar arteries are rare and are best differentiated from tumour by a combination of CT and radionuclide scanning.

Infarction in the distribution of the middle cerebral artery is most common and produces various scan patterns depending upon the location and extent of the obstruction and upon collateral circulation. A proximal carotid arterial obstruction with poor collateral circulation may involve the basal ganglia and parts of the cerebral cortex in all four lobes.

The radionuclide angiogram is most useful in the early stages of infarction when it may show diminished blood flow to the affected region before the static images become positive. Cowan et al [28] found this pattern in 23% of cases while in only 8% was the reverse true. The radionuclide angiogram is more often positive at all stages in the early evolution of infarcts. Often a so called 'flip-flop' phenomenon is observed (Fig. 89.14) i.e. decreased perfusion in the early arterial phase, equalization of activity during the capillary phase, followed by relatively increased activity during the venous phase. This variation in activity is thought to be caused by slower entry and washout of the tracer in the involved area due to collateral circulation.

Differences of 1 mm diameter of the internal carotid arteries are sufficient for detection by dynamic flow scanning [29].

Infarction is occasionally caused by thrombosis of the dural sinuses or major cortical veins, e.g. in mastoiditis, trauma, endocarditis and hypercoagulability states.

Hypoperfusion syndromes

Infarction may occur as a result of lowered blood pressure, anoxia or extracranial vessel occlusion despite normal cerebral vasculature. The two types of infarction generally encountered are *laminar cortical necrosis* and so called *'watershed'* infarction.

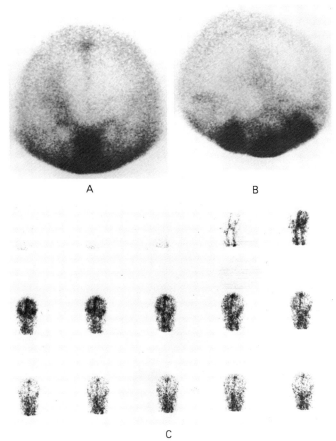

Fig. 89.14A, B & C Right middle cerebral artery occlusion and infarction (^{99m}Tc-DTPA). (A) Anterior. (B) Right lateral showing increased uptake. (C) Radionuclide angiogram showing 'flip-flop' phenomenon.

Laminar necrosis develops when brain anoxia occurs only long enough to destroy the most sensitive layers of the brain, usually layers 3 and 4. The layers superficial and deep to these remain viable. The resulting brain scan pattern varies depending upon the artery involved and upon the extent of necrosis. Hawes and Mishkin [30] described a crescentric pattern extending along the affected branches. Laminar necrosis is associated with cardiac and respiratory arrest, anaesthetic accidents, convulsions and even hypoglycaemia.

Watershed infarcts occur at the junction between major cerebral arterial distributions. Figure 89.15 shows a watershed infarct along the boundary between the right middle and anterior cerebral arterial distributions. These lesions follow the same pattern of evolution described above. The radionuclide angiogram is usually normal unless there have been previous strokes.

Haemorrhage

Approximately 12% of CVA's are caused by haemorrhage, either intracerebral or subarachnoid. Generally the static brain scans do not become positive before 7 to 10 days following the stroke. This fact and the excellent resolution

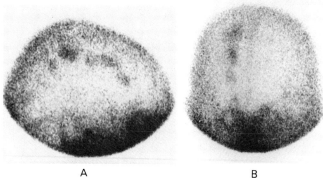

Fig. 89.15A & B 'Watershed infarct'. Multiple focal lesions along the margins of arterial distributions (A) Right lateral. (B) Anterior. Compare with Figure 89.11. This infarction followed cardiac arrest and resuscitation.

of these lesions by CT limit the role of brain scanning in their diagnosis.

Vascular anomalies

The two principal cerebral vascular anomalies are *aneurysms* and *vascular malformations*.

Vascular malformations of the central nervous system are of four types: arteriovenous malformations, capillary telangiectasia, cavernous angiomas and venous angiomas. The most common are arteriovenous malformations (AVM). They produce an early 'blush' of activity during the arterial phase of the radionuclide angiogram that persists into the capillary and venous phases (Fig. 89.16). Radionuclide angiography is also useful to follow AVMs and meningiomas after artificial embolization procedures[31].

Comparison with CT scanning

CT has greatly increased the radiologist's role in the diagnosis and differential diagnosis of stroke while diminishing the need for radionuclide scanning. The proportion of abnormal CT studies during the first 28 days of stroke is approximately the same as with radionuclide scans.

On the other hand, in many patients, the CT findings are equivocal, particularly if previous infarction has occurred. The low density lesions visualized on CT scans within the first 72 hours of infarction may develop into encephalomalacia causing a persistent low density, making the two indistinguishable. The important differentiation between recent and remote infarct is better made by radionuclide scanning. Furthermore, identical findings are found in the two studies in only about 45% of patients: the studies are more complementary than alternative. Intravenous contrast media used for CT may adversely affect the stroke patient.[32]

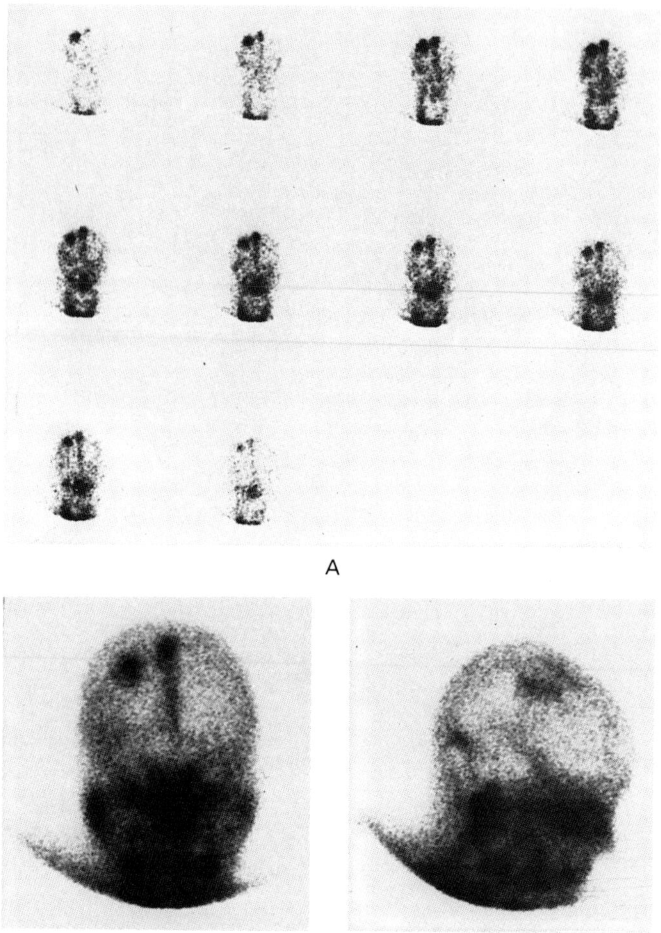

Fig. 89.16A, B & C Arteriovenous malformation. (A) Radionuclide cerebral angiogram showing arterial blush, which fades in the venous phase. (B) Early anterior. (C) Early right lateral. Note prominent draining veins.

RADIONUCLIDE CISTERNOGRAPHY

CSF physiology

CSF is produced by the choroid plexus, ventricular ependyma, and the arachnoid by both active secretion and passive diffusion, and flows out of the fourth ventricular foramina into the subarachnoid spaces. Some of the CSF flows downwards to bathe the spinal cord; the remainder ascends through the incisura, over the cerebral convexities, and drains by bulk flow through the arachnoid villi into the superior longitudinal sinus (Fig. 89.17). The rate of CSF production in adults is approximately 0.4 ml/minute and is largely independent of CSF pressure, a critical factor in the production of hydrocephalus. The chief clinical

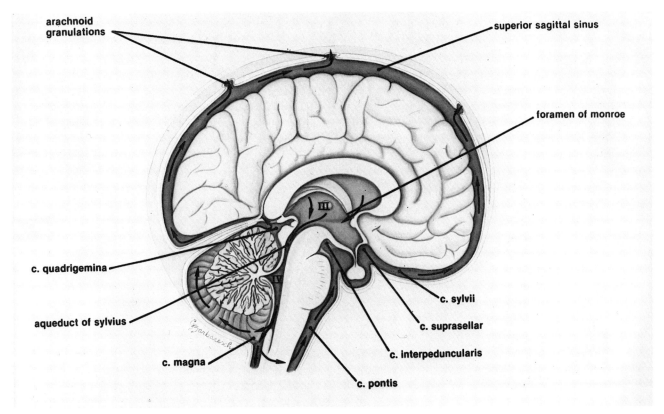

Fig. 89.17 Cerebrospinal fluid circulation.

Table 89.4 Properties of CSF tracers.

| Radiopharmaceutical | Usual dose | | Photon energy | CSF $T\frac{1}{2}$ effective hours | Radiation dose | | | |
	MBq	μCi	MeV		Spinal cord* mGy	rads	Whole body mGy	rads
^{131}I-HSA	4	100	0.364	24	60–180	(6–18)	1.7	(0.17)
^{99m}Tc-HSA	37	1000	0.140	5	20–50	(2–5)	0.3	(0.03)
^{111}In-transferrin	20	500	0.173, 0.247	21	70	(7)	2.6	(0.26)
^{111}In-DTPA or EDTA	20	500	0.173, 0.247	10	20	(2)	0.4	(0.04)
^{169}Yb-DTPA	20	500	0.177–0.198	12	60–250	(6–25)	0.7	(0.07)

* Surface dose to spinal cord at injection site in patients without CSF block

concerns of this 'third circulation' are with obstruction and leakage. The radionuclide tests discussed here involve the identification and localization of these two problems.

Techniques

Usually the radiopharmaceutical is injected into the lumbar subarachnoid space, although cisterna magna and intraventricular injections are occasionally required. Some acceptable radiopharmaceuticals, along with their properties and usual adult dosages are listed in Table 89.4. ^{111}In-DTPA and ^{99m}Tc-DTPA are the most commonly used.

A scintillation camera is preferred for serial cisternographic images. Positioning is simple and scintiphotos can be completed in 1 to 3 minutes. Good quality images are obtained with 30 000 to 50 000 counts.

The usual scanning sequence is 1, 3, 6, 24 and 48 hours after injection. Early scans are important because ventricular reflux, the hallmark of obstructive communicating hydrocephalus is usually visualized early if it occurs at all. This reflux is especially important with children and infants where the ascent of CSF through the head is more rapid. The 48-hour scans are of interest in delineating porencephalic and subarachnoid block in patients with a 'delayed clearance' pattern as in cerebral atrophy.

Hydrocephalus

Hydrocephalus is a pathologic increase in the CSF volume associated with enlargement of the ventricles.
1. *Obstructive hydrocephalus*

(a) Noncommunicating (the ventricles do not communicate with the subarachnoid space) — obstruction occurs between lateral ventricles and basal cisterns.
(b) Communicating — obstruction occurs in basal cisterns, cerebral convexities, or arachnoid villi.

2. *Nonobstructive hydrocephalus*
   (a) Generalized — due to cerebral atrophy (hydrocephalus ex vacuo)
   (b) Localized — due to porencephaly of any cause.

Both Hakim et al [33] and Ommaya et al [34] have described the pathogenesis of obstructive hydrocephalus. Some precipitating event such as haemorrhage, gliosis, infection or tumour blocks the CSF pathways. CSF formation continues undiminished, raising CSF pressure. As CSF volume increases and CSF pressure rises above venous pressure. intracranial venous vascular volume decreases. Ultimately, interstitial water and cellular lipids are lost as the ventricles continue to expand. Alterations in the ventricular ependyma develop, so that the capillaries in the deep periventricular white matter become the principal site of CSF absorption, causing an apparent reversal of normal CSF flow. If equilibrium is re-established before brain hypoxia develops, **'compensated hydrocephalus'** exists, often without symptoms. If ventricular expansion continues, however, progressive loss of brain substance occurs with characteristic progression of symptoms.

The cisternographic changes observed in hydrocephalus are best understood by considering the *normal* pattern (Figs 89.18 & 89.20). By 1 to 3 hours, the basal cisterns are visualized. Only the cisterna magna and quadrigeminal cistern are distinctly visualized. The pontine, interpeduncular, and suprasellar cisterns cannot be separately distinguished. By 3

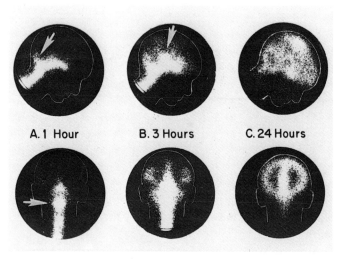

Fig. 89.18 Normal cisternogram showing right lateral (top) and posterior views. At 1 hour the cisterna magna [arrows] and basal cisterns are filled. By 3 hours the large quadrigeminal cistern [arrow] is visible and activity is entering the sylvian fissures. In the posterior view the interhemispheric fissure is well defined. By 24 hours activity is distributed completely over the convexities and has largely cleared from the basal cisterns.

to 6 hours, activity has entered the sylvian and interhemispheric fissures. By 24 hours, the activity surrounds the hemispheres. Because of radiopharmaceutical diffusion into the cerebral cortex, images after 24 hours increasingly reflect cerebral tissues rather than CSF spaces and this residual tracer clears slowly. At *no* time is activity normally seen within the ventricles.

The changes in the cisternographic pattern found in hydrocephalus relate only to the presence or absence of ventricular reflux and the relative rate of CSF clearance. In obstructive communicating hydrocephalus there is ventricular reflux and delayed clearance (Fig. 89.19). In noncommunicating hydrocephalus, the cisternographic pattern is normal or there may be delayed clearance, but there is no ventricular reflux.

Normal pressure hydrocephalus versus cerebral atrophy

After Hakim [33] first described the syndrome of normal pressure hydrocephalus (NPH), an enthusiastic effort was directed toward finding better methods for its diagnosis because it is one of the few treatable presenile dementias. NPH is not essentially different from obstructive communicating hydrocephalus with elevated pressure in regard to cause and cisternographic findings. Why the pressure is normal or only slightly elevated in NPH is not perfectly understood.

Massively enlarged ventricles may be seen with only slightly elevated CSF pressure. Short of spontaneous remission, the only possibility for reversal is by operative diversionary shunting. The symptoms associated with NPH are dementia, spastic gait and urinary incontinence, progressing to coma. CT shows ventricular dilatation with little cortical atrophy.

Bannister et al [35] first recognized the cisternographic pattern of ventricular reflux and delayed clearance. Ependymal (and/or choroid plexus) reabsorption draws CSF into the ventricle where it clears, although more slowly than by the normal convexity route. Obstruction can occur anywhere within the subarachnoid space, which accounts for the varying cisternographic patterns described in this disease. Obstruction at the level of the basal cisterns or the incisura is shown in Figure 89.19. The CSF resorptive area is considerably reduced, resulting in greatly enlarged ventricles. This pattern is most often associated with clinical improvement following diversionary shunting. If the mechanical block is higher over the convexity, a 'combination' pattern is seen (i.e. ventricular reflux and variable but delayed flow over the convexities). In this case, the prognosis following shunting is more difficult to predict. Individual patient circumstances determine whether the patient should be shunted.

Cerebral atrophy or hydrocephalus ex vacuo results from a loss of brain substance by degenerative processes rather than by pressure expansion. The symptoms associated with cerebral atrophy are often identical to those of normal pressure hydrocephalus. CT scans in atrophy demonstrate enlarged ventricles and dilated sulci and fissures (Ch. 85).

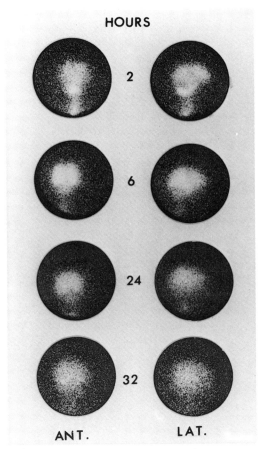

HOURS

2

6

24

32

ANT.   LAT.

Fig. 89.19 Communicating hydrocephalus with complete incisural block. Ventricular reflux is seen in all views. No activity ascends over the convexities. Note blurring of ventricular outline after 24 hours caused by diffusion of ^{111}In-DTPA into cerebral tissue.

The most common cisternographic pattern is normal or delayed tracer ascent without ventricular reflux. Transient ventricular reflux, when it occurs, does not usually persist at 24 hours.

Paediatric cisternography

In children, the normal cisternographic pattern is similar to that of adults (Fig. 89.20) except that CSF clearance is more rapid. Activity reaches the basal cisterns by 15 to 30 minutes and surrounds the convexities by 12 hours. In noncommunicating hydrocephalus, the usual sites of obstruction are the aqueduct and the outlets of the fourth ventricle. These infants require diversionary shunting. If a ventriculocisternal shunt is contemplated, the neurosurgeon must assure himself that the CSF pathways over the convexities are patent. These patients ordinarily have increased intracranial pressure and lumbar puncture should be avoided because of the danger of brain-stem herniation. The proper time to perform cisternography is after the pressure has been lowered by removal of ventricular fluid. If patients with noncommunicating hydrocephalus have

normal cisternographic patterns under these conditions, they may respond satisfactorily to ventriculocisternal shunts or ventriculocisternostomy [36]. Patients with delayed clearance or block after adjustment of CSF pressure require ventriculoatrial or ventriculoperitoneal shunts.

In communicating hydrocephalus, the same patterns seen in adults are found but these patients are better examined by CT.

Computerized tomography versus radionuclide cisternography

In most clinics, CT has largely replaced radionuclide cisternography as a screening test for hydrocephalus because of its clear delineation of CSF spaces. In presenile dementia, the principal diagnostic problems to be excluded are cerebral atrophy, tumours, chronic subdural haematomas, and NPH. CT is sensitive in detecting all of these with the possible exception of bilateral subdural haematoma, in which case hydrocephalus is not a consideration. Nevertheless, once the diagnosis of hydrocephalus has been made, the question of patient management remains. There is broad consensus among neurosurgeons that in the absence of significant CSF obstruction, the patient is not likely to benefit from shunting. It is in estimating CSF clearance capacity that radionuclide cisternography is most useful. The evaluation of CSF dynamics using CT and metrizamide iohexol or iopamidol is complicated by continuing concern for their toxicity. Radionuclide cisternography remains the procedure of choice for this purpose. If cerebral atrophy is clearly demonstrated by CT, there is little indication for cisternography. However, in the case of significant ventricular dilatation without atrophy, cisternography may be of value. Those patients with ventricular reflux and delayed clearance, especially with low subarachnoid blocks (Fig. 89.19) are probably candidates for CSF drainage studies to test clinical response to lowered CSF pressure.

Shunt patency studies

Once the hydrocephalic patient has been shunted, regular examinations are required to assure shunt patency. Usually a diagnosis of shunt patency and adequate CSF flow is easily made by examination of the patient and inspection of the subcutaneous CSF reservoir. If the patient is alert and asymptomatic and the reservoir readily rebounds after compression, the shunt is probably functioning well. In cases of obvious neurological deterioration with increased intracranial pressure and sluggish or unresponsive reservoirs, shunt replacement is usually required, and the final diagnosis of blocked shunt should be made in the operating room. However, the clinical diagnosis of shunt adequacy may require additional diagnostic information. If serial CT scans are available, sudden dilatation is a reliable indication of a blocked shunt.

Several methods of determining shunt patency have been devised, but the most reliable employ radionuclides. A simple method of measuring CSF shunt flow involves the

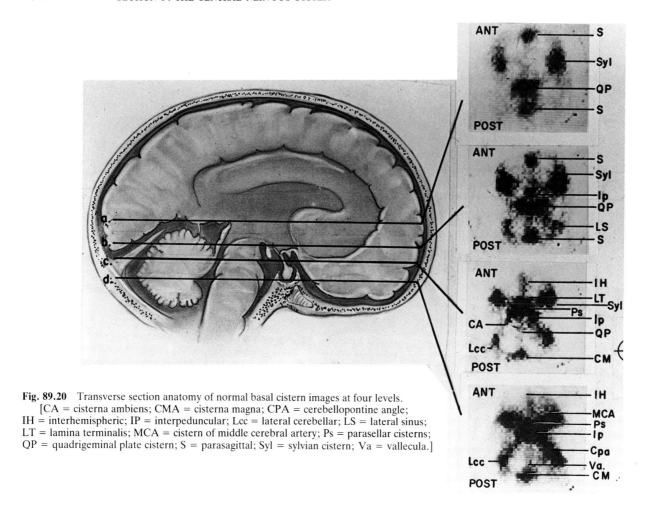

Fig. 89.20   Transverse section anatomy of normal basal cistern images at four levels.
[CA = cisterna ambiens; CMA = cisterna magna; CPA = cerebellopontine angle; IH = interhemispheric; IP = interpeduncular; Lcc = lateral cerebellar; LS = lateral sinus; LT = lamina terminalis; MCA = cistern of middle cerebral artery; Ps = parasellar cisterns; QP = quadrigeminal plate cistern; S = parasagittal; Syl = sylvian cistern; Va = vallecula.]

injection of a small amount of radiopharmaceutical, usually ^{99m}Tc-DTPA or pertechnetate, directly into the subcutaneous shunt reservoir. A scintillation camera is used to image the shunt system and to measure the tracer clearance from the reservoir. The clearance half-time is then determined and flow of CSF through the reservoir is determined from the relationship:

$F = \lambda V$ [where F = CSF shunt flow in ml/minute, $\lambda = 0.693/T_{\frac{1}{2}}$, which is determined from the time activity curve, and V = reservoir volume [37].]

Figure 89.21 shows brisk clearance from a 16-mm Pudenz reservoir. The scintiphoto is confirmatory evidence of an unobstructed distal ventriculoatrial catheter. The peritoneal end of the ventriculoperitoneal shunt can be visualized for qualitative evidence of shunt function and to rule out encystment of the abdominal catheter tip which may cause symptomatic obstruction.

Lumboperitoneal shunts are less commonly used because of serious spinal complications, yet they are occasionally encountered. Function can be judged by injecting a nondiffusible tracer into the lumbar intrathecal space and scanning the lower abdomen.

CSF rhinorrhoea

Although relatively uncommon, CSF rhinorrhoea poses a difficult diagnostic problem. Occasionally it is difficult to establish that the rhinorrhoea is of spinal fluid origin and it is especially difficult to identify the exact site of leak before surgery. Nuclear diagnostic techniques are most successful in proving the origin, and occasionally in pinpointing the probable leak site.

Most cases of CSF rhinorrhoea result from head trauma, although spontaneous leaks also occur.

A nondiffusible radiopharmaceutical is injected into the lumbar intrathecal space, after which nasal pledgets are placed on the anterior and posterior turbinates bilaterally and the activity counted. Even 'nondiffusible' tracers quickly reach the blood stream and then appear in the mucous secretion. Cotton pledgets should be carefully weighed and their radioactivity measured. The results are compared with serum specimens drawn at the same time and expressed in terms of counts/fluid gram. This method will then account for normal nasal radioactivity as well as differences in pledget size and absorption. Note: Serum to CSF ratios under 1.5 should not be interpreted as evidence of CSF rhinorrhoea.

When the patient is actively leaking, scintillation scanning is used to localize the actual leak site [38]. ^{99m}Tc-HSA or ^{111}In-

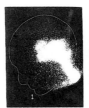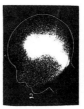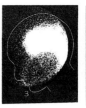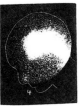

Fig. 89.22 Far left. scintiphotos 3 hours after lumbar injection of ^{99m}Tc-albumin showing ventricular reflux and abnormal accumulation of activity beneath the suprasellar cistern.

Panel 2 — After induction of leaking, small amount of activity is noted in nasal region.

Panel 3 — A trace of activity is seen a few minutes later coming from the region of the ethmoid sinus and sella.

Panel 4 — 10 minutes afterward leak tract no longer visible.

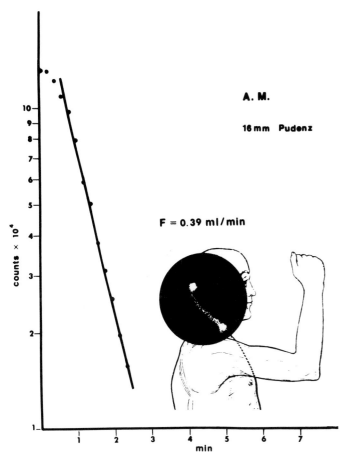

A. M.

16 mm Pudenz

F = 0.39 ml / min

Fig. 89.21 Graph of a shunt reservoir activity following injection of 3.7 MBq ^{99m}Tc-pertechnetate into a 16-mm Pudenz reservoir in a ventriculoperitoneal shunt system. The study demonstrates normal CSF flow of 0.39 ml/minute.

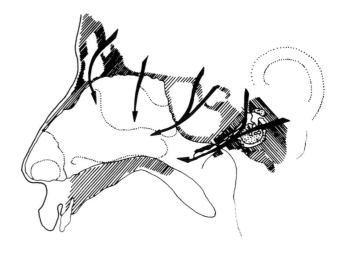

Fig. 89.23 Schematic diagram indicating several possible routes of CSF rhinorrhea. (After DiChiro [38]).

DTPA is injected in large doses (80 to 110 MBq) to achieve high counting rate and maximum resolution. The patient is injected in the lumbar space, then kept recumbent for 3 to 4 hours until scans show activity well cephalad and forward in the basal cisterns. The patient is then seated upright with head down to induce nasal leaking. Images are taken with the head in the lateral position until the leak tract is visualized. Often this tract is evident only transiently (Figs 89.22 & 89.23).

Radionuclide ventriculography

The injection of radiopharmaceuticals directly into the cerebral ventricles has occasional applications, especially where access is easy, as in children with open fontanelles and adults with existing burr holes or shunt reservoirs:

1. Radionuclide ventriculography may aid in assessing the patency of ventriculocisternal shunts.

2. The communication of porencephalic cysts or of an encysted temporal horn with the lateral ventricles may be made more easily by radionuclide techniques than by contrast ventriculography.

3. Documenting a communication between the lateral ventricles and a posterior fossa cyst may be useful in determining the shunting procedure to be undertaken. While contrast ventriculography is generally required in these cases, the radionuclide ventriculogram may indicate the CSF communication and dynamics more effectively.

BIBLIOGRAPHY

REFERENCES

1. Raimondi A S 1966 Ultrastructure and the biology of human brain tumours. Prog Neurol Surg 1:1–63
2. Reese T S, Karnovsky M J 1967 Fine structural localization of a blood-brain barrier to exogenous peroxidase. J Cell Biol 34:207–217

3. Bakay L 1967 Basic aspects of brain tumour localization by radioactive substances: review of current concepts. J Neurosurg 27:239–245

4. Ryerson T W et al 1978 A quantitative clinical comparison of three ^{99m}Technetium labelled brain imaging radiopharmaceuticals. Radiology 127:429–432

5. Oldendorf W H 1974 Lipid solubility and drug penetration of the blood-brain barrier. Proc Soc Exp Biol Med 147:814–816

6. Uszler J M et al 1975 Human CNS perfusion scanning with ^{123}I-iodoantipyrine. Radiology 115:197–200

7. Kuhl D E, Barrio J R, Huang S-C 1982 Quantifying local cerebral blood flow by N-isopropyl-p-[^{123}I] iodoamphetamine (IMP) tomography. J Nucl Med 23:196–203

8. Holmes R A, Golle R 1969 Appearance of the transverse sinus by brain scanning. Am J Roentgenol 106:340–343

9. Rosenthal L, Ambhanwong S, Stratford J 1969 Observations on the effect of contrast material on normal and abnormal brain tissue using radiopertechnetate. Radiology 92:1467–1472

10. Menter F A 1979 Manifestations of drug toxicity. Curr Probl Diagn Radiol 13:55

11. Schall G L, Quinn J L 1971 Diagnosis of central nervous system disease. In: Blahd W (ed) Textbook of nuclear medicine. McGraw Hill New York

12. Conway J J 1972 Radionuclide imaging of the central nervous system in children. Radiol Clin North Am 10:291–300

13. Cushing H, Eisenhardt L 1928 Meningiomas: their classification, regional behavior, life history and surgical end-results. Thomas, Springfield

14. Alderson P O, Gado M H, Siegel B A 1977 Computerized cranial tomography and radionuclide imaging in the detection of intracranial mass lesions. Semin Nucl Med 7:161–173

15. Baker H L, Hauser O W, Campbell J K 1980 National cancer institute study; evaluation of computed tomography in the diagnosis of intracranial neoplasms. Radiology 136:91–96

16. Mikhael M A, Mattar A G 1976 Sensitivity of radionuclide brain imaging and computerized transaxial tomography in detecting tumors of the posterior fossa. J Nucl Med 18:26–28

17. Buell U et al 1978 Computerized transaxial tomography and cerebral serial scintigraphy in intracranial tumors — rates of detection and tumor-type identification. J Nucl Med 19:476–479

18. Watson N E et al 1980 A comparison of brain imaging with gamma camera, single-photon emission computed tomography, and transmission computed tomography. J Nucl Med 21:507–511

19. Davis D O, Potchen E J 1970 Brain scanning and intracranial inflammatory disease. Radiology 95:345–352

20. Crocker E F et al 1974 Technetium brain scanning in the diagnosis and management of cerebral abscess. Am J Med 56:192–201

21. Jordan C E, James A E, Hodges F J 1972 III: Comparison of cerebral angiogram and the brain radionuclide image in brain abscess. Radiology 104:327–331

22. Gize R W, Mishkin F S 1970 Brain scans in multiple sclerosis. Radiology 97:297–299

23. Weisbaum S D, Garnett E S 1980 Brain scan in Schilder's disease. J Nucl Med 14:291–292

24. Furuse M et al 1978 Adrenoleukodystrophy. Radiology 126:707–710

25. Cowan R J, Maynard D, Lassiter K R 1970 Technetium-99m pertechnetate brain scans in the detection of subdural haematoma. A study of the age of the lesion as related to the development of a positive scan. J Neurosurg 32:30–34

26. Razzak M A, Mudarris F, Christie J H 1980 Sensitivity of radionuclide brain imaging and computerized transaxial tomography in detecting subdural haematoma. Clin Nucl Med 5:154–158

27. Matsuda H, Maeda T, Tonami N, Hisada K, Mori H 1981 Three types of abnormal scan patterns in posterior cerebral artery infarction. Clin Nucl Med 6:38–41

28. Cowan R J et al 1973 Value of the routine use of the cerebral dynamic radio-isotope study. Radiology 107:111–116

29. Alker G J et al 1981 False positive dynamic imaging of the cerebral circulation due to a congenital anomaly. Clin Nucl Med 6:532–536

30. Hawes D R, Mishkin F S 1972 Brain scans in watershed infarction and laminar cortical necrosis. Radiology 103:131–134

31. Curl F D et al 1972 Radionuclide cerebral angiography in a case of bilateral carotid-cavernous fistulae. Radiology 102:391–392

32. Kendall B E, Pullicino P 1980 Intravascular contrast injection in ischaemic lesions. II. Effect on prognosis. Neuroradiology 19:241–243

33. Hakim S, Venegas J G, Benton J D 1976 The physics of the cranial cavity, hydrocephalus and normal pressure hydrocephalus: mechanical interpretation and mathematical model. Surg Neurol 5:187–210

34. Ommaya A K, Metz H, Post K O 1972 Observations on the mechanics of hydrocephalus. In: Harbert J C et al (ed) Cisternography and hydrocephalus. Thomas, Springfield. p 57

35. Bannister R G, Gilford C, Kocen R 1967 Isotope encephalography in the diagnosis of dementia due to communicating hydrocephalus. Lancet 2:1014–1017

36. Milhorat T H 1972 Hydrocephalus and the cerebrospinal fluid. Williams and Wilkins, Baltimore, p 183

37. Harbert J C, Haddad D, McCullough D C 1974 Quantitation of cerebrospinal shunt flow. Radiology 112:379–387

38. DiChiro G, Reames P M 1964 Isotope localization of cranionasal cerebrospinal fluid leaks. J Nucl Med 5:376

SUGGESTIONS FOR FURTHER READING

Davson H 1967 Physiology of the cerebrospinal fluid. Little Brown, Boston

DeLand 1976 F H Cerebral radionuclide angiography, Saunders, Philadelphia

Harbert J C 1976 Radionuclide techniques in the evaluation of cerebrospinal fluid shunts. CRC Crit Rev Diagn Imaging 9:207–228

McCullough D C, Harbert J C 1972 Pediatric radionuclide cisternography. Semin Nucl Med 2:343–352

Pollay M, Curl F 1967 Secretion of cerebrospinal fluid by the ventricular ependyma of the rabbit. Am J Physiol 213:1031–1038

10 The Face: Orbit; Teeth; ENT

Editor: Ronald G. Grainger

Contents
90 The orbit *J. Vignaud, O. Bergès, M. L. Aubin, E. Chadrycki, I. F. Moseley*
91 Maxillofacial radiology *James McIvor*
92 Dental radiology *James McIvor*
93 The ear, nose and throat *Thomas Powell*

90 The orbit

J. Vignaud, O. Bergès, M. L. Aubin, E. Chadrycki, I. F. Moseley

Anatomy

Techniques of examination
  Conventional radiology
  Computed tomography
  Ultrasound
  Angiography
  Contrast examination of the lacrimal system

Orbital pathology
  Orbital malformations
  Orbital trauma
  Investigation of suspected intraorbital foreign bodies
  Inflammatory diseases
  Vascular lesions
  Orbital space occupying lesions

Intraocular abnormalities
  Lesions of the anterior segment
  The vitreous
  Retinal lesions
  Choroidal lesions

ANATOMY [1]

The walls of the orbit (Fig. 90.1)

The orbit is a pyramidal cavity, with its base lying anteriorly, surrounded by a strong bony rim in continuity with the walls.

The roof is fragile, and irregular, due to the convolutional impressions of the cerebral frontal lobes, from which it is separated by the meninges. The supraorbital recess of the frontal sinus invaginates its anterior part, and the trochlea, or pulley, of the superior oblique muscle lies anteromedially on the orbital roof.

The medial wall, or lamina papyracea, which is very thin, separates the orbital contents from the nasal fossa anteriorly, the ethmoid air cells and, posteriorly, the anterior portion of the sphenoid sinus. An anterior depression, the lacrimal fossa, houses the lacrimal sac.

The floor of the orbit is also thin; it is traversed from back to front by the infraorbital nerve, which runs, at first in a groove, and then in a canal which opens at the antero-superior border of the maxillary antrum. This latter is separated from the orbit by the orbital floor.

The lateral, strongest wall of the orbit, formed by the malar and the greater wing of the sphenoid, separates the orbital contents from the temporal fossa.

Several foramina open into the orbit. The optic canal (Fig. 90.2), lies between the two roots of the lesser wing of the sphenoid, running obliquely at 35° to the midsagittal plane and 35° craniocaudally with respect to the orbitomeatal line. Through it pass the optic nerve and ophthalmic artery. The optic canals are usually bilaterally symmetrical, but slight asymmetry may occur: agenesis of the inferior root of the lesser wing gives a 'keyhole' appearance; there may be a separate canal inferiorly for the ophthalmic artery.

The superior orbital fissure, between the greater and lesser wings of the sphenoid bone, communicates with the anterior part of the cavernous sinus. Through it pass the ocular motor nerves (III, IV, VI), the lacrimal, frontal and nasal branches of the first division of V, the ophthalmic veins and an arterial connection between the middle meningeal and ophthalmic arteries. Slight asymmetry of the superior orbital fissures is frequent.

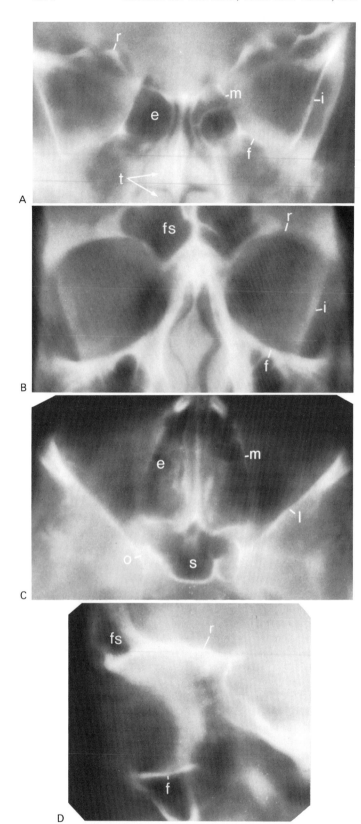

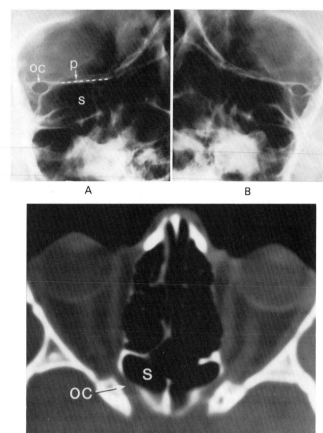

Fig. 90.2 Optic canal. (A) & (B) Conventional oblique anteroposterior projections (right and left). (C) Axial CT (wide window). [oc = optic canal; p = planum sphenoidale; s = sphenoid sinus].

The inferior orbital fissure lies between the lateral and inferior walls, separating the middle cranial fossa from the maxillary antrum; emissary veins pass through it.

A fibrous covering, the periorbita, lines the inner surface of these bony walls, and is continuous with the intracranial dura mater. It closes the inferior orbital fissure.

The orbital contents (See Fig. 90.4)

These include the eye (or globe), the optic nerve, extraocular muscles (including the levator palpebrae superioris), lacrimal gland, vessels and nerves, all of which are surrounded by orbital fat.

The globe is approximately spherical, with a normal anteroposterior diameter of 22 mm. It is covered, from without, by the tough sclera (whose transparent anterior portion forms the cornea), the richly vascular choroid and the retina. Its contents include the lens, iris and ciliary body. The anterior chamber is bounded by the cornea, the anterior surface of the iris and the central portion of the lens, while the posterior chamber lies between iris and lens; these chambers contain the aqueous. The retrolental portion of the globe is filled by the vitreous.

Fig. 90.1 Tomography of the normal orbit. (A) & (B) Frontal projections (postero-anterior). (C) Submentovertical. (D) Lateral projections. [e = ethmoid sinus; fs = frontal sinus; f = floor of orbit; i = innominate line; l = lateral wall of orbit; m = medial wall; o = optic canal; r = roof of orbit; s = sphenoid sinus; t = turbinates].

The thick optic nerve, with a transverse diameter of about 4 mm, is a direct anterior extension of the brain and is thus covered by meninges, with a subarachnoid space containing cerebrospinal fluid, between them.

Four rectus muscles (superior, medial, inferior and lateral), connected by an aponeurosis, form the muscle cone, separating extra- and intraconal spaces. These muscles originate on the inferior root of the lesser wing of the sphenoid and from the annulus of Zinn. Superior and inferior oblique muscles encourage oblique gaze; the levator palpebrae superioris muscle lies directly above the superior rectus.

The lacrimal gland lies anteriorly on the superolateral surface of the globe. At the inner canthus, superior and inferior lacrimal canaliculi run into a common canaliculus, which opens into the lacrimal sac and drains via the nasolacrimal duct into the nasal cavity.

TECHNIQUES OF EXAMINATION [2]

Conventional radiography (and tomography)

A complete study of the orbit includes occipitofrontal projections at 35° to 50° to the orbitomeatal line (see Ch. 83 for a general discussion on skull radiography); a lateral projection although superimposing right and left sides is useful, particularly for the planum and body of the sphenoid bone. The submentovertical projection may also be helpful. Supplementary techniques for foreign body localization are described on page 1883.

For the optic canal (Fig. 90.2), an oblique posteroanterior projection (OM + 35°, sagittal plane at 35°) is the most useful. Axial tomography (Fig. 90.3), using the same projection, or in the submentovertical plane, may also be employed. Plain films should always be obtained first, as they may give valuable diagnostic information. With current techniques, however, it would seem that conventional tomography is of value only when CT is not available.

Computed tomography (CT) [3,4] (Figs. 90.3 & 90.4)

High spatial resolution CT affords excellent demonstration of the orbit and its contents, particularly the optic nerve and extraocular muscles. The detailed internal anatomy of the globe is better examined with ultrasound.

CT sections should be thin (1 to 3 mm) and contiguous, so that images can be reconstructed in coronal, sagittal and oblique planes, without further irradiation of the patient. The plane of the axial sections is chosen by means of the digital radiographic facility (scout film or scanogram), so as to pass through the neuro-ocular plane, i.e. the plane which includes the lens, optic nerve and optic canal when the eye is in the primary position; its landmarks are the centre of the orbit anteriorly and the tuberculum sellae posteriorly (approximately OM − 10°). The eyes should be stationary during scanning. Direct coronal sections and sagittal sections may be performed on some machines, but with the latest scanners, reformatted images are generally acceptable.

'Physiological studies', with the eyes in various directions of gaze, may be of interest, but their use is limited by considerations of irradiation dose (Fig. 90.4) [5].

Intravenous contrast medium is useful to demonstrate the degree of vascularization of the lesion, as well as the vessels and the dural sheath of the optic nerve (it should, however be noted that there is no blood-tissue barrier in the orbit).

The bony structures surrounding the orbit may be very satisfactorily studied using a wide CT window (Fig. 90.2).

Ultrasound [6] (Fig. 90.5)

Frequencies of 7 to 12 MHz are optimal for the eye, orbit, and periorbital region. A and B modes are generally used in clinical examinations, the former for measurement of the eye, optic nerve and extraocular muscles, and investigation of the borders, internal structure, reflectivity and attenuation characteristics of a lesion (see Ch. 4 for a general discussion of techniques). The B mode demonstrates the size, shape and position of a lesion and may also be used for assessment of motion, mobility and internal structure.

C and M modes and Doppler techniques are less commonly used.

Angiography

Orbital phlebography

Use of this method is now almost restricted to investigation of orbital varices, or occasionally of lesions involving the cavernous sinus. Techniques and normal anatomy are discussed in Chapter 83.

Arteriography [7] (Fig. 90.6)

Since the orbit is fed by arteries arising from both the internal and external carotid arteries, both arteries must be studied, usually by selective catheterization. Lateral and anteroposterior projections are commonly used; submento-

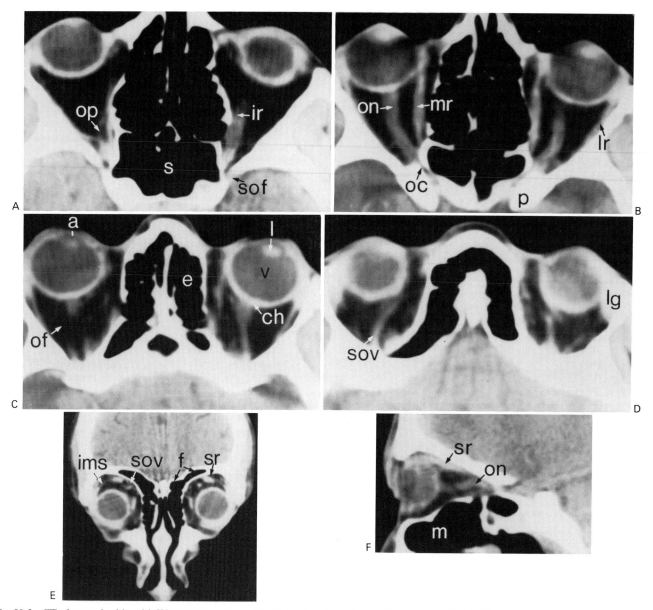

Fig. 90.3 CT of normal orbit, with IV contrast medium. (A-D) Axial sections, from below upwards. (E) & (F) Coronal and sagittal sections. [ch = choroid; e = ethmoid sinus; f = frontal sinus; l = lens; lr = lateral rectus muscle; m = maxillary antrum; mr = medial rectus muscle; oc = optic canal; on = optic nerve; op = ophthalmic artery; p = anterior clinoid process; ims = intermuscular septum; lg = lacrimal gland; s = sphenoid sinus; sov = superior ophthalmic vein].

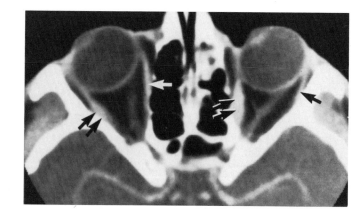

Fig. 90.4 Axial CT in right lateral gaze. The right lateral and left medial rectus muscles [double arrows] are contracted, while the left lateral and right medial rectus muscles [single arrows] are relaxed.

Fig. 90.5 Normal ultrasound of orbit. (A) B mode. (B) A mode.
[a = anterior chamber; f = retrobulbar fat; l = lens; n = optic nerve;
r = retina; v = vitreous].

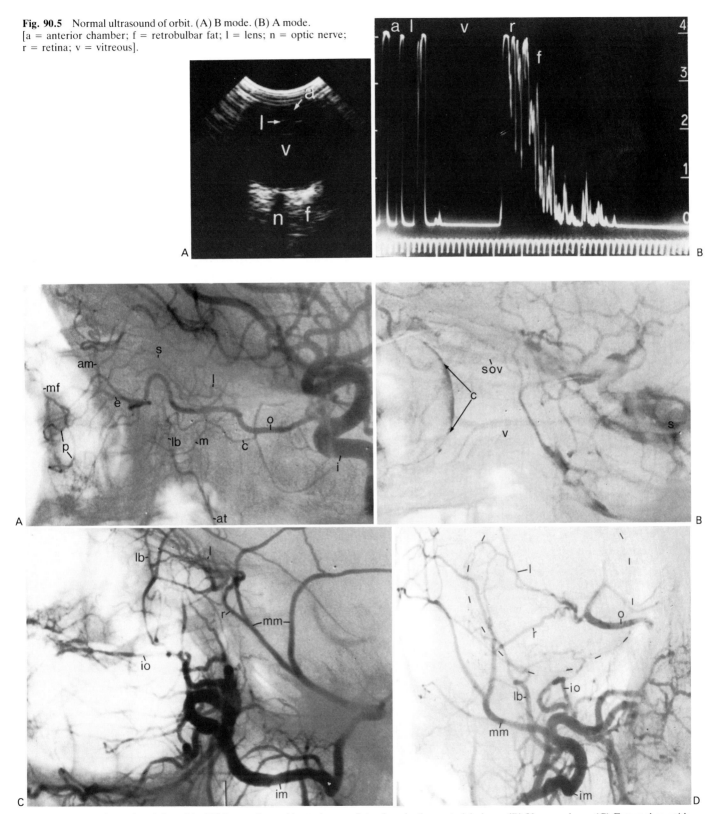

Fig. 90.6 Arteriography of the orbit. (A) Internal carotid arteriogram, lateral projection, arterial phase. (B) Venous phase. (C) External carotid arteriogram, lateral projection, arterial phase. (D) External carotid arteriogram as (C), anteroposterior (right orbit). [am = anterior meningeal artery; at = anterior deep temporal artery (lb = lacrimal branch); c = ciliary artery; cc = choroidal crescent; e = anterior ethmoidal artery; i = internal carotid artery; im = internal maxillary artery; io = infraorbital artery; l = lacrimal artery; m = inferior and medial muscular artery; mf = medial frontal artery; mm = middle meningeal artery; o = ophthalmic artery; p = palpebral arteries; r = recurrent meningeal artery; s = supraorbital artery; sov = superior ophthalmic vein; v = vortex veins]. (The orbital margin is dotted in D.).

vertical projections may also be employed. Direct magnification, using a fine (0.1 to 0.2 mm) focus, and photographic subtraction, enables demonstration of vessels down to 200 μm to be demonstrated.

Arterial, capillary and venous phases are obtained. The first demonstrates the ophthalmic artery, which usually arises from the carotid siphon, coursing under the optic nerve in the optic canal, and through the posterior third of the orbit. It then loops around the nerve, usually passing lateral to it (80% of cases), and finally straightens to emerge from the muscle cone anteriorly. The ophthalmic artery gives branches to the muscles, the choroid (ciliary arteries), optic nerve, retina (central retinal artery), ethmoid sinus and adjacent dura mater, and to the lacrimal gland.

In the capillary phase in the lateral projection, a fine crescentic shadow, representing the choroid, delineates the posterior portion of the globe.

Branches of the external carotid artery also supply the orbit [8], especially the middle meningeal (which may indeed be the sole or principal supply of the ophthalmic artery) [9], a lacrimal artery and the deep temporal artery.

The superior and inferior ophthalmic veins (Ch. 83), while draining the orbit, also receive blood supply from the nasal fossae and face; they are therefore better seen on external carotid angiography.

Contrast examination of the lacrimal system (dacryocystography) (Fig. 90.7)

After instillation of topical anaesthetic into the conjunctival sac, a fine, flexible catheter is introduced into a canaliculus (the superior when possible), and a small quantity of water soluble iodinated contrast medium is injected continuously during tomography.

Bilateral injection enables comparison with the normal side or, if abnormalities are bilateral (a not uncommon finding), simultaneous demonstration of the two sides. For

good visualization of the lacrimal system, tomography is superior to plain films and demonstrates better the anatomy of the surrounding structures.

ORBITAL PATHOLOGY

Orbital malformations

Development of the globe starts at the third week of gestation and by the sixth week of intrauterine life the main structures are formed. However, maturation continues until the end of gestation, and even into the postnatal period.

Development of the facial skeleton is linked to that of the brain and eye. It originates from the first branchial arch, which gives rise to the superior and inferior facial buds, separated by the facial sulci. The confluence of the maxillary, mandibular and nasal buds forms the face, sulci between the nasal and superior mandibular buds forming the lacrimal sac. The globe develops between the superior maxillary and frontal buds.

Malformations affect the orbital contents and/or walls, and may be due to hereditary conditions, chromosomal aberrations or acquired disorders of development.

Anophthalmia, absence of the eye, is extremely rare, and usually associated with lethal conditions. *Microphthalmia*, like anophthalmia often part of a syndrome of first and second branchial arch anomalies, is frequently the consequence of an acquired defect (rubella, toxoplasmosis, etc.); (Fig. 90.8) but may be developmental (Fig. 90.9). Plain radiographs may show small or abnormally shaped orbits, microcephaly, and/or intracranial calcifications.

Cyclopia is a rare malformation associated with aplasia of the frontal bud, and a complex neural malformation. A single eye lies in a single midline orbit.

The position of the orbits may be abnormal. *Hypotelorism* (reduced interorbital diameter) is related to hypoplasia of the ethmoid bones, while *hypertelorism* is found in all malformations associated with hypertrophy of the frontal buds. These abnormalities may be solitary, but are frequently found in complex malformations.

Ocular ultrasonography is invaluable for the assessment of eyes with corneal abnormalities or opaque media which prevent ophthalmological evaluation. In *aniridia* (absence of the iris), the frequent association of nephroblastoma should be excluded by ultrasound or urography. Radiological confirmation of absence of the lens is not required unless the cornea is opaque. *Subluxation* of the lens occurs in many complex malformations, notably Marfan's syndrome and homocystinuria.

Congenital cataract may be isolated, but occurs in syndromes such as chondrodystrophia punctata, Lowe's syndrome rubella and Down's syndrome. Ultrasonography may be helpful for analysis of the position and form of the

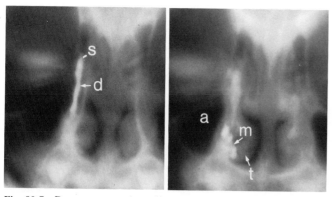

Fig. 90.7 Dacryocystography, with tomography (anteroposterior). The lacrimal sac [s] and the nasolacrimal duct [d] are normal in calibre, and the water soluble contrast medium passes freely into the inferior meatus [m]. [a = maxillary antrum; t = inferior turbinate].

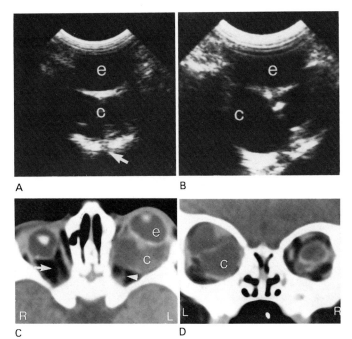

A   B

C   D

Fig. 90.8 Congenital (rubella) malformations of the eye and optic nerves. (A) & (B) B-mode ultrasound of the *left* orbit. (C) & (D) axial and coronal CT. On the right side, microphthalmos is associated with a very thin optic nerve [arrows]; note subluxation of the lens, which has a cataract. On the left, microphthalmos is associated with a colobomatous cyst [c] of the optic nerve. Both imaging techniques demonstrate the relationship of the cyst to the eye [e] and the optic nerve [arrowhead]. There is proptosis and the orbit is enlarged on the left.

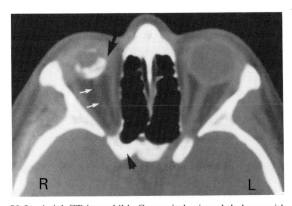

Fig. 90.9 Axial CT in a child. Congenital microphthalmos with choroidal calcification [arrow], a hypoplastic optic nerve [small arrows], a narrowed optic canal [arrowhead] and a small orbit on the right. The left side is normal.

abnormal lens, and may also show associated anomalies of the posterior segment. CT shows increased density of the lens, and may also reveal ocular or optic nerve dysplasia.

Congenital glaucoma (Fig. 90.10) is manifest in early life by photophobia and buphthalmos (enlargement of the globe). It may be associated with other ocular abnormalities, particularly in cases of neurofibromatosis, Sturge-Weber syndrome and Lowe's syndrome.

In cases of *leukoria* (opacity of the vitreous), ultrasonography, by showing reflection echoes representing synchisis scintillans and asteroid hyalosis in the midvitreous, allows

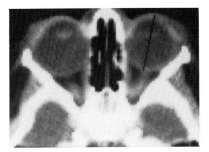

Fig. 90.10 Congenital glaucoma; axial CT. Note increased diameter of the eyes (buphthalmos) and relative posterior displacement of the lens, due to accumulation of aqueous.

differentiation of a persistent hyperplastic primary vitreous from retinal dysplasia or a retinoblastoma.

Septo-optic dysplasia (Ch. 86) is a syndrome of hypoplasia of the anterior optic pathways. CT is the simplest method of assessment of this condition, since all its components may be shown in a single study.

A *colobomatous cyst* results from lack of closure of the inferior portion of the globe at the optic disc.

Complex malformations

The syndrome of the first branchial arch is due to an abnormality of development between the seventh and eighth weeks of intrauterine life. Abnormalities include hypoplasia of the jaws; malformations of the temporomandibular joint, the teeth and the pinna or external auditory canal; supernumerary cartilages or blind fistulae along a line joining the ear and the lateral angle of the mouth; malformations and/or malposition of the globe and the eyelids. These vary from minor hypoplasia to total aplasia. The most important syndromes, which are described in more detail elsewhere, include the Treacher-Collins syndrome, Goldenhar syndrome, oculomandibulofacial dysplasia, oculovertebral dysplasia and otocephalia.

Median or paramedian clefts of the lids may be seen.

The *craniofacial dysostoses*, including Apert's syndrome, Crouzon's disease and Greig's syndrome include hypertelorism; brain malformations may co-exist. Since palpebral colobomas may be associated with meningocele or meningoencephalocele, careful assessment of the skull base by plain films or CT is of great value, especially when corrective surgery is planned.

The phakomatoses

Neurofibromatosis

The characteristic sphenoid dysplasia is discussed elsewhere (Ch. 86), as is plexiform neuroma (Ch. 86). Enlargement of the optic canal in this condition can be the result of the bony dysplasia, a tumour (optic nerve glioma or nerve sheath meningioma) or, rarely, chronic raised intracranial pressure. CT is of prime value in assessment of the plain film findings.

Tuberous sclerosis

Retinal phakomas are flat, discoid lesions, which are often multiple; they may bulge into the vitreous, where they can be visualized by ultrasonography. Microphthalmia and orbital coloboma may coexist.

Sturge-Weber disease

The ocular manifestation of this condition is the choroidal angioma, usually present on the same side as the skin lesion; it can give rise to congenital glaucoma, buphthalmos or retinal detachment. Ultrasonography demonstrates a thickening of the choroid; calcification may be evident. In advanced cases, microphthalmia is frequent.

Von Hippel-Lindau disease

A common ocular finding is the angioma located peripherally in the retina, which may be detectable ultrasonically.

Orbital Trauma

Fractures involving the orbit usually involve the facial bones more widely. They are discussed in detail in Chapters 86 and 91.

Injuries to the soft tissues are usually caused by direct trauma. Except for the globe, these structures are the field of CT, although ultrasound may offer complementary information, particularly concerning the optic nerve. Conventional tomography is useful only if there are associated bony lesions or foreign bodies.

Ocular trauma may take the form of contusion or concussion, with or without rupture of the outer coats, and direct injury, simple or penetrating, with possible foreign bodies. Localization of foreign bodies is discussed below. Hyphema (bleeding into the anterior chamber) may resolve spontaneously or lead to complications such as vascular infiltration of the cornea, recurrence or hypertony (raised intraocular pressure).

Ultrasonography shows scattered echoes in the inferior or dependent portion of the chamber. When haemorrhage is more extensive, ultrasonography is the best method of assessing the more posterior structures. The lens may be partly or totally subluxed anteriorly or posteriorly (Fig. 90.11); it may develop a contusional cataract, with an intact capsule, or it may rupture, liberating lenticular material into the vitreous or anterior chamber.

Vitreous haemorrhages also prevent fundoscopy; ultrasound can demonstrate the shape, size, position and mobility of such haemorrhage, but its chief contribution is to show the retina and sclera (Fig. 90.12). In a traumatized eye, increased thickness of the choroid is a frequent finding, but haemorrhage is difficult to distinguish from solid choroidal tumours

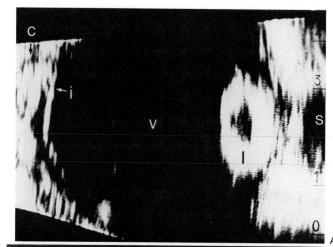

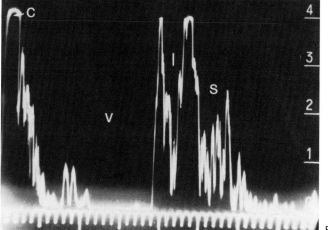

Fig. 90.11 Traumatic subluxation of the lens. Ultrasound (A) B mode, (B) A mode. The lens [l], which has a cataract, lies at the posterior pole of the globe; it produces posterior shadowing [s]. [c = cornea; i = iris; v = vitreous].

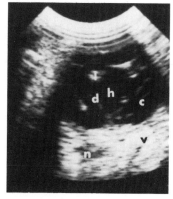

Fig. 90.12 Post-traumatic lesions (B mode ultrasound). [c = choroidal detachment; h = vitreous haemorrhage; l = posterior luxation of lens material; d = retinal detachment; n = optic nerve; v = dilated intraconal veins].

or lesions of the retina. Retinal detachment must be excluded, and the ultrasonic examination may have to be repeated a number of times if any doubt persists, particularly when opaque media prohibit fundoscopy. The appearances are described on page 1894. It is also possible to show retinal oedema ultrasonically.

Rupture of the anterior segment is usually detected clinically. Rupture of the posterior segment can be demonstrated as discontinuity of the posterior wall, by means of ultrasound. Careful examination is necessary if the abnormality is not to be overlooked.

Phthisis bulbi — atrophy of the globe with thickening of the walls, sometimes accompanied by scleral and lenticular calcification — can occur as the late result of trauma or infection. Calcification may be visible on plain radiographs, and CT or ultrasound will demonstrate a dense shrunken globe.

Shearing injuries of the optic nerve at the disc, the result of severe ocular trauma, may be shown by ultrasound, as may haematoma and oedema of the nerve and/or sheath. B mode demonstrates an enlarged nerve, and A mode permits measurement of the diameters of the optic nerve and the haematoma. With grosser injuries, in which the nerve is sectioned, the discontinuity may be appreciated at CT, but in the acute phase detail is often obscured by haematoma. CT is the method of choice for the demonstration of retrobulbar haematomas, which may be seen to lie free in the retrobulbar space, inside or outside the muscle cone, in a muscle, or subperiosteally.

Investigation of suspected intraorbital foreign bodies

Imaging techniques will be required to answer the following questions:
— is there a foreign body?
— where is it, relative to the globe and optic nerve?
— what is its nature; is it magnetic?

Techniques which can be employed and are often used in combination include conventional radiography (including bone-free and non-screen techniques), CT, ultrasound and magnetism (the Berman locator).

Conventional radiography

A foreign body will be shown on plain films only if it is of sufficient radio-opacity; this will depend on its nature, its size and the density of the surrounding structures. It should be remembered that glass is generally radio-opaque.

The following projections are obtained for detection of the foreign body: occipitofrontal (OM – 35°), and a lateral centred on the orbit, both with the eyes in the primary

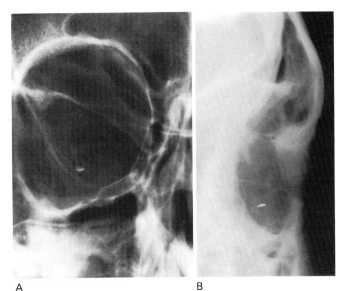

A   B

Fig. 90.13 Plain film localization of a foreign body. (A) OF and (B) lateral projections.

position (Fig. 90.13). To these may be added tangential bone free, craniocaudal and lateral projections of that part of the globe anterior to the orbital margins (for which dental films are used).

Further investigation then depends on the results of these views.
1. If no foreign body is shown, it may be too small or of insufficient radio-opacity. Ultrasound examination is then carried out, possibly in association with CT.
2. If the foreign body is shown on the standard films, but not on the bone-free films, it lies behind the anterior third of the globe, is of dense material and at least 0.3 mm in diameter. It may be intra or extraocular, but precise localization is possible.
3. If the foreign body is seen only on the bone-free films, it lies in the anterior third of the eye, or in the lids, but is poorly radio-opaque. Precise localization is by means of ultrasound. CT is rarely necessary.
4. If the foreign body is visible on all four films, it is anterior and dense. Localization is by ultrasound.

Localization techniques [2]

The 'eye-moving' technique consists of radiographs in occipitofrontal and lateral projections, with the head stationary, and different directions of gaze: up, down, left and right (Figs. 90.14 & 90.15). If the foreign body lies within the globe, it will be seen to move; should it move with the gaze, it is anterior to the centre of rotation, while if it shows contrary motion, it is posterior. Small but undoubted movements indicate a central position, and should be differentiated from the lack of movement seen with an extraocular foreign body. It should, however, be noted that some very heavy intraocular fragments do not move with the eyes, while the rare foreign body lying in Tenon's capsule or within one of the extraocular muscles adjacent to the globe, will move with it.

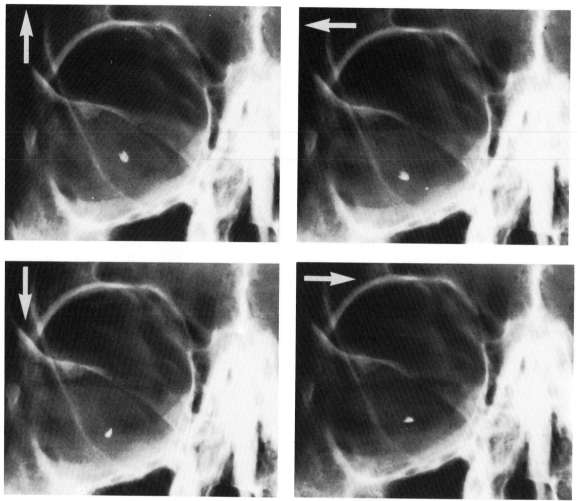

Fig. 90.14 'Eye moving' radiographs, taken in different directions of gaze (indicated by the arrows). The particle has a different shape on each film but does not move significantly: it is within the globe, near its equator.

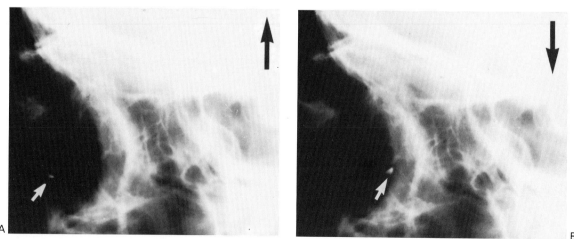

Fig. 90.15 'Eye moving' method, lateral projection. When the foreign body does not move in the frontal projection, a lateral is usually helpful. Here, it moves contrary to the direction of gaze, and therefore lies peripherally in the globe, near its equator. (A) Looking upwards. (B) Looking down.

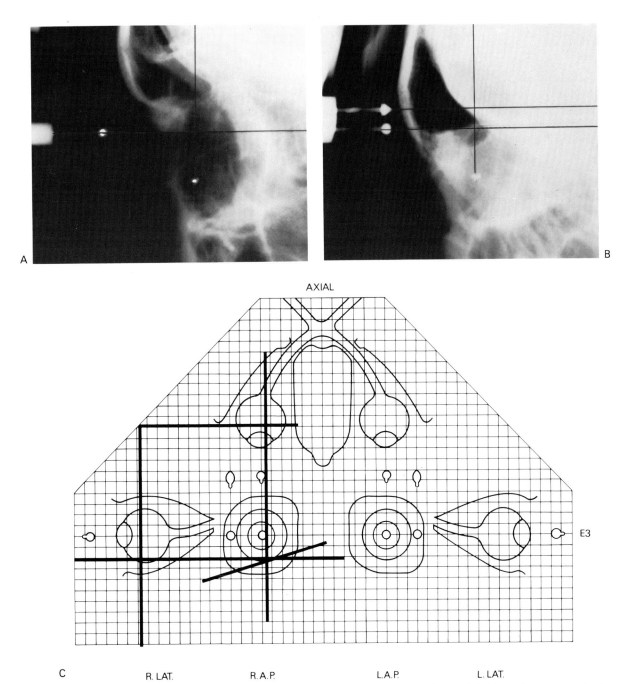

Fig. 90.16 Geometrical localization (Sweet's method). (A) true lateral: cone and sphere are superimposed. (B) Off lateral: cone and sphere are separated. (C) Chart showing the foreign body relative to the orbital structures in three planes.

Geometrical techniques are based on measurement of the distance between known landmarks and the foreign body in two projections. A diagram representing the presumed position of the foreign body relative to the eye, can then be drawn in anteroposterior and axial planes (Fig. 90.16).

Ultrasonic localization is now widely used. Both A and B modes can be employed, and the M mode may reveal the magnetic character of the foreign body if it moves under magnetic influence. If plain radiographs have shown the foreign body, its position relative to the globe can be shown

precisely by ultrasound, which demonstrates it as a punctate, highly reflective echo, with occasionally a posterior cone of absorption.

This technique is however, of limited utility in cases ·of very small foreign bodies lying in the posterior part of the globe, especially within the sclera. Serial axial sections are first performed then, when the fragment is located, a section perpendicular to the first is obtained. The axial dimension of the globe has been measured and a diagram showing the site of the foreign body relative to the coats of the globe can

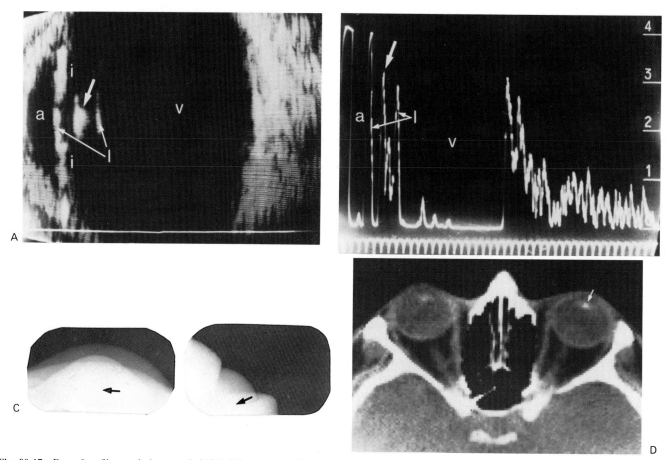

Fig. 90.17 Bone-free films and ultrasound. (A) & (B) ultrasound (B and A modes). (C) Axial and lateral bone-free projections. (D) CT. Bone-free projections confirms that the foreign body is anterior, within the eye. Ultrasound shows it to lie within the lens, while CT shows only increased density in the affected lens. [arrows = foreign body; a = anterior chamber; i = iris; l = lens (anterior and posterior surfaces); v = vitreous].

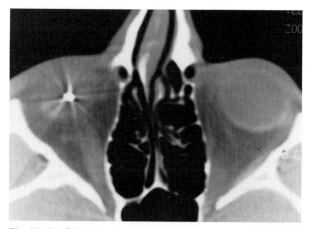

Fig. 90.18 CT. A foreign body, dense enough to cause artefacts, lies near the inferior margin of the globe.

then be drawn. It may be compared with that obtained by geometrical techniques. The M mode may be useful in showing movement in a pulsatile magnetic field, indicating the magnetic nature of the foreign body.

Ultrasonography may also demonstrate luxation of the lens, vitreous haemorrhage, retinal detachment or rupture of the sclera.

If conventional radiography has not revealed a foreign body, ultrasound may be particularly helpful in demonstrating a nonopaque fragment. These generally lie in the anterior portion of the eye and can therefore be localized precisely relative to the anterior chamber, iris and ciliary body (Fig. 90.17).

CT is used when plain films and ultrasound have been insufficient, when the foreign body is shown to lie within the orbit, but outside the globe, when there is a doubt as to its nature or location, or when multiple fragments are present (in the latter context, stereoradiography or conventional tomography may also be of value) (Fig. 90.18). During the CT study, the eye must be immobile. CT is excellent for precise localization of extraocular foreign bodies; since most modern machines have a facility for measuring distances, a scale diagram can be drawn showing the exact location of a foreign body in three dimensions.

A magnetic detector (Berman locator) based on the principle of mine detectors, can be used to indicate whether the foreign body is magnetic.

Inflammatory diseases

Endocrine exophthalmos (Fig. 90.19)

By far the most frequent cause of endocrine exophthalmos (and indeed the commonest cause of proptosis) is hyperthyroidism (Graves' disease); primary hyperadrenalism, long-standing steroid therapy or acromegaly can also produce exophthalmos. The following discussion applies to thyroid eye disease.

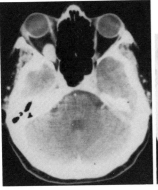 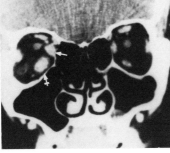

A   B

Fig. 90.19 Graves' disease. (A) & (B) Axial and coronal CT. It is difficult to determine the nature of the orbital mass shown in (A), but the coronal section confirms hypertrophy of the inferior [crossed arrow] and medial [arrow] rectus muscles.

Thyroid ophthalmopathy is the result of endocrine and immunological disturbances. The combined effects of thyroid stimulating hormone and long acting thyroid stimulator (a gamma-globulin) lead to overproduction of hydrophylic mucopolysaccharides, producing oedema of the orbital tissues, and proptosis.

There is hypertrophy of the fat, oedema of the interstitial tissue of the conjunctiva and fatty infiltration and degeneration of the extraocular muscles, which may eventually become fibrotic. Proptosis is bilateral in 70% of cases, but even in unilateral proptosis, the diagnosis of thyroid disease must always be considered [10]. The proptosis is axial if all muscles are involved, and reducible; there is retraction of the upper lid. The exophthalmos may become malignant, with complete, irreducible protrusion of the globe, oedema of the lids and conjunctival chemosis.

Diagnosis depends on the clinical features and laboratory tests, but the latter may be normal. In such cases, radiology can be contributory, since the differential diagnosis will include vascular and neoplastic causes of exophthalmos, as well as orbital granuloma (see below).

Plain radiographs are generally normal, but in advanced cases, the orbits may be enlarged. CT is the modality of choice [11,12]; axial and coronal images may be required when the diagnosis is doubtful, or for pre or postoperative assessment. Proptosis may be assessed by CT, but clinical measurement usually suffices. The extraocular muscles are characteristically enlarged. All muscles may be affected, but often only one or two are abnormal. The inferior and medial rectus muscles are most commonly involved. Swelling of muscles on the side opposite the clinically affected eye is highly suggestive of the diagnosis. The swelling affects the body of the muscles, whereas in orbital granuloma, the anterior tendinous portions are also involved.

In some cases, muscle swelling is not marked, but proptosis appears to be due mainly to hypertrophy of the orbital fat, which is increased in amount in the intra- and extraconal spaces, particularly anteriorly.

The calibre of the optic nerve may be reduced when the nerve is stretched by the expanded muscles or fat. In advanced cases, the lamina papyracea shows a concavity due to the raised intraorbital pressure.

Ultrasound can be used to demonstrate the same changes as CT, but generally less graphically. It is also less satisfactory for assessment of compression of the optic nerve at the orbital apex.

Infections

Cellulitis is a diffuse infection of the orbit, often streptococcal. It may be confined to the tissues anterior to the orbital septum, or involve the whole orbit [13]. Orbital abscess is rare; it may be located either within the orbital soft tissues, or subperiosteally. Osteomyelitis, septic thrombophlebitis of the venous sinuses and cerebral veins, meningitis, encephalitis and subdural or cerebral abscess may occur. The most frequent sources of infection are sinusitis, trauma (with or without a foreign body) (Fig.90.20), skin infections or bacteraemia.

Plain films often demonstrate opaque sinuses; bone destruction due to osteomyelitis is much less common.

CT is the most valuable technique [14]. It enables assessment of the extent of infection and shows possible abscess formation. Clinical examination of the acutely infected orbit may be very restricted. The following abnormalities may be shown: in preseptal cellulitis, swelling of the lids and preseptal soft tissues; in orbital cellulitis, oedema of the preseptal tissues, proptosis, diffuse swelling and loss of outline of the retrobulbar structures. When an orbital abscess is present, to these changes may be added a more or less well defined mass, showing capsular contrast enhancement. If the abscess is subperiosteal, it will be more circumscribed, lying outside the muscle cone and displacing the overlying muscle, which may be swollen; opacity of an adjacent sinus, with possible destruction of its walls, may be evident. A foreign body may be present. The CT study should include the entire head to exclude intracranial complications.

In dacryocystitis, the lacrimal system may be obstructed at any site, most commonly the inferior portion of the

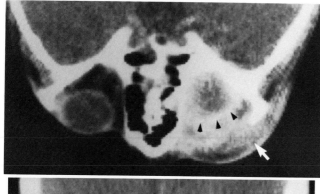

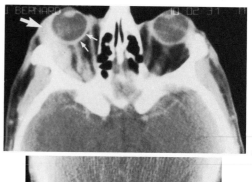

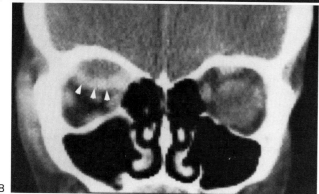

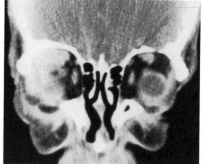

Fig. 90.20   Orbital granuloma due to foreign body. (A) & (B) Axial and coronal CT. A mass [arrowheads] occupies the superior part of the orbit; it is inhomogeneous. Its margins are well defined and show contrast enhancement. There is marked proptosis and swelling of the upper lid [arrow].

lacrimal sac, which is dilated. Knowledge of the size of the sac is useful in planning surgery.

Parasitic infections. Retrobulbar hydatid cysts are the most frequent. CT shows a spherical mass of low attenuation, occasionally with enhancement of its walls after intravenous contrast medium. Several vesicles may be seen infiltrating the orbital tissues. Curvilinear calcification is sometimes visible.

Idiopathic orbital granuloma ''pseudotumour''
(Fig. 90.21)

The term 'orbital granuloma' is reserved for a poorly under-stood group of inflammatory conditions in which no systemic or local cause can be identified [15]. This group thus excludes thyroid eye disease and infections.

The aetiology is unknown and clinical, radiological and indeed pathological diagnosis is often difficult. Histologi-cally, there is infiltration by lymphocytes and plasma cells of one or more of the orbital structures. In order of frequency, the lacrimal gland, extraocular muscles, sclera, optic nerve and fat are affected, usually on one side only. The patient presents with a painful proptosis and/or ophthalmoplegia; decreased visual acuity is not uncommon.

Plain films are usually normal. Typically, CT shows swelling of the lacrimal gland, and swelling and loss of definition of the extraocular muscles, including their anterior

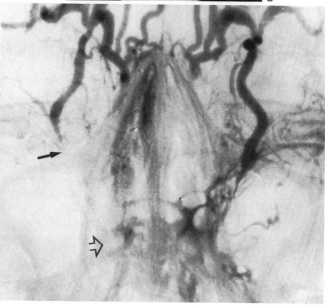

Fig. 90.21   Orbital pseudotumour. (A) & (B) axial and coronal CT. There is an extraconal mass and the lacrimal gland is swollen [arrow]. Note contrast enhancement of the choroid [small arrows]. The coronal section shows swollen muscles. (C) Phlebography shows typical attenuation of the superior ophthalmic vein on the right, which is occluded near the superior orbital fissure [arrow]. The cavernous sinus fills by crossflow [open arrow].

portion [16,17,18]. The sclera [18] and optic nerve may show similar changes, and the contrast between the retrobulbar structures and the orbital fat is reduced, due to an increase in density of the latter. All the involved structures may show intense abnormal contrast enhancement. When these changes are associated with the typical clinical picture in a patient with a normal thyroid function, the diagnosis of granuloma is strongly suggested.

Other conditions: myositis, metastatic or primary tumours of muscles and orbital oedema associated with a caroticocavernous fistula, must be considered. Differential diagnosis is more difficult when only the lacrimal gland is affected; absence of bone erosion favours the diagnosis of granuloma.

In practice, the test of the diagnosis is rapid, sustained improvement with systemic steroid therapy.

Specific granulomatous diseases

Sarcoidosis

The most common orbital manifestation of this condition is infiltration of the lacrimal glands (parotid and submandibular glands may also be affected, giving the picture of Mikulicz's syndrome).

Wegener's granuloma [19]

The orbit is usually affected when disease spreads from the adjacent paranasal sinuses. Uni- or bilateral retrobulbar masses may be present.

Amyloidosis

Orbital involvement is rare; well defined masses or diffuse infiltration may be seen.

Histiocytosis X may also cause lacrimal gland or retrobulbar infiltrates or masses. The association with bone lesions is suggestive.

Optic neuritis

This condition, causing loss of vision, with or without pain, in one or both eyes, may be of toxic, infective or inflammatory origin. Multiple sclerosis is a common cause. When the clinical picture is in doubt, CT may be useful in excluding a compressive cause for the visual loss [20]. Rarely, an affected optic nerve is expanded and shows pathological contrast enhancement. Of more positive diagnostic value in multiple sclerosis is cranial CT showing the characteristic paraventricular low density cerebral lesions. MRI is even more useful than CT, but both techniques are helpful in excluding other diseases (Chs 5 and 85).

Vascular lesions

Orbital varices (Fig. 90.22)

Varicose veins may develop within the orbit, involving one or, more commonly, a number of veins. They may become very extensive, and, after thyroid disease, varices are one of the commonest causes of proptosis. Usually developmental in origin, they are sometimes associated with facial or, more rarely, intracranial venous malformations.

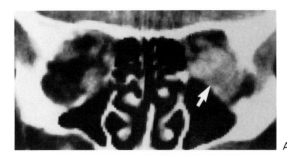

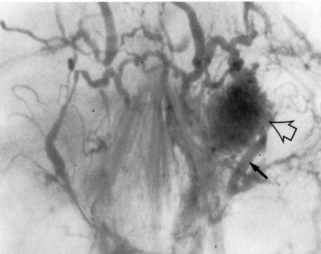

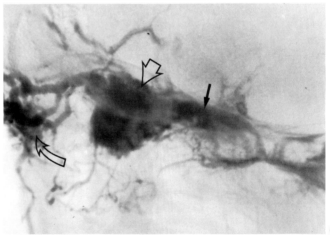

Fig. 90.22 Orbital varix. (A) Coronal CT. (B) & (C) Orbital phlebogram, anteroposterior and lateral projections. Axial CT showed no abnormality, but the coronal section reveals a retrobulbar mass [arrows], more evident in the prone position. Phlebography opacifies a varix [open arrow] in relation to the third portion of the superior ophthalmic vein [arrow]. Note also cutaneous varices [curved arrow].

Proptosis, increased on bending, straining or assuming the prone position, is characteristic. Abnormal veins may be visible beneath the lids. Plain radiographs demonstrate small, rounded areas of calcification, representing phleboliths, in about one third of cases. The orbit may be expanded. The combination of clinical and plain film features establishes the diagnosis in many cases. CT which is carried out in prone position, is of limited value; it shows a more or less extensive, amorphous, nodular or serpiginous mass, sometimes containing phleboliths. There is, of course, marked contrast enhancement. Ultrasonography is quite specific, showing a soft, echo-free lesion which increases in size with the Valsalva manoeuvre.

Orbital phlebography may be carried out if the diagnosis is in doubt, or if cosmetic surgery is planned. Because of the slow flow within the ectatic veins, a prolonged sequence, sometimes up to 30 seconds, may be required. Nevertheless, the varices are often only partially opacified [21].

Arterial lesions

Intraorbital aneurysms are extremely rare. Arteriovenous fistulae (Fig. 90.23) may arise as the result of malformations, following trauma, or apparently spontaneously. They may lie within the orbit or, more commonly, in the region of the cavernous sinus. Only the orbital manifestations are discussed here; the other features are described in Chapters 85 & 86.

Plain films may demonstrate enlargement of the superior orbital fissure by a dilated superior ophthalmic vein. The density of the affected orbit may be increased on the occipito-frontal film, due to soft tissue swelling. Hypertrophied vascular grooves, or evidence of trauma may also be evident.

Ultrasound examination shows a dilated, poorly echogenic, compressible superior ophthalmic vein. The M-mode demonstrates pulsation, evidence of venous arterialization, while Doppler studies reveal an arterial waveform, fading during a Valsalva manoeuvre and then returning after a short delay with lesser amplitude.

CT demonstrates enlargement of the superior ophthalmic vein (and sometimes of the inferior ophthalmic vein); the extraocular muscles may be swollen.

If the diagnosis is evident on clinical examination, these investigations are redundant: angiography is required for assessment and planning treatment.

Orbital space-occupying lesions

Tumours of vascular origin

These represent up to 15% of primary retrobulbar tumours and comprise: capillary angioma, cavernous haemangioma, haemangioendothelioma (benign or malignant) haemangiopericytoma (benign or malignant), vascular leiomyoma and lymphangioma.

The *capillary angioma* is a tumour of early childhood. It forms a soft, bluish mass, which may involve any part of the orbit, including the eyelid. Ultrasonography shows it as a diffuse lesion with small, irregular echoes, its pattern being similar to that of lymphoma, sarcoma or granuloma.

CT is also nonspecific, demonstrating a diffuse lesion with marked contrast enhancement.

Arteriography confirms the diagnosis, showing a highly vascular mass and enables identification of the feeding

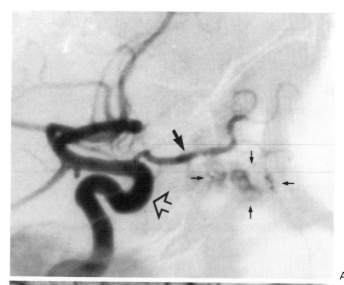

A

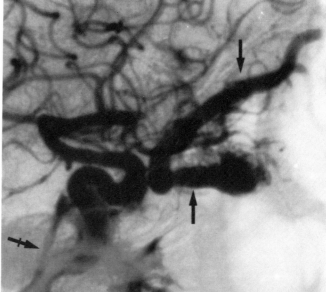

B

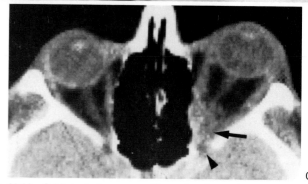

C

Fig. 90.23 Orbital arteriovenous malformation. Internal carotid arteriogram, lateral projection, arterial (A): and late (B) phases: The AVM [small arrows] is fed by the inferior and medial muscular branch of the ophthalmic artery [arrow]. [open arrow = internal carotid artery]. Venous drainage is to the superior and inferior ophthalmic veins (arrows in B) and the inferior petrosal sinus [crossed arrow]. The malformation was also supplied by branches arising from the infraorbital artery, entering the orbit via the inferior orbital fissure. (C) Axial CT. The superior orbital fissure [arrowhead] is enlarged and there is a mass [arrow] at the orbital apex.

vessels, which may arise from the ophthalmic and/or external carotid arteries. However, it is performed only if surgery is considered, since these lesions usually regress with growth of the child.

Cavernous haemangioma, the commonest primary retrobulbar tumour, is a slow growing, well-defined, rounded or lobulated mass consisting of large vascular spaces surrounded by a firm capsule (Fig. 90.24). Plain films may rarely demonstrate phleboliths; enlargement of the orbit is more common.

These lesions have a specific 'honeycomb' ultrasound pattern of alternating weak and strong echoes, corresponding to their structure. CT, the investigation of choice, reveals a well defined, homogeneous, rounded tumour, usually lying within the muscle cone, lateral to the optic nerve, and enhancing with intravenous contrast medium.

Arteriography may show small arterial tufts at the border of the tumour, but paradoxically, the haemangioma is frequently not opacified, probably because of the very slow flow in the cavernous spaces [22].

Haemangioepithelioma, haemangiopericytoma and vascular leiomyoma are rare tumours, without specific radiological features, while lymphangioma is a benign diffuse tumour involving the orbit and adjacent part of the face, seen mainly in children.

Tumours of the lacrimal gland [23] (Fig. 90.25)

The lacrimal gland gives rise to benign tumours of various types (all rare), mixed tumours and malignant tumours including carcinoma and lymphoma.

Mixed tumours represent about half of lacrimal gland neoplasms, and are slow growing, well encapsulated tumours presenting in early middle age. Malignant transformation

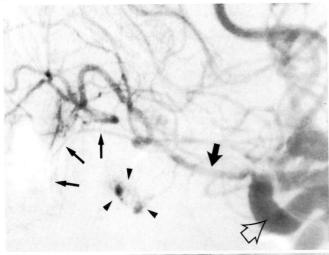
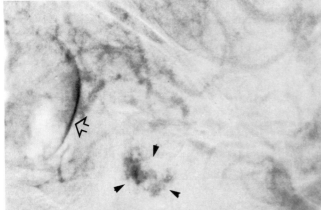
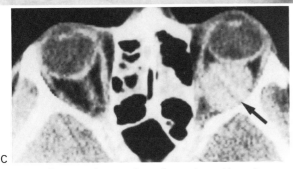

Fig. 90.24 Cavernous haemangioma. Internal carotid arteriogram. lateral projection, (A) arterial and (B) venous phases. Partial opacification of the lesion [arrowheads]; note mass effect on a muscular artery [arrows] and on the choroidal crescent (open arrow in B). [Open arrow = internal carotid artery; broad arrow = ophthalmic artery]. (C) Axial CT. An enhancing intraconal mass [arrows] displaces the globe forwards.

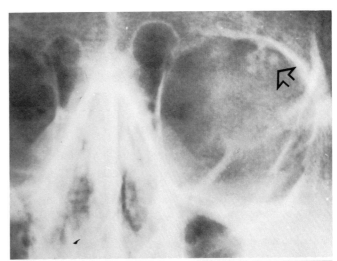
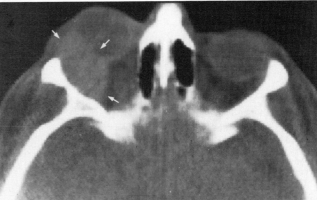

Fig. 90.25 Mixed tumour of lacrimal gland. (A) Occipito-frontal skull radiograph. (B) Axial CT. Calcification is seen on the plain film in the superolateral portion of the orbit, anteriorly; the roof is minimally excavated [arrow]. CT shows an enlarged gland displacing the eye forward.

may, however, occur, with rupture of the capsule and infiltration of the neighbouring soft tissues and bone. Differential diagnosis is from inflammatory conditions, which are more often bilateral, and dermoid cysts lying in the position of the lacrimal gland.

Plain films and tomography may reveal a focal enlargement of the orbit superolaterally, well defined in cases of mixed tumours; irregular destruction, and calcification within the mass are suggestive of malignancy.

CT shows the gland to be increased in size; it is usually well defined, although less so in cases of carcinoma. In general, CT does not differentiate adequately between mixed tumours and carcinomas.

The features which suggest malignancy on plain films, also apply in the case of CT. In inflammatory conditions, such as orbital granuloma, other structures are often seen to be involved. Ultrasound does not contribute to differential diagnosis; arteriography is similarly unrewarding.

Dermoid cysts most typically arise adjacent to the lacrimal gland, at the superolateral angle of the orbit anteriorly and are therefore considered here. They may, however, be encountered elsewhere, at the superomedial angle, for example. The cyst is a slowly growing tumour of aberrant dermoid tissue, which characteristically causes a well defined, rounded erosion of the bone, with a fine cortical margin; the bone may be expanded. CT confirms the diagnosis, showing material of relatively low density within the cyst; a fat-fluid level may be present.

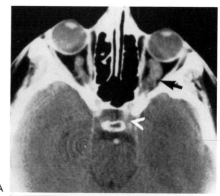

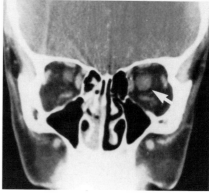

Fig. 90.26 Glioma of the left optic nerve. (A) & (B) Axial and coronal CT. The left optic nerve is thickened [arrow]. Extension to the chiasm [arrowhead] was better shown in other sections.

Tumours of nerve

Neural tumours may arise from the optic nerve (or its dural sheath) or from the peripheral nerves within the orbit.

Optic nerve glioma[24] (Fig. 90.26) arises from glial cells: astrocytes and oligodendrocytes. It may develop in any part of the optic pathway from nerve to tract; only tumours of the nerve are considered here. This tumour is seen most often in children aged 5 to 10 years; neurofibromatosis is a common association. Clinical features include decreased visual acuity and irregular constriction of the fields, proptosis and papilloedema, which progresses to optic atrophy. Papilloedema may be due to raised intracranial pressure when the tumour involves the chiasm and obstructs the foramina of Monro.

Plain films and tomograms may be normal at presentation; the most frequent abnormality is rounding and increased diameter of the optic canal, often with thinning of the bony margins. This is a significant finding because it indicates involvement beyond the intraorbital portion of the nerve.

CT is the examination of choice, and shows a fusiform expansion of the optic nerve, whose density is the same or slightly greater than that of a normal nerve. Enhancement with intravenous contrast medium is very variable. Coronal images permit comparison with the contralateral nerve, and confirm that the tumour arises from, and not alongside the nerve. The CT study should include the entire optic pathways, to exclude intracranial extension.

Ultrasound can demonstrate clearly the enlarged optic nerve. However, absorption of echoes is marked, so that assessment of the posterior extent of the tumour is difficult. Anterior bulging of the optic disc, or indeed, of the whole posterior portion of the globe, pushed forward by the tumour, may be evident. In the A-mode, the echoes are of moderately high amplitude (40 to 60% of those of the sclera); they are very regular[25].

Angiography is rarely indicated, even when the diagnosis is questionable[26]. It demonstrates increased diameter of the loop made around the nerve by the ophthalmic artery and, occasionally, a faint tumour blush. Differentiation from optic nerve sheath meningioma is not always possible.

Meningioma of the sheath of the optic nerve (Fig. 90.27) develops from meningoblastic rests in the dura mater and grows around the optic fibres, compressing but not infiltrating them. It generally presents in adult life, with axial proptosis, decreased visual acuity and a constricted field or central scotoma.

Plain films, including tomograms, are unrewarding in the majority of cases. The optic canal is usually normal if the meningioma only arises from the nerve sheath; it may however be widened by the tumour or narrowed due to hyperostosis. Calcification may be visible, overlying the optic canal, or along the optic nerve.

At ultrasonography, the lesion has reflectivity similar to that of optic nerve glioma, but with less well defined borders; calcification may be detected.

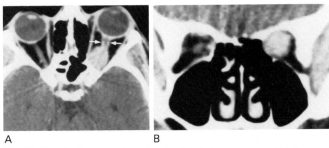

Fig. 90.27 Meningioma of the sheath of the left optic nerve. (A) & (B) Axial and coronal CT. The tumour involves the sheath of the nerve [arrows], while the nerve itself is seen as a less dense core within the mass.

CT is once again the procedure of choice, giving a good demonstration of the site and shape of the tumour, and showing its relationship to the surrounding structures [27]. Before intravenous contrast medium, the optic nerve appears diffusely thickened and dense; it shows marked contrast enhancement, more intense than in the case of optic nerve glioma. Calcification is not infrequent, and may be obviously circumferential. A careful study of the intracranial end of the optic nerve is important to exclude an intracranial extension.

Arteriography sometimes demonstrates a tumour blush, which may be dense, but is often virtually normal, except in advanced cases, when the calibre of the ophthalmic artery is increased if the tumour is markedly hypervascular; its loop around the nerve may be widened.

Generalized expansion of the optic nerve simulating a meningioma at CT examination may be seen in papilloedema whatever its cause, due to expansion of the subarachnoid space around the nerve [28]. The increased density seen with meningioma is however absent. A-mode ultrasound demonstrates the widening of the sheath [29].

Tumours arising from the other orbital nerves may be divided into schwannomas, which develop from the sheath of the nerve, and neurofibromas, whose site of origin is the nervous elements themselves.

Schwannomas may arise from any peripheral nerve. They are generally benign. Round or ovoid, they are well encapsulated and do not adhere to surrounding structures. Plain films may demonstrate enlargement of the orbit, and occasionally of the superior orbital fissure. CT shows a rounded mass of soft tissue density, lying inside or outside the muscle cone, and enhancing after intravenous contrast medium, thus resembling a cavernous haemangioma. Ultrasound shows no characteristic features; angiography, rarely indicated, may show dilated vessels and a tumour blush.

Neurofibromas may have identical appearances in all modalities. Plexiform neurofibroma is a particular variety seen in neurofibromatosis, involving the nerves of the orbit and often also the adjacent soft tissues, which are thickened. CT shows the generalized intra and periorbital soft tissue thickening, which can be impossible to distinguish from soft tissue hemihypertrophy, which also occurs in this condition. Some degree of sphenoid dysplasia is not uncommonly present, and

other manifestations of neurofibromatosis may be evident. Ultrasonography is not characteristic.

Malignant tumours

Primary and secondary malignant tumours occur within the orbit. Those of vascular and lacrimal gland origin have already been mentioned.

Various types of sarcoma and reticulosis represent 80% of primary malignant tumours of the orbit. They cause rapidly progressive proptosis, with diplopia. Anterior segment changes are not uncommon and compression of the optic nerve is frequent. The orbit is also a frequent site of metastatic disease; the tumours involve the soft tissues and/or bony walls. In children, neuroblastoma and in the adult, breast, lung, thyroid and gastrointestinal cancers are the most common.

Plain films and/or tomography may demonstrate irregular erosion of bone, highly suggestive of the diagnosis. Masses shown by CT are without specific features and, in the absence of bone changes, the diagnosis of malignancy is difficult. Diffuse involvement of all the retrobulbar structures is suggestive, but may be seen in, for example, granulomatous disease. The relatively common tumour of childhood, *rhabdomyosarcoma*, is particularly misleading: increase of the size of all or part of a muscle, with well defined borders, maybe seen in the early stages. The tumour may be adjacent to a muscle or may simulate an enlarged lacrimal gland.

At an advanced stage, these malignant tumours invade the entire retrobulbar space, the orbital walls and the neighbouring structures.

Reticuloses and lymphoma do not produce characteristic CT abnormalities. Differential diagnosis from granuloma may be particularly difficult, since a therapeutic trial of steroids may reduce the symptoms due to a malignant tumour as well as to granuloma, although remission is usually temporary.

Ultrasound is similarly unrewarding in this context. All these malignant tumours belong to Coleman's infiltrative group [6], showing an irregular anterior border, heterogeneous internal structure, weak reflectivity and poor visualization of the posterior border due to marked acoustic absorption.

Rare intraorbital tumours

Myxoma, fibroma and myoblastoma are all rare tumours. CT shows a well defined retrobulbar mass, but histological diagnosis depends on biopsy. Intraorbital meningioma, arising from aberrant meningoblasts in the orbital fat is described, but is extremely rare [30].

Neighbouring tumours

Tumours arising in surrounding structures (paranasal sinuses, nasopharynx, middle or anterior cranial fossae) may invade the orbit.

INTRAOCULAR ABNORMALITIES

Examination of the internal structure of the globe is generally the province of ultrasonography [31].

Congenital and traumatic lesions are discussed in the appropriate sections (pp. 1880 and 1882).

Lesions of the anterior segment

Ultrasound is useful in cases of corneal or lenticular opacity, not only for the demonstration of these abnormalities, but also to assess any associated lesions (vitreous haemorrhage, retinal detachment, choroidal effusion). A and B-modes can be useful to differentiate between subcapsular, cortical or nuclear cataracts. When calcification is dense, it may be detected on plain radiographs. If lens implantation is planned, ultrasound is used to exclude associated abnormalities such as retinal detachment which might contraindicate operation, and to measure accurately the anteroposterior diameter of the globe.

The vitreous

In an emmetropic eye, the vitreous is echo-free, but in myopia or senile vitreous degeneration, weak echoes appear best detected with the A-mode. Ophthalmoscopy is inadequate for assessment of these lesions. With a minimal recent haemorrhage into the posterior vitreous, echoes of low amplitude are detected on the detached hyaloid membrane, while if the bleeding is more marked, the form and pattern of the echoes vary considerably, often suggesting bands or masses. Real-time B-mode scanning with eye movement enables identification of the site of the lesions: if they lie in the solid portion of the vitreous, movement is rapidly attenuated, whereas in the liquid portion, movements are greater, more rapid and slowly attenuated; this distinction is of prognostic and therapeutic significance.

Unresorbed vitreous haemorrhage can lead to organization of the retina due to vitreous retraction, or retinitis proliferans. Ultrasonography is useful when vitrectomy is planned, providing complementary information in difficult cases and aiding identification of ocular lesions e.g. luxation of the lens, preretinal membranes, detachment. These lesions may influence the operative technique.

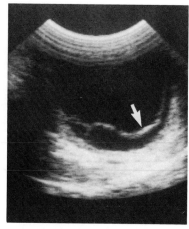

Fig. 90.28 Retinal detachment. B-mode ultrasound. A membrane [arrow] is seen within the vitreous, attached to the optic disc and the ora serrata. In real time it showed slow, undulating after movements; its high reflectivity is characteristic of a detached retina.

Retinal lesions (Fig. 90.28)

Detachment of the retina is frequent after ocular trauma and in high myopia, due to traction on the retina by the vitreous. The degree is variable; its extent may be very limited, or total, extending from the disc to the ora serrata. The detached segment is more or less mobile, with slow and sinuous movements, particularly at first. CT demonstrates some cases, but ultrasound is the method of choice. The A mode permits detailed study of the subretinal space for serous fluid, blood or crystalline cholesterol debris.

Eventually, the detached retina becomes thickened or retracted, with a 'T' or triangular appearance from optic disc to ora serrata.

Secondary detachment due to, for example, choroidal melanoma, must be excluded. Retinopathies, including the diabetic type, may show increased thickness of the retina, together with decreased echogenicity.

In the B-mode, subretinal haemorrhage is manifest as an echogenic zone, well limited anteriorly by the retina, which may be poor in echoes superiorly and more dense inferiorly as the solid elements fall to the dependent portion.

Retinoblastoma (Fig. 90.29)

This highly malignant lesion is the most common intraocular tumour of childhood. Some cases are hereditary, as an autosomal dominant of incomplete penetration, and are often bilateral. Young children are most at risk: 85% of these tumours are detected before 3 years of age. The tumour may grow into the vitreous, and then seed into the aqueous. In about one quarter of cases, there is extension into the subretinal space, producing retinal detachment and with a risk of haematogenous metastasis (to bones, lung and liver).

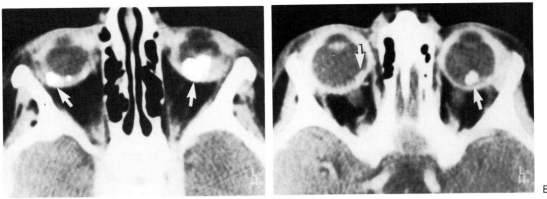

Fig. 90.29 Bilateral retinoblastoma. (A) & (B) Axial CT. Several calcified masses are visible on both sides and there is contrast enhancement of the outer coats of the globes. There is no evident extention to the optic nerves, which appear normal in size.

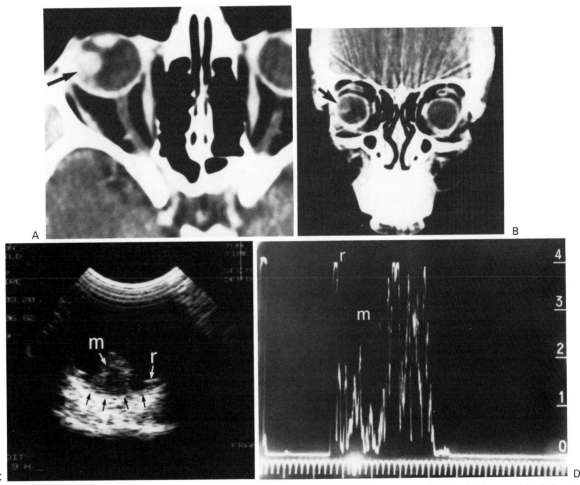

Fig. 90.30 Malignant melanoma. (A) & (B) Axial and coronal CT. (C) & (D) B and A mode ultrasound. CT and Ultrasound both demonstrate an upper temporal intraocular tumour. CT shows contrast enhancement, while ultrasound reveals its moderately echoic, heterogeneous nature, with choroidal excavation. [m = melanoma; r = retinal detachment; arrows = choroidal excavation].

When the choroid is involved, orbital extension is frequent. Of particular importance is extension into the optic nerve, often localized to the region of the posterior scleral foramen, but sometimes as far as the chiasm; cerebral and meningeal spread can then occur. Typically, a young child presents with a blind 'cat's eye' due to white retrolental tumour.

Ultrasound shows an intraocular mass, ranging from a small, solid tumour to a large, irregular, often mushroom-shaped, inhomogeneous, sometimes cystic tumour with calcification, perhaps with an associated retinal detachment. Although calcification can be seen on plain radiographs in up to 75% of cases, it is better assessed by CT, which demonstrates uni- or bilateral lesions, sometimes multifocal, thickening the outer wall of the globe, often calcified. Contrast enhancement is variable. The main value of CT is detection of orbital and intracranial extension [32]. Postoperative assessment is important because local recurrence is not rare, but differentiation from granulomatous or more acute inflammatory changes is difficult.

Choroidal lesions

Choroidal detachments have characteristic ultrasound appearances: they extend to the equator of the globe, forming an acute angle at the posterior wall, which appears thin relative to the detached retina and choroid. Ultrasound is of value in excluding an underlying tumour.

Malignant melanoma (Fig. 90.30)

This highly malignant neoplasm arises in the choroid and is the commonest uveal tract tumour, and the commonest primary intraocular tumour in adults, presenting usually between 50 and 60 years of age.

Ultrasonography is of great value, since tumours greater than 1 mm in diameter should be shown and differential diagnosis is possible when the diameter exceeds 2.5 mm. A and B modes are complementary, revealing the characteristic features: a moderately echogenic tumour (10 to 60% of scleral peaks), solid, immobile, but with rhythmic pulsations indicating its vascularity. The size, shape and position of the lesion can be assessed, and certain characteristic features may be evident: choroidal vascularization or excavation, frequently with posterior shadowing. Retinal detachment and posterior scleral infiltration may also be present.

CT shows only relatively large tumours. The findings are characteristic but not specific: a focal, dense thickening of the posterior wall of the globe, with contrast enhancement. The technique is more valuable for the detection of the posterior extension to the optic nerve or retrobulbar space.

Metastatic tumours to the choroid are frequent at necropsy, but often clinically silent. Their radiological features are nonspecific.

Choroidal angiomas are strongly reflective on B-scanning, and are seen as small echogenic masses bulging towards the vitreous. In the A-mode, the peaks are relatively high in comparison with the retinal peaks.

BIBLIOGRAPHY

REFERENCES

1. Wolff E 1968 Anatomy of the eye and orbit. Lewis, London
2. Lloyd G A S 1975 Radiology of the orbit. Saunders, London
3. Hesselink J R et al 1982 Computed tomography of the paranasal sinuses and face. Part I: normal anatomy; Part II: pathologic anatomy. J Comput Assist Tomogr 6:559–577
4. Tadmor R. New P J F 1978 Computed tomography of the orbit with special emphasis on coronal sections. Part I: Normal anatomy; Part II: Pathologic anatomy. J Comput Assist Tomogr 2:24–44
5. Isherwood I, Pullen B R, Ritchings R T 1978 Radiation dose in neuroradiological procedures. Neuroradiology 16:477–481
6. Coleman D J, Lizzi F L, Jack R L 1977 Ultrasonography of the eye and orbit. Lea and Febiger, Philadelphia
7. Hayreh S S 1962 The ophthalmic artery: III. Branches. Br J Ophthalmol 46:212–247
8. Lasjaunias P, Brismar J, Moret J, Théron J 1978 Recurrent cavernous branches of the ophthalmic artery. Acta Radiol 19:553–560
9. Moret J, Lasjaunias P, Théron J, Merland J J 1977 The middle meningeal artery. Its contribution to the vascularisation of the orbit. J Neuroradiol 4:225–248
10. Brismar J, Davis K R, Dallow R L, Brismar G 1976 Unilateral endocrine exophthalmos. Diagnostic problems in association with computed tomography. Neuroradiology 12:21–24
11. Cabanis E A, Iba Zizen M T, Guillaumat L 1979 Diagnostic tomodensitométrique des exophtalmies basedowiennes. A propos de 60 observations. Bull Mem Soc Fr Ophthalmol 91:263–276
12. Enzmann D, Donaldson S S, Kriss J P 1979 Appearance of Graves' disease on orbital computed tomography. J Comput Assist Tomogr 3:815–819
13. Goldberg F, Bernes A S, Oski F A 1978 Differentiation of orbital cellulitis from preseptal cellulitis by computed tomography. Pediatrics 62:1000–1005
14. Zimmerman R A, Bilaniuk L T 1980 CT of orbital infection and its cerebral complications. Am J Roentgenol 134:45–50
15. Blodi F C, Gass J D M 1968 Inflammatory pseudotumour of the orbit. Br J Ophthalmol 52:79–93
16. Enzmann D, Donaldson S S, Marshall W H, Kriss J P 1976 Computed tomography in orbital pseudotumor (idiopathic orbital inflammation) Radiology 120:597–601
17. Nugent R A, Rootman J, Robertson W D, Lapointe J S, Harrison P B 1981 Acute orbital pseudotumors: classification and CT features. Am J Roentgenol 137:957–962
18. Bernardino M E, Zimmerman R D, Citrin C M, Davis D C 1977 Scleral thickening: a CT sign of orbital pseudotumor. Am J Roentgenol 129:703–706
19. Vermess M, Haynes B F, Fauci A S, Wolff S M 1978 Computer assisted tomography of orbital lesions in Wegener's granulomatosis. J. Comput Assist Tomogr 2:45–48
20. Levine H L, Ferris E J, Lessel S, Spatz E L 1975 The neuroradiological evaluation of 'optic neuritis'. Am J Roentgenol 125:702–716
21. Vignaud J, Clay C, Bilaniuk L T 1974 Venography of the orbit. An analytical report of 413 cases. Radiology: 110:373–382
22. Dilenge D 1974 Arteriography in tumors of the orbit. CRC Crit Rev Clin Radiol 5:213–250
23. Lloyd G A S 1981 Lacrimal gland tumours: the role of CT and conventional radiology. Br J Radiol 54:1034–1038
24. Pásztor E, Remenár L 1978 Optic nerve gliomas. 1. Clinical diagnosis and pathology. Acta Neurochir 41:191–203

25. Dallow R L 1975 Evaluation of unilateral exophthalmos with ultra-sonography: analysis of 258 consecutive cases. Laryngoscope 85:1905–1918
26. Moseley I F, Bull J W D 1975 Computerised axial tomography, carotid angiography and orbital phlebography in the diagnosis of orbital space occupying lesions. In: Salamon G (ed) Advances in cerebral angiography. Springer, Berlin, pp 364–369
27. Lloyd G A S 1982 Primary orbital meningiomas. Clin Radiol 33:181–188
28. Cabanis E A, Salvolini U, Rodallec A, Menichelli F, Pasquini U, Bonnin P 1978 Computed tomography of the optic nerve. Part II. Size and shape modifications in papilledema. J Comput Assist Tomogr 2:150–155
29. Skalka W S 1977 Ultrasonography of the optic nerve. In: Smith J L (ed) Neuro-ophthalmology update. Masson, Paris, 119–130
30. Karp L A, Zimmerman L E, Borit A, Spencer W 1974 Primary orbital meningiomas. Arch Ophthalmol 91:24–28
31. Aubin M L, Vignaud J 1978 Computerised tomography of the eye: a study of 62 pathologic cases. Neuroradiology 16:456–457
32. Danziger A, Price H I 1979 CT findings in retinoblastoma. Am J Roentgenol 133:695–697

SUGGESTIONS FOR FURTHER READING

Aron Rosa D, Doyon D 1974 Etude radiologique des exophtalmies tumorales d'origine orbitaire et endocrinienne. Clin Ophtalmol 3:145–156
Arger P H 1977 Orbit roentgenology. Wiley, New York
Gyldensted C, Lester J J, Fledelius H 1977 Computed tomography of orbital lesions. A radiological study of 144 cases. Neuroradiology 13:141–150
Hanafee W N, Dayton G O 1970 The roentgen diagnosis of orbital tumors. Radiol Clin North Am 8:403–412
Guillot P, Saraux H, Sedan R 1966 L'Exploration neuroradiologique en ophtalmologie. Masson, Paris
Jacobs L, Weisberg L A, Kinkel W R 1980 Computerized tomography of the orbit and sella turcica. Raven Press, New York
Jones I S, Jakobiec F A 1979 Diseases of the orbit. Harper and Row, Hagerston
Lombardi G 1967 Radiology in neuro-ophthalmology. Williams and Wilkins, Baltimore
Moseley I F, Sanders M D 1982 Computerized tomography in neuro-ophthalmology. Chapman and Hall, London
Salvolini U, Menichelli F, Pasquini U 1977 Computer assisted tomography in 90 cases of exophthalmos. J Comput Assist Tomogr 1:81–100
Vignaud J, Clay C, Salvolini U, Bilaniuk L T 1982 Radio-ophtalmologie Vol 16 of Fischgold H (ed) Traité de radiologie. Paris, Masson

91 Maxillofacial radiology

James McIvor

Fractures
Benign cysts
Benign tumours
Ameloblastoma and other odontogenic tumours
Odontomes
Non-neoplastic bone lesions
Miscellaneous radiolucent lesions of the jaws
Malignant tumours
Fibro-osseous lesions
Infection and associated conditions
Differential diagnosis of radiolucent and radio-opaque
   bone lesions
Abnormalities of growth and development
The temporomandibular joint
Salivary glands
Soft tissue calcification

FRACTURES

Fractures of the maxilla

Maxillary fractures are still classified according to the system of Le Fort who defined three principle patterns of fracture, after a series of macabre experiments carried out on cadavers at the beginning of the 20th century (Fig. 91.1).

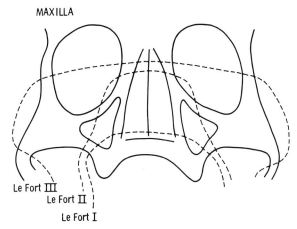

Fig. 91.1 Diagram of the fracture lines in Le Fort I, II and III fractures.

In a Le Fort I fracture (Fig. 91.2), the tooth-bearing part of the maxilla becomes separated from the rest of the maxilla by fractures through the medial and lateral walls of the maxillary sinuses, and by a fracture through the lower part of the nasal septum.

The Le Fort II fracture (Fig. 91.3) is more extensive and the separated fragment is pyramidal. The apex of the pyramid is the lower part of the nasal bones, and the fracture lines run inferiorly and laterally through the medial and inferior walls of the orbits, and then through the lateral walls of the maxillary sinuses. The nasal septum is fractured at a variable level.

In the Le Fort III fracture (Fig. 91.4 & 91.5) there is complete craniofacial disjunction. The fracture line runs through the nasal bones as in the Le Fort II fracture, and then

1899

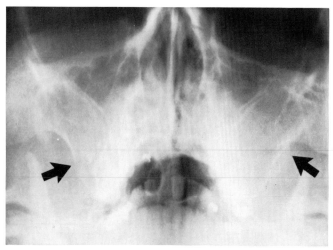

Fig. 91.2 Le Fort I fracture. The fractures of the lateral walls of the maxillary sinuses have been arrowed. The fractures of the medial walls cannot be seen on this projection.

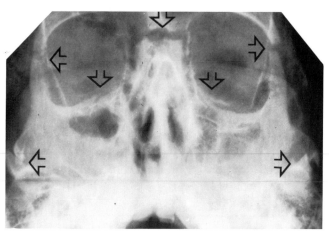

Fig. 91.4 Combined Le Fort II and Le Fort III fractures. There are fractures of the nasal bones, lateral orbital margins, inferior orbital margins and zygomatic arches. All have been marked with arrows.
There is a fluid level in the right maxillary sinus and there is opacification of the left maxillary sinus.

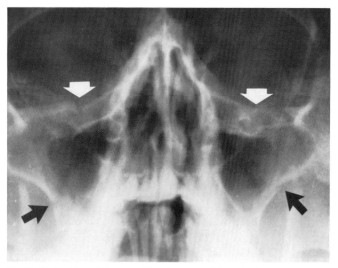

Fig. 91.3 Le Fort II fracture. The fractures of the inferior margins of the orbits and of the lateral walls of the maxillary sinuses have been arrowed. The fracture of the nasal bones is not visible on this projection.

posteriorly and laterally through the medial and lateral walls of the orbits, and through the zygomatic arches. The nasal septum is fractured superiorly.

In practice many fractures do not fit these descriptions exactly; for instance, there may be a Le Fort II fracture on one side and a Le Fort III on the other, or a Le Fort I or II fracture may coexist with a Le Fort III (Fig. 91.4 & 91.5). However, the Le Fort classification is still in general use, as it allows these complicated fractures to be described in a few words, and has the additional advantage of grouping them according to the pattern of subsequent surgical management. In Le Fort I and II fractures the detached maxillary fragment is usually wired to the zygomatic arches, but if these are fractured, as in a Le Fort III fracture, it is necessary to resort to a more complicated type of pin and rod fixation to the skull vault.

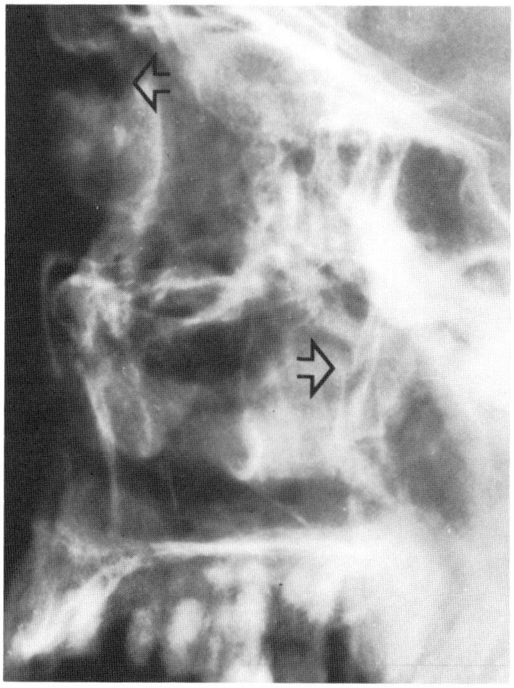

Fig. 91.5 Lateral view of fractures shown in Figure 91.4. There is a fracture of the nasal bones with wide separation [arrow] and there are fractures of the posterior walls of the maxillary sinuses [arrow].

Fractures of the zygoma

The zygomatic bone contributes to the lateral and inferior margins of the orbit, the lateral wall of the maxillary sinus, and the anterior end of the zygomatic arch. Consequently, a fracture of the zygomatic bone results in fractures at these regions (Figs. 91.6 & 91.7). It is often impossible to see all four fractures on a single occipitomental film but the presence of even one fracture line should raise the suspicion of other fractures, and is an indication for further radiographs.

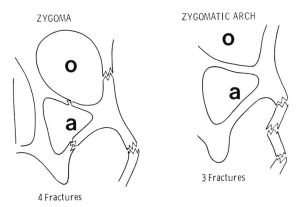

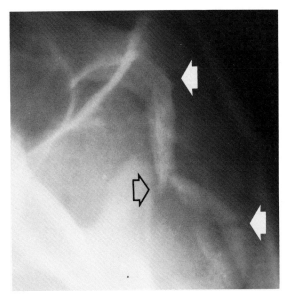

Fig. 91.6 Diagram of the usual site of fracture of the zygoma and of the zygomatic arch. [0 = orbit, a = antrum].

Fig. 91.8 Fracture of the zygomatic arch. The three fractures have been arrowed.

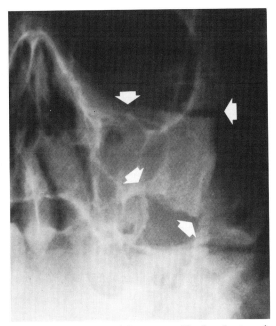

Fig. 91.7 Displaced fracture of the zygoma. The four fractures have been arrowed.

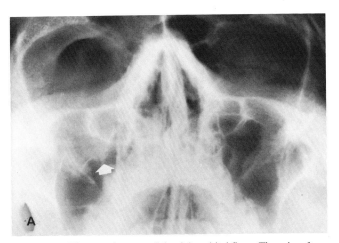

Fig. 91.9A Blow-out fracture of the right orbital floor. There is soft tissue shadowing in the upper part of the right maxillary sinus [arrow] but no fracture is visible.

The zygomatic arch may be fractured in association with a fracture of the zygoma as described above, or it may be fractured as a result of direct trauma, when it may fracture in three places (Figs. 91.6 & 91.8).

There are fractures in this region in Le Fort II and III fractures as already described.

Blow-out fractures of the orbital floor

A 'blow-out' fracture of the orbital floor is an uncommon sequel to blunt trauma applied to the front of the orbit. The orbital rim remains intact, but the temporary increase in pressure within the orbit causes the thin floor to fracture and the soft tissues of the orbit to herniate through the defect into the maxillary sinus.

This may show as a soft tissue shadow in the upper part of the maxillary sinus on an occipitomental radiograph

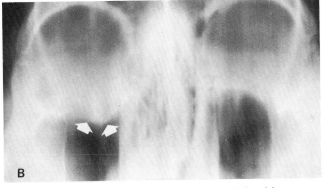

Fig. 91.9B Tomogram of the same case, showing displaced fractures of the thin bony floor of the orbit [arrows].

(Fig. 91.9A), but the fractured orbital floor rarely shows on plain films.

The clinical importance of this fracture is that the inferior rectus and oblique muscles may become attached to the orbital floor by fibrous tissue, which results in permanent limitation of upward movement of the eyeball and in diplopia on looking upwards.

If a blow-out fracture is suspected, tomography of the orbital floor is indicated and will demonstrate any fractures which are present. (Fig. 91.9B). CT scanning in the coronal plane has been used to demonstrate blow-out fractures of the orbital floor, and will demonstrate soft tissue displacement and herniation more accurately than conventional radiographic tomography.

Indirect signs of maxillary fractures

There are three radiological abnormalities which are often due to maxillary fractures, but which also occur in other conditions. Their presence in patients with a history of facial trauma should increase the suspicion that a fracture is present, and should be an indication for further films.

Soft tissue swelling is a common and nonspecific sign which is almost invariably present if there is a recent fracture.

Opacification of the maxillary sinus is usual in fractures which involve its wall (Le Fort I, II and III fractures, zygomatic fractures) and a fluid level is occasionally seen. These abnormalities should suggest haemorrhage into the sinus.

Soft tissue emphysema is a rare but useful sign, as it provides positive evidence of a fracture involving the nasal cavity, or one of the paranasal sinuses [1]. It may show as multiple small radiolucent areas in the soft tissues, or the air may enter the orbit to outline the eyeball (Fig. 91.10).

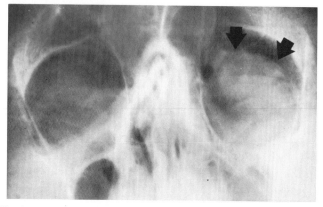

Fig. 91.10 Soft tissue emphysema of the left orbit outlining the upper margin of the eyeball. There is an undisplaced fracture of the left zygoma which cannot be identified on this film.

Radiographic demonstration of maxillary fractures

Fractures of the maxilla and zygoma can be difficult to demonstrate radiologically, particularly if there is no displacement. The initial films should consist of an occipi-

tomental and a 30° occipitomental, taken PA if possible, as this provides better bony detail.

A lateral film of the facial bones is also useful, as it usually shows a step in the posterior wall of the maxillary sinus if the maxilla is fractured (Fig. 91.5).

Tomography of the orbits is indicated if there is any suspicion of a blow-out fracture of the orbital floor, or if there is any indication that the orbital contents have herniated through a fracture (Fig. 91.9B).

The zygomatic arches show reasonably well on occipitomental projections, but an underpenetrated submentovertical view provides the clearest demonstration.

Fractures of the teeth and of the alveolar bone are best shown on intraoral dental films.

Fractures of the mandible

Fractures of the mandible are classified according to the site of fracture (Fig. 91.11). The most common sites are the condylar neck (Fig. 91.12), the angle (Fig. 91.13) and the body (Fig. 91.14 & 91.15), but fractures can occur elsewhere (Fig. 91.16), and fractures at any site may be comminuted (Figs. 91.15 & 91.17).

Undisplaced fractures of the body and angle are classified as being 'horizontally favourable' if the fracture line runs inferiorly and anteriorly, as the muscles attached to the fragments tend to pull them together. Conversely, a fracture running posteriorly and inferiorly is described as 'horizontally unfavourable', as the fragments tend to be pulled apart by the muscles inserted into them (Fig. 91.18).

Fractures through the tooth-bearing part of the mandible are almost invariably compound into the mouth (Figs. 91.14 & 91.15).

The mandible, like the pelvis, is commonly fractured at two sites, as the bone is U-shaped and is held quite firmly at both ends by the capsules of the temporomandibular joints. For instance, a fracture of the body on one side is often accompanied by a fracture of the condylar neck on the other.

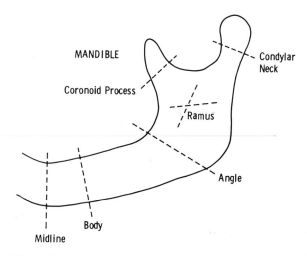

Fig. 91.11 Diagram of the common sites of fracture of the mandible.

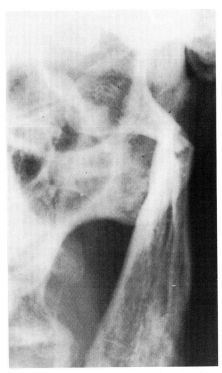

Fig. 91.12   Fracture of the condylar neck of the mandible.

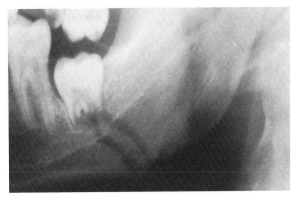

Fig. 91.13   Horizontally unfavourable fracture through the angle of the mandible. The two radiolucent lines repesent fractures through the inner and outer plates.

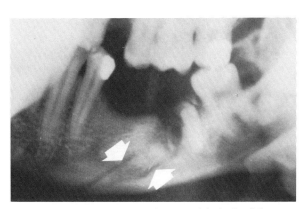

Fig. 91.14   Horizontally favourable fracture of the body of the mandible. The fracture lines through the inner and outer plates have been marked with arrows.

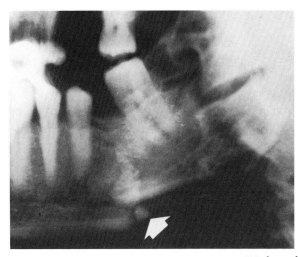

Fig. 91.15   Comminuted fracture of the body of the mandible [arrow] with some displacement.

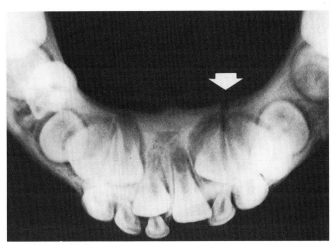

Fig. 91.16   Undisplaced fracture of the anterior part of the mandible in a child [arrow]. The fracture showed only on the intraoral occlusal film.

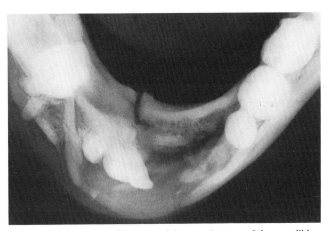

Fig. 91.17   Comminuted fracture of the anterior part of the mandible on an intraoral occlusal film.

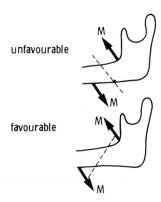

Fig. 91.18 Diagram of the fracture lines in horizontally favourable and unfavourable fractures of the body of the mandible. [M] indicates the direction of muscle pull on the anterior and posterior fragments.

Radiographic demonstration of mandibular fractures

Undisplaced fractures of the mandible can be difficult to demonstrate and may not show on plain films until a few days after the injury, when there will be some resorbtion at the fracture site.

The initial films should consist of a PA view of the facial bones, plus oblique views of both sides of the mandible, and if the patient is able to cooperate, a panoramic radiograph of the mandible is often helpful.

If an anterior fracture is suspected, a rotated PA film and an intraoral occlusal film are indicated. Fractures of the condyles and condylar necks are best shown on the half axial (Towne's) view. Fractures of the teeth and alveolar bone show most clearly on intraoral dental films.

In a few cases it will be necessary to resort to tomography of suspicious areas.

BENIGN CYSTS

General considerations

Benign cysts of the jaws differ pathologically from benign cysts occurring in other bones, as they are almost invariably of dental origin. They are common lesions which usually present clinically when they rupture into the oral cavity and become infected, with the result that the radiological features of infection are often superimposed on the radiological features of a simple cyst. In particular the cortical margin round the cyst is often incomplete due to infection.

In general, benign cysts and tumours displace the roots of adjacent teeth without resorbing them, although large lesions can cause some resorbtion. Malignant tumours, however, tend to resorb the roots of adjacent teeth without displacing them.

Benign cysts can become very large before they present clinically, mandibular cysts may extend from the condylar neck to the incisor region and maxillary cysts can expand into the maxillary sinus (see Fig. 91.20C).

The surgical treatment of benign cysts is usually curettage, followed by primary closure, but large cysts are occasionally marsupialised into the oral cavity. As in other bone lesions the final diagnosis depends on a combination of the clinical, radiological and histological features.

Dental cyst

An *apical dental cyst* (apical periodontal cyst) is the most common cyst of the jaws, and accounts for almost half of all radiolucent jaw lesions. It develops at the root apex of a nonvital permanent tooth, and can present at almost any age above 20 years (Fig.91.19 & 91.20). The pulp may be necrotic due to infection or trauma, or it may have been removed prior to root treatment.

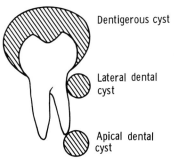

Fig. 91.19 Diagram of the sites of a dentigerous cyst, lateral dental cyst and apical dental cyst.

An apical dental cyst develops as a result of necrosis within a granuloma, so the radiological features of an apical granuloma merge with those of a small cyst. If the diameter of a corticated radiolucent area at the apex of a tooth exceeds 1 cm it is probably a cyst. Large cysts expand the cortical outline of the maxilla or mandible, and maxillary cysts may expand into the maxillary sinus.

The bony margin is corticated and continuous unless the cyst has become infected, or a pathological fracture is present when the cortical outline may be incomplete. Some cysts appear multilocular radiologically, but they are always unilocular at operation. The roots of adjacent teeth are often displaced, (Figs. 91.20A & B) and are very occasionally eroded (less than 5%).

The lining consists of thick, stratified, squamous epithelium which rarely shows evidence of keratinisation.

A **lateral dental cyst** (lateral periodontal cyst) is a rare lesion which develops lateral to the root of a dead or living tooth (Fig. 91.19). It has the same radiological features as an apical dental cyst, except that it is situated alongside a tooth, and not at its apex.

A **residual dental cyst** (residual periodontal cyst) is an apical or lateral dental cyst which was left behind when the tooth

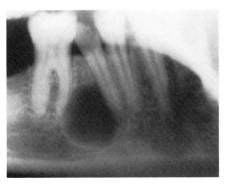

Fig. 91.20A Apical dental cyst arising from a carious lower right second premolar and displacing the root anteriorly. The cortical margin is largely intact.

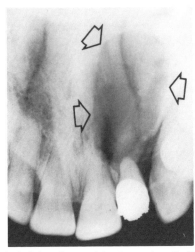

Fig. 91.20B Apical dental cyst arising from a heavily filled and non-vital upper left second incisor and displacing the root apex anteriorly. The cortical margin of the cyst has been destroyed by infection.

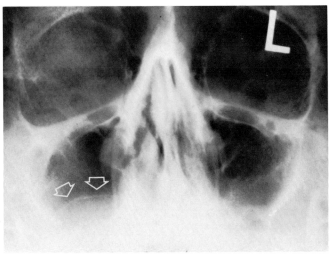

Fig. 91.20C Occipitomental projection of a large residual dental cyst which has expanded into the right maxillary sinus. The radio-opaque line at the upper margin of the soft tissue shadow [arrows] indicates that the lesion has originated outside the maxillary sinus and expanded into it.

from which it developed was extracted (Fig. 91.19). It is, therefore, more common in the older age groups. These cysts can become very large (Fig. 91.20C) and have the same radiological features as apical dental cysts, except that they occur in edentulous areas of the jaws.

Dentigerous cyst

A dentigerous cyst develops from the enamel forming tissue (enamel organ) of a developing permanent tooth. This produces the characteristic radiological appearance of a corticated radiolucent area surrounding the crown of an unerupted tooth (Figs. 91.19, 91.21 & 91.22).

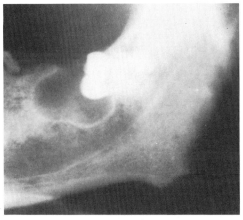

Fig. 91.21 Small dentigerous cyst around the crown of a horizontally impacted unerupted lower third molar. There is a root fragment anterior to the cyst.

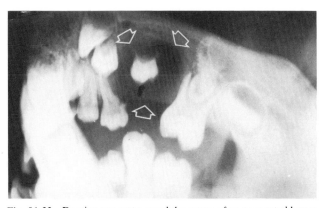

Fig. 91.22 Dentigerous cyst around the crown of an unerupted lower right second premolar. The radiolucent area [arrows] lacks a cortical margin as it has been destroyed by infection.

These cysts usually present during the second decade and commonly develop around the crowns of lower third molars. The cortical outline is continuous in the absence of infection. Adjacent teeth are often displaced, but their roots are rarely resorbed. Dentigerous cysts can become very large and may develop a multilocular appearance, but they are always unilocular at operation.

The lining of an uninfected cyst consists of thin, regular, stratified, squamous epithelium, with occasional keratinisation, but if the cyst has become infected, the lining will resemble that of a dental cyst.

Fissural cysts

An **incisive canal cyst** (nasopalatine cyst) arises within the incisive canal of the maxilla. The diagnosis can be made with some confidence if the diameter of the incisive canal measures more than 2 cm and should be suggested if the diameter exceeds 1.5 cm. The margin is smooth, corticated and continuous unless infection has supervened. These cysts usually present as painless, palatal swellings (Fig. 91.23).

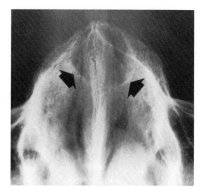

Fig. 91.23   Incisive canal cyst or nasopalatine cyst [arrows].

The lining of an uninfected cyst consists largely of stratified squamous epithelium, but ciliated columnar epithelium is sometimes present.

A **globulomaxillary cyst** is an uncommon fissural cyst which develops at the junction between the premaxilla and maxilla, where it appears as a corticated radiolucent area between the roots of the lateral incisor and the canine teeth. There may be some separation of the roots, but there is never any resorbtion. The cortical margin is continuous unless infection has occurred.

The lining may consist of nonkeratinising stratified squamous epithelium, keratinised squamous epithelium or ciliated columnar epithelium.

Median mandibular and median palatal cysts are extremely rare fissural cysts, which appear radiologically as corticated radiolucent areas in the midline of the mandible and palate.

Odontogenic keratocyst [2]

Odontogenic keratocysts (or primordial cysts) occur most commonly in the ramus of the mandible (Fig. 91.24), and are often associated with a missing lower third molar. However, they can arise from any tooth-bearing part of the jaws.

The diagnosis depends entirely upon the histological appearance of the lining, which consists of a thin layer of

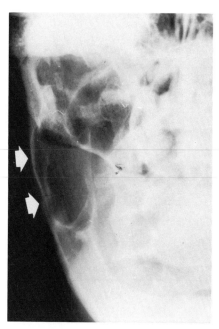

Fig. 91.24   Odontogenic keratocyst expanding the outer plate of the right ramus of the mandible [arrows].

keratinised, stratified, squamous epithelium. Microscopic daughter cysts are occasionally seen beyond the bony margin of the main cyst, and this may account for the relatively high incidence of recurrence after simple curettage (10 to 20%).

The cortical margin is usually smooth, but may be scalloped and is continuous unless infection has developed. Large odontogenic keratocysts will expand the maxilla or mandible, and sometimes have a multilocular appearance radiologically. They resemble a wide range of radiolucent lesions including dental cysts and benign solid tumours.

Multiple odontogenic keratocysts are a feature of Gorlin's syndrome (p. 1837).

Nonepithelial bone cyst [3]

The nonepithelial bone cyst (solitary bone cyst, haemorrhagic bone cyst, traumatic bone cyst, unicameral bone cyst) is almost invariably located in the body of the mandible below the premolar and molar teeth. They are rare lesions which are usually discovered incidentally in young adults.

Radiologically nonepithelial bone cysts differ from other benign cystic lesions, as they have no corticated margin and rarely cause expansion. They appear as irregular defects in the trabecular pattern of the mandible. They are invariably asymptomatic and never become infected (Fig. 91.25).

These lesions should not really be classified as cysts, as they have no epithelial lining. The pathology is uncertain, and it has been suggested that they are bone infarcts, or even a normal anatomical feature. The usual management is exploration and curettage, as this confirms the diagnosis. A few untreated 'cysts' have been seen to heal spontaneously on follow-up radiographs.

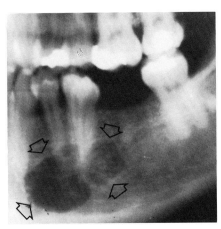

Fig. 91.25 Nonepithelial bone cyst of the mandible adjacent to the roots of the lower premolar teeth. The margin is irregular and not corticated [arrows].

BENIGN TUMOURS

General considerations

Benign tumours of the jaws are relatively rare and are much less common than benign cysts. The radiological abnormalities produced by benign tumours are broadly similar to those of simple cysts. However, tumours are more likely to be multilocular than benign cysts, are more likely to resorb teeth and occasionally calcify.

Tumours of bone and cartilage

The **giant cell tumour** (osteoclastoma) is an uncommon tumour of the jaws, and like giant cell tumours elsewhere, usually occurs in adults between 20 and 40 years. Radiologically it appears as an expanding multilocular lesion with a scalloped margin. Recurrence after excision is quite common.

The **giant cell reparative granuloma** is peculiar to the jaws and has the same radiological features as a giant cell tumour. However, it occurs in a younger age group (10 to 25 years) and, although it grows more rapidly than a giant cell tumour, it rarely recurs after removal.

Ivory osteomas and **osteochondromas** occasionally arise from the maxilla and mandible, and have the same features as in other bones. Multiple ivory osteomas are a feature of Gardner's syndrome (p. 1838).

The **chondroma** is a rare tumour of the maxilla, which usually develops after the age of 40 years. It appears as an area of bone destruction and has the unusual radiological feature of eroding the roots of teeth without displacing them. Complete excision is difficult, and recurrence is common.

There have been a few reports of **osteoid osteoma** in the maxillofacial region.

Tumours of soft tissue

The **fibromyxoma** [4] is a rare tumour of children and young adults, and appears radiologically as a multilocular expanding lesion.

The **ossifying fibroma** of the jaws is a rare tumour which seems to be a different pathological entity from the similarly named tumour of other bones and which is sometimes classified as a type of fibrous dysplasia. It begins as a radiolucent area with a corticated margin, and often erodes the roots of adjacent teeth without displacing them. The unusual radiological feature of this tumour is that areas of dense calcification subsequently develop within the radiolucent area, and can be quite extensive (Fig. 91.26). Recurrence after removal is common.

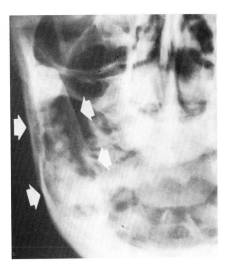

Fig. 91.26 Partially calcified ossifying fibroma expanding the right ramus of the mandible [arrows].

Haemangioma [5] of the mandible is an extremely rare tumour which appears radiologically as a multilocular radiolucency with occasional ring opacities in the soft tissues due to calcified phleboliths. Its importance lies in the fact that it usually results in torrential haemorrhage if the teeth are extracted from the affected bone, and the diagnosis should always be considered as a possibility for any multilocular radiolucent lesion in the mandible.

A **neurilemmoma** or **neurofibroma** rarely arises from the inferior dental nerve, and can cause widening of the inferior dental canal.

There have been a few reports of **fibromas, lipomas** and **ganglioneuromas** developing in the maxillofacial region.

AMELOBLASTOMA AND OTHER ODONTOGENIC TUMOURS

Ameloblastoma [6]

Ameloblastoma (adamantinoma) is a remarkably well known tumour despite the fact that it accounts for only 1 to 2% of tumours in the maxillofacial region. It appears as an expanding radiolucent lesion, usually in the mandible (Fig. 91.27), which often erodes the roots of adjacent teeth without displacing them. It is frequently multilocular and is probably the most common multilocular lesion to occur in the jaws.

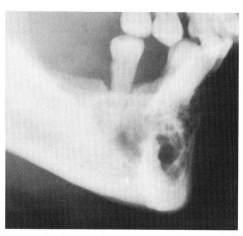

Fig. 91.27 Ameloblastoma in the anterior part of the mandible with a typical multilocular appearance.

Recurrence is common after simple curettage, so the tumour should be removed along with a margin of apparently normal bone. These tumours are slow growing and can reach an enormous size. Ameloblastoma is a locally invasive tumour, and its behaviour has been compared to that of a basal cell carcinoma. Pulmonary metastases have been reported in a few cases [7].

They usually present in early adult life, but can occur at any time after the age of 12 years.

Other odontogenic tumours

Adenomeloblastoma and **ameloblastic fibroma** are rarer than ameloblastomas, and occur in a slightly younger age group. They have the same radiological features as ameloblastomas and appear as expanding radiolucent lesions.

The **calcifying epithelial odontogenic tumour** [8] is an even rarer tumour, which is unusual radiologically in that there are multiple small areas of calcification within the enlarging radiolucency.

ODONTOMES

The term 'odontome' is best reserved for an abnormal growth of calcified dental tissue, which behaves like a hamartoma rather than a neoplasm. It stops growing when the individual stops growing. Many tumours of dental origin which used to be described as odontomes have since been reclassified according to the terminology used in general pathology.

Composite odontomes contain more than one dental tissue, and commonly present during adolescence as they delay or prevent the eruption of permanent teeth. Simple odontomes contain only one dental tissue. All odontomes are rare.

A **complex composite odontome** is a mass of enamel, dentine and cementum which shows as a dense radio-opacity with an irregular, but clearly defined margin (Fig. 91.28). Sometimes

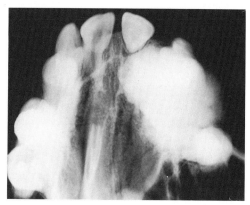

Fig. 91.28 Complex composite odontome in the upper premolar and molar regions which appears as a very dense radio-opacity with a well defined lobulated margin.

there are small radiolucencies within this radio-opaque mass due to small cysts. This lesion usually occurs in the molar regions, but can occur anywhere in the dental arch.

A **compound composite odontome** is a mass of small 'denticles', most of which contain enamel, dentine and cementum (Fig. 91.29). It is more common anteriorly than posteriorly. Multiple compound composite odontomes have been described in association with Gardner's syndrome.

An **enameloma** (or enamel pearl) is a small nodule of enamel which occasionally forms at the neck of a tooth.

Dentinomas are extremely rare, and there is some doubt about their existence as a pathological entity. They have the radiological appearance of a complex composite odontome, and tend to occur posteriorly.

A **cementoma** is a mass of cementum which can develop at the apex of an erupted tooth or in an edentulous area. These curious lesions are initially radiolucent, but soon develop

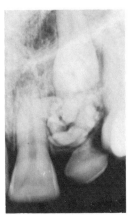

Fig. 91.29 Compound composite odontome situated between the erupted upper left deciduous lateral incisor and its permanent successor. It appears as a mass of 'denticles' or small deformed teeth.

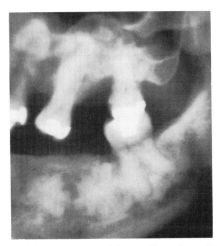

Fig. 91.30 Multiple cementomas of the maxilla and mandible showing as ill-defined opacities surrounded by a radiolucent margin in some places.

irregular areas of calcification (Fig. 91.30) and can eventually become completely radio-opaque. They rarely cause expansion of the bony cortex and are often multiple. There is some doubt about the pathological classification of this lesion, which is thought to be a type of fibrous dysplasia by some authorities.

Dilated composite odontomes and **germinated composite odontomes** are abnormally formed teeth, and have been described under that heading in Chapter 92.

NON-NEOPLASTIC BONE LESIONS

Idiopathic sclerosis (bone island, enostosis)

Irregular areas of bone sclerosis (bone islands) are common

in the tooth-bearing parts of the maxilla and mandible. They may be single or multiple, and can be quite extensive [9] in the mandible. They are usually situated adjacent to the roots of erupted teeth but can occur in edentulous areas. Their margins are usually irregular but are sometimes clearly defined. In some cases there is a precipitating factor such as chronic infection or traumatic dental extractions, but most cases are idiopathic.

Although idiopathic sclerosis is common, it is sometimes necessary to perform a biopsy to confirm the diagnosis and exclude a sclerotic tumour or sclerosing osteomyelitis.

Retained root fragments due to incomplete dental extractions are probably the commonest cause of radio-opacities in the tooth-bearing parts of the jaws and are frequently asymptomatic. They can usually be distinguished from bone islands by the presence of a radiolucent root canal within the opacity.

Torus palatinus and torus mandibularis

Torus palatinus and torus mandibularis are common non-neoplastic bony outgrowths which develop in adults of all ages. Radiologically there is progressive thickening of the cortex, due to laying down of subperiosteal lamellar bone. Torus palatinus arises from the midline of the hard palate posteriorly and torus mandibularis, which is usually bilateral, arises from the inner tables of the mandible in the premolar region (Fig. 91.31).

They are sometimes mistaken for ivory osteomas which they resemble radiologically, but their anatomical position should indicate the diagnosis. They are occasionally removed or surgically reduced in size if they make it impossible to fit satisfactory dentures.

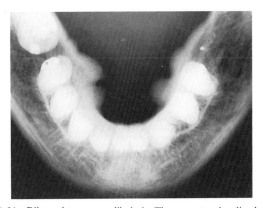

Fig. 91.31 Bilateral torus mandibularis. There are two localized areas of thickening of the inner tables of the mandible in the premolar region on both sides.

MISCELLANEOUS RADIOLUCENT LESIONS OF THE JAWS

The **Stafne bone cavity** [10] is an anatomical anomaly and not

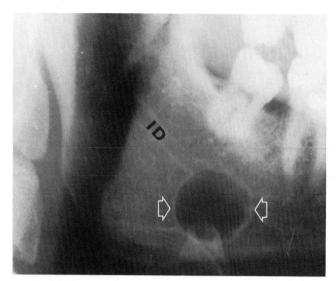

Fig. 91.32 Stafne bone cavity with the characteristic appearance of a corticated defect in the posterior part of the mandible below the inferior dental canal [I.D.].

a tumour. Radiologically it appears as a round or oval corticated defect in the posterior part of the mandible, below the inferior dental canal (Fig. 91.32).

Histiocytosis X (eosinophilic granuloma) is a rare cause of radiolucency in the maxillofacial region and usually develops in childhood or early adult life. The radiolucent area may be small (Fig. 91.33) or large, and as the teeth are not resorbed they appear to 'float' in the soft tissues. There is no cortical margin in the early stages but a cortex may develop if the lesion stops growing or regresses. Large lesions are often multilocular. The main differential diagnosis is malignancy and the diagnosis depends upon biopsy.

The **brown tumour of hyperparathyroidism** occasionally occurs in the jaws, and appears as an expanding radiolucent

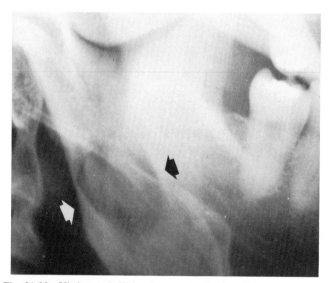

Fig. 91.33 Histiocytosis X showing as a noncorticated, but well defined defect [arrows] in the trabecular pattern of the ramus of the mandible.

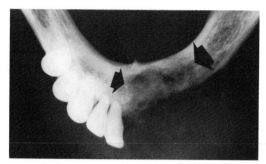

Fig. 91.34 Brown tumour of hyperparathyroidism. There is an irregular defect in the anterior part of the mandible [arrows].

area with an ill-defined margin and with erosion of the roots of adjacent teeth (Fig. 91.34). Hyperparathyroidism may also result in widespread resorbtion of the lamina dura of all the teeth, and if this radiological abnormality is present, the diagnosis can be made with reasonable confidence. Chronic renal failure can result in similar changes, and like renal osteodystrophy in other bones, also causes patchy sclerosis [11].

MALIGNANT TUMOURS

Carcinoma

Carcinoma is the most common malignancy of the maxillofacial region, and usually presents in the middle aged and elderly with pain, anaesthesia and loosening of teeth. Most tumours are squamous cell carcinomas or adenocarcinomas. They usually arise from the oral mucosa, and rapidly invade the underlying bone, but occasionally develop within the mandible or maxilla.

Radiologically these lesions are purely destructive, and show little evidence of bone expansion or of subperiosteal new bone formation. The margin of the lesion is very irregular (Fig. 91.35) and erosion of the roots of adjacent teeth is common.

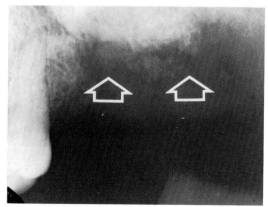

Fig. 91.35 Carcinoma of the upper alveolus. There is irregular destruction of the alveolar crest with loss of its normal cortical margin [arrows].

Osteogenic sarcoma [12,13]

Osteogenic sarcoma is the most common malignant tumour of the jaws in young adults, and usually presents between 15 and 30 years with pain, local anaesthesia and loosening of the teeth.

Radiologically it appears as an ill-defined area of bone destruction, which is often associated with resorbtion of the roots of adjacent teeth and with thickening of their periodontal membranes. In a few cases, sclerosis is more marked than bone destruction, and these tumours are said to have a slightly better prognosis.

However, the most striking radiological abnormality is the presence of subperiosteal new bone, which may have a lamellar (onion skin) or spiculated (sun ray) appearance and which is often very extensive (Figs. 91.36A & B).

Histologically the tumour is always much more widespread than the radiological abnormalities suggest and radical excision offers the only hope of a permanent cure.

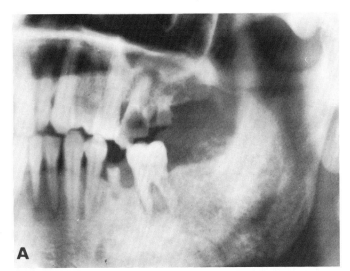

Fig. 91.36A Osteogenic sarcoma of the mandible with irregular bone destruction in the molar region, thickening of the periodontal membrane of the lower first molar and new bone formation in the soft tissues anterior to the ramus.

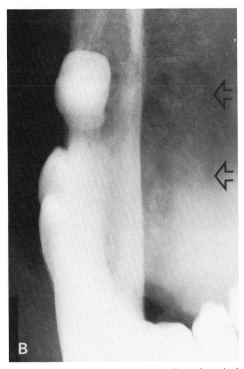

Fig. 91.36B Occlusal view of the same case to show the spiculated (sun ray) appearance of subperiosteal new bone arising from the inner aspect of the mandible [arrow].

Metastatic tumours and rare primary tumours

Metastatic carcinoma rarely affects the maxillofacial region, but when it does the primary tumour is usually situated in the breast, bronchus, colon or kidney. Radiologically there may be a single ill-defined area of bone destruction, or multiple coalescing radiolucent areas scattered throughout the maxillofacial bones (Fig. 91.37). Occasionally a single metastasis lodges in the inferior dental canal and widens it.

In most cases there is radiological evidence of widespread bone metastases in these patients, and it is most unusual to see lytic areas in the mandible in the absence of similar abnormalities in the skull vault. As in other bones, radiolucent metastases may become sclerotic after chemotherapy.

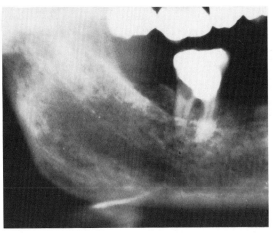

Fig. 91.37 Metastatic carcinoma of the breast. There are multiple small radiolucencies scattered throughout the ramus and body of the mandible.

Multiple myeloma may result in multiple radiolucencies in the mandible in the absence of similar radiolucent areas in the skull vault.

Burkitt's lymphoma [14] is very common in some parts of Africa, where it affects children of all ages. Radiologically it is a purely destructive lesion in the maxilla or mandible with patchy radiolucencies in the trabecular bone, destruction of the cortex, rapid resorbtion of the lamina dura and destruction of the developing teeth. It is usually accompanied by massive soft tissue swelling.

Metastatic neuroblastoma and **retinoblastoma** occasionally involves the maxillofacial region in children with widespread disease.

Ewing's tumour [15] and various other sarcomas have also been reported in the maxillofacial region as primary tumours.

Malignant lymphoma (e.g. lymphosarcoma, reticulum cell sarcoma etc.) can occur in the maxillofacial region usually in patients with extensive metastases.

FIBRO-OSSEOUS LESIONS [16]

Fibrous dysplasia

Fibrous dysplasia is usually monostotic in the maxillofacial region, but can be a feature of polyostotic fibrous dysplasia, or even of Albright's syndrome. It is more common in the maxilla than the mandible, and presents as painless bony swelling, usually in adolescence but sometimes earlier or later.

Fibrous dysplasia begins as an expanding radiolucent lesion, which does not cross suture lines, but can deform them. Sclerotic areas soon develop within the radiolucency, and these gradually enlarge and coalesce until there is dense,

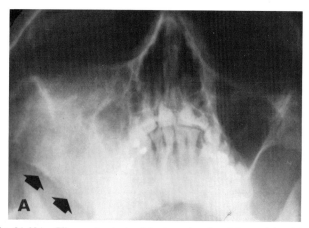

Fig. 91.38A Fibrous dysplasia of the lateral wall and floor of the right maxillary sinus. The bone is expanded and shows dense homogeneous opacification [arrows]. This feature is sometimes described as the 'ground glass' appearance.

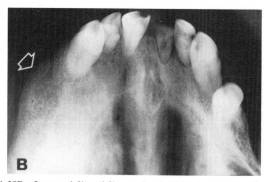

Fig. 91.38B Intraoral film of fibrous dysplasia in the right maxilla of a different case. There is thickening of the individual trabeculae resulting in an 'orange peel' appearance.

homogeneous opacification of the expanded bone (Fig. 91.38A), sometimes described as the 'ground glass' appearance.

Nonscreen intraoral films will sometimes show generalized thickening of the individual bone trabeculae, and this appearance, which has been compared to 'orange peel', is virtually diagnostic of the disease (Fig. 91.38B).

The teeth in the affected bone are often displaced and this can result in malocclusion. The eruption of developing teeth is usually delayed or prevented.

Fibrous dysplasia is occasionally complicated by chronic infection, which adds the radiological feature of patchy rarefaction and subperiosteal new bone formation to the existing generalized expansion and sclerosis. The resulting radiological appearance can resemble a sclerotic type of osteosarcoma or sclerosing osteomyelitis.

The condition usually becomes static in early adult life but the abnormalities which have developed do not regress. Treatment is aimed at reducing the facial deformity by surgical reduction of the enlarged bone or bones, and the operation may have to be repeated if growth continues.

Paget's disease (osteitis deformans) [17]

Paget's disease affects the maxilla more frequently than the mandible and is usually bilateral. In most cases it is preceded by Paget's disease of the skull vault.

As in other bones, the earliest radiological features are expansion and a loss of normal trabeculae. The trabeculae

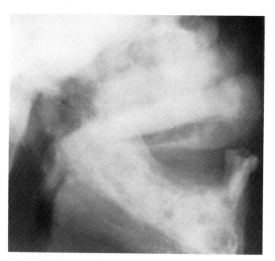

Fig. 91.39 Paget's disease of the maxilla and mandible. The maxilla is enlarged and contains coalescing areas of patchy sclerosis due to multiple cementomas. The mandible is expanded and has a coarse trabecular pattern with patchy sclerosis.

which remain behind become thickened, which results in the characteristic coarse trabecular pattern. Areas of dense bone sclerosis may develop later, and in the tooth-bearing parts of the jaws, masses of cementum may develop adjacent to the roots of teeth (hypercementosis) or in edentulous areas (multiple cementomas). These abnormalities are illustrated in Fig. 91.39.

Cherubism (familial intra-osseus swellings of the jaws) [18]

Cherubism is a rare disorder characterized by painless enlargement of both sides of the mandible which usually develops between two and four years. The condition runs a benign course and the swellings often regress a few years later. There is a family history in most cases which suggests that it is transmitted as an autosomal dominant. The pathological classification is uncertain but it is usually considered to be a type of fibrous dysplasia.

Radiologically there are expanding multilocular radiolucent areas on both sides of the mandible, with absence of the developing teeth in the radiolucent areas.

INFECTION AND ASSOCIATED CONDITIONS

Pyogenic osteomyelitis of the mandible

Acute osteomyelitis is usually precipitated by local conditions, such as periapical dental infections, dental extractions or a fracture. Considering the frequency of periapical infection, osteomyelitis is surprisingly rare. The infecting organism is usually a staphylococcus.

Acute osteomyelitis in children may complicate severe infections such as measles and typhoid, and is presumably a blood-borne infection in these cases. It may also be a complication of local pyogenic infections such as tonsillitis. Osteomyelitis is more common in systemic conditions such as malnutrition, diabetes mellitus, agranulocytosis and sickle cell anaemia. The incidence of infection is higher after radiotherapy and in osteopetrosis.

As in other bones, the radiological features do not appear until the clinical symptoms of pain, tenderness and soft tissue swelling have been present for a few days. The earliest change is an ill-defined area of rarefaction in the trabecular bone, or rarefaction of the lamina dura of a recently

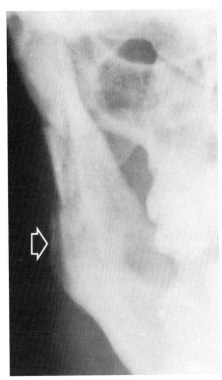

Fig. 91.41 Osteomyelitis of the body and ramus of the mandible with a periosteal reaction laterally [arrows].

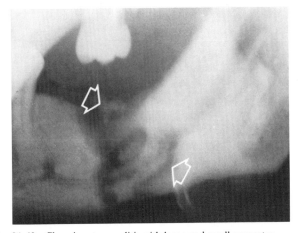

Fig. 91.42 Chronic osteomyelitis with large and small sequestra [arrows] plus a pathological fracture through the body of the mandible.

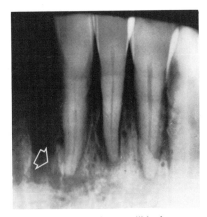

Fig. 91.40 Early osteomyelitis of the mandible due to recent extraction of a lower incisor tooth. There is a defect in the lamina dura around the socket of the extracted tooth [arrow] and patchy osteoporosis in the adjacent bone.

extracted tooth. The rarefaction rapidly progresses to more extensive bone destruction (Fig. 91.40), with resorbtion of the lamina dura of adjacent teeth. Subperiosteal new bone formation soon develops in most cases (Fig. 91.41).

Sequestra are inevitable, unless the appropriate antibiotic is given early, and appear as opacities lying in cavities (Fig. 91.42). A pathological fracture may occur if the mandible is seriously weakened (Fig. 91.42).

Chronic osteomyelitis [19] may follow acute osteomyelitis and has similar radiological features, with patchy osteoporosis, patchy sclerosis and sequestra lying in cavities. However, subperiosteal new bone is a relatively uncommon feature.

Garré's osteomyelitis (subperiosteal sclerosing osteomyelitis) presents as a tender bony swelling with intraoral sinuses, and often responds satisfactorily to antibiotics and conservative surgery. The infecting organisms are usually Gram-positive cocci which suggest that it is a subacute form of pyogenic osteomyelitis and not a separate pathological entity.

The dominant radiological feature is the formation of dense subperiosteal new bone. There is also patchy sclerosis in the underlying bone, patchy rarefaction and sequestrum formation.

Osteoradionecrosis is the name given to a particularly intractable form of chronic osteomyelitis, which may be a sequel to radiotherapy. Radiotherapy itself rarely produces any radiological change in the bone pattern of the maxilla or mandible, but very high doses occasionally result in rarefaction or sclerosis.

The most important complication of therapeutic radiation to the maxillofacial region is an increased susceptibility to osteomyelitis of the mandible. The radiological abnormalities produced by this infection are widespread patchy sclerosis, with areas of rarefaction and multiple sequestra. The disease often spreads throughout the mandible and is extremely difficult to control. It can be fatal.

Actinomycosis [20] is essentially a soft tissue infection, but cervicofacial actinomycosis occasionally spreads to the mandible, and results in chronic osteomyelitis.

Tuberculous osteomyelitis occurs rarely and is usually a sequel to dental extractions in a patient with open tuberculosis. Radiologically it appears as an irregular area of bone destruction.

Tertiary syphilis can result in a gumma (commonly in the hard palate) or in a low grade osteomyelitis. Radiologically these lesions are destructive, with little new bone formation.

Caffey's disease (infantile cortical hyperostosis)

Caffey's disease usually affects the mandible and is characterized by subperiosteal new bone formation in an infant during the first five months of life (Fig. 91.43). It also affects other bones, particularly the ribs, clavicles, radii and ulnae. As the subperiosteal new bone is not resorbed immediately, mandibular asymmetry is a common sequel and occasionally persists into adolescence and adult life, producing malocclusion of the teeth.

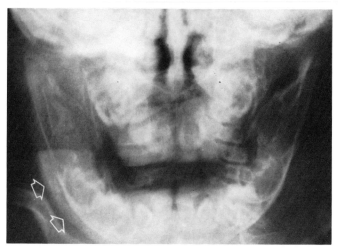

Fig. 91.43 Caffey's disease in an infant of three months showing a periosteal reaction on the right side of the mandible [arrows]. The crowns of the developing deciduous teeth are just beginning to calcify in the radiolucent dental crypts.

The differential diagnosis is infective osteomyelitis, and in young premature infants, rickets [21].

Osteomyelitis in infants

This uncommon infection is probably of haematogenous origin as it appears during the first three months of life before the teeth have erupted. Clinically it presents as an acute systemic illness with fever and gastrointestinal upset. It is much more common in the maxilla than in the mandible.

Radiologically, there is extensive destruction of bone with exfoliation of the developing teeth, sequestrum formation and occasional subperiosteal new bone.

The differential diagnosis in the mandible is infantile cortical hyperostosis.

It can result in partial anodontia due to loss of developing teeth, and to permanent asymmetry of the mandible if the infection destroys the epiphyseal cartilage of the condylar neck.

DIFFERENTIAL DIAGNOSIS OF RADIOLUCENT AND RADIO-OPAQUE BONE LESIONS

It is rarely possible to make an accurate pathological diagnosis of a radiolucent or radio-opaque lesion in the maxillofacial region on the radiological appearances alone. As in bone lesions elsewhere, the final diagnosis usually depends upon a combination of the clinical, radiological and histological abnormalities, together with the appropriate biochemical and immunological tests in some cases.

Table 91.1 is intended to be used as check list to ensure that most diagnostic possibilities have been considered [22,23].

Table 91.1 *Differential diagnosis of radiolucent and radio-opaque bone lesions*

	Radiolucent	Radio-opaque
Common	Alveolar abscess	Root fragment
	Periodontal abscess	Idiopathic sclerosis
	Apical granuloma	(bone island)
	Dental cyst	Torus mandibularis
	Dentigerous cyst	Torus palatinus
	Fissural cyst	Hypercementosis
Uncommon	Odontogenic keratocyst	Fibrous dysplasia (late)
	Nonepithelial cyst	Cementoma (late)
	Ameloblastoma	Ossifying fibroma (late)
	Fibrous dysplasia (early)	Paget's disease (late)
	Cementoma (early)	Complex composite
	Ossifying fibroma (early)	odontome
	Paget's disease (early)	Compound composite
	Pygonic osteomyelitis	odontome
	Giant cell tumours	
Rare	Carcinoma	Osteogenic sarcoma
	Osteogenic sarcoma	Garré's osteomyelitis
	Fibromyxoma	Osteoradionecrosis
	Metastatic carcinoma	Ivory osteoma
	Burkitt's lymphoma	Osteochondroma
	Metastatic lymphoma	Calcifying epithelial
	Histiocytosis X	odontogenic tumour
	Stafne bone cavity	Osteoid osteoma
	Cherubism	Treated metastatic
	Nonpyogenic infections	carcinoma
	Hyperparathyroidism	Albers-Schonberg
	Rare odontogenic tumours	disease
	Chondroma	Renal osteodystrophy
	Haemangioma, lymphangioma	
	Neurofibroma, neurilemmoma	
	Fibroma, lipoma	
	Ewing's tumour	
	Rare sarcoma	

ABNORMALITIES OF GROWTH AND DEVELOPMENT

Abnormalities of the facial bones

Cleft palate is the most common developmental anomaly of the maxillofacial region. The diagnosis is clinical and should be made at birth. If the cleft extends anteriorly through the alveolar bone on one or both sides, there will be displacement of the upper anterior teeth, and occasional absence of the lateral incisors. The maxilla often fails to grow normally during childhood, which results in relative mandibular protrusion in adult life.

In the **Pierre Robin syndrome** the mandible is extremely small, resulting in a 'bird face' deformity. The larynx is usually underdeveloped and cleft palate is common.

Hypertelorism (Greig's occular hypertelorism) is recognised clinically by the wide space between the eyes. It may be accompanied by incomplete development of the alveolar arches of the maxilla, with subsequent malocclusion in adult life, and by partial anodontia of the maxillary teeth.

In the **Treacher-Collins' syndrome** (mandibulofacial dysostosis, first arch dysplasia), the striking facial abnormalities are the antimongoloid tilt of the eyes, small deformed ears and a small mandible. Radiologically the zygomatic arches are absent or incomplete, and there is underdevelopment of the maxilla and of the mandible.

Crouzon's disease (craniofacial dysostosis) results in occular hypertelorism with underdevelopment of the maxilla leading to relative mandibular protrusion. The nose has a characteristic 'parrot beak' appearance, and there is usually craniostenosis of some, or all of the skull sutures.

Generalized skeletal abnormalities

These rare conditions are often due to an autosomal dominant gene, so there is frequently a history of similarly affected relatives.

Cleidocranial dysostosis affects the development of bones which ossify from membrane, and the development of the teeth. The maxilla is underdeveloped resulting in mandibular protrusion. There are always multiple dental abnormalities, the principle ones being prolonged retention of the deciduous teeth, failure of their permanent successors to erupt, abnormally shaped teeth, supernumerary teeth and partial anodontia. Skull radiographs show open fontanelles in adult life, and multiple Wormian bones at the sutures. The clavicles are absent or underdeveloped, the scapulae are small, the ribs are short and angled downwards, and the pubic symphysis remains deficient in adult life (Ch. 74).

Achondroplasia affects the bones which ossify from cartilage; consequently the skull base is underdeveloped and this results in relative mandibular protrusion in adult life. Eruption of the maxillary teeth is often delayed, and there is frequently malocclusion of the teeth which have erupted. The most significant abnormalities occur in the long bones, lumbar spine and pelvis resulting in dwarfism, spinal stenosis and lumbar lordosis (Ch. 74).

Multiple neurofibromatosis (Von Recklinghausen's disease) can result in asymmetrical growth of the facial bones and in localized bone defects (Ch. 74).

In **Gorlin's syndrome** (multiple basal cell naevi syndrome) multiple odontogenic keratocysts develop in the maxilla and mandible during childhood. The more significant abnormality is the appearance of multiple basal cell carcinomas, during the second decade. Bifid ribs are common.

Gardner's syndrome (Fitzgerald-Gardner syndrome) is a variant of familial polyposis of the colon, and is accompanied by multiple ivory osteomas of the skull and facial bones, including the mandible.

Albers-Schönberg disease (osteopetrosis, marble bone disease) results in generalised bone sclerosis, which affects the maxillofacial region as well as the rest of the skeleton. In addition, there is thickening of the lamina dura around the teeth, and an increased susceptibility to osteomyelitis of the mandible after dental extractions (Ch. 74).

Acromegaly results in continued growth of the facial bones including the alveolar arches, and this results in gradual and increasing spacing of the teeth. The mandible grows more than the maxilla which can result in gross mandibular protrusion (Fig. 91.44). The pituitary fossa is enlarged, the skull vault is thickened and there is often enlargement of the frontal sinuses. The tongue is sometimes enlarged and this can be shown on a lateral film of the facial bones [24].

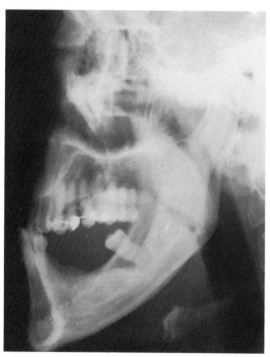

Fig. 91.44 Acromegaly. The mandible is excessively large resulting in mandibular protrusion and malocclusion. There are spaces between some of the upper teeth due to continued maxillary growth. The pituitary fossa is enlarged.

THE TEMPOROMANDIBULAR JOINT

Anatomy

The temporomandibular joint is a synovial joint, which is divided into upper and lower compartments by a fibrocartilaginous disc. These compartments usually form separate synovial spaces, but may communicate through perforations in the disc.

Two types of movement occur, first a simple hinge movement of the mandibular condyle in the glenoid fossa and, second, forward translation of the mandibular condyle, which may pass over the maximum convexity of the articular eminence in normal asymptomatic joints. The disc is attached to the mandibular condyle by the joint capsule and moves with it, as some fibres of the lateral pterygoid muscle are inserted into the disc itself.

Arthritis

The **pain-dysfunction syndrome** is the clinical diagnosis which is most frequently applied to patients with temporomandibular joint pain. The typical patient is aged 20 to 30 years and female. The symptoms are usually unilateral and often resolve after a year or two even without treatment. The aetiology is uncertain, and there are many theories including malocclusion of the teeth, muscle spasm and internal derangement of the joint.

In most cases the joint appears normal on plain radiographs, but there is sometimes narrowing or widening of the joint space which would fit with muscle spasm or disc displacement. In a few cases there is irregularity or even erosive changes in the articular surface of the mandibular condyle (Fig. 91.45).

Arthrotomography [25,26] of the temporomandibular joint is a fairly recent development which may rationalize the diagnosis and treatment of patients with the pain-dysfunction

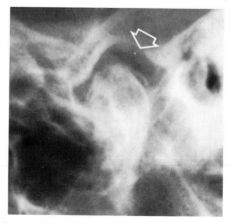

Fig. 91.45 Pain-dysfunction syndrome. The temporomandibular joint space is widened posteriorly [arrow] and there is some irregularity of the anterior articular surface of the condyle.

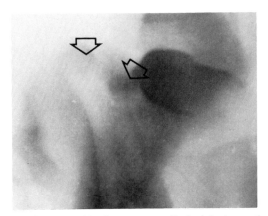

Fig. 91.46 Erosive arthritis of temporomandibular joint in a patient with rheumatoid arthritis. There are large irregular erosions of the condyle and of the anterior aspect of the condylar neck [arrows].

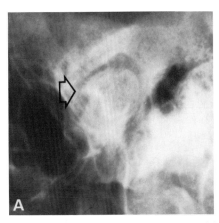

Fig. 91.47A Degenerative arthritis. There is narrowing of the joint space anteriorly with slight sclerosis. A small osteophyte arises from the anterior margin of the articular surface of the condyle [arrow].

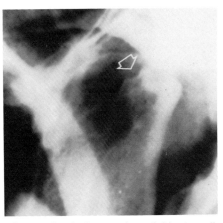

Fig. 91.47B Presumed early degenerative arthritis. A small erosion arises from the anterior aspect of the articular surface of the mandibular condyle [arrow].

syndrome by demonstrating internal derangement when it is present. Recent papers have shown that the disc may be fixed anteriorly or posteriorly instead of moving with the condyle, and have suggested that the symptom of 'clicking' is due to the condyle passing over the edge of the disc. Kinking of the disc has been demonstrated in a few cases, and it has been suggested that disc perforations are always pathological.

The examination is technically difficult as it requires the upper and lower joint compartments to be separately injected with contrast medium.

Inflammatory arthritis is uncommon, but can be a feature of connective tissue diseases such as rheumatoid arthritis and psoriasis. Erosions develop in the articular surface of the condyle and they can be very extensive (Fig. 91.46). The glenoid fossa remains radiologically normal.

Infection is an even rarer cause of inflammatory arthritis. It is usually due to local spread of infection from mandibular osteomyelitis or otitis media and results in destruction of the articular surfaces of the condyle and glenoid fossa.

Erosions of the mandibular condyle have been reported in patients on *prolonged haemodialysis*.

Degenerative arthritis (osteoarthritis) [27] can occur in the elderly, and eventually results in the same abnormalities as osteoarthritis in other synovial joints, namely narrowing, sclerosis and osteophyte formation. The sclerosis is confined to the mandibular condyle and osteophytes arise only from the anterior margin of the condyle (Fig. 91.47A). The articular surface of the glenoid fossa remains normal.

However, osteoarthritis of the temporomandibular joint is radiologically unusual in that these changes may be preceded by erosions of the articular surface of the condyle, even when there is no evidence of a generalized inflammatory arthritis or of local infection (Fig. 91.47B).

Injury

Fractures of the condylar neck are common (Fig. 91.12) and rarely involve the temporomandibular joint. The condyle itself and the glenoid fossa are occasionally fractured in severe trauma, and this results in haemarthrosis.

Ankylosis of the temporomandibular joint may follow infective arthritis or traumatic haemarthrosis. As these disorders usually occur in childhood, most cases are complicated by hypoplasia of the mandibular condyle due to the epiphyseal cartilage of the condylar neck having been damaged at the same time. Tomography is usually required to confirm the absence of a joint space, and to demonstrate bony ankylosis between the temporal bone and the mandibular condyle (Fig. 91.48).

Dislocation of the temporomandibular joint is a clinical diagnosis and not a radiological one as the condyle often moves anterior to the maximum convexity of the articular eminence in normal individuals. The role of radiology in such cases is to exclude a fracture or some other pathology such as a bone tumour.

Recurrent dislocation may be a feature of Marfan's syndrome and of the Ehlers-Danlos syndrome.

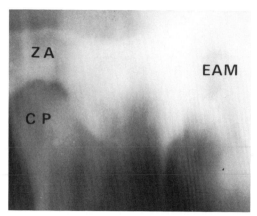

Fig. 91.48 Complete bony ankylosis of the left temporomandibular joint. The tomogram shows no evidence of a joint space. ZA = Zygomatic arch, EAM = External auditory meatus, CP = Coronoid process of the mandible.

The patient had injured the mandible in a fall at the age of nine years.

Developmental abnormalities

Aplasia or hypoplasia of the mandibular condyle may be unilateral or bilateral. Unilateral hypoplasia is usually a sequel to trauma or infection, and is often accompanied by ankylosis of the joint. Bilateral hypoplasia tends to be associated with a developmental anomaly such as the Treacher-Collins syndrome, the Pierre Robin syndrome or arthrogryposis multiplex congenita.

Unilateral hypoplasia results in gross asymmetry of the mandible and of the maxilla, due to reduced growth on that side. Bilateral hypoplasia results in a 'bird face' contour with a very small mandible.

Hyperplasia of the mandibular condyle is a rare condition of unknown aetiology, which develops at puberty and which is always unilateral. There is generalized enlargement of the condylar head which is often misdiagnosed as a bone tumour.

Hyperplasia of the coronoid process of the mandible is another rare abnormality of growth, which limits mandibular opening, and which is sometimes misdiagnosed as a tumour.

In **Hurler's syndrome** (gargoylism) the articular surface of the condyle is usually concave instead of convex, and this abnormality is specific for the syndrome [28].

SALIVARY GLANDS

General considerations

The parotid, submandibular and sublingual salivary glands are symmetrically placed round the oral cavity. The parotid glands are situated between the posterior borders of the rami of the mandible, and the upper ends of the sternomastoid muscles. Each gland drains through a single (Stensen's) duct, the orifice of which is situated in a papilla lateral to the crown of the second upper molar.

The submandibular glands are situated below the mylohyoid muscle, and medial to the posterior part of the body of the mandible. The submandibular duct (Wharton's) runs upwards from the gland until it reaches the posterior border of the mylohyoid muscle, when it turns forward in the floor of the mouth to open through a small papilla situated on either side of the lingual frenum, behind the lower incisor teeth.

The sublingual glands are situated anteriorly in the floor of the mouth above the mylohyoid muscle, and each gland opens into the oral cavity through several small ducts.

Surgical excision of the submandibular gland is usually the treatment of choice for a tumour, or for chronic infection, and the operation has few complications. Although the parotid gland can be surgically removed, the operation is usually reserved for malignant tumours, owing to the risk of damaging the facial nerve.

Sialography

The duct systems of the parotid and submandibular glands can be demonstrated by injecting contrast into the main duct from the mouth. The examination should be preceded by *plain radiographs* which will show radio-opaque calculi if they are present.

Cannulation of the parotid ducts is usually straightforward, but the orifices of the submandibular ducts can be extremely difficult to identify and cannulate, and a cut down procedure has been described for use in difficult cases [29]. It is often helpful to dilate the duct orifice with a series of lacrimal duct dilators before cannulation. Salivation may be induced by sucking a Vitamin C tablet.

The simplest and oldest technique is to pass a blunt needle into the duct orifice, but most radiologists now prefer to use a specially designed cannula, which consists of a tapered needle with a side hole, attached to a length of soft polythene tubing. A thin plastic catheter may also be used to cannulate the duct.

Contrast medium may be oil based (e.g. Lipiodol) or water based. The advantage of the more viscous oily contrast is that it remains in the duct system for a few minutes after removing the cannula, and this is usually long enough for the necessary films to be taken, but it has the serious disadvantage of remaining in the soft tissues for months, or years, if the main duct has been ruptured during cannulation, or if the injection pressure is excessive.

Water based contrast medium (e.g. Conray 280 or 420) is safer, as extravasation, although painful, is temporary. However, it is necessary to take films with the cannula still occluding the duct, as nonviscous water soluble contrast will be washed out of a normal gland in less than a minute by the normal flow of saliva.

0.5 ml of contrast medium is usually sufficient to outline the duct system, but films should be taken sooner if the patient complains of discomfort. Water soluble contrast will sometimes opacify the whole gland, as well as the duct system (see Fig. 91.57), and this is probably due to reflux of contrast into the acini. However, if the parenchymal opacification persists after the duct system has emptied, it is almost certainly due to rupturing the acini by excessive injection pressure. This complication can be avoided if the *hydrostatic technique* [30] is used; instead of injecting the contrast by hand, the barrel of an open syringe is suspended vertically about 20 cm above the duct orifice, and contrast medium is allowed to run into the duct under gravity.

Delayed radiographs should be taken 10 minutes after the needle or cannula has been removed, and if there is still contrast medium within the ducts it indicates duct obstruction or reduced function.

Sialography has a useful role in the diagnosis of chronic or recurrent swellings of the parotid or submandibular glands. It has no value in assessing the sublingual glands as each gland has multiple ducts, which are too small to cannulate; and it is of limited value in the diagnosis of painful swellings, as the examination is technically difficult in these cases, and can increase the pain considerably.

Sialography will demonstrate radiolucent calculi, sialectasis, duct strictures, abscess cavities, tumours and lacerations due to trauma.

Calculi

Calculi are more common in the submandibular region (Figs. 91.49, 91.50, 91.51 & 91.53) than in the parotid region (Fig. 91.52), and are usually a sequel to infection or stasis. Most calculi are radio-opaque.

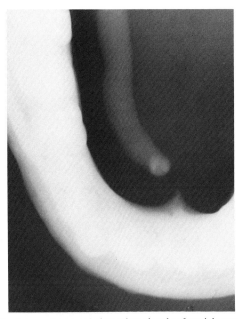

Fig. 91.50 Intraoral occlusal view taken shortly after sialography showing a single radio-opaque calculus occluding the anterior end of the submandibular duct. The cannula had been removed ten minutes earlier.

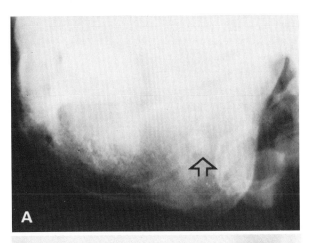

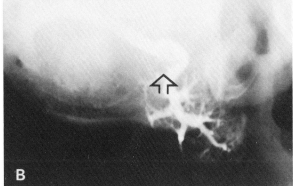

Fig. 91.51A & B Calculus (at the posterior end of the submandibular duct) which is radio-opaque on the preliminary film (A), and relatively radiolucent on the film taken after the duct system had been opacified with contrast medium (B). The is generalized dilatation of the intraglandular ducts and of the main duct due to stenosis of the duct orifice.

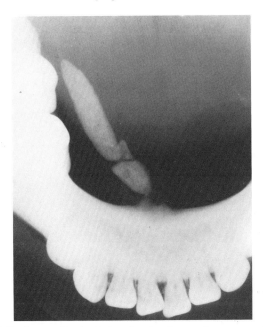

Fig. 91.49 Intraoral occlusal view showing three radio-opaque calculi in the submandibular duct.

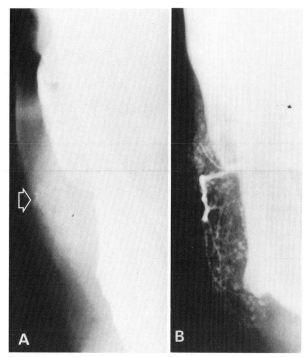

Fig. 91.52A & B   There are multiple small calculi within the right parotid gland [arrow] which show on the preliminary film (A). The sialogram film (B) shows widespread sialectasis and obscures the calculi indicating that they are situated within the sialectatic cavities. The duct system is normal.

Radio-opaque calculi in the submandibular duct are readily shown on intraoral occlusal films (Figs. 91.49 & 91.50), and calculi within the gland itself are shown by a lateral oblique film of the mandible (Fig. 91.51A).

Radio-opaque calculi in the parotid duct lateral to the ramus of the mandible can usually be demonstrated on a PA film, but small calculi situated anteriorly in the duct are best shown on an intraoral film which has been placed against the inside of the cheek. Radio-opaque calculi in the parotid gland itself will usually show on a PA film (Fig. 91.52A), or on a lateral oblique film of the mandible.

Once a calculus has formed it tends to cause stasis, which predisposes to recurrent infection, sialectasis, duct strictures and further calculus formation.

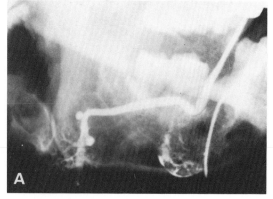

Fig. 91.53A   Submandibular sialogram showing two sialectatic cavities in the upper part of the gland and slight dilatation of the intra-glandular ducts.

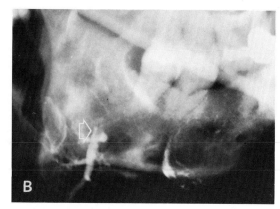

Fig. 91.53B   Delayed film showing a small radiolucent calculus [arrow] obstructing the main intra-glandular duct. There appears to be slight narrowing of the duct above the calculus and generalised dilatation below.

Duct strictures

Most strictures of the main ducts and of the intraglandular ducts are due to infection or calculi, and tend to predispose to recurrent infection, sialectasis and calculus formation. (Fig. 91.53B).

However, strictures at the orifices of the parotid ducts are often due to the habit of cheek biting, and strictures at the anterior ends of the submandibular ducts may be due to trauma from an ill-fitting denture.

Sialography will demonstrate strictures quite clearly and will often show dilatation of the duct system behind the stricture.

Sialectasis

Sialectasis describes a radiological appearance and simply indicates that sialography has demonstrated multiple cavities within the gland. The terms 'punctate' or 'globular' are sometimes used to describe small regular cavities measuring less than 2 mm in diameter, and the term 'cavitary' to describe larger cavities with irregular walls. A cavity which exceeds 5 mm in diameter is likely to be an abscess.

Infective sialectasis can produce any of these abnormalities, and is usually accompanied by calculus formation in the larger intraglandular ducts (Fig. 91.53), or in the main drainage duct (Fig. 91.50). Occasionally there are multiple calculi in the sialectatic cavities within the gland (Fig. 91.52). Duct strictures are common, and there may be calculi in the dilated duct system behind the stricture.

Sjögren's syndrome and other connective tissue diseases [31] are also associated with sialectasis. Most patients with Sjögren's syndrome have sialectasis and in some there is also dilatation of the main ducts (Fig. 91.54).

Similar abnormalities have been described in association with a wide variety of connective tissue disorders such as rheumatoid arthritis, systemic lupus erythematosus, anky-

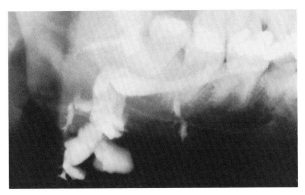

Fig. 91.54 Sjögren's syndrome. There is gross sialectasis of a submandibular gland with dilatation of the main duct.

losing spondylitis, Reiter's disease, polyarteritis nodosa and scleroderma. The incidence of sialographic abnormalities in patients with these conditions and without any clinical evidence of Sjögren's syndrome, has been estimated at 5 to 15%.

Childhood sialectasis [32,33] is a rare condition associated with intermittent tender swelling of one, or both parotid glands, which can develop at any age after 5 years, and which usually resolves at puberty. It is probably due to recurrent bacterial infection, and streptococcus has been cultured in a few cases. However, other causes such as virus infection, allergy and even duct obstruction have been suggested. The term congenital sialectasis has been used to describe this condition in the past, but is rarely used now.

The sialographic appearances are characteristic. There is generalized punctate sialectasis, with multiple small cavities measuring 1 to 2 mm in diameter (Fig. 91.55). The duct system is invariably normal and there is no evidence of calculi.

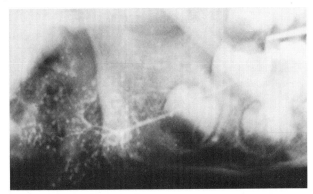

Fig. 91.55 Childhood sialectasis of the parotid gland. There is generalized punctate sialectasis with a normal duct system and no evidence of calculi.

Tumours

Salivary gland tumours can develop at any age, and usually present as a painless swelling. They are more common in the parotid than in the submandibular glands. The overall

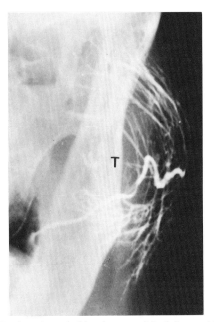

Fig. 91.56 Benign pleomorphic adenoma of the left parotid gland displacing the intraglandular ducts but not occluding them. The site of the tumour has been marked 'T'.

incidence of malignancy is 10 to 20%, being higher in the submandibular gland than in the parotid.

The typical sialographic appearance of a benign tumour is a duct-free area within the gland, surrounded by displaced ducts which are crowded together (Fig. 91.56). If parenchymal opacification has occurred, the tumour will appear as a well-defined filling defect.

Malignant tumours may have a similar appearance on sialography, but can narrow or occlude the intraglandular ducts without displacing them, and may produce an irregular parenchymal filling defect (Fig. 91.57).

The pathological classification of these tumours is complex. The benign pleomorphic adenoma is by far the most common tumour, and accounts for more than half of

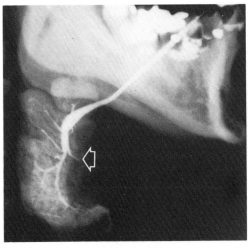

Fig. 91.57 Adenocarcinoma situated anteriorly in a submandibular gland. There is occlusion of the intraglandular ducts in the anterior part of the gland [arrow] and there is an irregular defect in the gland parenchyma.

all salivary gland tumours. Most other benign tumours are classified as monomorphic adenomas, and this group includes Warthin's tumour.

Malignant tumours are usually adenocarcinomas, the commonest type being muco-epidermoid carcinoma and adenoid cystic carcinoma (cylindroma). Although slow growing, malignant tumours of the salivary glands have a poor prognosis and the 10-year survival rate has been reported as less than 50%.

Isotope scanning with 1 to 2 mCi ^{99m}Tc-pertechnetate will outline normally functioning parotid, submandibular and sublingual glands as the isotope is excreted in the saliva like iodine. Most tumours produce an area of reduced uptake, the size of which depends upon the size of the tumour. The exception is Warthin's tumour, a rare type of adenoma, which concentrates the isotope and which therefore appears as an area of increased uptake or as a 'hot spot'.

CT scanning [34,35] has been combined with sialography in the assessment of space occupying lesions within the parotid gland. It will define the extent of a tumour more accurately than conventional sialography; it will often distinguish between benign and malignant tumours, and it is sometimes able to demonstrate the relationship of the tumour to the facial nerve.

Ultrasound will distinguish between solid tumours and fluid collections such as abscess cavities and cysts.

Trauma

Laceration of the main parotid duct, or of one of its larger intraglandular branches, occasionally results from penetrating facial injury, and is a very rare complication of surgery. Sialography will show extravasation of contrast medium from the duct system into the soft tissue (Fig. 91.58).

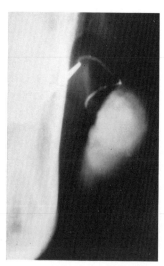

Fig. 91.58 Extravasation of contrast medium from the left parotid duct into the soft tissues. The duct had been damaged at surgery two weeks earlier.

SOFT TISSUE CALCIFICATION

Calcification is common in lymphoid tissue, and is presumably a sequel to old infection in most cases. The usual sites are the tonsil (Fig. 91.59) and the lymph nodes of the neck.

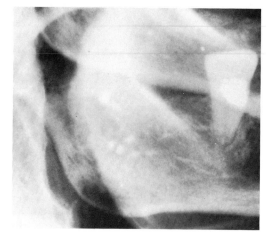

Fig. 91.59 Small areas of calcification in the tonsil.

Calculi are not uncommon in the *parotid and submandibular glands* and may be an incidental radiological finding.

Calcification is occasionally seen in the walls of the facial and lingual *arteries* in patients with hypercalcaemia or renal failure.

Small ring opacities are rarely seen in the subcutaneous tissues of the face, and may be due to *phleboliths* in a haemangioma (Fig. 91.60) or to multiple miliary *osteomas of the skin* [36].

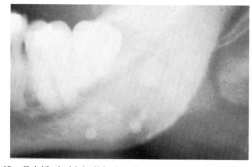

Fig. 91.60 Calcified phleboliths in a haemangioma of the cheek.

Small areas of subcutaneous calcification have been reported in *Gorlin's syndrome* and the *Ehlers-Danlos* syndrome.

BIBLIOGRAPHY

REFERENCES

1. Smith S N, Nortje C J 1980 Surgical emphysema following on undisplaced fractured zygoma. Br J Oral Surg 18:202–204
2. McIvor J 1972 The radiological features of odontogenic keratocysts. Br J Oral Surg 10:116–125
3. Steidler N E, Cook R M, Reade R C 1979 Aneurysmal bone cysts of the jaws. Br J Oral Surg 16:254–261
4. Killey H C, Kay L W 1964 Fibromyxomata of the jaws. Br J Oral Surg 2:124–130
5. Hayward J R 1981 Central cavernous haemangioma of the mandible. J Oral Surg 39:526–532
6. McIvor J 1974 The radiological features of ameloblastoma. Clin Radiol 25:237–242
7. Jephcote C M J 1981 Ameloblastoma with pulmonary metastases. Br J Oral Surg 19:38–43
8. Franklin C D, Pindborg J J 1976 The calcifying epithelial odontogenic tumour: A review and analysis of 113 cases. Oral Surg 42:753–765
9. Bhaskar S N 1968 Multiple enostosis: report of 16 cases. J Oral Surg 26:321–326
10. Adra N A, Barakat N, Melhem R E 1980 Salivary gland inclusions in the mandible: Stafne's idiopathic bone cavity. Am J Roentgenol
11. Kelly W H, et al 1980 Radiographic changes of the jawbones in end stage renal disease. Oral Surg 50:372–381
12. Finkelstein J B 1970 Osteosarcoma of the jaw bones. Radiol Clin North Am 8(3):425–443
13. Carrington G E, Scolfield H H, Conryn J, Hooker S P 1967 Osteosarcoma of the jaws. Analysis of 56 cases. Cancer 20:377–391
14. Burkitt D P, Wright D H 1970 Burkitt's lymphoma. Churchill Livingstone, Edinburgh
15. De Santis L A 1978 Radiographic findings of Ewing's sarcoma of the jaw. Br J Radiol 51:682–687
16. Schmamon A, Smith I, Ackerman L V 1970 Benign fibro-osseous lesions of the mandible and maxilla. Cancer 26:303–312
17. Cooke B E D 1956 Paget's disease of the jaws 15 cases. Ann R Coll Surg Engl 19:223–240
18. Khosla V M, Korobkin M 1970 Cherubism. Am J Dis Child 120:458–461
19. Johannsen A 1977 Chronic sclerosing osteomyelitis of the mandible. Radiographic differential diagnosis from fibrous dysplasis. Acta Radiologica: Diagnosis 18:360–368
20. Fradis M, Zisman D, Podoshin L, Wellisch G 1976 Actinomycosis of the face and neck. Acta Otolaryngol 102:87–89
21. Thomas P S 1978 The 'mandibular mantle' a sign of rickets in very low birth weight infants. Br J Radiol 51:93–98
22. Eversole L R, Rovin S 1972 Differential radiographic diagnosis of lesions of the jaw bones. Radiology 105:277–284
23. Killey H C, Kay L W, Seward G R 1977 Benign cystic lesions of the jaws. Their diagnosis and treatment. 3rd edn. Churchill Livingstone, Edinburgh p 170, Table A1
24. Ardran G M, Kemp F H 1972 The tongue and mouth in acromegaly. Clin Radiol 23:434–444
25. Katzberg R W, Dolwick M F, Helms C A, Mopens T, Bales D J, Coggs G C 1980 Arthrotomography of the temporomandibular joint. Am J Roentgenol 134:995–1005
26. Doyle T 1983 Arthrography of the temperomandibular joint: a simple technique. Clinical Radiology 34:147–153
27. Kreutziger K L, Mahan P E 1975 Temperomandibular degenerative joint disease. Oral Surg (Part 1) 40:165–182; (Part II) 40:297–319
28. Horrigan W D, Baker D M 1961 Gargoylism: A review of the roentgen skull changes with a description of a new finding. Am J Roentgenol 86:473–477
29. Friedlander A M 1976 Cut down sialography of the submandibular gland. J Oral Surg 34:555
30. Blair G S 1973 Hydrostatic sialography. Oral Surg 36: 116–130
31. Whaley K, Blair S, Low P S, Chisholm D M, Dick W C, Buchanan W W 1972 Sialographic abnormalities in Sjogren's syndrome, rheumatoid arthritis and other arthritides and connective tissue diseases. Clin Radiol 474–482
32. Jones H E 1953 Recurrent parotitis in children. Arch Dis Child 28 182–186
33. Maynard J D 1965 Recurrent parotid enlargement. Br J Surg 52: 784–789
34. Som P M, Biller H F 1980 The combined CT sialogram. Radiology 135:387–390
35. Stone D N, Mancuso A A, Rice D, Hanafee W N 1981 Parotid C T sialography. Radiology 138: 393–397
36. Carney R G, Radcliffe C E 1981 Multiple miliary osteomas of skin. Arch Dermat and Syph 64:483–486

SUGGESTIONS FOR FURTHER READING

Archer W H 1975 Oral and maxillofacial surgery. 5th edn Saunders, London
Beeching B 1981 Interpreting dental radiographs. Update, London
Bhaskar S N 1977 Synopsis of oral pathology. Mosby, USA; Kimpton,; London
Gorlin R J, Pindborg J J 1976 Syndromes of the head and neck. 2nd edn. McGraw Hill, New York
Ingram F L 1965 Radiology of the teeth and jaws. 2nd edn. Arnold, London
Killey H C, Kay L W, Seward G R 1977 Benign cystic lesions of the jaws. Their diagnosis and treatment. 3rd edn. Churchill Livingstone, Edinburgh
Kruger G O Textbook of oral and maxillo facial surgery. Mosby, USA
Lucas R B 1976 Pathology of tumours of the oral tissues. 3rd edn. Churchill Livingstone, Edinburgh
Kornblut A D, de Fries H O 1979 Malignant disease of the oral cavity. The Otolaryngological Clinics of North America. Saunders, USA
Manashil G B 1978 Clinical sialography. Thomas Springfield, Illinois
Mason D K, Chisolm D M 1975 Salivary glands in health and disease. Philadelphia Saunders
Pindborg J J, Kramer I R H 1971 Histological typing of odontogenic tumours, jaw cysts and allied lesions. WHO Geneva
Rowe N L, Killey H C 1968 Fractures of the facial skeleton. 2nd edn. Churchill Livingstone, Edinburgh
Sarnat B G, Laskin D M, Krugman W M 1980 The temporomandibular joint. 3rd edn Krogman, Springfield, Illinois
Sedano M O, Sauk J J, Gorlin R J 1978 Oral manifestations of inherited disorders. Butterworths, London
Stafne E C, Gilbilsco J A. Oral roentgenographic diagnosis. 5th edn. Saunders, Philadelphia
Taybi H 1982 Radiology of syndromes. 2nd Ed Year Book, Chicago
Trapnell D H Bowerman J 1973 Dental manifestations of systemic disease. Butterworths, London
Worth H M 1963 Principles and practice of radiologic interpretation. Year Book, Chicago
Zarb G A, Carlsson G E 1979 Temporomandibular joint function and dysfunction. Munsksgaard, Copenhagen

92 Dental radiology

James McIvor

Radiography
Anatomy of teeth and supporting structures
Developmental anomalies of teeth
    Defective calcification
    Abnormally shaped teeth
    Supernumerary and supplemental teeth
    Anodontia and partial anodontia
Eruption of teeth
    Normal eruption
    Abnormal eruption
Dental caries
Pulpitis and periapical infection
Periodontal disease
    Periodontal abnormalities associated with systemic
        disease
Fractures of the teeth and alveolar bone
Resorption of teeth

RADIOGRAPHY

Non-screen 'dental' films placed in the mouth have excellent resolution, and are particularly good at showing early carious lesions in the teeth, and the earliest bony changes of periapical and periodontal infection. The disadvantages are that the field size is small, and that the dose of radiation is relatively high.

Cassette films cover a much larger area but even so, it usually requires several films to demonstrate the upper and lower dental arches. Although small carious lesions and small bony abnormalities are not very well shown, the resolution is quite adequate for most bone lesions, such as cysts, tumours, infections and fractures.

Panoramic radiographs of the jaws have the great advantage of showing both dental arches on one film, and modern equipment will also show the lower parts of the maxillary sinuses, the whole of the mandible and the temporomandibular joints.

Modern panoramic machines are specialized tomographic units which take a curved 'slice' through the dental arches. The shape of the slice is fixed, and this results in poor definition if the shape of either dental arch is unusual, and is a common problem in the incisor region.

The dose of radiation is slightly higher than for a single cassette film.

In general, the bone detail is not as good as on conventional cassette films.

ANATOMY OF TEETH AND SUPPORTING STRUCTURES

The normal adult has 32 teeth, each quadrant having 2 incisors, 1 canine, 2 premolars and 3 molars. (Fig. 92.1). Adult teeth are usually designated by number counting from the

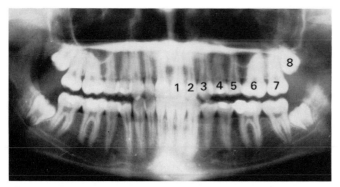

Fig. 92.1 Panoramic film of a normal adult aged eighteen years, in which the teeth in the left upper quadrant have been labelled. The third molars are unerupted.

midline, and the quadrant is indicated by two arms of a cross. Thus, the upper left canine, which is third from the midline, is described as ⌊3 and the lower right first molar, which is sixth from the midline, is described as ⁶̄ .

The permanent dentition is preceded by 20 deciduous teeth, there being 2 incisors, 1 canine and 2 molars in each quadrant (Fig. 92.2). These are designated by capital letters starting from the midline instead of numbers as in the permanent dentition. Thus, the upper left canine is described as ⌊C, and the lower right first molar as D̄ .

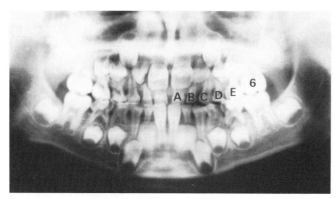

Fig. 92.2 Panoramic film of a normal child aged six years, in which the teeth in the left upper quadrant have been labelled. The deciduous teeth are all erupted, as are the first permanent molars.

Each tooth (Fig. 92.3) is composed largely of dentine, a living material with the radiodensity of lamellar bone and with a similar proportion of calcified inorganic material (70%). The intraoral part of the tooth or crown has a covering of enamel, the hardest and most radio-opaque tissue in the body, with a calcified inorganic content of 97%. Metallic fillings are more radio-opaque than enamel.

The root is covered with a thin layer of cementum, which has the same radiodensity as dentine, and which is too thin to show on a radiograph. This is surrounded by the periodontal membrane, which is clearly visible as a radiolucent line outlining the root, and beyond this lies the lamina dura which forms a continuous radio-opaque line around the root, and which is continuous with the lamina dura of the adjacent teeth at the level of the alveolar crest.

The pulp of the tooth appears radiolucent as it consists of soft tissues. Each tooth contains a pulp chamber in the crown

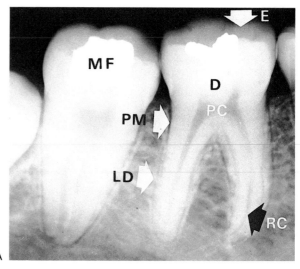

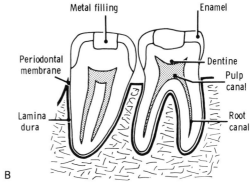

Fig. 92.3A & B (A) Labelled radiograph of a normal tooth and supporting structures. [E = enamel; D = dentine; PC = pulp canal; RC = root canal; PM = periodontal membrane; LD = lamina dura; MF = metallic filling].
(B) Line diagram of the radiograph.

which is continuous with one or more root canals. Each canal runs to the apex of a root where the blood vessels and nerves of the pulp communicate with those of the maxilla or mandible.

The part of a tooth which is nearest to the midline of the dental arch is described as 'mesial', and the part of the tooth furthest from the midline of the dental arch is described as 'distal'.

DEVELOPMENTAL ANOMALIES OF TEETH

Defective calcification

Dentinogenesis imperfecta (hereditary brown opalescent dentine) is a rare condition inherited as an autosomal dominant, which is sometimes associated with osteogenesis imperfecta. The teeth have short crowns and roots with small pulp chambers and narrow root canals (Fig. 92.4A). The

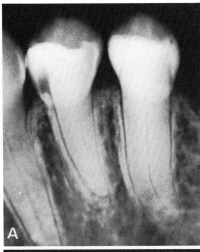

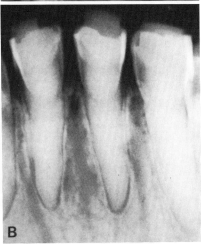

Fig. 92.4A & B Dentinogenesis imperfecta. The teeth have short crowns and roots with small pulp chambers and narrow root canals. The enamel appears normal on recently erupted teeth (A), but soon flakes off the incisal edges (B) and occlusal surfaces.

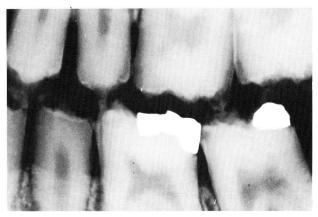

Fig. 92.5 Amelogenesis imperfecta. The enamel is normally calcified but extremely thin, and this gives the crowns a rectangular or square appearance.

enamel is normal when the teeth erupt, but soon flakes off due to inadequate support from the underlying poorly calcified dentine (Fig. 92.4B). The teeth become rapidly carious and periapical infection is common.

Amelogenesis imperfecta (hereditary enamel hypoplasia) is an even rarer condition, which is also inherited as an autosomal dominant. The enamel is normally calcified, but is extremely thin, and this results in the crowns having a rectangular or square appearance instead of the usual bulbous shape (Fig. 92.5). The incidence of caries is higher than in teeth with normal enamel.

Idiopathic enamel hypocalcification is another rare condition of unknown aetiology in which the enamel is normal in thickness, but is inadequately calcified. The enamel soon wears away and caries progress rapidly.

Morquio-Brailsford syndrome. The enamel is thin, poorly calcified, and tends to flake away from the underlying dentine.

Local enamel defects (enamel pits) may result from *severe childhood fevers*, such as measles and gastroenteritis, and are due to a temporary failure of enamel formation in the developing teeth.

Periapical dental infection of deciduous teeth can result in defects in the thickness and calcification of the enamel of their permanent successors.

Severe rickets in infancy may result in enamel hypocalcification, and *severe scurvy* can result in thin, hypocalcified dentine and in hypoplastic enamel due to inadequate development of the collagen matrix.

Hypophosphatasia, like severe rickets, results in hypocalcification of enamel and also causes premature loss of the deciduous teeth, due to defective cementum.

Hypoparathyroidism in infants and young children may cause hypoplastic enamel in the developing permanent teeth.

Fluorosis due to prolonged ingestion of water with a fluoride concentration exceeding 1 part per million, may result in pitting and discolouration of enamel.

Abnormally shaped teeth

Developmental anomalies of one or two teeth are common, and are rarely associated with more widespread abnormalities. The most common is the 'peg shaped' upper lateral incisor, which is obvious on clinical examination.

The term megadontia is sometimes applied to teeth which are unusually large, and the term microdontia to teeth which are abnormally small.

Gemination (geminated composite odontome, fusion) can occur anywhere in the dental arch, but is more common anteriorly (Fig. 92.6). It is usually the crowns of the affected teeth which are fused together.

Dens invaginatus (dilated composite odontome, dens in dente) results from invagination of the enamel into the

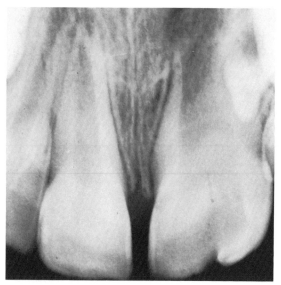

Fig. 92.6 Gemination or fusion affecting the upper left central and lateral incisors.

dentine during development, and produces an enamel lined cavity within the fully formed tooth (Fig. 92.7). The cavity communicates with the oral cavity and is the site of rapidly developing caries. The affected tooth, which is almost invariably an upper lateral incisor, is widened (dilated), and the radio-opaque enamel which covers the crown can be seen extending into the dentine.

Congenital syphilis results in abnormalities of the crowns of the developing permanent teeth. The upper incisors have notches in their incisal edges when they erupt six years later (*Hutchinson's teeth*), and the crowns of the developing first molars are small, with multiple irregular cusps (*Moon's molars*) when they erupt at the same time.

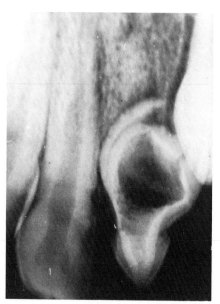

Fig. 92.7 Dens invaginatus of the upper left central incisor. The tooth is dilated and contains an enamel-lined cavity which communicates with the oral cavity.

The **Ellis-Van Creveld syndrome** and other ectodermal dysplasias are often associated with widespread dental abnormalities — usually small teeth with pointed crowns (*microdontia*) and *partial anodontia* (absence of some teeth).

Turner's syndrome (XO Syndrome) and **Down's syndrome** (Trisomy 21) may be associated with peg-shaped upper lateral incisors.

Dilaceration of the root of a permanent tooth may result from trauma during development but can occur spontaneously. It is usually seen in the upper anterior region where the angulation of the crown on the root produces a characteristic radiological appearance (Fig. 92.8).

Deformed roots in the permanent dentition may be a sequel to *hypoparathyroidism* in infancy, and are also a feature of *cleidocranial dysostosis*.

In **hypercementosis** (cementum hyperplasia) there is excessive formation of cementum around the root of an erupted tooth (Fig. 92.9). The condition often affects several adjacent teeth and the aetiology is unknown. Radiologically there is marked widening of the apical part of the root giving it a bulbous appearance, and the radiolucent line of the periodontal membrane can be seen outside the widened root.

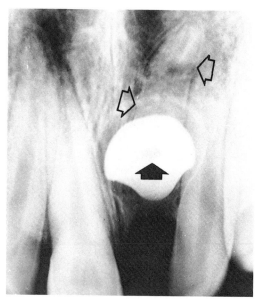

Fig. 92.8 Dilaceration of the root of the upper left permanent incisor. The root [open arrows] is normal in position, but the crown is angled posteriorly so that the root canal [solid arrow] appears as a small round radiolucency surrounded by dentine and enamel.

Hypercementosis should be distinguished from a cementoma which develops outside the periodontal membrane, and from the hypercementosis of Paget's disease, which is also situated outside the periodontal membrane.

Therapeutic radiation in childhood may arrest the normal development of permanent teeth and cause them to have small crowns and short pointed roots.

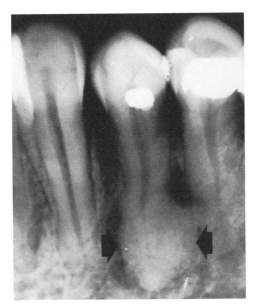

Fig. 92.9 Hypercementosis of the lower left first premolar. There is a mass of cementum around the root [arrows] giving it a bulbous appearance.

Supernumerary and supplemental teeth

Supernumerary teeth are extra teeth which do not resemble any normal tooth. They are usually multiple and are most common in the premaxillary region, where their presence often delays the eruption of the upper permanent incisors (Fig. 92.10).

Supplemental teeth are normally formed extra teeth, and they can occur anywhere in the dental arches.

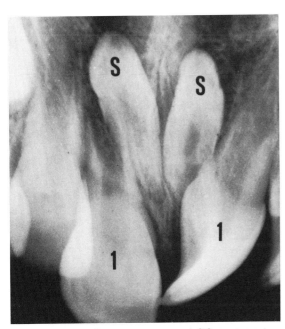

Fig. 92.10 Two inverted supernumerary teeth [S] are situated between the roots of the upper central incisors [1] and have resulted in rotation of the upper left first incisor.

Supernumerary and supplemental teeth are a feature of cleidocranial dysostosis and have been reported in Gardner's syndrome.

Predeciduous teeth in the new born are rare, as are post permanent teeth in adults.

Anodontia and partial anodontia

It is not uncommon for the upper lateral incisor or lower third molar (Fig. 92.11) to be absent in otherwise normal individuals.

Partial anodontia (absence of many teeth) and **complete anodontia** (total absence of teeth) occur rarely, and there is often a *family history* in affected individuals (Fig. 92.12). Partial anodontia may be associated with a generalized *ectodermal dysplasia* such as the Ellis-Van Creveld Syndrome.

Therapeutic radiation in early childhood can result in complete failure of odontogenesis in the irradiated area and is a very rare cause of partial anodontia.

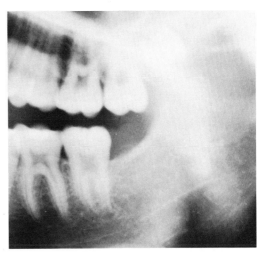

Fig. 92.11 The lower left third molar is absent.

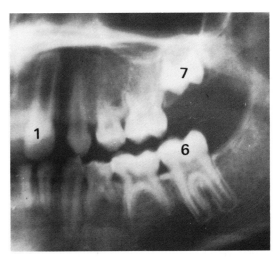

Fig. 92.12 Partial anodontia in a child aged 10 years. There are only three permanent teeth on the left side, and they have been appropriately numbered. Most of the deciduous teeth are still present.

Infective osteomyelitis in infancy is a rare cause of partial anodontia and is more likely to affect the maxilla than the mandible.

ERUPTION OF TEETH

Normal eruption

The deciduous teeth begin to erupt at 6 months and should all be present by 2½ years. The approximate times of eruption are listed below; in general the lower teeth appear slightly sooner than the upper teeth.

A	Central incisors	6–8 months
B	Lateral incisors	8–10 months
C	Canines	16–20 months
D	First molars	12–16 months
E	Second molars	20–30 months

The permanent teeth start to appear at the age of 6 years and should all be present by 20 years. The lower teeth erupt 6 to 12 months earlier than the uppers. The approximate times of eruption are as follows.

1	Central incisors	6–8 years
2	Lateral incisors	7–9 years
3	Canines	9–12 years
4/5	First and second Premolars	10–12 years
6	First molars	6–7 years
7	Second molars	11–13 years
8	Third molars	17–21 years

In general, the roots are incompletely formed when the permanent teeth erupt and take a further 2 years to develop fully.

Abnormal eruption

Delayed eruption of one or two permanent teeth is usually due to *insufficient space* in the dental arches. It commonly affects the upper canine which has to fit into a space between the lateral incisor and first premolar, and the lower third molar which has to fit behind the second molar and in front of the ramus of the mandible. These unerupted teeth which may come to lie obliquely or horizontally are usually described as 'impacted'.

The high incidence of impacted upper canines (Fig. 92.13) and lower third molars (Fig. 92.14) in developed countries is probably due to the crowns of the teeth being too large for the size of the dental arches. The size of each tooth is determined genetically and is fixed, whereas the normal growth of the jaws depends to some extent upon muscle activity, such as vigorous chewing. This is not required for

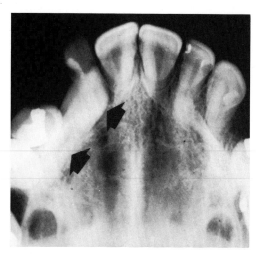

Fig. 92.13 Unerupted impacted upper right canine lying horizontally in the palate [arrows].

highly refined diets, as a consequence of which the jaws may not develop fully and the dental arches are often too small for a full complement of 'normal' sized teeth.

Eruption of normal teeth may be delayed or prevented by *local pathological conditions*, such as supernumerary teeth, cysts, tumours or odontomes.

If a *cleft palate* extends anteriorly through the dental arch, the eruption of the upper anterior teeth is usually delayed.

Cleidocranial dystostosis (Fig. 92.15) and *achondroplasia* are often associated with delayed eruption and noneruption of the permanent teeth.

A few permanent teeth will sometimes fail to erupt in the absence of any local or generalized abnormality, and there is frequently a *family history* of this condition in affected individuals.

Eruption depends on normal circulating levels of thyroxine and growth hormone. It is therefore delayed in *hypopituitarism* and *hypothyroidism* and is premature in patients with *gigantism*. Eruption is late in *progeria*.

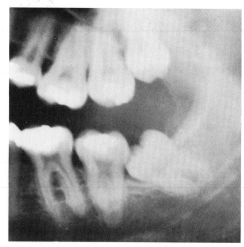

Fig. 92.14 Impacted lower left third molar.

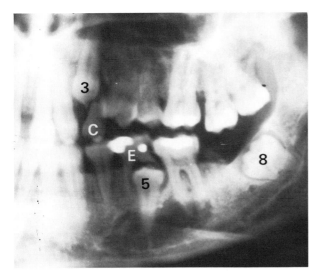

Fig. 92.15   Noneruption of three permanent teeth [numbers] with prolonged retention of two deciduous teeth [letters] in an adult with cleidocranial dysostosis.

The bony defect adjacent to the roots of the lower second premolar and lower first molar has the appearance of a nonepithelial cyst (haemorrhagic bone cyst).

DENTAL CARIES

Dental caries is a destructive process which affects the enamel and dentine of erupted teeth. The initial lesion is caused by Gram-negative bacilli which form acid below a dental plaque on the flat surfaces of adjacent teeth (Fig. 92.16 — interstitial caries), or on the irregular occlusal surfaces of molars and premolars (Fig. 92.17 — pit and fissure caries).

The earliest radiological change is a small defect in the enamel surface due to decalcification. This defect is difficult to demonstrate at first, but when the carious process has penetrated the enamel and reached the dentine, the defect is usually obvious.

The destruction of dentine progresses much more rapidly than the destruction of enamel, and is soon apparent as a radiolucent area within the crown (Figs. 92.16 & 17). If unchecked, the process continues until the crown of the tooth is completely destroyed (Fig. 92.18).

Bacterial invasion of the pulp (pulpitis) and periapical infection are inevitable sequelae of advanced caries.

'Radiation caries' is the term given to the high incidence of dental caries which often follows therapeutic radiation to the maxillofacial region in adults. It is almost certainly due to a reduction in salivary flow, and not to any alteration in the structure of the teeth which are, of course, fully formed in early adult life.

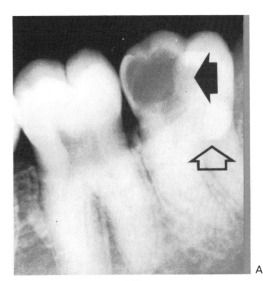

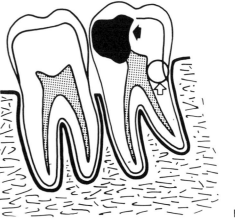

Fig. 92.17   (A) Advanced caries [solid arrow] originating from the occlusal surface and extending as far as the pulp chamber. The small defect in the enamel of the occlusal surface is not visible. The open arrow points to an enameloma or enamel pearl.

(B) Line diagram of the radiograph.

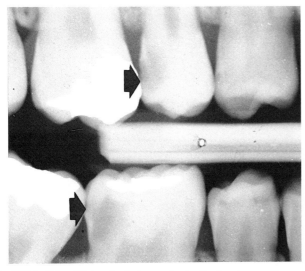

Fig. 92.16   Interstitial caries in two molar teeth, showing small defects in the enamel [arrows] with extensive destruction of the underlying dentine.

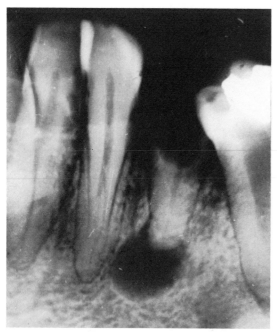

Fig. 92.18 Complete destruction of the crown of the lower first premolar due to advanced caries. There is a well defined radiolucent area at the root apex which has the typical appearance of an apical granuloma.

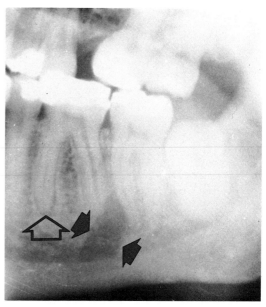

Fig. 92.19 There is a defect in the lamina dura over the apex of the mesial root of the lower first molar [open arrow]. This is an early feature of periapical infection.

There is a poorly defined radiolucent area at the apex of the distal root of the same tooth, which has the typical features of a chronic alveolar abscess [solid arrows].

PULPITIS AND PERIAPICAL INFECTION

Pulpitis itself produces no radiological abnormalities, but if it is a sequel to dental caries, as is usually the case, the caries will be apparent radiologically.

An **acute alveolar abscess** produces no radiological change in the alveolar bone in its early stages, and in this respect, it is similar to acute osteomyelitis. There may be slight thickening of the periodontal membrane of the affected tooth due to inflammatory oedema, but this is rarely obvious. After the infection has been present for seven to ten days, a small defect becomes apparent in the lamina dura over the root apex (Fig. 92.19), and a small area of rarefaction develops in the periapical alveolar bone.

A **chronic alveolar abscess** may follow an acute abscess, or may begin as a low grade infection. The radiological abnormalities do not appear until the infection has been present for at least seven days, and in the early stages are similar to those of an acute abscess. The defect in the lamina dura and the area of periapical rarefaction soon develop into a small, irregular radiolucency adjacent to the root apex (Fig. 92.19).

A **periapical granuloma** sometimes develops as a result of a long standing chronic periapical infection, and appears radiologically as a well defined radiolucent area at the root apex (Fig. 92.20). Histologically, a granuloma consists of granulation tissue and chronic inflammatory cells.

An **apical dental cyst**, the commonest cyst of the maxillofacial region, develops if an apical granuloma undergoes central necrosis and liquefaction, and this happens quite frequently. There are no definite radiological criteria which indicate that a cyst has developed, but if the diameter of a periapical radiolucent area exceeds 1 cm, it is more likely to be a cyst than a granuloma. Another difference is that a growing dental cyst has a corticated margin, whereas the bony margin of a granuloma is rarely corticated.

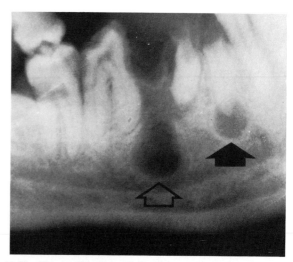

Fig. 92.20 The small round radiolucent area with the corticated margin [solid arrow] is typical of an apical granuloma.

The larger radiolucent area with no cortical margin [open arrow] is a small residual dental cyst, the cortical margin having been destroyed by infection.

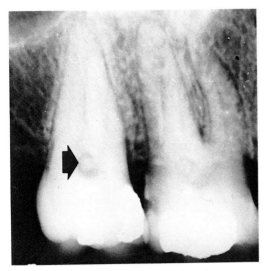

Fig. 92.21 Small pulp stone in the pulp chamber of an upper molar.

Pulp stones can develop in the pulp chamber of any tooth, but they are most common in the molar regions (Fig. 92.21). They may be a sequel to chronic inflammation, but their aetiology is uncertain. They are asymptomatic.

PERIODONTAL DISEASE

Radio-opaque *calculus* plays an important role in the aetiology of inflammatory periodontal disease, and is commonly deposited around the necks of the lower incisors (Fig. 92.22) and upper molars. It results in inflammation of the soft tissues at the necks of the teeth (gingivitis) and

resorption of the cortical and trabecular bone of the alveolar crest (Fig. 92.22).

A **periodontal pocket** forms when the periodontal membrane is destroyed, and appears radiologically as widening of the radiolucent periodontal membrane and destruction of alveolar bone (Fig. 92.23A & B). The radiolucent space contains infected necrotic material. Pockets are usually multiple and show most clearly between the teeth on intraoral radiographs.

An **acute periodontal abscess** causes slight generalized widening of the periodontal membrane and rarefaction of the surrounding alveolar bone. These signs are often difficult to detect and take seven to ten days to develop.

A **chronic periodontal abscess** results in a small area of bone destruction adjacent to the root of the affected tooth. In

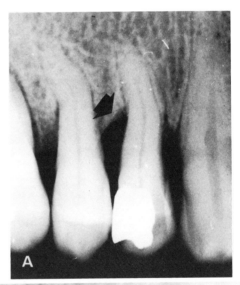

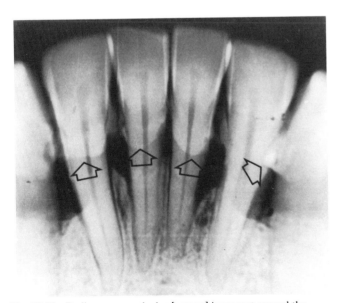

Fig. 92.22 Radio-opaque calculus [arrows] is present around the necks of the lower incisor teeth. There is considerable resorption of the underlying alveolar bone.

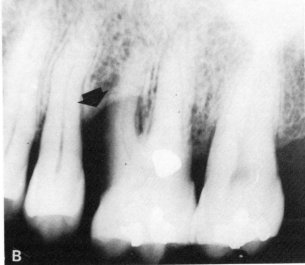

Fig. 92.23 (A) Deep periodontal pocket [arrow] with apparent widening of the periodontal membrane.
(B) Deep periodontal pocket [arrow] between the upper left second premolar and upper first molar teeth.

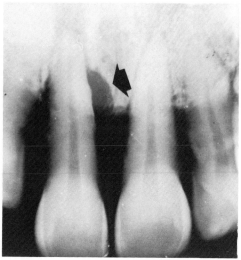

Fig. 92.24 Chronic periodontal abscess [arrow] adjacent to the root of an upper right central incisor. There is extensive resorption of bone around the adjacent teeth indicating advanced periodontal disease.

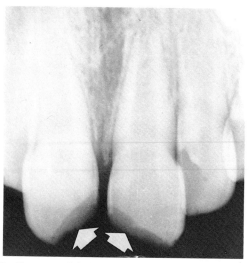

Fig. 92.25 Fractures of the incisal edges of the crowns of both upper central incisors [arrows].

addition, there may be localized widening of the periodontal membrane or a defect in the lamina dura (Fig. 92.24).

In **atrophic periodontitis** (or periodontosis) the pockets appear in the absence of calculus or inflammation and are usually situated in the upper anterior region at first. Apart from the absence of calculus and the position of the pockets, the radiological abnormalities are similar to those of inflammatory periodontal disease.

Periodontal abnormalities in association with systemic disease

The incidence of inflammatory periodontal disease is higher in *diabetes mellitus* and *pregnancy*.

Scleroderma (progressive systemic sclerosis, acrosclerosis) results in thickening of the periodontal membranes of all the teeth.

Osteopetrosis (Albers-Schönberg disease, marble bone disease) and *infantile hypoparathyroidism* may cause generalised thickening of the lamina dura, and *hyperparathyroidism* often results in rapid resorption of the lamina dura.

FRACTURES OF THE TEETH AND ALVEOLAR BONE

Fractures of the crown are caused by direct trauma, and occur most frequently in the upper incisor region (Fig. 92.25). They may be associated with fractures of the roots and with fractures of the facial bones. Fractures which extend into the pulp chamber result in pulpitis and periapical infection. Detached fragments of the crown may be driven into the adjacent soft tissues, particularly the lips.

Root fractures are caused by trauma to the crown, and are most common in the upper incisor region (Fig. 92.26). They show best on intraoral films and may be multiple. The pulp often undergoes partial or complete necrosis, and periapical infection is a common complication. Root fractures may result from attempted dental extractions and the fragments can be displaced into the maxillary sinus in the upper molar region (Fig. 92.27), or into the soft tissues.

Alveolar fractures may follow blunt trauma as in road traffic accidents, but can also follow an attempted dental extraction, especially in the upper molar region where the maxillary sinus often extends below the level of the root apices and weakens the alveolar bone (Fig. 92.28).

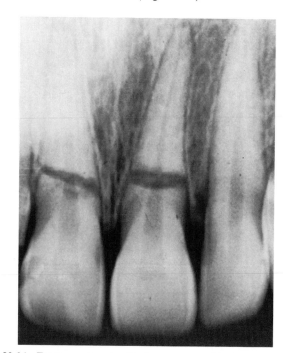

Fig. 92.26 Fractures of roots of both upper central incisors.

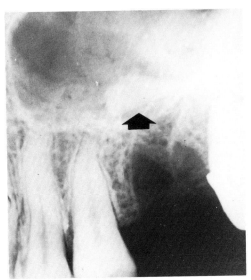

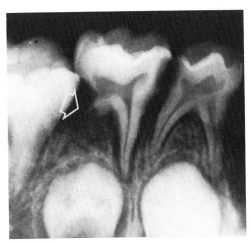

Fig. 92.29 Physiological resorption of the distal root [arrow] of the lower right second deciduous molar due to eruption of its permanent successor.

Fig. 92.27 Two roots [arrows] of the upper left first molar have been displaced into the left maxillary sinus in the course of an attempted extraction. Note empty root sockets.

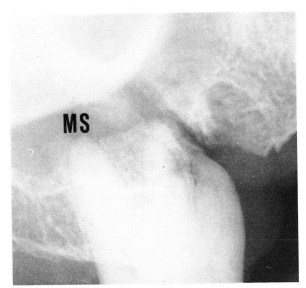

Fig. 92.28 Alveolar fracture extending into the maxillary sinus [MS] which occurred during the attempted extraction of an upper molar tooth.

RESORPTION OF TEETH

The roots of deciduous teeth are normally resorbed before the teeth are lost (Fig. 92.29), but ankylosis to the alveolar bone can occur — particularly if the permanent successor is missing.

The roots of traumatised, nonvital and infected teeth are frequently resorbed, and the roots of unerupted teeth are occasionally resorbed even in the absence of infection.

Malignant and locally invasive tumours frequently resorb the roots of teeth without displacing them. Benign cysts and tumours occasionally cause root resorption, but are much more likely to cause displacement.

Enlargement of the pulp chamber (internal resorption) may follow trauma even if the tooth is not fractured and remains vital. Rarely it occurs in the absence of any history of injury, when it is described as idiopathic internal resorption.

BIBLIOGRAPHY

SUGGESTIONS FOR FURTHER READING

Bhaskar S N 1979 Radiographic interpretation for the dentist, 3rd edn. Mosby, USA; Kimpton, London.
Barr J H, Stephens R C 1980 Dental radiology. Basic concepts and their application to clinical practice. Philadelphia, Saunders, Philadelphia
Cohen B, Kramer I R H 1976 Scientific foundations of dentistry. Heinemann, London
Dixter C, Langlais R P, Lichty G C 1980 Paediatric radiographic interpretation. Exercises in dental radiology, Vol 3. Saunders, Philadelphia
Glickman I 1976 Clinical periodontology, 5th edn. McGraw Hill, New York
Gorlin R J, Pindborg J J 1976 Syndromes of the head and neck, 2nd edn, McGraw Hill
Ingram F L 1965 Radiology of the teeth and jaws, 2nd edn. Arnold, London
Langlais R B, Kasle M J 1978 Intra-oral roentgenographic interpretation exercises in dental radiology Vol 1. Saunders, Philadelphia
Langlais R B, Bentley K C 1979 Advanced oral roentgenographic interpretation. Exercises in dental radiology Vol 2. Saunders, Philadelphia
Shafer W G, Hine M K, Levy B M 1974 A textbook of oral pathology, 3rd edn. Saunders, Philadelphia
Smith N J D 1980 Dental radiography. Blackwell Scientific Publications, Oxford
Stafne E C, Gilbilsco J A 1976 Oral roentgenographic diagnosis, 5th edn. Saunders, Philadelphia
Strahan J D, Waite I M 1978 A colour atlas of periodontology. Wolfe, London
Trapnell D M, Bowerman J 1978 Dental manifestations of systemic disease. Butterworth, London
Taybi H 1982 Radiology of syndromes. 2nd edn. Year Book, Chicago
Worth H M 1963 Principles and practice of oral radiologic interpretation. Year Book, Chicago
Wuehrmann A H, Manson-Hing L R 1977 Dental radiology, 4th edn. Mosby, USA; Kimpton, London

93

The ear, nose and throat

Thomas Powell

The nose and paranasal sinuses
    Methods of radiological examination
    Anatomy
    Abnormalities of development
    Infection, inflammation and allergy
    Tumours
    Trauma

The ear
    Methods of radiological investigation
    Anatomy
    Tomography
    Infective and inflammatory disease
    Tumours
    Trauma
    Congenital abnormalities

The pharynx
    Methods of radiological examination
    Anatomical features
    Inflammatory and related lesions
    Benign tumours
    Malignant tumours
    Cervical dysphagia
    Foreign bodies

The larynx
    Methods of radiological examination
    Radiological anatomy
    Tumours
    Infective and inflammatory disease
    Trauma
    Laryngocele
    Recurrent laryngeal nerve paralysis
    Extrinsic displacement and compression

Diagnostic radiology has always been important in otorhino-laryngology and has contributed much to the understanding and management of diseases of the ear, nose and throat. During the past 40 years the pattern of ENT disease has changed and there is no longer such a preponderance of infective abnormalities. The development of the operating microscope and the revolutionary improvement in endoscopic equipment have altered the diagnostic approach, with a resulting change in the importance of some radiological examinations.

At the present time, the still developing techniques of CT and interventional radiology continue to alter the relative importance of different aspects of the radiological contribution in otorhinolaryngology.

The nose and paranasal sinuses

METHODS OF RADIOLOGICAL EXAMINATION

The principal radiological techniques are listed in Table 93.1. Whenever the demonstration of the presence of fluid is important, the examination should be carried out using a horizontal X-ray beam. An antiscatter grid (either moving Potter Bucky or stationary of at least 40 lines/cm) is necessary except when the field size can be limited to a circle of less than 8 cm. Omission of the grid results in a reduction in the radiation dose. Table 93.1 indicates the principal anatomical features shown in each projection and the main diagnostic applications. The list is, however, by no means exhaustive and individual difficult cases may require modifications to these projections and techniques.

Table 93.1 *Radiography of the paranasal sinuses*

Radiographic projection and technique	Anatomical features displayed	Applications
Occipitomental (Water's view). Posteroanterior with canthomeatal line extended 45°, no angulation of incident ray.	Maxillary antra, frontal sinuses, sphenoid sinuses (with mouth open), zygomatic bone.	Survey view of paranasal sinuses for infection, allergy, tumour and trauma.
Occipitofrontal (Caldwell view). Posteroanterior with canthomeatal line extended 10°, no angulation of incident ray.	Frontal sinuses, orbits, nasal cavity, maxillary antra (lateral walls), ethmoid sinuses.	Survey views of frontal and ethmoid sinuses, nasal cavity, detection of erosion in lateral wall of maxillary antrum.
Lateral	Frontal, maxillary and sphenoid sinuses (both sides superimposed), nasal cavities and nasopharynx.	Examination of posterior choanae for polypi, examination of sphenoid sinuses, assessment of bone thickness in the walls of the frontal sinus, detection of cysts in the floor of the maxillary antra.
Submentovertical (axial) Anteroposterior. Head hyperextended with canthomeatal line parallel to film, no angulation of incident ray.	Ethmoid and sphenoid sinuses, maxillary antra, nasopharynx.	Assessment of posterior spread of sinus malignancy.
Oblique. Posteroanterior, head rotated 40° and the canthomeatal line extended 30°	Posterior ethmoid sinuses, optic canals.	Examination of posterior ethmoid sinuses on each side separately.
Tomography Coronal Occipito frontal position	Paranasal sinuses and nasal cavity	Examination of the sinuses for mucocele, malignancy, trauma, including blow-out injuries, investigation of CSF rhinorrhoea.
Tomography Sagittal	Paranasal sinuses, postnasal space	Investigation of CSF rhinorrhoea.
Tomography Submentovertical (axial)	Ethmoid and sphenoid sinuses, optic canals.	Investigations of malignancy and mucocele of the ethmoid and sphenoid sinuses.
CT Horizontal and coronal sections	Paranasal sinuses, orbits and adjacent soft tissue planes.	Investigation of bone destruction and soft tissue spread associated with sinus malignancy.

ANATOMY

The paranasal sinuses are, as their name implies, all closely related to the nasal cavity. They are named after the bones in which they lie and consist of the frontal, sphenoid, ethmoid, and maxillary sinuses (sometimes called maxillary antra). They are lined by ciliated columnar epithelium with mucus secreting glands.

The cilia are more numerous nearer the ostia of the sinuses and promote drainage of the mucus secretions. The paranasal sinuses develop as invaginations of the mucous membrane of the nasal cavity into the surrounding bones. None of the paranasal sinuses is visible at birth as they are small and contain secretions.

Maxillary antra

The maxillary antra appear within a few weeks of birth and enlarge throughout childhood. Apart from the alveolar recess inferiorly which only develops completely with the eruption of the permanent dentition, the sinuses have reached their adult configuration by about the age of 14 years. The adult maxillary antrum is a large cavity lying in the body of the maxilla, triangular when viewed in the posteroanterior plane and quadrilateral in the lateral projection. The roof is formed by the floor of the orbit and contains a ridge for the infraorbital canal which conducts the infraorbital nerve and vessels. The floor of the antrum is formed by the alveolar process of the maxilla. This region is poorly defined in infancy and childhood due to the overlying developing teeth, and does not pneumatize fully until the second dentition has completely erupted (Fig. 93.1). The medial wall of the maxillary antrum is formed by the lateral wall of the nasal cavity. Laterally, the maxillary antrum extends for a variable distance into the zygomatic bone forming the zygomatic recess. Below this the lateral wall is relatively thin and often shows a defect due to the superior dental vessels which may simulate a fracture. The maxillary antrum drains into the middle meatus of the nasal cavity (q.v.).

Though the antra may vary in size in different individuals, they are almost always symmetrical. Septa may occur within the antrum and may be partial or complete, the latter type being associated with separate ostia for the two chambers. A posterior ethmoidal cell may at times enlarge and encroach on the medial wall of the maxillary antrum, and may occupy a considerable proportion of its volume. Anatomically separate ethmoidal and antral cells of these types are not necessarily involved in infection of the adjacent

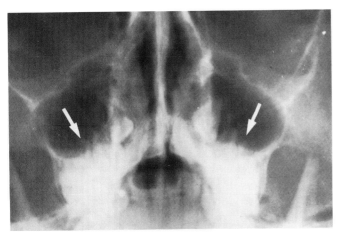

Fig. 93.1 Maxillary antra in patient aged 6 years. Note the incomplete pneumatization of the alveolar recesses.

cells and conversely may be infected when the other antral compartments are spared.

Frontal sinuses

The frontal sinuses appear rather later than the maxillary antra. At birth rudimentary frontal sinuses are present anterior to the ethmoids and although they enlarge in this situation in the first two years of life, they remain invisible on the radiograph. They cannot usually be demonstrated radiographically until the age of two years at which time they have begun to extend into the vertical plate of the frontal bone. At the same time pneumatisation of the orbital plate is occurring, and the frontal sinuses continue to enlarge to reach adult size at about the age of 14 years. The frontal sinus drains via the frontonasal duct into the middle meatus of the nasal cavity (q.v.).

The frontal sinuses in the adult consist of irregular cavities lying between the inner and outer tables of the frontal bone with a variable extension upwards and backwards. They are closely related above and behind to the cranial cavity and below it to the orbit and nose. The anterior wall is sub-

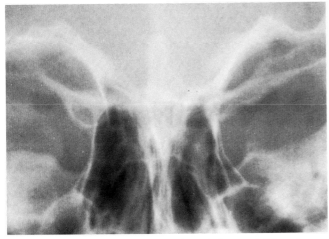

Fig. 93.2 Congenital absence of the frontal sinuses. Adult patient.

cutaneous. The frontal intersinus septum is usually asymmetrical in relation to the midline and the two frontal sinuses are, unlike the maxillary antra, usually asymmetrical. The size of the frontal sinus varies considerably in different individuals, and one or both may be completely absent. (Fig. 93.2) The absence of both may be associated with a persistent metopic suture. Very large frontal sinuses may be developmental, but are also associated with acromegaly. The frontal sinuses tend to be larger in men than in women. Relatively thick anterior and posterior walls may lead to an apparent loss of translucency on the radiographs. Errors in diagnosis from this may be avoided by noting the wall thickness on the lateral or submentovertical projections.

Ethmoid sinuses

The ethmoid sinuses develop and reach maturity at about the same time as the frontal sinuses. They lie in the lateral masses of the ethmoid bone between the orbits and the lateral wall of the upper half of the nasal cavity. On each side there are up to 20 ethmoid cells classified radiologically into anterior and posterior groups. They are variable in distribution, and may extend into the frontal, maxillary, and sphenoid bones. Such ethmoid cells lying outside the confines of the ethmoid bone are referred to as 'agger ethmoidal cells'. Occasionally such cells may appear to be part of the maxillary or frontal sinuses (Fig. 93.3).

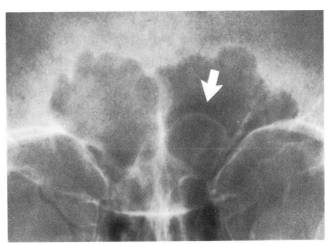

Fig. 93.3 Agger ethmoidal cell bulging up into left frontal sinus.

Sphenoid sinuses

The sphenoid sinus cannot be recognized radiologically until about the age of 3 years. It enlarges progressively to reach adult size at about the time of puberty, but its eventual size varies considerably in different individuals. In some cases there is complete pneumatization of the body of the sphenoid with extensions into the greater wing and even into the occipital bone; only rarely is there complete failure of pneumatization. The intersinus septum is often asymmetrically placed. The normal adult sphenoid sinus is related superiorly to the pituitary fossa, anteriorly to the ethmoid sinus, and inferiorly to the floor of the sphenoid bone and the roof of the nasopharynx.

When interpreting radiographs of the paranasal sinuses, it is important to bear the following in mind:

1. The relative lack of radiolucency of the paranasal sinuses in infancy
2. The changes in shape which take place in the sinuses as they grow to their adult configuration
3. The developmental variations described above
4. Apparent abnormalities of aeration of the sinuses due to the thickness of their bony walls. The thickness of overlying soft tissues should also be taken into account, e.g. facial swelling after injury may simulate an opaque sinus
5. Apparent abnormalities of radiolucency of the sinuses resulting from inaccuracies of radiographic projection, particularly obliquity.

When these factors have been taken into account, a radiograph of a normal paranasal sinus shows an area of relative radiolucency with a clearly defined bony margin. The mucosal lining of a normal sinus is thin and is not usually visible.

The nasal cavity

The nasal cavity consists of paired passages passing between the external nose anteriorly and the nasopharynx posteriorly. The roof is formed by the cribriform plate of the ethmoid and the floor by the hard palate. A central septum divides the nasal cavity into two halves, most of the septum being bony, though there is a small cartilaginous portion which projects forward into the external nose. The nasal septum usually bulges a little to one side or the other, only marked displacements being pathological and symptomatic. The lateral wall of the nasal cavity is complex with contributions from the ethmoid, palatine, lachrymal and maxillary bones.

Projecting from the lateral wall on either side are the three turbinates. The largest is the inferior turbinate, the free edge of which is curved down and back on itself into a scroll-like configuration. The space below and lateral to the inferior turbinate is known as the inferior meatus. The middle turbinate is less complex in structure than the inferior turbinate. The space lying between it and the inferior turbinate is known as the middle meatus. The frontonasal duct draining the frontal sinus opens anteriorly into the middle meatus and the ostium of the maxillary antrum lies at about its mid point. The superior meatus lies above the middle turbinate and receives the drainage of the ethmoid and sphenoid sinuses. Projecting into it is the relatively small superior turbinate which divides the cavity into the superior meatus proper and the spheno-ethmoidal recess.

The nasal cavity is lined by mucus secreting columnar epithelium and its complex internal anatomy, particularly of the inferior meatus allows a large mucosal surface area, warming the incoming air and trapping particulate material.

ABNORMALITIES OF DEVELOPMENT

Underdevelopment of the paranasal sinuses

There are marked individual variations in the extent to which the paranasal sinuses develop, though these variations are much more apparent in the frontal and sphenoid sinuses than they are in the maxillary antra and ethmoids. In particular, the frontal sinuses are often hypoplastic or absent, some cases being associated with persistence of the metopic suture into adult life.

Abnormally small paranasal sinuses may be found in hypoplastic states of the skull base and facial skeleton. These include cleidocranial dysostosis, craniofacial dysostosis, pycnodysostosis, progeria (Werner's syndrome), some cases of achondroplasia and mucopolysaccharidosis, and hypothyroidism. Hypoplasia or absence of the frontal sinuses is common in Down's syndrome [1]. Unilateral hypoplasia of the skull due to craniostenosis is usually associated with underdevelopment of the frontal sinus on the affected side. The bone marrow hyperplasia found in the severe haemoglobinopathies such as sickle cell anaemia and thalassaemia may cause gross encroachment on the paranasal sinuses, particularly the maxillary antra.

Arrested development of the maxillary antra may occur as a result of antral infection in infancy or childhood, in which case the sinuses have a permanently immature configuration with no extension lateral to the infraorbital foramen (Fig. 93.4).

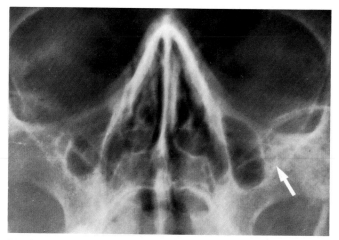

Fig. 93.4 Hypoplasia of the maxillary antra. They have an infantile configuration with the infraorbital foramen [arrow] lying lateral to the midpoint of the lateral wall of the antrum.

Overdevelopment of the paranasal sinuses

Symmetrical overdevelopment of the paranasal sinuses is a frequent finding in acromegaly, particularly affecting the frontal sinuses, causing the characteristic supra-orbital prominence. Unilateral overdevelopment of the paranasal sinuses, particularly affecting the frontal and ethmoid sinuses may be seen in agenesis or atrophy of one cerebral hemisphere due to birth injury where unilateral enlargement of the mastoid air cells may also be seen.

Choanal atresia

Congenital occlusion of the posterior nares is an uncommon condition causing nasal obstruction in infants and young children. The nature and time of presentation depends upon whether the occlusion is partial or complete, and whether it involves one or both sides of the nose. The obstruction may be membranous or bony, the latter being far more common. Externally, some asymmetry of the face and nose is common and the palate may show a high arched appearance.

Infantile cases are usually bilateral, and present with breathing difficulties, particularly during feeding. Unilateral atresia may present much later, even in adult life.

Radiological appearances

It is unusual to be able to make a diagnosis of choanal atresia on the plain film, though this may be suspected because of hypoplasia and diminished translucency of the affected half of the nasal cavity seen on the posteroanterior film (Fig. 93.5A). Only rarely can the obstructing bony septum be seen, even though it may in some cases exceed 1 cm in thickness.

A definitive diagnosis of choanal atresia is made by introducing contrast medium, e.g. oily propyliodone, through a fine catheter into the nasal cavity with the patient in the supine position. The contrast medium runs into the most dependent part of the nasal cavity outlining the obstruction of the posterior choana. Radiographs are then obtained in the lateral projection (Figs. 93.5B & 6).

Postnasal obstruction in the neonate or young infant is most often due to choanal atresia though rare cases of postnasal polypi and lymphoid hyperplasia are seen even at this age. Cases presenting in older children should be distinguished from tumours in the nasopharynx and postinflam-

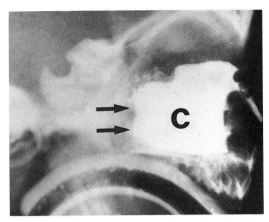

Fig. 93.6 Choanal atresia in a neonate. The atresia plate [arrows] is identified by contrast medium in the nasal cavity [C].

matory stenosis. The latter is now very rare, but used to be a complication of tonsillectomy and of diphtheria.

Displacement of the nasal septum

The nasal septum is characteristically a midline structure in infancy but as growth occurs, displacement to one or other side is usual. Severe displacement may be due to unbalanced growth between the walls of the nasal cavity and the septum, and should be distinguished from displacement of the nasal septum due to tumours such as polypi.

INFECTION, INFLAMMATION AND ALLERGY

This is by far the largest group of diseases of the nose and paranasal sinuses. An individual patient may suffer at various times from each of the three disease states. Infection in nonallergic individuals occurs, and is often precipitated by an acute upper respiratory infection. Infection may also occur in patients with allergic rhinitis and sinusitis, the oedematous mucosa causing obstruction to the drainage of the paranasal sinuses. Any other cause of obstruction, such as trauma or congenital deviation of the nasal septum may predispose to infection. Infection of the maxillary antra sometimes occurs due to dental root sepsis, and may follow dental extraction. Loss of a dental root fragment into the antrum is always followed by infection. Once sinus disease is established it tends to recur, because of damage to the ciliated columnar epithelium. Treatment is normally directed to the elimination of infection, the suppression of allergic responses, the drainage of retained secretions and the relief of obstruction.

Radiological examination should consist of an occipitomental projection, with the addition of the occipitofrontal and lateral when necessary. Conventional tomography may

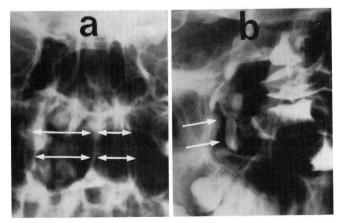

Fig. 93.5 Choanal atresia, adult patient, (A) hypoplasia and opacity of the left side of the nasal cavity, (B) atresia shown by contrast medium in nasal cavity [arrows].

be of value in doubtful cases, and CT is indicated where there is reason to suspect orbital or intracranial extension of the infective process [2]. The principal finding is a loss of radiolucency of the affected sinus, the pattern taking various forms as described below. A doubtful loss of radiolucency cannot be resolved by comparison with the opposite side, since bilateral disease is often present.

A-mode ultrasound examination is a simple and inexpensive technique. Normal sinuses can be distinguished from those containing fluid, and from those filled with solid contents [3]. Thermography may be useful in the diagnosis of acute inflammatory processes in the frontal or maxillary sinuses.

Sinusitis

Acute inflammatory disease of the paranasal sinuses, whether precipitated by infection or by allergy (vasomotor rhinitis), results in swelling of the mucosa. The maxillary antra are most frequently affected, followed by the frontal sinuses. Isolated inflammatory disease in the ethmoid and sphenoid sinuses is uncommon, such infections usually being found in patients with antral and frontal sinusitis. Ethmoid sinusitis is seen most often in children and teenagers, and may be complicated by orbital cellulitis.

The affected maxillary antrum shows swelling of its mucosa, which in simple infection tends to parallel the antral walls (Fig. 93.7). In contrast, in allergic sinusitis the mucosa may show a scalloped appearance, and polypi may be seen in some patients. Swelling of the mucosa may become so marked as to reduce the lumen to a narrow slit (Fig. 93.8) and may in some cases completely obliterate the antral cavity. Complete radio-opacity of a paranasal sinus may also be caused by obstruction with resulting retention of secre-

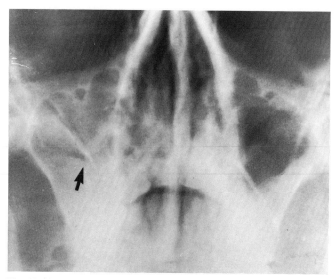

Fig. 93.8 Acute maxillary sinusitis. Severe mucosal thickening [arrow] on the right almost obliterating cavity. Slight mucosal thickening on the left.

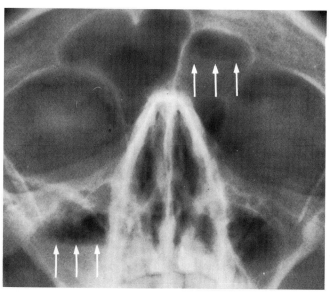

Fig. 93.9 Acute maxillary and frontal sinusitis showing fluid levels [arrows].

tions. These may form a fluid level if air is also present, a common finding in infective sinusitis, though much less often seen in allergy. Fluid levels are most frequently seen in the maxillary antra, but are also found in the frontal sinuses (Fig. 93.9). A horizontal X–ray beam is necessary for their demonstration, and they may be confirmed by tilting the head or turning the patient into the lateral decubitus position, in which case the fluid level alters in position (Fig. 93.10). Time should be allowed for the often viscous fluid to gravitate into the new position.

If the radiological features in the sinuses do not indicate whether a primary infective or allergic origin is likely, further evidence may be found in appearance of the mucosa over the turbinates, which is commonly swollen in allergic rhinitis but normal in simple infections. The simultaneous involvement

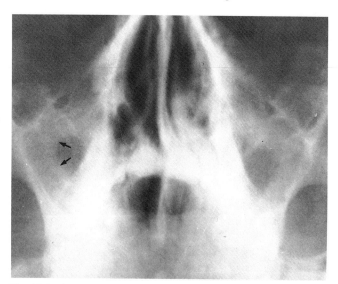

Fig. 93.7 Acute maxillary sinusitis. Bilateral mucosal thickening which parallels the antral walls [arrows].

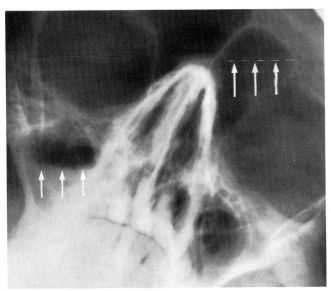

Fig. 93.10 Fluid levels confirmed by tilting the patient to the left (Same patient as Fig. 93.9).

of several or all of the sinuses is a feature of allergy rather than infection.

Concurrent sinusitis and orbital cellulitis in patients with a depressed immune response may indicate an opportunistic infection such as aspergillosis or mucormycosis [4].

Chronic sinusitis

In some patients, complete radiological clearing of acute inflammatory changes may take place, though clinically it is often found that such patients are subject to further attacks. However, some cases appear to progress to a more chronic form of sinusitis showing persisting mucosal swelling, occasionally associated with some thickening or sclerosis of the bony walls of the sinus. The presence of polypi suggests that the persisting abnormality is of allergic origin. Chronic sinusitis is most commonly seen in the maxillary antra and frontal sinuses. Chronic infection of the ethmoid and sphenoid sinuses is uncommon and is usually associated with frontal sinusitis.

Complications of sinusitis

Osteomyelitis

Both acute and chronic sinusitis are occasionally complicated by osteomyelitis, though antibacterial chemotherapy has greatly reduced the incidence. In some cases bone infection is precipitated by sinus surgery. As in the case of osteomyelitis in the long bones, the clinical features precede the radiological changes, and a clinical diagnosis should therefore be made and treatment commenced without waiting for radiological confirmation. The radiological features of acute osteomyelitis include blurring or loss of the sinus outline with surrounding reduction in bone density and trabecular

pattern. Radionuclide studies using ^{99m}Tc polyphosphate or other bone seeking agents may be of value in the diagnosis of sinus related osteomyelitis prior to the development of radiological changes [5].

Epidural and cerebral abscess

A rare but dangerous complication of frontal sinusitis is the spread of sepsis posteriorly to the dura with the development of an abscess. An infective thrombophlebitis may result, and may lead to a cerebral abscess, particularly in the frontal lobe. Metastatic foci of osteomyelitis may develop in other parts of the skull.

Computed tomography is indicated for the investigation of an extradural, subdural, extradural or intracerebral abscess. Contrast enhancement should be used in order to demonstrate the vascular capsule of the abscess. If CT is not available, radionuclide brain scanning is useful for the investigation of a possible cerebral abscess.

Mucocele

Obstruction of the ostium of a paranasal sinus causes the secretions to accumulate and to fill the sinus. There is increase in pressure, with expansion of the sinus and erosion of its walls. Most mucoceles result from inflammatory or allergic mucosal swelling, but occasionally the obstruction is due to injury or tumour. Mucoceles are found most commonly in the frontal sinus, because the long frontonasal duct is particularly vulnerable to obstruction by mucosal swelling. Less frequently mucoceles occur in the ethmoid cells, and are also seen occasionally in the sphenoid and maxillary sinuses. Maxillary sinus mucoceles are less rare than has been stated in the past [6]. A spheno-ethmoidal mucocele is an ethmoid mucocele which has expanded into the sphenoid sinus.

Frontal sinus mucocele

Frontal sinus mucocele presents as a supraorbital swelling, or with proptosis, sometimes painful. Radiologically there is enlargement of the sinus with blurring of its outline and loss of its characteristic scalloped superior margin. The enlargement affects both the orbital and frontal components of the sinus, and there is bulging of the intersinus septum to the opposite side. Despite the fact that the sinus is full of secretions, it often shows increased radiolucency due to pressure atrophy of its walls [7] (Fig. 93.11). The orbital margin may be deformed or destroyed, and this may be the most obvious radiological feature. Doubtful cases may be resolved by tomography, particularly in the lateral plane [8]. CT shows the characteristic expansile and destructive nature of the lesion and is of particular value in the determination of the intra-orbital and intracranial extension [9].

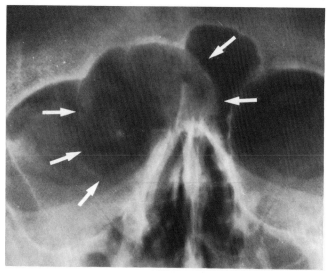

Fig. 93.11 Frontal sinus mucocele. Note radiolucency despite mucus contents. Marked extension into the right orbit produced severe proptosis.

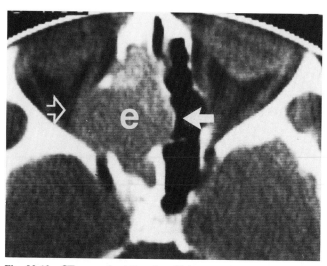

Fig. 93.13 CT scan of orbito-ethmoidal mucocele. The mucocele [e] has expanded across the midline to bulge into the right ethmoid air cells [solid arrow], and into the orbit displacing the medial rectus and optic nerve [open arrow].

Ethmoid sinus mucocele

The presenting feature is a palpable mass at the inner canthus, but radiological detection is more difficult than with frontal sinus mucocele [10]. They usually arise from the anterior ethmoidal cells (the relatively rare mucoceles arising from the posterior ethmoid expand into the sphenoid sinus and are described as spheno-ethmoidal mucoceles). The radiological features include loss of radiolucency of the ethmoid cells, disappearance or intraorbital displacement of the lateral wall of the ethmoid sinus (Fig. 93.12), destruction of the ethmoid septa, and expansion into the frontal sinus (fronto-ethmoidal mucocele). In doubtful cases coronal tomography is of value, but CT is more definitive in outlining the expansion of an ethmoid mucocele both within the ethmoid labyrinth and into the orbit (Fig. 93.13).

Empyema

An empyema is a paranasal sinus filled with pus and may result either from an acute sinusitis, or due to infection of a pre-existing mucocele. In the first case the radiological features are those of an acute sinusitis with complete loss of radiolucency. Some loss of definition of the wall of the affected sinus may suggest the correct diagnosis. More often the diagnosis is made on a clinical basis, in that the patient is more ill than would be expected in a simple acute sinusitis, and the affected sinus is more painful.

An empyema complicating a mucocele usually shows only the radiological features of the mucocele itself (Fig. 93.14), but peripheral contrast enhancement of a mucocele on CT is evidence of active infection [2].

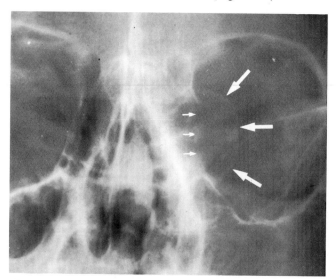

Fig. 93.12 Orbito-ethmoidal mucocele. Lateral wall of anterior ethmoidal cells bulging into orbit [arrows]. Absence of lateral ethmoidal wall in its normal situation [small arrows].

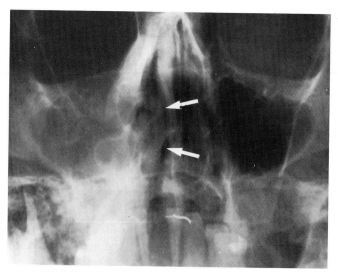

Fig. 93.14 Infected mucocele (empyema) of right maxillary antrum. Antrum is opaque and its medial wall bulges into the nasal cavity [arrows]. Note soft tissue swelling over right side of nose.

Cysts

A localised sessile dome-shaped swelling in the mucosa of a paranasal sinus may be due to a cyst (Fig. 93.15). These may be of the secretory variety (mucus retention cysts) or the nonsecreting type (degenerative cysts). Occasionally secretory cysts are large and may produce pressure deformity of the antral wall, but the majority of cysts of both types are small and cannot be distinguished radiologically. Both tend to occur as a sequel to a previous episode of infection and may radiologically be confused with polypi. They are often seen arising from the floor of the maxillary antrum, as shown on occipitomental and lateral projections.

Cysts of dental origin (dentigerous and radicular cysts) may bulge upwards into the antrum, originating from the dental roots related to the alveolar recess. In particular, dentigerous cysts may become very large and may occupy the whole maxillary antrum. If standard sinus films show a cyst arising from the lower part of a maxillary antrum of suspected dental origin, occlusal films and an orthopantomogram may be helpful.

A globulomaxillary cyst is of developmental origin, and is due to incomplete fusion of the premaxilla and maxilla. Radiologically there is characteristic displacement of the canine and lateral incisor teeth (Fig. 93.16).

Polyposis

Allergy may be complicated by polyposis which may affect both the paranasal sinuses (particularly the maxillary antra) and the nasal cavity. Polypi are pedunculated mucosal swellings containing only sparsely cellular oedematous tissue and covered by normal epithelium.

Most polypi arise from the mucosa of the nasal fossae. They may grow to fill completely the nasal cavity and may extend into the posterior choana and nasopharynx. Radiologically the nasal cavity is completely opaque and is sometimes expanded with atrophy of its walls (Fig. 93.17). In cases showing expansion of the nasal cavity, there may be an accompanying enlargement of the ethmoid cells [11].

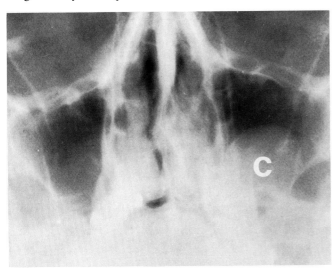

Fig. 93.15   Nonsecreting cyst [C] of left maxillary antrum.

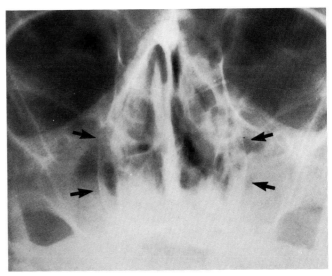

Fig. 93.17   Nasal polyposis. Nasal cavity is markedly widened with thinning of its lateral walls [arrows].

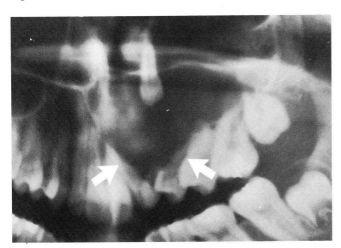

Fig. 93.16   Globulomaxillary cyst. Lateral incisor tooth is displaced medially and first premolar is displaced laterally [arrows]. The canine tooth is displaced markedly upwards.

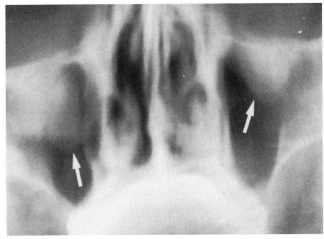

Fig. 93.18   Maxillary sinus polyposis [arrows].

Polypi in the maxillary antra appear as rounded soft tissue shadows (Fig. 93.18) which are often multiple, and which may fill the antrum causing complete radio-opacity. An antral polyp may grow through the ostium of the sinus into the nasal cavity, and may enlarge to present in the posterior choana. These are termed antrochoanal polyps. They may be visible on lateral soft tissue radiographs of the naso-pharynx (Fig. 93.19). A submentovertical projection is also useful in their demonstration. The ipsilateral maxillary antrum is characteristically radio-opaque.

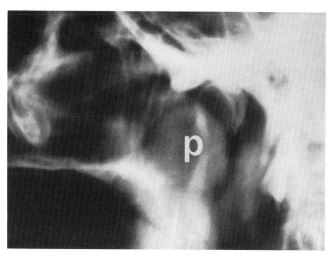

Fig. 93.19 Antrochoanal polyp [p] — lateral projection.

Specific inflammatory lesions

Diseases in this category are rare in the developed countries. Destructive inflammatory lesions may occur in the nasal cavity and maxillary antra due to *tuberculosis, syphilis, yaws* and *leprosy*.

Clinical and histological involvement of the nose in *sarco-idosis* occurs commonly. Radiological changes in the nasal bones similar to the cystic appearances found in the hands in sarcoidosis have been described, but are rare.

TUMOURS OF THE NOSE AND THE PARANASAL SINUSES

Benign tumours

Benign tumours of the nasal cavity are comparatively rare. *Papilloma* and *angioma* may occur, but are usually small and do not show any radiological features. In some patients they present clinically with epistaxis, which may be severe, and in these circumstances selective angiography of the internal maxillary artery may be successful in demonstrating the bleeding point. The haemorrhage may then be controlled by embolization of the feeding vessel. In some cases of intrac-table epistaxis, the bleeding may be found to arise from the anterior ethmoidal artery and these are not generally amenable to embolization.

Neurofibroma also occurs occasionally in the nasal cavity, but produces no characteristic change other than the pres-ence of a soft tissue mass associated with pressure atrophy of the walls of the nasal fossae.

Benign tumours of the paranasal sinuses include *fibroma, angioma,* epithelial (inverted) *papilloma, epidermoid* (choles-teatoma), *osteoma* and *osteochondroma, osteoclastoma,* and *osteoid osteoma* [13].

Osteoma

Osteomas are the commonest benign tumours affecting the paranasal sinuses and show a predominantly male sex distri-bution. They are of two types: the more common ivory osteoma, which consists of hard dense bone and the much rarer cancellous osteoma. They are found most often in the frontal sinus, but ethmoid sinus osteomas also occur quite commonly. Maxillary and sphenoid sinus osteomas are rare.

Radiologically an ivory osteoma appears as a dense well defined mass having a round or lobulated outline (Fig. 93.20). The affected sinus is otherwise normal in appearance, unless the osteoma obstructs its ostium, in which case retention of secretions occurs and a secondary mucocele may be formed. A cancellous osteoma shows an opacity which is of little more than soft tissue density.

The majority of osteomas are relatively small, but very large tumours can occur, which fully occupy the affected sinus causing erosion of its walls and encroachment on the orbit and cranium (Fig. 93.21).

An infrequent complication of ethmoid osteoma is the development of cerebrospinal fluid rhinorrhoea or the entry of air into the cranium due to erosion of the floor of the anterior fossa. (Fig. 93.22).

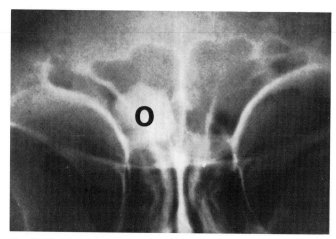

Fig. 93.20 Frontal sinus osteoma. A homogeneous dense mass lies in the right frontal sinus [O], which is otherwise normal. Incidental finding.

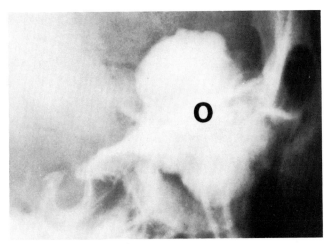

Fig. 93.21 Large ethmoid sinus osteoma [O]. The tumour occupies much of the ethmoid sinus and bulges up into the cranium. Patient presented with proptosis.

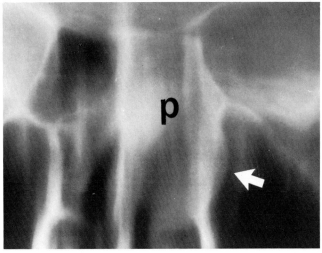

Fig. 93.23 Epithelial (inverted) papilloma [p]. Tumour in upper part of nasal cavity has obstucted or invaded ethmoid sinus and is bulging into the upper part of the maxillary antrum [arrow].

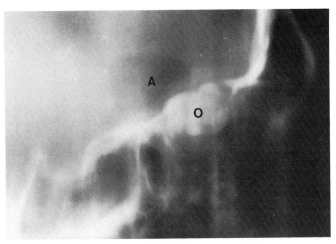

Fig. 93.22 Ethmoid sinus osteoma [O]. Tomogram shows erosion of floor of the anterior cranial fossa and the associated dura producing an aerocele [A]. Patient presented with headache. Air was also present in the cerebral ventricles.

thinning of its walls. The features erroneously suggest a mucocele or even a carcinoma.

The difficulty of distinguishing pressure atrophy of bone from true malignant invasion in epithelial papilloma makes biopsy necessary in most cases to exclude malignancy.

Leontiasis ossium

This term is used to describe the clinical appearance due to an overgrowth of the facial skeleton with encroachment on the paranasal sinuses. It has a number of pathological causes, including *fibrous dysplasia*, *Paget's disease*, and a low grade periostitis. Radiologically there is thickening of the facial bones with encroachment on the lumen of the maxillary antra (Fig. 93.24). As the disease progresses, the facial skeleton becomes increasingly deformed, with invasion of the orbit. Biopsy may be necessary to establish the histological nature.

Epithelial (inverted) papilloma

This is an uncommon benign tumour arising from the mucous membrane of the nasal cavity, and less commonly from the paranasal sinuses. It occurs predominantly in males. There is a tendency to recurrence after removal and malignant change occasionally takes place.

The radiological features usually consist of a nasal mass with opacification of the paranasal sinuses [14]. The nasal mass tends to show features similar to those found in nasal polyposis with expansion of the nasal cavity and thinning of its wall (Fig. 93.23). Bone destruction does not generally occur. The ostia of the paranasal sinuses on the side of the lesion may be obstructed, in which cases the affected sinuses become opaque. An inverted papilloma may however arise in the maxillary antrum, producing a tumour which completely occupies the affected sinus with expansion and

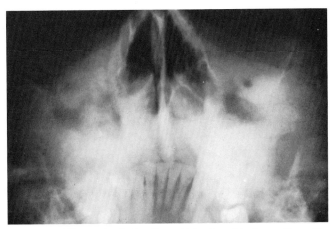

Fig. 93.24 Fibrous dysplasia. Gross thickening of both maxillae with encroachment on the maxillary antra.

Miscellaneous tumours

There are a number of uncommon benign tumours which may affect the paranasal sinuses. *Fibromas*, seen occasionally in the frontal sinuses are small polypoid lesions, not distinguishable from other causes of a polyp. *Neurofibromas* may occur, and may be large with gross distortion of the facial skeleton. *Ossifying fibromas* are large tumours which expand to obliterate the affected sinus and cause much facial deformity (Fig. 93.25). *Chondroma, osteochondroma* and *haemangioma* occur rarely.

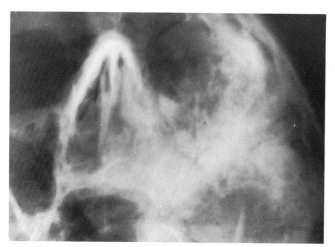

Fig. 93.25   Ossifying fibroma of left maxillary antrum. Large ossifying tumour has obliterated left antrum and is invading the left orbit. There was severe facial deformity.

A *cholesteatoma* (epidermoid) occurs occasionally in the maxillary antra and may grow to fill the cavity of the affected sinus with expansion of its walls. The radiological features suggest a mucocele. CT may be of value in distinguishing the lower attenuation value due to the fat content of a cholesteatoma.

Meningoceles and *encephaloceles* may occasionally present in infancy as soft tissue masses in the nasal cavity. A frontal meningocele may present in older children or adolescents showing a circumscribed midline bone defect associated with absence or hypoplasia of the frontal sinuses. The features may suggest a mucocele both clinically and radiologically.

Malignant tumours of the paranasal sinuses

The majority of malignant tumours of the paranasal sinuses are of epithelial origin. Most arise in the maxillary antra, though ethmoid carcinoma is also quite common. Malignant tumours are rare in the frontal and sphenoid sinuses.

Tumours of connective tissue and bony origin also arise in the paranasal sinuses, but occur much less frequently. They include *fibrosarcoma, myxosarcoma,* and *osteosarcoma. Plasmacytoma* and *melanoma* may be seen occasionally. Metastases may show features indistinguishable from primary tumours of the paranasal sinuses.

Carcinoma

These form the majority of malignant tumours affecting the paranasal sinuses. They arise from the mucosa of the sinus and may be columnar celled or squamous in type, the latter as a result of metaplasia of the epithelium. Carcinoma of the paranasal sinuses tends to occur in middle-aged and elderly patients, affecting males more frequently.

The radiological features consist of a soft tissue mass which partly or completely fills the air space of the affected sinus. Bone destruction may occur followed by extension of the tumour into the adjacent structures. The bone destruction is irregular, and is not associated with sclerosis. Expansion of a sinus, as seen in benign tumours and mucoceles, is rarely present in carcinoma.

Carcinoma of the maxillary antrum

This is a slow growing tumour presenting with pain, nasal obstruction and epistaxis. Radiological examination should include occipitofrontal, occipitomental, lateral and submentovertical projections; conventional tomography in the coronal plane is of value, together with CT where available. The diagnosis may be suspected on standard sinus radiographs showing the presence of radio-opacity with bone destruction (Fig. 93.26). The destructive changes may be overlooked on plain radiographs, particularly when they

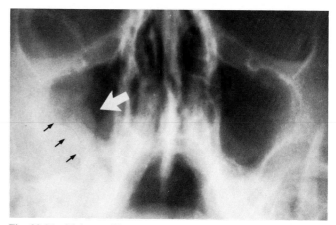

Fig. 93.26   Right maxillary sinus carcinoma. A lobulated mass bulges into the antral cavity [large arrow] destruction of the lateral antral wall [small arrows].

involve the medial wall which is often poorly seen even in normal subjects. Destructive changes in the lateral wall are more easily seen, particularly on the occipitofrontal projection (which is otherwise not a particularly useful view of the maxillary antra). Conventional tomograms of the maxillary antra in the coronal plane improve the detection of bone

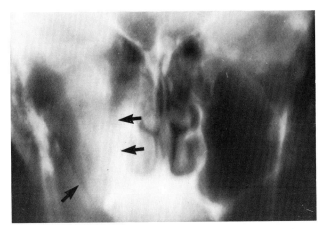

Fig. 93.27 Carcinoma of right maxillary antrum. Tomogram showing complete loss of radiolucency with destruction of lateral and medial walls [arrows].

erosion [15], but are less useful for the detection of the soft tissue extent of the lesion outside the antrum (Fig. 93.27). For this purpose the use of CT has greatly enhanced the accuracy of radiological diagnosis [2,16,17]. The extent of bone destruction is better defined, particularly of the anterior wall; but minimal bony changes may not be detected because of partial volume effect. Soft tissue limits are demonstrated with an accuracy which cannot be achieved by conventional methods. When the outline of the tumour cannot be clearly shown, it may be suspected because of obliteration of the normal fascial planes. Possible tumour extension into such important areas as the infratemporal fossa, the orbit, the pterygopalatine fossa, the nasopharynx and the cranial cavity may be assessed by CT (Fig. 93.28) [18]. Areas of necrosis and abscess formation may also be seen. Neither conventional radiography nor CT will necessarily distinguish between the soft tissue opacity produced by the tumour and that which is due to obstruction and infection secondary to the tumour. Contrast enhanced examinations are not usually of value in the assessment of maxillary sinus carcinoma. For most purposes, horizontal sections are adequate, but invasion of the orbit and through the hard palate is better assessed on coronal sections. These are better obtained by direct

methods, as computer generated coronal reconstructions lack sufficient detail.

Quite apart from the diagnostic value of CT in patients with carcinoma of the maxillary antrum, the determination of the soft tissue limits of the tumour enables the radiotherapist to plan treatment with much greater precision than can be achieved using conventional tomographic methods [19]. The response of such tumours to radiotherapy may also be monitored by the use of CT [18].

CT has superceded conventional methods of axial tomoraphy. Although useful diagnostic information can be obtained by conventional axial tomography, in many patients the necessary degree of hyperextension of the neck cannot be obtained because of the age of the patient or because of respiratory difficulty. Angiography, though employed in the past for the determination of the extent of maxillary sinus carcinoma, is also now largely obsolete.

Radiological methods, including CT, do not distinguish benign tumours from early malignant lesions, before the development of bone erosion, or before soft tissue extension beyond the affected sinus has taken place. For this purpose biopsy remains essential.

Carcinoma of the ethmoid sinus

The radiological approach is in general similar to that described above. The most useful views are the occipitofrontal, axial, and oblique projections (Fig. 93.29). The detection of early ethmoid carcinoma is difficult, as the destruction of its thin bony walls and septa may easily be overlooked. The detection of early destructive changes is enhanced by tomography in the coronal plane. As with the maxillary sinus, CT is of great value. Ethmoid sinus carcinoma tends to spread into the orbit (often causing proptosis), into the nasal cavity, into the opposite side of the ethmoid and nose, and into the cranium. All these features are well shown on CT (Fig. 93.30) [18]. Coronal sections may be valuable, particularly for the assessment of orbital encroachment and intracranial spread.

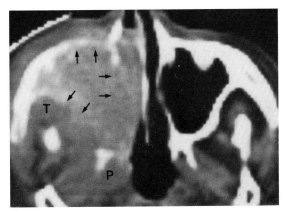

Fig. 93.28 CT scan showing carcinoma of left maxillary antrum. Destruction of anterior, medial and lateral antral walls. Tumour is present in the infratemporal fossa [T] and lies posterior to the pterygoid plates which are partly destroyed [P].

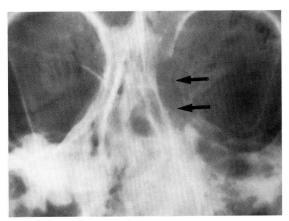

Fig. 93.29 Carcinoma of the left ethmoid sinus. A large tumour occupies the ethmoid cells with opacity of the nasal cavity and left maxillary antrum. Left lateral wall of ethmoid sinus is destroyed [arrows].

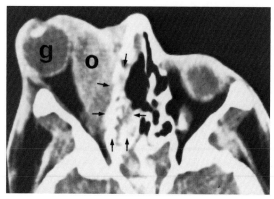

Fig. 93.30 CT scan showing left ethmoid carcinoma. Ethmoid air cells [arrows] are opaque. Tumour extends into orbit [O]. There was marked proptosis: note displacement of globe [g]. (Reproduced by kind permission of Dr J. Husband, The Royal Marsden Hospital, London).

Carcinoma of the frontal and sphenoid sinuses

These tumours are comparatively rare. Carcinoma of the frontal sinus causes early obstruction. The radiological changes produced are due to a combination of malignant and infective changes and may be indistinguishable from infection occurring alone, unless there is obvious bone destruction.

Carcinoma of the sphenoid sinus produces opacity with bone destruction, spread tending to occur either downwards and forwards into the sphenoethmoidal recess or upwards into the pituitary fossa. It may be difficult in some cases to determine whether the radiological abnormality is due to a sphenoid sinus carcinoma, to upward spread of a naso-pharyngeal carcinoma, to invasion of the sphenoid by a pituitary tumour, or to a chordoma.

Malignant tumours of the nasal cavity

Many tumours presenting in the nasal cavity are extensions of primary lesions arising in the maxillary or ethmoid sinuses. Primary malignant tumours of the nasal cavity occur less frequently. Most are squamous in type, but adenocarcinoma and melanoma also occur, and chondrosarcoma may arise from the nasal septum.

Radiologically a soft tissue mass is seen in the nasal cavity, with destruction of the nasal septum or lateral wall of the nasal cavity. The destruction may be difficult to detect and again coronal tomography may be helpful. CT may also be very useful. (Fig. 93.31).

TRAUMA

Fractures of the facial skeleton involving the paranasal sinuses are outside the scope of this section and are dealt with elsewhere (Chapter 91) together with orbital blow-out injuries involving the antra and ethmoid sinuses. Foreign bodies in the paranasal sinuses most commonly result from road traffic accidents, both glass and metallic fragments entering the antra on occasion. Foreign bodies also occur due to the displacement of a tooth root during extraction, or the loss of an amalgam fragment or a broken reamer into the antral cavity. A tooth root may enter the antrum, sometimes because of an unusually close relationship between the root of the affected tooth and the floor of the antrum. A fistula between the antrum and the mouth may form and is always complicated by infection of the antrum. Both the defect and the tooth fragment may be shown by tomography, either using standard tomographic methods, the orthopantomograph or CT.

Intranasal foreign bodies are common, particularly in childhood where they are usually due to the introduction of small plastic toys or buttons. Both patients and their physicians may insert packs of gauze or cotton wool and may forget to remove them subsequently. These foreign bodies are initially radiolucent but acquire an external deposit of calcium phosphate and carbonate causing the production of a radio-opaque mass in the nose called a rhinolith.

Barotrauma

Exposure of an individual to rapid changes in atmospheric pressure may cause a traumatic sinusitis associated with thickening, often polypoid, of the antral mucosa. Complete opacity of the antrum is not uncommon. The change in atmospheric pressure may also force infected material from the nasal cavity into the sinus producing a simple infective sinusitis.

Wegener's granulomatosis and midline lethal granuloma

These are histologically similar diseases characterised by a multifocal necrotizing angiopathy. Granulomatous masses

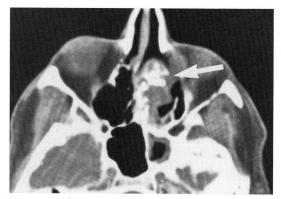

Fig. 93.31 CT scan showing chondrosarcoma of left nasal cavity. Note calcification [arrow]. (Reproduced by kind permission of Dr J. Husband, The Royal Marsden Hospital, London).

form in the nose and paranasal sinuses, particularly the maxillary antra, initially causing loss of radiolucency, and subsequently associated with cartilage and bone destruction. In Wegener's granulomatosis, there is usually involvement of the lungs and kidneys.

The ear

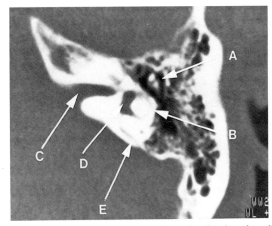

Fig. 93.32 CT scan of right temporal bone showing incudomallear joint [A], lateral semicircular canal [B], internal auditory meatus [C], vestibule [D], vestibular aqueduct [E]. (Reproduced by kind permission of Medicamundi).

METHODS OF RADIOLOGICAL INVESTIGATION

The principal methods of radiological examination are indicated in Table 93.2 together with the anatomical features demonstrated, and the clinical applications. The list is by no means exhaustive and an individual approach is often necessary for a particular case. Because the structures to be examined are so small, adequate radiological examination requires the use of fine grain film-screen combinations and the finest possible anode focal spot consistent with the necessary radiographic output. For maximum detail, the incident beam should be coned to a circle of 5 to 8 cm. This achieves a marked improvement in image quality due to a reduction in scattered radiation, making a grid unnecessary and achieving a reduction in radiation dose.

For tomographic examination of the ear, it is better to use apparatus capable of a complex (pluridirectional) tomographic movement (polytomography). The complex motion does not reduce the effective thickness of the tomographic section, but the structures which are out of the plane of interest are more completely blurred, and fewer artefacts result. The resulting sections are therefore much more easy to interpret.

Many standard projections of the ear display the area of interest, either partly or completely within the outline of the orbit. In all such cases a great reduction in the radiation exposure to the lens and cornea can be achieved by using the appropriate alternative posteroanterior projection i.e. with the eye closer to the film. This is of particular importance when multiple exposures are to be obtained for a tomographic examination. The corneal dose received during an anteroposterior tomographic examination of the petrous bone may exceed 10 cGy [20]. The use of the posteroanterior projection may achieve a 90% reduction in the corneal dose, and with careful control of the examination minimizing the total number of radiographic exposures, a corneal dose for the whole examination may be reduced to less than 0.1 cGy. The use of lead eye shields may enable some anteroposterior radiographs to be obtained with protection of the eye but many useful projections of the petrous bone are partially or completely perorbital. Lead eye shields for tomographic examinations may cause artefacts.

As in the case of the paranasal sinuses, CT is of increasing importance in the radiological examination of the ear. The improved resolution performance of recent scanners is essential for this purpose. The resolution obtained is capable of clear demonstration of the bony labyrinth and auditory ossicles [21] (Fig. 93.32). With further design improvements, high resolution CT could completely replace conventional polytomography for evaluating the petrous bone [22].

ANATOMY

The temporal bone consists of three main portions, the squamous, tympanic, and petromastoid with the styloid process arising from the underside of the latter. It contains, in close anatomical relationship, the complex transducers for hearing and balance.

The external ear

The external ear consists of the pinna and the external auditory meatus. The external meatus is cartilaginous in its lateral half, continuous with the cartilage of the pinna. The inner half is bony and lies within the petrous temporal bone. It is bounded medially by the tympanic membrane which is attached to an annular groove, the tympanic ring. The external meatus is related anteriorly to the temporomandibular joint and posteriorly to the mastoid and antrum. Below and behind the external meatus, lies the jugular bulb from which it is separated by bone which varies in thickness in different individuals. In infancy the external auditory meatus is relatively short.

Table 93.2 *Radiographic examination of the temporal bone*

Radiographic projection and technique	Anatomical features displayed	Applications
Lateral oblique: lateral projection 15° or 30° caudal angulation of incident ray.	Mastoid, external meatus middle ear and attic, lateral sinus plate.	Survey view for pneumatization, cholesteatoma
Supraorbital: posteroanterior with canthomeatal line perpendicular to film. 30° caudal angulation of incident ray. (Towne-Vincent)	Internal auditory meatus, cochlea, mastoid and antrum.	Survey view of mastoids, and of mastoid antrum for cholesteatoma; suspected acoustic neuroma.
Submentovertical (base, axial view) canthomeatal line parallel to the film, no angulation of incident ray.	External auditory meatus, middle ear, cochlea and internal auditory meatus, mastoid, pharyngotympanic tube.	Survey view of mastoid and middle ear. Assessment of anterior extent of cholesteatoma.
Perorbital (occipitofrontal) Canthomeatal line perpendicular to the film, no angulation of incident ray.	Internal auditory meatus, cochlea, vestibule and semicircular canals, tympanic cavity, external auditory meatus.	Survey view of inner ear. Suspected acoustic neuroma, trauma.
P.A. oblique (Stenver's) Canthomeatal line perpendicular to the film, head rotated 45°, 5° cranial angulation of incident ray.	Mastoid tip, petrous bone, including internal auditory meatus, vestibule and semicircular canals.	Survey view of inner ear. Suspected acoustic neuroma. Assessment of mastoid tip air cells.
Transorbital (Guillen) Canthomeatal line perpendicular to film, head rotated 10° towards the side to be examined, no angulation of incident ray.	Similar to those seen on straight perorbital view. Medial wall of middle ear cavity is tangential and ossicles are shown.	Demonstration of middle ear cavity and ossicles.
Subaxial (70° occipitomental) Canthomeatal line 35° extension; 35° caudal angulation of incident ray.	Posterior surface of temporal bone, jugular foramen.	Suspected glomus jugulare tumour
Tomography: coronal (posteroanterior) in cochlear plane	External auditory meatus middle ear and ossicles, epitympanic recess, cochlea, oval window, genu of facial canal	Investigation of congenital anomalies; suspected attic cholesteatoma; trauma; tumours.
Tomography: coronal (posteroanterior) in vestibular plane	Vestibule, lateral and superior semicircular canal, horizontal part of facial canal, internal auditory canal.	Investigation of suspected acoustic neuroma, attic cholesteatoma; suspected erosion of lateral semicircular canal; congenital anomalies; trauma; tumours.
Tomography: lateral in plane of middle ear	Ossicles and epitympanic recess, antrum and mastoid, vertical part of facial canal, lateral semicircular canal, styloid process.	Suspected dislocation of ossicles, attic cholesteatoma, trauma, tumours.
Tomography: lateral in plane of vestibule	Vestibule, promontory, common crus of posterior and superior semicircular canals, vestibular aqueduct.	Investigation of trauma, otosclerosis, Ménières disease.
Tomography: lateral in plane of internal auditory canal	Internal auditory canal	Suspected acoustic neuroma, trauma.
Computed tomography (CT)	Detailed sectional images of ear including anatomy of bony labyrinth and ossicles. Intracranial structures adjacent to the temporal bone.	Investigations of congenital anomalies, suspected destructive processes including cholesteatoma, benign and malignant neoplasms, suspected tumours in the cerebellopontine angle including acoustic neuroma, trauma.
Angiography	Dependent on selective study performed.	Investigation of chemodectomas, and other causes of pulsatile tinnitus.
Positive contrast cisternography (iophendylate or metrizamide)	Cerebellopontine angle	Suspected acoustic neuroma
Air cisternography (with CT)	Cerebellopontine angle	Suspected acoustic neuroma.

The middle ear

The tympanic membrane separates the external ear from the middle ear or tympanic cavity, which communicates anteroinferiorly with the nasopharynx by means of the pharyngotympanic tube (Eustachian tube) and posterosuperiorly by means of the aditus ad antrum with the mastoid air cell system.

The medial wall of the tympanic cavity has a projection in its upper part due to the lateral semicircular canal, which divides the cavity into a lower part or tympanic cavity proper and an upper part, the epitympanic recess (attic). Below the lateral semicircular canal, the basal turn of the cochlea produces a further anatomical feature, the promontory. Traversing the middle ear cavity are the three bony ossicles (malleus, incus and stapes). The ossicles may be visualized on lateral, perorbital and basal radiographic projections, but detail of the anatomical relationships can only be made out on tomographic sections in the coronal and sagittal planes. The incudomallear joint is seen in sagittal section, the two ossicles having the characteristic appearance of a 'molar tooth'. The relationship of the ossicles as they traverse the middle ear cavity is seen on coronal sections; the malleus and incus are clearly seen but the stapes is often difficult to visualize.

The mastoid air cells

Arising from the posterior aspect of the epitympanic recess is a short channel called the aditus ad antrum, leading to the mastoid antrum itself which is a cavity of variable size forming the first part of the mastoid air cell system. The normal antrum is the shape of an inverted truncated cone with a 'maximum' transverse diameter of 6 mm and a maximum height of 11 mm. However, much larger antra than this are occasionally seen, sometimes only on one side [23]. The anatomical features of the mastoid antrum are well seen in the lateral oblique, submentovertical and supraorbital projections. An apparently large antrum on the supraorbital (Towne) projection may be due to an anteriorly placed dominant lateral sinus.

The extent of the mastoid air cell system is variable, usually involving the mastoid process, the lateral part of the petrous, and a limited part of the squamous portion of the temporal bone. In some individuals, pneumatisation may be much more extensive with air cells occupying the whole of the petrous bone including the apex and sometimes extending into the parietal and occipital bones. There is also a great variation in the size of individual air cells, a normal mastoid containing both large and small cells.

At birth the petromastoid is composed of diploic bone. Pneumatization commences in early infancy and the mastoid antrum may be recognizable by the age of 4 months. Pneumatization proceeds to reach maturity at about the time of puberty. Variations in the degree of pneumatization occur both as features of normal development and as a result of infection in infancy and childhood. A common pattern of such arrested development is the diploic or infantile mastoid where only small cells are formed immediately above and posterior to the middle ear, the mastoid process containing only diploic bone. The sclerotic mastoid is frankly pathological in nature and will be referred to below.

The inner ear

The inner ear consists of a series of membranous sacs, lying within a protective bony capsule, the bony labyrinth. This is composed of dense cortical bone rendering it clearly visible on radiographs in many projections. It is particularly easy to see in childhood where the remainder of the petromastoid is diploic in nature, and stands out in sharp contrast to its surroundings in an extensively pneumatized adult mastoid. It consists of three components, the vestibule, cochlea and semicircular canals.

The vestibule is well seen on perorbital and Stenver's projections as a small oval cavity lying in close relationship to the lateral end of the internal auditory meatus below the semicircular canals and above the cochlea. The lateral semicircular canal, seen on perorbital projections extends horizontally from the vestibule to project into the upper part of the middle ear cavity at the junction of the cavity proper and the epitympanic recess. The superior semicircular canal, seen on Stenver's projection, extends upwards from the vestibule to produce a prominence on the anterosuperior surface of the petrous, the arcuate eminence. The posterior semicircular canal, seen on the supraorbital projection extends horizontally backwards from the vestibule, its lateral limb being closely related to the aditus ad antrum.

The cochlea is a snail-shaped structure with its apex anteriorly. It is seen in Stenver's, supraorbital, and perorbital projections and may also be recognized on the axial view.

Facial nerve canal

The facial nerve has a complex course as it passes through the temporal bone (Fig. 93.33). The first part of the facial

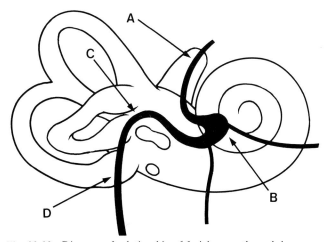

Fig. 93.33 Diagram of relationship of facial nerve through bony labyrinth showing its course in the internal auditory meatus [A], the genu [B] lying above the cochlea, below the lateral semicircular canal [C] and then turning down to descend [D] to emerge at the stylomastoid foramen.

nerve lies in the superior compartment of the internal auditory meatus. It then enters a bony canal which arises from the anterior wall of the superolateral part of the internal auditory meatus, to negotiate a sharp curve first forwards and then laterally and backwards above the cochlea to reach the medial wall of the middle ear cavity. This is the genu or second part of the facial nerve canal. The third part passes backwards and slightly downwards in the medial wall of the middle ear cavity below the lateral semicircular canal. On reaching the posterior limit of the medial wall of the middle ear cavity, the fourth part of the facial nerve canal passes downwards to emerge at the stylomastoid foramen.

Internal auditory meatus

This important channel in the petrous bone transmits the 7th cranial nerve (facial) and the two divisions of the 8th cranial nerve (acoustic and vestibular). It is well seen on perorbital, supraorbital and Stenver's projections and is also visible on the axial view. Tomography is generally carried out in the coronal plane supplemented by lateral tomograms in problem cases. On coronal tomograms it appears as a tubular structure showing a slight fusiform expansion in its lateral half. Height measurements are generally made at the point of maximum diameter, and length measurements from the posterior lip of the porus acousticus internus to the thin bony plate defining the medial margin of the vestibule (Fig. 93.34).

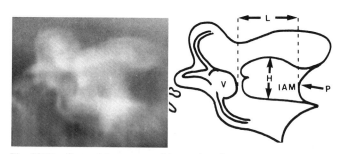

Fig. 93.34 Coronal tomogram of internal auditory meatus showing measurement end points. Note vestibule [v] and posterior lip of porus [p].

The average height is 4 mm (range 2 to 8 mm) and the average length is 8 mm (range 4 to 12 mm) [24]. In any one individual, the right and left meatus should not differ by more than 1 mm in height and 2 mm in length [25] (note that many types of pluridirectional tomographic apparatus produce magnification).

Anatomically the meatus is divided into two compartments, the upper containing the facial and superior vestibular nerves; and the lower the acoustic and inferior vestibular nerves. The septum dividing the meatus is attached to a bony ridge at its lateral end which is clearly seen on coronal tomograms, the crista falciformis.

Further methods of examining the internal auditory meatus include angle cisternography using iophendylate (Myodil), metrizamide or air. High definition CT is necessary for the metrizamide and air techniques.

TOMOGRAPHY OF THE EAR

Detailed radiological assessment of the middle ear and bony labyrinth requires the use of tomography. An understanding of the anatomy in two basic planes is crucial.

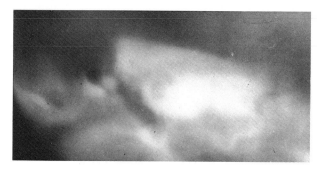

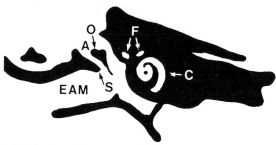

Fig. 93.35 Coronal tomogram right temporal bone in cochlear plane showing external auditory meatus [EAM], scutum [S], ossicles [O] lying in the attic [A]; facial canal [F], and cochlea [C].

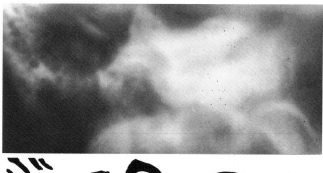

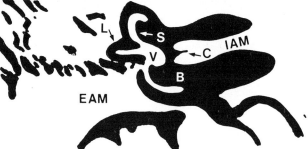

Fig. 93.36 Coronal tomogram of right temporal bone in vestibular plane showing external auditory meatus [EAM], lateral semicircular canal [L], part of superior semicircular canal [S], vestibule [V], basal turn of cochlea [B], crista falciformis [C] and internal auditory meatus [IAM].

Coronal tomography is very important. The so called cochlear plane refers to a coronal section through the middle of the cochlea (Fig. 93.35). The section passes through the anterior part of the external auditory meatus, the medial end of the roof of which is sharply triangular in shape (the scutum or spur), separating the meatus at this point from the epitympanic recess. Immediately posterior to this is the aditus ad antrum. Medial to the scutum lies the incudomallear joint and the handle of the malleus can be seen passing downwards and medially indicating the position of the tympanic membrane. Inferomedially the middle ear cavity shows a triangular recess where it joins the pharyngotympanic tube.

The vestibular coronal plane lies approximately 4 mm posterior to the cochlear plane (Fig. 93.36). The section is in the plane of the posterior part of the external auditory canal and shows the posterior part of the scutum. The vestibule and lateral semicircular canal are seen, and section passes through the internal auditory meatus.

With these two planes as anatomical reference points, further tomographic sections may be obtained to demonstrate points of particular interest such as the posterior lip of the porus acusticus internus and the facial nerve canal (see below).

The applications of lateral tomography are fewer but reference to two anatomical planes may be found useful. A sagittal section in the plane of the epitympanic recess shows the incudomallear joint with the parallel relationship of the

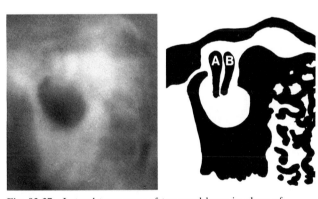

Fig. 93.37 Lateral tomogram of temporal bone in plane of incudomallear joint showing malleus [A] incus [B]. Note so called molar tooth appearance.

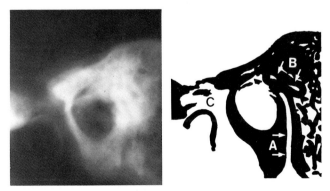

Fig. 93.38 Lateral tomogram of temporal bone in plane of facial nerve canal [A], also showing lateral semicircular canal [B] and temporomandibular joint [C].

handle of the malleus anteriorly and the long process of the incus posteriorly (the so called molar tooth) (Fig. 93.37). At a point 3 mm medial to this, a sagittal section passes through the lateral semicircular canal. Beneath this, the facial nerve canal is seen passing backwards and turning downwards to emerge at the stylomastoid foramen between the styloid and mastoid processes (Fig. 93.38).

INFECTIVE AND INFLAMMATORY DISEASE

Acute otitis media and mastoiditis

In most cases, acute infection of the middle ear and mastoid occurs as a complication of upper respiratory tract infection via the Eustachian tube. In childhood this may occur as a complication of one of the acute infectious fevers. Rarer causes of acute mastoiditis include haematogenous infection and direct injury.

Pathologically there are two types of acute otitis media and mastoiditis. The secretory type is of lesser severity and leads to few complications: it may be of allergic rather than infective origin. Acute suppurative otitis media is more severe, and is more frequently accompanied by acute mastoiditis. Complications are more common, and spread of sepsis outside the middle ear and mastoid may occur.

Radiological examination is not often undertaken in uncomplicated otitis media, but there are recognizable features. A loss of radiolucency of the Eustachian tube and the middle ear cavity occurs, seen on the submentovertical projection. There is also opacity of the mastoid antrum with blurring of its outline. Extension of infection to the mastoid causes loss of translucency of the mastoid air cells, beginning in the periantral region and spreading peripherally. These abnormalities are most easily detected in the lateral oblique projection (Fig. 93.39) but comparison of the two sides on the

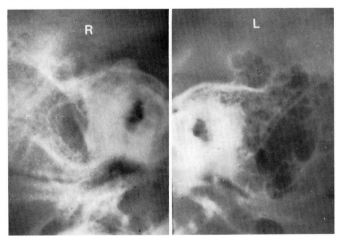

Fig. 93.39 Acute right mastoiditis. Lateral oblique radiograph showing opaque mastoid air cells. Normal left mastoid for comparison.

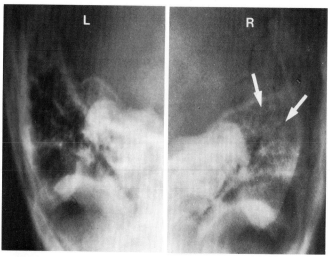

Fig. 93.40 Acute right mastoiditis. Supra-orbital projection showing opaque right mastoid air cells [arrows] compared with normal cells on left side.

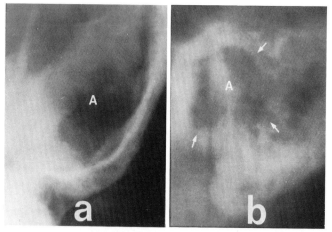

Fig. 93.41 Acute mastoiditis with abscess. [a] Stenver's projection showing loss of outline of mastoid air cells [A]. (b) Tomogram showing abscess cavity [A] with fairly well defined margin [arrows] showing no sclerosis.

supra-orbital view is also useful (Fig. 93.40). The changes of acute mastoiditis are much easier to see in a cellular mastoid than in the infantile diploic type, where tomography may be needed for its recognition. Persistent acute infection causes progressive decalcification of the mastoid cell walls due to hyperaemia. This process may continue to complete break-down of the cell walls with the development of a mastoid abscess, detection of which may be difficult because of the preceding decalcification. Abscess formation tends to commence in the air cells immediately posterior to the mastoid antrum best localized by tomography (Fig. 93.41). Its position may be of considerable clinical importance since a close relationship to the sinus plate may predispose to lateral sinus thrombosis, and close proximity to the tegmen tympani may lead to an extradural abscess. Temporal lobe abscess may also occur. In patients with pneumatization of the whole of the petrous bone including the apex, spread of infection medially may cause an apical petrositis with lateral rectus palsy (Gradenigo's syndrome).

Acute mastoid infection may also spread forwards into the external auditory meatus and downwards into the soft tissues of the neck (Bezold's abscess).

Antibiotic therapy has made all these complications rare except in neglected cases. Antibiotics may however simply mask the symptoms, and radiological examination may demonstrate a progressive destructive inflammatory process — the 'antibiotic mastoid'.

Chronic suppurative otitis media and mastoiditis

As with chronic infection in the paranasal sinuses, this may follow an acute attack of otitis media and mastoiditis, or may occur without any such history. Some cases may be due to inadequate treatment, but may occur despite apparently adequate antibiotic therapy.

A continuing low grade infective process leads to the progressive obliteration of the mastoid air cell system with reactive sclerosis (Fig. 93.42). The time taken for this to develop varies, but may occur in less than a year. Chronic mastoiditis may be complicated by abscess formation and sequestra. These features may be difficult to recognize because of the associated mastoid sclerosis, and tomography may be useful. Radiological distinction from a cholesteatoma (see below) may be difficult but the margin of an abscess is less well defined. An abscess complicating chronic mastoiditis may lead to extradural and intracerebral sepsis.

The most common serious complication of chronic infection of the middle ear and mastoid is the development of a cholesteatoma.

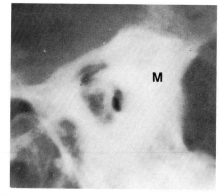

Fig. 93.42 Chronic mastoiditis. Dense sclerosis of mastoid air cells [M].

Cholesteatoma

Radiological examination of the mastoid for postinfective complications should not be attempted unless accurate information is available as to the previous surgical history of the patient. The changes following mastoidectomy, including enlargement of the aditus, and partial or complete removal of the mastoid air cell system, may on occasion mimic the destructive changes of a cholesteatoma. A fully healed mastoidectomy cavity will usually show a more clearly defined sclerotic margin.

Radiological examination of the postoperative mastoid may be carried out in the investigation of residual infection, cholesteatoma formation, sequestrum formation, and fistula of the lateral semicircular canal (see below).

Acquired cholesteatoma

Most cholesteatomas arise in the attic (epitympanic recess). They may extend down into the middle ear cavity causing displacement or destruction of the ossicles, and sometimes causing erosion of the lateral semicircular canal with the production of a labyrinthine fistula. The less common antral cholesteatoma may develop in this site or may occur due to posterior extension of an attic cholesteatoma.

Radiologically a cholesteatoma shows a well defined area of bone destruction with a thin or absent marginal line of sclerosis. The presence of a cholesteatoma is easier to recognize in a sclerotic mastoid (Fig. 93.43). The occurrence of a cholesteatoma in a cellular mastoid is unusual, but it can occur, and may be overlooked[27] (Fig. 93.44).

On a lateral oblique radiograph, an attic cholesteatoma shows enlargement of the attic. Large lesions show an

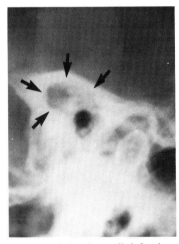

Fig. 93.43 Sclerotic mastoid showing well defined cavity due to cholesteatoma [arrows].

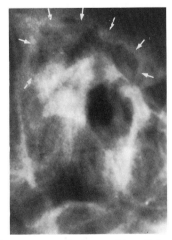

Fig. 93.44 Cholesteatoma cavity [arrows] in cellular mastoid.

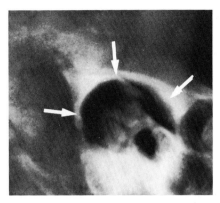

Fig. 93.45 Large atticoantral cholesteatoma [arrows]. Bony labyrinth visible with unusual clarity through thinned lateral wall.

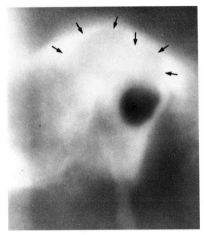

Fig. 93.46 Atticoantral cholesteatoma. Lateral tomogram showing well defined cavity expanding the attic and antrum [arrows]. The margin shows no sclerosis. Note absence of ossicles.

unusual clarity of the bony labyrinth visible through the thinned walls of the attic (Fig. 93.45). Lateral tomograms are sometimes helpful (Fig. 93.46).

Large cholesteatomas are well seen on lateral oblique, perorbital, supraorbital, Guillen and Stenver's projections. However, the multiplicity of radiographic projections used in the past for the demonstration and delineation of cholesteatoma have largely been superceded by polytomography.

The features of a cholesteatoma include:-
1. the enlargement of the attic together with erosion of the scutum, and upward extension towards the tegmen tympani (Fig. 93.47).
2. displacement or destruction of the ossicular chain;
3. erosion of the facial nerve canal;
4. erosion of the lateral semicircular canal with production of a labyrinthine fistula (Fig. 93.48).

This diagnosis should be made with caution, and only when the canal appears eroded on two adjacent tomographic sections 1 mm apart. False positive diagnoses are common[28], and are probably due to the plane of the section lying behind or in front of the apex of the canal.

Despite the diagnostic accuracy of polytomography in the diagnosis of cholesteatoma[29], there is still a conflict of

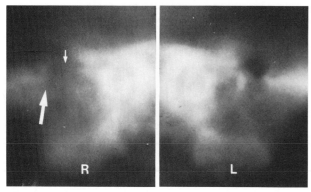

Fig. 93.47 Right attic cholesteatoma. Coronal tomograms showing erosion of scutum [large arrow] and opaque attic with absent ossicles [small arrow]. Normal left side for comparison.

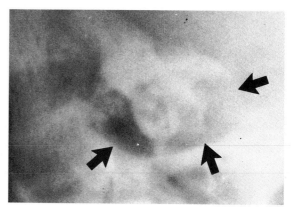

Fig. 93.49 Congenital cholesteatoma of petrous apex. Extensive destruction of petrous apex [arrows] partly sparing the bony labyrinth.

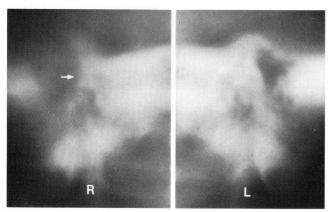

Fig. 93.48 Right attic cholesteatoma with erosion of the lateral semicircular canal [arrow]. Normal left side for comparison.

opinion concerning the role of radiology. Some feel that radiology is superfluous; others feel that it is indispensible. Certainly, most cholesteatomas may be diagnosed by direct examination. For these patients a lateral oblique radiograph is adequate, demonstrating not only the cholesteatoma but the extent of pneumatization of the mastoid, and the relationship of the lateral sinus and middle fossa dura. The most valuable contribution of diagnostic radiology is in those cases where the diagnosis is in doubt, particularly where the tympanic membrane is obscured by a large aural polyp, or when complications are suspected.

The introduction of high resolution computed tomography for the investigation of the petrous bone has reopened the question of what can be contributed by radiological methods in the management of cholesteatoma [26]. In addition to demonstrating the characteristic bone erosion, CT is of particular value in showing ossicular displacement and destruction, and in the demonstration of the soft tissue mass of the cholesteatoma. The attenuation values of such masses tend to be significantly lower than those associated with other inflammatory or neoplastic masses in the middle ear [26].

Congenital cholesteatoma (epidermoid)

Congenital cholesteatomas may be found in all the bones of

the skull and even within the cranial cavity. In the context of the ear they occur in the cerebellopontine angle, in the petrous apex, in the jugular fossa and in the middle ear cleft. In the cerebellopontine angle they may resemble other tumours found in this site, but may show a fluffy outline with air and a scalloped appearance with Myodil. CT may show a nonenhancing mass of low attenuation [26]. Cholesteatoma of the petrous apex often produces a large area of bone erosion (Fig. 93.49).

Cholesteatoma arising in the jugular fossa may resemble a glomus tumour, but the marked vascularity of the latter on angiographic studies is diagnostic. Congenital cholesteatomas of the middle ear and mastoid are difficult to distinguish from acquired cholesteatomas in the same site, particularly as the significance of an apparently minor previous episode of otitis media may be uncertain. The congenital variety is probably rare [26].

Otosclerosis

This is a disease of unknown origin characterized by the production of foci of new bone formation, most commonly in the region of the vestibular and cochlear windows (the so called fenestral type) or more rarely in the cochlea itself (the cochlear type). The disease is twice as common in females as in males and in many cases appears to be genetically determined. In 80% of cases there is bilateral involvement. It is characterized by progressive hearing loss of early onset, eventually causing severe but rarely total deafness.

Pathologically there is an initial hypervascular phase in which decalcification occurs, subsequently followed by sclerosis and thickening of the affected bone. The region of the vestibular window is most frequently affected, and may cause obliteration of the window with associated fixation of the footplate of the stapes. The cochlear window is also affected and foci deep to these windows may infiltrate the labyrinthine capsule, encroaching on the lumina of the cochlear coils, the semicircular canals and the internal auditory meatus [30].

Plain radiography is of little value in the diagnosis of otosclerosis. Polytomography in the coronal plane may be diagnostic but more specialized projections have been advocated [30].

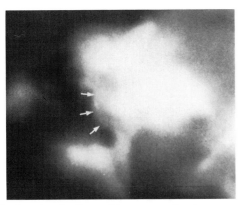

Fig. 93.50 Otosclerosis. Coronal tomograms showing severe decalcification of the promontory [arrows] in initial hypervascular phase of otosclerosis.

In the initial hypervascular phase of otosclerosis, decalcification may render the anatomy of the bony labyrinth almost unrecognizable (Fig. 93.50.) Subsequent sclerosis and thickening of the bony capsule leads to narrowing or obliteration of the windows, thickening of the promontory and of the bony walls of the vestibule. Localized foci may be seen bulging from the medial wall of the tympanic cavity.

The diagnosis of fenestral otosclerosis is usually clinical, but a definite diagnosis of the cochlear type can only be made by radiological methods, and surgical confirmation is not possible.

The radiological features of otosclerosis may resemble those seen in so called tympanosclerosis where there is reduction in size of the tympanic cavity and calcific thickening involving the ossicles secondary to long standing chronic otitis media.

Menière's disease

This disease is characterized by episodic vertigo, progressive deafness and tinnitus. The exact pathophysiology is not known but is probably associated with an imbalance of production and absorption of endolymph. Since the endolymph passes from the labyrinth via the vestibular aqueduct, radiological investigations have been directed towards the

demonstration of this structure. Detailed tomographic studies of the petrous temporal bone have shown abnormal narrowing or obliteration of the vestibular aqueduct in more than 40% of cases [31]. Whether the disease is caused by this narrowing, or whether a pre-existing narrowing predisposes to Menière's disease remains uncertain.

Radiologically the vestibular aqueduct is shown in sagittal sections in the plane of the common crus of the superior and posterior semicircular canals (Fig. 93.57). From a clinical point of view, the importance of demonstrating this finding is uncertain, but radiological investigations are indicated to exclude other causes of the presenting clinical syndrome, the most important of which is acoustic neuroma [32].

TUMOURS OF THE EAR

The external ear

Benign exostoses involving the external meatus are common, particularly in cold water swimmers. They are demonstrated in the lateral oblique projection or by sagittal tomography, and may be seen to reduce the lumen of the external meatus to a narrow slit. They may cause obstruction with secondary infection presenting as an acute mastoiditis.

Malignant tumours include basal and squamous cell *carcinoma* and are characterized radiologically by progressive bone destruction, often very extensive and showing little or no reactive sclerosis. More rarely a *melanoma* may produce a similar appearance.

A nonmalignant hyperplasia of the epithelium with retention of the desquamated debris (*keratosis obturans*) may also present clinically with obliteration of the lumen of the external meatus and may show radiological enlargement of the bony meatus [33].

The middle ear

Chemodectoma

These benign tumours arise from chemoreceptor tissue in the jugular fossa and in the middle ear. They are identical in histological appearance with carotid body tumours. Clinically they are of two types: glomus tympanicum tumours involving the middle ear and the mastoid without evidence of jugular bulb involvement, and the more common glomus jugulare tumour involving the jugular bulb and vein and sometimes extending intracranially and into the middle ear and mastoid area [34].

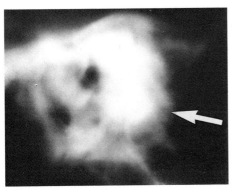

Fig. 93.51 Vestibular aqueduct [arrow]. Lateral tomograms showing normal appearances. This anatomical feature may be absent in patients with Menière's disease.

Glomus jugulare tumours

These tumours are more common in women. They present with tinnitus, often pulsatile in type, with variable involvement of the 9th, 10th and 11th cranial nerves and sometimes with deafness. Clinically, there may be a haemorrhagic aural polyp, or a red bulging tympanic membrane. There may be a resemblance to the appearance seen in dehiscence of the jugular bulb, where the jugular vein bulges into the floor of the middle ear.

Glomus tumours are not malignant, but are locally invasive. They are relatively radio-resistant, and surgical management is complicated by the very vascular nature of the tumour.

Radiological investigation is directed towards demonstrating the tumour vascularity and the associated bone destruction. An enlarged jugular fossa may be shown on the subaxial (70° occipitomental) projection supplemented if necessary by tomography (Fig. 93.52). A large jugular fossa is not however itself evidence of a glomus tumour, since marked asymmetry may occur, the right fossa usually being larger than the left. The normal jugular fossa however retains its cortical outline. Bone destruction begins in the region of the jugular fossa, but may involve the middle ear and external auditory canal, the petrous apex, the floor of the posterior cranial fossa including the hypoglossal foramen, and the foramen magnum.

CT will also identify bone destruction, and contrast enhancement will show any associated intracranial extension of the lesion. Carotid arteriography with subselective catheterization of the ascending pharyngeal and occipital branches of the external carotid may demonstrate an extensive tumour circulation (Fig. 93.53), the detail of which is much improved by subtraction films [35]. Angiography is carried out, not only for diagnostic purposes, but in order to perform therapeutic embolization of the tumour. This is of value both as a method of treatment in the inoperable case, and for preoperative reduction of the blood supply prior to surgical resection [36].

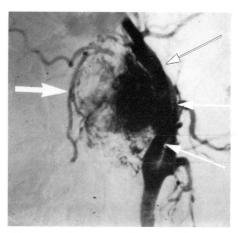

Fig. 93.53 Glomus jugulare tumour. Subtracted lateral carotid angiogram showing extensive tumour circulation [large arrow], displacing the internal carotid artery forwards [arrows]. (Same patient as Fig. 93.52).

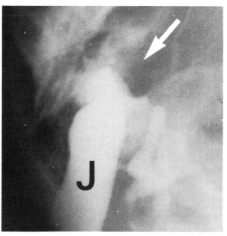

Fig. 93.54 Glomus jugulare tumour. Jugular venogram showing jugular vein [J]. Filling defect in jugular fossa [arrow]. No filling of the lateral sinus. (Same patient as Figs. 93.52 & 53).

Angiography is also of value in the exclusion of other causes of pulsatile tinnitus, including congenital and acquired arteriovenous fistulae, persistent primitive arteries, other vascular tumours, and carotid stenosis [37].

Percutaneous retrograde jugular venography [38] is now performed less often in view of the availability of CT, and the proven value of selective arteriography. In glomus tumours a filling defect may be seen in the jugular bulb, often producing complete obstruction, with nonfilling of the lateral sinus (Fig. 93.54). The tumour may extend down into the upper part of the internal jugular vein.

Malignant tumours of the middle ear

Apart from rare cases of *sarcoma*, most malignant tumours of the middle ear are due to *squamous carcinoma* or less commonly *adenocarcinoma*. A high proportion of cases are associated with chronic suppurative otitis media. Radio-

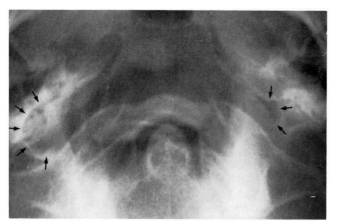

Fig. 93.52 Glomus jugulare tumour. Note the much enlarged right jugular fossa [arrows], compared with the opposite normal side [arrows].

logical investigation is indicated to determine the extent of bony infiltration and destruction, and in order to aid the planning of radiotherapy [39]. There is often extensive bone destruction which may involve both the squamous and the petromastoid. The bony labyrinth is relatively resistant to destruction and may be spared in an otherwise extensively destroyed petrous bone. The bone destruction may be shown on plain films, but is more precisely demonstrated by conventional tomography and CT. Invariably there is associated infection with loss of radiolucency of the mastoid air cells.

Tumours of the petrous bone

Apart from erosion due to extrinsic tumours such as *acoustic neuroma*, primary *benign* and *malignant tumours* of the petrous bone are rare. Primary *cholesteatoma* is described above. Deposits may occur in *histiocytosis* X, and *plasmacytoma* may occur either as a localized lesion, or as part of a general myelomatosis. Secondary *metastatic deposits* may occur, and direct invasion may take place from tumours of the nasopharynx. Localized bone overgrowth may occur in the temporal bone as a result of an *osteoma* and reactive hyperostosis due to a *meningioma* may be seen. *Fibrous dysplasia* may produce bony thickening and sclerosis in the temporal bone. *Paget's* disease may occur and may be of the sclerosing type or the osteoporotic type (osteoporosis circumscripta).

The most important tumours affecting the petrous bone are those which arise in the cerebellopontine angle, including 8th nerve tumours and meningioma [40].

8th nerve tumours

Tumours arising from the 8th cranial nerve are relatively common, accounting for about 8% of all intracranial tumours, and 90% of tumours arising in the cerebellopontine angle. They occur mainly in patients aged 30 to 50 years, and present with tinnitus and progressive deafness, with associated vestibular disturbances and an absent corneal reflex due to 5th nerve involvement. Facial weakness due to compression of the 7th cranial nerve is also sometimes found. Histologically there are two types, the more common Schwannoma derived from the nerve sheath, and the rarer neurofibroma, which may be associated with generalized neurofibromatosis. 8th nerve tumours usually lie with the main tumour mass intracranially, but part of the lesion is often within the internal auditory meatus, and rarely the whole tumour may be intrameatal.

Routine radiographic examination of the internal auditory meatus should be carried out in the perorbital projection. In doubtful cases, the supraorbital and Stenver's projections may be useful, but tomography is essential for the detection of early bone erosion. Very thin tomographic sections are undesirable, as the vestibule and porus acousticus internus should be seen on the same section for measurement of meatal length.

The radiological features [41] consist of:
1. Widening of the internal auditory meatus (more than 2 mm greater than the opposite side is very suggestive of an acoustic neuroma)
2. Shortening of the internal auditory meatus (more than 3 mm is significant)
3. Alteration in the shape of the meatus with the development of a trumpet shaped flaring medially (Fig. 93.55)
4. Erosion of the crista falciformis
5. Erosion of the tip of the petrous bone

In addition to the diagnostic features in the internal auditory meatus, evidence of raised intracranial pressure may be seen i.e. decalcification of the floor and dorsum of the sella turcica.

CT scanning with contrast enhancement is undoubtedly the investigation of choice for the diagnosis of extrameatal lesions. Tumours of the 8th cranial nerve are generally either isodense or minimally hyperdense, but usually show moderate or marked contrast enhancement (Fig. 93.56) Displacement of the 4th ventricle may be shown and there may be secondary hydrocephalus.

If a bone window setting is used, erosion of the meatus may be detected. There are many references to the use of CT in the identification of 8th nerve tumours [42,43], but the diagnosis of the small acoustic neuroma, i.e. less than 1.5 cm, may require the use of ancillary techniques [44].

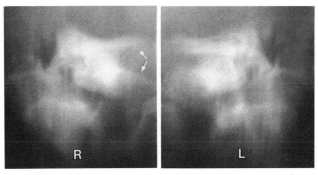

Fig. 93.55 Right acoustic neuroma. Coronal tomograms showing expansion of right internal auditory meatus [arrows]. Normal left side for comparison.

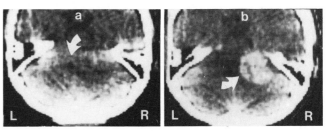

Fig. 93.56 Right acoustic neuroma. (A) CT scan before enhancement shows displaced fourth ventricle [arrow] but no density changes. (B) After enhancement a well defined mass is seen in the cerebellopontine angle [arrow].

Radionuclide examinations are now rarely used, except in centres without facilities for CT scanning. Brain scanning using ⁹⁹ᵐTc pertechnetate will show an area of high uptake in the cerebellopontine angle in cases of 8th nerve tumours. The smallest lesions diagnosable by this technique are larger than those shown by CT using modern apparatus [45].

The diagnosis of the small acoustic neuroma

Small intrameatal 8th nerve tumours present early clinically and may show radiological abnormalities of the internal auditory meatus at an early stage. Small lesions in the region of the porus are less easy to detect and contrast methods may be of value. The older techniques of air encephalography and cerebellopontine angle cisternography using iophendylate (Myodil) are now obsolescent, though they remain of some value in centres having no access to high definition CT.

Iophendylate cisternography [46] is performed by the injection of 1 to 2 ml of the contrast medium into the lumbar sac. The patient, lying in the lateral decubitus position with the side to be examined downwards and the head turned 15° towards the table top, is tilted 45° head down and maintained in this position for about 2 minutes. In this position the contrast medium surrounds the porus acousticus internus, and will normally enter the internal auditory meatus. After bringing the patient back to the horizontal position, radiographs are taken in the perorbital and axial projections. An acoustic neuroma in the porus will prevent filling of the internal auditory meatus, and shows as a filling defect within the contrast medium (Fig. 93.57).

Failure to fill the meatus may be due to an intrameatal neuroma, but is not necessarily abnormal, since filling is sometimes prevented by anatomical factors such as arachnoid redundancy and adhesions, a narrow meatus and a prominent loop of the anterior inferior cerebellar artery. Nonfilling is therefore an equivocal finding, but a normal examination satisfactorily excludes a neuroma, and by using a low volume of contrast medium, very small tumours may be detected.

Water-soluble contrast media may be used instead of iophendylate, either in a relatively high dose with conventional radiography and tomography, or in a much lower dose using CT. This technique is however much less reliable than CT air cisternography because of the difficulties in resolving small changes in attenuation values in close vicinity to the dense bone of the petrous apex. Beam hardening effects and partial volume artefacts contribute to these problems.

The same problems do not apply to the relatively large differences in attenuation values resulting from the use of air as a contrast medium, and in centres where high definition CT is available, CT air cisternography and meatography have superceded the older methods. [47,48] Resolution of detail on the best scanners is such that the 7th and 8th cranial nerves can be individually demonstrated, not only in the cerebellopontine angle, but within the internal auditory meatus. The anterior inferior cerebellar artery is also sometimes shown. The volume of air required is only 5 ml introduced by lumbar puncture, and the resulting morbidity is therefore very small. This factor, together with the simplicity and accuracy of the method, makes it the technique of choice at the present time for the detection of a small acoustic neuroma. [49]

Axial CT scans are obtained, and an acoustic neuroma shows as a mass of soft tissue density bulging into, and outlined by air within the cerebellopontine angle (Fig. 93.58).

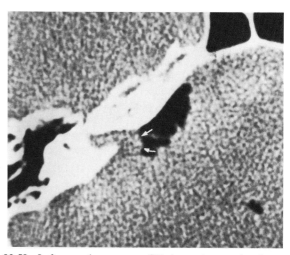

Fig. 93.58 Left acoustic neuroma. CT air meatogram showing a small tumour outlined by air [arrows]. (Reproduction by kind permission of Dr I. Glaves, Scarborough Hospital, England).

Meningioma

A meningioma occurring in the cerebellopontine angle may present radiological features similar to those seen in acoustic neuroma, with erosion of the petrous bone including the porus, and with similar CT appearances. The internal auditory meatus is not usually affected however.

TRAUMA TO THE EAR

Foreign bodies

The commonest cause of a foreign body in the ear is an

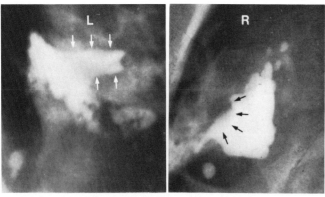

Fig. 93.57 Small right acoustic neuroma. Angle cisternogram using iophendylate showing nonfilling of right internal auditory meatus and the outline of a 6 mm tumour [arrows]. Normal left side for comparison showing good filling of internal auditory meatus [arrows].

industrial accident involving the entry of a small fragment of hot molten metal (slag) into the middle ear. Secondary infection is common. Radiological examination is necessary for the determination of the presence of a foreign body and for its localization.

Fractures of the temporal bone

Fractures of the temporal bone are less common than those which involve the vault of the skull. Clinically they may present with an aural discharge of blood or cerebrospinal fluid, deafness, or facial paralysis.

Fractures may be extralabyrinthine or labyrinthine in type. Extralabyrinthine fractures are commonly due to an extension of a vault fracture involving the squamous temporal bone into the tegmen tympani, sometimes involving the epitympanic recess and external meatus but sparing the bony labyrinth. Such fractures may cause leakage of cerebrospinal fluid.

Fractures involving the labyrinth are of two types:
1. Longitudinal fractures running parallel to the long axis of the petrous bone. In addition to the involvement of the labyrinth they also cross the medial wall of the tympanic cavity where injury to the facial nerve may occur. Medially the fracture may extend into the middle or into the posterior cranial fossa.
2. Transverse fractures of the petrous bone commonly extend forward from the region of the jugular fossa to cross either the internal auditory meatus or the bony labyrinth. A complete sensorineural deafness is a feature of such fractures.

Radiological examination should consist of a full examination of the skull in posteroanterior, lateral, half-axial and submentovertical projections, the lateral being carried out with a horizontal X–ray beam to detect fluid levels in the sphenoid sinus, and the presence of subarachnoid air in the cranial cavity. Tomography of the clinically affected petrous bone should then be carried out in the lateral and coronal planes [50]. Fracture lines are visible not only at the time of the injury but may remain visible for many years.

Indications for detailed radiological investigation include the evaluation of patients suffering from post-traumatic deafness and facial paralysis, and the presence of cerebrospinal fluid leakage through the ear or nose (leaking cerebrospinal fluid discharging through the pharyngotympanic (Eustachian) tube may cause the patient to complain of rhinorrhoea).

Post-traumatic deafness

Transverse fractures of the petrous bone extending through the internal auditory meatus or bony labyrinth cause complete and permanent sensorineural deafness. Such fractures are best shown on coronal tomography (Fig. 93.59).

Conductive deafness presenting after head injury may be due to injury to the ossicular chain. This is more commonly found in association with longitudinal fractures but dislocations and displacement of the ossicles may also occur in the absence of any fracture. The commonest types involve dislocation of the incudomallear and incudostapedial joints. The

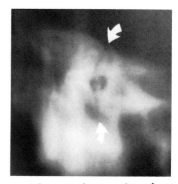

Fig. 93.59 Transverse fracture of petrous bone [arrows]. Coronal tomogram showing vertical transverse fracture passing downwards through petrous bone at lateral end of internal auditory meatus. Complete sensorineural deafness.

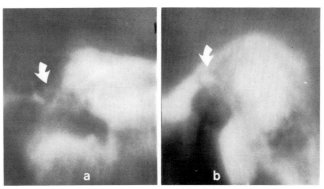

Fig. 93.60 Incudomallear dislocation. (a) Coronal tomogram in cochlear plane showing absence of normal ossicular shadow. (b) Lateral tomogram in plane of incudomallear joint showing only the mallear component.

incus itself is particularly vulnerable to displacement because of its relative lack of anatomical support. Dislocations of the incudostapedial joint are difficult to recognize. Dislocations of the incudomallear joint are best seen on lateral tomograms: the normal 'molar tooth' appearance of the joint lying within the epitympanic recess is lost (Fig. 93.60) [51].

Displacement of the incus may be shown on coronal tomograms. High definition CT is a recent and valuable method for the demonstration of the anatomy of the ossicles [22], and is likely to be of great value in the assessment of trauma to the ear, including ossicular dislocation [49].

The diagnosis of ossicular dislocation is of particular importance in the management of post-traumatic deafness since it represents one of the few remediable causes of this condition.

Facial paralysis

The facial nerve may be injured by transverse fractures crossing the internal auditory meatus, by labyrinthine fractures involving the facial nerve in the region of the genu, and longitudinal fractures of the petrous bone involving the medial wall of the middle ear and injuring the horizontal portion of the facial nerve as it passes backwards beneath the lateral semicircular canal. A slightly more posterior fracture may involve the descending portion of the facial nerve as it

passes down to emerge at the stylomastoid foramen. Identification of a fracture in this site is of particular clinical
importance, since lesions of this part of the facial nerve may
be repaired surgically. The facial nerve may also be injured
during mastoid surgery.

Leakage of cerebrospinal fluid

CSF otorrhoea and rhinorrhoea may occur following a head
injury causing a fracture of the petrous bone. Leakage
through the ear will occur where there is a dural tear associated with a fracture extending into the external auditory
meatus. Such fractures most commonly involve the anterior
part of the tegmen tympani and extend into the floor of the
middle cranial fossa. Fractures involving the epitympanic
recess, but with an intact tympanic membrane and external
meatus cause the leaking cerebrospinal fluid to pass down the
pharyngotympanic tube and enter the nasal cavity.
Depending on the position of the patient, rhinorrhoea may
occur. Such cases sometimes present after an interval of
months or even years after the injury. Tomography is
necessary for the demonstration of the site of injury (Fig.
93.61). Surgical repair of the dural defect is required, since
spontaneous closure does not usually take place.

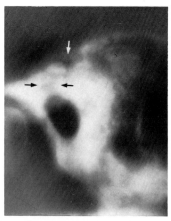

Fig. 93.61 Persistent thecotympanic fistula. Lateral tomograms
showing fistulous tract [black arrows]. Note small aerocele [white
arrow]. Patient had recurrent meningitis and CSF rhinorrhoea 3 years
after a head injury.

CONGENITAL ABNORMALITIES
OF THE EAR

Congenital abnormalities of the ear occur infrequently. The
commonest types are those in which there is hypoplasia or
atresia of the external auditory meatus, often associated with
malformations of the middle ear. Deformities of the pinna
are sometimes, but not invariably associated. Apart from the
thalidomide syndrome, there is no particular association
between congenital anomalies of the external and middle
ear, and those anomalies involving the inner ear, which has
a different embryological origin.

External and middle ear anomalies

Anomalies of the external and middle ear range from minor
distortions of the ossicles, to major involvement with hypo-
plasia of the external meatus and middle ear cavity. Frey's
classification [52] is useful:
Group 1 Solitary malformations of the ossicles.
Group 2 Hypoplasia of the external meatus with a bony
        atresia plate often associated with malformed ossi-
        cles but with a middle ear cavity of normal size.
Group 3 A more severe hypoplasia or atresia of the external
        meatus with a larger atresia plate with malformed
        ossicles and a hypoplastic middle ear cavity.
Group 4 Complete atresia of the external meatus with a
        large atresia plate often associated with absence of
        the middle ear cavity and ossicles.
Group 5 Atypical malformations.
    Polytomography is necessary for the radiological demon-
stration of congenital anomalies of the external and middle
ear. High definition CT may also be of value.
    The normal external auditory meatus is aligned with its
longitudinal axis approximately in the horizontal plane. The
hypoplastic meatus is aligned with a downward slope as it
passes laterally and tends to be short and conical in form.
The atresia plate which forms the medial end is composed

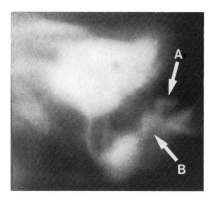

Fig. 93.62 Atresia of external auditory meatus. Coronal tomograms.
The external meatus is short and conical. Bony atresia plate is shown
[B]. Ossicles [A] are fused to atresia plate. Tympanic cavity and inner
ear are normal in appearance.

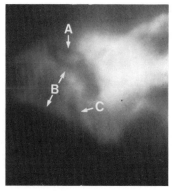

Fig. 93.63 Atresia of external auditory meatus. Ossicles [A] lie in
rather hypoplastic attic. Atresia plate [B] is very thick. Facial nerve
canal [C] is anteriorly placed in cochlear plane.

of bone which is usually 1 to 4 mm in thickness. The ossicles are fused to the inner aspect of the atresia plate, and are often deformed, the malleus and incus being fused into a bony mass (Fig. 93.62). More severe degrees of atresia may show an absent external meatus, with a very thick atresia plate, pneumatized by extension of the mastoid air cells forward. In such cases the temporomandibular joint is placed more posteriorly than usual.

The radiological examination should aim to determine the thickness of the atresia plate, the size and shape of the tympanic cavity, the state of the ossicular chain, the degree of pneumatization of the mastoid antrum and air cells, the route of the facial nerve canal (which may lie more anteriorly than normal) (Fig. 93.63) and the relationship of the temporomandibular joint to the facial nerve canal and middle ear (the temporomandibular joint may lie more posteriorly and at a higher level than normal) [53]. The position of the carotid canal and jugular fossa are also of importance since they may lie unexpectedly close to the middle ear cavity.

Deformities of the external and middle ear may form part of a more complex embryological maldevelopment as for example in the Treacher-Collin's syndrome (mandibulofacial dysostosis). In such cases the middle ear cavity is small due to encroachment by the atresia plate, high jugular bulb and a low tegmen tympani. There are many such complex congenital syndromes involving the ear [54].

Congenital anomalies of the inner ear

Severe or complete deafness is the usual mode of presentation. In the Mundini deformity, the normal $2\frac{3}{4}$ turns of the cochlea are reduced to $1\frac{1}{2}$ turns. In more severe forms, there may be hypoplasia or absence of the cochlea, which is often associated with a narrow internal auditory meatus. Aplasia and deformities of the semicircular canals also occur, and are occasionally associated with fistulous communications between the theca and the tympanic cavity resulting in recurring attacks of meningitis [55] (Fig. 93.64). Congenital dilatation of the internal auditory meatus may be mistaken for pathological enlargement caused by an acoustic neuroma but such cases are usually bilateral (Fig. 93.65).

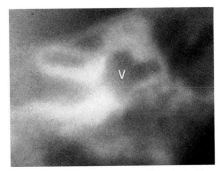

Fig. 93.64 Congenital deformity of labyrinth. Coronal tomogram showing dilatation of vestibule and lateral semicircular canal [V]. Internal auditory meatus is rather narrow. Patient presented with recurrent meningitis.

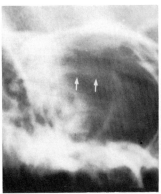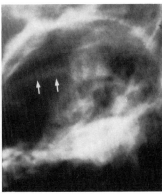

Fig. 93.65 Congenital dilatation of the internal auditory meatus. Perorbital projections clearly show the roof of the meatus on each side [arrows]. The floor is rather indistinct.

As with deformities of the external and middle ear, tomography is necessary for the adequate radiological examination of the inner ear [56].

The pharynx

METHODS OF RADIOLOGICAL EXAMINATION

The principle methods of radiology of the pharynx are indicated in Table 93.3. Radiological examination of the pharynx is complementary to the use of indirect or direct endoscopy. In some patients radiological examination may be indicated because the patient is nervous, and cannot adequately tolerate an endoscopic examination. However, when adequate endoscopy can be carried out, it is more accurate than radiodiagnostic techniques in the diagnosis of lesions involving only the mucosa or projecting into the lumen. Endoscopy cannot however assess the deeper extent of an invasive or destructive lesion, for which radiological examinations are particularly indicated.

Conventional radiological methods including plain films and tomography demonstrate only the soft tissue outlines of the pharynx. Additionally there may be evidence of the extension of nasopharyngeal lesions into the nasal cavity and paranasal sinuses, and bone destruction may be detected in the base of the skull, the posterior part of the facial skeleton, and the upper cervical spine. Nasopharyngography may show the outline of pharyngeal lesions more clearly.

Until the introduction of CT, it was not possible to assess the extent to which a nasopharyngeal lesion had invaded the soft tissue planes of the pharynx. Detailed CT anatomic

Table 93.3 *Radiological examination of the pharynx*

Radiographic projection and technique	Anatomical features displayed	Applications
Lateral views (a) During quiet breathing with mouth open (b) During forced expiration with mouth closed and nose held. (Xerography is of value)	Posterior ends of nasal conchae, soft tissue and bony walls of pharynx, hard and soft palate, tongue, epiglottis.	Demonstration of tumours of nasopharynx, and associated bone erosion. Tumours of the palate, tongue and epiglottis.
Submentovertical (base, axial): canthomeatal line parallel to film. No angulation of incident ray.	Lateral pharyngeal walls. Base of skull, mastoids.	Tumours arising from lateral walls of pharynx. Demonstration of associated erosion of the skull base, and mastoid infection.
Tomography in lateral projection	For separation of soft tissue planes seen on lateral radiograph.	For improved demonstration of tumours and associated bone erosion.
Computed tomography (CT)	Horizontal and coronal sections of soft tissues	Improved demonstration of soft tissue. Limits of pharyngeal tumours for therapy planning.
Pharyngography using aqueous or oily propyliodone	Outlines of walls of nasopharynx including lateral recesses.	Improved demonstration of pharyngeal tumours.
Barium swallow (with video or cine recording for subsequent analysis)	Oropharynx and hypopharynx	Analysis of functional disorders of swallowing. Demonstration of pharyngeal pouches and tumours of hypopharynx.
Angiography	Dependent on vessel selected	Demonstration of vascular tumours including juvenile angiofibroma and carotid body tumours.

studies of the fascial and muscular planes of the pharynx [57] have enabled a much more accurate determination of the limits of pharyngeal tumours to be obtained.

ANATOMICAL FEATURES

The pharynx is subdivided into the nasopharynx which lies between the posterior choanae and the lower border of the soft palate; the oropharynx which extends from the lower margin of the soft palate to the level of the hyoid bone; and the hypopharynx, extending from this point to the upper margin of the cricoid cartilage, where it merges with the oesophagus.

The posterior wall of the pharynx is shown as a soft tissue shadow anterior to the cervical vertebrae. As it curves backwards and downwards below the body of the sphenoid the soft tissue posterior wall is of variable thickness and may have a rather poorly defined edge. The thickness of the posterior wall becomes less as it passes downwards and between C2 and C4 it lies approximately parallel to the spine about 3 mm in front of the vertebrae. Below this level it becomes thicker approaching 1 cm in thickness in the postcricoid region but not exceeding the AP diameter of one vertebral body at this point. The soft tissue thickness of the wall of the nasopharynx and of the upper part of the oropharynx is much greater in infancy and childhood, and may not achieve an adult configuration until about 25 years. The increased thickness is due to hyperplastic lymphoid tissue which is often seen in the young. The lymphoid tissue is composed of localized aggregations on the lateral walls of the oropharynx — the pharyngeal tonsils; smaller aggregations on the posterior surface of the back of the tongue, the lingual tonsils; and numerous aggregations present throughout the wall of the nasopharynx and the upper part of the oropharynx and extending into the soft palate. The latter when enlarged are described as adenoids. The lymphoid tissue surrounding the pharynx at this point is sometimes referred to as Waldeyer's ring.

The anterior boundary of the oropharynx is formed by the posterior third of the tongue, which in the normal resting position shows crenated mucosal folds which may mimic a tumour. These may be flattened to some extent by a slight protrusion of the tongue. Below the tongue lies the epiglottis from which the aryepiglottic folds stretch downwards and backwards forming the anterior margin of the hypopharynx.

The outline of the posterior and lateral walls of the pharynx can also be identified in the axial projection, but detailed axial anatomy is seen much more clearly on CT. By this means four distinct fascial planes are identified: the prevertebral fascia, the pharyngobasilar fascia, the carotid sheath and the buccopharyngeal fascia. These fascial planes are identified as the boundaries between the muscles of the pharynx and the intervening fat. The invasive characteristics of different tumours may disturb these soft tissue planes in recognizably different ways [58].

INFLAMMATORY AND RELATED LESIONS

Adenoids

The lymphoid tissue of the naso- and upper oropharynx referred to above is much larger in infancy and childhood than in the adult. The common inflammatory hypertrophy of childhood is referred to as 'adenoids' in which enlargement may occur to a degree which completely obstructs the nasopharynx, the patient characteristically breathing through the mouth. In such cases clinical examination is definitive, but a lateral radiograph will demonstrate the hypertrophied soft tissues in the posterior part of the nasopharynx (Fig. 93.66).

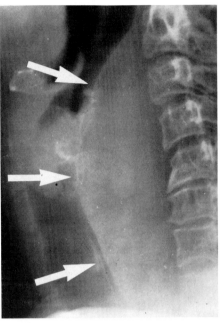

Fig. 93.67 Retropharyngeal abscess. A large soft tissue swelling displaces the trachea and larynx forwards. The abscess followed an endoscopy.

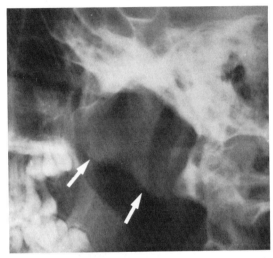

Fig. 93.66 Adenoids. Patient aged 11 years showing lobulated soft tissue mass in the nasopharynx.

In some cases there may be difficulty in deciding whether the adenoidal soft tissue pad is of a normal thickness or whether there is hypertrophy. In such cases, reference may be made to tables giving the average and range of normals at differing ages [59]. The decision as to whether to manage an individual case by conservative or surgical means is based on clinical factors, such as the degree of obstruction and the occurrence of infection in the middle ear and mastoid, rather than on the absolute size of the adenoid pad as seen on radiological examination.

Pharyngeal abscess

Abscesses in the soft tissues adjacent to the pharynx may be parapharyngeal, usually secondary to tonsillar infection or perforation by foreign bodies, or retropharyngeal when the abscess is usually due either to an associated vertebral osteitis or to spread of infection from suppurating cervical lymph nodes. In these cases the infection may be of tuberculous origin. Rarely a retropharyngeal abscess may be a complication of endoscopy (Fig. 93.67). Radiological exam-

ination is indicated, not for the diagnosis of the presence of an abscess, but for determination of its cause. The lateral radiograph of the neck shows a soft tissue mass separating the posterior pharyngeal wall from the spine. On erect films gas with a fluid level may occasionally be seen and rarely a radio-opaque foreign body may be noted. It is often of low density since small meat and fish bones are often poorly calcified. Erosion or destruction of a cervical vertebra may be seen in cases where the abscess is secondary to tuberculous or pyogenic osteitis. Vertebral subluxation may be seen particularly in the infant and does not necessarily imply a spinal origin of the abscess, as laxity of the spinal ligaments secondary to infection may cause some degree of vertebral instability. Calcification may be visible in cervical lymph nodes in cases of tuberculous infection, or may be seen in the abscess itself.

BENIGN TUMOURS OF THE PHARYNX

Juvenile angiofibroma

This is a highly vascular benign tumour of the nasopharynx showing a marked tendency to infiltrate soft tissue planes, but not usually destructive although soft tissue and bone displacement may occur. It occurs almost exclusively in adolescent males and is said to regress spontaneously on rare occasions. Juvenile nasopharyngeal angiofibroma presents clinically with nasal obstruction and epistaxis. Cranial nerve involvement is occasionally present. Clinical examination shows a sessile globular mass arising from the roof of the nasopharynx. Histologically the lesion is a highly vascular benign hamartoma arising from the mucoperiosteum on the underside of the body of the sphenoid. Biopsy is hazardous due to the danger of massive haemorrhage. Radiological examination is indicated to assess the size and extent of the lesion, to determine its blood supply and sometimes to reduce its vascularity by embolization.

The lateral radiograph shows a soft tissue mass arising from the roof of the nasopharynx, often extending forward as far as the nasal cavity and the posterior walls of the maxillary antra (Fig. 93.68). Characteristically the tumour tends to produce displacement and pressure erosion of bone rather than true invasion, though this may also occur in some cases. Pressure effects may be noted in the sphenoid, hard palate, and pterygoid plates. In addition, extension forward may cause pressure on the posterior walls of the maxillary antra, with anterior bowing [60]. Extension into the nose may cause expansion of the nasal fossae, mimicking benign nasal polyps, though the expansion caused by the latter is rarely so marked. Extension upwards into the sphenoid sinus is seen, and intracranial extension occurs in some cases.

These pressure effects are well shown by conventional tomography but the extent of soft tissue infiltration can only be determined with accuracy by CT in the horizontal plane, supplemented if necessary by coronal sections. Forward extension of the tumour may be seen into the nasal cavity, the pterygomaxillary fissure, the pterygopalatine fossa, into the paranasal sinuses via their ostia, and through the orbital fissures [61] (Fig. 93.69).

CT also shows the typical displacement of bony structures rather than the irregular bony erosion characteristic of malignant tumours. Characteristically nasopharyngeal angiofibromas extend forward, thus leaving the carotid sheath region intact [57]. Opacity of the paranasal sinuses is not

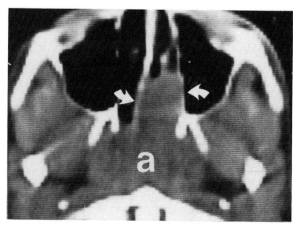

Fig. 93.69 Juvenile angiofibroma. CT scan showing tumour mass [a] extending forwards into the right nasal cavity producing slight displacement of the nasal septum and the medial wall of the maxillary antrum [arrows].

necessarily due to tumour invasion as the presence of a mass in the nasal cavity may cause obstruction of the ostia of the sinuses.

Angiographic studies show a very vascular tumour, supplied in most cases by the internal maxillary artery and by the ascending pharyngeal artery (Fig. 93.70). Cases with intracranial extension may derive a blood supply from dural branches of the internal carotid artery [62].

Therapeutic embolization is now an established method of management, primarily as a preoperative procedure for the reduction of intraoperative blood loss [63]. When carrying out such procedures it is important to exclude anatomical communications between the internal and external carotid systems in order to avoid the potentially dangerous complication of escape of emboli into the intracranial circulation.

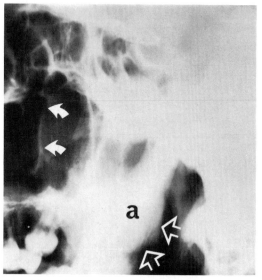

Fig. 93.68 Juvenile angiofibroma. The tumour [a] lies beneath the body of the sphenoid. Its lower margin bulges backwards and downwards into the oropharynx [open arrows] while its anterior margin displaces the posterior wall of the maxillary antrum slightly forwards [solid arrow].

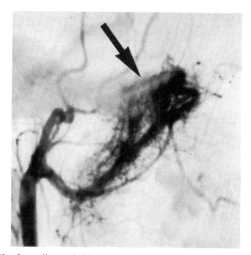

Fig. 93.70 Juvenile angiofibroma. Subtracted external carotid angiogram showing marked tumour circulation supplied by the internal maxillary artery. (Same patient as Fig. 93.68).

Chordoma

This is a benign, locally invasive tumour which arises from notochordal remnants. Although they may occur anywhere

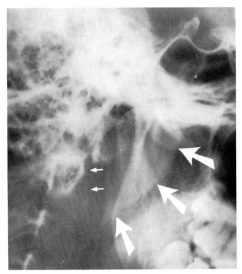

Fig. 93.71 Chordoma. Soft tissue mass bulging into nasopharynx [solid arrows]. Destructive changes in the body of C2 [small arrows].

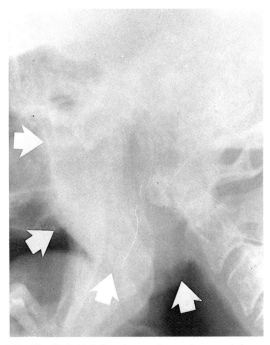

Fig. 93.72 NonHodgkin's lymphoma of nasopharynx. A large soft tissue mass is present obstructing the posterior choanae.

along the line of the primitive notochord, most are found either in the sacrum or in the region of the clivus arising either in the basiocciput or basisphenoid. The latter may produce a tumour mass which extends predominantly into the cranium, but occasionally in infants presents with a nasopharyngeal mass. Cranial nerve palsies and brain stem compression may occur and in the case of nasopharyngeal tumours there may be dysphagia.

The tumour is characterized by a destructive lesion in the region of the clivus sometimes associated with calcification. A large soft tissue mass may be present in the nasopharynx and these features may be seen on a lateral radiograph (Fig. 93.71). Tomography may be of value in delineating the area of calcification and bone destruction, and CT may also be useful. Contrast enhancement on CT sometimes occurs. Myelography is helpful on occasion for the demonstration of any intracranial or intraspinal component.

Craniopharyngioma

Cystic masses arising from Rathke's pouch remnants are most commonly found in the suprasellar region. Occasionally however a craniopharyngioma may present, usually in infancy, with a nasopharyngeal soft tissue mass.

MALIGNANT TUMOURS OF THE NASOPHARYNX

Apart from occasional cases of *fibrosarcoma*, the majority of malignant tumours in the nasopharynx are either due to a *lymphoma*, *lymphoepithelioma*, or *carcinoma* usually of the squamous type. Lymphomas of the nasopharynx are gener-

ally of the nonHodgkin's variety and present with a large soft tissue mass in the nasopharynx (Fig. 93.72) which may or may not be associated with lymphadenopathy. Secondary infection may occur in the mastoids due to obstruction of the pharyngotympanic tube. Bone destruction is not usually a feature.

Nasopharyngeal carcinoma

Nasopharyngeal carcinoma tends to occur in rather older patients than lymphoma, and is commoner in males. Some cases present with a large mass which may be associated with pain and cranial nerve lesions, but in other cases the presenting feature may be enlargement of cervical lymph nodes, the primary nasopharyngeal tumour being discovered later on clinical examination. Radiological examination should include the lateral and submentovertical projections and sagittal tomography is of value in the demonstration of bone destruction. Nasopharyngography is useful for the demonstration of early tumours on the lateral wall of the nasopharynx (Fig. 93.73) [64].

The radiological features on plain films with tomography include a soft tissue mass in the nasopharynx; this is usually best seen on the lateral projection but a mass arising from the lateral wall may be seen better on the axial view (Fig. 93.74). Destruction of the bony base of the skull is a common feature (Fig. 93.75) and the tumour may penetrate into the cranium via the foramina. Hyperostosis is also sometimes seen in the base of the skull (Fig. 93.76) [65]. The mastoids are frequently opaque due to obstruction of the pharyngotympanic tube. There is occasional opacity of the paranasal sinuses, usually due to secondary infection rather than invasion.

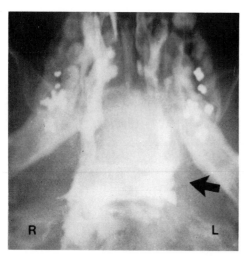

Fig. 93.73 Nasopharyngeal carcinoma. Nasopharyngogram showing an asymmetric appearance due to early tumour on the left side of the nasopharynx.

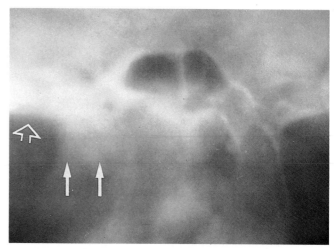

Fig. 93.76 Nasopharyngeal carcinoma. Tomogram showing hyperostosis of the base of the skull [open arrow] and destruction of pterygoid plates [arrows].

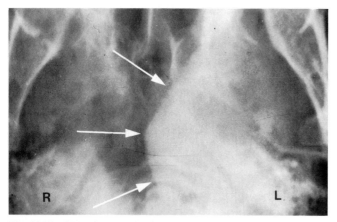

Fig. 93.74 Nasopharyngeal carcinoma. Base view showing large soft tissue mass arising from the left side of the nasopharynx.

CT in the horizontal and coronal planes is of great value in the assessment of nasopharyngeal carcinoma. It is superior to any other modality in the clarity, ease and accuracy of imaging of small masses in this area [66]. In addition to showing the soft tissue tumour and the bone destruction, CT also demonstrates the ability of nasopharyngeal carcinomas to penetrate the fascial planes of the walls of the nasopharynx. Lesions which appeared clinically to be confined to the mucosa have been shown on CT to be associated with deeper infiltration (Fig. 93.77). Intracranial extension secondary to penetration of the base of the skull by the primary tumour is also well shown by CT (Fig. 93.78).

Malignant tumours of the oropharynx

Apart from occasional cases of sarcoma, tumours of the oropharynx are generally due to carcinoma, the squamous type occurring more frequently than the adenocarcinoma. The commonest site of origin is the anterior wall including the base of the tongue. They may be predominantly infiltrative, in which case there is little radiological evidence of their presence, but a mass may be seen on the lateral radiograph in the case of proliferative lesions. Radiological distinction must be made from the marked irregularity of this part of the tongue which is occasionally a normal feature. Oropharyngeal tumours arising from the posterior pharyngeal wall (Fig. 93.79) are often exophytic, but occasionally resemble retropharyngeal abscesses in this site.

Malignant tumours of the hypopharynx

Malignant tumours of the aryepiglottic fold and piriform fossa are considered with supraglottic carcinomas of the larynx. Carcinoma of the *postcricoid* region presents with dysphagia. The radiological features include a postcricoid soft tissue mass which may cause anterior displacement of

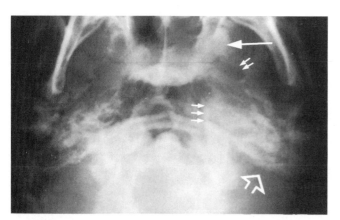

Fig. 93.75 Nasopharyngeal carcinoma. Destruction of the base of the skull in region of foramen lacerum [3 arrows], enlargement of foramen ovale [2 arrows], destruction of pterygoid plates [single arrow] and opaque mastoid [open arrow].

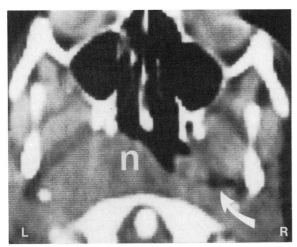

Fig. 93.77 Nasopharyngeal carcinoma. CT examination shows tumour mass [n] bulging into the left side of the nasopharynx. The parapharyngeal space is invaded. Normal parapharyngeal space shown on the right side [arrow].

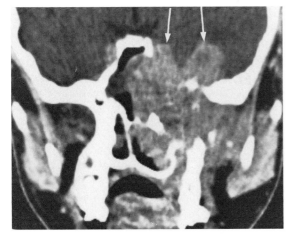

Fig. 93.78 CT scan showing intracranial extension [arrows] of malignant nasopharyngeal tumour (angiosarcoma). (Reproduced by kind permission of Dr J. Husband. The Royal Marsden Hospital, London).

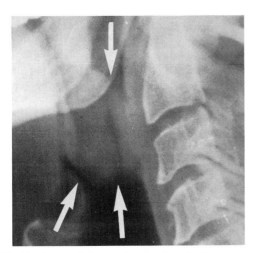

Fig. 93.79 Carcinoma of the oropharynx. Exophytic tumour mass arising from the posterior oropharyngeal wall (arrows).

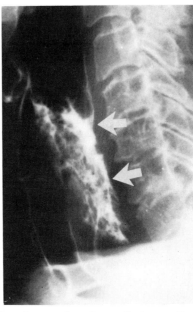

Fig. 93.80 Hypopharyngeal carcinoma. Barium swallow examination showing irregular stricture in the postcricoid region [arrows]. Note aspiration of barium into the trachea.

the larynx. Barium swallow examination shows an irregular stricture in the postcricoid region often accompanied by some aspiration of barium into the larynx and trachea (Fig. 93.80). Radiological distinction should be made from an extensive laryngeal carcinoma invading the hypopharynx. These cases show gross laryngeal abnormalities whereas it is unusual for a postcricoid carcinoma to cause laryngeal invasion, though displacement commonly occurs.

CERVICAL DYSPHAGIA

Dysphagia localized to the cervical region is a common presenting complaint. Only a small minority of patients presenting in this way are found to have a postcricoid carcinoma of the oesophagus (see above). Of the remainder, some prove to have no demonstrable radiological abnormality. These patients, whose complaint is often described as being like a lump in the throat, are described as suffering from *globus*. Occasionally a cause for this complaint is found in the lower oesophagus, but in most cases no underlying abnormality can be found.

The remainder of these patients consist of a group of inter-related abnormalities having either or both a functional and an anatomical basis. They include various protrusions from the lateral wall of the pharynx including the rare true diverticula, pseudodiverticula (pharyngoceles) and pharyngeal 'ears', posterior pharyngeal diverticula (Zenker's), cricopharyngeus spasm, and postcricoid webs [67].

Pharyngeal protrusions

A diffuse bulge of the lateral wall of the piriform fossa, sometimes referred to as a pharyngocele is associated with occupations such as glass blowing and the playing of wind instruments [67], and may also be seen in association with upper oesophageal obstruction. Small protrusions or 'ears' extend laterally usually at a rather higher level and are in most cases an incidental finding appearing only transiently on contrast swallow examination. True diverticula are rare. They arise from the lateral wall of the piriform fossa and may result either from increased pressure due to upper oesophageal obstruction or may be due to a congenital weakness in the lateral wall of the hypopharynx, possibly as a result of incomplete obliteration of 2nd, 3rd or 4th branchial cleft (Fig. 93.81). There may be some clinical and radiological resemblance to a laryngocele (see below). A pharyngeal diverticulum is demonstrated by a contrast swallow examination; increasing the intrapharyngeal pressure by forced expiration against partially closed lips (a modified Valsalva manoeuvre) is helpful in demonstrating these lesions. Laryngoceles are not opacified by this technique but are shown by laryngography. Occasionally a true pharyngeal diverticulum may result from an acquired weakness following tonsillectomy.

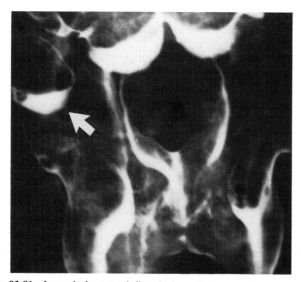

Fig. 93.81 Lateral pharyngeal diverticulum. Barium swallow examination (frontal view) showing right sided diverticulum. (Film during Valsalva manoeuvre).

Posterior pharyngeal diverticula (Zenker's diverticula)

Zenker's diverticula are a common cause of upper oesophageal dysphagia which may be severe. Food collects in the diverticulum where it stagnates and subsequent regurgitation may cause an unpleasant taste and smell; there may be aspiration with choking episodes. Occasionally the diverticulum becomes large enough to form a palpable mass in the neck, usually on the left side.

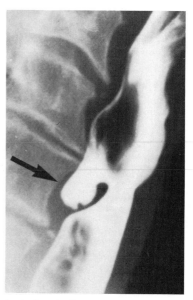

Fig. 93.82 Zenker's diverticulum. Barium swallow examination showing small posterior pharyngeal pouch.

The diverticulum arises posteriorly through an area of weakness (Killian's dehiscence) between the oblique and transverse fibres of the inferior constrictor of the pharynx (cricopharyngeus). It is possible to show both radiologically and by manometric methods that there is impaired relaxation of the cricopharyngeus thus causing the formation of a pulsion diverticulum (Fig. 93.82). The diverticulum enlarges downwards initially displacing the oesophagus forwards but large diverticula extend posterolaterally usually on the left side and may extend down into the mediastinum. A fluid level behind the upper oesophagus is a common radiological feature of a large posterior pharyngeal diverticulum.

Cricopharyngeus spasm

In the act of swallowing, contraction of the pharyngeal constrictors is accompanied by a simultaneous relaxation of the cricopharyngeus muscle which forms the upper oesophageal sphincter. Failure of the cricopharyngeus to relax may cause dysphagia and may present as an isolated abnormality (sometimes described as cricopharyngeal achalasia), or may be accompanied by the formation of a Zenker's diverticulum (see above).

Postcricoid web

A thin shelf-like mucosal projection arising usually from the anterior wall of the oesophagus is described as a web (Fig. 93.83). They occur more commonly in women and are a frequent cause of upper oesophageal dysphagia. Optimal demonstration requires cine radiography in the AP and lateral projection. It is necessary to instruct the patient to swallow a large mouthful of the barium suspension as the web may fail to appear when only a small bolus is swallowed.

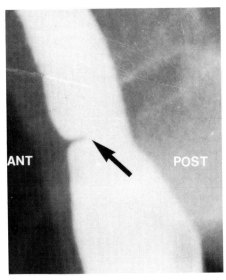

Fig. 93.83 Postcricoid web. Barium swallow examination showing thin shelf-like mucosal projection anteriorly.

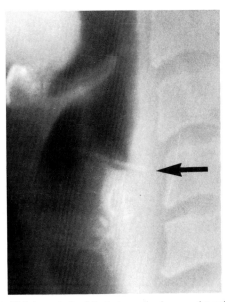

Fig. 93.84 Fish bone lodged just above the laryngeal vestibule.

It is apparent that in some cases they are a transient phenomenon present for only part of the time during which the cervical oesophagus is filled with barium [68], and it is for this reason that cine radiography is desirable for their demonstration. Posterior webs are seen occasionally and multiple webs also occur. There is an association with iron deficiency anaemia (sideropenic dysphagia) in which the hypopharyngeal mucosa shows a diffuse abnormality. There is also an association with neuromuscular incoordination of the act of swallowing and with malignancy in the hypopharynx or oesophagus [67].

It is possible that only a proportion of webs are actually responsible for the dysphagia in the patients in whom they are found. In other patients, the presence of the web may simply be associated with another more important abnormality. Although there is increased incidence of postcricoid carcinoma in patients with webs [69], the malignant lesion does not necessarily occur at the same site. This indicates that the web is not in itself precancerous but may indicate the presence of an abnormal mucosa with concomitant malignancy [67].

FOREIGN BODIES

The impaction of a foreign body in the pharynx is a frequent occurrence. They are most commonly found in the tonsillar fossae, the valleculae and in the postcricoid region. Meat and fish bones are a common cause and may be recognisable on a plain lateral radiograph (Fig. 93.84) but many such foreign bodies are too small or too poorly calcified to be visible. If perforation occurs, a retropharyngeal abscess may result with characteristic radiological features. In infancy and childhood small toys and coins may be swallowed usually impacting in the postcricoid region.

The larynx

METHODS OF RADIOLOGICAL EXAMINATION

Plain radiography

Survey views of the larynx are usually taken in the lateral position as the larynx is not then obscured by any other structures. For most purposes a single lateral film will suffice, but phonating 'ee' throws the laryngeal ventricles into relief and enables a better assessment of the anterior commissure to be made.

Anteroposterior radiographs tend to be unsatisfactory due to the obscuring shadows of the cervical spine. It is possible, however, to demonstrate the air space of the larynx using high kV (125 to 150) together with a 2 mm brass filter. Films taken by this technique show markedly reduced bone contrast with unimpaired air to soft tissue contrast.

Xerography

Much improved delineation of the detail of the soft tissues and cartilages of the larynx may be obtained on xerograms [70]. Improvement is due to the edge enhancement effect, a special characteristic of xerography whereby even small differences in radiodensity between adjacent structures may be depicted as a distinct line at the interface. The ossified laryngeal cartilages are also very clearly shown

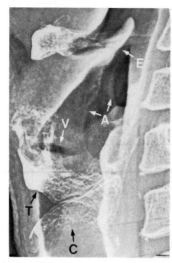

Fig. 93.85 Lateral laryngeal xerogram. Cricoid cartilage [C]. Thyroid cartilage [T], epiglottic [E], aryepiglottic folds [A], ventricle [V].

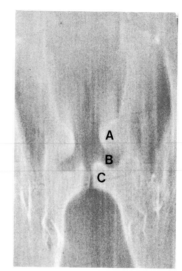

Fig. 93.86 Normal frontal xerotomogram. Vestibular fold [A], ventricle [B] and vocal fold [C]. (Figs. 93.85 & 86 reproduced by kind permission of Dr S. S. Amar, Nottingham General Hospital).

(Fig. 93.85). Xerography may be used in tomographic examinations (Fig. 93.86), and the clear and detailed images obtained are very suitable for radiotherapy treatment planning [71].

Tomography

Tomographic examination of the larynx is carried out using a linear technique in order to obtain a short exposure time. The examination is carried out in the anteroposterior position and enables the outline of the laryngeal soft tissues to be clearly seen free of confusing shadows due to the cervical spine. It is carried out without discomfort to the patient, and is a good method for the demonstration of tumours of the larynx.

Laryngography

The patient is prepared by withholding food and fluid for 4 hours and is then sedated (e.g. Diazepam). Atropine is given to reduce secretions and the hypopharynx and larynx are anaesthetised using a topical spray of lignocaine. A soft polythene catheter is then passed through the nose and positioned with its tip above the epiglottis. Aqueous or oily propyliodone (Dionosil) are then instilled through the catheter to coat the larynx with the contrast material. The patient is instructed to breath quietly and if adequate anaesthesia has been obtained, there will be little or no coughing. Excessive quantities of contrast medium should be avoided as they tend to flood the lower lobe bronchi causing segmental pulmonary collapse; 5 to 8 ml is usually adequate.

Radiographs are then obtained with the larynx at rest, with

Table 93.4 *Radiological examination of the larynx*

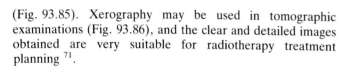

Radiographic projection and technique	Anatomical features shown	Applications
Lateral: at rest, mouth open, tongue slightly protruded.	Epiglottis, aryepiglottic folds, laryngeal cartilages.	Survey views of larynx for tumours. Trauma, foreign body, stenosis, inflammation.
Lateral: phonating	Anterior commissure, laryngeal ventricles	Assessment of anterior cord tumours.
Lateral: xerography	As above	For improved soft tissue detail.
Tomography: anteroposterior at rest and phonating	Detail of soft tissues and cartilaginous structures of larynx and subglottic space	Detailed assessment of laryngeal tumours and other causes of hoarseness.
Laryngography	Anatomical detail of larynx including mucosa	As for tomography. Mucosal detail is superior.
Barium swallow	Hypopharynx and upper oesophagus	Investigation of dysphagia, suspected extrinsic compression or invasion from laryngeal tumours.
Computed tomography (CT)	Cross sectional anatomy of larynx	Accurate delineation of laryngeal tumours for radiotherapy planning; trauma.

the patient phonating, and performing the Valsalva manoeuvre [72].

The anatomical detail displayed by means of laryngography is similar to that shown on good quality tomograms though the mucosal relief is clearer and superficial mucosal lesions can only be shown by this method.

Cine radiography

High speed cine radiography is of value in the evaluation of functional disorders of swallowing and of phonation.

Computed tomography

The use of computed tomography (CT) in the evaluation of diseases of the larynx, particularly tumours is a comparatively recent development. Horizontal sections are obtained and are of value in the delineation of submucosal tumour extent, invasion of the pre-epiglottic space, and cartilage displacement or invasion [73]. Spread across the anterior or posterior commissure is also apparent. CT does not demonstrate lesions confined to the mucosa and does not distinguish tumour from oedema. Movement artefacts may cause practical difficulties. The methods of radiological examination are summarised in Table 93.4.

RADIOLOGICAL ANATOMY

The larynx lies in the neck opposite the 3rd to the 6th cervical vertebrae, rather higher in children and in females than it is in adult males. The adult larynx is considerably larger in males and is different in shape. The supporting framework of the larynx is provided by nine cartilages; the epiglottis, thyroid and cricoid, and paired arytenoid, corniculate and cuneiform cartilages.

On the lateral projection, the epiglottis is seen as a leaf-like soft tissue shadow extending upwards and backwards from a point just below the base of the tongue separating the valleculae in front from the vestibule of the larynx behind. The aryepiglottic folds are seen passing downwards and backwards from the epiglottis. The vestibular and vocal folds can be seen separated by the radio-lucency of the laryngeal ventricle (seen on films in phonation).

The laryngeal cartilages are not visualized unless they become ossified. Ossification is common, variable in extent and commences in early adult life. It begins in the posterior free edge of the thyroid cartilage to spread upwards into the laminae and into the superior and inferior cornua. The cricoid cartilage, shaped like a signet ring with the impressing component of the ring posteriorly, commonly shows ossification which tends to commence in the posterior quadrate lamina of the cartilage. It lies immediately below the thyroid cartilage and is united below to the first ring of the trachea.

The arytenoid cartilages are often densely ossified, even in the absence of ossification in the thyroid and cricoid cartilages. They may be seen lying posteriorly immediately above the lamina of the cricoid and give attachment anteriorly to the vocal folds. The corniculate cartilages are small, lying immediately above the arytenoids, and the cuneiforms lie in the lower part of the aryepiglottic fold. Like the epiglottis, they are composed of yellow elastic cartilage and rarely ossify.

The anatomy of the cavity of the larynx as seen on a coronal section tomogram or anteroposterior laryngogram extends from the laryngeal entrance between the two aryepiglottic folds to the level of the upper ring of the trachea. Projecting into this cavity are two pairs of folds: the upper pair are known as the *vestibular or ventricular folds* and the lower pair are called the *vocal folds*. Between them lies the ventricle or sinus of the larynx. The portion of the larynx above the vestibular folds is the vestibule of the larynx. The symmetrical concavity of the lower surfaces of the vocal folds as they are continuous with the upper part of the trachea is an important anatomical feature and tends to be lost or flattened on the affected side in the presence of injury or damage to the recurrent laryngeal nerve.

TUMOURS OF THE LARYNX

The diagnosis of laryngeal tumours is usually made on clinical evidence by direct or indirect laryngoscopy and biopsy. Radiological examinations are of value to determine the extent of the lesion and to influence the planning of surgical or radiation therapy. Radiological examination is of particular importance for:
1. The examination of nervous or apprehensive individuals and children who cannot adequately tolerate endoscopy
2. The examination of the larynx in the presence of large lesions preventing distal visualization
3. The examination of the subglottic space
4. The assessment of invasion of the laryngeal cartilages and the soft tissue surrounding the larynx. Conventional tomography and more recently CT are of particular importance for this purpose [73,74,75]. CT gives a better demonstration of submucosal tumour invasion, spread into the pre-epiglottic space, and displacement and invasion of the laryngeal cartilages [73].

Carcinoma of the larynx

This is the commonest type of laryngeal tumour. They are classified according to their site of origin into glottic tumours, arising from the vocal folds; supraglottic tumours arising from the epiglottis, the aryepiglottic folds, the vestibular folds and laryngeal ventricle; and subglottic growths arising usually from the lateral wall of the subglottic space and excluding those which arise from the inferior surface of the vocal folds. Morphologically, laryngeal tumours are exophytic, ulcerative or infiltrative. Premalignant leukoplakia and hyperkeratosis may occasionally be recognized by laryngography.

Glottic tumours

More than two thirds of cases of carcinoma of the larynx arise in the vocal folds. The lesion most commonly arises in the anterior two thirds of the vocal fold and occurs less frequently in the anterior commissure. Lesions of the vocal folds are readily visualized both by tomography and laryngography (Fig. 93.87) but radiological examination is of particular value in determining the presence of subglottic extension of the lesion (Fig. 93.88). Carcinoma arising in the anterior commissure is less amenable to direct examination as the region may be partly obscured by the epiglottis. Such

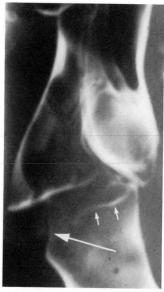

Fig. 93.89 Carcinoma of the vocal fold extending to the anterior commissure. Lateral laryngogram showing failure of filling of the anterior part of one of the laryngeal ventricles [small arrows], with an anterior tumour [long arrow].

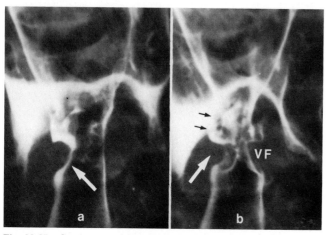

Fig. 93.87 Carcinoma of the larynx (frontal view). (a) Enlarged fixed right vocal fold [arrow]. Left fold is retracted and not visible. (b) Phonation film showing left vocal fold [VF]. Abnormality on the right side is less conspicuous but deformity of the right vocal fold is still visible with ulceration in the ventricle [small arrows].

lesions sometimes present late with extensive prelaryngeal infiltration. Lesions of the anterior commissure are more easy to see by laryngography (Fig. 93.89) than by tomography, though large growths can be seen on the plain radiographs. Tumours of the anterior commissure are also well seen by CT [73].

It is important to determine whether there is invasion of the thyroid cartilage, since the prognosis is significantly worse in such cases. Clinically, although some pain may be present, it is not uncommon to find that cartilage erosion has occurred without symptoms. Large areas of erosion may be seen on a plain lateral radiograph but tomography is also of value (Fig. 93.90). Comparison of the two thyroid laminae on

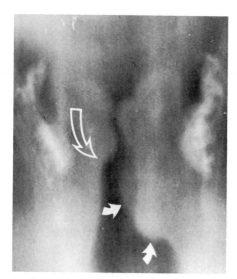

Fig. 93.88 Carcinoma of the larynx. Tomograms showing extensive subglottic extension of the tumour of the left vocal fold [solid arrows]. Note the normal subglottic angle on the right side [open arrow].

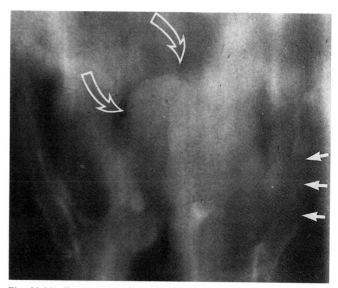

Fig. 93.90 Erosion of thyroid cartilage. Coronal tomogram shows a large supraglottic tumour mass [open arrows]. There is a 1.5 cm defect in the left thyroid ala [solid arrows].

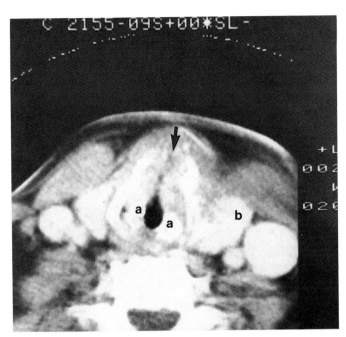

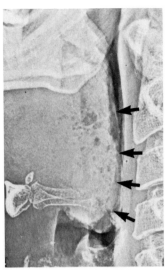

Fig. 93.92 Carcinoma of the epiglottis. Lateral xerogram showing a supraglottic tumour mass destroying the epiglottis and extending up to the base of the tongue. (Reproduced by kind permission of Dr S. S. Amar, Nottingham General Hospital).

Fig. 93.91 CT of larynx. A tumour in the anterior commissure has perforated the thyroid cartilage [solid arrow]. The arytenoids [a] are densely calcified. Tumour spreading along the outside of the right thyroid ala has displaced the upper pole of the thyroid [b]. (Reproduced by kind permission of Dr C. A. Parsons, the Royal Marsden Hospital, London).

the coronal section tomograms may be misleading, because of anatomical variations and assymmetry [77]. Infiltrated cartilage appears mottled and the edges of the areas of destruction may appear serrated. CT is more sensitive than either clinical examination or conventional radiology in the detection of cartilage erosion (Fig. 93.91) [73].

Supraglottic tumours

Carcinoma of the epiglottis may be of the invasive or the exophytic type, the latter often reaching a considerable size before diagnosis. Infiltrative lesions may spread anteriorly to the vallecula, the base of the tongue and the pre-epiglottic space (Fig. 93.92). An adequate radiological assessment can usually be obtained from the lateral radiograph, supplemented by laryngography with fluoroscopy for the assessment of mobility of the epiglottis.

Tumours arising in the aryepiglottic folds may spread to involve the piriform fossa, the laryngeal surface of the epiglottis and the vestibular folds (Fig. 93.93 & 94). Posterior extension may result in dysphagia. Lesions of the vestibular folds are assessed by tomography or laryngography (Fig. 93.95). If dysphagia is present, a barium swallow may be of value. Tumours arising in the anterior half of the vestibular folds spread into the base of the epiglottis and to the opposite side of the larynx, but do not tend to spread down to involve the vocal folds. Tumours arising in the posterior part of the vestibular folds may infiltrate deeply and involve the arytenoid cartilages and the aryepiglottic folds. Tumours arising from the laryngeal ventricle tend to spread rapidly

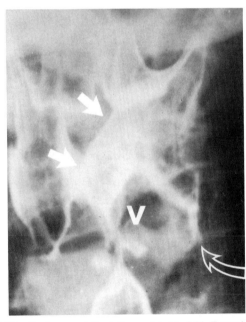

Fig. 93.93 Carcinoma of the left aryepiglottic fold. Frontal laryngogram shows large tumour arising from and obliterating the outline of the left aryepiglottic fold [solid arrows]. There is swelling of the left vestibular fold [v] and partial obliteration of the left piriform fossa [open arrow].

both upwards and downwards and may be indistinguishable from growths arising in adjacent structures.

Subglottic tumours

Subglottic tumours generally arise on the lateral wall of the subglottic space and may be examined by tomography or laryngography. They may be of proliferative or invasive types.

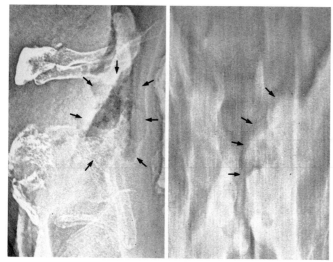

Fig. 93.94 Carcinoma of left aryepiglottic fold. Lateral xerogram and frontal xerotomogram clearly show tumour [arrows]. Reproduced by kind permission of Dr S. S. Amar; Nottingham General Hospital).

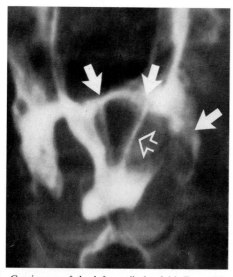

Fig. 93.95 Carcinoma of the left vestibular fold. Frontal laryngogram shows a large tumour arising from the left vestibular fold [solid arrows] with preservation of the left aryepiglottic fold [open arrow]. There is partial obliteration of the left piriform fossa.

The detection of tumours recurrent after radiotherapy is complicated by the frequent persistence of oedema for long periods after radiotherapy. Infection with perichondritis also makes the diagnosis of recurrent malignancy by radiological methods almost impossible.

Other malignant tumours of the larynx

Apart from carcinoma, malignant tumour of the larynx is rare. Many types of sarcoma may involve the larynx, the fibrosarcoma being most common and chondrosarcoma occurring occasionally. Extramedullary plasmacytoma may

occur tending to form polypoid tumour masses in the larynx. Initially these remain localized to the larynx and require only local treatment, but myelomatosis eventually develops in the majority of cases.

Benign tumours and cysts of the larynx

Compared with malignant tumours, benign tumours and cysts of the larynx occur infrequently.

Laryngeal papilloma

These benign columnar cell tumours occur in infants and in adults. The infantile type presents with respiratory distress which may be severe, with feeding difficulties and dysphonia. The lesions are often multiple and may almost fill the air space of the larynx and extend below the level of the glottis. Radiologically they may be shown on plain lateral radiographs, but xeroradiography is preferable. Radiological examination is important since laryngoscopy is technically difficult in small infants.

The condition is important because of the respiratory obstruction which occurs, but there is no tendency to malignant change.

Laryngeal papilloma in adults, despite a similar histological appearance, may be premalignant. Radiological diagnosis may be made by tomography, laryngography or xeroradiography (Fig. 93.96).

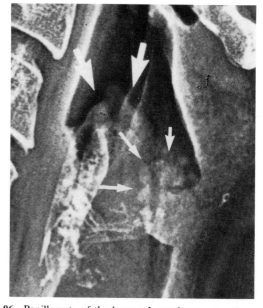

Fig. 93.96 Papillomata of the larynx. Lateral xerogram showing papilloma lying in the laryngeal vestibule [solid arrows] and in the region of the anterior commissure [small arrows]. (Reproduced by kind permission of Dr I. H. Gravelle, University Hospital of Wales, Cardiff).

Laryngeal cysts

Like papilloma, cysts of the larynx may also present in infancy and in adult life. Congenital cysts are very rare and present with severe respiratory obstruction in infancy. Radiographic examination shows obliteration of the air cavity of the larynx with ballooning of the pharynx above the lesion. The soft tissue mass of the cyst may be visible radiologically. Laryngeal cysts in adults are relatively common and the majority occur in the epiglottis. They are best demonstrated on lateral radiographs. The so called ventricular cyst is an internal laryngocele (see below).

Other benign tumours

Chondromas of the larynx are rare but can be distinguished from other laryngeal masses if they contain calcification. *Fibromas* may present as small sessile lesions on the cords indistinguishable from early malignant lesions. *Haemangioma* and *neurofibroma* may occur, but are extremely rare.

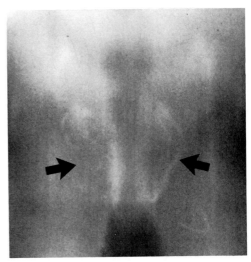

Fig. 93.97　Laryngeal stenosis. Coronal tomograms shows severe stenosis of the larynx. There is marked medial displacement of both thyroid cartilages [arrows]. Stenosis resulted from prolonged intubation following a drowning accident.

INFECTIVE AND INFLAMMATORY DISEASE OF THE LARYNX

Radiological examination is seldom required in inflammatory and infective disease processes affecting the larynx. Radiological changes are usually confined to soft tissue swelling with narrowing of the air space and loss of the normal soft tissue outlines. These changes are often very marked in the epiglottis. Tuberculous laryngitis may occur but is rarely recognized radiologically: ulcerative lesions may be visible on laryngography. Diptheritic laryngitis was common in the past, but has been virtually eliminated in developed countries. Acute allergic responses may present as laryngeal oedema.

TRAUMA TO THE LARYNX

Injuries to the larynx may result from blunt or penetrating injuries. Foreign bodies may enter the larynx. The injury may be confined to oedema and haematoma formation, but fractures of the laryngeal cartilages and of the hyoid bone may occur, occasionally with dislocation of the arytenoid cartilages. Resolution of the post-traumatic changes may lead to fibrosis with stricture formation. Iatrogenic injury to the larynx may result from prolonged intubation and laryngeal stenosis may occur as a result (Fig. 93.97).

Radiological evaluation may be carried out by plain radiography, tomography including CT, and xerography[78].

LARYNGOCELE

A laryngocele is an air-filled diverticulum arising from the laryngeal ventricle. A small extension normally arises from the anterior superior aspect of the laryngeal ventricle called the appendix of the ventricle. Laryngoceles arise by an increase in size of the appendix, probably as a result of congenital weakness. They may be classified into internal, external, and combined types (Fig. 93.98)[79]. If the laryngocele is contained within the larynx, medial to the thyroid cartilage, it is described as an internal laryngocele. The air-containing space lies within the ventricular fold which becomes enlarged, often causing some obstruction to the airway. (This type is sometimes referred to as a ventricular cyst). More commonly, however, the laryngocele enlarges upwards above the thyroid cartilage, to lie in relation to the thyrohyoid membrane. At this point it may penetrate the thyrohyoid membrane at the site of entry of the superior laryngeal vessels to lie under the thyrohyoid muscle. This type, described as an external laryngocele, presents as a soft swelling in the neck lateral to the larynx. Although bilateral laryngoceles have been described, most cases are unilateral. Infection may occur, particularly in the internal type, giving rise to a laryngopyocele.

A radiological diagnosis can often be made simply by obtaining standard anteroposterior and lateral radiographs or xerographs, but tomography may be necessary particularly for the diagnosis of the internal type (Fig. 93.99). The external laryngocele appears as a sharply defined oval or round radiolucent area protruding into the soft tissues of the neck lateral to the hyoid and the thyroid cartilage. There may be clinical and radiological confusion with a lateral pharyngeal diverticulum, as both may be distended by the Valsalva

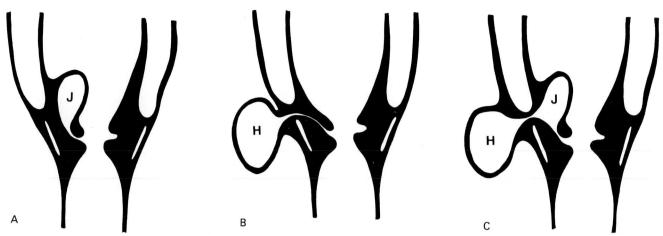

Fig. 93.98 Types of laryngocele. (a) Internal laryngocele. An air filled sac [J] arises from the laryngeal ventricle and bulges into the vestibule. (b) External laryngocele. The air filled sac [H] lies entirely outside the larynx. (c) Combined type. There are internal [J] and external [H] laryngoceles which communicate with one another and with the laryngeal ventricle.

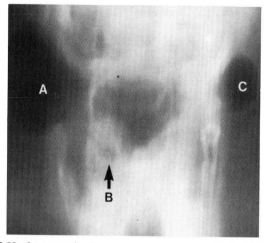

Fig. 93.99 Laryngocele. Tomogram showing an air filled sac [A] due to an external laryngocele seen lying in the right side of the neck, communicating with a smaller sac [B] due to an internal laryngocele lying in the vestibular fold. Small left sided external laryngocele [C].

manoeuvre. However, when the patient relaxes, the lateral pharyngeal diverticulum usually collapses, whereas the laryngocele remains distended. The laryngocele can sometimes be emptied by gentle external pressure. In addition, barium swallow examination will produce mucosal coating of a pharyngeal diverticulum, but not of a laryngocele.

An internal laryngocele is best demonstrated by tomography as it may be obscured by the spine on the anteroposterior radiograph. The radiological features consist of an air-containing space lying within an enlarged vestibular fold. If the laryngocele is large, there is usually displacement of the larynx to the opposite side with partial obstruction of the vestibule of the larynx. An internal laryngocele may also be shown on the lateral radiograph when it appears as a clearly defined radiolucent area lying in the anterosuperior aspect of the larynx which may extend from the level of the laryngeal ventricle to the hyoid bone.

RECURRENT LARYNGEAL NERVE PARALYSIS

Clinical methods are usually employed in the diagnosis of vocal cord paralysis. If the cords cannot be seen, a radiological examination can be carried out. This is most simply achieved by television fluoroscopy which, without the use of contrast agents, will readily demonstrate the vocal cords and will show the loss of movement on the affected side. Plain radiographs however often fail to show the vocal cords and tomography is more diagnostic. Coronal tomograms show some thickening of the affected side of the larynx with enlargement of the ventricle and flattening of the subglottic angle. The paralysed vocal cord may not be recognized on the phonation film, but will remain in an unchanged position on the resting film (Fig. 93.100).

There are numerous causes of recurrent laryngeal nerve paralysis. It occurs most frequently on the left side because of its long intrathoracic course and may result from tumours,

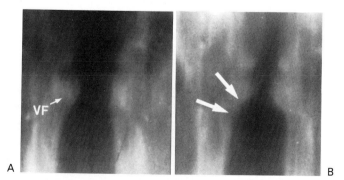

Fig. 93.100 Recurrent laryngeal nerve paralysis. (A) On quiet respiration the vocal fold [VF] lies in the adducted position. (B) Phonation. Note the relatively obtuse subglottic angle [arrows] compared with the normal side.

aneurysms, and following surgical procedures in the mediastinum and thyroid. Unilateral vocal cord paralysis in infancy may present with respiratory obstruction.

EXTRINSIC DISPLACEMENT AND COMPRESSION OF THE LARYNX

A mass in the neck may displace the trachea and larynx to the opposite side. Lymphadenopathy due to *Hodgkin's* disease is a common cause.

Thyroid tumours may cause marked displacement and compression of the trachea may occur. Compression is usually most marked in association with malignant thyroid swellings (Fig. 93.101) and with Riedel's thyroiditis. Malignant thyroid swellings may also extend between the trachea and the oesophagus causing oesophageal compression and displacement. Other rarer causes of tracheal and laryngeal displacement include *branchial cysts* and *chemodectomas* of the carotid body.

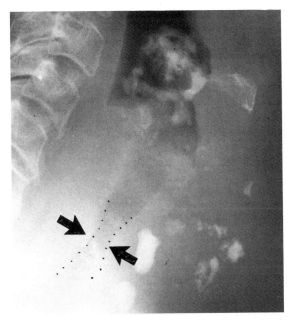

Fig. 93.101 Carcinoma of the thyroid. Lateral projection showing severe tracheal stenosis [arrows] associated with the large partly calcified thyroid mass.

BIBLIOGRAPHY

REFERENCES

1. Spitzer R, Robinson M I 1955 Radiological changes in teeth and skull of mental defectives. Br J Radiol 28:117–127
2. Bilaniuk L T, Zimmerman R A 1982 Symposium on neuroradiology: computed tomography in evaluation of the paranasal sinuses. Radiol Clin North Am 20:51–66
3. Edell S L, Isaacson S 1978 A-Mode ultrasound evaluation of the maxillary sinus. Otolaryngol Clin North Am 11:531–540
4. Centeno R S, Bentson J R, Mancuso A A 1981 CT scanning in rhinocerebral mucormycosis and aspergillosis. Radiology 140:383–389
5. Greyson N D, Noyek A M 1978 Nuclear medicine in otolaryngological diagnosis. Otolaryngol Clin North Am 11:541–560
6. Som P M, Shugar J M A 1980 Antral mucoceles: a new look. J Comput Assist Tomogr 4:484–488
7. Jackson A R 1977 Bone thinning in frontal mucoceles. Br J Radiol 50:181–184
8. Potter D G 1972 Tomography of the orbit. Radiol Clin North Am 10:21–38
9. Price H I, Danziger A 1980 Computerised tomographic findings in mucoceles of the frontal and ethmoid sinuses. Clin Radiol 31:169–174
10. Lloyd G A S, Bartram C I, Stanley P 1974 Ethmoid mucoceles. Br J Radiol 47:646–651
11. Lloyd G A S 1971 Axial tomography of the orbits and paranasal sinuses. Br J Radiol 44:373–379
12. Merland J J, Melki J P, Chiras J, Riche M C, Hadjean E 1980 The place of embolization in the treatment of severe epistaxis. Laryngoscope 90:1694–1704
13. Zizmor J, Noyek A M 1968 Cysts and benign tumours of the paranasal sinuses. Semin Roentgenol 3:172–201
14. Rothfield P, Shapiro R, Lasser A, Kent D 1977 Epithelial (inverted) papilloma: a correlated radiological histological study. Clin Radiol 28:530–544
15. Dodd G D, Collins L C, Egan R L, Herrera J R 1959 The systematic use of tomography in the diagnosis of carcinoma of the paranasal sinuses. Radiology 72:379–392
16. Hesselink J R, New P F J, Davis K R, Weber A L, Robertson G H, Taveras J M 1978 Computed tomography of the paranasal sinuses and face: part II pathological anatomy. J Comput Assist Tomogr 2:568–576
17. Jing B S, Goepfert H, Close L G 1978 Computerised tomography of paranasal sinus neoplasms. Laryngoscope 88:1485–1503
18. Forbes W St C F, Fawcitt R A, Isherwood I, Webb R, Farrington T 1978 Computed Tomography in the diagnosis of diseases of the paranasal sinuses. Clin Radiol 29:501–511
19. Jeans W D, Gilani S, Bullimore J 1982 The effect of CT scanning on staging of tumours of the paranasal sinuses. Clin Radiol 33:173–179
20. Chin F K, Anderson W B, Gilbertson J D 1970 Radiation dose to critical organs during petrous tomography. Radiology 94:623–627
21. Shaffer K A, Haughton V M, Wilson C R 1980 High resolution computed tomography of the temporal bone. Radiology 134:409–414
22. Lloyd G A S, du Boulay G H, Phelps P D, Pullicino P 1979 The demonstration of the auditory ossicles by high resolution CT. Neuroradiology 18:243–248
23. Tillit R, Wilner H I, Conner G H, Eyler W R 1970 The large mastoid antrum. Radiology 94:619–624
24. Valvassori G E, Pierce R H 1964 The normal internal auditory canal. Am J Roentgenol 92:1232–1241
25. Lin S R, Lee K F, Stein G N 1973 Asymmetrical internal auditory canals. Arch Otolaryngol 98:164–169
26. Phelps P D, Lloyd G A S 1980 The radiology of cholesteatoma. Clin Radiol 31:501–512
27. Buckingham R A, Valvassori G E 1970 Tomographic and surgical pathology of cholesteatoma. Arch Otolaryngol 91:464–469
28. Rovsing H, Jensen J 1968 Tomographic visualisation of labyrinthine fistula. Radiology 90:261–267
29. Brunner S, Sandberg L E 1970 Tomography in cholesteatoma and chronic otitis media. Arch Otolaryngol 91:560–567
30. Jensen J, Rovsing H, Brunner S 1966 Tomography of the inner ear in otosclerosis. Br J Radiol 39:669–672
31. Valvassori G E, Clemis J D 1976 Abnormal vestibular aqueduct in cochleovestibular disorders. Adv Otorhinolaryngol 24:100–105
32. Wilbrand H F 1976 Tomography in Menières disease — why and how. Morphological, clinical and radiographic aspects. Adv Otorhinolaryngol 24:71–93
33. Lagundoye S B, Martinson F D, Fajemisin A A 1975 Tomography of the petrous bone in keratosis obturans. Br J Radiol 48:170–175
34. Britton B H 1974 Glomus tympanicum and glomus jugulare tumours. Radiol clin North Am 12:543–551

35. O'Callaghan J, Timperley W R, Ward P 1979 The CT scan and subtraction angiography in chemodectomas. Clin Radiol 30:575–580

36. Kendall B, Moseley I 1977 Therapeutic embolisation of the external carotid arterial tree. J Neurol Neurosurg Psychiatry 40:937–950

37. Holgate R C, Wortzmann G, Noyek A M, Makerewicz L, Coates R M 1977 Pulsatile tinnitus: the role of angiography. J Otolaryngol 6:49–62

38. Hitselberger W E, Witten R M 1969 Jugular Venography. Arch Otolaryngol 89:167–169

39. Phelps P D, Lloyd G A S 1981 The radiology of carcinoma of the ear. Br J Radiol 54:103–109

40. Goldman A M, Martin J E 1970 Tumours involving the temporal bone. Radiol clin North Am 8:387–402

41. Valvassori G E 1969 The abnormal internal auditory canal. The diagnosis of acoustic neuroma. Radiology 92:449–459

42. David K R, Parker S W, New P F J et al 1977 Computed tomography of acoustic neuroma. Radiology 124:81–86

43. Thompson J L G 1978 Computerized axial tomography in posterior fossa lesions. Clin Radiol 29:1–8

44. Valvanis A, Schubiger O, Wellauer J 1978 Computed tomography of acoustic neuromas with emphasis on small tumour detectability. Neuroradiology 16:598–600

45. Burrows E H 1969 Scintigraphic diagnosis of acoustic neurofibromas. Br J Radiol 48:1000–1006

46. Valvassori G E 1972 Myelography of the internal auditory canal Am J Roentgenol 115:578–586

47. Valvanis A, Dabir K, Hamdi R, Oguz M, Wellauer J 1982. The current state of the radiological diagnosis of acoustic neuroma. Neuroradiology 23:7–13

48. Phelps P D, Lloyd G A S 1982 High resolution air CT meatography: the demonstration of normal and abnormal structures in the cerebellopontine cistern and internal auditory meatus. Br J Radiol 55:19–22

49. Taylor S 1982 Symposium on neuroradiology: the petrous temporal bone (including the cerebello-pontine angle). Radiol Clin North Am 20:67–86

50. Wright J W 1974 Trauma to the ear. Radiol Clin North Am 12:527–532

51. Potter G D 1973 Trauma of the ear. Otolaryngol clin North Am 6:401–412

52. Frey K W 1965 Die Tomographie der Labyrinthmissbildungen. Fortsch Geb Roentgstrahl 102:1–13

53. Phelps P D, Lloyd G A S, Sheldon P W E 1977 Congenital deformities of the middle and external ear. Br J Radiol 50:714–727

54. Fitz C R, Harwood-Nash D C F 1974 Radiology of the ear in children. Radiol Clin North Am 12:553–570

55. Phelps P D, Lloyd G A S 1978 Congenital deformity of the internal auditory meatus and labyrinth associated with cerebrospinal fluid fistula. Adv Oto-rhino-laryng 24:51–57

56. Phelps P D, Lloyd G A S, Sheldon P W E 1975 Deformity of the labyrinth and internal auditory meatus in congenital deafness. Br J Radiol 48:973–978

57. Mancuso A A Bohman L, Hanafee W, Maxwell D 1980 CT of the nasopharynx — normal and variants of normal. Radiology 137:113–121

58. Bohman L, Mancuso A, Thompson J, Hanafee W 1981. CT approach to benign nasopharyngeal masses. Am J Roentgenol 136:173–180

59. Samuel E, Lloyd G A S 1978 Clinical radiology of the ear, nose, and throat, 2nd Edn. Lewis, London p 224

60. Holman C B, Miller W E 1968 Juvenile nasopharyngeal fibroma. Am J Roentgenol 94:292–298

61. Duckert L G, Carley R B, Hilger J A 1978 Computerized axial tomography in the preoperative evaluation of an angiofibroma. Laryngoscope 88:613–618

62. Wilson G H, Hanafee W N 1969 Angiographic findings in 16 patients with juvenile angiofibroma. Radiology 92:279–284

63. Roberson G H, Price A C, Davis J M, Gulati J 1979 Therapeutic embolization of juvenile angiofibroma. Am J Roentgenol 133:657–663

64. Johnson T H, Green A E, Rise E N 1967 Nasopharyngography — its technique and uses. Radiology 80:1166–1169

65. Wastie M L 1972 The value of tomography in carcinoma of the nasopharynx. Br J Radiol 45:570–574

66. Carter B L, Karmody C S 1978 Computed tomography of the face and neck. Seminars in Roentgenology 8:257–266

67. Schwartz E E, Tucker J A, Holt G P 1981 Cervical dysphagia: pharyngeal protrusions and achalasia. Clin Radiol 32:643–650

68. Ekberg O 1981 Cervical oesophageal webs in patients with dysphagia. Clin Radiol 32:633–641

69. Lindvall N 1953 Hypopharyngeal carcinoma in sideropenic dysphagia. Acta Radiol (Diagn) Stockh 39:17–37

70. Noyek A M, Steinhardt M I, Zizmor J 1978 Xeroradiography in otolaryngology. Otolaryngol Clin N Am 11:445–456

71. Julian W L, Noscoe N J, Berry R J 1981 Xerographic tomography of the larynx. Clin Radiol 32:577–583

72. Powers W E, McGee H H Jr, Seaman W B 1957 Contrast examination of the larynx and pharynx. Radiology 68:169–178

73. Parsons C A, Chapman P, Counter R T, Grundy A 1980 The role of computed tomography in tumours of the larynx. Clin Radiol 31:529–533

74. Jing B S 1975 Roentgen examination of laryngeal cancer: a critical evaluation. Can J Otolaryng 4:64–73

75. Archer C R, Sagel S S, Yeager V L, Martin S, Friedman W H 1981 Staging of carcinoma of the larynx: comparative accuracy of CT and laryngography. Am J Roentgenol 136:571–575

76. Mancuso A A, Calcaterra T C, Hanafee W N 1978 Computed tomography of the larynx. Radiol Clin N Am 16:195–208

77. Hateley W, Evison G, Samuel E 1965 The pattern of ossification in the laryngeal cartilages: a radiological study. Br J Radiol 38:585–595

78. Greene R, Stark P 1978 Trauma of the larynx and trachea, Radiol Clin N Am 16:309–320

79. Giovanniello J, Grieco V, Bartone N F 1970 Laryngocele. Am J Roentgenol 108:825–829

SUGGESTIONS FOR FURTHER READING

Bilaniuk L T, Zimmerman R A 1982 Computed tomography in evaluation of the paranasal sinuses. Radiol Clin North Am 20 (1):51–66
An up to date summary of the present status of C.T.

Di Guiglielmo L 1977 Xerography in otolaryngology. Exerpta Medica, Amsterdam.
Mainly an atlas, but beautifully illustrated.

Glazer H S, Mauro M H, Aronberg D J, Lee J K T, Johnston D E, Sagel S S 1982 CT of laryngoceles. Am J Roentgenol 140:549–552

Greene R, Stark P 1978 Trauma of the larynx and trachea. Radiol Clin North Am 16 (2):309–320

Guinto F C Jr, Himadi G M 1974 Tomographic anatomy of the ear. Radiol Clin North Am 12 (3):405–417
The clearest available account of the anatomy of a complex region.

Jing B S 1978 Malignant tumours of the larynx. Radiol Clin North Am 16 (2):247–260

Littleton J T, Shaffer K A, Callahan W P, Durizch M L 1981 Temporal bone: comparison of pluridirectional tomography and high resolution computed tomography. Am J Roentgenol 137:834–845

Lloyd G A S, Phelps P D 1982 The investigation of petro-mastoid tumours by high resolution CT. Br J Radiol 55:483–491
These authors have contributed much to the CT literature relating to the ear.

Mafee M F, Kumar A, Yannias D A, Valvassori G E, Applebaum E L 1983 CT of the middle ear in the evaluation of cholesteatoma and other soft tissue masses. Comparison with pluridirectional tomography. Radiology 148:465–472

Momose K J, Macmillan A S Jr 1978 Roentgenologic investigation of the larynx and trachea. Radiol Clin North Am 16 (2):309–320

Phelps P D, Lloyd G A S 1983 Radiology of the ear. Blackwell Scientific Publications, Oxford
Modern account well illustrated with many examples of the application of high resolution CT.

Samuel E, Lloyd G A S 1978 Clinical radiology of the ear, nose and throat, 2nd edn. Lewis, London
Becoming somewhat dated in some respects, but nevertheless useful and comprehensive, albeit lacking significant CT.

Swartz J D 1983 High resolution computed tomography of the middle ear and mastoid. Part 1: Normal radio-anatomy including normal variations. Radiology 148:449–454

Swartz J D, Goodman R S, Russel K B, Ladenheim S E, Wolfson R J 1983 High resolution computed tomography of the middle ear and mastoid. Part 3: Surgically altered anatomy and pathology. Radiology 148:461–464

Swartz J D, Goodman R S, Russel K B, Marlow F I, Wolfson R J 1983 High resolution computed tomography of the middle ear and mastoid. Part 2: Tubo-tympanic disease. Radiology 148:455–459

Taylor S 1982 The petrous temporal bone (including the cerebello-pontine angle). Radiol Clin North Am 20 (1): 67–86
An up to date account including high quality CT.

Unger J D, Shaffer K A 1980 Ear, nose and throat radiology. Saunders, Philadelphia
Light, stimulating and readable.

Valvassori G E, Potter G D, Hanafee W N, Carter B L, Buckingham R A 1982 Radiology of the ear, nose and throat. Saunders, Philadelphia
Authoritative, up to date and well illustrated account.

Zizmor J 1978 An atlas of otolaryngologic radiology. Saunders, Philadelphia

SECTION

11

Angiography Interventional Radiology and Other Techniques

Editor: David J. Allison

Contents
94 Arteriography *David J. Allison*
95 Phlebography *Anne P. Hemingway*
96 Digital subtraction angiography *Thomas F. Meaney, Meredith A. Weinstein*
97 Vascular ultrasound *H. Meire*
98 Interventional radiology *David J. Allison*
99 Radiology in oncology *Colin Parsons*
100 Nuclear medicine in oncology *William D. Kaplan*
101 Paediatric nuclear medicine *H. Theodore Harcke*
102 Paediatric ultrasonography *Constantine Metreweli*
103 Ultrasonography of the infant brain *Keith Dewbury*

94 Arteriography

D. J. Allison

History

Technique
  Equipment
    Needles, wires, catheters & sheaths
    Contrast media
    Injection apparatus
    Radiographic apparatus
  Methods
    Introduction
    Patient preparation
    Contraindications
    Anaesthesia
    Arterial puncture & catheterization
    Selective catheterization
    Aftercare
    Radiographic considerations
    Special techniques
  Complications
    Contrast medium related complications
    Adverse drug reactions
    Puncture site complications
    Catheter-related and general complications

Vascular disorders
  Congenital abnormalities
  Vascular malformations
    Predominantly arterial lesions
    Capillary or small vessel malformations
    Venous (cavernous) haemangiomas
  Arteriovenous fistula
  Aneurysms
    Congenital aneurysms
    Infective aneurysms
    Degenerative aneurysms
    Dissecting aneurysms
    Post-stenotic aneurysms
    Traumatic aneurysms
    Post-inflammatory aneurysms
    Cirsoid aneurysms
  Atheroma
    Medial sclerosis
  Arteritis
    Infective arteritis
    Necrotizing arteritis

Giant cell arteritis
Takayashu's arteritis
Thromboangiitis obliterans
Stenosis, thrombosis and embolism
  Stenosis
  Fibromuscular hyperplasia
  Standing waves
  Thrombosis
  Leriche syndrome
  Subclavian steal syndrome
  Embolism
Ischaemia
Haemorrhage
Tumours
  Diagnosis
  Localization
  Site of origin
  Operability
  Treatment
Trauma
Arterial embolization
Percutaneous transluminal angioplasty

Regional arteriography
  Head and neck
    Arch aortography
    Common carotid arteriography
    External carotid arteriography
    Internal carotid arteriography
  Thorax and abdomen
    Thoracic aortography
    Cardiac and pulmonary arteriography
    Bronchial arteriography
    Lumbar aortography
    Pelvic arteriography
    Renal arteriography
    Gastrointestinal arteriography
  The upper extremity
  The lower extremity
  The endocrine organs
    Pituitary gland
    Parathyroid glands
    Adrenal gland
    Pancreas

HISTORY

The medical and scientific significance of the ability to visualize vascular structures radiographically was recognized from the earliest days of radiology. In January 1896, just one year after Roentgen had delivered his historic manuscript reporting the discovery of X–rays to the Physical Medical Society of Wurzburg, Haschek and Lindenthal produced a radiograph showing the injected vessels of an amputated hand [1]. During the next two decades detailed X–ray studies were obtained of the vascular systems in animals and man for anatomical purposes by workers in both Europe and America [2], and it is astonishing to reflect on the fact that the first X–ray atlas of the arterial tree was published (in England) as long ago as 1920 [3]. During the 1920s attention turned to obtaining arteriograms *in vivo*, and substances such as Lipiodol, strontium bromide, sodium iodide and Selectan were used in man to obtain peripheral arteriograms and venograms, aortic and pulmonary arteriograms, and even cerebral arteriograms. Portuguese workers such as Egas Moniz, Reynaldo dos Santos and Lopo de Carvalho were pre-eminent among the pioneers of human arteriography [4], and the extent of their contribution has not been sufficiently acknowledged by many of those who have followed in their footsteps. The significance of the work they did was not lost on their contemporaries, however; when Moniz returned to Portugal after presenting his epoch-making paper entitled 'arterial encephalography, its importance in the localization of brain tumours' to the Academy of Medicine in Paris in 1928, he received a saluation from the combined professors of the Medicine Faculty at the railway station! [5]. Another pioneer in the field of arteriography was Forssmann who was particularly interested in techniques for visualizing the heart and pulmonary vessels [6]. In 1928 after practising on a cadaver, he passed a catheter from his own antecubital vein into the right atrium, a procedure that not only paved the way for all subsequent development in cardiac catheterization, but must also surely be remembered as one of the most courageous feats of self-experimentation in modern medicine.

In the early days of arteriography vessel exposure by incision was required for vascular catheterization and though this technique is still used in certain circumstances (see below), percutaneous arterial puncture is the preferred method in most cases. Percutaneous puncture was used at first simply to introduce contrast medium directly through a needle into a vessel, and this technique was used successfully for translumbar aortography as long ago as 1929 [7]. It was even used for thoracic aortography by Nuvoli in 1936 [8], and was applied to many other more accessible vessels. A major advance came with the introduction of percutaneous techniques for the introduction of catheters into blood vessels [9,10] and the *percutaneous catheter replacement technique of Seldinger* [11] introduced in 1953 soon became (and remains) the most widely used method of angiographic catheterization. As arterial puncture and catheterization techniques developed, together with improvements in contrast media and catheters and the introduction of rapid film-changers, it

became possible to obtain high quality arteriograms of all the principal vascular beds in the body. Arteriography rapidly occupied a vital place in diagnostic medicine and became not only a indispensable investigation in branches such as vascular surgery, cardiac surgery and neurosurgery, but played no small part in influencing the actual direction of development of these and other specialities.

During the 1970s it seemed that arteriography, having reached its apparent zenith, was about to face a slow decline in importance as many of its roles were supplanted by less invasive and, for the most part, easier imaging techniques such as ultrasound, isotope studies, computerized tomography, and, more recently, magnetic resonance imaging. While it is true that arteriography will probably never regain the dominant position it once held in many fields of diagnosis, there are three recent factors which seem certain to secure it an important place in radiology for many years to come. The first of these is the development of digital vascular imaging (DVI), also known as digital subtraction angiography (DSA). This technique, described in detail in Chapter 96, enables high quality vascular images to be obtained using only very small volumes of intra-arterial contrast medium. For many purposes sufficient detail of the arteries can be obtained using only an intravenous injection of contrast medium. The second important factor influencing modern arteriographic practice is the introduction of a new generation of contrast media. These media, described in detail in Chapter 7, do not give the sensation of intense heat or pain that conventional contrast agents induce when injected into vessels. They also cause less damage to the vascular endothelium and have fewer systemic toxic effects than the older agents. Finally, a development which seems certain to assure a place for the angiographer in our departments of the future is the advent of interventional vascular radiology. Interventional radiology is described in detail in Chapter 98 where it can be seen that many of its techniques (notably selective perfusion, embolization and angioplasty) depend upon good arteriographic technique for their success. With increasing specialization in radiology it seems inevitable that the arteriographer of the future will be called upon to perform these interventional procedures, and there is probably no branch of radiology that will make greater demands on the clinical judgement and technical expertise of the radiologist.

TECHNIQUE

Equipment

1. Needles, wires, catheters and sheaths

Needles

There are many different arterial puncture needles available commercially and some common examples are shown in Figure 94.1. Most conform to a fairly standard manufacturer. Detailed dimensions can be obtained from specialist texts [2] or the various manufacturers' specification sheets, but most needles used in adults are approximately 1.2 mm in outside diameter and accept a standard 0.038 inch guide wire. The length of the needle is usually between 7 cm and 12 cm. Smaller needles are used in children, and larger needles (o.d. 1.6 mm; length 20 cm) are used for translumbar aortography.

Guide wires

A wide variety of guide wires is commercially available (Fig. 94.2A). The basic requirement of a wire is that it should be stiff enough to carry a catheter across a percutaneous track into a vessel without buckling, yet at the same time be flexible enough to pass along curves and bends in the vascular system with the minimum possible trauma. It is particularly important that the tip of the wire is soft and flexible; it is this first segment of wire that is most likely to cause damage as it is advanced through the arterial lumen,

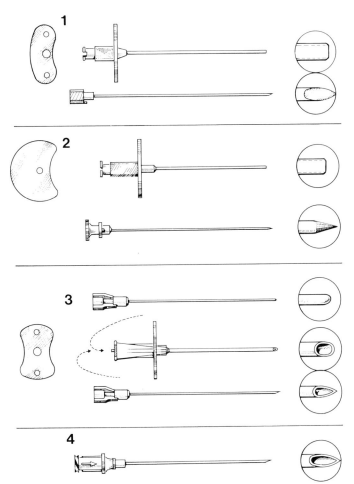

Fig. 94.1 Some examples of arterial puncture needles in common use:

1. Disposable needle with solid, bevelled-tip, central stylet
2. 'Pencil-point' needle
3. Disposable three-piece needle incorporating hollow, bevelled-tip stylet and blunt, solid stylet
4. Simple one-piece disposable needle with bevelled tip.

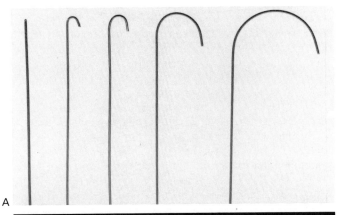

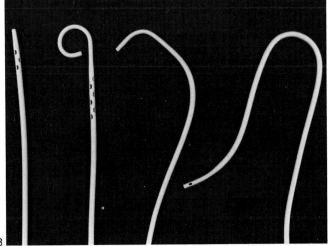

Fig. 94.2A & B Some examples of guide-wires (A) and catheters (B) in common use. (A) The curved wires shown ('J' wires) vary in radius of curvature from 1.5 mm to 15 mm. (B) Some of the many different available catheter shapes are illustrated. From left to right: straight 'flush'; 'pig-tail'; 'cobra'; and 'side-winder'. Note the side-ports on some of the catheters.

basic design, which incorporates an inner obturator or stylet with an outer needle or cannula. The inner stylet can be removed when the needle is in the lumen of the artery and replaced with a guide wire of appropriate diameter. In some needles the central stylet is sharp and the outer cannula blunt so that the latter can be safely advanced in the vessel with minimal risk of damage to the vascular wall once the sharp stylet has been removed. In other needles there is a sharp outer needle with a central blunt obturator which can be passed beyond the tip of the needle. In some systems both the cannula and its stylet are sharp and in yet others there is a flexible outer sheath of Teflon or similar material which can be left in the artery when all the rigid metal parts have been removed. The 'pencil point' needle has a pointed central stylet and a blunt cannula; it is a very useful needle for the beginner to use (see below). The *dimensions* of needles vary enormously according to the needle type, the purpose for which it is to be used and the and the first few centimeters of most guide wires are made more flexible than the rest of the wire. Standard wires vary in diameter from 0.025–0.038 inches though very fine and very thick wires are available for specialized techniques. The length of most standard wires is between 100–150 cm, but very long wires (*exchange* wires) of 260 cm may be used when it is desirable to exchange a catheter for one of a different shape while keeping the tip of the wire in a selected vascular site. Guide wires with a straight tip cannot always be advanced through tortuous or diseased arteries without damaging the intima. For this reason it is sometimes necessary to use a *J-shaped wire* [12,13,14] (Fig. 94.2A). The tip of such a wire can be straightened in order to introduce the wire through a percutaneous needle; once the tip escapes from the needle lumen, however, it adopts the J-configuration which creates a smooth, curved leading end to the wire. This is much easier to negotiate around a sharp bend in a vessel than a straight wire, and it is also much less likely to embed itself in a plaque of atheroma, possibly causing dissection or perforation of a vessel. Several different diameters of J-curve are available (Fig. 94.2A). Only the wires with a J of radius 3 mm or less, however, are intended to form a complete 'J' within the vessel lumen as described above. The larger diameter wires are simply used to direct the tip of an advancing catheter into a selective vessel when this is proving difficult with the catheter alone. *Tip-deflecting* and *variable stiffness* wires have a moveable core which can be manipulated inside the wire to change the shape or stiffness of the end of the wire; they are sometimes used in selective techniques or interventional procedures, as are *heavy duty* wires which are more resistant to buckling forces than conventional wires. *Teflon-coated* wires [15] are thought to reduce the risk of clotting and, having a low friction coefficient, are the preferred wires to use with polyurethane catheters. The smoothness and integrity of a guide wire is essential to the safety of the vascular procedure being performed and it is hardly necessary to point out that a kinked or otherwise damaged wire should never be used.

Catheters

Most modern catheters are made of polyethylene, polyurethene or Teflon and are radio-opaque. Some catheters incorporate wire meshwork into their wall to give superior strength and torque-control. A discussion of the *pros* and *cons* of the different catheter materials is beyond the scope of this chapter, but in general terms the type of material influences the stiffness and flexibility of the catheter, its ability to be shaped at different temperatures, the smoothness of its walls and its friction coefficient, its ability to be tapered and its general 'handling' characteristics.

Catheters may have a single hole (or 'port') at the end (for very selective injections), an end-hole together with side-holes, or a blocked end with side-holes only. The holes are clustered near the tip of the catheter to concentrate the bolus of contrast delivered. There are several reasons for having side-holes in a catheter: they increase the rate at which contrast medium can be injected through the catheter; by dispersing the direction of exit of contrast medium from the catheter they reduce the 'jet' effect of the injection thereby preventing recoil of the catheter tip; and they minimize the risk of dissection of the artery for if one or more of the ports are not lying freely in the lumen of the vessel the contrast medium can still escape through the exposed ports. Extra ports can be made in the catheter using a commercially available punch but care should be taken if this is done not to weaken the catheter unduly nor to place a port on the outer curve of a shaped catheter which would allow the inadvertent passage of a guide wire through the hole instead of the catheter lumen.

Catheters come in a variety of sizes and shapes (Fig. 94.2B). Catheters intended principally for abdominal use are usually 60–80 cm in length; those intended for use in the thorax or carotid territories 100–120 cm. The external diameters of different catheters are usually referred to in French Sizes. The sizes used most commonly in adult diagnostic work are 5F–7F. In children smaller sizes may be used, and in interventional work larger sizes are occasionally needed for some angioplasty procedures. For specialized selective work a *co-axial* system may be used where a small catheter (e.g. 3F) is passed down inside a larger catheter (e.g. 7F), and in interventional work various *balloon catheters* are used. Some of these are *flow-guided* and some have *detachable* balloons for embolization. A number of catheter manipulating instruments exist which allow the catheter tip to be deflected in one or more planes to achieve a super-selective position. The value of these *steerable catheters* is generally overrated and experienced angiographers do most of their selective work with simple pre-shaped catheters. Generally speaking it is good practice to use the smallest diameter catheter feasible for any particular study to minimize the risk of arterial damage by the procedure [2,16]. The smaller the catheter, however, the lower the rate at which contrast medium can be injected, and the torque control of smaller catheters is usually appreciably inferior to that of larger catheters. Recent advances in catheter technology have improved both the torque control and delivery rate of smaller catheters and this, together with the introduction of digital vascular imaging which greatly reduces the need for large contrast doses, will almost certainly accelerate the trend towards the use of smaller gauge catheters in vascular work.

The shape of a catheter is very important (Fig. 94.2B). *Straight* catheters with multiple side-ports are used for rapid injection into large vessels such as the aorta. *'Pig-tail'* or similarly shaped catheters are also used for general injections into large arteries such as the thoracic or lumbar aorta, pulmonary artery, and the cardiac cavities where the risk of subintimal or subendocardial injection is thereby minimized and good mixing achieved to avoid contrast 'streaming'. The *cobra* and *sidewinder* shapes shown in Figure 94.2B are useful for a variety of selective examinations (see below), and many other shapes have been described for particular types of arteriography, particularly in the carotid and coronary circulations. Note that the sidewinder catheter illustrated in Fig. 94.2B is shaped like a shepherd's crook and it is in this configuration that the catheter is mostly used for the selective catheterization of aortic branches. The catheter is straightened outside the body for introduction into the vascular system over a guidewire in the normal way; the tip is temporarily introduced into a branch vessel (usually the left subclavian), the catheter is allowed to fold at the pre-shaped 'knuckle' and the whole catheter then advanced so that the free limb is withdrawn from its sidebranch. The catheter is then available in its sidewinder configuration for the selective catheterization of any other chosen branch (see Figs. 94.14 and 94.17). The 'turning' of the catheter can be performed in vessels other than the left subclavian (e.g. opposite common iliac) but most operators are most consistently successful using the subclavian technique. When used in the carotid arteries a sidewinder catheter can often be introduced directly into the common carotid vessels without the preliminary turning procedure described above.

Some radiologists still like to shape their own catheters for a particular purpose using a heat source such as a steam kettle.

Sheaths and dilators

Instead of exchanging arterial catheters over a guide wire, some operators prefer to work through a sheath, particularly if several changes of catheter are envisaged during a procedure. The flexible sheath is itself introduced into the artery over a guide wire by means of a tapered *introducer*. The introducer is then removed and replaced by a catheter. Some sheaths have a haemostatic valve which prevents the reflux of blood between the catheter and sheath. Although sheaths obviate frictional trauma to the wall of the artery during catheter manipulation they require a larger hole in the artery than does the catheter alone, and they can be inadvertently dislodged from the artery by a backward movement of the catheter. This may at first pass unobserved during fluoroscopy resulting in haemorrhage or haematoma.

The sheath introducer can be used on its own as a *vessel dilator*. When polyurethane catheters are used it is essential to dilate the arterial puncture site prior to insertion of the catheter as polyurethane cannot be tapered to a fine tip. Dilatation of the puncture site is also helpful prior to the introduction of a catheter into a groin which is fibrotic owing to a previous procedure, inflammation or trauma.

Dilators are now supplied with Luer fittings and can be used alone for arterial injection into the iliac or femoral arteries. They are longer and more flexible than a needle, yet shorter and more convenient than a catheter.

Injections made through needles, dilators or other short sheaths should always be made through intermediate connecting tubing. This reduces the radiation dose to the operator during a hand injection, and minimizes the risk of the intra arterial cannula becoming dislodged during either a hand or a mechanical injection. All taps used on intra arterial needles, cannulae or catheters should have interlocking fittings to minimize the risk of inadvertent disconnection.

2. Contrast media

For arteriography we ideally require a medium that gives good contrast, possesses a low viscosity (for rapidity of injection) and is non-toxic. The early contrast agents unfortunately exhibited a number of toxic side-effects and one of the best-known examples of this is given by the substance known as thorotrast (thorium dioxide). Thorotrast was an excellent contrast medium but instead of being excreted from the body it was stored in the reticuloendothelial system and, as a radioactive substance, it ultimately induced malignant tumours. The plain film appearances of a patient who had been studied with thorotrast were very characteristic (see Fig. 54.1), and the opacities in the spleen could be seen even many years after the original arteriogram.

The contrast media that have been in almost universal use for angiography during the past decade such as the sodium and methylglucamine diatrizoates and metrizoates are now being superseded by a new generation of low osmolality media such as iohexol, iopamidol and ioxaglate which are subjectively more pleasant for the patient and are less toxic in many ways than previous media. For more detailed information concerning the various contrast media the reader is referred to Chapter 7.

3. Injection apparatus

Contrast medium injected at hand pressure will produce adequate opacification of the smaller vascular beds, but it is necessary to use a pressure injector when injecting into large vessels with rapid flow such as the aorta, pulmonary artery, coeliac axis, etc. Various injectors are available commercially and some of these have extremely sophisticated control systems which give wide ranges of possible pressure and flow, different shaped injection pressure curves, and automatic exposure timing devices which can trigger radiographic exposures at the most appropriate instant in the injection sequence. Digital vascular imaging may reduce the requirement of automatic injections in some circumstances owing to the enhanced imaged quality such systems provide; in a department with only conventional imaging equipment, however, it is not possible to provide a proper arteriographic service without a rate-controlled automatic pressure injector.

4. Radiographic apparatus

Good equipment is a vital factor in producing good arteriograms. When contrast medium is injected into vessel with rapid flow it is necessary to take rapid serial films in order to obtain the necessary information. This is particularly true when a pathologically high flow exists as in, say, an arteriovenous fistula when it will be impossible to delineate the anatomy of the abnormal vessels unless a rapid filming sequence is possible. Where very rapid changes are occurring, as in the heart, *cine radiography* is necessary, but for most other arteriography a rapid series of cut films is adequate. Several types of automatic cut-film changer are available and some of these allow speeds of up to six films a second.

Many radiologists now prefer to take *smaller format* rapid sequence films using a 105 mm or similarly sized camera, and the most modern systems include a *digital subtraction* facility (Chapter 96). A high power tube is necessary for angiography and the design of the stand and table is very important. Ideally it should not be necessary for the patient to move once a catheter has been manipulated into the desired position yet it may be essential to obtain views in different projections. Modern tables allow re-orientation of the tube and film-changer through a very wide range of movement while the patient remains still. A *moving top* table permits successive exposures to be made at different centering points while the table carries the patient across the tube axis. This means that films of the aorta, pelvis and legs can be obtained from a single aortic injection. On the most modern stands even this function can be carried out without any movement of the patient.

A *video recorder* is a useful item of equipment that permits the instant review of fluoroscopic recordings. It is particularly valuable in cardiac angiography and in interventional radiology.

It is very easy to waste film and expose the patient to an unnecessarily high dose of radiation during arteriography. Filming sequences should be carefully planned to make only those exposures that will contribute definite diagnostic information. The unnecessary use of very rapid serial exposures is one of the commonest errors in arteriography.

Methods

1. Introduction

The risks associated with modern arteriography are extremely small. Arteriography is still nevertheless an 'invasive' procedure and it should never be undertaken unless the radiologist is satisfied that the likely benefits justify the potential risks. An arteriogram should never be done simply because it has been scheduled or 'routinely requested' by a clinical team; mistakes inevitably occur and the radiologist responsible for the procedure should be satisfied in every case that proper indications exist for the particular study requested. The arteriographer should also be quite clear before starting as to what information is required from the procedure; this ensures that the correct studies and projections are obtained, and allows rational decision-making during the procedure if something unexpected is shown or a problem arises.

2. Patient preparation

Informed consent should be obtained for arteriography. A doctor, preferably the responsible radiologist or a member of the radiology department, should see the patient before the procedure to explain what is to be done, check that no contraindications to the study exist, check the appropriate pulses and ensure that adequate premedication is arranged. The groin should be shaved if a femoral approach is to be used. It has been the usual practice for patients to be on 'nil by mouth' for an appropriate period prior to the procedure to avoid the risk of aspiration during a possible contrast reaction or other serious accident. It is now the policy in many departments, however, only to stop solid foods and to permit free oral fluids unless general anaesthesia or heavy premedication is being used. Whatever regimen is adopted adequate measures should be taken to avoid dehydration during the procedure and the recovery period.

3. Contraindications

There are very few absolute contraindications to arteriography but there are many factors which considerably increase the hazards of the technique. Always check that a patient is not *pregnant* before arteriography as the radiation dose may be considerable. If arteriography is essential in a pregnant patient the dose to the fetus should be minimized by protection, field collimation and careful choice of filming sequences. Caution should be exercised in patients on *anticoagulant* therapy or with other *bleeding diatheses*. Arteriography should be avoided if possible in such cases; if it is essential then all possible steps should be taken to correct or improve the coagulation defect before and during the procedure if this is clinically acceptable. Percutaneous *translumbar aortography* should not be performed in patients with a significant coagulation defect, as the bleeding site cannot be controlled. Other factors which increase the risk of bleeding from an arterial puncture site include systemic hypertension and disorders predisposing to increased fragility of the vessel wall such as Cushing's syndrome, prolonged steroid treatment and rare connective tissue disorders such as certain types of the *Ehlers-Danlos syndrome*. Arteriography may be necessary in a patient with a suspected or known previous adverse reaction to contrast medium and this problem is discussed in Chapter 7. Arteriography can require larger doses of contrast medium than any other radiological procedure, and particular care must be exercised in infants, dehydrated or shocked patients; patients with serious cardiac or respiratory disease; patients in hepatic or renal failure; and other patients with serious metabolic abnormalities.

4. Anaesthesia

Most arteriography is now performed under local anaesthesia, though general anaesthesia is necessary for babies and young children; confused, difficult, or very nervous patients; and some complex and interventional procedures. Although general anaesthesia can be more pleasant for the patient than local anaesthesia and reduces motion artefact on the radiographs it nevertheless adds to the risks of arteriography. This is not only because of the (small) risks inherent in general anaesthesia, but also because it masks the patient's subjective symptoms and reactions. These may provide the radiologist with immediate warning of a mishap such as the subintimal injection of contrast medium or the inadvertent wedging of the catheter tip in a small artery; a warning which may well prevent more serious injury. When local anaesthesia is to be used the patient should be sedated with a suitable premedication. This should contain an analgesic as most procedures cause some discomfort, and it is not only kinder to the patient to make the study as painless as possible, but it makes for appreciably better angiography. A suitable premedication for a 70 kg adult is papaveretum (Omnopon) 20 mg i.m., and lorezapam 2 mg orally 1 hour prior to the procedure.

It is important that the arterial puncture site should be adequately anaesthetized. After cleansing the skin with a suitable preparation 5–10 ml of 1–2% lignocaine is infiltrated around the artery. It is usually possible to insert the local anaesthetic posterior to the artery as well as anterior to it, which makes the arterial puncture much less uncomfortable for the patient. If the puncture site is inadequately anaesthetized arterial spasm may make selective catheterization very difficult because of the lack of free catheter movement.

5. Arterial puncture and catheterization

There are four principal techniques for arteriography:

a. percutaneous needle puncture of an artery
b. percutaneous catheterization of an artery
c. catheterization through an arteriotomy ('cutdown')
d. digital subtraction arteriography following the venous injection of contrast medium

a. Percutaneous needle puncture

It is possible to opacify arteries in many areas of the body using a direct percutaneous needle puncture. Although the general trend among radiologists is undoubtedly away from this method towards transfemoral catheter techniques, it is nevertheless important for the angiographer to be competent in needle puncture because it may be difficult or impossible in some patients to obtain access to a particular part of the vascular tree in any other way.

The common carotid and vertebral arteries can be punctured in the neck using an anterior approach to obtain arteriogram of the carotid and vertebro-basilar systems; the subclavian, axillary or brachial arteries can be punctured for upper limb arteriography, the abdominal aorta (high or low) for lumbar, pelvic and leg arteriography; and the femoral artery for single leg studies.

Percutaneous studies in the head and neck and upper limb have been largely supplanted by the transfemoral catheter method except in special circumstances, but *translumbar aortography* and *femoral arteriography* are still performed routinely in many centres. Femoral studies are now usually performed using a flexible needle sheath or a vessel dilator

rather than a rigid needle, however, to reduce the risk of vessel injury and needle dislodgement. The technique of femoral puncture is described below under percutaneous catheterization.

Translumbar aortography (Figs. 94.3, 94.4) is performed with the patient lying prone and may be done under local anaesthesia (with adequate sedation and analgesia) or general anaesthesia. Before the procedure the radiologist should check whether the patient has a bleeding diathesis or

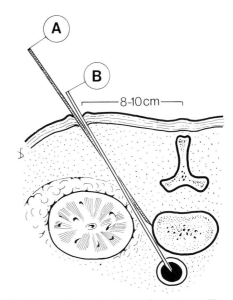

Fig. 94.3 Technique of translumbar aortic puncture. The needle has engaged the vertebral body (A): it is then withdrawn a little and reintroduced at a steeper angle (B) to pierce the aorta (patient prone).

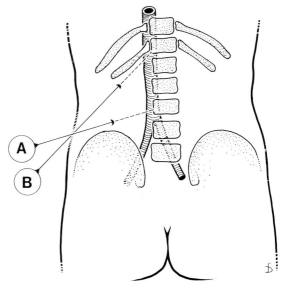

Fig. 94.4 Standard (A) and high (B) translumbar aortic punctures (patient prone).

is severely hypertensive, and examine the control film for signs of calcification in the wall of an *aortic aneurysm*. Aneurysms should not be punctured and it is also inadvisable to puncture a previous *aortic vascular graft*. Puncturing Dacron or other graft material is to be avoided principally because of the risk of infection but also for fear of damaging a functioning anastomosis. It is also possible to dislodge the pseudointima which lines a Dacron graft and cause vascular occlusion. The needle is inserted through a small skin incision into the left flank at a point midway between the lower costal margin and the iliac crest and approximately 10 cm from the midline in the average adult. The needle is advanced at an angle of approximately 45° from the vertical plane until it enters the aorta at the level of L3. It is common practice first to engage the vertebral body with the needle tip, then partially to withdraw and advance the needle at a steeper angle until it slides along the lateral margin of the body and into the aorta (Fig. 94.3). When a free, spurting backflow of arterial blood is observed test injections of contrast medium are made under fluoroscopic control to check the position of the needle (and avert the risk of aortic dissection) before proceeding to a full study. 60 ml of urografin 76% or its equivalent injected over 3–4 seconds will normally opacify the lower aorta, pelvic vessels and limb vessels satisfactorily, though considerable adjustments to the volume and rate of injection will need to be made in individual patients depending on the state of the vascular tree. If the lower aorta is blocked or aneurysmal, or it is particularly desirable to visualize other aortic branches (e.g. the renal arteries) a *high translumbar puncture* is made. For this the needle is inserted 1–2 cm higher in the flank and angled in a cephalic direction to hit the aorta at T12 (Fig. 94.4). Remember when doing this that other structures such as the pericardium and pleura are not too far away from the tip of the needle!

Guidance from the vascular surgeon concerning the presence and location of bruits in the aorta and iliac vessels may aid in the proper selection of radiological technique. A bruit, for example, in the abdomen may indicate a stenosis of the abdominal aorta and suggest the use of a high approach.

The principal specific complications of translumbar aortography are retroperitoneal bleeding and aortic dissection though rarer problems such as vertebral disc or bone infection, pericardial bleeding, pneumothorax, chylothorax and pancreatitis have all been reported. The great majority of cases of intimal dissection produced by the technique settle spontaneously and require no more than careful observation.

b. Percutaneous arterial catheterization

The great majority of arterial catheters are inserted into the femoral artery at the groin. The skin is shaved (on the ward preferably!), cleansed and the artery palpated to select the site of puncture before local anaesthetic is injected. Various anatomical descriptions are given regarding the site at which to puncture; in the author's experience the best place is where the artery can be most easily palated irrespective of the relationship of this point to the inguinal skin crease.

Since this is usually the point where the artery crosses the pubic bone it is also the easiest point at which to achieve haemostasis afterwards. After local anaesthesia a small scalpel incision is made in the skin (large enough to accommodate the anticipated catheter), the skin being temporarily drawn laterally during the incision to avert the risk of a scalpel injury to the arterial wall. A pair of fine artery forceps is inserted into the incision and used to create a tunnel through the subcutaneous tissues down to the artery. This manoeuvre is particularly important in large or obese patients for it not only facilitates catheterization but it reduces the risk of a post-operative haematoma: any escaping blood emerges through the incision and is immediately apparent, instead of collecting subcutaneously. The technique employed for puncturing the artery is a matter of personal preference. A reliable way is to feel the artery with the middle and index fingers of one hand (the left in most people) and insert the needle (held in the other hand) between the two palpating fingers. Gentle pressure with the needle will alter the pulse as detected by the lower (index) finger giving reassurance as to its correct alignment. The needle is held angled forwards (Fig. 94.5) and passed right through the artery (but see below for alternative technique). The central stylet is then withdrawn, the needle angled slightly more towards the horizontal, and then withdrawn at an even rate, assisted by gentle rotatory movements to avoid any sudden jerking. When the tip of the needle is safely in the arterial lumen there will be a free, spurting backflow of blood from the hub. While the needle is held steady with one hand the soft tip of a guide wire is threaded through the needle into the artery. When a sufficient length of wire is inside, the needle is removed and firm manual pressure maintained on the puncture site until the needle has been exchanged for a catheter or dilator (Fig. 94.5). The guide wire is removed when the tip of the catheter is in a satisfactory position and the catheter is then flushed free of blood with heparinized-saline (v.i.). At the end of a correctly conducted insertion procedure there should be no bleeding around the catheter which will move freely and painlessly through the puncture site when manipulated. Many radiologists prefer to puncture only the anterior wall of the vessel to minimize the trauma to the vessel. The puncture to both vessel walls does not, however, seem to increase the risk of complications [16,17] as these are usually caused by the subsequent manipulations with guide wires and catheters. Protagonists of the 'right-through' technique (of which the author is one) consider it to be a more consistently reliable method of getting the needle tip safely into the lumen of the vessel. If a guidewire does not pass freely into the arterial lumen it should not be forced: this technique is *never* successful and usually causes an intimal dissection. If there is good backflow of blood the reason for failure of the wire to pass freely may be either that the needle is angled sharply towards one wall of the blood vessel or that the wire is passing into a small branch vessel such as the superficial circumflex iliac, deep circumflex iliac or inferior epigastric artery. A number of manoeuvres may help including fluoroscopy, gently repositioning of the angle of the needle, or changing to a J-wire. A *gentle* injection of contrast medium is possible to help ascertain the nature of the problem but

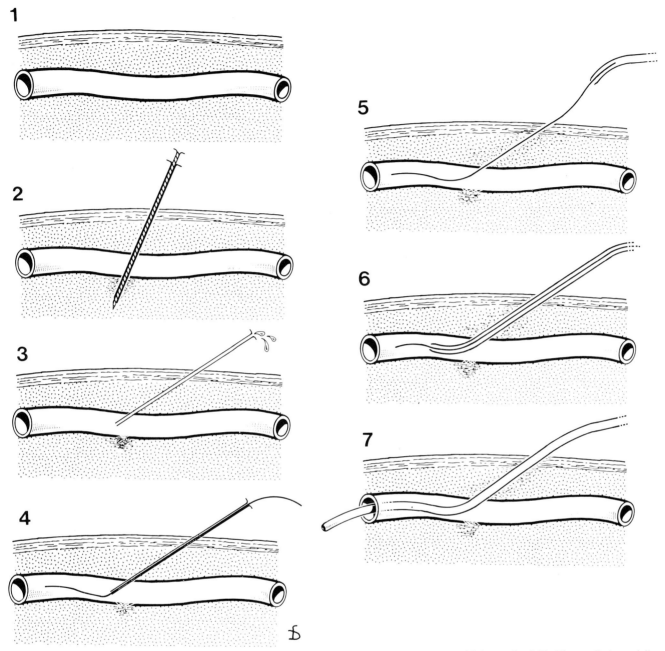

Fig. 94.5 One of the commonly-used techniques of percutaneous arterial catheterization. The artery (1) is transfixed (2). The needle is partially withdrawn and re-angled (3). A guide-wire is passed into the needle during free back-flow of blood (3,4); the needle removed and a catheter or introducer inserted over the wire (5,6). When the catheter is safely within the arterial lumen and wire is withdrawn (7).

only if good backflow is present. If there is poor backflow then the needle may be positioned near an atheromatous plaque or a stenosis, may be only partially in the lumen, or may have caused an intimal dissection. In these circumstances discretion is usually the better part of valour and it is wise to start again with a fresh puncture. In difficult cases remember that there is usually a femoral artery in the opposite leg! Better two groin punctures than a dissection or a large haematoma.

The catheter is flushed with a heparinized-saline solution throughout the procedure to prevent clotting. Various concentrations of heparin are used in different centres; the author uses 5000 iu heparin/litre normal saline. During an average procedure it would be unusual for a patient to receive much more than about 1000–2000 iu in this way; if for some reason this amount is significantly exceeded the usual precautions should be observed regarding the use of anticoagulants (enquiry as to ulcer history etc), and the clinical team informed. It is generally better to give a firm hand flush intermittently, than to maintain a continuous slow flush infusion. This technique not only leaves the proximal end of the catheter free for manipulation but is also more effective since a slow infusion may only clear the proximal holes of a catheter with multiple side-ports; clot forms in the end-port and the more distal side-ports which is then blown out into the vascular system when a pressure contrast injection is performed!

c. Arteriotomy

It is sometimes preferable to expose an artery by formal cutdown and catheterize it through an arteriotomy than to attempt the percutaneous technique. This is often done for cardiac procedures in infants [18], and some cardiologists still use the *Mason Sones* cutdown technique in adults (Chapter 35). In peripheral arteriographic procedures brachial arteriotomy is used by some radiologists in preference to an axillary puncture for the introduction of catheters when an arm approach is required, and in patients with coagulation problems an arteriotomy can be a safer method of access than a percutaneous puncture.

d. Digital subtraction angiography. DSA, DVI

Although digital enhancement techniques can of course be used to improve the images of conventional arteriograms (Fig. 94.6), they can also be used to avoid the need for an arterial puncture in some circumstances. Contrast medium is injected into a peripheral or central vein and provides sufficient vascular detail during its passage through the arterial side of the circulation to give diagnostic information (Fig. 94.7 and see Fig. 94.64). The subject of digital vascular imaging is covered in Chapter 96.

6. Selective catheterization

By manipulating a catheter under fluoroscopic control it is possible to insert the catheter selectively into various branches of the vascular system such as the renal artery, coeliac axis, axillary artery, etc. Different catheter shapes are available (Fig 94.3.) each of which is suitable for a particular manoeuvre or for catheterizing certain arterial branches. Some radiologists like to shape their own catheters using a hot-water bath or steam but a wide variety of pre-shaped catheters can be obtained commercially and these are adequate for most purposes.

Superselective catheterization (also referred to, paradoxically, as *sub* selective) refers to the catheterization of small subsidiary arteries which themselves arise from named branch arteries. Examples of arteries which can be catheterized in this way include the pancreatico-duodenal arteries, the jejunal or ileal branches of the superior mesenteric artery and individual branches of the external carotid artery such as the lingual or superior thyroid arteries, etc. Superselective catheterization is being increasingly used for *embolization* procedures (Chapter 98).

7. Aftercare

When an arteriographic study is completed the catheter is withdrawn and firm manual pressure applied to the puncture site for 5–10 minutes. The radiologist should be absolutely satisfied that bleeding has stopped before the patient leaves the angiography suite. The wound site is then checked at regular intervals by the nursing staff who should also record pulse and blood pressure observations for a reasonable period following the procedure and check that distal pulses remain palpable. Pressure pads, sand bags and other accoutrements are generally a waste of time. It is much better to be able to see the puncture site than to cover it up. If bleeding does not stop from a puncture site, press for a longer period! Almost all post-catheterization bleeding can ultimately be controlled by local pressure unless the artery has been torn or there is a coagulation abnormality.

An adequate record of the procedure should be entered in the patient's case notes. This should include the date; the name of the operator; the puncture site; the catheter size; the studies performed; the names and doses of anaesthetic agents; the volumes and concentrations of contrast medium and other drugs administered; preliminary findings; any complications during the procedure; the integrity or otherwise of the pulse peripheral to the puncture site at the end of the procedure; and the post-procedural nursing instructions. These notes are important not only for patient

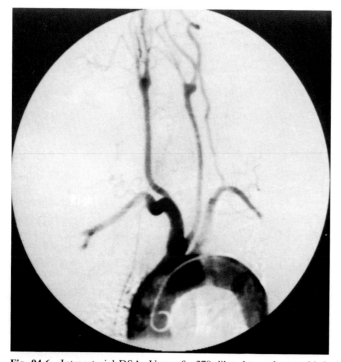

Fig. 94.6 Intraarterial DSA. Urografin 270 diluted to only one-third of its normal iodine concentration has been injected into the aortic arch, and a digitally-enhanced study obtained.

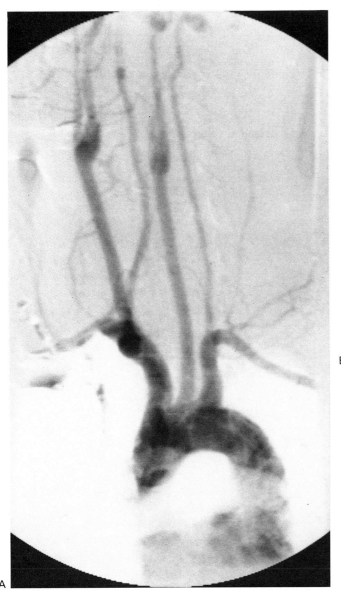

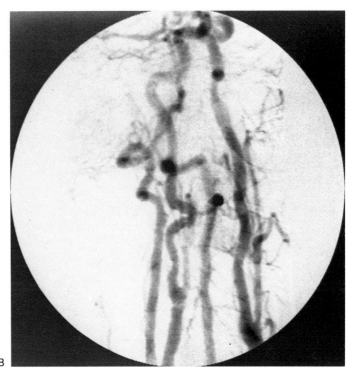

Fig. 94.7A & B   Intravenous DSA. Undiluted non-ionic contrast medium (iohexol 350) has been injected into a peripheral arm vein. Digital enhancement gives good images of the neck arteries (A). An arm vein injection in a different patient (B) shows detail on a magnified image of the carotid bifurcations and syphons.

care but also as a medico-legal record, and they should be comprehensive and accurate. Arteriography is most safely performed on an in-patient basis, the patient remaining on bed rest overnight following the procedure.

8. Radiographic considerations

Good radiography is a vital factor in arteriography. A control film should always be obtained so that the correct exposure factors can be established and the film accurately centred. The radiographs should be carefully collimated to the field of interest and exposed during arrested respiration when the study involves regions affected by respiratory movement. It is best to choose a point to stop respiration that lies in the *normal* respiratory cycle; an unusually vigorous respiratory movement (e.g. 'take a deep breath and hold') may dislodge a catheter which has only a tenuous hold on its selective position!

9. Special techniques

Subtraction films

Subtraction films may help by showing the arteries free of confusing shadows cast by non-vascular structures such as bone. They are particularly useful in the head and neck. A subtraction film is made by exposing a radiograph of the area of interest immediately prior to the injection of contrast medium. A reversed image of this radiograph (the subtraction *mask*) is then superimposed on subsequent radiographs showing opacified vascular structures so that the mask obscures all non-vascular detail. A final image showing only the opacified vessels can then be obtained (subtraction *print*). Figure 94.8 shows a conventional arteriogram together with its subtraction print.

Digital subtraction techniques in which the process is performed electronically, are rapidly superseding the manual method described above.

Pharmacoangiography

Selective catheterization techniques permit the local delivery

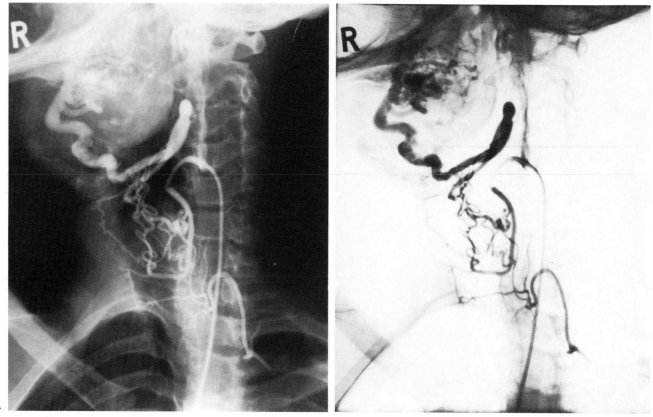

Fig. 94.8A & B   'Manual' subtraction technique. A superior thyroid artery is shown feeding a lingual arteriovenous malformation. In the standard film (A) many non-vascular strictures are visible and the injected vessels appear white. On the subtraction print (B), most of the non-vascular strictures have been eliminated and the vessels are shown in black.

of potent pharmacological agents to local vascular territories. There have been four principal areas of application: vasoconstrictor agents, vasodilator agents, fibrinolytic agents and chemotherapeutic agents.

Vasoconstrictor agents

Vasoconstrictors such as adrenaline [19,20,21], vasopressin [22,23] or angiotensin [24] can be injected for diagnostic or therapeutic purposes. In diagnostic procedures the rationale is that the vasoactive drug affects normal vessels more than tumour vessels leaving the latter less constricted and more conspicuous. There is no doubt that tumours can be diagnosed with greater accuracy by this method, particularly in the kidney [25,26] but advances in other imaging techniques have reduced the importance of this branch of arteriography and it is not routinely performed in most centres. The *therapeutic* use of vasoconstrictor agents is discussed in Chapter 98.

Vasodilator agents [20]

These have also been used both diagnostically and therapeutically. In diagnosis they have been employed to give improved parenchymal opacification of certain organs, and to demonstrate better the venous phase of an arteriogram, especially the portal vein during coeliac and mesenteric studies. The therapeutic applications are discussed in Chapter 98. Dilator drugs which can be administered in this way include tolazoline, histamine, papaverine, reserpine and prostaglandins.

The trans-catheter infusion of *fibrinolytic* and *chemotherapeutic* agents is discussed in Chapter 98.

Magnification angiography

Radiographic magnification has been employed to obtain improved visualization of small vessels [21,27,28,29,30]. The method requires careful attention to radiographic details (focus-object-film distances), a fine-focal spot tube with a large current-carrying capacity, and minimal movement artefact. The clinical yield from magnification arteriography has proved somewhat limited, and the method has been used principally for research studies, particularly in the renal, pulmonary and cerebral circulations.

Complications

The principal complications of arteriography are listed in Table 94.1.

Table 94.1 Complications of arteriography

1. **Contrast medium-related complications**

   Minor adverse reactions

   Major adverse reactions and death

   Local vascular changes (effects on blood cells, viscosity, vascular tone; results of extravasation, etc.)

   Systemic vascular changes (effects on blood volume, osmolality, etc.)

   Individual organ toxicity (heart, kidney, brain, etc)

2. **Adverse reactions to local anaesthetic or other drugs**

3. **Puncture site complications**

   Haemorrhage (external bleeding or haematoma)

   Intramural or perivascular injection of contrast medium

   Vascular thrombosis (dissection, local trauma)

   Peripheral embolization from puncture site

   Vascular stenosis or occlusion

   Aneurysm or pseudoaneurysm formation

   AV fistula

   Local sepsis

   Damage to nerves

   Damage to other local structures

4. **Catheter-related and general complications**

   Catheter thrombus embolism

   Air embolism

   Gauze embolism

   Dissection, perforation or rupture of vessels

   Organ ischaemia or infarction secondary to spasm, dissection or embolism

   Interventional accidents (Chapter 98)

   Fracture and loss of guidewire or catheter fragments

   Knot formation in catheters

   Inadvertent injection of toxic material (e.g. skin cleansing lotion)

   Inadvertent over-heparinization

   Vaso-vagal reaction

1. Contrast medium-related complications

The many possible adverse effects of contrast media together with details of their prevention and treatment are discussed in Chapter 7. It is anticipated that the general introduction of low osmolality and non-ionic media will reduce considerably the incidence of contrast-related problems in arteriography.

2. Adverse drug reactions

Apart from contrast medium reactions adverse or idiosyncratic effects may be caused by local anaesthetic agents or other drugs given during the procedure.

3. Puncture site complications

Haemorrhage

Haemorrhage may occur from the puncture site and may cause external blood loss or a subcutaneous haematoma which can result in extensive bruising (Fig. 94.9). Excessive

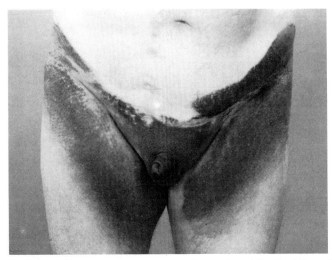

Fig. 94.9 Extensive groin haematomas in a patient following bilateral femoral artery catheterization.

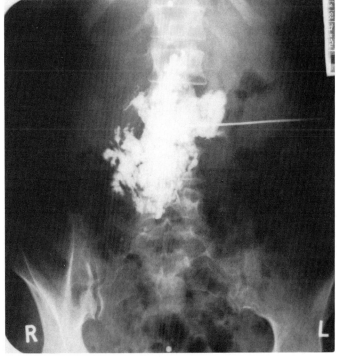

Fig. 94.10 Contrast extravasation. A translumbar aortogram needle is seen in the left flank. Its tip, unfortunately, lies outside the aorta.

bleeding is usually the result of bad technique. Particular caution is necessary in patients with a bleeding diathesis or hypertension and following the use of ballon catheters in transluminal angioplasty. If inexplicable continued bleeding occurs check that inadvertent *over-heparinization* has not occurred. This can be corrected if necessary by the administration of protamine sulphate (10 mg counteracts the effects of 1000 international units of heparin).

Bleeding following a translumbar aortogram is usually retroperitoneal though cases of intraperitoneal, pleural and pericardial haemorrhage have been described. Some cases require transfusion, but surgical intervention is fortunately rarely necessary. Care should be taken not to give too much protamine; remember that the action of heparin is relatively short-lived.

Intramural and perivascular contrast injection

Contrast may be inadvertently injected into the wall of a vessel or outside the vessel (perivascular). In most cases little harm (apart from pain) results from a perivascular injection, but it is possible to dissect and occlude an artery with a *subintimal* injection of contrast medium. *Never inject into a needle or catheter that does not exhibit free back flow.* Figure 94.10 shows the perivascular injection of contrast medium during a translumbar aortogram and Fig. 94.11 an example of an aortic dissection (produced by the same operator on his next case!).

Vascular thrombosis

Vascular thrombosis can result from severe trauma to the vessel at the puncture site or from subintimal contrast injection. It is also possible that thrombus wiped off the outside of the arterial catheter during its extraction forms a nidus for thrombus at the puncture site. Vascular trauma at the puncture site can be minimized by good technique. Never use force to introduce a wire into a vessel; if it does

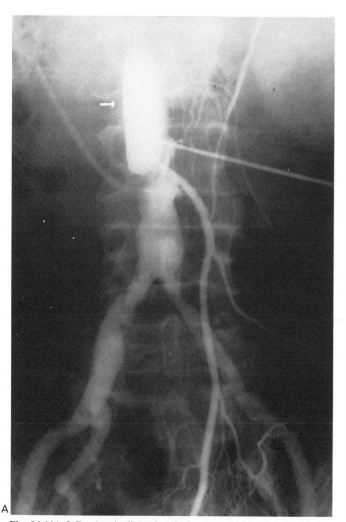
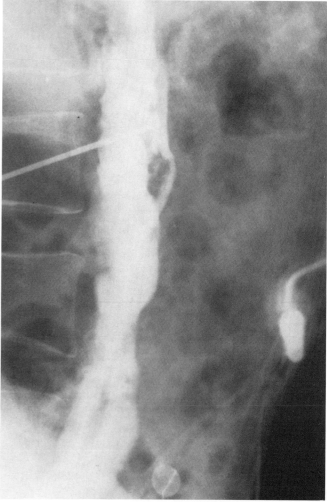

Fig. 94.11A & B   Aortic dissection during translumbar aortography. On the AP film (A) there is a very dense opacity with a suspiciously straight edge (arrows): features highly suggestive of a dissection. A lateral film (B) shows an intimal flap near the needle tip. Persistent staining of a localized area of vessel wall with contrast medium after an injection usually indicates that a dissection has occurred.

not pass easily something is wrong! It is often better for the inexperienced operator to start again with a fresh needle puncture than to persist with one that is causing problems. A ten minute delay with a successful outcome is always preferable to a dissection and/ or groin haematoma.

Peripheral embolization

Peripheral embolization from the puncture site probably occurs to a minor degree in many cases, but clinically obvious embolization is rare.

Local vascular complications

Vascular complications such as false aneurysm (pseudo-aneurysm) or AV fistula formation, and late stenosis or occlusion can all result from arterial procedures. Good technique is the best preventative measure.

Local sepsis

Local sepsis may occur following an arterial puncture and this factor is particularly important if early surgery is comtemplated. The utmost care should be taken to observe sterile precautions and when a study is performed in a patient with local skin contamination (e.g. open wound, ileostomy etc), a protective adhesive sheet such as 'Steridrape' helps to keep the operative field uncontaminated.

Injury to local structures

Injury to local structures such as nerves, joints and bones is rarely of clinical significance. Occasionally damage to branches of the femoral nerve gives rise to areas of cutaneous anaesthesia or paraesthesia in the thigh. These normally recover completely.

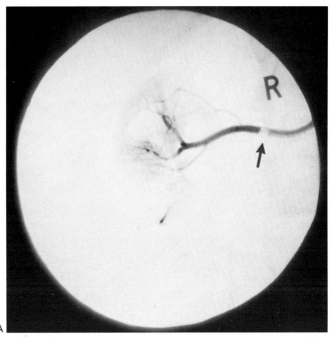

A

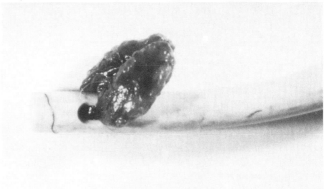

B

Fig. 94.12A, B Catheter thrombus. During a renal arteriogram (A) a filling defect was noted at the catheter tip (arrow). On cautious withdrawal of the catheter a thrombus was found protruding from the side-ports (B). Note the fragment of gauze thread on the catheter tip: this was incorporated in the clot and presumably caused it. Care should always be taken when handling swabs in association with wires or catheters.

4. Catheter-related and general complications

Catheter thrombus embolism

Thrombus can form in or on a catheter (Fig. 94.12) and be ejected into the vascular system. This is always undesirable, and in areas such as the cerebral or coronary circulations is extremely dangerous. Catheters should be flushed assiduously during all arteriographic procedures (see p. 1995) to prevent thrombus formation. Some radiologists routinely employ systemic heparinization for arteriography [31]. Other types of embolism that may occur are *air embolism* (usually from incorrectly loaded pressure injectors) and *thread embolism* from fragments of gauze swab (Fig. 94.12). Therapeutic (deliberate!) embolization is discussed in Chapter 98.

Vascular injuries

Vascular injuries distant from the puncture site may be produced by the catheter or guide wire, or by the intramural injection of contrast medium or saline. If there is ever any doubt about whether a needle or catheter tip is in a satisfactory position, contrast medium should always be injected in preference to saline. Under fluoroscopic control, it is then possible to stop the injection immediately if any extravasation or other mishap is apparent. The commonest injury is dissection of the tunica intima from the tunica media and this complication is far more likely to occur in previously diseased vessels than in normal vessels. The intima forms a raised flap (Fig. 94.13 and see Fig. 94.40) which may

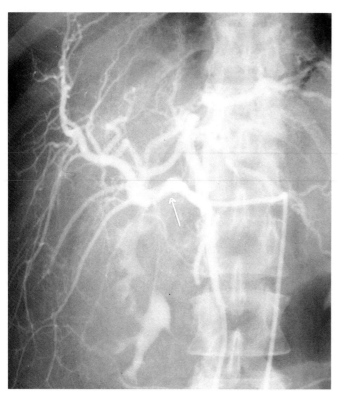

Fig. 94.13 Hepatic artery dissection. An intimal flap has been raised (arrow) which is partially occluding the vessel lumen.

completely occlude the vessel. It is also possible to perforate vessels with a guide wire or to rupture them when a forced injection is made through a catheter wedged into a vessel of the same calibre.

Organ injuries

Apart from those related to the effects of contrast medium, (Chapter 7), organ injuries are normally caused by ischaemia during arteriographic procedures. This may occur through wedging of the catheter so that the normal flow to an organ is obstructed; dissection of the feeding artery; spasm, thrombosis or rupture of the feeding artery; or embolism. The ischaemia resulting from one of the above events may have no observable clinical sequelae, may result in temporary or permanent functional abnormalities in the affected organ or system, or may cause infarction of the organ. The clinical importance of these accidents depends very much on the vascular territory in which they occur; complete occlusion of a carotid, coronary or renal artery is likely to have disastrous consequences whereas occlusion of, say, an hepatic artery may not necessarily produce any adverse effects.

Interventional accidents

There is a higher risk of inadvertent damage to vessel or organs during interventional vascular procedures than during conventional diagnostic studies. These problems are discussed in Chapter 98.

Guide-wire fracture

Occasionally fragments of guide-wire or catheter may become detached within the vascular system. Catheters may also become knotted during over-enthusiastic manipulation procedures. Special interventional techniques exist for dealing with these problems (Chapter 98). With good technique they should not occur in the first place.

Injection accidents

Tragedies have occurred when toxic substances have been inadvertently injected into blood vessels. Skin cleansing fluids should always be removed from the instrument trolley immediately after the puncture site has been prepared. Drugs should always be double-checked before injection through a catheter, and particular care is necessary with heparin which is available in solutions which are considerably different in their concentration.

Vaso-vagal reactions

Vagally mediated reactions may occur during arteriography in response to either the injection of contrast medium, or to the discomfort and psychological effects of the procedure. Bradycardia is a prominent feature of such reactions which must be distinguished from acute allergic responses to the contrast medium or local anaesthetic. The incidence of vaso-vagal reactions is considerably reduced if proper premedication is employed.

VASCULAR DISORDERS

Although many of the previous functions of arteriography have now been replaced by other imaging modalities, arteriography remains an indispensable diagnostic tool in modern medicine and a wide variety of indications exists for its use. Many of the disorders investigated by means of arteriography are common to different parts of the vascular tree, and it is convenient to consider these disorders in general terms before looking at the arteriography of regional vascular beds.

Congenital abnormalities

Congenital anomalies of the vascular tree are common, but only a few are of clinical or radiological significance. Important congenital vascular lesions affecting the central nervous system are considered in Chapter 85, and abnormalities of the heart, upper aorta (including coarctation) and pulmonary arteries in Section III.

In the lower thoracic aorta one or more anomalous arteries may arise to supply a *sequestrated lung segment* (Fig. 94.14). This anomaly may be discovered at any age, and is commonly associated with recurrent pulmonary infection in the affected lung which is partially, or completely separated from the normal bronchial tree. Radiographically the lesion is seen more commonly on the left than the right [32] and the arteriographic findings establish the diagnosis beyond doubt.

In the lumbar aorta coarctation may occur (Fig. 94.15) and is commonly associated with stenosis or occlusion of the branch arteries arising at the level of the coarctation [33]. Rarely complete occlusion of the aorta is present with enlarged collateral vessels in the lumbar and/or mesenteric territories. Infrarenal coarctation may be of the hypoplastic form, with diffuse narrowing of the lower aorta and/or iliac vessels. Hypoplasia of the abdominal aorta is said to have been first recognised in 1733 by John Baptist Morgagni in a 33-year-old monk [34,35]. 'But on the internal surface of the great artery, from the superior branches quite to the emulgents were beginnings of future ossification. This artery, though in a body of tall stature, was scarcely thicker than a finger of moderate size: and the other sanguiferous vessels, also, were narrow in the same proportion.'

Since that time many authors have noted that hypoplasia of the distal aorta and proximal iliac vessels is usually associated with premature and severe atherosclerosis. Despite the fact that Morgagni first noted the disorder in a monk it is much commoner in females than males and various factors have been postulated as causing it. These include congenital rubella, embolization from the heart, trauma, fibromuscular dysplasia, Buerger's disease, premature atheroma (i.e. atheroma causing narrowing, rather than the commoner view of hypoplasia leading to atheroma through altered stress patterns), diabetes mellitus, smoking, radiation in childhood and the contraceptive pill (though the latter causes seem improbable in Morgagni's monk!). A good anatomical argument for a congenital aetiology in at least some of these cases is put forward by Arnot and Louw [35]. They suggest that the anomaly is caused by excessive fusion of the two embryonic dorsal aortas around the twenty fifth day of intrauterine life, and point out in favour of this fusion theory that in many cases there is a single lumbar trunk at the L4 or L5 level which subsequently divides into right and left lumbar arteries.

The combination of hypoplasia and premature atherosclerosis frequently leads to occlusive symptoms at an early age. A common angiographic feature is an 'hourglass' stenosis [36] between the renal arteries and the

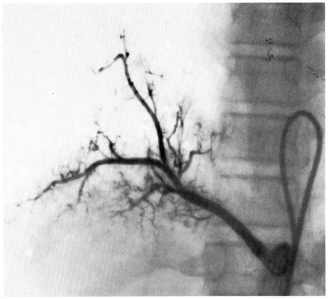

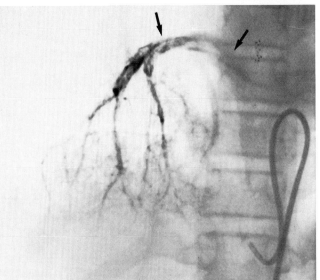

Fig. 94.14A & B Sequestrated lung segment. The artery supplying the anomalous segment arises directly from the aorta (A). In the last phase of the study (B) the draining vein is shown proceeding towards the left atrium (arrows). (Illustration by courtesy of Dr Anne Hemingway)

bifurcation (Fig. 94.16), and complete occlusion of the aorto-iliac region ultimately occurs.

Congenital anomalies of the branches of the abdominal aorta are frequent [37,38]. The coeliac and superior mesenteric arteries are linked embryologically and persistence of part or all of this link (the ventral longitudinal anastomosis) results in a variety of anomalies. There may be a single coeliac-mesenteric trunk arising from the aorta; separate coeliac and superior mesenteric arteries with a major connecting vessel (*arc of Buhler*); and part or all of the hepatic arterial system may arise from the superior mesenteric artery. The variations of arterial supply to the liver are important to both the

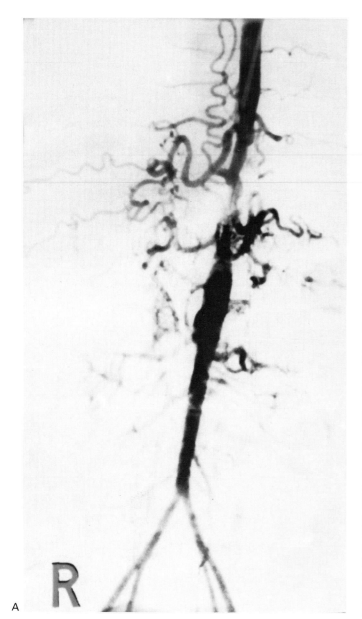

A

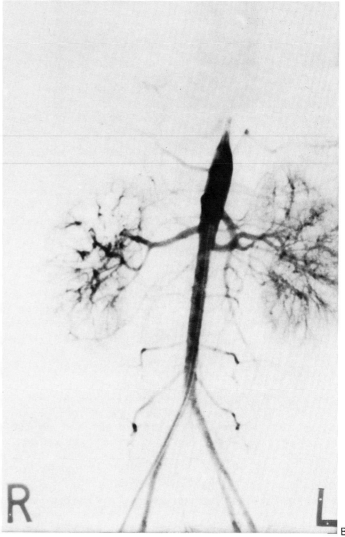

B

Fig. 94.15A & B Congenital abdominal coarctation in a child. An aortogram (A) shows the high stenosis with large collateral vessels feeding into the visceral branches below the obstruction. Attempted transluminal angioplasty failed owing to the rigidity of the stenosis (B), but a surgical graft was successfully inserted subsequently.

surgeon and the embolizing radiologist: in approximately 20% of patients the right hepatic vessels arise partially or completely from the superior mesenteric artery and in a similar percentage the left hepatic artery is partially or completely replaced by a branch from the left gastric artery (see Fig. 94.66). In 2.5% of patients all the principal hepatic vessels arise from the superior mesenteric artery (Fig. 94.17).

Variations in the arterial supply to the kidneys are common owing to the complicated embryological development of these organs. Over 20% of kidneys examined arteriographically have more than one artery [39] and some have three or even four. The additional arteries (which may be looked on as branches of persistent lateral splanchnic arteries) [40] arise from the mid or lower aorta but may also come from the aortic bifurcation or the iliac arteries. Horseshoe kidneys and ectopic kidneys usually have multiple or anomalous arteries. Multiple renal arteries are sometimes referred to as *accessory* arteries, a misleading term which suggests that they provide an extra or 'reserve' blood supply to the organ. This is not so: every renal artery supplies its own portion of the kidney which is likely to become ischaemic if that branch is damaged. Multiple renal arteries are clinically and radiologically important for several reasons; firstly, if a selective renal arteriogram has been performed the non-opacified zone supplied by another artery may be mistaken for a pathological entity by the inexperienced operator (Fig. 94.18 and see Fig. 94.29). Secondly, when pathology is being sought in the kidney (e.g. tumour, arterial

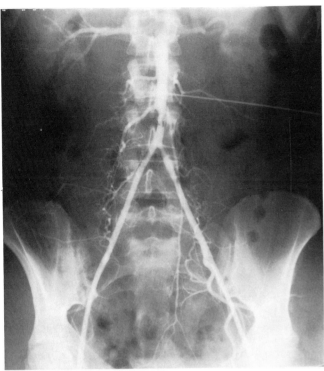

Fig. 94.16 Translumbar aortogram in an adult female showing an 'hour-glass' stenosis just above the aortic bifurcation. Note the small calibre of the lower aorta and the iliac vessels (Illustration by courtesy of Dr P. Finn).

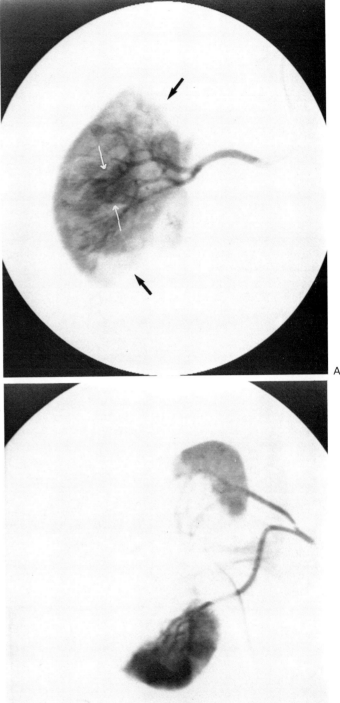

Fig. 94.18A & B Multiple renal arteries. When the principal renal artery is opacified (A) filling defects are seen in the nephrogram at the upper and lower poles (black arrows). These appearances are characteristic of areas supplied by unopacified supernumerary arteries and should not be mistaken for pathology. The opacity or 'blush' indicated by the white arrows is a renal cortical rest, not a tumour. The upper and lower poles of the kidney were opacified by a separate injection into a second artery (B).

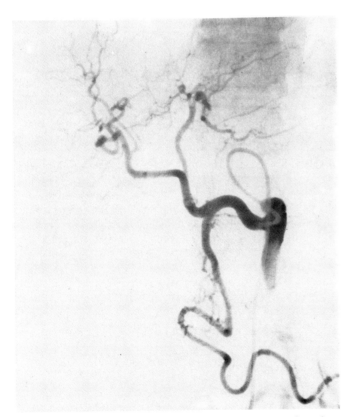

Fig. 94.17 Replaced common hepatic artery. The common hepatic vessel is shown arising from the superior mesenteric artery instead of from the coeliac axis.

stenosis, etc.), *all* the renal arteries present should be identified and studied or the pathology may be missed. Finally, the surgeon contemplating a renal procedure may wish to know the number and distribution of the renal arteries, especially if renal transplantation is being considered. The presence of more than one renal artery may mean that a kidney is unsuitable as a donor organ. Arteriography may confirm the congenital absence of a kidney (*agenesis*) when other methods (e.g. urography) have failed to explain the absence of renal tissue [41]. It is not usually possible for the angiographer to differentiate between *congenital hypoplasia* and lesions acquired in intrauterine life or early childhood as being the cause of a very small kidney [39]. It has been suggested that in acquired disease the origin of the renal artery retains its width [42]. It seems certain that true congenital hypoplasia is an extremely rare entity, and that most 'congenitally' small kidneys are probably the end-result of chronic atrophic pyelonephritis starting in early infancy [43].

In the upper limb there are few arterial anomalies of radiological importance. Occasionally the brachial artery divides into its radial and ulnar branches higher than usual which may be important if a brachial puncture or arteriotomy is contemplated.

In the lower limb the principal blood supply in the embryo is the axial artery, a branch of the umbilical (internal iliac) artery. The importance of this artery diminishes during development and the external iliac and femoral arteries become the dominant vessels. In normal indivuduals the axial system is represented by the inferior gluteal artery and the artery to the sciatic nerve (arteria comitans nervi ischiadici). Occasionally the external iliac artery and femoral artery may be absent or hypoplastic (Fig. 94.19) and an enlarged *primitive sciatic artery* (i.e. axial artery) supplies the lower extremity. Vascular malformations consitute an important subgroup of congenital anomalies. They are considered below.

Vascular malformations (arteriovenous malformations, angiomas, haemangiomas)

The subject of blood vessel tumours is a complex one with bewildering terminology and a variety of pathological and surgical classifications. While true neoplasms of vascular endothelium exist, and while many benign and malignant tumours derived from other tissues exhibit abnormal vascularity, we are principally concerned under this heading with lesions consisting of benign collections of abnormal blood channels. From the arteriographer's point of view there are three principal categories of vascular malformation (which do not necessarily correspond to any histopathological classification):

Predominantly arterial or arteriovenous lesions
(arteriovenous malformations, plexiform angiomas)

These are usually clinically pulsatile and there may be a bruit on auscultation. Radiologically there are enlarged tortuous feeding arteries which communicate more or less directly with dilated veins (Figs. 94.20, 94.21). There is usually rapid flow through such lesions and a fast filming sequence is necessary when they are being studied. Although presumably congenital in origin the malformations may remain relatively quiescent for years until a stimulus such as local trauma, puberty or pregnancy activates their growth which may then be extremely rapid. Although they are histologically benign they may cause a number of problems such as local bleeding, trophic changes, distal ischaemia, pain and disfigurement. If large they may cause death through haemorrhage, compression of vital structures or cardiac failure secondary to the massive AV shunting that can develop through their abnormal vascular channels. In some patients the lesions are very small and remain virtually unchanged throughout life. When the lesions are large or multiple they may be associated with local gigantism and present as overgrowth of a foot, hand or entire limb.

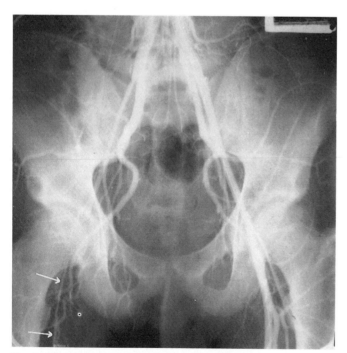

Fig. 94.19 Hypoplasia of the external iliac artery. The primitive sciatic artery is visible in this case (arrows) but is not unduly enlarged. In some individuals the sciatic artery may be as large as a femoral artery and be the principal vessel of supply to the limb.

Capillary or small vessel malformations

Malformations affecting predominantly the capillaries or very small vessels (arterioles and venules) are difficult to

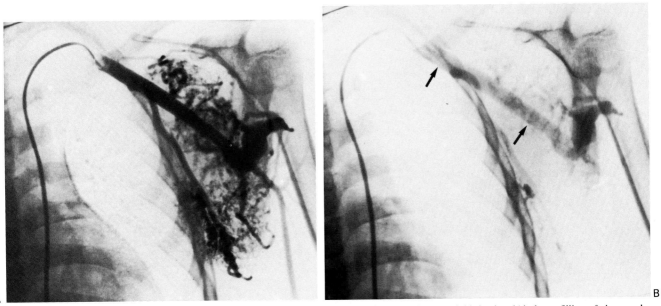

Fig. 94.20A & B   Arteriovenous malformation of the scapula in a 10 year old boy. A subclavian arterial injection (A) shows filling of abnormal vascular spaces around the scapula. A few seconds later venous filling is seen. (arrows, B).

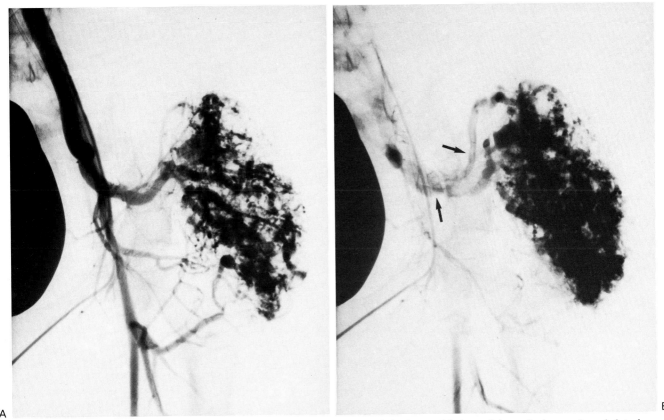

Fig. 94.21A & B   Arteriovenous malformation of the buttock in a 17 year old girl. (A) The arterial phase of the study shows enlarged gluteal feeding vessels. (B) Prominent early-filling veins are visible only two seconds later (arrows).

demonstrate radiologically and for the most part do not require investigation (e.g. the skin capillary naevus or 'port wine' stain). There are however one or two notable exceptions. *Angiodysplasia* is ectasia of small vessels in the mucosa and submucosa of the caecum and ascending colon. The lesions of angiodysplasia may be demonstrated by mesenteric angiography (see Fig. 94.76) and are clinically important as a cause of obscure gastrointestinal bleeding (see p. 2042). The lesions of Osler-Weber-Rendu disease (hereditary haemorrhagic telangiectasis) may also be shown by arteriography (Figs. 94.22 & 94.73) but this is not usually of any particular diagnostic value unless embolization of a bleeding lesion is contemplated.

Venous (cavernous) haemangiomas

Cavernous angiomas consist of collections of dilated veins and abnormal venous channels. Clinically they are non-pulsatile, can easily be compressed and are gravity-dependent. Angiograms of such lesions are usually disappointing: the study frequently appears normal in the arteriogram phase, there is no significant increase in flow and the only abnormal finding may be some abnormal venous staining in the late films. *Venography* is usually the best way of demonstrating the lesion if a clinical indication exists for doing so, or digital subtraction angiography from the arterial side if this facility is available.

The angiomas described in association with dyschondroplasia (Maffucci's syndrome), and other rare disorders are usually predominantly venous in nature. They may show on plain radiographs when they contain phleboliths, but arteriography in such cases is unrewarding and meddlesome.

Arteriovenous fistula

An abnormal communication between an artery and a vein causes rapid shunting of blood between the high and low pressure circulations. Such a fistula is sometimes seen in vascular malformations, may occur spontaneously or secondary to tumour, aneurysm, inflammation or necrosis, but is most frequently post-traumatic in origin. The most obvious example of a spontaneous AV fistula is that of the carotico-cavernous fistula, which presents with pulsating exophthalmos (Chapter 86). A traumatic fistula may result from a gunshot or stab wound, or any other penetrating injury (Fig. 94.23). Many such penetrating injuries are perpetrated by the medical profession! Examples include the iatrogenic AV fistulae that may occur in the liver and kidney following biopsies or interventional procedures; in the hip, spine and other sites following orthopaedic operations; in the groin following femoral arteriography and in the neck following carotid or vertebral punctures.

Closure of a haemodynamically significant arteriovenous fistula results in an immediate and dramatic bradycardia. This is called *Branham's sign* [44] and is diagnostically useful since temporary digital compression of the fistula elicits bradycardia [45]. The same phenomenon may be observed if effective compression can be applied to the 'arterial' type of AV malformation. An arteriovenous fistula can lead to high output cardiac failure and such a lesion should be treated once diagnosed. Good arteriography is important in demonstrating the anatomy of the abnormal communication and requires a fast injection of an adequate volume of contrast medium with early rapid serial filming. Some of these lesions can be treated by interventional methods, which, in certain sites, may obviate difficult or dangerous surgery.

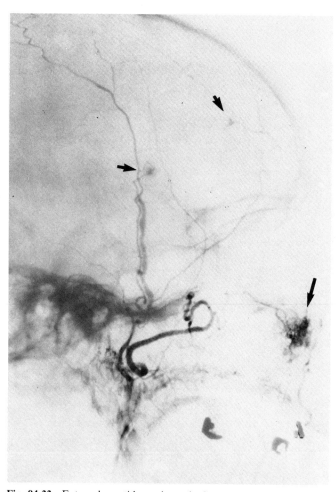

Fig. 94.22 External carotid arteriography in a case of *Osler-Weber-Rendu disease* with epistaxis. Telangiectases are visible in the scalp vessels (short arrows), and a large lesion is seen in the nasal septum (long arrow). The latter lesion was embolized and this successfully controlled the nasal bleeding.

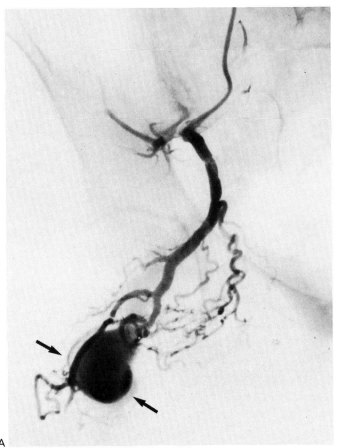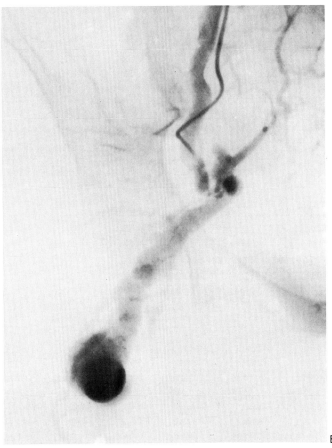

A   B

Fig. 94.23A & B Arteriovenous fistula in the buttock following a penetrating injury in a road accident. (A) A selective gluteal arteriogram shows a false aneurysm at the site of injury (arrows). (B) The contrast medium passes rapidly into a dilated vein.

Aneurysms

An aneurysm is a sac filled with blood in direct communication with the interior of an artery. A *true* aneurysm is due to local dilatation of the artery whereas a *false* aneursym is a sac with walls formed of condensed connective tissue which communicates with the lumen of the artery through an aperture in its wall. *Ectasia* of an artery is dilatation which is not sufficiently pronounced to merit the term aneurysmal and is often widespread whereas an aneurysm is usually localised to a specific site in an artery which may otherwise be relatively normal. Aneurysms may be classified into the following types:

1 Congenital
2 Infective
3 Degenerative
4 Dissecting
5 Post-stenotic
6 Traumatic
7 Post-inflammatory (arteritic; necrotic)
8 Cirsoid

1. Congenital aneurysms

It is always difficult to know whether an aneurysm is truly congenital or has arisen secondary to a disease process. It is thought that many of the aneurysms arising in the cerebral circulation (Chapter 85) are congenital in origin ('berry' aneurysms), especially as they may occur in association with other cardiovascular anomalies; other aetiological factors, however, such as hypertension and atheroma are probably also important.

2. Infective aneurysms

Aneurysms may arise as a result of direct or indirect damage to the arterial wall by microorganisms. One of the best known examples is a syphilitic aneurysm which is usually fusiform and affects the proximal aorta (Chapter 40) though arteries anywhere in the body can be affected. Syphilitic aneurysms are now relatively rare in the developed countries where early diagnosis and treatment of the disease is available. Aneurysms also result from bacterial endocarditis and may affect any of the larger arteries, especially the femoral and superior mesenteric vessels. These aneurysms can grow very rapidly in size and usually require early surgical treatment to obviate rupture. Non-syphilitic infective aneurysms are commonly referred to as *mycotic aneurysms* (see Fig. 94.85); strictly speaking this term is a misnomer as they are usually due to bacterial, not fungal, infections [46].

3. Degenerative aneurysms

One of the commonest causes of aneurysms is so-called degenerative arterial disease which refers to vascular damage by atheromatous changes in the vessel wall. Generally speaking the incidence of these aneurysms is greater in advancing age, in patients with co-existent hypertension and in men compared to women. Atheromatous aneurysms may occur anywhere in the body but common sites include the abdominal aorta, the iliac, femoral and popliteal arteries, visceral arteries (especially the splenic artery), and cerebral arteries; they are sometimes multiple. Aneurysms may be visible on the plain radiograph if they become calcified and *curvilinear calcification* is a characteristic feature (Fig. 94.24). The aneurysms may be fusiform (Fig. 94.25) but if stretching occurs asymmetrically in a weak section of the arterial wall, a *saccular* aneurysm may be formed (Fig. 94.26). A saccular aneurysm is more liable to rupture than a fusiform aneurysm. Aneurysms commonly contain thrombus which may break off and cause peripheral embolization. The arteriographer should be aware of the possibility that an aneurysm contains clot for two reasons: firstly, the lumen of an aneurysm as demonstrated at arteriography may

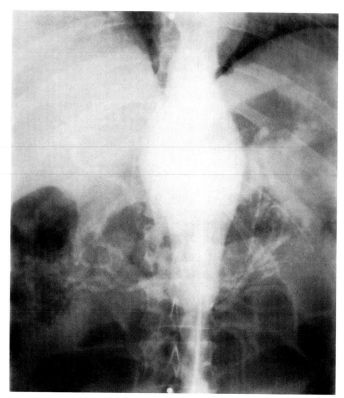

Fig. 94.25　Fusiform abdominal aneurysm.

not be the true lumen of the aneurysm but simply a passage through a large lining thrombus. Indeed, the apparent lumen of a large aneurysm may be similar in calibre to the normal artery. The true size of the aneurysm may be better shown by ultrasound or CT (Fig. 94.27). Secondly, great caution is necessary if a catheter is passed through an aneurysm because of the risk of fragmenting the contained thrombus. A low lumbar aneurysm can be studied by a high TLA or by a catheter passed down from the arm. If a femoral approach is preferred or is essential, the aneurysm should be gingerly traversed with a J-wire and the injection made at a point safely above the aneurysm. Aneurysms may also occur in the arteries and veins involved in *arteriovenous malformations* (see Fig. 94.86).

4. Dissecting aneurysms

Haemorrhage occurs into the tunica media of the vessel (usually the aorta), and splits the wall of the vessel for a variable extent. The blood contained within the split may opacify at arteriography and show as a false lumen. The true lumen may be severely compromised or completely obstructed. The dissection sac frequently spirals around the aorta so that opacification of the true lumen may give the appearance of a twisted tape. The inner layer of the split wall may appear as a thin radiolucent line separating the true from the false lumen if both are opacified (Fig. 94.28). Sometimes the blood in the false lumen bursts back into the true lumen

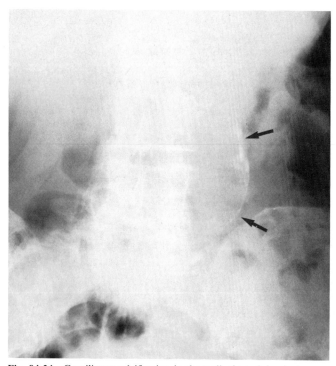

Fig. 94.24　Curvilinear calcification in the wall of an abdominal aneurysm (arrows).

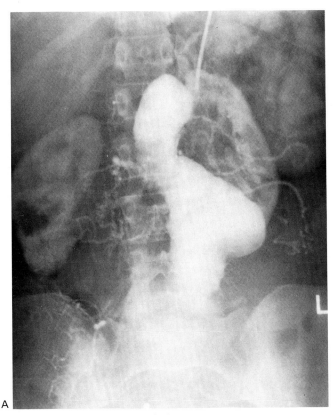
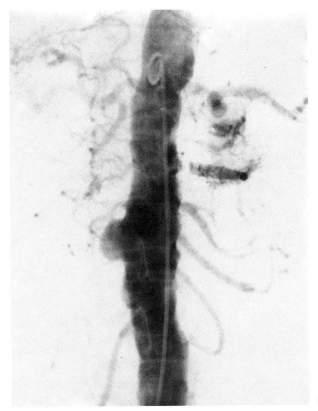

Fig. 94.26A & B Saccular abdominal aneurysms.

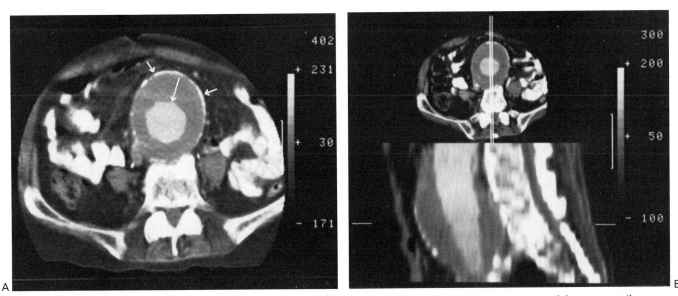

Fig. 94.27A & B CT scan of an abdominal aneurysm. (A) The contrast enhancement shows blood in the patent lumen of the aneurysm (long arrow), while the true calibre of the aneurysm is defined by the calcification seen in the arterial wall (short arrows). Note the erosion of the vertebral body by the aneurysm. (B) A sagittal reconstruction gives a 'lateral' view of the aneurysm.

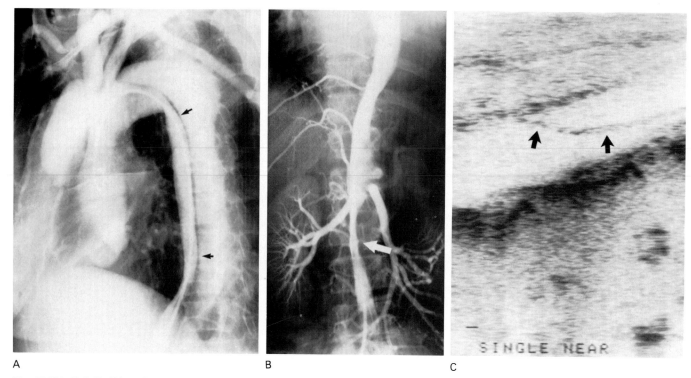

A   B   C

Fig. 94.28A, B & C   Dissecting aneurysm. (A) A Thoracic aortogram shows the inner layer of the dissection sac as a radiolucent line (arrows). (B) The abdominal aorta of the same patient shows the 'twisted cape' sign (arrow). (C) An ultrasound scan shows the dissection flap (arrows).

through a second aperture giving a so-called *double-barrelled* aorta.

Dissecting aneurysm occurs most commonly in hypertensive patients and there is an increased risk of the condition in Marfan's syndrome. The dissection starts most commonly in the arch of the aorta (Chapter 40) and may extend proximally to the heart or distally down into the abdomen. Branch vessels such as the neck vessels, renal, mesenteric and iliac vessels may all become involved by the dissection and may be acutely obstructed by the process.

DeBakey [47] defines three principal types of dissecting aortic aneurysm: Type I, the commonest begins in the ascending aorta just above the aortic valve and extends around the arch into the descending aorta; Type II (typical of Marfan's disease) involves only the ascending aorta; Type III begins just beyond the origin of the left subclavian artery and extends caudally in the descending aorta, usually involving the abdominal aorta as well. Retrograde dissection may also occur back around the arch into the ascending aorta.

Dissecting aneurysm is a dangerous condition with an extremely high mortality [48]. The role of the radiologist is to confirm or refute the clinical diagnosis, and, if a dissection is present, to determine its site and extent as this information will critically affect the surgical management. The plain chest radiograph may suggest the diagnosis, particularly if recent previous films are available for comparison. The shape of the aortic knuckle is lost as the aorta distends towards the left and gives an abnormal mediastinal contour. Occasionally a

soft tissue mass separates the calcified rim of an aortic knuckle from its pleural reflection, but this is an unreliable sign. A pleural effusion may also be present. The most useful radiological investigations are CT scanning and arteriography. The investigation of dissecting aneurysm is discussed more fully in Chapter 40.

We are reminded by Abrams [48], that aortic dissection is not new and is no respecter of rank: he quotes from an article by Nicholls [49] describing the post-mortem of George II entitled *Observations concerning the body of his late majesty*. 'The aorta was dilated and showed a transverse fissure an inch and a half long, through which some blood had lately passed under the external coat and formed an elevated ecchymosis.'

5. Post-stenotic aneurysms

The walls of a blood vessel immediately distal (downstream) to an area of narrowing are subjected to abnormal stresses owing to the flow turbulence generated by the obstructing lesion. This may result in a post-stenotic dilatation or aneurysm (Fig. 94.29). Common examples include the vascular dilatation found distal to an aortic coarctation or pulmonary stenosis, and the aneurysm that may occur distal to a subclavian obstruction at the thoracic inlet. The subclavian artery may be compressed at this site by a cervical rib, an abnormal first rib, or muscular and fibrous bands associated with the scalenus anticus or medius muscles (the

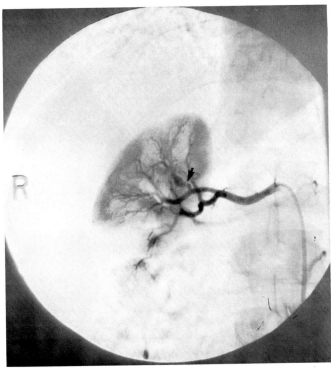

Fig. 94.29 Post-stenotic aneurysm. There is a stenosis of a branch artery in the kidney (arrow). Distal to the stenosis the artery is aneurysmally dilated. Note the defect in the lower pole nephrogram indicating the presence of a second (unopacified) renal artery.

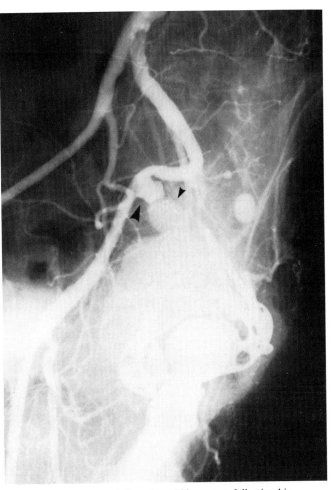

Fig. 94.30 Aneurysm of the external iliac artery following hip replacement. The exothermic reaction of the bone cement (small arrowhead) used in the prosthesis has caused an aneurysm in the neighbouring vessel (large arrowhead).

'scalene syndrome'). The compression may only occur in certain positions and arteriograms of this region should include studies with the arm in both neutral and elevated positions. Subclavian aneurysms commonly contain thrombus and may cause symptoms attributable to recurrent digital embolization. It should be emphasized that the chance radiographic finding of an anomalous or cervical rib does not merit further investigation in the absence of clinical symptoms.

6. Traumatic aneurysms

These are frequently false aneurysms and occur at sites of vascular injury (Fig. 94.23). A variety of different types of trauma can produce an aneurysm including penetrating, cutting, crush and stretching injuries, and thermal injuries (Fig. 94.30).

7. Post-inflammatory aneurysms (arteritis; necrotizing vasculitis)

Aneurysms may occur following weakening of the vessel wall by inflammation. This may be secondary to surrounding local infection as in pancreatitis (Fig. 94.31), or may result from an inflammatory process within the vessel itself such as arteritis. Some of the *collagen disorders* are characterized by

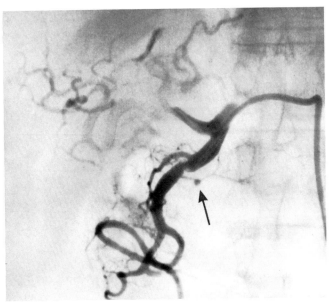

Fig. 94.31 Pancreatic aneurysm. A selective gastroduodenal arteriogram reveals a small aneurysm in the head of the pancreas (arrow). The patient suffers from chronic pancreatitis.

a necrotizing vasculitis which can in some cases lead to the formation of small aneurysms or *microaneurysms*. In polyarteritis nodosa such microaneurysms can be demonstrated by arteriography in a proportion of cases, and may assist in establishing the diagnosis [50]. The aneurysms are most easily shown in the hepatic and renal circulations (Fig. 94.32). Radiologically similar microaneurysms can occur in 'mainline' drug addicts, HbAs positive patients (?link with drug abuse), transplanted kidneys during rejection [51], in association with atrial myxoma, and, rarely, in other collagen diseases such as systemic lupus erythematosus.

In *Behçet's disease* aneurysms may occur [52,53] and can become very large. They are found in the aorta and large vessels but may also occur in the peripheral vessels and the pulmonary circulation. Rupture of one of these aneurysms is a cause of sudden death in Behçet's disease.

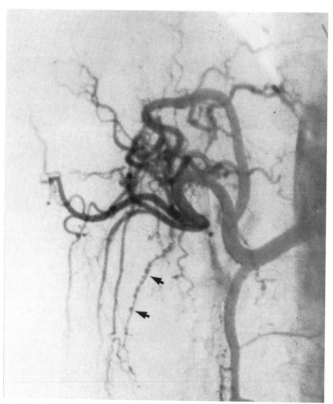

Fig. 94.32 Polyarteritis nodosa (PAN). The classical microaneurysms are seen in this hepatic arteriogram (arrows).

8. Cirsoid aneurysm

This is the surgical term applied to a pulsatile mass of abnormal, dilated, intercommunicating arteries and (sometimes) veins, the so-called 'bag of worms'. Most occur in the scalp in association with the frontal or temporal arteries and may arise following local trauma. They gradually increase in size and may rupture. The entities covered by the term prob-

ably include congenital arteriovenous malformations, traumatic AV fistulae, and traumatic aneurysms. They are always conspicuous lesions arteriographically, and some can be treated by embolization.

Atheroma

Atheroma (atherosclerosis) is a disorder of the arterial wall causing irregularity and narrowing of the vascular lumen which may lead to distal ischaemia. Thrombosis and occlusion may occur, or weakening of the vessel wall with dilatation or aneurysm formation. The disease is characterized by the accumulation of lipid deposits in the intima. The soft, porridge-like material from which the disease takes its name (*athere*: gruel) may be discharged into the lumen leaving an atheromatous ulcer on the wall which may be the starting point for thrombus or embolus formation. The lesions of atheroma may calcify and be visible on the plain radiograph (Fig. 94.33). There are other causes of arterial calcification visible on the plain radiograph. These include disorders giving rise to a raised serum calcium, notably hyperparathyroidism (primary and secondary; Fig. 94.34A); diabetes; Werner's syndrome (a rare condition of premature ageing); arteriovenous malformations; aneurysms and medial sclerosis.

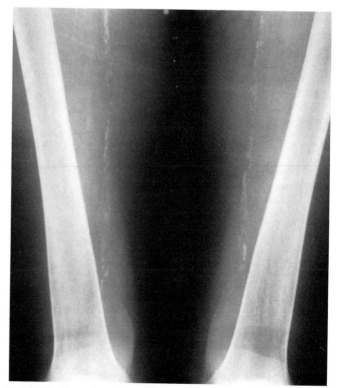

Fig. 94.33 Extensive calcification in atheroma of the superficial femoral arteries.

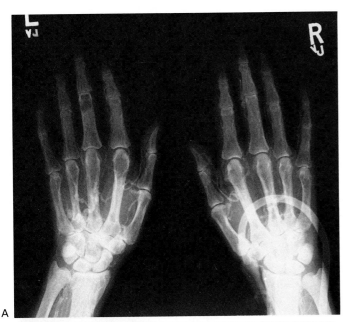

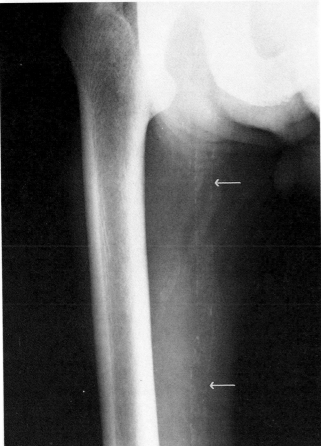

Fig. 94.34A & B Two examples of arterial calcification:
(A) Hyperparathyroidism (Note the osteitis fibrosa cystica).
(B) Monckeberg's medial calcific sclerosis (arrows).

The incidence of atheroma increases with advancing age and is commoner in men than pre-menopausal women; in the older age groups the incidence is approximately equal.

Atheroma is a major cause of death and disability, and its investigation accounts for a substantial proportion of all arteriograms performed. The sites in which atheroma is of particular clinical importance include the carotid and cerebral arteries (see Chapter 85), the coronary arteries (see Chapter 35), the abdominal aorta and its renal and visceral branches, and the iliac and lower extremity vessels. Atheroma is rare in the pulmonary arteries unless pulmonary hypertension is also present. Atheroma tends to be deposited on the posterior wall of vessels, particularly in the aorto-iliac region, and the lumen may be severely compromised without this being evident on a single AP projection; oblique or lateral views may be necessary in appropriate cases.

The presence of atheroma in a vessel makes the job of the arteriographer more difficult and dangerous. It may be awkward or impossible to negotiate a catheter or wire through a lumen lined with irregular clumps of atheroma, and the tip of the catheter may elevate plaques of atheroma leading to vascular dissection or occlusion, or dislodge unstable thrombus leading to embolism. The radiologist should always approach an atheromatous vascular tree with caution, and remember that the purpose of diagnostic arteriography is to acquire necessary information without harming the patient. Some useful tips for the more experienced operator on negotiating difficult arteries are to be found in the superbly illustrated book by Ring and McLean [54].

Medial sclerosis

In *Monckeberg's medial calcific sclerosis* (medial degeneration) the medium-sized muscular arteries, particularly of the limbs, become tortuous, hard and calcified: 'pipe-stem arteries'. The calcification may be very extensive (Fig. 94.34B) but there is no significant luminal narrowing unless (as is often the case) there is co-existent intimal atheroma. Bone may eventually form in the calcified areas which are initially patchily distributed in rings or plaques but later become continuous.

Arteritis

A variety of inflammatory disorders may affect blood vessels and many of these produce changes that can be discerned radiologically. In the acute stages of an arteritis arteriography may be normal or may show irregularity of the lumen of vessels, variation in the calibre of vessels, thrombus or occlusion. In the later stages, depending on the balance of progression or healing in the disease, the arteriogram may show stenoses or long segments of arterial narrowing; dilatation, ectasia or aneurysm formation; occlusions; or a return to normal appearances. In many cases, the arteriographic findings in arteritis are non-specific as they can be produced by a number of different disorders.

Infective arteritis

Infective arteritis such as syphilis can lead to aneurysm formation (p. 2009).

Non-specific arteritis may occur as a result of injury by bacterial toxins, ionizing radiation, chemicals, etc. It usually affects small arteries which are not individually demonstrable arteriographically. A general reduction in the vascularity of the affected organ or region may sometimes be seen.

Necrotizing arteritis

Necrotizing arteritis occurs in a number of collagen diseases. In many of these the changes are at a microscopic level and are not usually demonstrable arteriographically (e.g. *Churg-Strauss syndrome*). Microaneurysms and changes in vessel calibre may be seen, however, notably in polyarteritis nodosa [50].

Giant cell arteritis (temporal arteritis)

Giant cell arteritis produces changes in vessel calibre that can be demonstrated by selective arteriography of the superficial temporal artery and other arteries [55,56]. The diagnosis,

however, is made on the basis of clinical findings and arterial biopsy, and arteriography is not necessary [56].

Takayashu's syndrome [57]

Takayashu's syndrome (syn. pulseless disease; aortic arch syndrome; young female arteritis; giant cell aortitis). This is a rare disorder described by the Japanese ophthalmologist, Takayashu. There is thickening of the wall of the aorta and the origins of its main branches, particularly in the neck, leading to stenosis, thrombosis and occlusion of vessels. The radial pulse is frequently absent. The disease may also affect the pulmonary arteries and other vessels (Fig. 94.35). Although the disease was originally described in young women similar changes have been reported in order patients and both sexes. The radiological changes are described in Chapter 40.

Thromboangiitis obliterans (Buerger's disease)

This is a condition in which thrombotic occlusion of the vessels, usually in the legs, causes ischaemia leading to gangrene of the toes and feet. It occurs characteristically in young males, is strongly associated with smoking, and was thought by Buerger and others to be an inflammatory disorder of the vessels with consequent thrombosis [58,59]. Many consider that Buerger's disease is not a separate pathological entity, but simply represents a type of atheromatous disease with peripheral thrombosis [45,60,61]. Whatever the truth of the matter there is little doubt that some patients with ischaemic symptoms show an arteriographic pattern of vascular occlusion which is more peripheral than is

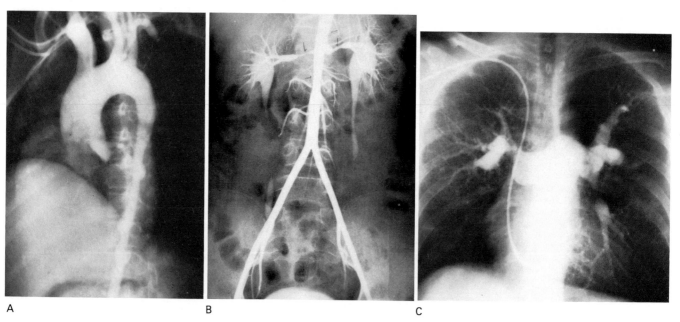

A   B   C

Fig. 94.35A, B & C   Takayashu's disease. (A) Severe narrowing of the thoracic aorta. (B) In a different patient the abdominal aorta and renal arteries are affected. (C) The pulmonary vessels can be involved. (Figures by courtesy of Dr. Lenny Tan: Singapore).

commonly seen in atheromatous disease, and with apparently healthy arteries above the level of the occlusion [62]. Spiral or 'corkscrew' collateral vessels are said to be a characteristic feature of the disorder.

Behçet's disease [52,53] may involve both veins and arteries. The venous manifestations of the disease are common and predominantly related to thrombophlebitis. Two principal types of involvement have been described in the arteries: an *occlusive* form of disease affecting peripheral vessels (simulating non-arteritic peripheral vascular disease), and an *aneurysmal* form which can affect any of the arteries but characteristically involves the aorta or other large vessels Chapter 40.

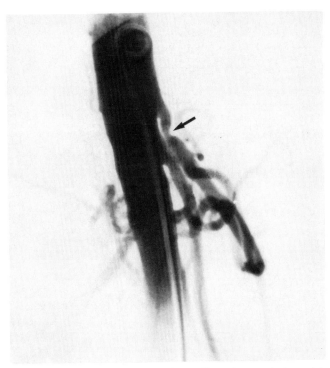

Fig. 94.36 Lateral aortogram showing coeliac axis stenosis (arrow) in a patient with visceral angina.

Stenosis, thrombosis and embolism

Stenosis

Stenosis or narrowing of an artery can be congenital or acquired in origin. Some examples of congenital stenoses such as coarctation of the thoracic and abdominal aorta have already been alluded to. They may also occur in the pulmonary arteries and in some of the abdominal vessels such as the coeliac axis and the renal arteries. Rarely, congenital stenoses occur in the extremities such as in the *popliteal entrapment syndrome* [62], where the popliteal artery is compressed as it passes through an anomalous muscle insertion.

Acquired stenoses of vessels are due in the vast majority of cases to atheromatous disease. Other causes include trauma, arteritis, fibrosis at the site of a surgical anastomosis, previous ligation, extrinsic compression or encasement by tumour, and rarely, arterial wall cysts. Some cases of mesenteric ischaemia are thought to be due to compression of the coeliac axis by an abnormal arrangement of fibres of the diaphragmatic crura. The coeliac territory 'steals' blood via collaterals from the superior mesenteric artery causing so-called *visceral angina*. The same symptoms can be caused by acquired atheromatous stenoses of the coeliac and mesenteric vessels. Investigation of visceral angina is best done by *lateral aortography* with rapid early serial filming. This may show stenosis of one of the major visceral vessels (Fig. 94.36).

Fibromuscular hyperplasia

Fibromuscular hyperplasia [43,63,64,65,66], also known as fibromuscular dysplasia or medial dysplasia is an interesting condition of unknown aetiology. Arteries affected by the condition may show a variety of histological changes including intimal fibrous stenosis, medial fibromuscular stenosis, subadventitial fibroplasia and periarterial fibrous stenosis. There are several subclassifications based on the

relative preponderance of these changes. The condition presents most commonly in young adult females and frequently affects the renal arteries. It can however affect other arteries including the mesenteric and cephalic vessels [43] and, rarely, the extremities [62]. There is an association with cerebral aneurysms [43]. Arteriographically, fibromuscular hyperplasia classically causes an irregular beaded appearance of the affected vessel caused by areas of stenosis alternating with sacculated or sometimes even aneurysmal segments (Fig. 94.37). This appearance has been variously described as a 'string of sausages', 'string of beads' or 'string of pearls', (an interesting range of descriptions which must presumably reflect either the respective social classes or the leisure interests of the various radiologists concerned!). The areas of stenosis may be very severe and cause ischaemia which in the renal arteries may lead to hypertension (cf renal arteriography p. 2033) or occlusion. Frequently the condition does not present as a fully developed 'string of pearls', but as a more modest localized stenosis. Patients with neurofibromatosis have an increased incidence of fibromuscular dysplasia.

Standing waves

The 'string of beads' appearance described above should not be confused with the so-called 'bead phenomenon' [67] which also goes under various other descriptions such as standing waves, *Perlschnuraterie*, stationary arterial waves, static shock phenomenon, corrugated artery and accordion artery. These terms refer to the regular symmetrical contractions

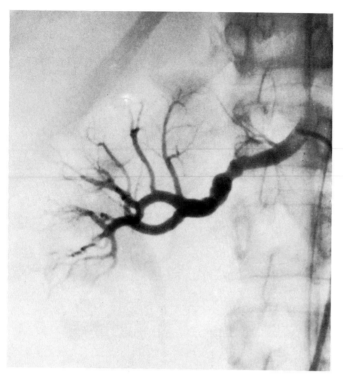

Fig. 94.37   Renal arteriogram showing the 'string of pearls' appearance of fibromuscular dysplasia.

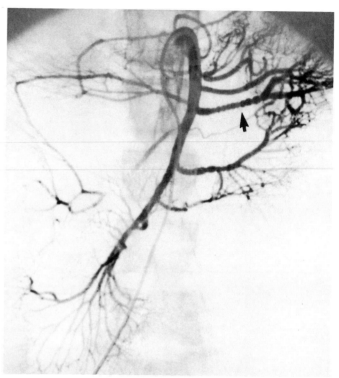

Fig. 94.38   'Standing waves' in a jejunal artery (arrow).

along a segment of artery (Fig. 94.38) that are occasionally seen during an arteriogram, particularly in the lower extremity. Their aetiology is unknown but they are of no pathological significance. It has been suggested that they are caused by longitudinal muscular contractions in the arterial walls [68].

Thrombosis

Arterial thrombosis causing occlusion may occur as a result of many different processes including atheromatous disease, trauma, inflammation, tumour, blood disorders and others. Arteriography is employed (when it affects clinical management) to determine whether thrombosis is present when it is suspected clinically, and to determine if possible its extent. One of the most important causes of thrombosis is atheromatous disease and the investigation of the stenoses and thomboses produced by the condition in the carotid (Chapter 85), coronary (Chapter 35) and aortoiliac-femoral systems comprises a major part of arteriography. In the abdominal aorta, iliac vessels and lower limb vessels the processes of stenosis and thrombosis reduce the vascular supply to the lower extremities and cause *intermittent claudication*. As further reduction in flow occurs the patient suffers *rest pain* and ultimately the ischaemia leads to *gangrene*. When the blood flow through a vessel is slowly compromised a *collateral* circulation is established which

takes over the supply function of that vessel; the ultimate thrombosis of the vessel may then be a clinically unimportant event. If a vessel becomes occluded suddenly, however, by an acute thrombosis or embolism, the symptoms and signs of ischaemia are very much worse and the situation may require rapid surgical treatment. It is important for the arteriographer when investigating these conditions to know the origins and courses of potential collateral routes and ensure that they have been adequately demonstrated; knowledge about the existence or the integrity of such collateral vessels may considerably influence clinical management. Thrombosis of the superficial femoral artery is a common event (Fig. 94.39). A collateral pathway is usually established between the profunda system and the popliteal system, though these may also become occluded in advanced disease. When a common or external iliac vessel is blocked (Fig. 94.40) collateral pathways usually develop between the gluteal and obturator branches of the internal iliac (hypogastric) artery and the lower limb vessels. In the case of a common iliac occlusion collaterals develop from the opposite iliac system, from the lumbar and sacral arteries, and from the inferior mesenteric system via its superior haemorrhoidal connections with the pudendal system.

Complete occlusion of the lower aorta may occur (Fig. 94.41) and lumbar and visceral collaterals are then of vital importance. Occlusion of the lower aorta usually extends upwards to the renal arteries and commonly stops at that point. Total occlusion *above* the renal and visceral arteries is very rare [69].

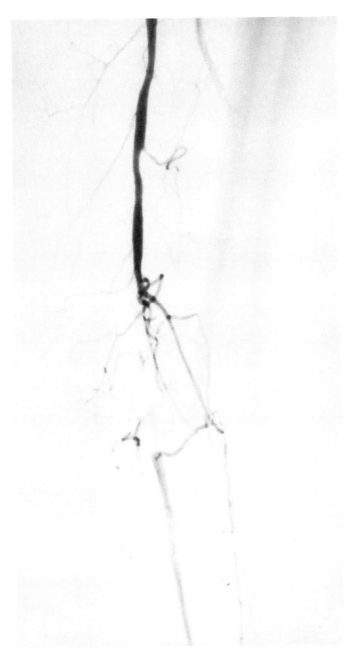

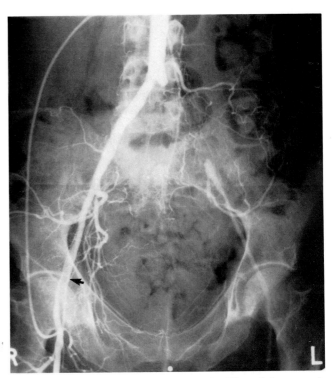

Fig. 94.40 Common iliac occlusion. Note the filling of the external iliac vessel via lumbar and gluteal collaterals. Note also the dissection produced in the right external iliac artery by the catheterization procedure (arrow).

Fig. 94.39 Thrombosis of the superficial femoral artery. Note the collateral vessels supplying the distal patent segment.

Leriche syndrome

Leriche [70] described a syndrome of complete obliteration of the aortic bifurcation occuring predominantly in young adult males and including the feature of absent thigh and leg pulses, weakness of the lower extremities without claudication, and inability to maintain an erection. The term *Leriche syndrome* is now more loosely applied to a spectrum of clinical symptoms and signs referable to either complete or partial aorto-iliac obstruction.

Stenosis of major abdominal aortic branches such as the mesenteric or renal vessels may cause *visceral angina*

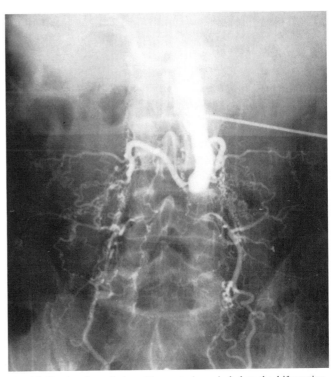

Fig. 94.41 Aortic occlusion. The aorta is occluded at the bifurcation. Note the massive enlargement of the lower lumbar arteries which are the principal collateral vessels in this patient.

(p. 2017) in the former case, and deterioration of renal function and/or hypertension in the latter. The effects of *thrombosis* of these vessels depends greatly on whether it is an acute or acute-on-chronic event. If an adequate collateral circulation exists the immediate effect of thrombosis may be slight. Sudden thrombosis, however, may lead to organ infarction which, in the case of the superior mesenteric system, is usually fatal.

Subclavian steal syndrome

Atheromatous lesions occur in the upper limb vessels, but are much less frequently the cause of clinical symptoms than lesions affecting the arteries of the lower extremity. Severe stenosis or thrombotic occlusion of the proximal subclavian artery may occur, however, and this sometimes produces the phenomenon of 'subclavian steal'. In this disorder the arm obtains its blood supply by reverse flow down the ipsilateral vertebral artery (whose origin lies distal to and unaffected by the subclavian stenosis). The blood comes from the opposite vertebral artery or from the circle of Willis and it is postulated by some that this syphonage of blood from the vertebro-basilar system may be sufficient to produce symptoms of cerebral insufficiency in some cases. 'Subclavian steal' is well demonstrated by arch aortography which should include films exposed sufficiently late to demonstrate the delayed passage of opacified blood *down* the vertebral artery and into the arm of the affected side (Fig. 94.42).

Embolism

Embolism is the impaction in the vascular system of undissolved material brought there by the blood stream. Emboli may be composed of thrombus, fat, gas, amniotic fluid, tumour fragments, tissue fragments, parasites, pus, or external artefacts introduced either accidentally or deliberately (c.f. therapeutic embolization). Thrombus is the commonest form of embolus and on the arterial side of the circulation may originate in the left atrium due to fibrillation, on damaged mitral and aortic valve cusps, on the endocardium following myocardial infarction, within aneurysms of the heart or vessels, and on atheromatous plaques and ulcers. A very rare form of arterial embolization is *paradoxical embolization*. This occurs when a clot on the venous side of the circulation passes through a patent foramen ovale or other septal defect and enters the arterial system. For this

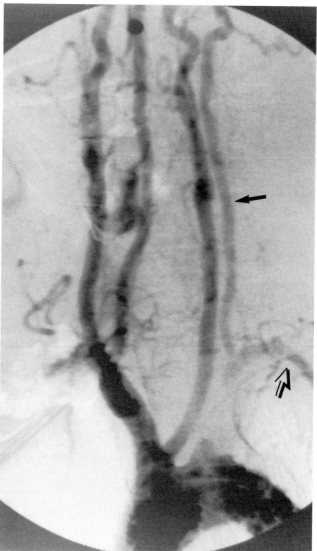

Fig. 94.42A & B The 'subclavian steal' phenomenon. An intravenous (arm vein) DSA shows the aortic arch (A). Note the occluded stump of the left subclavian artery (arrow). A few seconds later (B) the left vertebral artery fills from *above downwards* (solid arrow), and the subclavian artery distal to the vertebral origin becomes opacified (hatched arrow).

to happen of course the pressure in the right atrium has to exceed that in the left atrium. An embolus may lodge anywhere in the arterial system, the bigger the embolus the more proximal being the site of its impaction. The clinical effects of an embolus obviously depend on the vascular bed obstructed; an embolus into the cerebral circulation may cause a stroke or death, whereas an embolus into, say, a small muscle vessel or the liver may pass unnoticed. A large embolus may occasionally obstruct the aortic bifurcation ('saddle' embolus), and a typical site for a smaller embolus to lodge in the lower limb is in the popliteal artery.

Arteriography will normally establish the site of occlusion by an embolus and this is an important factor in determining the best surgical approach when operative intervention seems necessary. In some centres selective intra-arterial strepto-kinase infusion is employed in the treatment of some types of acute thrombosis or embolism [71] (Chapter 98).

Ischaemia

Ischaemia refers to an insufficiency in the supply of blood to an organ or region of the body. The clinical effects vary with the site and degree of vascular insufficiency, but typical manifestations of ischaemia include pain, trophic changes, temperature changes, deterioration or loss of function in the affected organ, and, in severe or progressive instances, infarction of tissue. There are many different causes of ischaemia and arteriography is used to investigate the condition in a number of ways:

1. It can identify the site, extent and sometimes the nature of an organic vascular obstruction. This is a most important function of arteriography which is indispensable to the clinical management of cardiac disease, peripheral vascular disease, etc.

2. It can often confirm or refute a clinical suspicion of significant vascular insufficiency. A good example of this is the investigation of suspected mesenteric angina (p. 2017).

3. It may establish whether ischaemia is due to an organic vascular lesion when other causes of vascular insufficiency could account for the clinical picture. An example of this might be the demonstration of a subclavian stenosis in a case of Raynaud's phenomenon.

4. Pharmacoangiography can be used to investigate whether ischaemia is due to vasomotor disturbances, or organic vascular disease.

5. It can demonstrate whether ischaemia can be corrected surgically by displaying the 'run-off'.

Haemorrhage

Arteriography is used in both the localization of haemorrhage and its treatment. The technique is particularly valuable in gastrointestinal bleeding (Fig. 94.43 and see p. 2040), but can be used in the investigation of many types of haemorrhage including epistaxis (Fig. 94.22), haemoptysis, renal tract bleeding and bleeding following trauma. Interventional techniques (Chapter 98) can be used to control bleeding by the infusion of drugs or therapeutic embolization.

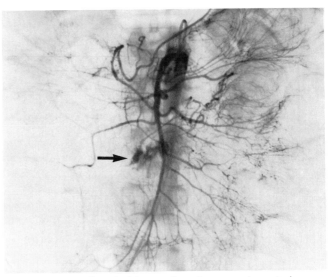

Fig. 94.43 Gastrointestinal haemorrhage from an enteroenteric anastomosis. A superior mesenteric arteriogram in an actively bleeding patient shows contrast medium leaking from the region of a previous surgical anastomosis (arrow).

Tumours

For many years arteriography has proved extremely useful in the investigation of tumours and suspected tumours. Much of the information previously acquired by arteriography in this area of diagnosis can now be obtained less invasively (and often more accurately) by techniques such as ultrasonography, nuclear medicine, computerized tomography and magnetic resonance imaging. For certain types of lesion, however, and in particular clinical circumstances, arteriography remains an important tool in tumour investigation and management, and it is important for every radiologist to be aware of the potential applications of the technique. It should also be remembered that the sophisticated imaging modalities that are supplanting the role of arteriography in this field are not universally available, nor are they likely to be in the foreseeable future. Arteriography is used in five ways in the investigation and management of tumours:

1. Diagnosis
2. Localization
3. Site of origin
4. Operability
5. Treatment

1. Diagnosis

The presence of a tumour can often be established or confirmed by arteriography, and the radiological features demonstrated by the study may assist in differentiating a tumour from other space-occupying lesions (e.g. cyst, abscess), may sometimes point to the benign or malignant nature of the lesion, and, occasionally, may suggest a specific histological diagnosis.

The radiologist looks for three radiological features when assessing an arteriogram of a tumour or suspected tumour: displacement, pathological circulation and encasement.

a. Displacement of normal arteries and veins (Fig. 94.44 & 94.45). As the tumour grows it distorts surrounding vessels and in many cases the approximate size and shape of the tumour can be ascertained from the vessels swept around it. This feature alone does not clinch the diagnosis of a solid tumour; similar appearances may occur with cystic lesions.

b. Pathological circulation is a term used to describe the abnormal vascularity that may occur within or adjacent to a solid tumour (Figs. 94.45, 94.46). It covers a spectrum of different appearances. There may be changes in the calibre

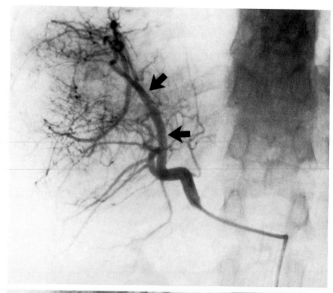

A

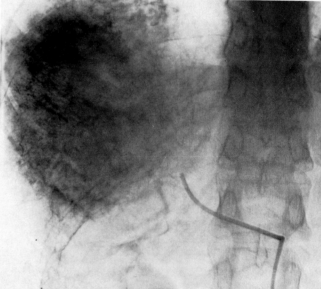

B

Fig. 94.45A & B Hepatic arteriography in a case of massive liver metastasis. (A) Arterial phase: The tumour deposit is displacing the hepatic artery (arrows). (B) Parenchymal phase: There is a dense 'blush' in the large tumour deposit.

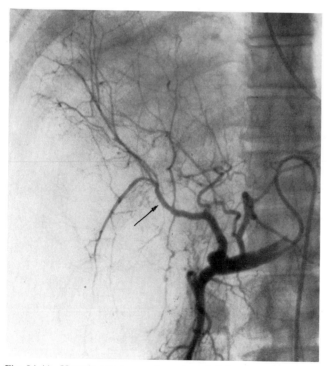

Fig. 94.44 Hepatic arteriogram in a case of cholangiocarcinoma. The tumour is arteriographically avascular but has produced a curved displacement of the right hepatic artery (arrow).

of vessels; abrupt occlusions; increased tortuosity; abnormal vascular spaces or 'lakes' that may fill in either the arterial, capillary or venous phase of the study; arteriovenous communications, and even aneurysms (Fig. 94.47). In some tumours there is an abnormally dense appearance on arteriography owing to its increased vascularity in comparison with the surrounding normal tissue, but no demonstrable morphological abnormalities in the vessels. These tumours characteristically opacify in the capillary phase of a study — the so-called *tumour blush* (Fig. 94.48 and see Figs. 94.55 & 94.91). It should be emphasized that the presence of a pathological circulation does not necessarily imply that a tumour is malignant. Some benign tumours may show very bizarre vascular appearances.

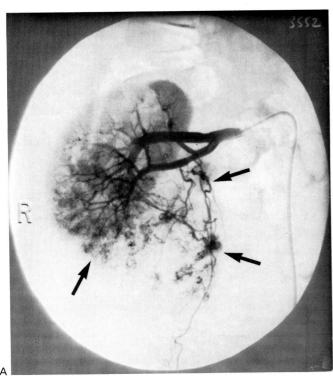

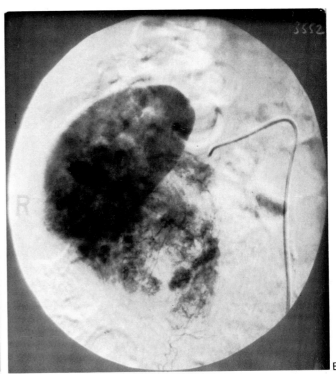

Fig. 94.46A & B Pathological circulation in a renal cell carcinoma. (A) Arterial phase: Abnormal vessels are seen in a tumour growing from the lower pole of the kidney (arrows). (B) Nephrogram phase: The tumour contains irregular areas with abnormal vasculature and dense tumour 'blushes'. Compare the appearance of the tumour with that of the normal nephrogram in the upper pole.

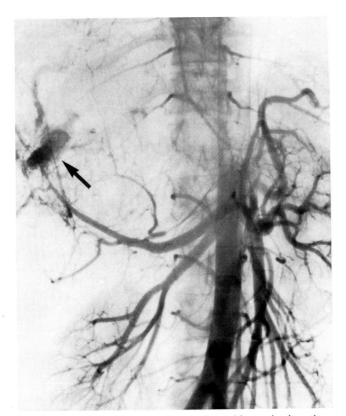

Fig. 94.47 Hepatic arteriogram in a patient with massive hepatic secondary deposits from a rhabdomyosarcoma of the heart. There is a large aneurysm in the tumour circulation (arrow).

c. Encasement is a term that describes the narrowing or cuffing of a vessel by a surrounding tumour mass (Fig. 94.49). Early encasement may produce very subtle changes in calibre that must be looked for carefully. In the late phase of an arteriogram, encasement of the adjacent *veins* may also be demonstrated. Encasement is an important sign for it usually (though not invariably) indicates the presence of a *malignant* tumour, and it may also influence the *operability* of tumours in certain sites.

2. Localization

In some circumstances the diagnosis of a tumour is virtually certain on the basis of clinical and biochemical evidence, but the location of the tumour is unknown. This situation occurs with functioning endocrine tumours such as parathyroid adenomas, and pancreatic apudomas. Arteriography is sometimes employed to localize such tumours for the surgeon.

3. Site of origin

Despite the accuracy of cross-sectional imaging techniques in demonstrating the site and extent of tumours it is occasionally impossible to determine the site of origin of a tumour, particularly if it is large and invading adjacent structures. This situation is relatively uncommon but arises most often with large tumours in the liver, stomach, adrenal,

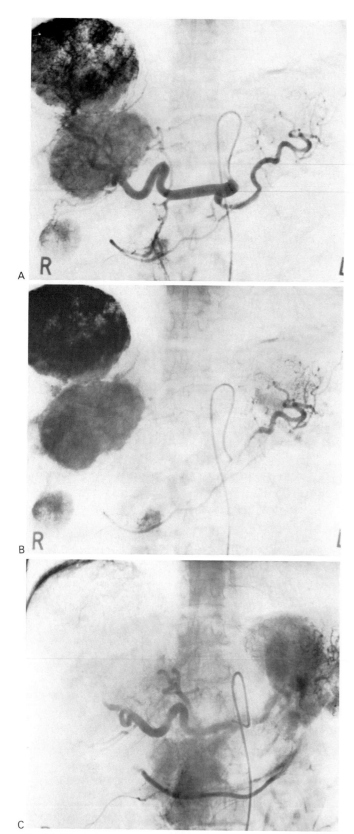

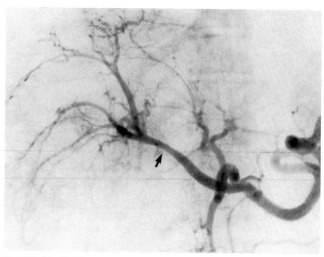

Fig. 94.49 Carcinoma of the gall bladder. The tumour has produced displacement and encasement (arrow) of the right hepatic artery.

Fig. 94.48A, B & C Malignant glucagonoma deposits in the liver. (A) Coeliac arteriogram showing three large secondary tumours in the liver. (B) The tumour blush is very dense in the capillary phase of the study. (C) The lesions have been embolized.

kidney, pancreas and retroperitoneum. An arteriogram in such a case will frequently identify the vessels supplying the lesion and give a valuable clue as to its site of origin; this may assist the surgeon in planning an operative strategy (see Fig. 94.59).

4. Operability

An important function of arteriography in tumour management is in the assessment of the potential *operability* of a lesion. Arteriography demonstrates the vascular supply to a tumour together with any local anomalies of the arterial tree that may influence the surgical approach to a tumour. It also shows whether arterial or venous encasement or invasion has occurred and whether the tumour has compromised the blood supply to neighbouring vital organs; factors that may indicate to the surgeon that a tumour is irresectable or that special arrangements may be necessary to make resection possible (e.g. vascular bypass, assistance from other surgeons with special skills, unusual transfusion requirements, tourniquets, hypothermia, etc.). Arteriography may reveal secondary tumour deposits which previous investigations have failed to demonstrate. This is most likely to happen in the case of liver metastases which, if vascular in nature, can be shown by arteriography when only a few millimeters in diameter (Fig. 94.50). Knowledge about the presence or absence of secondary tumour in the liver may profoundly influence the clinical management of an abdominal tumour.

Caution should be exercised in interpreting hepatic arteriograms performed in patients who have had previous percutaneous techniques performed (PTC, biopsy, biliary drainage etc). A small arterio-portal fistula may cause a parenchymal blush which can easily be mistaken for a tumour deposit (see Fig. 51.38, p. 982).

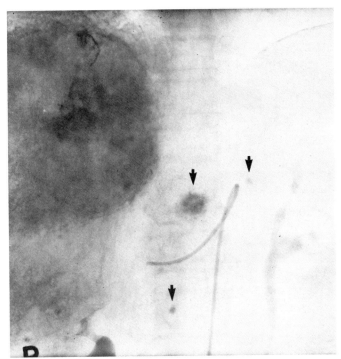

Fig. 94.50 Selective hepatic arteriography in a patient with metastatic tumour deposits in the liver. The large right lobe tumour was shown on CT, but the small deposits in the left lobe (arrows) were only demonstrated on this vascular study.

5. Treatment

Arteriographic techniques may be used in the treatment of tumours. Regression of some benign primary tumours has been reported after selective (wedged) arteriography alone [72], but the most common therapeutic applications are *selective infusion* techniques and *embolization* techniques. These are discussed in Chapter 98.

Trauma

Arteriography may be used to assess organic or vascular injury after trauma (including iatrogenic trauma). In blunt or crushing injuries (particularly to the abdomen) arteriography may demonstrate the extent of visceral and vascular trauma to the liver, spleen, kidney or bowel. In *deceleration injuries* arteriography may show damage to the thoracic aorta and in penetrating injuries throughout the body arteriography may show either early or late vascular pathology. In *orthopaedic injuries* the ultimate fate of a limb may depend more on the extent of any associated vascular injury than the skeletal injury. Arteriography is used to investigate suspected vascular injury or insufficiency (Fig. 94.51, 94.52).

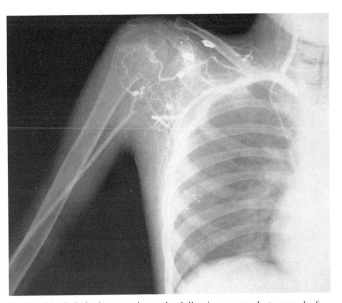

Fig. 94.51 Subclavian arteriography following a gun-shot wound of the shoulder. The axillary artery has been severed; circulation to the arm is maintained via collateral vessels around the shoulder joint.

Iatrogenic trauma may take many forms. Percutaneous or operative biopsy techniques in organs such as the liver or kidney can cause bleeding or arteriovenous fistulae that may need investigation or treatment by angiographic techniques; surgery of almost any kind may cause vascular problems in which arteriography may be helpful or indispensable in making subsequent management decisions (Fig. 94.53).

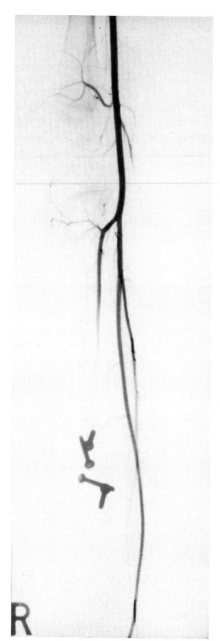

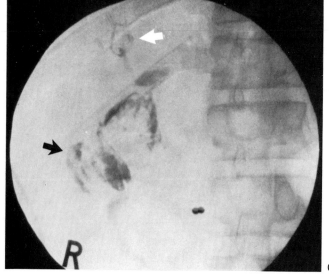

A

B

C

Fig. 94.52 Lower limb arteriography in a case of non-union of a tibial fracture. The anterior tibial artery does not fill for more than a few centimetres from its origin. The region of the fracture (screws) is only supplied by a small twig from the posterior tibial artery.

Fig. 94.53A, B & C Superior mesenteric arteriography in a case of post-surgical bleeding. The patient has had a choledocho-jejunostomy and an entero-enterostomy. Active bleeding is shown on the initial study (A) from the region of the choledocho-jejunostomy (arrow). A selective jejunal arteriogram (B), shows detail of the bleeding artery, and a late film in the same study (C) shows extravasated contrast medium in both the biliary tree (white arrow) and the bowel lumen (black arrow).

Arterial embolization

There are a number of clinical situations (e.g. bleeding) in which it is desirable to reduce or abolish the blood supply to an organ or region. In many cases this can be achieved most efficiently and safely by the use of percutaneous trans-catheter embolization techniques which are discussed in detail in Chapter 98.

Percutaneous transluminal angioplasty

Vascular disease commonly results in symptoms or signs attributable to ischaemia of the affected organ or region. In a number of cases it is possible to alleviate this ischaemia by percutaneous techniques designed to increase the effective lumen of the vessels supplying the affected region. These techniques (which commonly obviate surgery) are described in detail in Chapter 98.

REGIONAL ARTERIOGRAPHY

In this section the techniques and special problems relating to arteriography are considered. For purposes of brevity the general points above concerning the indications for arteriography, complications, etc. are not repeated for each vascular territory; these are mentioned again only when some particular aspect requires emphasis. Where rates and volumes are given for injections of contrast medium, it should be assumed that these will be considerably lower if digital subtraction techniques are being used.

1. Head and neck

Arch aortography

Arch aortography is most safely performed with a pig-tailed catheter. This is situated in the ascending aorta so that during injection the partially unfolded tip remains clear of the aortic valve. The flow in this region is higher than in any other artery in the body, so a large volume of contrast medium needs to be injected at an adequate rate. Typical factors in an adult would be 60 ml Urografin 370 (or equivalent) at 30 ml/s with a very rapid, early filming sequence. The aorta arches posteriorly and to the left in the superior medias-tinum, so is best demonstrated in the right posterior oblique projection (left anterior oblique) in which it lies parallel to the film; obviously other projections may be necessary in particular cases and it is the usual practice to obtain both oblique views in most patients. On a single projection a vascular stenosis or other significant pathology may be missed completely.

Arch aortography may be used to examine the aorta in cases of suspected aneurysm, aortitis or dissection; for 'cardiac' problems such as aortic valve or root disease; congenital anomalies such as vascular rings and coarctation (Chapter 40); and for problems affecting the origins of the great vessels. The place of aortography in the investigation of transient ischaemic attacks and other neurological conditions is discussed in Chapter 83. In the investigation of the subclavian arteries an arch study may show proximal disease, and is the best way of demonstrating the existence of a *subclavian steal phenomenon* (Fig. 94.42).

Common carotid artery

The common carotid artery can usually be selectively catheterized with a 'headhunter'-shaped catheter (Fig. 94.2B); in difficult cases a shepherd's crook or 'sidewinder' (Fig. 94.2B) is nearly always successful; other shapes are also available. A common carotid arteriogram may be requested by the vascular surgeon or neurologist seeking information about occlusive disease at the carotid bifurcation prior to possible surgery (Fig. 94.54). Another, rarer, indication is the investigation of a suspected *carotid body tumour* (chemodectoma, paraganglioma, chromaffinoma, potato tumour). This tumour may be mistaken clinically for an aneurysm, but the arteriogram is diagnostic (Fig. 94.55); a densely vascular lesion lies at the carotid bifurcation splaying the origins of the internal and external arteries. Other vascular tumours in the neck include the *glomus jugulare tumour* (Fig. 94.56) seen usually at or near the base of the skull, and the very rare *vagal neuroma*. Although all these tumours are supplied by branches of the external carotid artery, a common carotid arteriogram gives the surgeon valuable information concerning the relationship of the lesion to the internal carotid artery and whether that vessel is displaced or compromised by the tumour.

External carotid arteriography

Selective external carotid arteriograms are relatively straightforward to perform in younger patients but can be difficult and dangerous in older patients with atheroma in the neck vessels. A 'headhunter' or similar catheter is suitable, and the artery is most easily selected when screening in the lateral position. This can be done using horizontal fluoroscopy with the patient supine, or using vertical fluoroscopy with the patient's head lateral and shoulders in the LAO. The normal external carotid system is easily opacified by a firm hand injection of 5–10 ml contrast medium (preferably non-ionic or low osmolality because conventional media cause severe

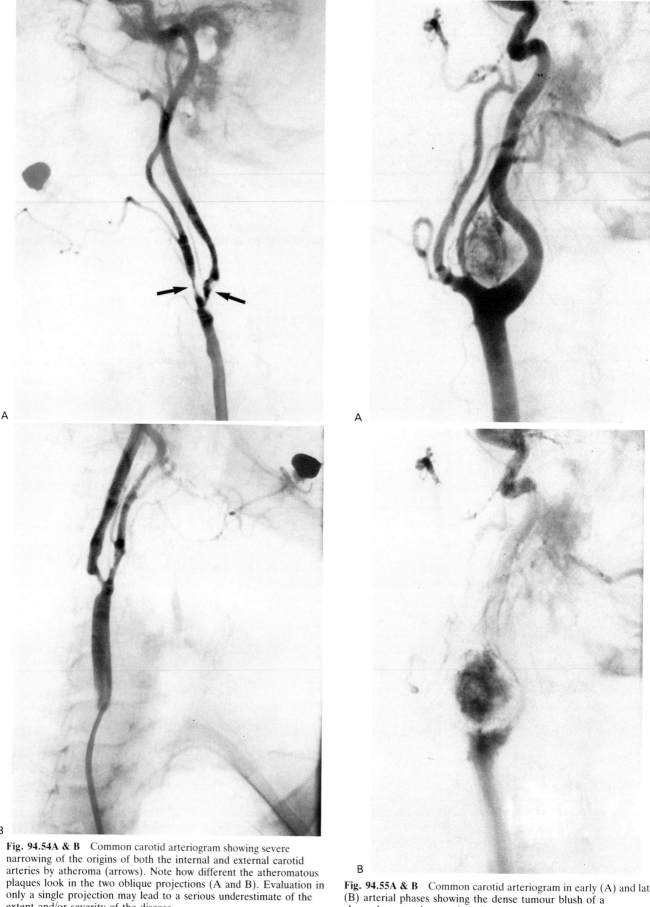

Fig. 94.54A & B Common carotid arteriogram showing severe narrowing of the origins of both the internal and external carotid arteries by atheroma (arrows). Note how different the atheromatous plaques look in the two oblique projections (A and B). Evaluation in only a single projection may lead to a serious underestimate of the extent and/or severity of the disease.

Fig. 94.55A & B Common carotid arteriogram in early (A) and late (B) arterial phases showing the dense tumour blush of a chemodectoma characteristically splaying the carotid bifurcation.

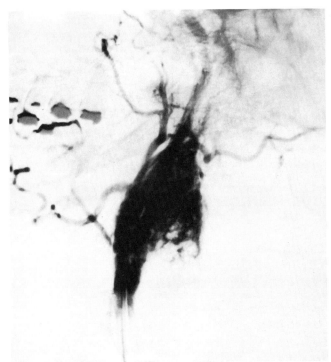

Fig. 94.56 Glomus jugulare tumour shown on carotid arteriography.

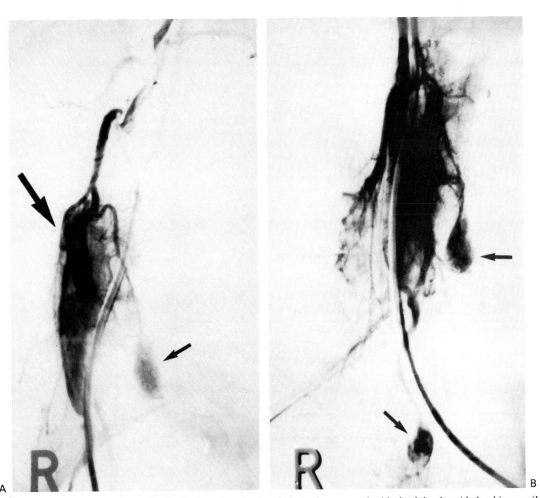

Fig. 94.57A & B Superior thyroid arteriography. In the lateral projection (A) the dense vascular blush of the thyroid gland is seen (large arrow) and a smaller blush indicates the site of a parathyroid adenoma (small arrow). In the AP projection (B) a less collimated view shows a second tumour lying in the thorax (arrows indicate sites of both tumours).

discomfort in this territory). The indications for selective external carotid studies are relatively few. They include the more exact assessment of the feeding vessels to tumours shown on common carotid studies (see above), especially if embolization is to be used in the pre-operative or definitive treatment of the lesion. One tumour in which selective studies are particularly helpful is the *juvenile angiofibroma* (nasopharyngeal fibroma), a highly vascular tumour which usually presents in the nasopharyngeal area of young males, and which is now often treated either definitively or pre-operatively by embolization. External carotid angiography is also used in some centres to assist in the diagnosis or embolization of *meningiomas*.

Arteriovenous malformations are particularly common in the external carotid territory and selective studies are essential to delineate the extent of these lesions and their vessels of supply. In addition to ipsilateral studies an antero-posterior filming sequence should always be obtained during contrast injection into the *contralateral* external carotid artery to demonstrate any collateral vessels crossing the mid-line. An ipsilateral *internal* carotid study may reveal unsuspected enlargement of the natural communications that exist between the internal and external systems: vitally important information for the surgeon or embolizing radiologist.

Epistaxis may be investigated by selective arteriography with a view to therapeutic embolization (Chapter 98).

Parathyroid adenomas [72,73] can be demonstrated by selective superior thyroid arteriography (Fig. 94.57) but they are usually located surgically or by other less invasive imaging techniques.

Readers interested in more detailed descriptions of arteriographic techniques in the external carotid system are referred to the beautifully illustrated book devoted to the subject by Djindjian and Merland [74].

Internal carotid arteriography

Internal carotid and cerebral arteriography is performed for the investigation and treatment of intracranial pathology and is described in Chapter 83.

2. Thorax and abdomen

Thoracic aortography

The investigation of the thoracic aorta is discussed in Chapter 40.

Cardiac and pulmonary arteriography

These important topics are dealt with in Chapters 24 and 33 respectively.

Bronchial arteriography

There has been a recent revival of interest in bronchial arteriography because of the possibility of localizing and controlling haemoptysis by therapeutic embolization in appropriate cases [75]. It is also possible to embolize hypertrophied bronchial arteries as part of a combined radiological and surgical corrective procedure in certain types of congenital cardio-pulmonary anomaly.

There is considerable variation in the way in which the bronchial arteries arise from the thoracic aorta [76,77,78]. The commonest arrangement is one main right artery from a common intercosto-bronchial trunk at about the level of T5, and two left bronchial arteries arising a little lower. Specially designed bronchial catheters are available, but other catheters can be used, their essential features being a reasonably tapered tip and a 'shepherd's crook' configuration. The bronchial arteries may communicate with radiculo-medullary branches supplying the spinal arteries, and it is safest to use a non-ionic contrast medium as transverse myelitis has been reported as a complication of simple arteriography, as well as following bronchial embolization. A hand injection of 3–5 ml contrast medium normally suffices to demonstrate the bronchial arteries (Fig. 94.58), and the injection sometimes causes coughing. Diagnostic bronchial arteriography is performed in cases of recurrent haemoptysis where no cause can be found by the usual investigations; in these cases an unusual cause such as an arteriovenous malformation may

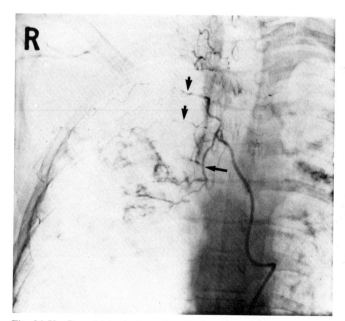

Fig. 94.58 Bronchial arteriography. An intercosto-bronchial trunk has been opacified with Iohexol. The bronchial artery is shown by a long arrow; intercostal arteries by short arrows.

be shown and it may be possible to embolize it. Emergency bronchial arteriography is performed in cases of life-threatening haemoptysis to locate and embolize the bleeding site in patients in whom surgery is impossible or inappropriate [75].

Lumbar aortography

The lumbar aorta is best opacified by an automatic pressure injection of contrast medium through a catheter passed up from a percutaneous femoral puncture. 50 ml of Urografin 370 (or equivalent) injected in 2 seconds gives adequate opacification in the average adult. The catheter should be a pig-tailed or a straight 'flush' catheter with side-holes. When there is atheroma affecting the aorta and iliac vessels the use of a J-wire will greatly facilitate the safe passage of the catheter to its desired position. A *preshaped* catheter (other than a pigtail) should never be used for aortography because of the risk of damage to the aortic intima, dislodgement of atheromatous plaques, or the inadvertent injection of a large volume of contrast medium at high flow into a small branch artery causing its rupture or dissection. If the femoral route is not available (e.g. severe iliac disease, previous Dacron graft etc), a *translumbar aortogram* may be performed (p. 1993); if a translumbar aortogram is contraindicated (or for preference in other centres) a catheter can be passed down to the lumbar aorta from an *axillary puncture* or *brachial arteriotomy*. It is hoped that as *intravenous digital subtraction angiography* becomes more widely available it will obviate the need for these arterial approaches to the lumbar aorta in a substantial proportion of patients.

Congenital lesions

Aortography may be needed to define the nature and extent of suspected congenital abnormalities in the aorta and its branches. These have been discussed in general terms above and Fig. 94.15 shows an example of a congenital abdominal coarctation. It may be necessary to examine the aorta both above and below the coarctation for the surgeon to be fully cognizant of the relevant anatomy and, in the case of a tight stenosis or complete occlusion, this may need a high TLA or an arm approach to the upper end of the lesion.

The wide congenital variation that exists in the arrangement of the blood supply to the kidneys has been described above and this is of particular practical importance in the assessment of potential renal donors (see p. 2036). Aortography is sometimes performed prior to surgery on a *horseshoe kidney* or a *pelvic kidney* to help define the number and origins of their arteries of supply.

Atherosclerosis

Lumbar aortography is most commonly performed for the assessment of aorto-iliac atherosclerosis and its sequelae (stenosis, occlusion, aneurysm) with a view to possible surgery (Figs 94.24, 94.40, 94.41). Valuable information for the surgeon will include: the site and extent of localized pathology (e.g. stenoses or aneurysms); the suitability or otherwise of the aorta above the lesions for possible grafting; the involvement by disease of major aortic visceral branches such as the coeliac, superior mesenteric and renal vessels, and the state of the distal arterial tree ('run-off').

Aortic branch disease

Aortography is the best way of demonstrating disease affecting the origins of the aortic branch arteries (e.g. mesenteric, renal). Not only does this give a more general demonstration of the state of the arteries but it obviates the risk of damage to an artery in which flow might already be precarious by the 'blind' use of a selective catheter (e.g. a selective renal catheter may damage an atheromatous plaque and convert a partial occlusion at the renal artery origin to a complete one). Going immediately to a selective study, furthermore, may result in a lesion being completely overlooked: a selective catheter may pass straight through a stenosis at the origin of a visceral vessel and demonstrate an apparently normal circulation in the territory concerned. The best view of a vessel is nearly always that obtained at right angles to its long axis; a study for suspected stenosis of the mesenteric vessels as in *visceral angina* should, therefore, always include a lateral aortogram (Fig. 94.36), while an aortogram for the investigation of *renal hypertension* is initially best performed in the AP projection. Sometimes the origin of a renal vessel may be concealed by the edge of the aorta in the true AP position because of the point at which it arises on the circumference of the vessel; if there is doubt about the integrity of the renal artery origin a slightly oblique view will usually resolve it.

Demonstration of the branches of the aorta is a necessary step in the evaluation of patients prior to surgery on thoraco-abdominal aneurysms.

Aortitis

Arteritis may occur in the aorta as in any other artery. Classical examples include syphilis (Chapter 40) and Takayashu's disease (Fig. 94.35 and Chapter 40), both of which affect the aorta more commonly in the thorax than in the abdomen. There are, however, other arteritides which may affect the lumbar aorta resulting in either occlusive changes or aneurysms: they include infection (often resulting in a *mycotic aneurysm* [79,80]; giant cell arteritis [81], Behçet's syndrome [52,53,82]; and other rare or ill-defined collagen disorders [83,84].

Tumours

With the increasing sophistication of other imaging modalities the role of aortography in the investigation of abdominal tumours has diminished considerably in recent years. When arteriography is now employed it is often as part of management (e.g. embolization, chemo-infusion) rather than diagnosis and this usually entails selective arterial work rather than general aortography. Aortography is, however, still used in tumour diagnosis in centres whether other modalities are unavailable, when the presence of a tumour is strongly suspected but it cannot be located by other means (e.g. ectopic phaeochromocytoma — see below), and in the occasional case where the organ of origin of a known tumour cannot be decided. Paradoxically this latter indication usually applies to very large abdominal tumours where CT and ultrasound may be unable to define normal anatomical boundaries owing to their distortion, compression or invasion by a mass. For instance, the surgeon may wish to know if a large right-sided mass originates in the kidney, adrenal gland or liver as this may affect his/her planning and management. Aortography may be helpful in this situation by suggesting which are the true arteries of supply to the lesion (Fig. 94.59). A problem that may arise here is the fact that some tumours acquire a 'parasitic' blood supply from adjacent organs as they enlarge, and this should be borne in mind when interpreting the aortogram with a view to deciding the organ of origin of a tumour. Acquisition of a 'foreign' blood supply in this way is a feature suggestive of malignancy, but this (as with many things in medicine!) is not invariable, particularly if there has been bleeding, infection or previous

surgery in the region of the tumour all of which may stimulate the development of unusual collateral sources of supply. Criteria for helping to decide between malignant and benign lesions at angiography have been discussed already (p. 2021); it has to be said that in many cases it is difficult or impossible.

Pelvic arteriography

The arteries of the pelvis are best demonstrated overall by a pressure injection of contrast medium into the aorta just above the bifurcation using a pig-tailed or straight catheter with side-ports. If necessary selective studies of particular arteries on either side of the pelvis can then be performed from the same puncture site. Ipsilateral catheterization of the internal iliac artery can usually be performed with a simple 'cobra' (femoro-visceral) catheter; if not, a sidewinder catheter is always successful (unless there is severe occlusive vascular disease). The contralateral internal and external iliac systems can be catheterized by passing a catheter over the aortic bifurcation and down the opposite common iliac vessel. If this is difficult because of an acute bifurcation, then the free limb of a sidewinder catheter will often reach selectively into either the internal or external system from the aortic bifurcation, a position that usually suffices for diag-

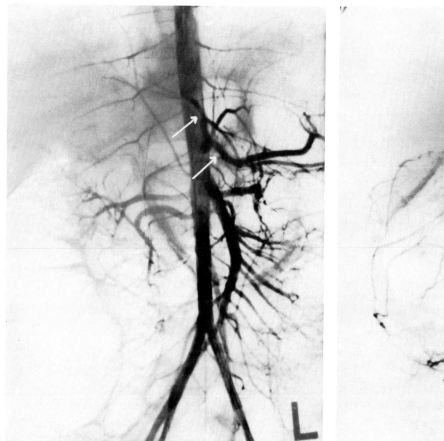

A

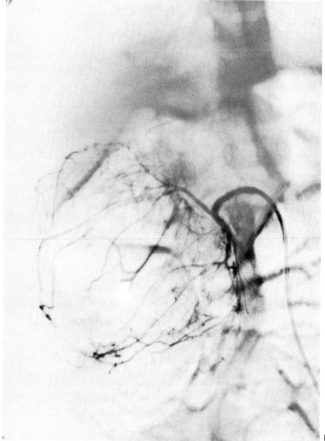

B

Fig. 94.59A & B   Wilms' tumour (nephroblastoma) (A) A flush aortogram shows a large mass displacing the hepatic artery (white arrows). (B) A selective renal arteriogram (lower pole vessel) shows the tumour to arise from the kidney. CT scanning did not resolve the site of origin of this large tumour which could have been hepatic, adrenal or renal.

nostic studies. If it is essential to get a catheter even further (e.g. for interventional purposes) the sidewinder catheter can be used to direct a suitable wire into the desired artery and then be exchanged for a conventionally curved catheter. A wire passed down into the opposite femoral artery from a catheter at the bifurcation can sometimes be pinioned at the groin by external pessure over the pubis so that it is not dislodged when the catheter is fed down the wire from the bifurcation.

Pelvic arteriography is most commonly performed as part of an aorto-iliac-femoral series in the assessment of occlusive vascular disease (Fig. 94.40). Other indications include the investigation of arteriovenous malformations in pelvic viscera and the gluteal region (a common site for these lesions: Fig. 94.60); the control of bleeding from the pelvic viscera or soft tissues by drugs or emboli in a variety of situations including tumour, trauma and post-surgical haemorrhage (Fig. 94.61); renal transplant arteriography (see below); and the investigation of pelvic tumours. With the use of other imaging modalities the latter indication for pelvic arteriography has become infrequent, but it is still used in special circumstances; an example includes the search for a pelvic phaeochromocytoma which may occur in the *organ of Zuckerkandl* or in other neuroendocrine tissue including the

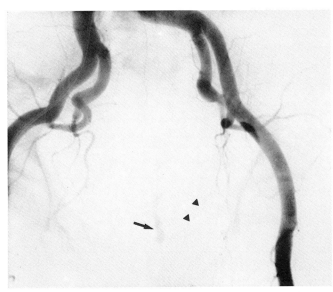

Fig. 94.61   Arteriography in acute haemorrhage. This patient bled profusely following a prostatectomy. Pelvic arteriography shows contrast extravasation in the prostatic bed (long arrow), from an internal pudendal branch (arrowhead). The pudendal artery was embolized.

wall of the bladder. One of the principal presenting symptoms of the patient whose tumour is shown in Figure 94.62 was his observation that micturition was followed by a pounding headache!

Renal arteriography

Advances in CT, ultrasound and isotope techniques have all contributed to a reduction in the need for selective renal angiography, but the procedure still remains one of the

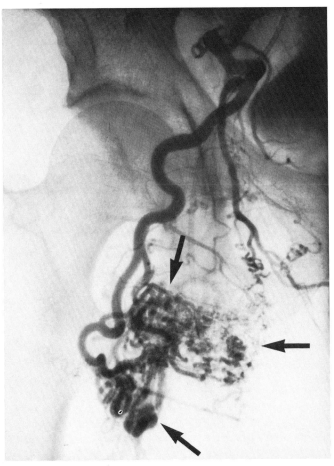

Fig. 94.60   Gluteal arteriogram in a case of arteriovenous malformation. Note the extensive abnormal vascularity of the lesion (arrows).

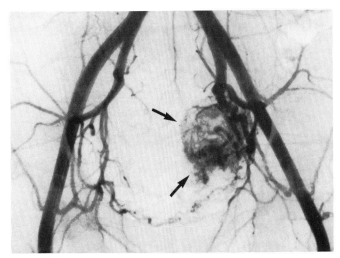

Fig. 94.62   Pelvic phaeochromocytoma. A pelvic arteriogram shows a dense tumour blush in a phaeochromocytoma (arrows) arising from the bladder wall.

commonest selective studies that the angiographer may be requested to perform.

In the majority of cases the radiologist is well advised to perform an *aortogram* prior to embarking on selective renal angiography. Obviously there are exceptions to this rule as when the dose of contrast medium is critically limited and only very restricted information is sought. In general, however, the aortic study provides a number of benefits: firstly, there is great variation in the number and arrangement of the renal arteries; a complete selective study (depending on the clinical context) may require selective examinations of all the arteries feeding a kidney. If a selective study is obtained of only the principal supplying artery the existence of another artery or arteries (which may contain or supply the pathological lesion) may remain unsuspected. Secondly, there may be bilateral renal pathology which was previously unsuspected, knowledge of which may significantly affect surgical management. Thirdly, (and this is particularly important if there is any question of therapeutic radiological intervention such as embolization or angioplasty which may put the vascular supply of one kidney at risk), it demonstrates the existence and gross functional integrity of the contralateral kidney prior to selective studies on the side of immediate interest.

The renal artery can usually be selectively catheterized with a simple curved catheter (Fig. 94.2B); if difficulty is experienced because of a particularly acute caudal angulation of the artery relative to the aorta, then a sidewinder shape may be necessary. For the superselection of individual branch arteries prior to interventional procedures it is usually necessary to use one or more different guidewires, and it is also very helpful to alter the angle of the renal artery relative to the aorta by asking the patient to assist with appropriate respiratory movements. When performing superselective studies remember that the ventral (anterior) branch of the renal artery is the predominant supply to the lower pole and the dorsal (posterior) branch is the predominant supply to the upper pole [85].

The average adult kidney can be opacified with 6–10 ml Urografin 290 (or equivalent) injected by hand or pump in 1–2 seconds. Kidneys with large tumours or vascular malformations may require much larger volumes by mechanical injection. Filming sequences in renal arteriography should always include rapid early radiographs to show the *arterial phase* of the study. The *nephrographic phase* immediately follows the arteriographic phase and consists of dense opacification of the renal substance due to contrast medium in both capillaries and nephrons. Radiographs in this phase are very important for the demonstration of certain types of pathology, as avascular lesions will appear as filling defects against the opacified renal tissue. The *venous phase* of the study shows filling of the renal veins and these are best seen 5–10 seconds after the start of the injection. Detailed descriptions of these phases are available in specialized texts [85]. Contrast media are, to a greater or lesser extent, nephrotoxic and the minimum necessary volume should be used during the procedure. Particular caution is necessary in the case of single kidneys, transplanted kidneys, interventional procedures, or in the presence of impaired renal function. Non-ionic media are to be preferred in such

cases and, ideally, should be used in all selective renal studies.

Congenital lesions

Congenital variations of vascular significance are discussed on p. 2005.

Tumours and cysts [86,87]

Ultrasonography is now the procedure of first choice in the investigation of suspected renal mass. Percutaneous cyst puncture, isotope studies and CT are also useful in appropriate cases (Chapters 56,60), and arteriography is now used as a complementary technique to one or more of these other methods in situations where there is continued doubt about the diagnosis, where the surgeon requires specific vascular information, or where embolization or perfusion therapy is contemplated.

Benign tumours

Simple cysts displace arteries, do not exhibit a pathological circulation, appear as a filling defect in the nephrogram phase and may be outlined by a ring of fine veins in the venous phase. In *polycystic* disease the main arteries are usually narrower than normal despite the increased size of the kidney, and in the parenchyma the arteries are elongated and follow the cyst contours. The nephrogram shows multiple filling defects.

Angiomyolipoma (hamartoma) is a rare tumour which can occur in isolation, or in association with tuberous sclerosis (epiloia, Bourneville's syndrome) when multiple tumours may be present. The tumour is interspersed with lipid deposits which appear radiolucent on radiographs and give patchy low attenuation values on the CT scan. The angiographic appearances of the tumour (which is usually very vascular) are bizarre and AV shunts and aneurysms may be present. The appearances may be mistaken for those of a renal cell carcinoma.

Adenomas may occur in the kidney, usually subcapsular in location; other benign lesions include *haemangiomas* and *fibromas*.

Pseudotumours of the kidney. Angiography may be helpful in distinguishing insignificant anatomical variations of renal shape and architecture from pathological entities. A *dromedary hump* is a normal bulge on the lateral surface of the (usually left) kidney that may be mistaken for a tumour. A *benign cortical* rest (cortical island, cortical infolding, focal hypertrophy, cortical hyperplasia), can cause alarm on the IVU. It displaces the calyces and looks like a tumour. At angiography the 'infolded' cortical tissue gives a dense blush in the nephrogram phase (Fig. 94.18). A DMSA isotope scan will show functioning renal tissue at the site of the cortical rest, while a true tumour produces a filling defect on the isotope study.

Malignant tumours

Wilms' tumour (nephroblastoma) This tumour usually occurs in children under five years of age, but can present later in life. It is bilateral in up to 10% of cases [62]. The tumour may grow to a very large size and usually (though not invariably) exhibits a pathological circulation at angiography (Fig. 94.59). The principal differential diagnosis in this age group is from a *neuroblastoma* which arises from the adrenal gland but may displace and invade the kidney. A Wilms' tumour usually causes more obvious distortion of the intrarenal architecture than a neuroblastoma.

Renal cell carcinoma (hypernephroma) This is usually a highly vascular tumour with a conspicuous pathological circulation (Fig. 94.46). A small proportion, however, (<10%), may be hypovascular. The venous phase of an arteriogram performed in a case of renal carcinoma should be carefully scrutinized for evidence of tumour in the renal vein as this finding may considerably influence subsequent management. Failure to visualize the main renal vein despite the injection of a large volume of contrast medium and prolonged filming suggests that the venous drainage may be compromised by tumour infiltration, thrombosis or compression [88]. The demonstration of a large venous collateral network is another feature suggesting that the renal vein is obstructed [89]. *Adrenaline* (epinephrine) has been used to help in the diagnosis. In doubtful cases 5–10 μg adrenaline is injected through the renal catheter in a few ml of saline, and contrast medium injected 10–30 seconds later. Adrenaline constricts normal vessels rendering the pathological tumour vessels more conspicuous. There is no doubt that this method is effective in demonstrating renal tumours more clearly [89]; radiologists vary, however, in their opinions concerning its value in diagnostic practice.

Urothelial tumours These may show some increased vascularity but do not exhibit the grossly pathological circulation commonly seen in renal cell carcinoma. Other malignant tumours include renal sarcoma, lymphoma, and metastases from other organs. All these tumours may exhibit varying degrees of vascularity.

Vascular abnormalities

The general angiographic features of the following vascular abnormalities have already been described earlier in this chapter.

Aneurysms may occur in the main renal artery, usually as a result of degenerative atherosclerotic disease but also as congenital lesions, as part of the spectrum of fibromuscular dysplasia, or following local trauma or inflammation [43]. The demonstration of multiple aneurysms affecting small or medium-sized vessels in the kidney is highly suggestive of polyarteritis nodosa (PAN) [43,50], and renal angiography is

sometimes performed to help establish this diagnosis if it is suspected clinically [50].

Arteriovenous malformations and fistulae. Congenital AVMs occur in the kidney and are usually easily identified at angiography because of their abnormal vessels, rapid flow and early venous filling. Embolization may be curative if it is technically possible. An arteriovenous fistula may occur as a feature of a congenital AVM, but may also result from trauma, surgery, percutaneous biopsy or nephrostomy, tumour or rupture of an aneurysm. Any of these fistulae may be associated with haematuria. This may be occult or may be massive and life-threatening. Embolization is the treatment of choice in many of these cases.

Renal artery stenosis. The commonest cause of main renal artery stenosis is arteriosclerosis (Fig. 94.63); other causes include fibromuscular hyperplasia (p. 2017) [43,63,64,65,66], congenital stenosis or coarctation [43,90], neurofibromatosis [43,91], and rarely, extrinsic compression. The latter can be caused by fibrous musculotendinous bands of the diaphragmatic crura or psoas muscle [43,92], by hilar tumours such as phaeochromocytoma [43,93] or lymphosarcoma deposits, or by pressure from a hydatid cyst or abdominal aortic aneurysm. Renal artery stenosis is an important condition because it may be the cause of hypertension. *Renovascular hypertension* probably accounts for only 5% of all cases of hypertension but its importance lies in the fact that it may be curable by either surgery or transluminal angioplasty.

A 'flush aortogram' should always be performed when investigating a case of suspected renal artery stenosis for the

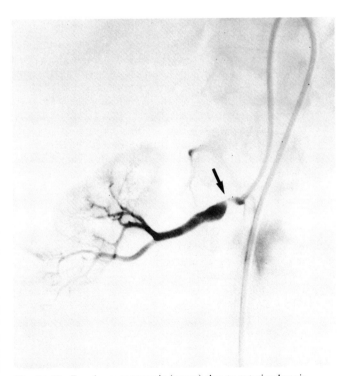

Fig. 94.63 Renal artery stenosis (arrow) due to arteriosclerosis.

reasons mentioned above (see 'aortic branch disease'). Selective studies should, in fact, be avoided unless the findings on aortography are diagnostically inadequate, equivocal, or raise a new question that can only be resolved by a renal arteriogram. Selective catheterization will of course also be necessary if a stenosis is revealed and it is the intention to proceed directly to angioplasty. A feature of longstanding renal artery stenosis is the collateral circulation that develops. The first three lumbar arteries are the principal collateral sources; others may include unnamed twigs from the aorta, the fourth lumbar artery, the internal iliac or gonadal vessels via periureteric channels, and the intercostal or adrenal arteries via capsular channels. The enlarged lumbar arteries in this situation can be mistaken for small or supernumary renal vessels.

Vascular studies in renal transplantation

1. The donor

Part of the preliminary assessment of the suitability of a *renal transplant donor* includes an aortogram to show the number and position of the arteries supplying the prospective transplant kidney, and to exclude disease in either this organ or the one that is to remain behind. The renal arteries are commonly among the first branches of the aorta to be opacified and an early, rapid film sequence will often help in the task of differentiating what is renal from what is not renal. The lumbar arteries can easily be mistaken for small supernumary renal vessels; helpful distinguishing points include the fact that the lumbar arteries normally (though not invariably) opacify somewhat later in the injection sequence than renal vessels, and they have a characteristic bend where they curve backwards alongside the vertebral body. Selective renal arteriography should never routinely be performed during a study of a potential renal donor because the risk (albeit small) of damaging a normal kidney in a normal person is quite unacceptable. In two situations, however, it may be justified: 1) if there is some doubt about the vascular anatomy of an otherwise suitable transplant kidney which would significantly affect surgical management and which can only be resolved by a selective study; and 2) if the initial aortogram reveals unsuspected pathology in either kidney that requires more selective angiographic evaluation.

2. The recipient

Transplanted kidneys are usually situated in the iliac fossa and the artery of the grafted organ anastomosed to the recipient's internal iliac (hypogastric) artery. Arteriography of the transplanted kidney may be requested in order to investigate either poor function of the organ (in the absence of overt urinary obstruction), or hypertension. The aim of the radiologist in this situation is to obtain the maximum information about the vascular supply to the kidney with the least risk to what is a very precious organ to the patient. Non-ionic contrast medium is used for preference and the safest preliminary approach (if DSA is unavailable or

inadequate) is a percutaneous femoral puncture on the side *opposite* to the transplant. A catheter is positioned just above the bifurcation and a pelvic aortogram obtained (Fig. 94.64B); alternatively, a catheter can be passed over the bifurcation into the common iliac artery. The best position to show the transplant artery is unpredictable and views in

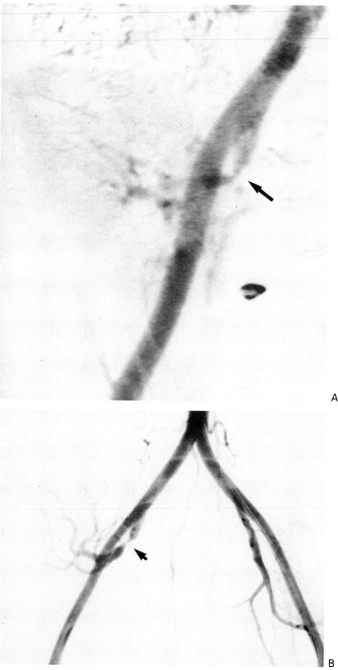

Fig. 94.64A & B Renal transplant artery stenosis. The transplanted kidney has been attached to the right internal iliac (hypogastric) artery by an end-to-end anastomosis. A stenosis (arrowed) of the artery supplying the transplant is shown by an intravenous (antecubital vein) DSA study (A), and by an intra-arterial catheter injection into the lower aorta (B) prior to a successful transluminal angioplasty.

different projections may be necessary to visualize the whole artery; video review of test injections is very helpful in selecting the most useful projections. Selective studies of the transplant artery may be necessary in some cases if the above arteriograms are inadequate and these can be done from either a contralateral or an ipsilateral approach. In a proportion of cases a stenosis may be demonstrated of the transplant artery (not necessarily at the site of the anastomosis). In some of these patients renal function is dramatically improved following angioplasty (Chapter 98) and hypertension (if present) may be cured or ameliorated. If DSA is available satisfactory views may be obtained from an IV injection (Fig. 94.64A). In other patients the arteriographic signs of rejection may be present [94]. These include the slow transit of contrast medium through the kidney, loss of visualization of the more periperal intrarenal arteries and loss of the cortical nephrogram. In some chronic cases marked irregularity and sudden tapering of the vessels is visible, and microaneurysms may be present [51].

Renal trauma

Arteriography may help in the assessment of renal damage following blunt or penetrating trauma. The filming sequence should include some rapid early radiographs to demonstrate a possible arteriovenous fistula and radiographs in the nephrographic phase to assess the integrity of the renal paranchyma. A delayed film will give a demonstration of the collecting systems. Information obtained from an arteriogram in this situation can considerably influence management, even as to whether or not an emergency nephrectomy may be necessary; in some circumstances arterial embolization may obviate surgery.

Miscellaneous conditions

In the past arteriography has been used in the assessment of a number of disorders for which it is no longer used (except in unusual circumstances) because of advances in other imaging methods, medical therapy and biopsy techniques. These conditions include pyelonephritis, xanthogranulomatous pyelonephritis, pyonephrosis, renal tuberculosis, and hydronephrosis. The interested reader is referred to specialist texts for details of the arteriographic appearances that have been described in these disorders.

Gastrointestinal arteriography

General points

The principal indications for arteriography of the gastrointestinal tract are the diagnosis and/or treatment of gastrointestinal bleeding; the localization, pre-operative assessment and/or treatment of gastrointestinal tumours (including hepatic and pancreatic lesions); the investigation of suspected mesenteric ischaemia [95] and, in combination with venous studies, the evaluation of the anatomy and flow dynamics of the portal system in portal hypertension.

Good arteriography requires an experienced radiologist, good equipment (which can take early, rapid films and late films), a mechanical injection pump, and an experienced radiographer. It is of course feasible to perform gastrointestinal arteriography on an occasional basis but the interpretation of a study is just as important as its technical execution, and there is no doubt that the diagnostic value and reliability of the various procedures are greatest in units where they are performed regularly. It is likely that the quality, comfort and safety of gastrointestinal arteriography will improve with the increased use of digital techniques and the newer contrast media. These factors, together with the increasing therapeutic role of arteriography, make it probable that the method will continue to play an important part in the management of gastrointestinal disorders: it is surprising how often, despite advances in other imaging methods, it is still an arteriogram that produces the definitive answer in a difficult diagnostic problem.

The three major vessels of supply to the gastrointestinal viscera are the coeliac axis, the superior mesenteric artery and the inferior mesenteric artery. Although all three vessels opacify during an aortic injection the radiographic detail on such a study is inadequate for diagnosis in most cases and it is usually desirable to perform selective arteriography of individual arteries or their branches. There are two exceptions to this: the first is when the origins of the vessels are being examined in a case of suspected mesenteric ischaemia: a lateral aortogram is then the study of choice at least as an initial manoeuvre (see above under 'Stenosis, thrombosis and embolization', p. 2017; and Fig. 94.36). The second is when a patient presents with bleeding due to an *aorto-duodenal fistula*. Selective arteriography may be completely normal in such a patient even in the presence of active bleeding; a lateral aortogram will confirm the diagnosis which should be considered particularly in a patient with a history of previous aortic surgery and gastrointestinal bleeding.

The choice of selective vessels to be studied, and the sequence of their investigation will depend on the clinical problem under investigation. In a patient with upper gastrointestinal bleeding, for instance, attention would clearly be focused on the coeliac and superior mesenteric territories rather than the inferior mesenteric.

The value of gastrointestinal angiography is very dependent on the nature of the pathology under investigation. Vascular tumours (Fig. 94.65) or malformations are usually easy to identify; other lesions such as ulcers which cause minimal angiographic changes in the vasculature are usually impossible to demonstrate unless they are actively bleeding during the procedure or have produced secondary changes such as aneurysms in the local vessels.

The coeliac axis [96]

The coeliac axis is the artery of the primitive foregut and through its three branches (left gastric, splenic and common hepatic) it supplies the stomach and upper duodenum, spleen, liver and pancreas (Fig. 94.66 and see Fig. 94.92). The coeliac stem arises from the front of the aorta at the level of L1; it can be catheterized with a femoral-visceral catheter (Fig. 94.2B), but a *sidewinder* catheter (Fig. 94.2B)

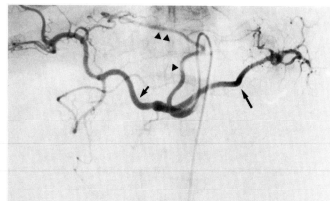

Fig. 94.66 Coeliac axis arteriogram using a 'sidewinder' catheter. The splenic (long arrow), left gastric (single arrowhead) and common hepatic arteries (short arrow) are well demonstrated. Note that the left gastric artery also gives rise to an accessory left hepatic artery (double arrowhead).

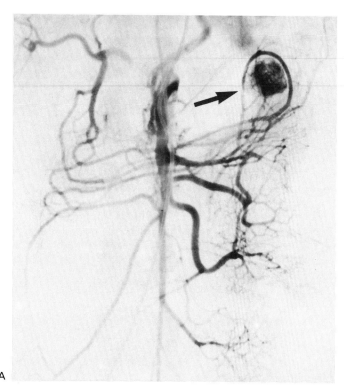

A

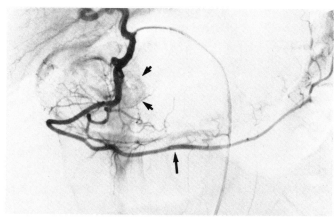

Fig. 94.67 Selective gastroduodenal arteriogram. The right gastro-epiploic artery (one of its terminal branches) is seen coursing round the greater curve of the gas-filled stomach (long arrow). A faint tumour blush (short arrows) reveals a pancreatic polypeptidoma situated in the head of the pancreas.

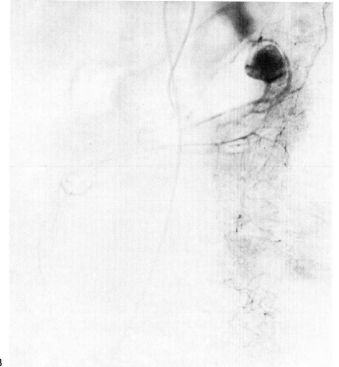

B

Fig. 94.65A & B Superior mesenteric arteriography showing the early (A) and late (B) arterial phases of the study. A very vascular leiomyoma is demonstrated in the upper jejunum (arrow).

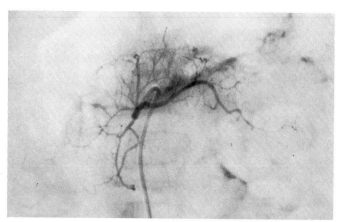

Fig. 94.68 Dorsal pancreatic arteriogram. The outline of virtually the whole pancreas is demonstrated by this selective injection into a large dorsal pancreatic artery (a branch of the splenic artery).

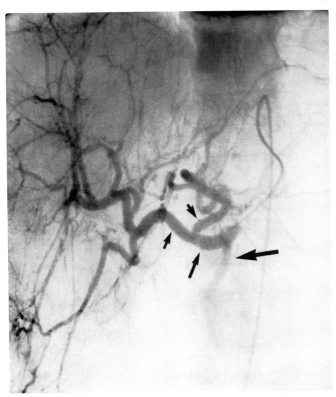

Fig. 94.69 Selective hepatic arteriogram. A sidewinder catheter has been positioned in the common hepatic artery with its tip just proximal to the origin of the gastroduodenal artery which is faintly opacified (large arrow). The proper hepatic artery (small arrow) divides into the right and left hepatic branches (short arrows).

is preferred by the author because it is less likely to be dislodged during a pump injection and can be further manipulated into the splenic or hepatic arteries in a high proportion of cases. Superselective studies of the left gastric, gastroduodenal (Fig. 94.67), dorsal pancreatic (Fig. 94.68) and hepatic vessels (Fig. 94.69) can be obtained with appropriate catheters.

Distension of the stomach and duodenum with carbon dioxide gas helps to reduce the number of confusing shadows produced by opacification of normal folded mucosa in these organs, and oblique views are necessary for the complete demonstration of the duodenum and pancreas.

The coeliac territory can normally be adequately opacified in the average adult by 30–50 ml Urografin 370 or equivalent delivered at 8–10 ml/s by a mechanical injector. Pump injections are also necessary for splenic or common hepatic arteriograms, but hand injections suffice for superselective studies. The radiographic filming sequence should extend sufficiently long to allow visualization of the portal venous system; an *indirect splenoportogram*. This occurs in 8–14 seconds after injection in most patients but may take longer in the presence of splenomegaly or portal obstruction (see Chapters 50 & 95).

Hepatic arteriography [97] is usually performed for the assessment of liver tumours (primary or secondary: see Figs. 94.44,

94.45, 94.48, 94.49), or hepatic bleeding. It is considered further in Chapters 50, 51 and 98).

Pancreatic arteriograpy [98] is now performed relatively infrequently. It was used for many years as a diagnostic tool in cases of suspected carcinoma and chronic pancreatitis, but there is considerable overlap in the angiographic appearances of these diseases and, in the light of other diagnostic advances, the diagnostic role of angiography has diminished in this area. There are three principal indications remaining for pancreatic arteriography:

1. The pre-operative assessment of tumours and cysts in the pancreas (usually already diagnosed by other methods) to define their relationship to vascular structures and, in the case of malignant lesions, their potential resectability. In practice this means excluding tumour encasement of major contiguous vessels, particularly the splenic vein.

2. As part of the investigation of haemobilia (see below: *gastrointestinal bleeding*).

3. To locate pancreatic endocrine tumours (see p. 2053: 'arteriography of the endocrine organs' in which the technique of pancreatic arteriography is discussed).

The superior mesenteric artery [96]

The superior mesenteric artery (SMA) supplies the bowel derived from the primitive mid-gut; from the mid-duodenum to the splenic flexure. It arises from the front of the aorta 1 cm below the coeliac axis and is easily catheterized selectively in most individuals with a sidewinder or femoral-visceral catheter. 30–50 ml 'Urografin 370' or its equivalent injected at 8–10 ml/sec from an automatic injector will opacify the SMA in the average adult (Fig. 94.70). In a large individual it may be impossible to include all the SMA territory on one field of view, and two runs may be necessary. Care should be taken to include the caecum and ascending colon in the radiographic field as these are likely sites for *angiodysplasia* to be found [99,100,101]. It is also important to continue filming up to 20 seconds after the contrast injection. This allows visualization of the superior mesenteric and portal veins, ensures that abnormal venous filling from tumours, malformations or angiodysplasia is demonstrated, and facilitates the detection of extravasated contrast medium in the bowel in cases of active bleeding (see Fig. 94.43).

Selective jejunal, inferior pancreatico-duodenal and middle/right colic arteriograms can be performed using a sidewinder catheter with its free limb down the SMA. Selective ileo-colic or ileal arteriograms, however, require a femoral-visceral (cobra-shaped) catheter which has been passed down the SMA trunk over a suitable guidewire (see Fig. 94.75).

The inferior mesenteric artery [96]

This is the artery of the hind gut, supplying the bowel from the splenic flexure to the rectum (Fig. 94.71). It arises from

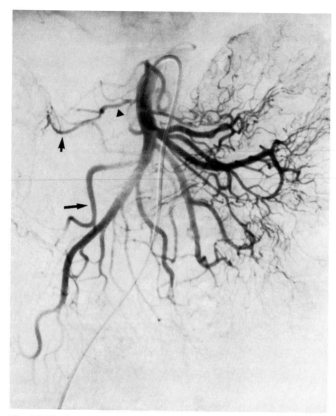

Fig. 94.70 Superior mesenteric arteriogram. The upper branches on the patient's left supply the jejunum, the lower branches the ileum. On the right are the middle colic artery (arrowhead) the right colic artery (short arrow) and the ileo-colic artery (long arrow). The continuation of the main arterial stem ultimately forms the left-hand limb of the ileo-colic anastomotic loop.

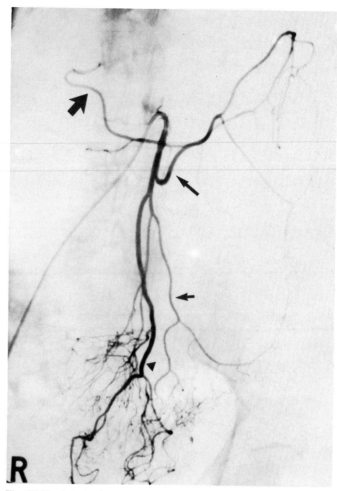

Fig. 94.71 Inferior mesenteric arteriogram showing superior left colic artery (long arrow), inferior left colic artery (short arrow), and superior rectal artery (arrowhead). Note the anastomosis between the superior left colic branches and the middle colic artery (broad arrow).

the front of the aorta 3–4 cm above the aortic bifurcation and is the most difficult of the three major visceral vessels to catheterize. A sidewinder catheter is one of the best catheters to use (Fig. 94.2B), and opacification of the vessel and its branches is usually achieved with a hand injection of 10 ml Urografin 370 or its equivalent. IMA arteriography is painful with conventional contrast media and low osmolality agents should be used for preference.

Because of the flexures of the sigmoid and splenic colon these areas are best viewed in the LPO and steep RPO projections respectively. The anastomoses between branches of the superior left colic artery (IMA) and middle colic artery (SMA) in the region of the splenic flexure represent one of the most tenuous areas of vascular supply in the alimentary tract (Griffiths' point [37]) and this region is one of the commoner sites at which ischaemic changes may be observed in conditions of mesenteric vascular insufficiency. When one of the major visceral vessels is obstructed by atherosclerotic disease, the region of bowel it normally supplies is fed by collaterals from other vascular territories. These collaterals may be very large (particularly if the SMA is blocked) and can present a bizarre appearance at angiography: [102] one of the best known is the *wandering artery of Drummond* which represents the communication between the vascular arcades along the mesenteric border of the colon [103].

Gastrointestinal bleeding [96,101,104,105,106,107,108]

One of the most important applications of gastrointestinal angiography is in the management of gastrointestinal bleeding. The technique is not only able to identify the site and likely cause of the bleeding in many cases, but, with the use of interventional techniques, may also provide the opportunity for stopping it without recourse to surgery [105,109,110]. There is no question, however, that the successful application of the method requires the services of a radiologist skilled in abdominal arteriography.

Endoscopy has rapidly become established as the principal investigative modality in the management of gastrointestinal bleeding (Chapters 45 and 48). It is widely available, easy to arrange, relatively non-invasive, allows biopsies to be obtained, provides a definitive diagnosis, often identifies a cause for bleeding even though the bleeding has temporarily stopped, and can be used to coagulate appropriate lesions. Arteriography should not normally be undertaken without a previous endoscopy and is used only when the latter is unsuccessful in locating the source of bleeding, or when therapeutic embolization seems indicated. Arteriography does, however, have some important advantages over endoscopy that are useful in certain clinical circumstances:

1. It can often precisely localize a bleeding site in regions inaccessible or relatively inaccessible to the endoscope, e.g. liver, pancreas, jejunum, ileum and afferent loops.

2. In a case of significant *active* bleeding good arteriography is almost certain to localize the site irrespective of its anatomical location [108].

3. Trans-catheter embolization has application to a much wider range of lesions than is endoscopic coagulation.

Barium studies (Chapters 43,44,46,47) may be helpful in cases of chronic or intermittent bleeding by revealing ulcers, tumours, etc. In acute bleeding, however, in a centre where facilities for both endoscopy and emergency angiography exist, there is little place for barium studies in diagnosis. Their interpretation is unreliable in the presence of blood clot, a lesion demonstrated is not necessarily the cause of bleeding, and the presence of barium in the abdomen may precludes the use of angiography (and therefore of embolization) for several days [101].

Isotope studies [111] (Chapter 3) may be valuable in the management of gastrointestinal bleeding, usually as a complementary technique to arteriography. Isotope methods are very sensitive in detecting blood loss from the gastrointestinal tract, but are less accurate than arteriography in localizing the site of bleeding. In many centres isotope studies are used to establish whether or not active haemorrhage is occurring before submitting the patient to arteriography in order precisely to define the bleeding site. The relative roles of isotope studies and arteriography in the management of bleeding depend very much on the facilities and expertise locally available.

Active bleeding Active blood loss is identified arteriographically by the extravasation of contrast medium into the bowel (or biliary) lumen (Figs. 94.43, 94.53, 94.72). It is said that a bleeding rate as low as 0.5 ml/min can be identified in this way [112]. Generally speaking, the more rapid the blood loss the greater is the chance of locating the site angiographically. The decision to perform an arteriogram in an actively bleeding patient who requires a laparotomy is not one to be taken lightly. The experience of the radiologist is a critical factor and the study should only be performed if there is a high expectation of a successful outcome in terms of accurate localization or interventional therapy. In some clinical situations (e.g. following previous surgery, suspected haemobilia, or suspected small bowel bleeding) the indications for emergency angiography will be much stronger than in others, and close cooperation between radiologist, physician and surgeon is important if the technique is to be used to best advantage. *Interventional techniques* for the control of gastrointestinal bleeding are discussed in Chapter 98.

Chronic bleeding There are a number of patients who have a history of chronic gastrointestinal bleeding (sometimes for many years) in whom no cause can be demonstrated despite intensive investigation by blood tests (to exclude a bleeding diathesis), searches for parasites, barium studies, endoscopy, isotope studies and sometimes even laparotomy. Selective arteriography may reveal a cause for bleeding in these patients. In the upper gastrointestinal tract causes of occult bleeding that may be shown include gastric or duodenal arteriovenous malformations, haemobilia due to aneurysms or vascular lesions in the liver or pancreas (Figs. 94.31 & 95.73) or even unsuspected portal hypertension without gross endoscopic changes. In the small bowel [113] typical causes

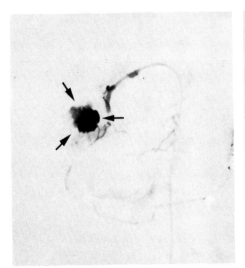
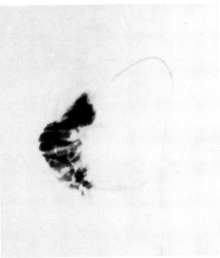
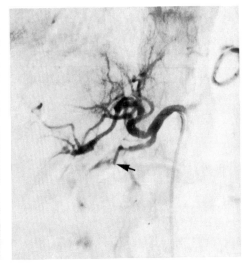

A   B   C

Fig. 94.72A, B & C   Selective gastroduodenal arteriogram. Active bleeding is in progress from a large duodenal ulcer (A). The arrows point to extravasated contrast medium in the ulcer base. (B) The contrast medium outlines the second part of the duodenum. (C) Post-embolization study. The occluded gastroduodenal stump is arrowed.

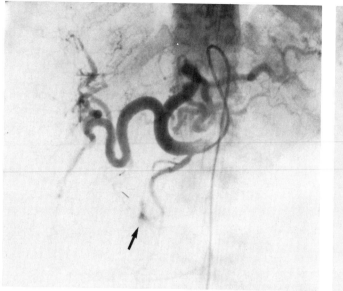 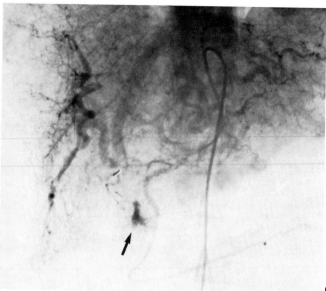

A   B

Fig. 94.73A & B   Common hepatic arteriogram in a patient with hereditary telangiectasia with unexplained gastrointestinal bleeding. A large telangiectasis is shown in the head of the pancreas (arrow). The lesion is more conspicuous in the late arterial phase of the study (B) and multiple smaller lesions are visible in the substance of the liver. Note that the lesion is within 1–2 cm of the surgical clips that mark the site of a previous duodenotomy undertaken during a previous laparotomy that failed to identify a cause for bleeding!

include Meckel's diverticulum (not usually shown at angiography), arteriovenous malformations (Fig. 94.74), and small vascular tumours (e.g. leiomyomas) that have remained undetected by previous imaging techniques. If a catheter can be selectively introduced into the branch supplying a small bowel lesion (Fig. 94.75), the patient can be transferred to the operating theatre with the catheter *in situ* so that per-operative angiography (or methylene blue injection) can be used to help localize the lesion for the surgeon.

Angiodysplasia [99,100,101,108]. In the large bowel the commonest cause of occult bleeding is angiodysplasia. This is a disorder affecting predominantly the middle-aged and elderly, though it may also occur in younger patients [114]. It consists of vascular ectasias in the microcirculation of the mucous and submucous layers of the bowel, and usually occurs in the caecum and ascending colon. The lesions can cause either acute or chronic bleeding and are difficult to detect owing to their small size (usually 3 mm diameter). At endoscopy they are visible as small spider-like lesions which are easily missed by the inexperienced operator, and they cannot be demonstrated on barium studies. At laparotomy the surgeon can neither see nor feel areas of angiodysplasia, and they cannot usually be found by the pathologist unless special localization techniques are used. Arteriographically angiodysplasia appears as one or more tiny lakes of contrast medium that usually lie on the anti-mesenteric border of the bowel. The lesions act as tiny shunts and early-filling, conspicuous veins may be seen draining the abnormal area (Fig. 94.76). Sometimes dozens of lesions are present, giving a diffuse hypervascular appearance to a large area of the caecum or ascending colon. The simple demonstration of a site of angiodysplasia at arteriography does not (unless it is

actively bleeding) prove that it is the source of haemorrhage. A high proportion of patients with chronic occult bleeding, however, in whom angiodysplasia is shown arteriographically and in whom no other cause for bleeding can be found at laparotomy will be cured by resection of the affected portion of bowel [108]. There is an association between angiodysplasia and *valvular heart disease* [115,116] and *Meckel's diverticulum* [117].

Portal hypertension [118,119]. Portal hypertension is an important cause of gastrointestinal bleeding and angiographic techniques may be used in three principal ways to assist in its investigation and management:

1. To determine the cause of hypertension if this is not already known (e.g. demonstration of an arterio-portal fistula; demonstration of an unusual site of venous obstruction).

2. To show the anatomy and flow dynamics of the portal venous system to assist the clinician in decisions concerning possible management (e.g. shunt surgery).

3. To apply interventional techniques to control bleeding in appropriate cases.

Portal hypertension and the techniques for its investigation are discussed further in Chapter 50; and interventional methods for control of variceal bleeding are described in Chapter 52.

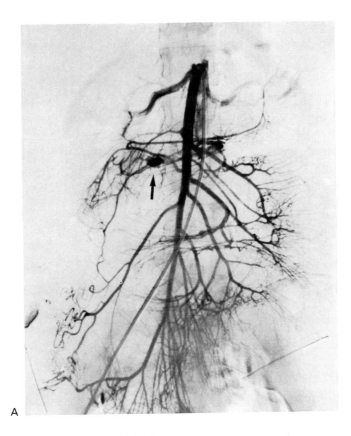

A

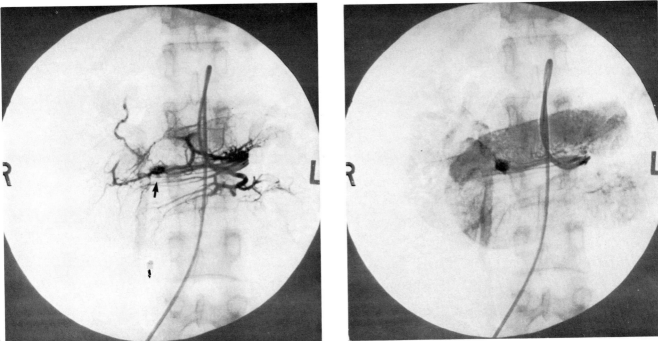

B

C

Fig. 94.74A, B & C   (A) A superior mesenteric arteriogram shows a vascular malformation (arrowed) in a patient with occult gastrointestinal bleeding. (B) A selective study shows the lesion to lie in the upper jejunum. (C) The capillary phase of the selective study allows precise localization of the malformation because the mucosal blush of the bowel outlines the first loop of the jejunum.

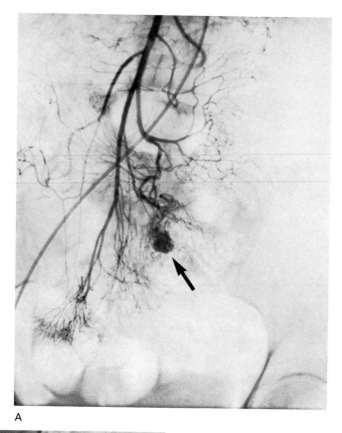

A

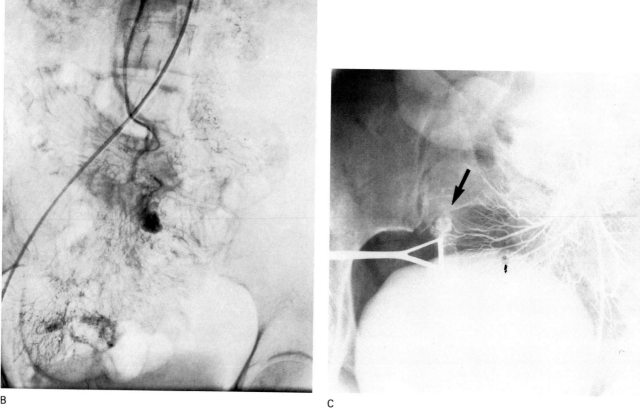

B   C

Fig. 94.75A, B & C   Superior mesenteric arteriogram (A) showing a vascular tumour in the upper ileum (arrow). (B) A catheter has been passed selectively into the vessel feeding the lesion. (C) A hand injection of contrast medium in the operating theatre reveals the precise location of the tumour for the surgeon.

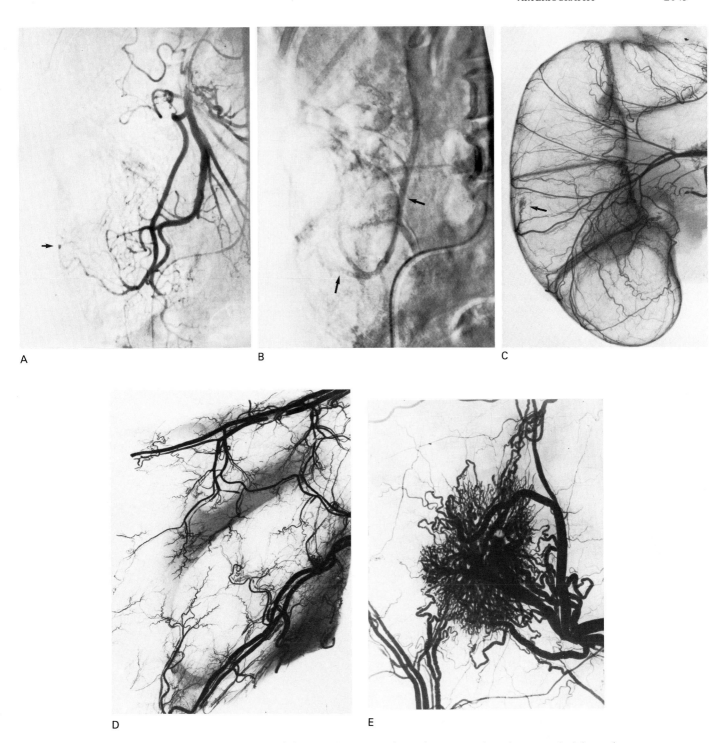

Fig. 94.76A, B, C, D & E Angiodysplasia of the colon. (A) A superior mesenteric arteriogram reveals a minute vascular lake on the antimesenteric border of the caecum (arrow). (B) The lesion acts as a shunt as evidenced by the early-filling conspicuous draining vein (arrows). (C) The affected segment of bowel is removed surgically and injected with a barium-gelatin mixture. The lesion is visible in the injected specimen (arrow). (D) Microradiograph of a section of the normal injected caecum (× 60). (E) Microradiograph of the area of angiodysplasia (× 60).

The upper extremity [120]

Arteriography of the arm can be performed by intravenous DSA, direct needle puncture of the subclavian, axillary or brachial artery, or through a catheter. Of the direct arterial methods the catheter approach is probably the least traumatic and most useful. A catheter passed from a femoral puncture site allows the proximal subclavian artery and the more distal vessels to be examined at the same procedure if necessary, and has the advantage of employing a percutaneous route that is familar to all angiographers — an important factor in avoiding morbidity in what is a relatively infrequent examination in most departments. Special axillary catheters are available but a femoral-cerebral catheter (head hunter) is perfectly adequate for studying the arm and in the average adult will reach almost to the elbow from an entry point in the groin. The subclavian artery is normally adequately opacified with an injection of 15–20 ml ioxaglate (or non-ionic medium of equivalent concentration) delivered over 3–4 seconds. Care should be taken not to damage the *vertebral* artery, especially if any automatic injector is being used. For more distal examinations of the brachial artery and beyond a hand injection of 10–15 ml contrast medium is sufficient. These volumes are subject to considerable variation according to the clinical circumstances, and will also be modified if DSA is available.

Conventional contrast media are very painful in the upper extremity, particularly the hand, and digital examinations were formerly performed under nerve block or general anaesthesia; this is no longer necessary with low osmolality media which are the agents of choice in this area. The indications for arteriography of the upper extremity are few in number. *Thoracic outlet syndromes* and other clinical manifestations of possible subclavian abnormalities will require a subclavian arteriogram (Fig. 94.77). Aneurysms (see Fig. 94.85) arteriovenous malformations (see below) and ischaemia subsequent to trauma or suspected embolus are other indications for an arterial study. Arteriography is occasionally performed to distinguish digital ischaemia due to *Raynaud's phenomenon* from organic disease due to peripheral embolization or arteritis secondary to inflammatory disorders [121]. In uncomplicated Raynauds disease the arteries may be constricted but remain morphologically normal; in cases of embolization abrupt local occlusions occur, and in arteritis occlusions and irregularities in vessel calibre may be demonstrated (Fig. 94.79). Arteriography is also occasionally used in the evaluation of soft tissue or bone tumours in the upper extremity, which are sometimes extremely vascular. With the increasing use of therapeutic

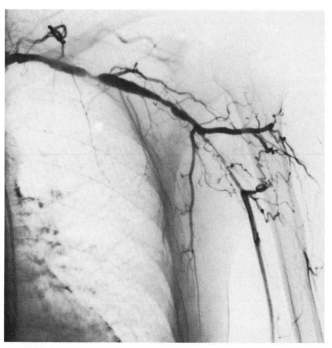

Fig. 94.77 Subclavian arteriogram in a patient with advanced untreated systemic lupus erythematosus. Note the irregularities in calibre of the vessels affected by arteritis. A segment of the axillary artery is almost occluded.

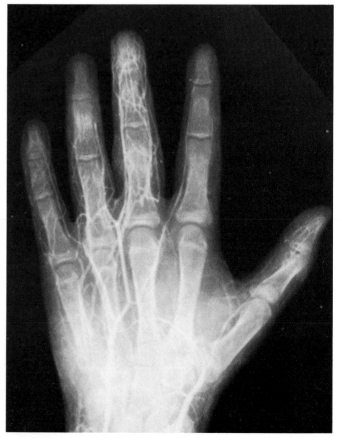

Fig. 94.78 Digital arteritis. Note the irregular calibre of the small vessels of the hand with occlusions and regions of hypovascularity.

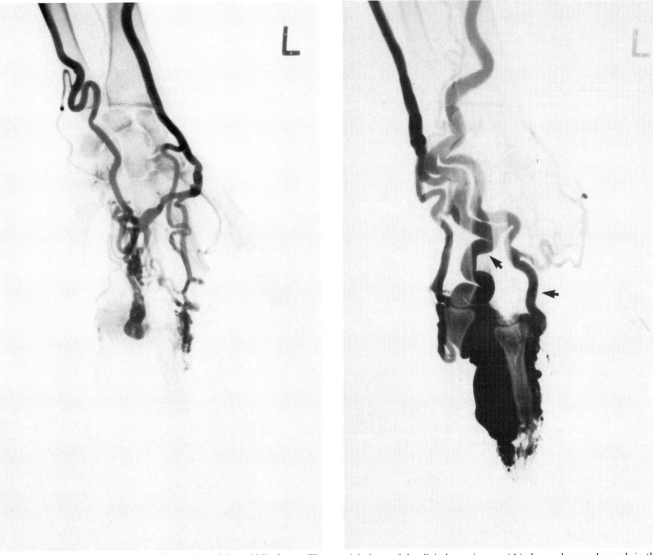

Fig. 94.79A & B   Arteriovenous malformation of the middle finger. The arterial phase of the digital arteriogram (A) shows abnormal vessels in the carpus fed by enlarged radial and ulnar vessels. One second later (B) a massive arterio-venous space in the middle finger has opacified and large veins (arrows) are seen draining the lesion. This study was performed under local anaesthesia from a femoral approach using a non-ionic contrast medium (Iohexol).

embolization arteriography is being employed more frequently in the study of *arteriovenous malformations* in the arm. These may be very unsightly, lesions on the hand (Fig. 94.80) carry a constant danger of bleeding from trauma (and may cause secondary digital ischaemia due to shunting), and large lesions can cause cardiac failure. Preliminary studies of an AVM are best obtained using the femoral catheter approach. When lesions below the elbow require selective catheterization for embolization, however, this is best done using a catheter (with miniature coaxial catheters if necessary) passed down from a brachial arteriotomy. Predominantly *venous* malformations may appear relatively normal on the arteriogram; sometimes *phleboliths* are present and are visible on the plain radiograph (Fig. 94.80 A,B).

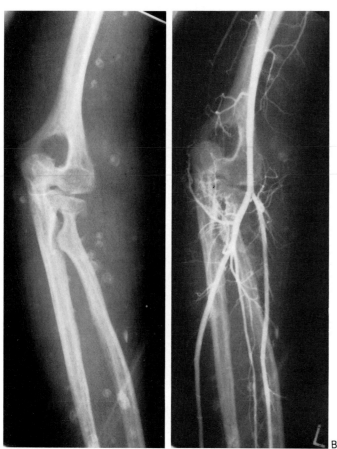

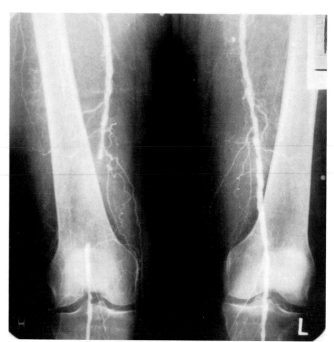

Fig. 94.80A & B (A) Multiple phleboliths are present in an extensive venous haemangioma of the arm. (B) The arteriogram appears normal in the arterial phase; there were some faintly opacified abnormal venous spaces in the late films of the study (not shown).

The lower extremity [45]

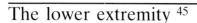

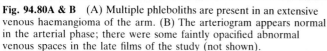

Arteriography of the leg can be performed by intravenous DSA, by direct needle puncture of a femoral artery or the aorta (TLA), or by a catheter which can be introduced using the femoral, axillary or brachial approach.

Femoral arteriography of a single leg is usually performed by puncturing the ipsilateral common femoral artery (if it is palpable) and injecting contrast medium through a needle or, preferably, a short flexible cannula which permits the patient to be repositioned without the risk of arterial dissection or

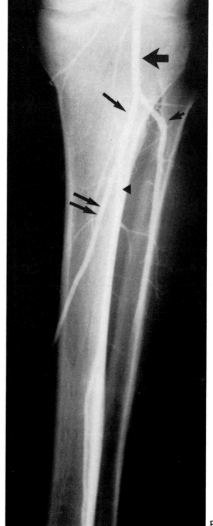

Fig. 94.81A & B (A) Superficial femoral and popliteal occlusion. This is a classical site. Note the popliteal artery filling via collaterals and the severe disease in the opposite femoral artery. (B) Normal 'run-off' (different patient). Note the anatomical arrangement of the vessels in the A–P projection: popliteal artery (broad arrow), anterior tibial artery (short arrow), common posterior tibial artery (long arrow), peroneal artery (arrowhead), posterior tibial artery (double arrow).

needle dislodgement. 20 ml ioxaglate or a non-ionic equivalent injected by pump or hand over 3–4 seconds is normally adequate for a femoral arteriogram; if a lower aortic injection is being made through a catheter a pump injection of 50 ml contrast medium over 4–5 seconds will be necessary. It is often very important for the vessels of the whole extremity to be visualized and if a moving-top table or moving stand is not available multiple injections may be necessary for this purpose. The timing of the radiographic exposures is important and will often need to be tailored to the individual case to allow for the considerable variations in vascular flow that exist in different patients with arterial disease. Many vascular surgeons prefer the radiologist to avoid puncturing the femoral artery at a point that may shortly be the site of a vascular graft or other surgical procedure; in such cases, and in those where the femoral artery is not palpable or information about more proximal vessels is also sought, a catheter study from the opposite leg to show the aorta, iliac vessels and both lower extremities is preferable. Where both femoral arteries are impalpable, a *translumbar aortogram* or a catheter study using an axillary or brachial approach can be performed if intravenous DSA

is unavailable or inadequate for the purpose. In cases where it is essential to puncture an artery that cannot be palpated (e.g. for the purposes of transluminal angioplasty) the site of the artery can be located by an ultrasound probe, intravenous DSA if available, or contrast medium injected into the aorta via an alternative access route.

It is important to obtain plain radiographs of the limb before injecting contrast medium as any calcification present in the arteries (see Fig. 94.33) may be invisible on the post-injection films. Failure to demonstrate calcified areas on preliminary films in this way may lead to serious errors of interpretation as such areas can be mistaken for contrast medium on the injected study.

Arteriography of the lower extremities may be necessary to investigate a wide variety of the vascular disorders described above; in the great majority of patients, however, it is used for the assessment of *occlusive vascular disease* secondary to atheroma, embolization or arteritis. Remember that many patients presenting with peripheral vascular disease have other complicating features which the angiographer should check on in case they affect the radiological procedure; they include factors such as cardiac

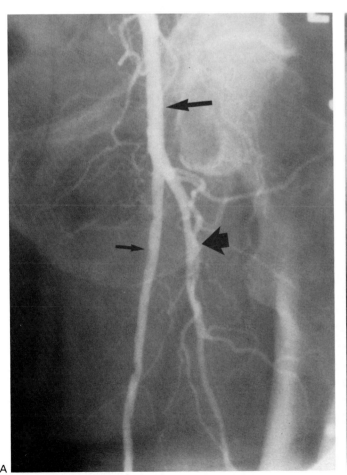
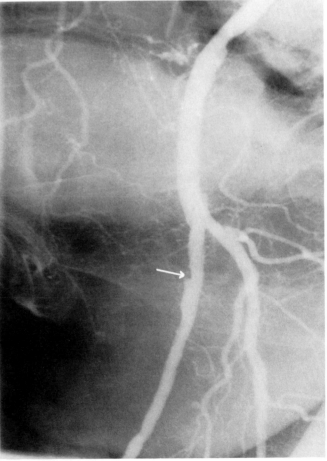

A   B

Fig. 94.82A & B   Views of the common femoral (long arrow), deep femoral (profunda: broad arrow) and superficial femoral (short arrow) arteries. (A) In the antero-posterior projection, the origin of the profunda vessel is concealed by the origin of the superficial vessel. (B) An oblique projection (same side raised) gives a good view of the profunda origin (in this case normal). Note how much worse the atheromatous plaque in the superficial femoral artery appears on the oblique projection (arrow).

disease, hypertension, renal impairment, diabetes and anti-coagulant therapy.

Other indications for lower limb arteriography include the investigation of aneurysms, trauma and arteriovenous malformations, and interventional procedures such as embolization and angioplasty (Chapter 98).

It is important for the angiographer to have a good working relationship with the vascular surgeon if the most useful information is to be obtained from lower limb arteriography. Knowledge of the requirements of the surgeon and of the possible surgical options available in any given case will help to ensure that essential views are not overlooked and unnecessary views not taken. In the case of occlusive vascular disease the surgeon will normally wish to see the full extent of the occluded or compromised segment (or segments) and be acquainted with the quality of the vascular supply both above and below the region of principal abnormality. In the case of femoral disease the state of the popliteal and lower limb vessels (the 'run-off') is often particularly important and in the present of a complete superficial femoral occlusion (Figs. 94.39 & 94.81) delayed films may be necessary to show these more distal vessels after they have filled via collaterals. The surgeon will wish to know which distal vessel or vessels are opacified and, in cases where reconstructive surgery below the knee is contemplated, whether the plantar arch is present and complete. The origin of the *profunda femoris* artery is not well seen in the AP projection and an oblique view (affected leg raised) will give valuable information (Fig. 94.82). The profunda is a very important contributor to the blood supply of the limb and its anatomy must be demonstrated in detail.

With the increasing popularity of percutaneous transluminal angioplasty in lower limb occlusive disease, many radiologists have established a working protocol with their surgical colleagues with respect to the management of

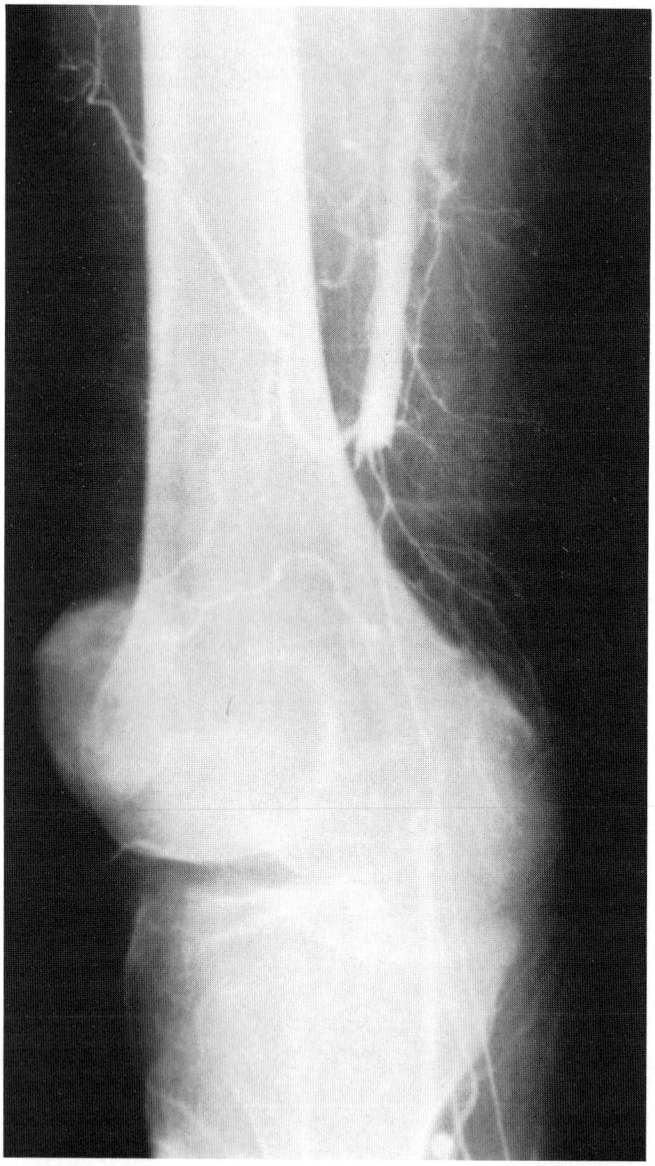

Fig. 94.83 Popliteal embolus. Contrast medium comes to an abrupt stop near the origin of the popliteal artery. Note the rounded filling defect due to the upper border of the intraluminal thrombus. The embolus frequently lodges more distally in the popliteal artery than in this example.

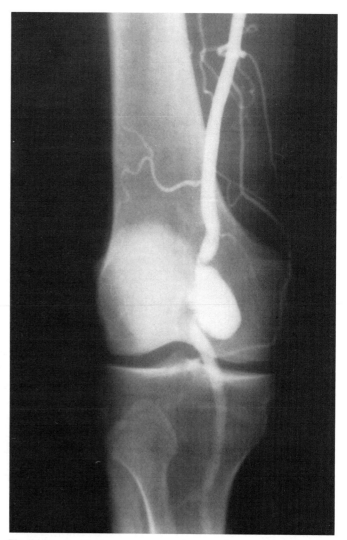

Fig. 94.84 Popliteal aneurysm secondary to atheromatous disease.

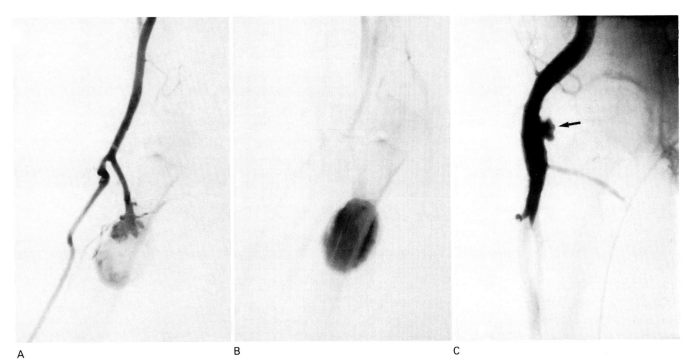

A   B   C

Fig. 94.85A, B & C Mycotic aneurysms of the limbs: (A) Mycotic aneurysm of the ulnar artery secondary to a local abscess. (B) Late film of same study. (C) Mycotic aneurysm of the common femoral artery (arrowed) secondary to infection related to hip surgery.

stenoses or occlusions revealed at angiography. If a lesion that appears to be suitable for treatment by angioplasty is demonstrated the operator proceeds to this without further consultation, thereby saving the patient a second procedure and (often) a separate arterial puncture.

Emboli, e.g. from the heart in a patient with fibrillation, many cause acute obstruction of a limb and require urgent investigation. Emboli frequently become impacted in the popliteal region where the sharp the sharp 'cut-off' of contrast medium on the arteriogram, lack of collateral filling and appropriate clinical history are virtually diagnostic (Fig. 94.83). Aneurysms may occur in the femoral and popliteal territory secondary to atheroma (Fig. 94.84), infection (Fig. 94.85) trauma or arteriovenous malformations (Fig. 94.86). The extent of the aneurysm may be greater than that suggested by the angiogram owing to the presence of thrombus within the lumen of the aneurysm. **Aneurysms** may be asymptomatic, cause pain, pulsation or local pressure symptoms, cause distal ischaemia secondary to the embolization of thrombus from the aneurysm, and may leak or rupture. A popliteal aneurysm is a rare cause of unilateral clubbing of the toes [122] and unilateral finger clubbing has been described in association with an aneurysm in the subclavian artery [123]. **Tumours** of the soft tissues or bones are

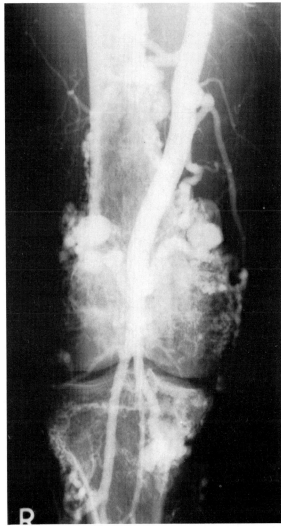

Fig. 94.86 Multiple aneurysms in a massive arteriovenous malformation around the knee joint.

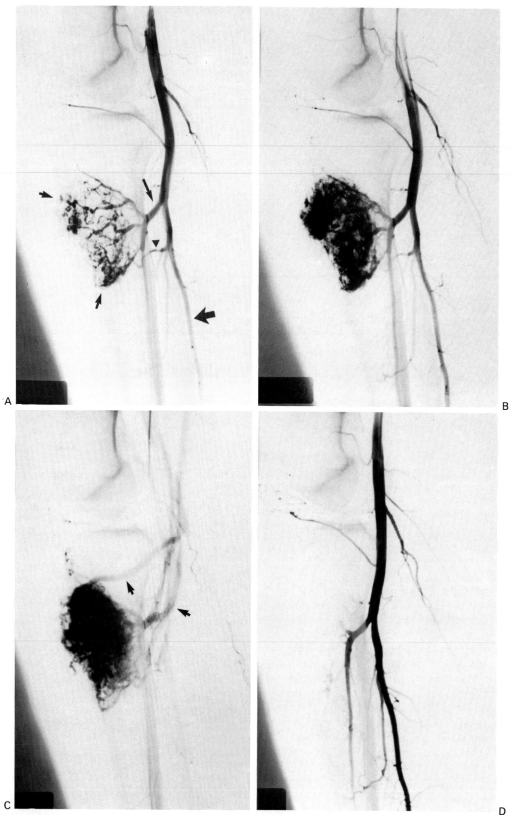

Fig. 94.87A, B, C & D   Haemangioma of the upper tibia. Early arterial lateral film (A/B) following a popliteal artery injection show the vascular tumour (short arrows) supplied by the *anterior tibial* artery (long arrow) and twigs from the *peroneal* artery (arrowhead). The *posterior tibial* artery is not involved (broad arrow). A few seconds later (C) large veins are seen draining the lesion (short arrows). After embolization a repeat arteriogram (D) shows abolition of the blood supply to the lesion.

occasionally examined by arteriography, particularly if embolization is being considered as a form of therapy. They are frequently extremely vascular (Fig. 94.87).

Buerger's disease (thromboangiitis obliterans) is said to affect the lower limb vessels of young males. It is discussed on p. 2016.

Vascular malformations occur in the lower limb as elsewhere in the body and may reach massive proportions (Fig. 94.86). They can cause local gigantism, trophic changes in the skin and bone, distal limb ischaemia, local haemorrhage and high output cardiac failure. Embolization is the most effective form of treatment in many cases (see Chapter 98). Traumatic *arteriovenous shunts* may occur following trauma or iatrogenic injury; a fast filming sequence is necessary to demonstrate the feeding and draining vessels as the flow through such lesions may be extremely rapid.

The endocrine organs

For many years arteriography played an important role in the investigation of certain endocrine disorders, principally as a technique for the localization of functioning tumours related to the parathyroid and adrenal glands, the sympathetic chain and the pancreas. Endocrine arteriography is for the most part a time-consuming occupation that requires a high order of angiographic expertise both for its execution and interpretation, and it is not surprising that in recent years its role has been steadily usurped by advances in less invasive and less operator-dependent modalities such as isotope imaging and CT. Indeed, many previously important investigations such as adrenal arteriography are now virtually obsolete. It is possible that the general trend away from arteriography may be slowed by developments such as DSA and non-ionic contrast media, but the advances in other localizing techniques are so impressive that any significant long-term role for arteriography in this field seems most unlikely.

The pituitary gland

Arteriography now plays virtually no part in the management of pituitary tumours. The *localization* of these tumours is obviously not a problem, and their pre-therapeutic assessment does not normally include angiography.

The parathyroid glands [72,73]

Parathyroid adenomas may be multiple and/or ectopic and in some patients their localization can be exceedingly difficult. A number of techniques for pin-pointing these tumours

are available and the 'best' method varies from institution to institution depending on the local techniques and expertise available. The great majority of parathyroid tumours can be found during surgical exploration of the neck by an experienced operator, and many surgeons do not request any form of pre-operative localization in uncomplicated cases. Radiological methods may be helpful to the less experienced surgeon in cases where a preliminary exploration has failed and when the tumour(s) lie in the mediastinum. Thallium and technetium subtraction isotope scanning, enhanced CT, venous sampling, arteriography and ultrasound are all methods in present use for localising parathyroid tumours. Arteriography occasionally reveals a tumour on an arch aortogram, but bilateral selective superior and inferior thyroid arteriography is usually required (Fig. 94.57). The technique is time-consuming and not without hazard since the thyro-cervical trunk (from which the inferior thyroid artery arises) gives branches of supply to the spinal cord which may be injured by high local concentrations of contrast medium such as occur during superselective injections. The advent of non-ionic contrat agents has clearly reduced this risk, and if DSA is available good images can be obtained with very small volumes of contrast medium; despite these factors the steady improvement in other imaging techniques, however, particularly isotope scanning and CT, make it unlikely that any significant resurgence of interest will occur in parathyroid arteriography except in centres with special experience in the technique or where other methods are unavailable.

The adrenal glands [124]

Arteriography was an important investigation for many years in the diagnosis of vascular adrenal tumours (Fig. 94.88) but is now rarely performed because most functioning adrenal tumours can be localized with either CT scanning or isotope techniques. The situation in which arteriography remains most useful is when adrenal CT scanning fails to reveal a tumour in a patient with a suspected phaeochromocytoma. In such a case the tumour or tumours may be found at a number of widely separated sites in the body in the location of sympathetic nervous tissue. These sites include the paraspinal region from the cervical region to the sacrum, the organ of Zuckerkandl, the pelvis and bladder, and the thorax (mediastinum). Venous sampling for catecholamines or MIBG isotope scanning (Chapter 55) may indicate the approximate location of such a tumour, and arteriography may then be the best technique for its precise localization (Fig. 94.89).

The pancreas [21,24,98]

The pancreas is the only remaining endocrine organ in which arteriography still has a significant role to play in the localization of tumours, with the exceptions mentioned above. Pancreatic endocrine tumours are derived from APUD cells (Amine Precursor Uptake and Decarboxylation) and are

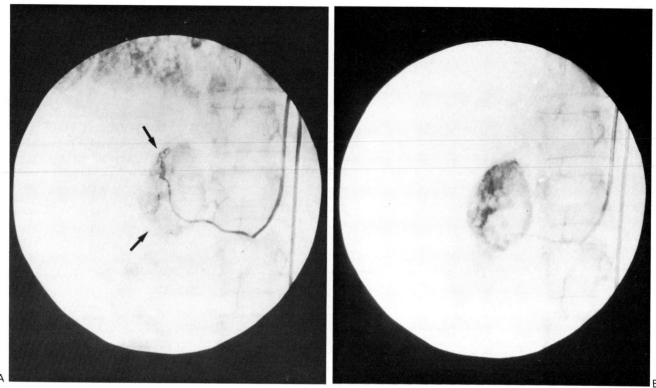

Fig. 94.88A & B   (A) Middle adrenal arteriogram showing a phaeochromocytoma (arrows). In the parenchymal phase of the study (B), the tumour blush shows a central defect due to partial necrosis of the tumour.

referred to as 'apudomas'. Depending on the predominant cell type the tumours produce one or more hormones such as insulin, glucagon, gastrin, 5-HT, somatostatin, pancreatic polypeptide and others. Many of these apudomas are too small to be demonstrated by enhanced CT scanning of the pancreas and there is as yet no satisfactory isotope scan available for their detection. The most useful localizing techniques at present are selective pancreatic arteriography and selective (portal) venous sampling. The majority of apudomas are vascular and show a dense capillary 'blush' after an arterial injection of contrast medium (Fig. 94.90, 94.91). The pancreas is supplied by vessels arising from the coeliac and superior mesenteric territory (Fig. 94.92) and an examination would normally include coeliac and superior mesenteric injections with selective splenic, hepatic and gastroduodenal studies. Superselective studies of the dorsal pancreatic and pancreatico-duodenal arteries may be necessary in the case of small tumours. The accuracy of pancreatic arteriography will probably be further enhanced by the use of intraarterial DSA and it seems likely to remain an important technique for the localization of endocrine tumours until a more sensitive 'non-invasive' method is developed.

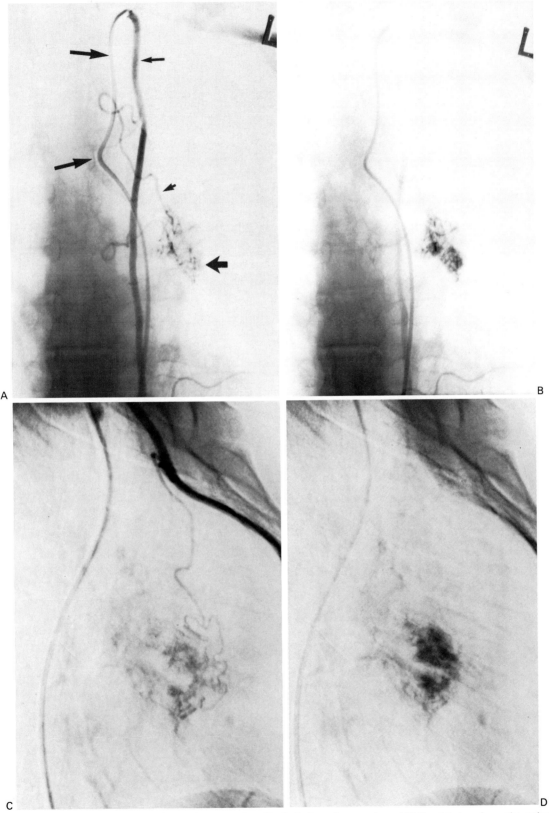

Fig. 94.89A, B, C & D   Internal mammary arteriogram in a case of mediastinal phaeochromocytoma (A) Frontal view shows the catheter (large arrows) in the aorta and subclavian artery. The internal mammary artery is opacified (small arrow), and the pericardiophrenic branch (arrowhead) supplies a tumour near the left hilum (broad arrow). The tumour is more conspicuous in a later film (B). Early (C) and late (D) films in the lateral projection show the exact position of the tumour in the chest.

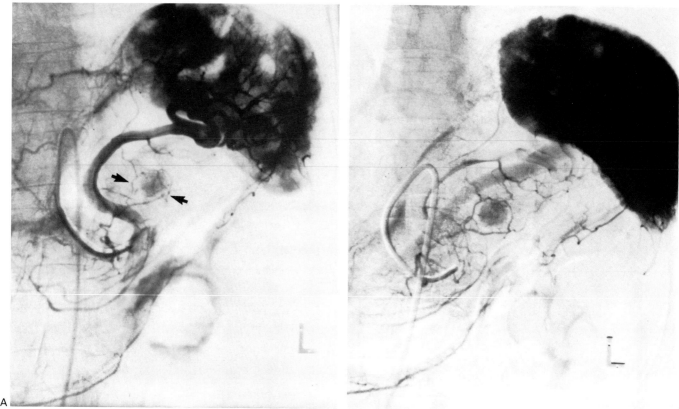

Fig. 94.90A & B   Splenic arteriogram. Early (A) and late (B) radiographs showing the characteristic 'blush' of a pancreatic insulinoma (arrows).

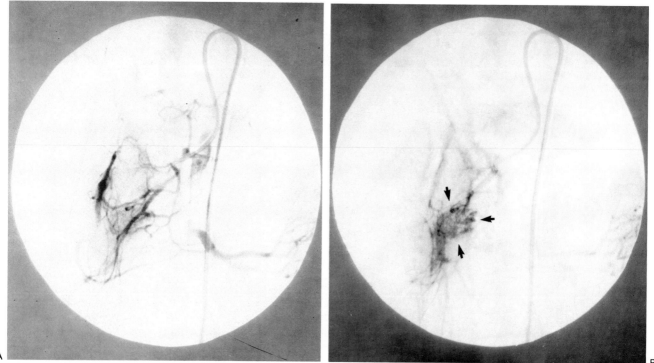

Fig. 94.91A & B   Selective inferior pancreatic-duodenal arteriogram (via superior mesenteric artery). Early (A) and late (B) films showing a small glucagonoma in the head of the pancreas (arrows).

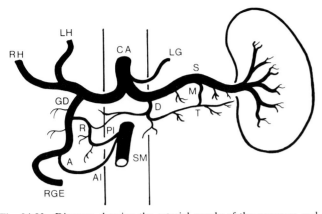

Fig. 94.92 Diagram showing the arterial supply of the pancreas and neighbouring structures. CA = Coeliac axis; LG = Left gastric artery; S = Splenic artery; M = Arteria pancreatica magna; D = Dorsal pancreatic artery; SM = Superior mesenteric artery; T = Transverse pancreatic artery; PI = Posterior inferior pancreaticoduodenal artery; AI = Anterior inferior pancreaticoduodenal artery; A = Anterior superior pancreaticoduodenal artery; R = Retroduodenal artery (posterior superior pancreaticoduodenal artery); GD = Gastroduodenal artery; RH = Right hepatic artery; LH = Left hepatic artery.

BIBLIOGRAPHY

REFERENCES

1. Haschek E, Lindenthal O T 1896 A contribution to the practical use of the photography according to Roentgen. Wien Klin Wschr 9:63
2. Abrams H L (ed) 1983 Introduction and historical notes. In: Angiography, 3rd edn. Little, Brown, Boston, ch 1, pp 3–13
3. Orrin H C 1920 The X-ray atlas of the systemic arteries of the body. Baillière, Tindall & Cox, London
4. Veiga-Pires J A and Grainger R G 1982 Pioneers in angiography. MTP Press, Lancaster
5. Goncalves A M 1982 Biography of Egas Moniz. Catalogo da exposicao itinerante da obra Egas Moniz e Reynaldo dos Santos. Publicacoes Ciencia e Vida Lda, Lisbon, p 77
6. Forssmann W 1931 Ueber Kontrastdarstellung der Hohlen des levenden rechten Herzens under der Lungenschlagader. Munchen Med Mschr 78:489–492
7. Dos Santos R, Lamas A, Pereira-Caldas J 1929 L'arteriographic des membres, de l'aorta et de ses branches abdominates. Bull Soc nat Chir 55:587
8. Nuvoli I 1936 Arteriografia dell' aorta toracica mediante puncture dell' aorta ascendente o del ventricolos. Policlinico Sez prat 43:227
9. Lindgren E 1950 Percutaneous angiography of the vertebral artery. Acta Radiol (Stockh) 33:389–404
10. Peirce E C, Ramey W P 1953 Renal arteriography: a report of a percutaneous method using the femoral artery approach and a disposable catheter. J Urol 69:578–585
11. Seldinger S 1953 Catheter replacement of the needle in percutaneous arteriography. Acta Radiol (Stockh) 39:368–376
12. Nebesar R A and Pollard J J 1966 A curved-tip guide wire for thoracic and abdominal angiography. Am J Roentgenol 97:508–510
13. Judkins M P, Kidd H J et al 1967 Lumen-following safety J-guide for catheterization of tortuous vessels. Radiology 88:1127–1130
14. Wholey M H 1968 A modified J-shaped wire for angiography. Br J Radiol 41:388–389
15. Judkins M P, Hinck V C, Dotter C T 1968 Teflon-coated safety guides. Am J Roentgenol 104:223–224
16. Kaude J, Grotemeyer P 1976 Catheterization techniques. In: Loose K E, van Dongen R J A M (eds) Atlas of angiography. Publishing Sciences Group, ch 2, pp 7–16
17. Kaude J 1975 Die Angiographic mit der Kathetermethode. Gefahren und Komplikationen. In: Loose K E (ed) Angiographic und ihre neuesten Erkenntrisse. Walter de Gruyter Verlag, Berlin, p 13
18. Boijsen E, Lundstrom N R 1968 Percutaneous cardiac catheterization and angiocardiography in infants and children. Am J Cardiol 22:572–575
19. Olin T B and Reuter S R 1965 A pharmacoangiographic method for improving nephrophlebography. Radiology 85:1036–1042
20. Allison D J 1983 Interventional Radiology. In: Steiner R E (ed) Recent advances in radiology and medical imaging 7 Churchill Livingstone, Edinburgh, ch 8, pp 139–170
21. Clouse M E, Costello P, Legg M A, Soeldre J S and Cady B 1977 Subselective angiography in locating insulinomas of the pancreas. Am J Roentgenol 128:741–746
22. Athanasoulis C A et al 1976 Angiography: its contribution to the emergency management of gastrointestinal haemorrhage. Radiol Clin North Am 14:265–280
23. Clark R A, Colley D P 1981 Pharmacoangiography. Semin Roetengol 16:42–51
24. Reuter S R, Redman H C 1977 Gastrointestinal angiography. W B Saunders, Philadelphia
25. Meiisel P, Apitzsch D E 1978 Atlas der Nierenangiographie. Springer-Verlag, Berlin
26. Vargha G Y 1981 Pharmacoangiography in the diagnosis of tumours. Akademiai Kaido, Budapest
27. Freeny P C, Lawson T L (eds) 1982 In: Radiology of the pancreas. Springer-Verlag, New York, p 475
28. Hilal S K, 1973 Small vessel angiography. CV Mosby, St Louis
29. Greenspan R H 1983 Magnification angiography. In: Abrams H L (ed) Angiography. Little, Brown, Boston, ch 9, pp 205–216
30. Allison D J, Stanbrook H S 1980 A radiologic and physiologic investigation into hypoxic pulmonary vasoconstriction in the dog. Invest Radiol 15:179–190
31. Wallace S, Medellin H, De Jongh D, Gianturco C 1972 Systemic heparinization for angiography. Am J Roentgenol 116:204–209
32. Abrams H L (ed) 1983 Additional applications of aortography. In: Angiography, 3rd edn. Little, Brown, Boston, ch 21, pp 467–483
33. Van Dongen R J A M (ed) 1976 Aortoiliac occlusive disease and abdominal aneurysms. In: Loose K E, van Dongen R J A M (eds) Atlas of angiography. Publishing Sciences group ch 5, p 123–163
34. Palmaz J C, Carson S N, Hunter G, Weinshelbaum A 1983 Male *hypoplastic* infrarenal aorta and premature atherosclerosis. Surgery 94 (1):91–94
35. Arnot R S, Louw J H 1973 The anatomy of the posterior wall of the abdominal aorta. South Afr Med J 47:899–902
36. DeLaurentis D A, Friedmann P, Wolferth C C, Wilson A, Naide D 1978 Atherosclerosis and the hypoplastic aortoiliac system. Surgery 83:27–37
37. Nebesar R A, Kornblith P L, Pollard J J, Michels N A 1969 Coeliac and superior mesenteric arteries. J & A Churchill, London
38. Michels N A 1955 Blood supply and anatomy of the upper abdominal organs, with a descriptive atlas. Lippincott, Philadelphia
39. Boijsen E 1983 Anomalies and malformations In: Abrams H L (ed) Angiography, 3rd edn. Little, Brown, Boston, ch 55, pp 1217–1230
49. Grays Anatomy, 31st edn., 1956. p 161
41. Hynes D M, Watkin E M 1970 Renal agenesis — roentgenologic problem. Am J Roentgenol 110:772–777
42. Templeton A W, Thompson J M 1968 Aortographic differentiation of congenital and acquired small kidneys. Arch Surg 97:114–117
43. Abrams H L (ed) 1983 Renal arteriography in hypertension. In: Angiography, 3rd edn. Little, Brown, Boston, ch 57, pp 1247–1297
44. Branham H H 1890 Aneurismal varix of the femoral artery and vein following a gunshot wound. Int J Surg 3:250

45. Bron K M 1983 Femoral arteriography. In: Abrams H L (ed) Angiography, 3rd edn. Little, Brown, Boston, ch 77, pp 1835–1875

46. McNeill-Love 1962 Blood and blood vessels. In: Bailey H, Love M (eds) A short practice of surgery. HK Lewis, London, pp 112–137

47. De Bakey M E, Cooley D A and Creech O 1955 Surgical considerations of dissecting aneurysm of the aorta. Ann Surg 142:586–612

48. Abrams H L (ed) 1983 Dissecting aortic aneurysm. In: Angiography, 3rd edn. Little, Brown, ch 20, pp 441–466

49. Nicholls F 1862 Observations concerning the body of his late majesty. Philos Trans R Soc Lond 52:265

50. Travers R L, Allison D J, Brettle R P, Hughes G R V 1979 Polyarteritis nodosa: a clinical and angiographic analysis of 17 cases. Semin in Arth & Rheum 8:184–198

51. Hemingway A P, Allison D J 1980 Renal aneurysms in rejected renal transplant. Br Med J 281:1640–1641

52. Adler O B, Rosenberger A 1984 Vascular aspects of Behcet's disease. Ann Radiol (Paris) 27:371–375

53. Enoch B A, Castillo-Olovares J L, Khoo T C L, Grainger R G, Henry L 1968 Major vascular complications in Behcet's syndrome. Postgrad Med J 44:453–459

54. Ring E J, McLean D J 1981 Interventional radiology. Little, Brown, Boston

55. Gillander L A 1969 Temporal arteriography. Clin Rad 20:149–156

56. Sewell J R, Allison D J, Tarin D, Hughes G R V 1980 Combined temporal arteriography and selective biopsy in suspected giant cell arteritis. Ann Rheum 39:124–128

57. Lande A, Bard R, Bole P, Guarnaccia M 1978 Aortic arch syndrome (Takayashusu's arteritis): arteriographic and surgical considerations. J Cardiovasc Surg 19 (5):507–513

58. Buerger L 1924 Circulatory disturbances of the extremities including gangrene, vasomotor and trophic disorders. Saunders, Philadelphia

59. McKusick V A, Harris W S, Ottesen O E, Goodman R M, Shelley W M, and Bloodwell R D 1962 Buerger's disease: a distinct clinical and pathologic entity. JAMA 181:5–12

60. Wessler S, Ming S C, Gurewich V and Freiman D G 1960 A critical evaluation of thromboangiitis obliterans: the case against Buerger's disease. New Eng J Med 262:1149–1160

61. Szilagyi D E, DeRusso F J, Elliot J P 1964 Thromboangitiitis obliterans: clinicoangiographic correlations. Arch Surg 88:824–835

62. Sutton D 1980 Arteriography. In: Textbook of radiology and imaging, 3rd edn. Churchill Livingstone, Edinburgh, pp 595–627

63. Kincaid O W, Davis G D, Hallerman F J, Hunt J C 1968 Fibromuscular dysplasia of the renal arteries: arteriographic features, classification and observations of natural history of the disease. Am J Roentgenol 104:271–282

64. McCormack L J, Poutasse E F, Meaney T F, Noto T J, Dustan H P 1966 A pathologic-arteriographic correlation of renal arterial disease. Am Heart J 72:188–198

65. Apitzsch D E (ed) 1978 Gefasserkrankungen der Niere. In: Atlas der Nierenangiographie. Springer-Verlag, Berlin, ch 4, pp 33–52

66. Hunt J C, Harrison E G, Kincaid O W, Bernatz P E, Davis G D 1962 Idiopathic fibrous and fibromuscular stenoses of the renal arteries associated with hypertension. Proc Mayo Clin 37:181–216

67. Loose K E (ed), Loose D A 1976 Upper and lower extremities. In: Atlas of angiography. Publishing Sciences Group, ch 4, pp 74–122

68. Ishikawa K, Mashima Y, Morioka Y, Hara K 1973 Accordion-like arterial shadows observed on the arteriogram. Angiology 24:398–410

69. Lipchik E O, Rob C G and Schwartzberg S 1964 Obstruction of the abdominal aorta above the level of the renal arteries. Radiology 82:443–446

70. Leriche R 1940 De la resection du carrefour aortoiliaque avec double sympathectomie lombaire pour thrombose arteritique de l'aorte: le syndrome de l'obliteration termino-aortique par arterite. Presse Med 48:601–604

71. Gallant T E, Athanasoulis C A 1982 Regional infusion of thrombolytic enzymes. In: Athanasoulis C A, Pfister R C, Greene R E, Roberson G H (eds) Interventional radiology. W B Saunders, Philadelphia, pp 374–378

72. Doppman J L 1983 Parathyroid angiography. In: Abrams H L (ed), Angiography, 3rd edn. Little, Brown, Boston, ch 43, pp 977–999

73. Krudy A G, Doppman J L, Brennan M F et al 1981 Detection of mediastinal parathyroid gland by computed tomography, selective arteriography and venous sampling: an analysis of 17 cases. Radiology 140:739–744

74. Djindjian R, Merland J J 1978 Superselective arteriography of the external carotid arteries (translated by Moseley I F). Springer-Verlag, Berlin

75. Wholey M H, Cooperstein L A 1982 Embolisation of bronchial arteries in patients with haemoptysis. In: Wilkins R A, Viamonte M Jr (eds) Interventional radiology. Blackwell Scientific, Oxford, pp 137–150

76. Cauldwell E W, Siekert R G et al 1948 The bronchial arteries: an anatomic study of 150 human cadavers. Surg Gynecol Obstet 86:395–412

77. Milne E 1971 Bronchial arteriography, 2nd edn. Little, Brown, Boston, pp 567–577

78. Pinet F, Froment J C 1983 Angiography and embolization of the thoracic systemic arteries. In: Abrams H L (ed) Angiography, 3rd edn. Little, Brown, Boston, ch 38, pp 845–867

79. Parkhurst G F, Dekker J E 1955 Bacterial aortitis and mycotic aneurysm of the aorta: a report of 12 cases. Am J Path 31:821

80. Weintraub R A, Abrams H L 1968 Mycotic aneurysms. Am J Roentgenol 102:354–362

81. Gelfand M 1955 Giant cell arteritis with aneurysmal formation in an infant. Brit Heart J 17:264–266

82. Hills E A 1967 Behçet's syndrome with aortic aneurysms. Brit Med J 4:152–154

83. Abrahams D G, Cockshott W P 1962 Multiple non-luetic aneurysms in young Nigerians. Brit Heart J 24:83–91

84. Lepow H, Chu F, Moren O 1958 Multiple aneurysmal formation — an elastic tissue defect. Am J Med 24:631–637

85. Boijsen E 1983 Anatomic and physiologic considerations. In: Abrams H L (ed) Angiography, 3rd edn. Little, Brown, Boston, ch 51, pp 1107–1122

86. Apitzsch D E (ed) 1978 Nierentumoren. In: Atlas der Nieren-Angiographic. Springer-Verlag, Berlin, ch 8, pp 117–162

87. Cormier J M, Hernandez C, Kieny R and Natali J 1976 Organography. In: Loose K E, van Dongen R J A M (eds), Atlas of angiography. Publishing Sciences Group, pp 207–267

88. Folin J 1967 Angiography in renal tumors: its value in diagnosis and differential diagnosis as a complement to conventional methods. Acta Radiol (Stockh) (Suppl 267) p 1–96

89. Abrams H L (ed) 1983 renal tumour versus renal cyst. In: Angiography, 3rd edn. Little, Brown, Boston, ch 52, pp 1123–1174

90. Halpern M, Finby N, Evans J A 1961 Percutaneous transfemoral renal arteriography in hypertension. Radiology 77:25–34

91. Itzchak Y, Katznelson D, Boichis H, Jonas A, Deutsch V 1974 Angiographic features of arterial lesions in neurofibromatosis. Am J Roentgenol 122:643–647

92. Lampe W T 1965 Renovascular hypertension: a review of reversible causes due to extrinsic pressure on the renal artery and report of three unusual cases. Angiology 16:677–689

93. Alvestrand A, Bergstrom J, Wehle B 1977 Phaeochromocytoma and renovascular hypertension. A case report and review of the literature. Acta Med Scand 202:231–236

94. Hollenberg N K, Harrington D P, Garnic J D, Adams D F, Abrams H L 1983 Renal angiography in the oliguric state. In: Abrams (ed) Angiography, 3rd edn. Little, Brown, Boston, ch 58, pp 1299–1325

95. Boley S J, Brandt L J, Sprayregen S 1983 Mesenteric ischaemia. In: Abrams (ed) Angiography, 3rd edn Little, Brown, Boston, ch 72, pp 1731–1750

96. Allison D J, Hemingway P 1983 Angiography of the gastrointestinal tract. In: Nolan D J (ed) Radiological atlas of gastrointestinal disease, John Wiley, New York, ch 9, pp 281–309

97. Ring E J 1983 Vascular disease of the liver. In: Herlinger H, Lunderquist A, Wallace S (eds) Clinical radiology of the liver. Marcel Dekker, New York, ch 29, pp 953–974

98. Freeny C, Lawson T L (eds) 1982 Radiology of the pancreas. Springer-Verlag, New York

99. Baum S, Athanasoulis C A, Waltman A C, Galdabini J, Schapiro R H, Warshaw A L, Ottinger L W 1977 Angiodysplasia of the right colon, a cause of gastrointestinal bleeding. Am J Roentgenol 129:789–794

100. Boley S J, Sammartano R, Adams A, DiBiase A, Keinhaus S, Sprayregen S 1977 On the nature and aetiology of vascular ectasias of the colon (degenerative lesions of ageing) Gastroenterology 72:650–660

101. Allison D J 1980 Gastrointestinal bleeding: radiological diagnosis. Br J Hosp Med 23:358–365

102. Michels N A, Siddarth P, Kornblith P L, Parke W W 1963 The variant blood supply to the small and large intestines: its importance in regional resection. J Int Coll Surg 39:127–170

103. Boijsen E 1983 Superior mesenteric angiography. In: Abrams H L (ed) Angiography, 3rd edn. Little, Brown, Boston, ch 69, pp 1623–1667

104. Baum S 1983 Arteriographic diagnosis and treatment of gastrointestinal bleeding. In: Abrams H L (ed) Angiography, 3rd edn. Little, Brown, Boston, ch 70, pp 1669–1700

105. Allison D J 1983 Role of angiography. In: Jewell D P, Shepherd H A (eds) Topics in gastroenterology 11. Blackwell Scientific, Oxford, ch 3, pp 27–35

106. Allison D J 1978 Therapeutic embolization. Br J Hosp Med 20:707–715

107. Reuter S R and Bookstein J J 1968 Angiographic localisation of gastrointestinal bleeding. Gastroenterology 54:876–883

108. Allison D J, Hemingway P, Cunningham D A 1982 Angiography in gastrointestinal bleeding. Lancet 2:30–33

109. Rosch J, Dotter C T, Brown M J 1972 Selective arterial embolization, a new method of control of acute gastrointestinal bleeding. Radiology 102:303–306

110. Goldman N L, Land W C, Bradley E L, Anderson L 1976 Transcatheter therapeutic embolization in the management of massive upper gastrointestinal bleeding. Radiology 120:513–521

111. Froelich J W, Winzelberg G G 1982 Radionuclide detection of gastrointestinal haemorrhage. In: Athanasoulis C A, Pfister R C, Greene R E, Roberson G H (eds) Interventional radiology. W B Saunders, Philadelphia, ch 9, pp 149–156

112. Nusbaum M, Baum S 1963 Radiographic demonstration of unknown sites of gastrointestinal bleeding. Surg Forum Vol 14:374–375

113. Thompson, J N, Hemingway P, McPherson G A D, Rees H C, Allison D J, Spencer J 1984 Obscure gastrointestinal haemorrhage of small bowel origin. Br Med J 288:1663–1665

114. Allison D J, Hemingway A P 1981 Angiodysplasia: does old age begin at 19? Lancet 2:979–980

115. Galloway S J, Casarela W K, Shimkin P M 1974 Vascular malformations of the right colon as a cause of bleeding in patients with aortic stenosis. Radiology 113:11–15

116. Boss E G, Rosenbaum G M 1971 Bleeding from the right colon associated with aortic stenosis. Am J Dig Dis 16:269–275

117. Hemingway A P, Allison D J 1982 Angiodysplasia and Meckel's diverticulum: a congenital association? Brit J Surg 69:600–602

118. Chuang V P, Lunderquist A, Herlinger H 1983 Portal hypertension. In: Herlinger H, Lunderquist A, Wallace S (eds) Clinical radiology of the liver. Marcel Dekker, New York, ch 25, pp 645–714

119. Athanasoulis C A 1982 Portal hypertension and bleeding varices. In: Athanasoulis C A, Pfister R C, Greene R E, Roberson G H (eds) Interventional radiology. W B Saunders, Philadelphia, ch 7, pp 90–114

120. Sutton D 1983 Arteriography of the upper extremities. In: Abrams H L (ed) Angiography, 3rd edn. Little, Brown, Boston, ch 79, pp 1923–1936

121. Laws J W, Lillie J G, Scott J T 1963 Arteriographic appearances in rheumatoid arthritis and other disorders Br J Radiol 36:477–493

122. Powell T 1984 (personal communication)

123. Poland A 1870 Statistics of subclavian aneurism. Guys Hospital Reports, 15:47–119

124. Bookstein J J 1983 The role of angiography in adrenal disease. In: Abrams H L (ed) Angiography, 3rd edn. Little, Brown, Boston, ch 61, pp 1395–1424

SUGGESTIONS FOR FURTHER READING

Abrams H L 1983 Angiography, 3rd edn. Little, Brown, Boston

Djindjian R, Merland J J 1978 Superselective arteriography of the external carotid artery (translated by Moseley I F). Springer-Verlag, Berlin

Freeny C, Lawson T L 1982 Radiology of the pancreas. Springer-Verlag, New York

Herlinger H, Lunderquist A, Wallace S (eds) 1983 Clinical radiology of the liver. Marcell Dekker, New York

Hilal S K 1973 Small vessel angiography. CV Mosby, St Louis

Loose K E, van Dongen R J A M 1976 Atlas of angiography, Thieme edition. Publishing Sciences Group

Meiisel P, Apitzsch D E 1978 Atlas der Nierenangiographie. Springer-Verlag, Berlin

Nebesar R A, Kornblith P L, Pollard J J, Michels N A. Celiac and superior mesenteric arteries. J & A Churchill, London

Neiman H L, Yao J S T 1985 Angiography of vascular disease. Churchill Livingstone, New York

Nolan D J 1983 Radiological atlas of gastrointestinal disease. John Wiley, New York

Reuter S R, Redman H C 1977 Gastrointestinal angiography W B Saunders, Philadelphia

95 Venography

Anne P. Hemingway

Technique
  Equipment
  Contrast Media
  Venous access and imaging
Complications
  Local complications
  Vascular complications
  Systemic complications

Regional venography
  Head and neck
    1. Cerebral venography
    2. Orbital venography
    3. Jugular venography
  Thorax and abdomen
    1. Superior vena cavography
    2. Inferior vena cavography
    3. Azygos and ascending lumbar venography
    4. Renal venography
    5. Hepatic venography
    6. Portal venography
    7. Gonadal venography
  Extremities
    1. Upper limb venography
    2. Lower limb venography
  Pelvic venography

Venous sampling and venography of the endocrine
    organs
  Venous sampling
  The endocrine organs
    1. Parathyroid glands
    2. Adrenal glands
    3. Pancreas

The ability to gain access to the systemic venous system has been important to physicians and surgeons for centuries. Venesection was for a long time the remedy for most ailments; and venepuncture for the purposes of diagnosis (haematological and biochemical analysis), therapy (intravenous infusions, blood transfusions) and monitoring (central venous pressure) is without doubt the most commonly practised 'invasive' technique in hospitals today.

Radiologists employ simple venepuncture as a means of delivering contrast media for such procedures as intravenous urography and contrast-enhanced CT scans. The development of safer intravascular contrast agents (Chapter 7), advances in catheter and needle technology (Chapter 94) and greatly improved imaging facilities, however, enable the radiologist to study by more elaborate techniques the anatomy, physiology and pathology of the venous system for both diagnostic and therapeutic purposes.

TECHNIQUE

Equipment

The exact equipment needed depends on the particular investigation to be performed and special requirements will be dealt with in the appropriate sections. If, however, a department wishes to offer a comprehensive range of venous investigations then a wide variety of needles, catheters and guidewires will be needed (see Chapter 94). Small needles (butterfly) are useful when repeated injections may be needed into a peripheral vein. Larger intravenous cannulae (Venflon) are useful for rapid bolus injections of contrast medium which may require a pressure injection pump; and the largest sizes (14G and 16G) allow the passage of guidewires and hence the possibility of an exchange to longer IV lines for central injection if required (see sections on digital subtraction angiography, Chapters 94 and 96).

Other special requirements for venous studies include a length of tubing attached to a pressure gauge through which a patient can blow when performing a Valsalva manoeuvre.

Two narrow, inflatable tourniquets are also required for peripheral venography.

Contrast media

The advent of low osmolality and non-ionic contrast media (Chapter 7) has significantly improved patient comfort and safety in all forms of vascular imaging including venography. Prior to the introduction of these new agents only ionic contrast agents were available and they are hyperosmolar solutions. These were irritant to the venous endothelium [1,2] and dangerous if they extravasated when injected peripherally. If ionic agents have to be used (due either to local financial constraints or because the newer agents have not received official approval) then it is advised that they are diluted to bring their osmolality closer to that of plasma [3]. Specific volumes and rates of injection for individual investigations will be discussed under the appropriate headings.

Venous access and imaging

The venous system may be studied by either direct puncture of the vein with antegrade or retrograde passage of catheters and/or contrast media, or indirectly by injecting the medium into the arterial system and imaging the venous return. Contrast medium can also be injected intraosseously and the venous drainage imaged.

1. Direct venography

This is the commonest means of opacifying the venous system. A needle or catheter is placed directly into the venous system to be imaged and contrast medium injected. This can be done using an *antegrade* approach, for example a needle inserted in the dorsum of the foot to demonstrate the calf veins; or a catheter placed in the iliac veins to demonstrate the inferior vena cava. Alternatively a catheter may be directed *retrogradely* into the venous system as in selective hepatic or renal venography to demonstrate flow from these organs; or in the femoral veins to assess valve competence.

2. Indirect venography

In this approach contrast medium is injected into the *arterial* system of the area being studied. Delayed films of the area are then obtained in order to image the venous return. This technique is used to great advantage for examining the portal venous system, for while it is possible to gain direct access to the portal venous system the latter method is more invasive, and requires greater technical expertise than the indirect approach. Other areas where indirect venography is used include the cerebral veins and the renal veins. The advent of digital subtraction angiography has greatly improved the accuracy of indirect venography and will probably widen the scope of the technique.

3. Intraosseous venography [4]

This technique involves the injection of contrast medium into the bone marrow cavity at a site distal to the venous system that is to be imaged. A needle is passed through the bone cortex into the marrow, a manoeuvre that may require considerable force and some exponents of the technique perform the procedure under general rather than local anaesthesia. The correct position of the needle is tested by aspirating blood, and then 10–30 ml of contrast medium is injected rapidly into the marrow cavity. The contrast drains via sinusoids and small veins into the deep venous system of the region.

Indications

The technique has been most widely used for leg venography. Injections are made into the malleoli or calcaneum for the calf, the tibial tubercle or femoral condyle for the thigh and into the greater trochanter to show the pelvic veins and inferior vena cava. The prostatic, vesical, pudendal, and presacral veins are demonstrated by injecting the pubic ramus. The internal and external spinal venous plexuses can be visualised by the injection of contrast medium into the spinous processes of the vertebrae, and an injection into the lower ribs delineates the azygos venous system [5]. The veins of the upper limb may be examined by injection into the olecranon process, the lower end of the radius and the acromion.

Complications [6] specific to this procedure include damage to structures adjacent to the bone being punctured, for example, the aorta, spinal cord or bladder. Any invasive procedure involving bone carries a risk of introducing infection and causing osteomyelitis, and the procedure therefore should always be performed under strict aseptic conditions. Fat embolism should be suspected if patients develop neurological symptoms after the procedure.

4. Digital subtraction angiography

This technique and its applications are discussed in Chapters 94 and 96. The ability to inject small volumes of contrast medium into the arterial system and then indirectly image the venous system will undoubtedly be increasingly exploited in departments with DSA facilities. It has the major advantage that both the arterial and venous systems of an organ can be studied with one injection of dilute contrast medium thereby increasing the safety of the procedure (and incidentally reducing its cost).

COMPLICATIONS

The complications that may occur following venography can be divided into three main groups. Those occurring locally at the site of injection, those occurring within the vascular system and systemic complications. Many of the complications of *arteriography* (Chapter 94, Table 94.1) also apply to venography.

Local complications

Pain may occur at the site of contrast injection for a number of reasons. Firstly, ionic, hypertonic contrast agents may cause local pain owing to irritation of the vessel.

Extravasation of contrast medium (Fig. 95.1) will also cause pain owing to both the irritant nature and the volume of medium injected.

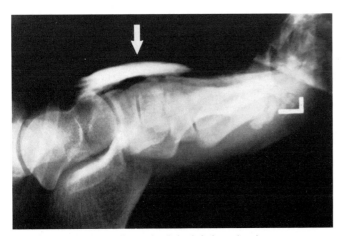

Fig. 95.1 A lateral radiograph of the left foot showing contrast medium which has extravasated into the soft tissues over the dorsum of the foot at the site of injection (arrow).

Pain has been reported in up to 65% of patients undergoing venography in a series by Lea Thomas[7]. In another series Bettman and Paulin noted that the incidence of this side effect was significantly reduced by the use of dilute contrast agents[8]. Extravasation of ionic contrast media into the skin has been reported to cause **tissue necrosis** and sloughing of skin[3,9,10]. The introduction of low osmolality and non-ionic agents will help minimize this risk. When injecting any substance careful attention should be paid to the patients's comments. *Severe* pain at the injection site should never be ignored as it does not occur if the needle is correctly positioned within the vein.

Vascular complications

1. Dissection of the vein being cannulated/catheterised may occur at the puncture site or distally due to catheter and/or guide wire manipulation.

2. Thrombophlebitis. There are a number of reports in the world literature which document the fact that following phlebography with hyperosmolar, ionic contrast media there is an increased incidence of thrombophlebitis in the limbs examined. The reported incidence of this complication ranges from 2.7%[11] to 33%[12]. The contrast medium is thought to cause an inflammatory reaction in the vessel wall with secondary thrombus formation[13]. These studies have been performed using ^{125}I-fibrinogen leg scans as an indicator of inflammation or thrombosis. Using this technique various groups[8,13,14,15] have shown that diluted ionic contrast agents show a much lower incidence of this complication, and that non-ionic contrast agents do not cause thrombosis. It is advisable to flush the contrast medium out of the veins at the end of the procedure with physiological saline[3].

3. Traumatic arterio-venous fistulae. When puncturing large veins, such as the femoral vein, subclavian vein or jugular vein difficulty may be encountered and the neighbouring artery may be punctured. Although this is usually of no significance there are reported cases of development of arterio-venous fistulae following such procedures[16].

Systemic complications

1. Contrast reactions (Chapter 7). As with any radiological investigation involving the administration of contrast medium there is an associated risk of an adverse reaction. These reactions appear to be less frequent with the newer non-ionic, low osmolar agents. Any risk of a reaction in a particular patient needs to be balanced against the risks of the condition being investigated. Atopic patients, and patients with a past history of contrast medium reactions can be covered with 24–48 hours of steroids prior to any necessary investigation with contrast medium (see Chapter 7).

2. Pulmonary embolism. Venography is most frequently performed to confirm the diagnosis of thrombosis. Calf and femoral vein clot, if loose, can be dislodged by manipulation of the leg and forceful injection of contrast. This complication is rare, but when deep vein thrombosis is demonstrated vigorous massage of the calf is inadvisable. Iliac vein, renal vein, hepatic vein and inferior vena caval clot can all be dislodged by manipulation of catheters and guidewires as well as by pressure injections of contrast medium.

3. Cardiac arrhythmias. Manipulation of catheters in the right side of the heart for any reason can cause arrhythmias. Injections of large volumes of contrast media in the right heart especially for pulmonary angiography may also cause dysrhythmias and continuous electrocardiographic monitoring is advised, particularly in patients being investigated for pulmonary embolic disease[3].

4. Air embolism. Because of the danger of air embolism in the venous system, care should be taken neither to inadvertently inject air into a vein nor to leave the lumen of any large-bore cannula or catheter open to the atmosphere.

Specific complications related to venography at various sites will be discussed under the appropriate sections in regional venography.

Regional venography

HEAD AND NECK

1. Cerebral venography (see Chapter 83)

The cerebral veins are usually visualised during the late phase of an arterial study (indirect venography). The advent of digital subtraction angiography has greatly facilitated this investigation. Small amounts of dilute contrast medium injected into the carotid or vertebral arteries or slightly larger volumes injected non-selectively into the arch of the aorta produce very good images of both the deep and superficial cerebral venous systems.

Cerebral venous occlusive disease [18] may cause infarction, intracerebral haemorrhage and raised intracranial pressure. There are a number of causes of this condition including infection, trauma, pregnancy, oral contraceptives, polycythaemia, dehydration and tumour invasion. On arteriography arterial flow may be normal or delayed. The venous phase of the study may show collateral or retrograde filling of veins and sinuses, or they may fail to opacify.

2. Orbital venograhy [19]

This technique is described in detail in chapter 83. The procedure is performed to visualise the orbital veins and the cavernous sinuses and its use is almost always restricted to the investigation of orbital varices and lesions involving the cavernous sinuses.

3. Jugular venography [19,20] (Chapter 83)

This technique can be used for visualization of the cavernous

sinuses, lateral sinuses, jugular bulb and jugular veins. The technique may be performed either by direct puncture of the internal jugular vein using the Seldinger technique or by retrograde catheterization of the jugular vein via the femoral vein.

THORAX AND ABDOMEN

1. Superior venacavography

Anatomy. The superior vena cava is formed by the junction of the two innominate (brachiocephalic) veins and then descends to the right of the ascending aorta to enter the right atrium at the level of the third costal cartilage. In its upper half it is covered by pleura on three sides, anteriorly, on the right and posteriorly. In its lower half it lies within the fibrous pericardium. Before it enters the pericardium it is joined from behind by the arch of the azygos vein [21,22].

Indications for superior venacavography include the investigation of the superior vena cava syndrome [23], the evaluation of mediastinal abnormalities, and the investigation of anatomical variants such as a left-sided superior vena cava. The technique may also be useful to follow up and to assess the adequacy of radiation or thrombolytic therapy [18].

Technique. The superior vena cava can be visualized either by the injection of contrast medium into arm veins, or by catheterization of the superior vena cava itself. In the former technique a needle or short cannula is placed in a large vein in the antecubital fossa. To be sure of obtaining good opacification of the superior vena cava this should be done bilaterally and simultaneous bolus injections of 30 ml contrast medium given. If obstruction of the superior vena cava is suspected the needles should be placed in the basilic veins in order that the axillary veins can be visualized and the extent of the obstruction assessed. Catheterization of the *superior vena cava* is normally carried out via one of the basilic veins. This can be done employing either a percutaneous puncture technique or a 'cut-down'. The catheter is advanced carefully under fluoroscopic control while repeated small injections of contrast medium serve to determine the site of any obstruction or thrombus. Once the catheter has reached the junction of the innominate veins contrast medium can be injected under pressure to delineate the superior vena cava (Fig. 95.2). If anatomical variants are suspected an approach from the left arm is advised as most variants occur on the left [21]. The superior vena cava can also be catheterized via the jugular veins or retogradely via the femoral vein if access from either arm is impossible.

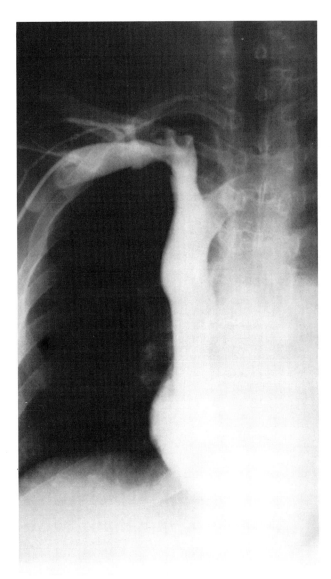

Fig. 95.2   Normal superior vena cava.

Table 95.1 Causes of superior vena cava syndrome

Mediastinal tumours

Common	Primary lung tumours
	Secondary lung tumours
	Lymphoma
Less common	Thyroid adenoma
	Neuroblastoma
	Plasmacytoma
	Thymoma
	Liposarcoma

Mediastinal fibrosis

Histoplasmosis
Tuberculosis
Sarcoidosis
Drug induced
Idiopathic

Aneurysms of ascending or descending aorta, or right subclavian artery

Luetic
Atheromatous
Dissecting

Thrombosis secondary to:

Central venous pressure monitoring or feeding lines
Ventriculo-atrial shunts
Transvenous pacing wires (Fig. 6)

Miscellaneous

Bronchogenic cysts
Behçets syndrome

been shown to be responsible in many cases. Tuberculosis, sarcoidosis, actinomycosis and cryptococcosis have all been reported in association with the syndrome [21]. The process is not usually rapid and so there is time for adequate collateral

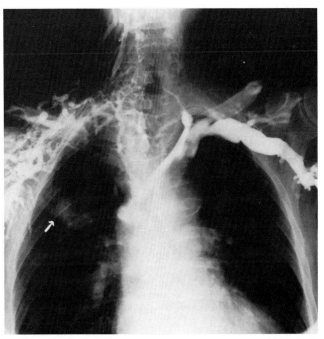

Fig. 95.3 Obstruction of the superior vena cava and brachiocephalic veins by mediastinal tumour deposits. Note the multiple collateral vessels and the primary bronchial tumour (arrow).

The superior vena caval syndrome [21,23] (Table 95.1).

This syndrome is characterised by cyanosis, swelling of the head, neck and arms, orbital oedema, proptosis and distension of veins on the neck and trunk. The commonest cause of the syndrome (approximately 90% of cases) is *mediastinal neoplasia*, usually primary or secondary lung tumours, and lymphoma (Fig. 95.3). The obstruction may be partial or complete and the severity of symptoms depends on both the rapidity of onset of the obstruction and the number of collateral vessels that have developed. Cavography will delineate the site of obstruction and its extent; it may also be useful in determining the potential resectability of tumours when obstruction is incomplete.

The most common benign cause of the superior vena cava syndrome is *mediastinal fibrosis* [24,25]. Histoplasmosis has vessels to develop. Symptoms may, therefore, be minimal or absent.

The original description of the syndrome was by Hunter in 1747 [26], in association with an *aortic aneurysm*. Luetic, atheromatous or dissecting aneurysms can all, if large enough, cause superior vena caval compression or obstruction.

The increasingly frequent use of both central venous catheters (for monitoring purposes and feeding) and transvenous pacing wires [27] has not been free of serious complications. *Thrombosis* of the vein used for access and the larger more central veins (Figs. 95.4, 95.5, 95.6) may occur, particularly if irritant fluids are injected via the catheter or if the line is left *in situ* for a long period.

Obstruction to any of the major veins which drain into the superior vena cava may occur as part of the *thoracic outlet*

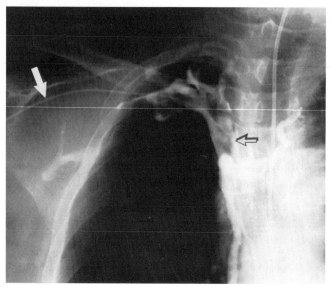

Fig. 95.5 Superior venacavogram showing fresh thrombus in the innominate vein and SVC (hatched arrow) which has occured following the insertion of a central feeding line (white arrow) for parenteral nutrition.

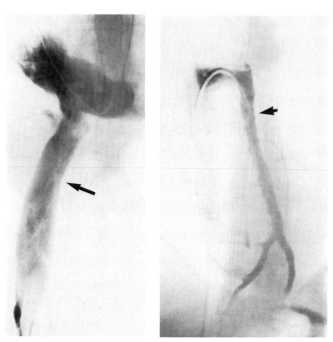

Fig. 95.4 Superior vena caval obstruction following thrombosis secondary to transvenous pacing. Multiple collateral vessels are seen in the neck following the injection of contrast medium into both antecubital fossae. The inferior vena cava (long arrow) and azygos vein (short arrow) are patent (reproduced by kind permission of the Editor of *Clinical Cardiology*).

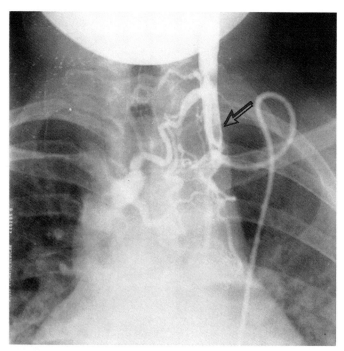

Fig. 95.6 Contrast medium has been injected into the subclavian vein through a Hickman line which had been difficult to insert. The patient had had a previous left-sided long line four years previously. The left innominate vein is occluded, and venous drainage is via collaterals. Fresh thrombus is seen in the jugular vein (arrow).

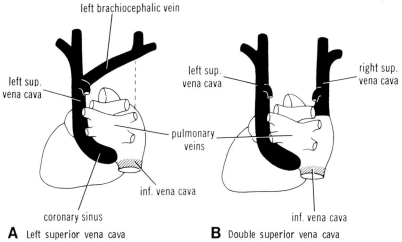

left brachiocephalic vein

left sup.
vena cava

left sup.
vena cava

right sup.
vena cava

pulmonary
veins

inf. vena cava

coronary sinus

inf. vena cava

A Left superior vena cava   **B** Double superior vena cava

Fig. 95.7   Persistent left superior vena cava (A) and double superior vena cava (B) (after Langman 1969) [32].

syndrome. Venography is a very sensitive method of ascertaining whether or not minor compression of thoracic outlet structures exists [28]. Other rarer causes of the syndrome are listed in Table 95.1.

Persistent left superior vena cava [29,30]

This congenital anomaly occurs in 0.3% of the population but occurs more frequently (4.3%) in patients with congenital cardiac disease. Although a left superior vena cava may occur in isolation it is more frequently found in association with a right superior vena cava. The left superior vena cava usually drains into the coronary sinus, though drainage into the left atrium has been reported (Fig. 95.7).

2. Inferior venacavography

A knowledge of the embryology of the inferior vena cava is useful in understanding its tributaries, anastomotic pathways and congenital anomalies [31,32]. In the young embryo paired *posterior cardinal veins* appear in the lower half of the body and join with the *anterior cardinal veins* from the head, neck and upper limb to form the *common cardinal veins* which drain into the sinus venosus. The *subcardinal veins* appear shortly afterwards along the medial aspect of the mesonephroi; they drain cranially into the posterior cardinal veins (Fig. 95.8A). As the mesonephroi enlarge the subcardinal veins take over their venous drainage and anastomose with each other (Fig. 95.8B). A new connection then develops between the right subcardinal vein and the right hepato-cardiac channel. This enlarges to become the hepatic

portion of the inferior vena cava. The left subcardinal vein then atrophies, with its distal portion persisting as the left gonadal vein. Blood from the left side then drains via the intersubcardinal anastomosis (left renal vein) to the right subcardinal vein which becomes the renal segment of the inferior vena cava (Fig. 95.8C). A third venous system develops, consisting of the *sacrocardinal veins* which drain the lower extremities and following the disappearance of the posterior cardinal veins they drain into the subcardinal system. The sacrocardinal veins form an anastomosis, which becomes the left common iliac vein and the portion of the left sacrocardinal vein proximal to this eventually disappears (Fig. 95.8D). A fourth venous system, composed of the *supracardinal veins*, begins to develop after the posterior cardinal veins become obliterated. The fourth to eleventh intercostal veins empty into the supracardinal veins. On the right the supracardinal veins along the terminal portion of the posterior cardinal vein form the azygos vein. On the left the supracardinal vein anastomoses with its right-sided partner and becomes the hemiazygos system. An anastomosis develops between the anterior cardinal veins (the left brachiocephalic vein). The second and third intercostal spaces drain via the left superior intercostal vein which in turn, drains into the left brachiocephalic vein. It is derived from the terminal portion of the left posterior cardinal vein and a part of the anterior cardinal vein. A similar vein on the right drains into the azygos system. The superior vena cava is formed by the right common cardinal vein and the proximal portion of the right anterior cardinal vein (Fig. 95.8E).

Abnormal venous drainage. Considering the complex nature of the development of the venous system it is not surprising that a number of variations are commonly encountered. A *double inferior vena cava* may occur at lumbar level (Fig. 95.9) when the left sacro-cardinal vein fails to lose its connection with the left subcardinal vein. The incidence of

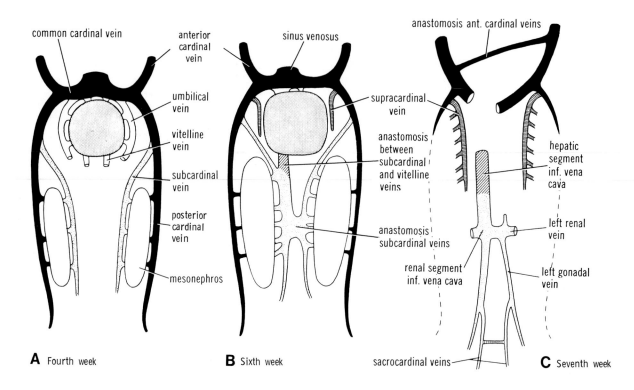

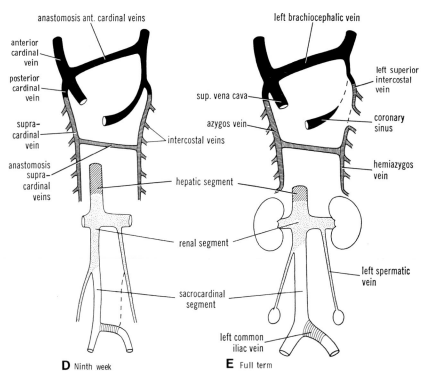

Fig. 95.8A, B, C, D & E   Diagrams showing the development of the inferior vena cava, the azygos vein and the superior vena cava in the embryo. A: fourth week; B: sixth week; C: seventh week; D: ninth week; E: full term. For details see text (after Langman, 1969) [32].

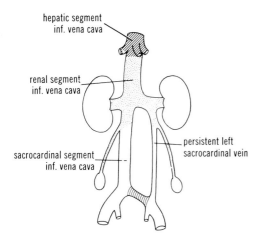

Double inferior vena cava

Fig. 95.9 Double inferior vena cava at the lumbar level owing to persistence of the left sacrocardinal vein (after Langman 1969) [32].

this anomaly varies between 0.2 and 3% [33]. The left common iliac vein may or may not be present. The cavae may be of equal size, but the right is usually larger. The left cava utilizes the renal vein for prerenal continuity with the right inferior vena cava. Failure of the right subcardinal vein to make its connection with the liver results in *absence of the inferior vena cava* (Fig. 95.10). Blood from the lower half of the body then drains via the azygos vein and superior vena cava to the heart. The hepatic vein enters the heart from below. This anomaly is usually associated with other cardiac abnormalities.

A persistent left sacrocardinal vein (left lumbar supra-cardinal vein) results in a *left-sided inferior vena cava* with an incidence of 0.2 to 0.5% [31,34]. The left inferior vena cava

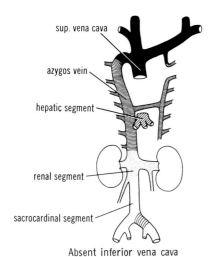

Absent inferior vena cava

Fig. 95.10 Absent inferior vena cava: the lower half of the body is drained by the azygos vein; the hepatic vein enters the heart at the site of the inferior vena cava (after Langman 1969) [32].

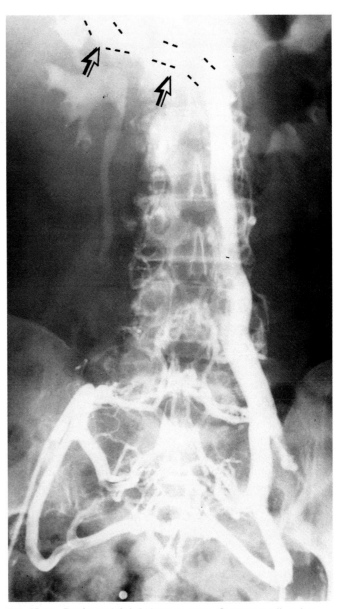

Fig. 95.11 Persistent left inferior vena cava. Contrast medium has been injected via the right femoral vein. The right IVC is absent; contrast medium has passed through the pelvic venous collaterals to the left iliac system and hence the left inferior vena cava. The cava drains into the left renal vein (arrows) and continues cranially as a normal right-sided IVC.

drains the left renal vein, crosses the spine and continues cranially as a normal right-sided inferior vena cava (Fig. 95.11).

For a more detailed account of the embryogenesis of these and other anomalies the reader is referred to the classifications by McClure and Butler [35] and Phillips [36].

Anatomy

The inferior vena cava (IVC) is a retroperitoneal structure

which arises posterior to the right common iliac artery from the junction of the right and left common iliac veins. It ascends posterior to the right gonadal artery, the transverse colon, root of the mesentery, duodenum and pancreas to enter the sulcus venae cavae on the posterior surface of the liver. The inferior vena cava then penetrates the diaphragm to enter the right atrium. The common iliac veins, lumbar veins, right gonadal vein, renal veins, right adrenal vein, phrenic vein and hepatic veins drain into the inferior vena cava.

Indications for inferior venacavography include: 1. assessment of extrinsic caval obstruction, 2. assessment of intrinsic caval obstruction, 3. assessment of patients before and after caval surgery for the prevention of pulmonary emboli to assess collateral channels, 4. investigation of tumours of the inferior vena cava, and 5. prior to the insertion of a caval umbrella (Chapter 98).

Technique

The first *in vivo* inferior venacavogram was performed by dos Santos [37] in 1935; he injected radio-opaque material via a saphenous vein cutdown. The technique has been greatly modified since then owing to the introduction of the Seldinger technique and developments in catheters, guide-wires and imaging systems. The inferior vena cava can be approached antegradely from the femoral veins or retrogradely via the arm or neck veins. The technique employed depends on the indication and area of interest, but the most commonly used approach is the one from the femoral vein. Puncture of the femoral vein has many similarities in technique to puncture of the femoral artery (see Chapter 94). The vein is not palpable, however, and the operator relies on the anatomical knowledge that the vein is just medial to the artery to achieve a successful puncture. The procedure is usually performed under local anaesthesia. The femoral artery is palpated and using the Seldinger technique the accompanying vein is transfixed. It is useful to ask the patient to perform a Valsalva manoeuvre during the puncture as this temporarily distends the vein. The central trochar is removed from the needle and a syringe containing a few ml of normal saline is attached to the cannula. This assembly is then slowly withdrawn, continuous suction being placed on the syringe. Using this technique entry into the venous lumen is instantly recognized by a backflow of venous blood into the saline-charged syringe. The syringe is then removed and a guide-wire inserted; a standard 3 mm J-wire is useful as a straight wire is liable to pass into venous tributaries such as the ascending lumbar vein. All precautions relating to the use of wires and introducer should be observed as described for arterial puncture in Chapter 94. Veins are very easily dissected by the misuse of catheters and guidewires. Following removal of the needle a catheter is advanced over the guidewire (a vessel dilator is needed prior to insertion of some pre-shaped catheters). If intravenous thrombus is suspected the catheter should be advanced under fluoroscopic control employing small injections (2–3 ml) of contrast medium. Once the catheter has been positioned satisfactorily

then 45–60 ml of contrast medium, e.g. Urografin 370 or Omnipaque 350, is injected over 3 seconds. Serial films are taken at two films a second for about 5 seconds followed by one film a second for 5–10 seconds depending on the indications for the procedure (Fig. 95.12). The procedure is performed in the antero-posterior and lateral projections. The advent of digital vascular imaging has meant that much smaller doses of contrast can be injected (20 ml of either Urografin 370 or Omnipaque 350 which has been previously

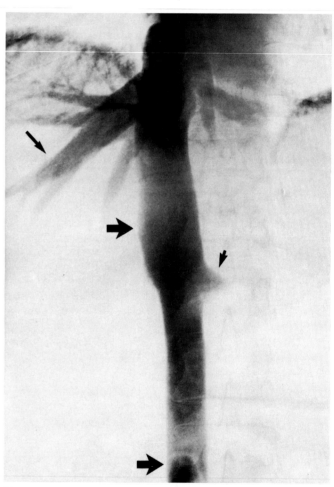

Fig. 95.12 Normal inferior vena cava (broad arrows); anteroposterior projection. Contrast medium has been injected via the right femoral vein. The patient has performed a Valsalva manoeuvre during the contrast injection and reflux has occurred into the hepatic veins (long arrow) and the left renal vein (short arrow).

diluted 1 in 4 with normal saline). Indeed it is possible, using DSA, to visualize the cava adequately from injection of contrast medium into a vein on the dorsum of the foot; in the investigation of venous thrombosis therefore, a cavogram can be performed at the same time as a peripheral venogram.

An approach from the arm may require a small cutdown or may be performed percutaneously. If the jugular vein is utilized, the Seldinger technique of puncture is employed, and care must be observed to avoid the potentially serious complication of air embolism.

Extrinsic obstruction of the inferior vena cava

Although in theory any of the structures which are related to the cava may impinge on it, only those of major clinical importance will be discussed here. Extrinsic compression may produce a number of effects on the cava and these have been summarized by Crumm and Hipona [38] (Table 95.2). Diffuse narrowing of the cava may occur in retro-peritoneal fibrosis and in diffuse neoplastic or inflammatory processes.

Table 95.2 Effects of extrinsic compression of the inferior vena cava

Angulation or displacement

Local narrowing

Distortion of contour

Blurring of margins

Changes in contrast medium density

Invasion of cava with thrombosis or occlusion

Liver enlargement due to tumour, inflammation, haemorrhage, cystic change or hypertrophy may cause compression, displacement or invasion of the inferior cava (Fig. 95.13). A characteristic appearance is found in the *Budd Chiari syndrome* (see Fig. 95.25) in which there can be quite marked hypertrophy of the caudate lobe of the liver which impinges on the inferior vena cava. Adrenal and renal neoplasms if large may cause extrinsic compression or displacement of the cava. Duodenal and pancreatic lesions may also produce a caval pressure deformity. Aortic aneurysms and aneurysms of the right iliac artery can compress the cava and may even erode into it causing an aortocaval fistula. This latter condition should be suspected in a patient who presents with a large, pulsatile abdominal mass, which may be painful and which has a loud murmur over it. The patient also has distended, pulsatile peripheral veins. The value of cavography in the assessment of abdominal lymphadenopathy in lymphoma has largely been superseded by CT.

The gravid uterus may, in the supine position, cause compression or complete obstruction of the inferior vena cava.

Intrinsic obstruction of the inferior vena cava

Intrinsic obstruction of the cava is usually a secondary phenomenon related to longstanding extrinsic compression and subsequent thrombosis [31]. Thrombus may also extend up from the ileofemoral region and occlude the lower inferior vena cava.

Tumours of the kidney may not only compress the inferior vena cava but may extend into the renal vein and inferior vena cava (Fig. 95.14), and cause caval obstruction. Tumour emboli may occur to the lungs. Renal vein thrombosis, which can occur in association with the nephrotic syndrome, may extend into and partially occlude the inferior vena cava (Fig. 95.15).

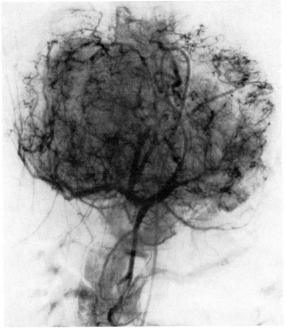
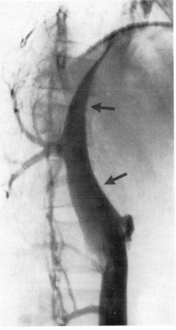
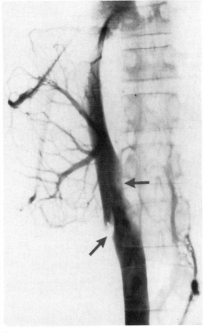

A   B   C

Fig. 95.13A, B & C   Inferior vena caval compression by a hepatoma. (A) hepatic arteriogram showing the vascular tumour. (B) lateral cavogram showing smooth posterior displacement and compression of cava (arrows). (C) AP projection showing abnormal filling of the intrahepatic veins due to compression of the principal veins (note their extensive intercommunication). The filling defects in the caval contrast (arrows) are produced by the influx of unopacified blood from the renal veins. This study suggested the cava was compressed and displaced but not invaded and the liver tumour was successfully resected.

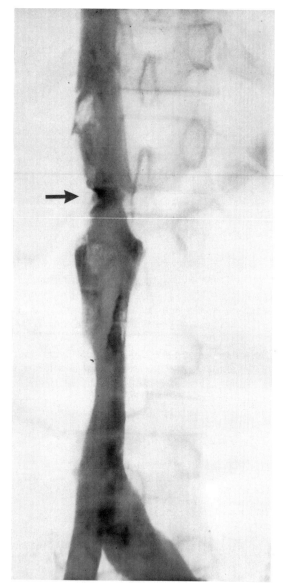

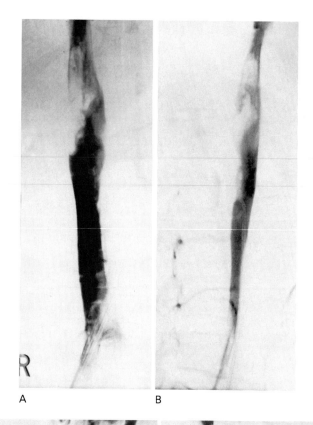

Fig. 95.14 Inferior venacavogram showing a lobulated filling defect (arrow) on the right due to extension of tumour from the right renal vein into the inferior vena cava.

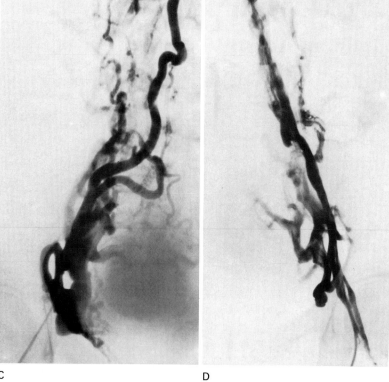

Fig. 95.15A, B, C & D Antero-posterior (A) and lateral (B) inferior venacavogram showing an extensive lobulated filling defect in the inferior vena cava due to extension of thrombus from the right renal vein into the cava. (C & D) Right and left femoral vein punctures showing the extensive collateral circulation that has developed following thrombosis of the IVC.

Similarly, *hepatic tumours* may extend into the hepatic veins and hence the inferior vena cava. *Inferior vena caval webs* have been described by Kimura et al [39], and are sometimes associated with the *Budd Chiari Syndrome* (see Fig. 95.25)

The inferior vena cava following surgery or therapeutic obstruction

Interruption of the inferior vena cava may be performed to prevent emboli from the legs and pelvis reaching the lungs.

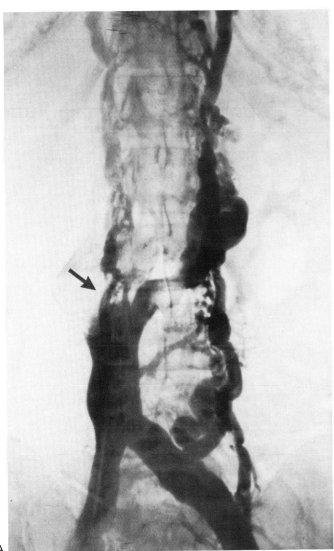

A

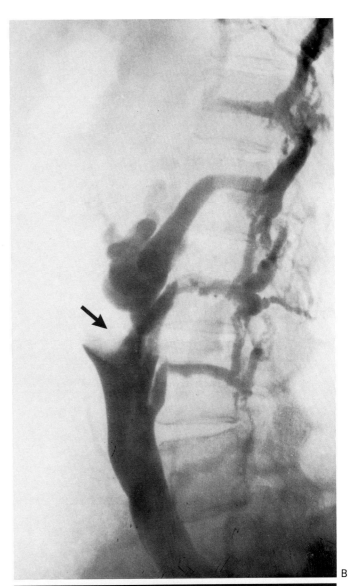

B

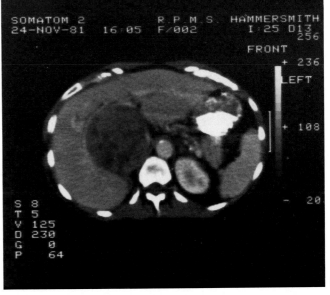

C

Fig. 95.16 Antero-posterior (A) and lateral (B) projections from an inferior venacavogram performed using a right femoral vein approach. The study shows occlusion of the cava (arrow) with upward drainage via large azygos and hemiazygos collateral veins. (C) CT scan in the same patient at the level of L3 showing a large tumour mass in the right para-aortic region anterior to the right kidney. This tumour was completely resected and histologically proved to be a leiomyosarcoma of the inferior vena cava. (Reproduced by kind permission of the editor of the British Journal of Radiology).

This can be performed surgically by ligation or percutaneously by the radiologist using an intracaval filter (see Chapter 98). Following caval interruption recurrent embolization may occur via collateral channels, especially the gonadal or ascending lumbar veins. Venography may be particularly valuable in identifying potential routes of recurrent embolization [4].

Tumours of the inferior vena cava

Leiomyoma, endothelioma, leiomyosarcoma (Fig. 95.16) and enchondroma are all primary tumours which have been found in the inferior vena cava, and all are rare [40,41]. The diagnosis is usually made at post-mortem, but there are some reports of resection in the literature. Developments in ultrasound and CT have facilitated the investigation of these lesions.

3. Azygos and ascending lumbar venography

The major systemic venous drainage in man is accomplished by the superior and inferior venae cavae. Obstruction of one or other or both of these major vessels is not incompatible with life, however, since venous drainage is maintained by collateral channels, of which the azygos and vertebral venous systems are the most important. The theory that these alternative venous systems are also of importance in the spread of disease was first propounded by Bateson in 1940 [42]. Although his ideas have been supported by the work of some other investigators [45], they are not universally accepted.

Anatomy

The *vertebral veins* are a complex network of veins that communicate transversely and longitudinally. At each vertebral level internal and external plexuses are present which drain into intervertebral veins and these communicate freely with vertebral veins at all levels. There is free communication between the vertebral veins in the sacral region and the iliac veins. The inferior vena cava communicates with the ascending lumbar trunk via the lumbar veins. The vertebral veins in the thorax drain into intercostal veins. In the lumbar region the lumbar veins drain into the ascending lumbar veins. On the right the ascending lumbar vein becomes the *azygos vein* as it enters the thorax, on the left it is continuous with the hemiazygos system. The azygos vein ascends in the thorax to the level of the fourth thoracic vertebra at which point it turns anteriorly and enters the superior vena cava (Figs 95.17, 95.18). In a small proportion of the population (0.5%), the azygos continues more laterally and enters the superior vena cava higher up, giving rise to an azygos lobe (see Chapter 8).

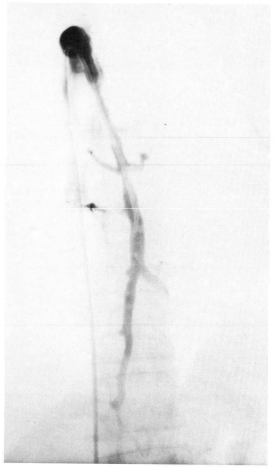

Fig. 95.17 Selective retrograde azygos venogram. A catheter has been passed from the right femoral vein into the superior vena cava and then passed over a guidewire into the azygos vein.

The *hemiazygos vein* crosses the vertebral column at about T8 or T9 to join the azygos vein. The accessory hemiazygos vein on the left is continuous with the hemiazygos below and the left superior intercostal vein above (Fig. 95.18). In 60% of the population the left renal vein connects with the hemiazygos system (Fig. 95.19).

The systemic venous network is subject to a number of congenital abnormalities such as interruption of the inferior vena cava, hypoplasia of the left innominate vein, persistent left superior vena cava and many others. In these anomalies the azygos and hemiazygos systems become the major channels for venous drainage. For a detailed account of this subject the reader is referred to Abrams [43].

Technique

A number of techniques are available for opacifying the azygos, hemiazygos and ascending lumbar venous systems. A needle or catheter may be placed in each femoral vein and contrast injected (30 ml over 3 seconds), whilst the inferior vena cava is externally compressed. Direct catheterization of

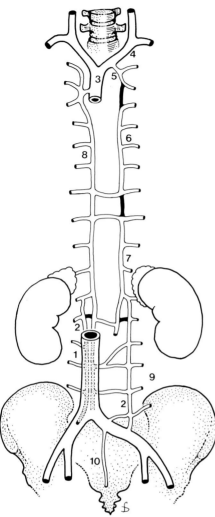

Fig. 95.18 Diagram of the azygos, hemiazygos and ascending lumbar veins (shaded segments = variable communications). Key: 1. Inferior vena cava. 2. Ascending lumbar veins. 3. Superior vena cava. 4. Left innominate (brachiocephalic) vein. 5. Left superior intercostal vein. 6. Superior hemiazygos vein. 7. Inferior hemiazygos vein. 8. Azygos vein. 9. Lumbar veins. 10. Median sacral vein.

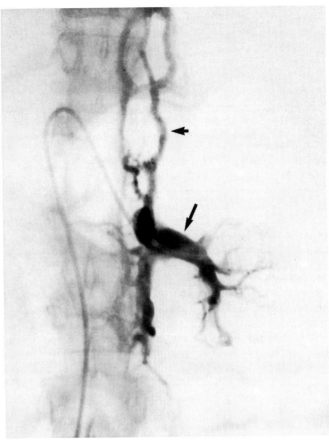

Fig. 95.19 Left renal venogram (long arrow) showing communication with the hemiazygos system (short arrow).

one or both ascending lumbar veins, however, gives optimal pictures of the azygos system [43]. Intraosseous venography may also be used [5]: in this method contrast medium is injected directly into the spinous processes of vertebrae in the lumbar region and into the posterior ribs in the thoracic region.

Indications

The indications for venography of the azygos and ascending lumbar veins are listed in Table 95.3 and causes of enlargement of the azygos vein in Table 95.4.

Table 95.3 Indications for azygos venography [43]

Anatomical variants
Caval obstruction
Unexplained cyanosis
Degenerative disc disease
Assessment of metastatic spread to spine
Carcinoma of the lung
Lymphoma

Table 95.4 Causes of azygos vein enlargement (greater than 5–7 mm)

Congestive cardiac failure
Portal hypertension
Obstruction or absence of inferior vena cava
Constrictive pericarditis

4. Renal venography [44,45]

Anatomy

Embryologically two renal veins on each side drain into the anastomoses between the subcardinal and sacrocardinal veins (see p. 2068). With the subsequent development of a definitive right-sided vena cava one vein on each side usually atrophies. On the left a single preaortic vein remains formed from an anastomosis between the anterior subcardinal veins. The adrenal and gonadal veins on the left also drain into this anastomosis. On the right one vein also atrophies, the remaining vein connecting directly with the inferior vena cava.

The intrarenal veins follow a similar pattern to the arteries. The arcuate veins, which drain the interlobular and medullary veins, run along the cortico-medullary junction. They communicate with each other and drain into interlobar veins and hence into lobar veins. The lobar veins unite anterior to the renal pelvis to form the main renal vein (Fig. 95.20).

The right renal vein lies antero-superior to the renal artery and has an average length of 32 mm. It is single in about 80% of the population; two to four separate veins are found in the remainder. In 6% of people the right gonadal vein drains into the renal vein [44]. The short length of the right renal vein and its anterior orientation means it is fore-shortened in the AP projection. The left renal vein is subject to more variations than the right, owing to its complex embryological development. It varies in length from 60–110 mm with an average of 84 mm [44]. It crosses the aorta to enter the inferior vena cava, and is related to the pancreas and third part of the duodenum. 86% of the population have a single preaortic vein, while in 2.4% a single retroaortic vein is found. In a further 7% the renal vein splits to form a circumaortic ring. Multiple veins with separate renal origin and caval entry are rare on the left. The left renal vein is joined superiorly by the adrenal vein and inferiorly by the gonadal vein. Both the left and right renal veins may contain valves, and these appear to be more common on the right. Their presence may hinder adequate retrograde venography [44].

Technique

The renal veins may be examined by direct catheterization or indirectly by late filming following an arterial injection. Direct renal venography may be accomplished using a pre-shaped catheter introduced, using the Seldinger technique, via the femoral vein. Either a femoral-visceral (Cobra) or femoral-cerebral B (sidewinder catheter) with end and side holes (see Chapter 94) may be used. If only the main renal vein is to be visualized a retrograde injection of 20–30 ml of contrast medium (e.g. Urografin 370 or Omnipaque 350) is injected over 2 seconds. If renal vein thrombus or tumour is suspected an inferior venacavogram should be performed before selective catheterization of the veins. In order to obtain detailed pictures of the intrarenal venous system it is frequently necessary deliberately to slow the intrarenal blood flow. This can be done by injecting 10 μg of adrenaline (epinephrine) into the renal artery through a selectively placed catheter; by temporarily occluding the renal artery with a balloon catheter, or by occluding the renal vein with a balloon catheter.

Indirect renal venography is accomplished by injecting contrast medium into the renal artery and taking delayed films. This technique required, until recently, the injection of quite a large volume of one of the ionic- hyperosmolar contrast agents which are directly nephrotoxic. The advent of the less toxic, non-ionic contrast agents and digital subtraction imaging have greatly improved both the safety and accuracy of this technique. It is now possible to inject 3 ml of contrast medium, diluted to a final volume of 10 ml with normal saline, via a renal artery catheter and using DSA accurately delineate not only the arterial supply but also the venous drainage of a kidney (Fig. 95.21).

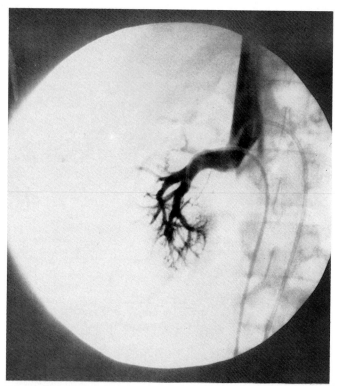

Fig. 95.20 Normal right-sided renal venogram. A catheter has been placed in the right renal vein and contrast medium injected. The catheter position is such that the lower pole veins have filled preferentially.

Indications

Renal vein thrombosis (RVT) (Fig. 95.22)

The causes of RVT are numerous (see Table 95.5) [44], and the condition occurs twice as often in men as in women. The rapidity of onset of the thrombosis governs the effect that it has on the kidney. If the occlusion occurs rapidly then haemorrhagic infarction may occur while gradual occlusion allows the development of a collateral circulation. The

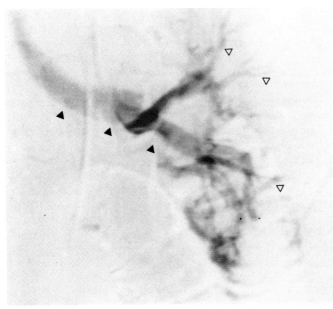

Fig. 95.21 Indirect renal venogram (DSA). 5 ml of Omnipaque 240 diluted with an equal volume of physiological saline was injected into the left renal artery and images acquired for ten seconds. The intrarenal (open arrowheads) and main renal (blocked arrowheads) veins are visualised.

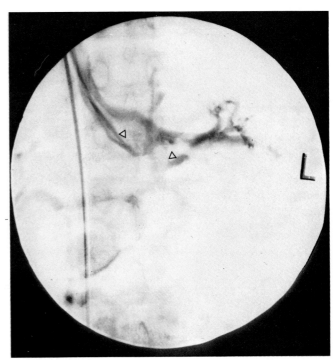

Fig. 95.22 Indirect renal venography using DSA. Following a renal arterial injection of contrast medium the renal veins are visualised. In this study large filling defects (arrowheads) indicate sites of thrombosis in the veins.

Table 95.5 Causes of renal vein thrombosis [44,46]

Children

    Diarrhoea and dehydration

Adults

Systemic disease	Amyloidosis
	Systemic lupus erythematosus
	Diabetes
Primary renal disease	Nephrosclerosis
	Chronic glomerulonephritis
	Membranous glomerulonephritis
	Tumour
	Papillary necrosis
External compression	Aneurysm
	Tumour
	Trauma

kidney responds initially by becoming congested and enlarged, but later it may atrophy. Clinically, patients develop the nephrotic syndrome, and one third may also suffer pulmonary embolism [44]. The diagnosis is made by selective renal venography and requires the visualization of intravascular thrombus. The risk of dislodging thrombus, by selective catheterization appears to be low [44,46], and accurate diagnosis is essential so that appropriate anticoagulant therapy can be instituted. Renal vein varices may occur as a sequel to RVT, and in patients with portal hypertension. In the series discussed by Abrams [44], all of the varices occurred on the left.

Investigation of renal tumours

In the presence of a large renal tumour it is valuable for the surgeon to know if there is tumour within the renal vein.

Manipulation of the vein at nephrectomy may cause massive tumour embolism to the lungs. A knowledge of its presence allows the surgeon to take appropriate precautions to prevent this happening.

Investigation of the non-functioning kidney

It is important to differentiate between renal agenesis, hypoplasia or a small kidney through disease.

Venography is the critical investigation in differentiating these conditions. Absence of a renal vein is pathognomic of renal agenesis [47,48].

Pre-operative assessment of renal veins

The left renal vein is used for the creation of splenorenal shunts in the management of portal hypertension. It is important for the surgeon to know pre-operatively if there is any anatomical variant present, such as a circumaortic ring or retroaortic vein. Venography is also valuable for assessing the patency of such shunts post-operatively (see Fig. 95.34). Following failed renal transplantation and removal of the kidney the radiologist may be asked to assess the patency of the iliac veins prior to a repeat transplantation.

For the renal venographic appearances found in a variety of benign renal conditions the reader is referred to Abrams [44]

5. Hepatic venography

Anatomy [49]

There are usually right, middle and left hepatic veins draining the liver. They enter the inferior vena cava either as a single trunk, or, more commonly, the right enters separately and the middle and left veins form a common trunk. The caudate and right lobes are also drained by several smaller veins which enter the IVC separately. The hepatic veins usually anastomose with each other within the liver.

Technique

The hepatic veins are usually catheterized retrogradely; the catheter may be passed from an arm vein, the jugular vein or femoral vein into the hepatic venous system. When catheterizing the hepatic veins from either an arm or jugular vein a pre-shaped catheter such as a general purpose catheter, a femoral-visceral (Cobra) or femoral-cerebral (Headhunter) catheter (see Chapter 94) is used. A femoral-cerebral III (sidewinder) or femoral-visceral (Cobra) catheter is most suitable for catheterization of the hepatic veins via the femoral vein. If venography is to be performed in association with pressure measurements an end-hole catheter should be used. It is frequently necessary to measure free and wedged hepatic venous pressure in the investigation of liver disease. Wedged hepatic venous pressure measurement requires that a catheter is impacted in a small branch of an hepatic vein. The catheter position is confirmed by the injection of contrast medium, and a dense stain is produced. Reports have indicated [50] that excess injection pressure may occasionally cause hepatocellular damage. Venography, with the catheter lying free in the hepatic veins, requires the injection of about 20–30 ml of contrast medium at a rate of 10–15 ml/s. Filling of the small hepatic venous radicles is assisted if the patient performs a Valsalva manoeuvre (Fig. 95.23).

Occasionally it is not possible to catheterize the hepatic veins retrogradely. In this situation direct transhepatic puncture of the hepatic veins can be performed (Fig. 95.24).

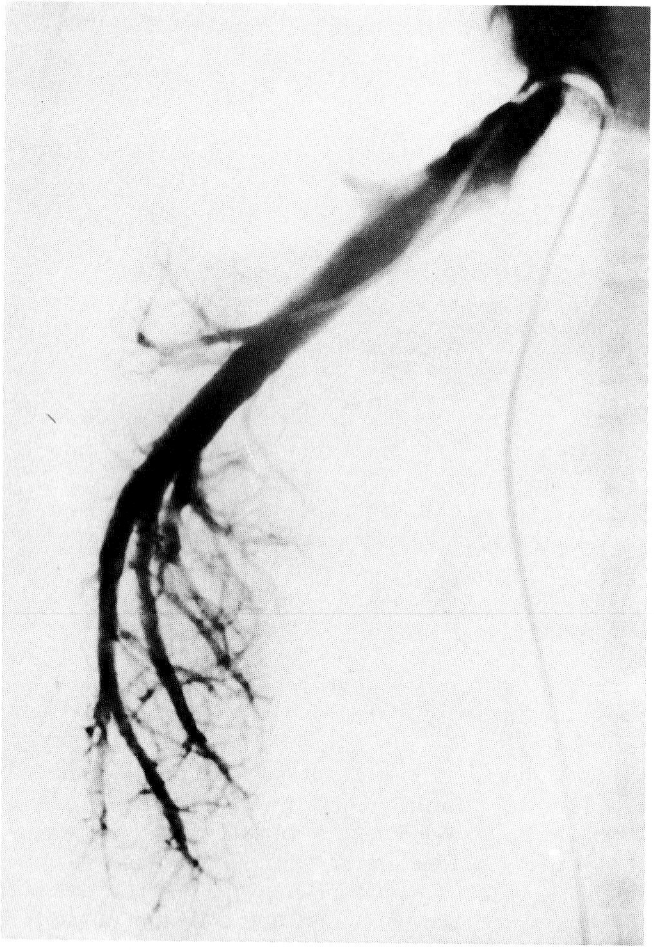

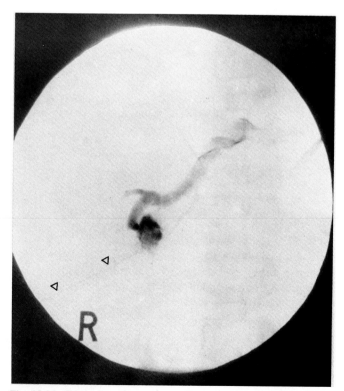

Fig. 95.23 Normal hepatic venogram. A femoral-cerebral III (Sidewinder) catheter has been passed from the femoral vein into the inferior vena cava and hence into the main right hepatic vein. Contrast medium has been injected into the hepatic vein while the patient performs a Valsalva manoeuvre. Small intrahepatic venous radicles are seen.

Fig. 95.24 Direct hepatic venogram. Retrograde right hepatic venography had been attempted but had failed. A Chiba needle (arrowheads) has been passed through the liver substance into a venous radicle. Contrast has been injected and a right hepatic vein has been opacified. A stenosis was demonstrated at the junction of the vein with the inferior vena cava.

Indications

Occlusion of the major hepatic veins (*Budd Chiari syndrome*) results in portal hypertension. The causes of hepatic vein thrombosis are listed in Table 95.6. The venographic appearances are characteristic and are said to

Table 95.6 Causes of hepatic vein thrombosis

Idiopathic
Contraceptive pill
Malignancy — hepatic   — renal
Thrombophlebitis migrans
Polycythaemia

resemble a 'spider-web' (Fig 95.25), this pattern is a result of the numerous small interconnecting collaterals which develop after the major veins are occluded. The inferior vena cava may show changes in this syndrome. The condition commonly appears to spare the caudate lobe which undergoes compensatory hypertrophy. It may become massively enlarged and cause compression of the inferior vena cava.

In *portal hypertension* it is frequently important to document portal venous pressure. It may not be technically possible to perform this directly in every patient. In these circumstances, the 'wedged hepatic venous pressure' gives an indirect measurement of portal venous pressure.

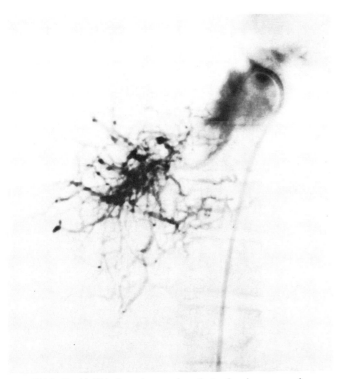

Fig. 95.25 Budd Chiari syndrome. A catheter has been passed retrogradely into a right hepatic vein. An injection of a small volume (5 ml) of contrast medium has outlined an extensive fine network of collateral vessels. This 'spider web' appearance is pathognomonic of the Budd Chiari syndrome.

Transjugular cannulation of the hepatic veins can be used as a route for liver biopsy in patients with poor coagulation or ascites (see Chapter 98).

6. Portal venography

Visualization of the portal venous system may be helpful in the diagnosis of portal hypertension and is essential for its proper management. It may also be of great value in the evaluation of other liver diseases and pancreatic disease (see below). The portal vein was first demonstrated by the direct injection of contrast medium into the main vein or one of its tributaries at laparotomy. This technique was devised by Blakemore and Lord in 1945 [51]. In 1951 Abeatici and Campi [52] demonstrated that contrast medium injected into the spleen flowed into the splenic and portal veins, and in the same year Leger [53] performed the first successful direct percutaneous splenoportogram in man. It was noted in the early 1950s that the portal vein was occasionally faintly visualized after the injection of contrast medium into the aorta [54], and in 1958 Odman [55] demonstrated the portal vein after injection of contrast medium into the coeliac axis. In recent years developments in contrast agents, equipment (especially DVI) and angiographic techniques have further improved the accuracy and safety of portography.

Anatomy

The portal venous system is illustrated diagrammatically in Figure 95.26.

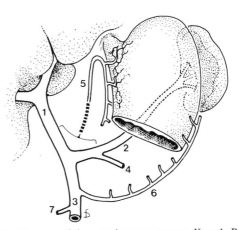

Fig. 95.26 Diagram of the portal venous system. Key: 1. Portal vein. 2. Splenic vein. 3. Superior mesenteric vein. 4. Inferior mesenteric vein. 5. Left gastric (coronary) vein. 6. Right gastro-epiploic vein. 7. Middle colic vein.

Technique

The portal venous system can be outlined in the following ways:

Direct methods — percutaneous splenoportography
transhepatic portography
per-operative mesenteric portography
transumbilical portography
transjugular portography
direct percutaneous
transabdominal portography

Indirect methods — arterioportography

Direct portography

Percutaneous splenoportography

Following the first successful use of this technique in man in 1957 [53], it was for many years the most widely used means of demonstrating the portal venous system. The patient is placed supine on the X-ray table and using fluoroscopy a safe puncture site is found. This should lie in the mid-axillary line and its exact position will depend on the size of the spleen. The puncture site is infiltrated with local anaesthetic. A needle and flexible cannula system (approximate French gauge 16) is then introduced quickly into the spleen during suspended respiration. The needle is directed cranially, medially and posteriorly towards the splenic hilum. Care must be taken not to direct the needle too far medially, however, as the major vessels at the hilum can be damaged by the needle tip. The needle is withdrawn quickly leaving the soft flexible cannula in the spleen, and if the tip lies within the splenic pulp there should be free backflow of blood. This method is safer than using a rigid needle alone as there is less risk of tearing the spleen during respiratory movements. Splenic pulp pressure can be measured through the cannula. The position of the catheter tip is ascertained by injecting a small volume of contrast medium. 30–50 ml of contrast medium is then injected rapidly into the splenic pulp and films of the area of interest are obtained at a rate of 1–2/s for 10–20 seconds. Great variation exists in the timing and film sequences required in different patients. Once satisfactory pictures have been obtained the cannula is removed. It may prove to be beneficial to embolize the cannula track, and this is most effectively done by injecting embolic material (Sterispon) down the cannula as it is withdrawn [56]. The procedure is contraindicated in a very small spleen and in the presence of markedly deranged coagulation or ascites.

Complications. The most hazardous complications of the procedure include haemorrhage and splenic rupture. The incidence of haemorrhage can be significantly reduced by embolization of the needle track [56]. A review of the literature has shown only four fatalities from haemorrhage in over 1200 studies [57]. Splenic rupture can occur if the procedure is performed in a very small spleen [58]. Some subcapsular extravasation of contrast medium may occur and cause pain which can last for a few hours. Injection of contrast medium into the peritoneum may cause pain but no serious sequelae have been reported.

Indications. Splenoportography is indicated to demonstrate the anatomy of the portal venous system, in the investigation of portal hypertension (see Chapter 50) and in any patient with signs or symptoms of obstruction of the portal vein such as oesophageal varices (Fig. 95.27) gastrointestinal bleeding of unknown cause and splenomegaly. Accurate delineation of the splenic and portal veins may also be needed when assessing the operability of hepatic and pancreatic tumours. The indications to perform this technique have declined dramatically with the improvements in indirect portography techniques.

Transhepatic portography [59]

This technique was first described by Bierman in 1952 [60]. Subsequent workers have modified the technique from simple needle puncture of an intrahepatic portal venous

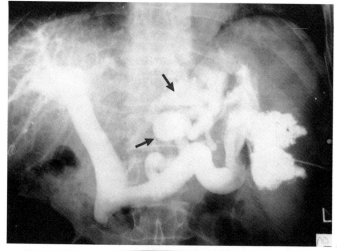

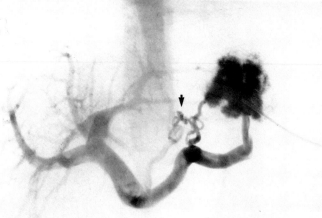

Fig. 95.27A & B (A) Direct splenoportogram. Contrast medium has been injected via a cannula into the splenic pulp. The splenic vein, portal and intrahepatic portal veins are visualised. Massive varicose dilatation of the left gastric vein is demonstrated (arrows).
(B) subtraction film in a different patient showing small left gastric varices (arrow).

radicle to sophisticated catheterization techniques. As in direct splenic puncture it is important that this procedure is not performed in the presence of deranged blood coagulation. The position of the portal vein can be outlined using either ultrasound or indirect splenoportography. It is also very useful to opacify the gallbladder prior to the procedure by giving oral cholecystographic contrast medium

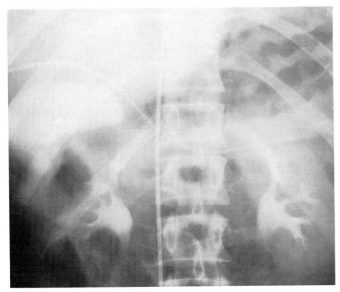

Fig. 95.28 Percutaneous transhepatic portal vein cannulation. An oral cholecystographic contrast agent was given on the day preceding the investigation to minimize the risk of inadvertent puncture of the gallbladder during the procedure.

the preceding day (Fig. 95.28). A puncture, performed under local anaesthesia, is usually made in the right mid-axillary line. The exact site is determined fluoroscopically and a sheathed needle is inserted into the portal vein during suspended respiration. The needle is withdrawn and the flexible sheath is slowly withdrawn using aspiration and entry into a portal radicle is confirmed by injecting a small volume of contrast medium. A guidewire is then passed through the sheath, along the portal vein. The guidewire is then kept in place and sheath is replaced with a longer, pre-shaped torque control catheter. The catheter can then be used for venography, venous sampling or embolization techniques. At the end of the procedure the catheter track can be embolized with Sterispon/gelfoam.

Complications [59] of the procedure include: haemorrhage from a liver surface into the peritoneum or within the liver substance into the biliary system; fistula formation (arterior-portal; arterio-biliary; arterio-venous); portal vein thrombosis; biliary peritonitis; puncture of the gallbladder or colon (Fig. 95.29A & B) particularly in very sick patients who are unable to suspend their respiration; pneumothorax; intrapleural bleed; pleural effusion and biliary-pleural fistula.

Indications. The major indication for this technique is for the embolization of gastric and oesophageal varices (see Chapters 52 and 98). The role that this technique has to play in the management of varices is controversial [61,62]. It seems likely that the principal remaining indication for this procedure is to provide a temporary respite for a patient with varices who is undergoing a course of sclerotherapy or awaiting a portosystemic shunt procedure. It may also be useful in the emergency management of a patient who has

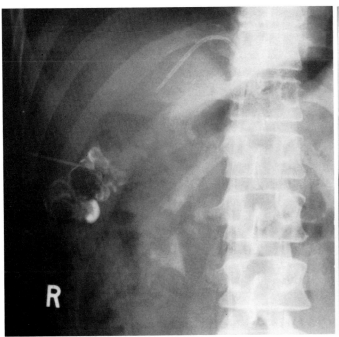

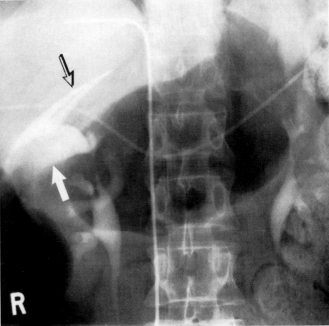

Fig. 95.29A & B Complications of percutaneous transhepatic portal cannulation: (A) the needle has entered the hepatic flexure of the colon. (B) a transhepatic catheter is safely in the portal vein. During preliminary attempts to puncture the portal vein contrast medium was injected into the gallbladder (white arrow) and into the subcapsular space (hatched arrow).

not yet been fully assessed. The effect of the procedure is variable, and rebleeding, due to the opening up of new collaterals, is common [62].

Transhepatic cannulation of the portal vein is also used for venous sampling procedures when a pancreatic hormone secreting tumour is suspected clinically, but cannot be localised by less invasive means [63]. Multiple samples are taken from the splenic, superior and inferior mesenteric veins, and also selectively from pancreatic veins. Simultaneous hepatic venous and arterial samples are also obtained to assess whether or not functioning hepatic metastases are present, and allow arterio-venous hormone gradients to be estimated.

Other *direct* methods of opacifying the portal venous system include per-operative mesenteric phlebography, transumbilical portography (Fig 95.30), transjugular portography (via the hepatic vein and liver), and direct transabdominal portography. Improvements in imaging technology and indirect portography have rendered these techniques largely obsolete.

Indirect portography [64] (arterioportography)

All of the direct methods of opacifying the portal venous system are associated with a small but definite incidence of morbidity. Indirect or arterioportography has not only the advantage of being less hazardous than many of the direct methods, but it can be combined with a study of the arterial

system as well. It is also possible by selective injections into the coeliac axis (or splenic artery), superior mesenteric artery and inferior mesenteric artery to opacify the mesenteric and splenic veins as well as the portal vein.

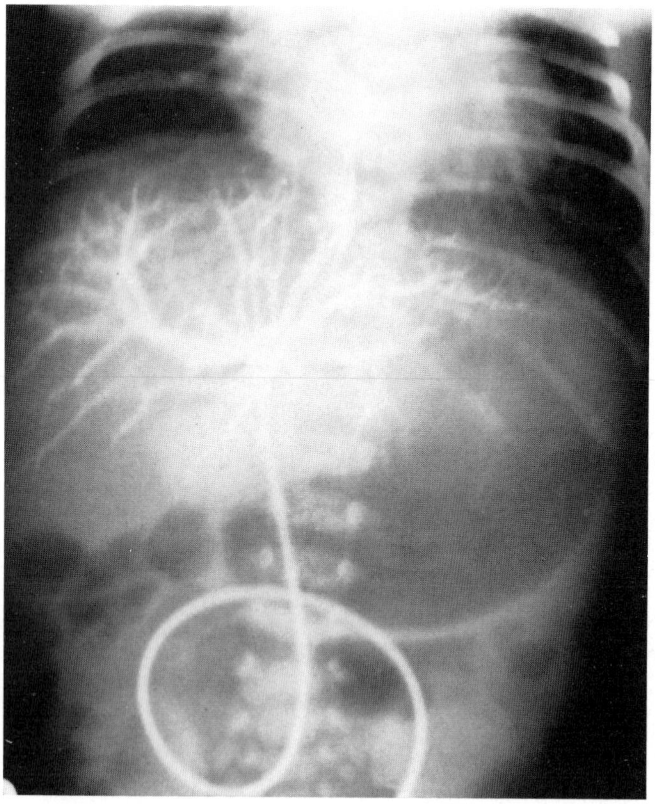

Technique — the coeliac axis, or superior mesenteric artery (or both) are selectively catheterised (Chapter 94) and films are taken for up to 40 seconds following the injection of contrast medium, for example 40–50 ml at 7–10 ml/s (Fig 95.31A & B). Larger quantities of contrast medium may be required in patients with splenomegaly. The radiographs that are taken following the injection of contrast medium should be centred so that the lower oesophagus is included on the film in order that varices are not missed. Oblique views may be needed to properly visualise the division into right and left intrahepatic branches. Some workers have reported the use of intra-arterial vasodilators administered just prior to contrast medium injection to improve portal vein visualization [64]. The advent of DSA/DVI (Chapter 96) has further improved the quality of images obtained via indirect injection methods. Fifteen ml of diluted (one part contrast '350' or '370' to two parts normal saline) contrast medium can be injected rapidly by hand and the portal vein, if patent, is readily visualized (Fig. 95.32). If the main splenic or portal veins are occluded, large collateral vessels may be demonstrated arising through the abdomen. If only one visceral artery is injected the portal vein may exhibit quite marked streaming and non-mixing of opacified and non-opacified blood (Fig. 95.33).

Indications — the major indications for arterioportography are listed in Table 95.7.

Table 95.7 Indications for arterioportography

Assessment of portal hypertension
Delineation and extent of varices
Evaluation of portosystemic shunts
Assessment of operability of hepatic or pancreatic neoplasms
Assessment of feasibility of therapeutic hepatic arterial embolization

Fig. 95.30 Trans-umbilical portal venogram in a neonate. The film is blurred because of the rapid respiratory movements.

The portal vein may be compressed or invaded in its extrahepatic or intrahepatic course. Intrahepatic portal venous abnormalities may be due to cirrhosis (see Chapter 50) where the mixture of necrosis, fibrosis and regeneration gradually impair circulation through the liver. Portal hypertension ensues, and varices may develop. Schistosomiasis is in many countries, the commonest cause of hepatic fibrosis and portal hypertension. Tumours, either primary intrahepatic or metastatic may compromise the intrahepatic portal veins. This abnormality may take the form of either invasion of the vein or compression and displacement of the vein (Fig. 95.34A & B). Portosystemic collateral vessels develop when the portal venous system is obstructed resulting in varices, but they are usually unable to decompress the system completely.

The portal venous system may also be compressed, or invaded in its extrahepatic course. *Cavernous transformation*

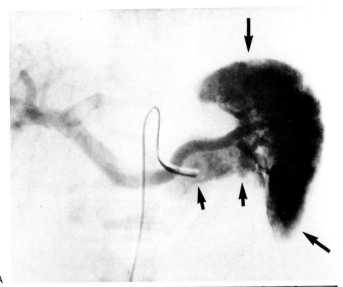

A

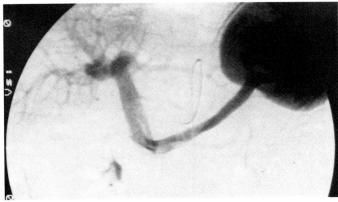

Fig. 95.32 Indirect splenoportogram using digital subtraction techniques. 15 ml of diluted contrast medium were injected into the splenic artery.

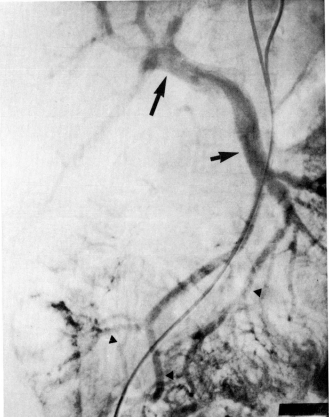

B

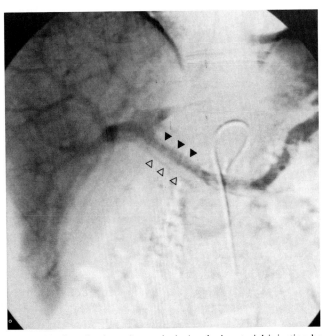

Fig. 95.33 Portal vein — 'streaming'. A splenic arterial injection has opacified the splenic blood. In the portal vein the splenic blood (solid arrowheads) is seen outlining the upper axial portion of the vein, while unopacified blood from the superior mesenteric system is occupying the lower axial portion of the vessel (open arrowheads).

Fig. 95.31A & B (A) Indirect splenoportogram. A catheter has been placed selectively in the splenic artery. Contrast medium has been injected and films taken to 20 seconds. The spleen (long arrows) and tail of the pancreas (short arrows) are both opacified with contrast medium. The splenic vein, main portal vein and intrahepatic portal venous radicles are seen. (B) Superior mesenteric venogram. Late films have been taken following an injection of contrast medium into the superior mesenteric artery. The mesenteric veins (arrowheads), superior mesenteric vein (short arrow) and portal vein (long arrow) are demonstrated.

of the portal vein usually occurs as a result of neonatal umbilical vein infection, often associated with the use of umbilical vein cannulae. The extrahepatic portal vein is thrombosed and multiple tortuous collateral vessels develop around the thrombosed vessels and drain portal blood into the intrahepatic portal radicles (Fig. 95.35). Abdominal sepsis later in life may also cause portal vein thrombosis and give rise to cavernous transformation. Calcification may occur in the portal vein as a result of previous thrombosis [64].

The extrahepatic portal vein may be compressed or invaded by tumours arising at or near the hilum of the liver.

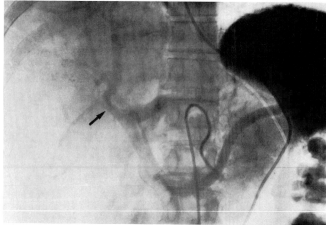

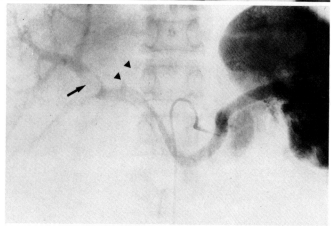

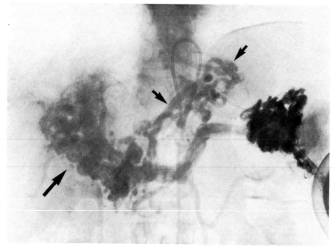

Fig. 95.35 A direct splenoportogram showing varices (short arrows) and cavernous transformation of the portal vein (long arrow).

Fig. 95.34A & B (A) An indirect splenoportogram showing narrowing of the right portal vein due to encasement by tumour (arrow). (B) An indirect splenoportogram showing a filling defect in the right portal vein due to invasion of the vein by tumour (arrow). The left portal vein is occluded by tumour (arrowheads).

Splenic vein occlusion can occur as a result of compression or invasion from pancreatic neoplasms, and chronic pancreatitis is associated with splenic vein thrombosis [65].

Portal hypertension is, in some patients, treated by creating a large portosystemic shunt in order to decompress the portal system (see Chapter 50). Pre-operatively portal venography is required to delineate anatomy, assess the size of the splenic vein and to check on the direction of flow within the portal venous system. As the left renal vein is frequently used to create the shunt renal venography is performed during the same procedure to exclude an anatomical variant which might modify the surgical procedure or render it impossible. Post-operatively assessment of the patency of a portosystemic shunt may be required. The spleen is frequently resected at operation and follow-up is therefore via the superior mesenteric artery and hence vein; or by retrograde catheterization of the shunt from the IVC or renal vein.

Invasion or compression of the portal vein usually renders a hepatic or pancreatic neoplasm inoperable. *Pre-operative angiography* may therefore be requested not only to delineate the arterial anatomy in relation to a tumour

but also to assess portal vein patency. Prior to the therapeutic embolization of hepatic tumours (see Chapter 98), careful arteriography is required and it is imperative to delineate the portal vein as to embolize the liver in the presence of complete portal vein occlusion can prove fatal.

7. Gonadal venography

Anatomy [66]

The testes and ovaries drain via a venous plexus into one to two main veins which then ascend in the retroperitoneal space. A single vein then drains on the left into the left renal vein, and on the right usually directly into the inferior vena cava (Fig. 95.36), although in a small percentage of people (6%) it may drain into the right renal vein. An important normal variant that may occur is that the left gonadal vein may communicate with the inferior mesenteric vein and thus drain via the portal as well as the systemic circulation (Fig. 95.37). This variation is particularly important if *embolization* of the gonadal vein is under consideration (chapter 98). Valves occur in the gonadal veins, more commonly on the right and more commonly in the ovarian than the testicular vein [66].

Technique

The gonadal veins are cannulated retrogradely. On the left a femoral-cerebral A (headhunter) catheter is the most useful shape and once the vein has been entered it can usually be manipulated, over a wire, some considerable distance along

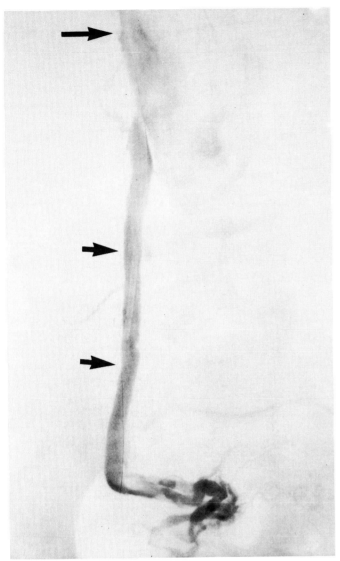

Fig. 95.36 Right ovarian venogram. The catheter has been passed from the IVC (long arrow) directly into the right ovarian vein (short arrows).

the vein. On the right a femoral-cerebral B (sidewinder III) shape catheter is very useful as the origin of the vein usually lies at a very acute angle with respect to the inferior vena cava. A long floppy-ended wire (Newton cerebral) is very useful in guiding the catheters down the veins, but great care must be taken not to dissect the vein or induce spasm by the injudicious use of wires. Contrast medium is injected by hand in volumes between 5 and 15 ml. The effect on venous filling of the patient performing a Valsalva manoeuvre should be assessed fluoroscopically prior to obtaining films as it varies considerably from individual to individual.

Indications

Testicular venography is usefully employed in the *location of undescended testicles* [67]. The descent of the testes into the

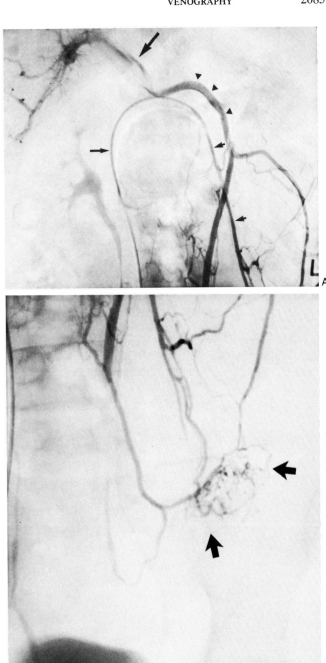

Fig. 95.37A & B (A) A catheter (arrow) has been passed from the IVC into the left renal vein and into the left testicular vein (short arrows). The contrast medium opacifies not only the gonadal vein but also the inferior mesenteric vein (arrow heads) and the portal vein (long arrow). (B) Lower projection of the same study. The mass of veins seen in the left iliac fossa (broad arrows) are not the pampiniform plexus of an undescended testis; they are *colonic* veins draining into the inferior mesenteric venous system.

scrotum may be arrested anywhere between the kidney and scrotum. The majority are found clinically to be in or close to the inguinal canal and if discovered early orchidopexy can be performed (Fig. 95.38). Testes which are found to lie intra-abdominally and cannot be restored to their normal position must be removed because of the greatly increased risk of their undergoing malignant change [67]. This policy still applies even if the diagnosis is not made until adult life. The technique of catheterization of the testicular veins is also extremely valuable in the non-surgical management of *varicoceles* [68]. The abnormal vein can be embolized with, for example, coils or detachable balloons. This technique is associated with a significant improvement in potency (see Chapter 98). Selective catheterization and *venous sampling* from the testicular or ovarian veins is of value in the diagnosis and localization of certain hormone-producing tumours when other tests have failed to localise a tumour to either the adrenal gland or gonads. In this instance blood samples can be obtained from both adrenal veins and gonadal veins and hormone levels assessed, thus permitting localization and lateralization. *Ovarian venography* is employed, as mentioned above for venous sampling techniques. It is also requested when clinically there is a suspicion of a venous malformation involving the ovaries and/or uterus.

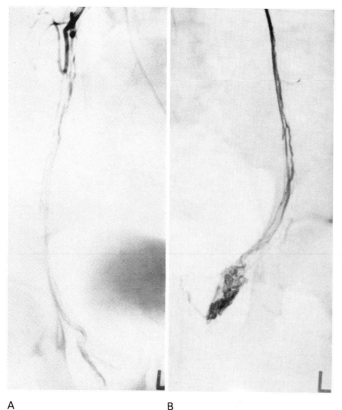

A   B

Fig. 95.38A & B (A) Right testicular venogram; the testis lies at the external ring (arrow). (B) left testicular venogram demonstrating the pampiniform plexus of veins (arrows) associated with an undescended testis in the inguinal canal.

EXTREMITIES

1. Upper limb venography [69]

Anatomy

As in the lower limb there is a superficial and deep system of veins, both of which drain into the axillary vein. Paired deep veins accompany the ulnar, radial and brachial arteries. The superficial veins drain most of the blood from the upper limb. Multiple intercommunicating veins lie in the subcutaneous tissue. Two major superficial veins, the *basilic* vein and the *cephalic* vein communicate at the antecubital fossa via the *median cubital vein*. The cephalic vein ascends on the lateral aspect of the arm to pierce the clavipectoral fascia and drain into the axillary vein. The basilic vein ascends medially and pierces the fascia of the upper arm to join the deep brachial veins to become the axillary vein. The axillary vein runs from the lower border of *teres major* to the outer border of the first rib where it continues as the subclavian vein. This vessel in turn is joined by the internal jugular vein behind the sternoclavicular joint to form the brachiocephalic or innominate vein. The right and left brachiocephalic veins unite to form the superior vena cava (see p. 2064).

Technique

The techniques for visualizing the SVC from the arm veins have already been discussed (p. 2064). When the veins of the arm itself are to be examined a butterfly needle, 19 or 21 gauge, is placed in a vein on the dorsum of the hand and contrast medium is injected. Care must be taken to avoid contrast extravasation. To opacify the deep veins a tourniquet should be placed on the arm just above the elbow, and inflated during the injection of contrast medium. The flow of contrast medium is assessed fluoroscopically and spot radiographs taken of areas of interest. The tourniquet is deflated to allow visualisation of the cephalic and basilic veins. It is important to opacify the basilic vein as failure to do so can give the false impression of axillary vein thrombosis [69]. Significant obstruction to the venous return from the arm can also be assessed by obtaining simple pressure measurements. The cannula used for introduction of contrast medium can be connected to a water manometer and a baseline pressure obtained. The measurement is repeated following exercise of the upper limb for two minutes. In a normal patient there will be no rise in pressure, whereas if there is a significant degree of obstruction the pressure will rise.

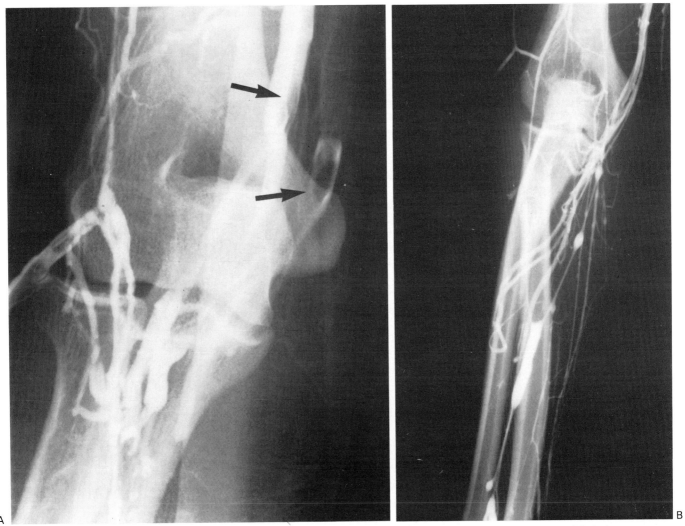

Fig. 95.39A & B (A) Arm venogram showing thrombus in superficial veins (arrows) following intravenous lines and drugs. (B) Arm venogram following administration of an irritant anaesthetic agent intravenously. Marked abnormalities of calibre are noted.

A

B

Indications

Venous thrombosis

Prior to the introduction of pacemakers and central venous feeding and monitoring lines, thrombosis of the veins of the upper limb was uncommon. Its incidence was estimated as being only 1–2% that of deep venous thrombosis of the lower limbs, but the increasing use of these vessels as a 'therapeutic route' has led to a significant increase in thrombosis of upper limb veins [70] (Fig. 95.39). Thrombosis of the axillary and subclavian veins only occasionally gives rise to pulmonary embolism (less than 10% of cases) [71]. Gangrene of the digits and hands has been reported as a rare complication of severe venous obstruction [72]. Causes of upper limb venous thrombosis are listed in Table 95.8.

Table 95.8 Causes of upper limb venous thrombosis (after Neiman and Yao 1985 [69])

Non-occlusive:	Intermittent compression of subclavian vein [69]
Occlusive:	Idiopathic
	Malignancy
	Trauma (clavicular fracture/dislocation)
	Radiation injury
	Transvenous pacemaker wire
	Central venous feeding/monitoring lines
	Irritant substances —
	anaesthetics, chemotherapy & antibiotics (Fig. 95.39A & B).
	Drug abuse — septic thrombophlebitis

2. Lower limb venography

Anatomy

The veins of the lower limb can be divided into deep and superficial systems. There are three pairs of deep veins in the calf which accompany the arteries. These veins unite just below the knee to form the popliteal vein which continues as the femoral vein, which accompanies the femoral artery. This in turn drains into the external iliac vein. Multiple superficial veins are present in the calf and are linked to the deep venous system via paired, valved communicating veins. The normal direction of flow is from the superficial to the deep system. The main superficial veins are the short and long saphenous veins. The short saphenous vein passes behind the lateral malleolus and continues along the posterior aspect of the calf to join the popliteal vein. The long saphenous vein passes anterior to the medial malleolus and postero-medial to the medial femoral condyle to drain into the femoral vein just below *Poupart's* ligament. Valves are present in all of the superficial, perforating and deep veins in normal subjects. They are more numerous distally. There are no valves in the common iliac veins or inferior vena cava.

Technique

Ascending venography

Where possible the procedure should be performed with the patient in an *erect or semi-erect position*. The leg being examined should be relaxed and non-weight bearing. A vein on the dorsum of the foot is cannulated using a 19 or 21 gauge butterfly needle. The needle tip should be pointing *towards* the toes as this improves deep vein filling. Many radiologists employ the use of a tourniquet placed just above the ankle to direct the flow of contrast into the deep veins [3]. There are, however, other authorities who feel that a tourniquet should *not* be used [73,74], except in exceptional circumstances, for example when there is such extensive deep venous thrombosis that without a tourniquet on the superficial veins fill, or when the opacification of numerous varicose veins would obscure a proper view of the deep veins. Similarly some workers also use a tourniquet placed just above the knee to delay emptying of calf veins and improve their filling.

After satisfactory positioning of the needle 60–100 ml of contrast medium (preferably a low osmolar or non-ionic medium) is injected as rapidly as possible *by hand*. The injection site must be scrutinised to detect any contrast medium extravasation. During injection of contrast medium the veins of the calf are examined fluoroscopically and spot radiographs taken in various projections. The popliteal, femoral and iliac veins are then examined and the opacification of these vessels may be enhanced by raising the calf, restoring the patient to the supine position, asking the patient to perform a Valsalva manoeuvre and releasing the tourniquet (if used) (Figure 95.40). If both legs are to be studied then this procedure is repeated on the opposite limb. It is possible to obtain adequate pictures of the external and common iliac veins in 95% of people by injecting 50 ml of contrast medium simultaneously into each foot with a thigh tourniquet in place. The tourniquets are deflated and the calves massaged (if clear of thrombus!) while radiographs are exposed over the pelvis and lower inferior vena cava [74].

Descending venography

A needle or short catheter is placed in the femoral vein using the Seldinger technique (see Chapter 94 and p. 2070). The examination is carried out with the patient in the erect or steep semi-erect position. Contrast medium is injected (10–15 ml) and the veins of the upper thigh are visualized fluoroscopically. Some reflux of contrast medium is normal due to gravity and the density of the medium. Reflux to the knee or below is, however, regarded as abnormal.

Intraosseous venography

This has been discussed above (see p. 2062).

Complications

The complications that may result from venography have been discussed on page 2063. The most common complication encountered during leg venography is *pain* caused by the contrast medium irritating the venous endothelium. The incidence and severity of pain can be significantly reduced by using sodium free or diluted ionic contrast media or preferably one of the new low osmolality or non-ionic media.

Extravasation of contrast medium into the tissues of the foot may cause a chemical cellulitis [10] and in 0.4% of cases this may progress to ulceration, tissue necrosis and gangrene [9,10]. The site of venepuncture should be constantly inspected throughout the procedure. If there is any swelling or complaint of pain the injection should be terminated immediately. Attempts to disperse the extravasated contrast by massage, warm compresses and dilution with physiological saline may be useful. The incidence of post-venographic *thrombosis* can be minimised by using non-ionic contrast medium; and by flushing the contrast medium from the veins with physiological saline at the end of the procedure. Some patients develop a *post-phlebographic syndrome* of pain, tenderness and erythema around the ankle joint which does not necessarily appear to be associated with the development of thrombosis. Like thrombosis, however, the incidence of this side effect can be reduced by using dilute or non-ionic contrast agents.

Contraindications to ascending phlebography [3] include known serious sensitivity to contrast medium, and severe local infection of the foot or ankle to be studied. Anti-

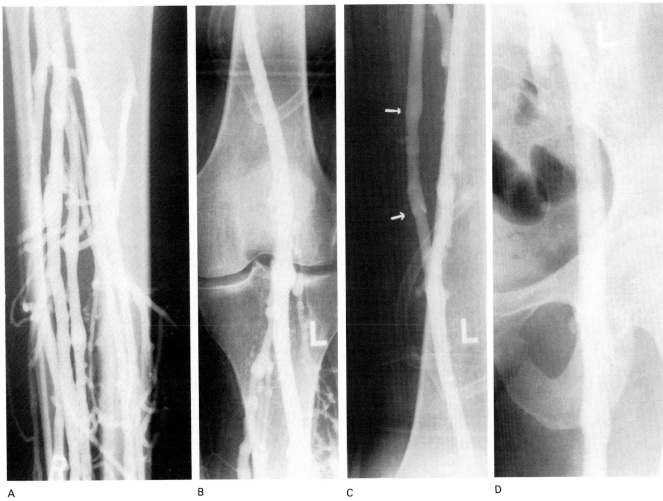

A   B   C   D

Fig. 95.40A, B, C & D   Ascending venography demonstrating:
(A) Normal calf veins.
(B) Normal popliteal veins.
(C) Normal popliteal and femoral veins (valves arrowed).
(D) Normal femoral and iliac veins (figure by courtesy of Helen Allison).

coagulants do not constitute a contraindication to the procedure.

Artefacts that can simulate pathology in lower limb venography are listed in Table 95.9.

Table 95.9 Artefacts simulating pathology during venography [10]

Arterial impressions

Non-filling of veins

Mixing defects

Entry of non-opacified blood

Overlying gas and bone shadows

Valve defects (turbulence)

Venturi effect

Air bubbles

Tourniquets

Previous surgery (e.g. venous plication)

Indications

Deep venous thrombosis

The diagnosis of deep vein thrombosis (DVT) is made by demonstrating the presence of constant filling defect(s) within the veins (Fig. 95.41). In fresh thrombus contrast is seen between the clot and the vein wall; whereas with old clot it may be adherent to the vein wall and therefore contrast is only seen above and below the thrombus but not around it. The non-filling of veins, the abnormal diversion of contrast flow or the abrupt termination of the contrast column are also signs which are suggestive but not diagnostic of deep vein thrombosis. Deep vein thrombosis may be treated conservatively with heparin or streptokinase. Loose clot may readily detach and cause pulmonary embolism. Extensive clot may require venous plication, surgical removal, or the insertion of an inferior vena caval filter to prevent pulmonary embolism. The causes of DVT are listed in Table 95.10. 25–30% of patients undergoing abdominal

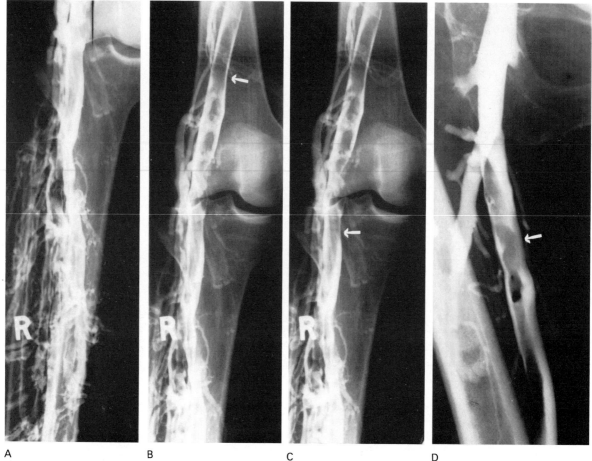

Fig. 95.41A–D Lower limb venogram. Extensive filling defects (arrows) due to thrombus are seen in the calf and popliteal veins and the femoral vein.

Table 95.10 Causes of deep vein thrombosis

Trauma	Polycythaemia
Surgery	Dehydration
Immobilization	Local infection
Contraceptive pill	
Malignancy	
Obesity	
Increasing age	

surgery and 40–60% of patients with either trauma or surgery to the hip joint or knee develop evidence of deep vein thrombosis [74,75]. DVT occurs in less than 1% of women taking the contraceptive pill; and in up to 30% of patients following myocardial infarction. The thrombosis is *bilateral* in 30% of cases clinically [76,77], and in 85% of cases at autopsy.

The post-phlebitic syndrome

Recanalization of veins affected by thrombus usually occurs but the valves are commonly damaged and become incompetent. Venous return is accomplished via these damaged veins and collaterals. Abnormally high venous pressures are transmitted to the superficial veins and ultimately skin discolouration and ulceration may occur around the ankle joint.

Varicose veins

Varicose veins (Fig. 95.42) occur in 4% of the adult population and can give rise to significant morbidity due to ulceration, haemorrhage, thrombosis and eczema [78]. Varicose veins are described as either primary or secondary in nature. Primary varicose veins affect the long and short saphenous veins and are frequently associated with incompetent perforating veins, the deep venous system is however normal. Secondary varicose veins on the other hand occur as a result of previous deep vein thrombosis. Less common causes of varicosities of the leg veins include arterio-venous malformations and congenital anomalies, such as the Klippel-Trenaunay syndrome [10]. The perforating veins contain valves which normally only permit flow from the superficial to deep system. In primary varicose veins there is only intermittent

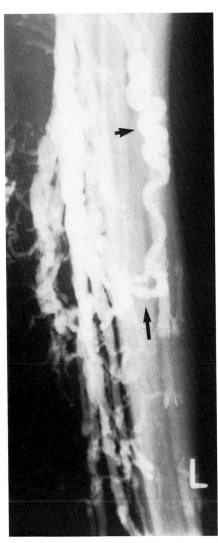

Fig. 95.42 Ascending venogram showing incompetent perforating veins (arrow) and superficial varicosities (short arrow).

reversal of the flow whereas in secondary varicose veins the flow is predominantly reversed due to the damaged deep system. Ascending phlebography can be employed to demonstrate the site(s) of incompetent perforators. A tourniquet is placed around the ankle and injection begins. Careful fluoroscopy will allow adequate identification of the level of incompetent vessels, and the technique can be repeated with the tourniquet moved progressively up the leg so that all of the vessels at fault can ultimately be identified. Early filming is essential because the rapid filling of varicosities frequently obscures the perforating veins. *Varicography* may be employed; this involves the direct puncture with a 21 or 23 gauge needle of a varix so that the perforator responsible can be identified and dealt with.

The Klippel-Trenaunay syndrome [79]

This consists of a cutaneous naevus of one lower limb,

varicose veins on the same side dating from infancy and hypertrophy of the limb. The deep veins may be hypoplastic or absent in which case the superficial veins cannot be stripped without further aggravating the condition. Venography can show the status of the limb veins (if any investigation or treatment seems appropriate or necessary).

PELVIC VENOGRAPHY

Anatomy

The femoral vein, after passing behind the inguinal ligament continues as the external iliac vein. This in turn is joined, at the level of the sacro-iliac joint, by the internal iliac vein. The common iliac veins then pass upward to unite to the right of the fifth lumbar vertebra to form the inferior vena cava. The inferior epigastric veins, circumflex iliac veins and pubic veins drain into the external iliac veins. The internal iliac (hypogastric) veins drain the gluteal, internal pudendal, pelvic visceral and sacral plexus veins.

Techniques

The external and common iliac veins can be demonstrated by means of ascending phlebography from a pedal injection; or by direct puncture at the groin. They can also be catheterized retrogradely using a catheter inserted from the contralateral groin, jugular vein or arm. The pelvic veins can also be selectively, retrogradely cannulated and opacified. Contrast medium is injected whilst the patient performs a Valsalva manoeuvre.

Indications

Thrombosis

It may be necessary to examine the pelvic veins to exclude venous thrombosis, particularly after pelvic surgery of any description.

Assessment of anastomoses

The pelvic veins, for example the sacral venous plexus or pelvic visceral veins, can provide valuable collateral pathways if the venous return on one side is either congenitally abnormal or becomes occluded.

Venous sampling and venography of the endocrine organs [63]

VENOUS SAMPLING

Venous sampling techniques are used to localise areas of abnormally increased hormone production. The techniques can be applied to virtually any site within the body in both the portal and systemic venous systems. Samples of blood are taken from known anatomical sites (identified fluoroscopically), numbered and plotted on a 'map' (Fig. 96.43). The samples are then analysed and the measured hormone levels also plotted on the map. Any abnormally high levels can than be localised.

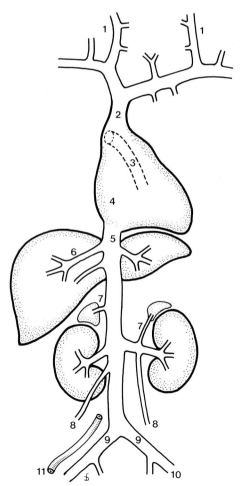

Fig. 95.43 Venous sampling map. Key: 1. Jugular veins. 2. SVC. 3. Azygos vein. 3. Right atrium. 5. IVC. 6. Hepatic veins. 7. Adrenal veins. 8. Gonadal veins. 9. Common iliac veins. 10. Femoral vein. 11. Femoral artery.

Technique

The procedure can be applied to both the systemic and portal venous systems. When sampling from systemic veins the venous system is usually entered at the groin using the Seldinger technique. A preshaped catheter with an end hole and two side holes close to the tip is used for sampling. The catheter is then guided to different sampling locations. The blood occupying the dead-space of the catheter is withdrawn and discarded. The sample is then taken, the volume of blood depending on local laboratory requirements. A very detailed knowledge of venous anatomy is needed to avoid incorrect localization of a sample.

When identifying the catheter position it is frequently necessary to inject a small volume of contrast medium. This may show that the cannulated vessel communicates freely with neighbouring vessels and therefore that a sample may reflect the venous drainage of quite a large anatomical area (Fig. 95.44). It is important for the operator not to aspirate blood too vigorously from small veins in order to avoid drawing in blood from neighbouring areas and therefore giving misleading results. Hormone production may fluctuate even during the course of a procedure and it may be necessary to take simultaneous arterial and venous samples so that the results are expressed as a ratio to correct for this effect.

The outcome of the technique is not only dependent on the radiologist but also on the clinicians who must ensure that the samples are correctly labelled and taken to the appropriate laboratory for analysis. There are a large number of possible sources of error in venous sampling and these are listed in Table 95.11.

Table 95.11 Sources of error in venous sampling

Operator errors:	Incorrect anatomical localization
	Incorrect rate of sample aspiration
	Failure to discard catheter 'dead space'

Variations in venous anatomy and flow patterns

Distortion of flow patterns by sampling catheter

Fluctuations in hormone production rate

Fluctuations in organ blood flow

Sample handling errors

Laboratory assay errors

Interpretation errors

Complications

Generally speaking venous sampling is a very safe procedure but the technique is theoretically subject to all of the general complications discussed on page 2063 and some specific complications should also be mentioned. The procedure can occasionally induce a sudden outpouring of hormone which may be dangerous (e.g. in a case of phaeochromocytoma). It is possible to infarct tissue, for example, the adrenal gland,

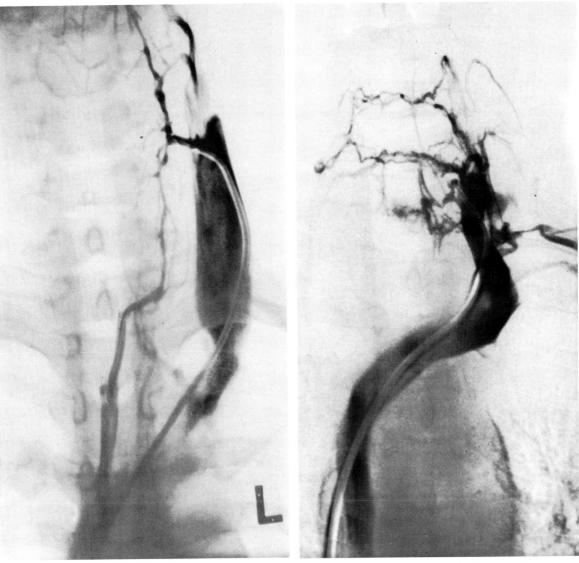

Fig. 95.44A & B   (A) Middle thyroid venogram showing filling of the superior, middle and inferior thyroid veins from a single injection. (B) Left internal jugular venogram in a patient who had undergone previous neck surgery. The main vein cannot be visualised and there are multiple collaterals.

if unnecessary force is used to either cannulate the vein or inject a test dose of contrast medium. Vigorous catheter manipulation in the right heart can lead to transient cardiac dysrhythmias.

Transhepatic portal venous sampling (see p. 2080 for description of technique and/or cannulation) carries a significant risk of complications, the most likely being haemorrhage. Embolization of the catheter track helps to minimize this risk.

THE ENDOCRINE ORGANS

1. The parathyroid glands [80]

Primary hyperparathyroidism is cured in more than 90% of patients by the first operation [81]. Localization techniques are therefore reserved in many centres for those patients in whom initial surgery is unsuccessful, or in whom hypercalcaemia recurs. In this group of patients, in whom there is little clinical doubt about the diagnosis, techniques such as isotope scanning (see Chapter 55) using thallium 201 and technetium 99 m, CT scanning, parathyroid angiography (see Chapter 94) and venous sampling may be useful. A knowledge of the normal venous anatomy is essential [82], but it must be remembered that previous surgery can cause significant distortion of the venous drainage patterns. The parathyroid glands drain into the internal jugular and innominate veins via the superior, middle and inferior thyroid veins. The inferior veins often unite to form a common trunk which drains into the left innominate vein. The thymic vein, which drains mediastinal structures, also drains into the left innominate vein. Mediastinal tumours are said to occur in some 20% of cases [83]. Samples are taken as selectively as possible from the inferior, middle and superior thyroid veins, as well as from the larger veins such as the jugular, sub-clavian, innominate and azygos veins. Thymic and left superior intercostal samples are also taken if possible. The samples are numbered and recorded on a map. Care is needed when obtaining a sample not to aspirate blood too enthusiastically as all the veins intercommunicate and blood can be drawn in from the contralateral side of the neck (Fig. 95.44). The accuracy of the technique in predicting the site of a tumour ranges 50–90% in different series [84,85,86,87].

2. The adrenal glands

Advances in imaging techniques such as CT and isotope scanning have considerably reduced the role of vascular studies in the diagnosis and localization of adrenal endocrine tumours. Adrenal venous sampling may still be useful in some patients, however, in whom the results of less invasive tests are negative or equivocal. In *hyperaldosteronism* it is important to know if the elevated hormone production is unilateral or bilateral. Unilaterally elevated hormone levels suggest an adenoma, whereas bilaterally elevated levels suggest hyperplasia [88]. In cases of suspected *phaeochromo-cytoma* venous sampling has proved to be an extremely accurate method for both the identification and exclusion of functioning tumours [89]. Phaeochromocytomas are ectopic in 10% and multiple in 10% of patients. Venous sampling is performed as one of the first investigations and directs further investigations to areas of raised hormone secretion [89,90]. As in all other sampling techniques multiple samples are taken, numbered and recorded on a map. Simultaneous arterial samples may be required so that results are given as ratios rather than absolute numbers. Prior to taking a sample contrast medium is injected to check true catheter position. An *adrenal venogram* may be performed in problem cases and this can add further information to that being obtained by other imaging modalities (Fig. 95.45A & B). Adrenal venography is not without hazard and the increasing accuracy of less invasive methods has now almost rendered the technique obsolete. Intra-adrenal extravasation of contrast occurs in about 4% of cases even when the operator is experienced. It seems to happen more often in those patients

with Cushing's syndrome and hyperaldosteronism due to 'fragile' veins. Following contrast medium extravasation the patient experiences worsening pain over about an hour. Pain requiring opiate analgesia and fever can last for 24 to 36 hours. This sequence of events is associated with ablation of gland function. This technique may be used deliberately to treat hormone secreting tumours of the gland (see Chapter 98). Contrast extravasation in one gland is an absolute contraindication to catheterizing the vein on the opposite side.

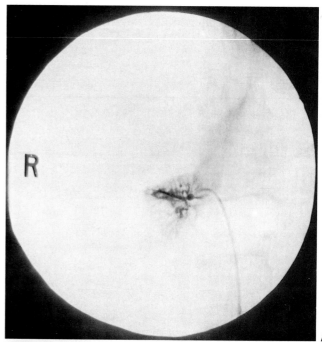

A

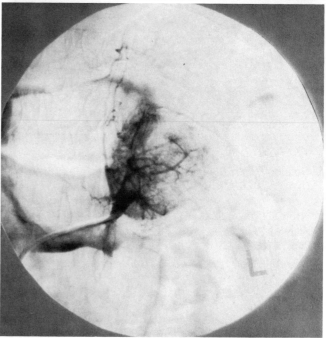

B

Fig. 95.45A & B   (A) Normal right adrenal venogram. (B) Left adrenal venogram showing a large vascular tumour, a phaeochromocytoma.

Iodine 131 MIBG (^{131}I-Meta-iodo-benzylguanidine) [91] is proving very useful in localizing phaeochromocytomas (see Chapter 55) and seems likely to supplant venous sampling as the best technique for locating ectopic tumours.

3. The pancreas [92]

Despite all the imaging modalities available for studying the pancreas, including angiography, CT, ultrasound, isotope studies, ERCP and other forms of contrast radiography, it remains exceedingly difficult to accurately and confidently diagnose many small primary tumours. The primary may be miniscule, but produce large amounts of hormone and give rise to the liver deposits which in the case of endocrine tumours are usually very hormonally active.

The pancreatic venous drainage is via the splenic, superior mesenteric and portal veins (Fig. 95.26). In order to perform venous sampling the portal vein has to be cannulated transhepatically. Simultaneous portal venous, systemic venous/hepatic, and mixed arterial samples are taken, mapped, labelled and sent to the appropriate laboratory. The hepatic vein samples allow the early detection of hormonally active metastases.

Pancreatic venous sampling is a technique that requires considerable expertise (Chapter 53) and is not without hazard [3] (Fig. 95.29). Its position in the sequence of diagnostic investigations in a case of suspected pancreatic endocrine tumour is not yet certain. Most radiologists agree that contrast-enhanced CT scanning is an effective and relatively non-invasive investigation which is scoring an increasingly high success rate in locating such tumours and should be one of the first-line investigations. If the CT scan is negative some investigators (including the author) proceed to selective pancreatic arteriography (Chapter 94) before submitting the patient to percutaneous portal venous sampling; others, however, believe the venous sampling technique to yield better results than arteriography.

It seems probable that advances in less invasive methods of investigation such as CT, DSA, MRI and isotope scanning (at present disappointing in the pancreas) will eventually render pancreatic venous sampling obsolete.

BIBLIOGRAPHY

REFERENCES

1. Mersereau W A, Robertson H R 1961 Observations on venous endothelial injury following the injection of venous radiographic contrast media in the rat. Journal of Neurosurgery 18:289
2. Ritchie W G M, Lynch R R, Stewart G J 1974 The effect of contrast media on normal and inflamed canine veins. Investigative Radiology 9:444–455
3. Allison D J 1981 Radiology in diagnosis of venous thrombo-embolism. In: Pitney W R (ed) Venous and arterial thrombosis. Churchill Livingstone, Edinburgh, pp 140–156
4. Sutton D 1980 Phlebography. In: Sutton D (ed) A textbook of radiology and imaging. Churchill Livingstone, Edinburgh, pp 635–636
5. Fischgold H, Adam H, Ecoiffier J, Plequet J 1952 Opacification of spinal plexuses and azygos veins by osseous route. J Radiol Electrol Med Nucl 33:37
6. Lea Thomas M, Tighe J R 1973 Death from fat embolism as a complication of intraosseous phlebography. Lancet 2:1415–1416
7. Lea Thomas M, MacDonald L M 1978 Complications of ascending phlebography. British Medical Journal 2:317–318
8. Bettman M A, Paulin S 1977 Leg phlebography: the incidence, nature and modification of undesirable side effects. Radiology 122:101–104
9. Spigos D G, Thane T T, Capek V 1977 Skin necrosis following extravasation during peripheral phlebography. Radiology 123:605–606
10. Lea Thomas M, Browse N L 1985 Venography of the lower extremity. In: Newman H L, Yao J S T (eds) Angiography of vascular disease. Churchill Livingstone, New York, pp 421–480
11. Athanasoulis C A 1972 Phlebography for the diagnosis of deep leg vein thrombosis. In: Fratontoni J, Wessler S (eds) Prophylactic therapy of deep vein thrombosis and pulmonary embolism. National Institutes of Health, Washington D C
12. Albrechtsson U, Olsson C G 1976 Thrombotic side effects of lower-limb phlebography. Lancet 1:723–724
13. Albrechtsson U, Olsson C G 1979 Thrombosis following phlebography with ionic and non-ionic media. Acta Radiologica (Diag) 20:46–52
14. Bettman M A, Salzman E W, Rosenthal D, Clagett P, Davies G, Nebesar R et al 1980 Reduction of venous thrombosis complicating phlebography. American Journal of Roentgenology 134:1169–1172
15. Berge T, Bergevist D, Efsing H O 1978 Local complications of ascending phlebography. Clinical Radiology 29:691–696
16. Farhat K, Nakhjavan F K, Cope C, Yazdanfar S, Fernandez I, Gooch A, Goldberg H 1975 Iatrogenic arteriovenous fistula: a complication of percutaneous subclavian vein puncture. Chest 67:480–482
17. Kido D K, Baker R A, Rumbaugh C L 1983 Normal cerebral anatomy. In: Abrams H L (ed) Abrams angiography, 3rd edn. Little, Brown, Boston, pp 231–271
18. Baker R A, Rumbaugh C L, Kido D K 1983 Pathology of cerebral vessels. In: Abrams H L (ed) Abrams angiography, 3rd edn. Little, Brown, Boston, pp 271–315
19. Rumbaugh C L, Kido D K, Baker R A 1983 Cerebral angiography. Technique, indications and hazards. In: Abrams H L (ed) Abrams angiography, 3rd edn. Ed Little, Brown, Boston, pp 219–231
20. Hanafee W N Dayton G O 1970 The roentgen diagnosis of orbital tumors. Radiologic Clinics of North America 8:403–412
21. Bettman M A, Steinberg I 1983. The superior vena cava In: Abrams H L (ed) Abrams angiography, 3rd edn. Little, Brown, Boston, pp 923–938
22. Grant J C B, Basmajian, J V 1965 Grant's method of anatomy, 7th edn. Williams & Wilkins Baltimore, pp 524
23. Lochridge S K, Kribbe W P, Doty D B 1979 Obstruction of the superior vena cava. Surgery 85:14–24
24. Mahajan V, Strimlau V, Van Ordstrand H S et al 1975 Benign superior vena cava syndrome. Chest 68:32–35
25. Dines D E, Bernatz P E, Pairolero P C, Payne W S 1979 Mediastinal granuloma and fibrosing mediastinitis. Chest 75:320–324

26. Hunter N 1747 History of aneurysm of aorta with some remarks on aneurysm in general. Med Observ Inquiries 1:323

27. Deanfield J E, Fox K M, Allison D J, 1982 Facial swelling: a complication of transvenous pacing. Clin Cardiol S:308–309

28. Lang E K 1983 Arteriography of thoracic outlet syndrome. In: Abrams H L (ed) Abrams arteriography, 3rd edn. Little, Brown, Boston, pp 1001–1018

29. Campbell M, Deuchar D C 1954 Left sided superior vena cava. British Heart Journal 16:423

30. Cha M E, Khoury G H 1972 Persistent left superior vena cava: Radiologic and clinical significance. Radiology 103:375–381

31. Ferris E J 1983 The inferior vena cava. In: Abrams H L (ed) Abrams angiography, 3rd edn. Little, Brown company, Boston, pp 939–975

32. Langman J 1969 Venous system. In: Langman J S (ed) Medical embryology, 2nd edn. E & S Livingstone, Edinburgh, pp 224–231

33. Hiisch D M, Chan K 1963 Bilateral inferior vena cava. JAMA 185:729–730

34. Seib G A 1934 The azygos system of veins in American whites and American negroes, including observations on the inferior caval venous system. Am J Phys Anthropol 19:39

35. McClure E F, Butler E G 1925 The development of the vena cava inferior in man. Am J Anat 35:331

36. Ferris E J, Hipona F A, Kahn P C, Phillips E, Shapiro J H (eds) 1969 Venography of the inferior vena cava and its branches. Williams & Wilkins, Baltimore

37. Dos Santos R 1935 Phlebographie d'une veine cave inferieure suture. J Urol Med Chir 39:586

38. Crummy A B, Hipona F A 1964 The aortic impression in inferior venacavography. Clin Radiol 15:130–131

39. Kimura C, Shirotani H, Hirooka M, Terada M H M, Iwahashi K, Maetani S 1963 Membranous obliteration of the inferior vena cava in its hepatic portion. J Cardiovasc Surg 4:87

40. Lawler G A, Leung A, Ali M H, Allison D J 1983 Leiomyosarcoma of the inferior vena cava. British Journal of Radiology 56:427–430

41. Cope J S, Hunt C J 1954 Leiomyosarcoma of the inferior vena cava. Arch Surg 68:752

42. Batson O V 1940 The function of the vertebral veins and their role in the spread of metastases. Ann Surg 112:138–149

43. Abrams H L 1983 The vertebral and azygos veins. In: Abrams angiography 3rd edn. Little, Brown, Boston, pp 895–921

44. Abrams H L 1983 Renal venography. In: Abrams angiography, 3rd edn. Little, Brown, Boston, pp 1327–1364

45. Anson B J, Daselar E H 1961 Common variations in renal anatomy, affecting blood supply, form and topography. Surgery, Gynecology & Obstetrics 112:439–449

46. O'Dea M J, Mal El R S, Tucker R M, Fulton R E 1976 Renal vein thrombosis. J Urol 116:410–414

47. Athanasoulis C A, Brown B, Baum S 1973 Selective renal venography in differentiation between congenitally absent and small contracted kidney. Radiology 108:301–305

48. Itzchak Y, Adar R, Mozes M, Deutsch V 1974 Renal venography in the diagnosis of agenesis and small contracted kidney. Clin Radiol 25:379–383

49. Reuter S R, Redman H C 1977 Vascular anatomy. In: Gastrointestinal angiography. W B Saunders, Philadelphia, pp 31–65

50. Casteneda-Zuruga W R, Jauregui H, Rysavy J A, Formanet A, Amplatz K 1978 Complications of wedge hepatic venography. Radiology 126:53–56

51. Blakemore A H, Lord J W Jr 1945 Technique of using vitallium tubes in establishing portocaval shunts for portal hypertension. Ann Surg 122:476

52. Abeatici S, Campi L 1951 Sur les possibilités de l'angiographie hepatique — la visualisation du systeme portal (recherches experimentales) Acta Radiol (Stockholm) 36:83–392

53. Leger L 1951 Phlebographie portale par injection splénique intraparenchymateuse. Mem Acad Chir 77:712

54. Rigler L G, Olfelt P C, Krumbach R W 1953 Roentgen hepatography by injection of a contrast medium into the aorta. Radiology 60:363

55. Ödman P 1958 Percutaneous selective angiography of the coeliac artery. Acta Radiol (Stockholm) (Suppl 59):1–168

56. Probst R Rysavy J A, Amplatz K 1978 Improved safety of spleno-

57. Anacker H, Deveris K, Linden G 1957 Leistungsfähigkeit und Grenzen der purkutanes Splenoportographie. Fortschr Roentgenstr 86:411

58. Bergstrand I 1983 Splenoportography. In: Abrams H L (ed) Abrams angiography, 3rd edn. Little, Brown, Boston, pp 1573–1604

59. Lunderquist A, Hoevels J, Owman T 1983 Transhepatic portal venography. In: Abrams H L (ed) Abrams angiography, 3rd edn. Little, Brown, Boston, pp 1505–1529

60. Bierman H R, Steinbach H L, White L P, Kelley K H 1952 Portal venepuncture: percutaneous transhepatic approach. Proc Soc Exp Biol Med 79:550

61. Lunderquist A Simert G, Tylen U, Vang J 1977 Follow-up of patients with portal hypertension and oesophageal varices treated with percutaneous obliteration of gastric coronary vein. Radiology 122:59–63

62. Sos T A 1983 Transhepatic portal venous embolization of varices: pros and cons. Radiology 148:569–570

63. Allison D J 1980 Therapeutic embolization and venous sampling. In: Taylor S (ed) Recent advances in surgery 10. Churchill Livingstone, Edinburgh, pp 27–64

64. Bron K M 1983 Arterioportography. In: Abrams H L (ed) Abrams angiography, 3rd edn. Little, Brown, Boston, pp 1605–1620

65. Camilleri M, Hemingway A P, Chadwick V S, Blumgart L H, Hodgson H J F, Allison D J 1982 Embolization of an intrapancreatic aneurysm. Br J Radiol 55:685–687

66. Ahlberg N E, Bartey O, Chidekel N 1966 Right and left gonadal veins, an anatomical and statistical study. Acta Radiol (Diagn) 4:593–601

67. Khan O, Williams G, Bowley N B, Allison D J 1982 Testicular phlebography in the localisation of the undescended testis. British Journal of Surgery 69:660

68. White R I Jr, Kaufman S L, Barth K H, Kadir S, Smyth J W, Walsh P C 1981 Occlusion of varicoceles with detachable balloons. Radiology 139:327–334

69. Neiman H L, Yao J S T 1985 Upper extremity venography. In: Neiman H L, Yao J S T (eds) Angiography of vascular disease. Churchill Livingstone, New York, pp 481–494

70. Campbell C B, Chandler J G, Tegtmeyer C J, Bernstein E F 1977 Axillary, subclavian and brachiocephalic vein obstruction. Surgery 82:816–826

71. Adams J T, McEvoy R K, DeWeese J A 1965 Primary deep venous thrombosis of the upper extremity. Arch Surg 91:29–42

72. Fontaine J R, Taverner D 1957 Gangrene of three limbs from venous occlusion. Ann Intern Med 44:549–554

73. Rabinor K, Paulin S 1983 Venography of the lower extremities. In: Abrams L H (ed) Abrams angiography, 3rd edn. Little, Brown, Boston, pp 1877–1921

74. Cohen S H, Ehrlich G E, Kauffman MS, Cope C 1973 Thrombophlebitis following knee surgery. J Bone Joint Surg 55A; 106–112

75. Heatley R V, Morgan A, Hughes L E, Okwonga W 1976, Preoperative or post-operative deep vein thrombosis. Lancet 1:437–439

76. Kakkar V V 1977 Fibrinogen uptake test for detection of deep vein thrombosis — a review of current practice. Semin Nucl Med 7:229

77. Browse N L, Thomas M L 1974 Source of non-lethal pulmonary emboli. Lancet 1:258–259

78. Widmer L K, Mal T and Martin H 1977 Epidemiology and Sociomedical importance of peripheral venous disease. In: Hobbs J T (ed) The treatment of venous disorders: a comprehensive review of current practice in the management of varicose veins and the postthrombotic syndrome. Lippincott, Philadelphia

79. Lea Thomas M, MacFie G P 1974 Phlebography in the Klippel-Trenaunay syndrome. Acta Radiol 15:43–56

80. Doppman J L 1983 Parathyroid angiography. In: Abrams H L (ed) Abrams angiography, 3rd edn. Little, Brown, Boston, pp. 977–999

81. Satava R M, Beatires O H, Scholz D A 1975 Success rate of cervical exploration for hyperparathyroidism. Arch Surg. 110:625–628

82. Doppman J L, Hammond W G 1970 The anatomic basis of parathyroid venous sampling. Radiology 95:603–610

83. Nathaniels E K, Nathaniels A M, Wang C 1970 Mediastinal parathyroid tumours: a clinical and pathological study of 84 cases. Annals of Surgery 171:165–170

portography by plugging off the needle track. American Journal of Roentgenology 131:445–449

84. Eisenberg H, Pallotta J, Sherwood L M 1974 Selective arteriography, venography and venous hormone assay in diagnosis and localization of parathyroid lesions. Am J Medicine 56:810–820
85. Davies D R, Shaw D G, Ives D R, Thomas B M, Watson L 1973 Selective venous catheterization and radio-immunoassay of parathyroid hormone in the diagnosis and localisation of parathyroid tumours. Lancet 1:1079–1082
86. O'Riordan J L H, Kendall B E, Woodhead J S 1971 Pre-operative localization of parathyroid tumours. Lancet 2:1172–1175
87. Powell D, Murray T M, Pollard J J, Cope O, Wang C, Potts J T 1973 Parathyroid localization using venous catheterization and radio-immunoassay. Archives of Internal Medicine 131:645–648
88. Horton R, Finc E 1972 Diagnosis and localization of primary aldosteronism. Annals of Int Med 76:885–890
89. Allison D J, Timmis B, Brown M 1983 Role of venous sampling in locating a phaeochromocytoma. British Medical Journal 28:1122–1124
90. Allison D J, Jones D H, Hamilton C A, Reid J L 1979 Selective venous sampling in the diagnosis and localization of phaechromocytoma. Clinical Endocrinology 10: 179–186
91. Sutton H, Wyeth P, Allen A P et al 1982 Disseminated malignant phaeochromocytoma: localization with iodine-133 labelled meta-iodobenzylguanidine. British Medical Journal 285:1153-1154
92. Lunderquist A, Owman T, Reichardt W 1983 Pancreatic venography. In: Abrams H L (ed) Abrams angiography, 3rd edn. Little, Brown, Boston, pp. 1467–1477

SUGGESTIONS FOR FURTHER READING

Abrams H L (ed) 1983 Abrams angiography, 3rd edn. Little, Brown, Boston
Chuang V P, Lunderquist A, Herlinger H 1983 In: Holinger H, Lunderquist A, Walllace S (eds) Clinical radiology of the liver. Part B. Marcel Dekker Inc, New York
Neiman H L, Yao J S T 1985 Angiography of vascular disease. Churchill Livingstone, New York
Pitney W R 1981 Venous and arterial thrombosis. Churchill Livingstone, Edinburgh, 1981

96 Digital subtraction angiography

Thomas F. Meaney and Meredith A. Weinstein

Equipment for digital subtraction angiography
Subtraction methods
Contrast material and delivery
Clinical applications
 Extracranial vascular studies
 Intracranial vascular studies
 Mediastinal masses
 Aortic dissection
 Thoracic aortic aneurysms
 Pulmonary arteriography
 Congenital heart disease
 Acquired heart disease
 Abdominal aorta
 Kidney and renal artery disease
 Extremities
Anticipated clinical utilisation

The concept of eliminating unwanted background from angiographic images was first described by Castellanos et al in 1937 [1] and applied clinically to a large number of patients beginning in 1938 by Robb and Steinberg [2]. The application of analogue film subtraction techniques was limited by a number of factors, including the exponential attenuation of X–rays which made the film subtraction process difficult and the general requirement for relatively large concentrations of intravenous contrast material to produce a satisfactory subtracted signal in the image. In the last few years, several technical developments in television, digital electronics, and image intensifiers have resulted in marked improvement in the electronic recording of images. Patient studies were carried out in relatively large numbers beginning in 1980 [3–6].

In addition to the advantages of the digital subtraction process, the technique afforded the additional advantage of a greater sensitivity to the detection of the iodine signal in blood vessels from relatively dilute concentrations of contrast material.

The major advantages of digital subtraction angiography (DSA) are ease of examination, reduced technical skills requirement, safety, informational content, rapidity of diagnosis, smaller volumes of contrast material for intra-arterial examinations, and cost. Some of these advantages are offset by disadvantages relating to the global intravenous injection of contrast material, motion artifacts producing misregistration, and sometimes unrealistic expectations on the part of the referring clinician.

In contrast to conventional angiography, DSA represents a method of examination which is relatively simple, rapid and with diagnostic rewards generally not attained by simpler examination methods. These factors have led to a rapid clinical acceptance of this method of investigation by both radiologists and the referring clinicians. The ability to perform arteriography on nonhospitalized patients has been a major driving force in the integration of DSA into clinical medicine. In the past, even though the initial clinical examination of a patient might indicate a vascular problem, indirect methods of study such as conventional radiography, ultrasound, etc. were generally employed to assist in the justification for an angiogram. DSA has largely removed the perceived necessity for carrying out such preliminary indirect examinations.

Substantial technical skills are required in the performance of conventional angiography, not only for the production of satisfactory angiograms, but also to ensure reduction of complications produced by manipulation of catheters through the cardiovascular system. While such skills may be present in angiographers practicing in smaller hospitals, the usual volume of conventional angiographic examinations is smaller, making maintenance of angiographic skills more difficult. Minimal technical skills are required for DSA carried out with intravenous injection of contrast material. A simple venepuncture and easily acquired knowledge concerning rates and volumes of contrast material injection and appropriate positioning for study of various blood vessels are all that is required in most cases. Passage of a catheter into the superior vena cava is a skill easily acquired by most radiologists without extensive angiographic training.

The two major categories of complications of conventional angiography are those associated with catheter manipulation and with the injection of contrast material. As noted above, catheter manipulation complications are essentially eliminated with intravenous DSA. Severe systemic reactions to contrast materials are very unusual (Ch. 7) in both conventional and intravenous digital subtraction angiography. In conventional angiography, there may be additional substantial complications resulting from selective or subselective injections of contrast material into sensitive organs such as the brain and kidney. This category of contrast complications is eliminated in intravenous DSA.

If the proper indication for DSA is selected, the informational content is often as satisfactory as conventional angiography for diagnosis and differential diagnosis. Stenotic, occlusive, embolic, and aneurysmal disease of the great vessels and their major branches are generally readily appreciated on DSA, subject to the limitations imposed by the patient's cardiac output and motion artifacts which may occur. In other disease processes in other parts of the body, the informational content may be considerably inferior to that of conventional angiography but sufficient to confirm or deny clinical suspicion of disease and warrant either no further investigation or indicate the need for conventional angiography.

In patients clinically suspected of problems of the cardiovascular system, a long delay often occurs between the initial patient examination, securing of a hospital bed, scheduling of a conventional arteriogram, and the reporting of the findings. Depending upon the organization of the DSA equipment, a DSA examination by intravenous injection can often be performed as rapidly as a blood count.

Because of the high contrast sensitivity of DSA, intraarterial injections of contrast material can be reduced considerably either in total volume or by using large volumes of diluted contrast. This has substantial advantages in certain regions of the body in patients with fragile clinical conditions who do not tolerate large amounts of contrast. Such examples include patients with severe central nervous system disease, renal failure, and patients with complicated congenital heart disease requiring multiple injections of contrast medium in order to delineate abnormalities. Another advantage is obtained in lack of or diminished pain in patients undergoing extremity arteriography with conventional ionic high osmolar contrast media.

Factors of cost may play a significant role in the clinical acceptance of the new technologies, and digital subtraction angiography, as compared with conventional techniques in many clinical settings, offers the substantial advantage of acquiring direct information regarding the vascular system that costs substantially less than conventional angiography.

There are a number of clinical disadvantages to digital subtraction angiography that should be emphasized.

Intravenous DSA uses the global injection of contrast material deposited either in a peripheral arm vein or the superior or inferior vena cava. As a consequence, not only the vessels of interest are opacified, but also those of no interest which may obscure the vessels under suspicion. As a consequence, considerable diagnostic skill is required; and, occasionally, diagnosis is rendered impossible because of *vessel overlap*.

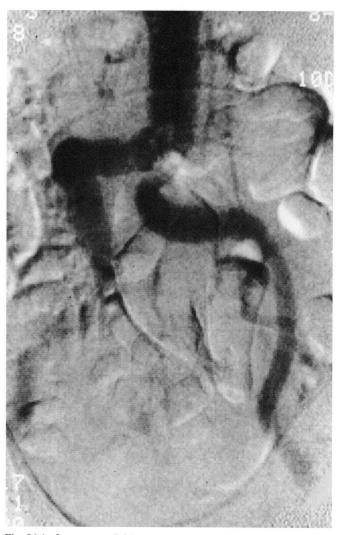

Fig. 96.1 Intravenous DSA examination of the lower abdominal aorta and iliac arteries degraded by the presence of peristaltic motion and producing an apparent abnormality involving the origin of the left common iliac artery.

Motion artifacts are responsible for the majority of unsatisfactory IV DSA examinations. The two major problems are caused by patient swallowing in the examination of the extracranial cerebral vessels and peristaltic motion in the case of abdominal examinations (Fig. 96.1). While various methods have been advocated to reduce these artifacts, none has been completely satisfactory. Often one can clinically anticipate those patients who are likely to have an unsatisfactory examination because of motion. Very ill, uncooperative patients are likely to have an unsatisfactory examination because of the artifacts caused by gross patient motion, and consideration should be given to excluding these patients from DSA examination.

The referring clinicians expect a satisfactory angiographic examination based on their experience with conventional selective arteriography. Education of referring physicians is required to indicate the percentage of satisfactory diagnostic examinations that is likely to be obtained in patients who are referred for DSA examination. While there are some variations in reported unsatisfactory examinations by intravenous DSA, one should not expect more than 85 to 90% technically satisfactory and diagnostic studies.

Equipment for digital subtraction angiography

Equipment for DSA consists of an X–ray generator preferably of high current capacity and with similar features to standard angiography systems. An X–ray tube with a high heat storage capacity is generally used because of heat dissipation requirements when multiple exposures are made over a short period of time. Image intensifiers used with such systems generally consist of cesium iodide phosphors with a choice of 10, 15, or 23 cm field. Some systems use larger intensifier tubes with input phosphor sizes up to 4.0 cm. These larger tubes have been advocated to provide a greater 'field of view' but may limit contrast sensitivity because of the larger angle of scatter acceptance and spatial resolution, unless the matrix number is proportionally increased.

Refinements in the television camera are advocated to provide better signal-to-noise ratio. The signal from the television camera is usually logarithmic, being amplified, digitized, and directed to two or more image memories for storage, integration and display. The memories are connected to and controlled by a computer equipped with digital disc, magnetic tapes, terminal, and operator's console. Some systems utilize analogue storage of the data (video tape); others utilize digital storage only, and some a combination of the two.

The field of view of the image intensifier may be digitized to matrices of varying sizes from 256×256 to 1028×1028, depending on the system.

Subtraction methods

Several digital subtraction methods are available. The most common, termed *mask-mode* subtraction, utilizes the last frame obtained before the injection of contrast material as the mask which is subtracted from all subsequent image frames. This is performed in real time. In actual practice, retrospective selection of the mask from a frame just before the appearance of contrast material will produce a better registration.

Another subtraction technique, termed *time-interval-difference imaging*, subtracts each succeeding frame from the previous one. This technique produces a series of images which show the change from one frame to the other.

A third method utilizes a *frame integration mode* which is employed when frames are generated from fluoroscopic-type doses to improve signal-to-noise ratio. In this scheme, the mask frame is subtracted from four to six frames after the arrival of contrast material with each frame averaged to a single image, which is then subtracted from the mask.

Irrespective of the type of system used, an essential requirement is the ability for *rapid remasking* of frame and contrast image. Only rarely is the initially acquired frame, before injection of contrast material, the most suitable for the subtraction process because of physiological or gross patient motion occurring between the initial frame and the arrival of contrast in the area of interest.

A number of clinical applications have been described [7] for obtaining *functional information*, particularly time/density curves from the angiographic images, a process which is greatly facilitated by the availability of digital information with a computer capable of utilizing software either generated de novo by the user, or derived from existing software packages, particularly emanating from nuclear medicine applications. A more detailed description of the physical parameters associated with the digital subtraction process lies beyond the scope of this chapter.

In a study of *radiation dose*, Pavlicek [8] found the average skin exposure to be 3700 mrads (9.55×10^{-4} C/kg) as compared with an average skin exposure of 23000 mrads (5.93×10^{-3} C/kg) in patients undergoing conventional examinations. In this same study, the dose to the bone marrow, thyroid, and lens of the eye were lower than in conventional angiography.

Contrast material and delivery

There are two commonly employed methods for intravenous injection of contrast material. The first consists of a *peripheral intravenous* injection of contrast material, usually into an antecubital vein, using a needle or, preferably, an intra-catheter of approximately 6 to 8 inches in length, with as large a catheter bore as feasible. We have used a 16-gauge catheter for such peripheral injections. The contrast material is delivered at the rate of 15 to 20 ml per second, and each injection consists of 40 ml of 30% contrast material followed by 20 ml of 5% dextrose and water or normal saline (layered in the same syringe). Prior to the injection of the bolus, a test injection of 3 ml is made, and the size of the vein and its relationship to tributaries is assessed by fluoroscopic observation. We have found that this technique of injection is satisfactory in the vast majority of patients.

Alternative injections on the venous side can be made either in the *superior or inferior vena cava* or right atrium. For such administrations, a No. 5 or No. 6 thin-wall French pigtail catheter is used with a bolus volume of 25 to 35 ml injected at the rate of 20 to 25 ml per second.

A recent study [9] has shown that comparable image quality can be obtained by the peripheral intravenous or central injection of contrast material for visualization of large and medium sized vessels. However, improved visualization of small vessels, such as intracranial arteries, is obtained from the central injection.

Depending on the patient's renal function, weight and age, four to five injections can be made. A major limiting factor in the concentration of the contrast material achieved in the area of interest is the patient's cardiac status. Poor cardiac output is believed to be a major factor but is often difficult to document in the angiographic setting.

Substitution of DSA as a receptor in place of conventional film/screen angiography may include all of the applications of conventional catheter angiography [40]. The safety of the examination is increased because less contrast material is often required. Weinstein et al [11] have shown that 18.5 g of iodine are usually injected in film/screen angiography of the aortic arch, whereas in intra-arterial DSA only 8.5 g is necessary.

The ability to reduce either the amount or concentration of conventional ionic contrast media results in significant pain reduction in certain arterial territories such as the extracranial carotid arteries or their branches, and those of the extremities.

This substantial clinical advantage will however need to be reassessed when the new low osmolar contrast media such as iohexol, iopamidol and ioxaglate become generally available. In most European countries and in South Africa, some or all of these new, more physiological but more expensive media are available for general use, but at the time of writing (February, 1984), they are still not released in the USA. Extensive experience (see Ch. 7) has shown that in all vascular territories, these low osmolar contrast media permit pain-free angiography even when using conventional injection volumes and concentrations and film-screen radiography.

Film-screen arteriography with low osmolar media at normal concentrations is as comfortable as intra-arterial DSA using conventional ionic media diluted 50 per cent.

Therapeutic embolization procedures are considerably reduced in time because sequential images can be produced in real time during the embolization. In angiography of the head and neck, even with magnetic tape and multiformat copies, costs can be reduced by between $40 to $100 per patient due to saving X–ray film costs.

It is recognized, of course, that spatial resolution of images obtained by intra-arterial DSA is considerably less than with film/screen conventional angiography. The smallest vessels that can be visualized with conventional film/screen angiography cannot be visualized with IA DSA, but this is of importance only in a limited number of cases.

The *framing rate* for performance of digital subtraction angiography is essentially identical to that used in standard, conventional angiography. Framing rates of 1 to 2 per second are adequate for most areas of the vascular system. The heart represents an exception under certain clinical conditions. In the evaluation of patients with congenital heart disease, a slower framing rate has been shown to be adequate in those with simple congenital heart defects where one has the opportunity to acquire semiquantitative information relating to recirculation. In studying the dynamics of the left ventricle, more accurate functional information can be obtained at higher framing rates.

CLINICAL APPLICATIONS

Extracranial vascular studies

The usual indications for intravenous DSA of the extracranial arterial circulation are patients with transient ischaemic attacks (TIA's), amaurosis fugax, completed strokes, signs and symptoms of basilar artery insufficiency, and asymptomatic neck bruits. The bifurcations of the common carotid arteries, the vertebral arteries, and the intracranial vessels are examined by DSA in these patients.

Right posterior oblique (RPO) and left posterior oblique (LPO) at 70° projections most frequently show the separate origins of the internal and external carotid arteries and without superimposition of the vertebral arteries (Fig. 96.2). After these views are obtained, additional views with greater or lesser degrees of obliquity are made until the separate origins of both the internal and external carotids are visualized without overlap. With accurate positioning, both carotid bifurcations can be included within an 11.25 cm image intensifier field. The smaller field decreases Compton's scatter and results in the utilization of the matrix over a smaller field of view. A 30° off-lateral view of the carotid siphons for evaluation of atherosclerotic disease of the internal carotid arteries and a study of the aortic arch can be obtained at the same sitting, depending upon contrast medium dose limitations.

The usual cause of a poor study in the carotid arteries is misregistration artifacts caused by patient swallowing. No satisfactory method has been devised to eliminate the patient's propensity to swallow. The ability to choose various masks to improve registration is essential in improving the number of satisfactory examinations. In addition, some systems provide the opportunity to reregister a misregistered image when a satisfactory mask cannot be obtained.

Chilcote et al [5] carried out a comparative study of IV digital subtraction angiography and conventional carotid arteriography in 100 patients in order to establish the accuracy and clinical usefulness of DSA. DSA examinations were rated as good or excellent in quality if the separate origins of the internal and external carotid arteries were well visualized without superimposition or

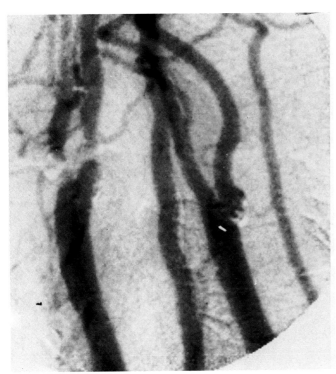

Fig. 96.2 DSA in the RPO projection separates the origins of the left internal and left external carotid arteries. The left internal carotid artery is moderately irregular and mildly narrowed at its origin. Calcification is seen in the posterior wall of the origin of the left internal carotid artery. Both vertebral arteries fill well.

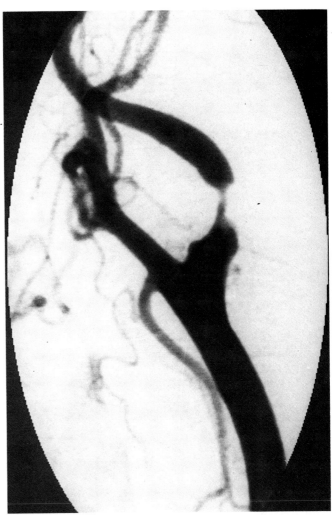

Fig. 96.3 Moderate to marked narrowing of the left internal carotid artery is well visualized after the intra-arterial injection of 5 ml of Conray 60 into the left common carotid artery.

overlap by the vertebral arteries and when the arterial contrast density was good or excellent. In only one of the 100 patients was a poor quality DSA examination the result of poor contrast density within the carotid arteries. In the comparative study, the quality of the DSA examination was good to excellent in 70% of patients.

Since that study, and with additional experience, this figure has increased to 85%. The reasons for this include the fact that in the comparative study, fewer injections of contrast material were made because the patients had already had a conventional angiogram. In addition, the comparative study considered an unsuccessful examination when the peripheral arm vein could not be catheterized, whereas this factor is now eliminated by introduction of a catheter via the femoral vein.

In the analysis of the comparison of the techniques when the carotid bifurcations were well visualized, the correlation with conventional digital angiography was excellent with a sensitivity of 95% and specificity of 99% with an overall accuracy of 97%. Although there is a substantial chance for misinterpretation when the bifurcations are not well visualized, this is immediately apparent, and no interpretation is made and an indication of the diagnostic uncertainty is given.

Small ulcerated arteriosclerotic plaques may be missed by digital subtraction angiography but they may also be difficult to detect by selective conventional angiography.

A number of workers have taken the position that examination of the carotid arteries and their bifurcations is more appropriate by selective, intra-arterial DSA (Fig. 96.3). Selective catheterization overcomes the potential problems with the intravenous route because overlap of vessels and a reduced concentration of contrast material at the site of interest are eliminated as factors which may degrade the quality of the examination. As compared with selective conventional (film/screen) carotid angiography, the use of DSA permits either a considerable (60 to 70%) reduction in the volume of contrast material or of the concentration required to produce diagnostic images. Considerable cost savings can be achieved by eliminating X–ray film in the examination. The disadvantages of selective catheterization and intra-arterial DSA are the usual requirement for hospitalization and the risk of complications either at the puncture site or dislodgement of atheromatous material during the catheterization procedure.

Intracranial vascular studies

Patients in this category usually have had previous CT examinations of the head. Intracranial IV. DSA is indicated in the evaluation of certain tumours, arteriovenous malformations, carotid fistulas, as well as occlusive dolichoectatic vascular disease. It also may play a significant role in the study of sellar and parasellar lesions (Fig. 96.4) and postoperatively to evaluate external carotid to internal carotid bypass operations (Fig. 96.5).

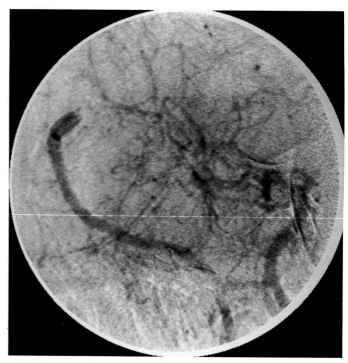

Fig. 96.5 A saphenous vein graft anastomosing the right external carotid artery to the right middle cerebral artery is seen to be widely patent. The middle cerebral artery was shown to fill well via this graft on subsequent images.

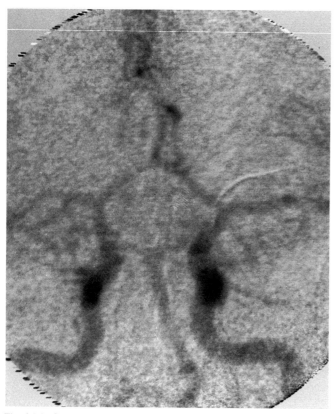

Fig. 96.4 Intracranial IV DSA after the injection of 40 ml of contrast material into the superior vena cava. The horizontal portions of both anterior cerebral arteries are elevated in this patient with a pituitary adenoma with suprasellar extension. The location of the internal carotid arteries relative to the sella turcica is well visualized prior to transphenoidal hypophysectomy.

The major disadvantage of intracranial DSA by the intravenous injection of contrast material is the simultaneous opacification of both carotid and vertebral arteries and their branches. Tailoring of the examination or using oblique views makes it possible to visualize areas of interest in most cases. The carotid siphons can be visualized with the 30° off-lateral view. For patients suspected of sellar and suprasellar lesions, the parasellar internal carotid arteries may be optimally visualized with a Waters' view. For evaluation of the basilar artery, the straight lateral and Waters' views are used. Spatial resolution can be improved by the use of a matrix of at least 512 × 512 and with the smallest image intensifier field of view that includes the area of interest.

Modic et al [12] have compared intravenous DSA with conventional angiography in the same patient and found that the fourth-order intracranial vessels were well visualized in all cases of conventional angiography, but infrequently with DSA. However, in 65% of their patients, DSA examination provided as much information as a conventional angiogram. DSA has virtually replaced conventional cerebral angiography for the preoperative evaluation of the juxtasellar carotid arteries prior to trans-sphenoidal surgery, because the large intracerebral vessels are well visualized with IV DSA.

Simultaneous opacification of vessels may be advantageous for evaluation of depression of the dural sinuses by parasagittal meningiomas, because the flow defects that occur in selective angiography from the mixture of opacified and unopacified blood are not present with DSA.

In most instances, DSA will not replace conventional angiography for the evaluation of arteriovenous malformations because of simultaneous opacification of vessels which increases the difficulty in determining which vessels are feeding the AVM. However, postoperative DSA represents a relatively noninvasive method for evaluating the success of surgery or therapeutic embolization of AVM.

Intra-arterial DSA following selective catheterization has been adopted by many for the study of intracranial disease. Improved visualization of the smaller arteries of the brain by intra-arterial injection (Fig. 96.6) offers

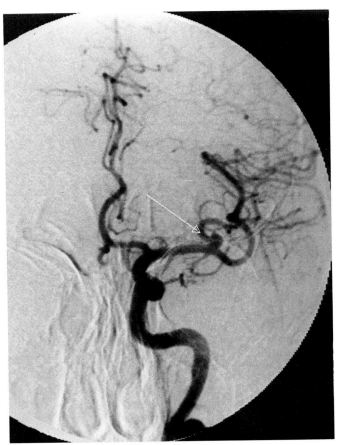

Fig. 96.6 An aneurysm of the trifurcation of the left middle cerebral artery is clearly seen after the intra-arterial injection of 6 ml of Conray 60 into the left internal carotid artery.

significant advantages over the intravenous route for many appplications of cerebral angiography.

Mediastinal masses

Following detection of a mass in the mediastinum by conventional radiological teachniques, the usual differential diagnostic process consists of obtaining various views of the mediastinum and tomography in an effort to delineate the specific characteristics of the mass and determine if the mass is vascular in origin. Often, the latter possibility is not resolved by conventional studies. CT, particularly with bolus contrast injection, has been helpful in the diagnosis of vascular abnormalities but can be less than satisfactory in some patients because of the difficulty of integrating the multiple cross-sections to characterize vascular structures positioned perpendicular to the plane of the CT sections. Conventional angiographic studies are often used to provide further help in the final diagnosis.

Digital subtraction angiography by intravenous injection provides a simple and convenient method to avert often lengthy and unrewarding specialized radiographic techniques. In the mediastinum, its application is directed to those patients presenting with masses where a clinical

history or physical examination does not provide enough information. In this group of patients, vascular abnormalities may consist of tortuous brachiocephalic vessels, saccular aneurysms of the thoracic aorta, and, more rarely, asymptomatic chronic dissections of the thoracic aorta. Congenital vascular abnormalities may be detected, such as the presence of a cervical aorta or anomalies of the origin of the brachiocephalic arteries.

Aortic dissection

The role of radiology in patients clinically suspected of aortic dissection consists of verification of the diagnosis, classification of the type of dissection, determination of its extent and involvement of major aortic branches. If intravenous digital subtraction angiography for suspected acute aortic dissection were used as an initial contrast examination and if it failed to resolve the diagnosis, performance of conventional angiography would be handicapped by the previous administration of contrast material for an intravenous DSA. However, IV DSA can provide a useful role in patients with known aortic dissections who are being managed medically in the determination of the stability of the dissection, or for postoperative evaluation (Fig. 96.7). Similarly, patients with clinical findings suggesting a remote aortic dissection may be satisfactorily examined by intravenous DSA.

The use of intra-arterial DSA by catheterization techniques can provide a rapid and convenient method for studying patients with acute or chronic aortic dissection. The ability to use smaller amounts of contrast material provides an opportunity for making more contrast injections than would be possible with standard film/screen angiographic techniques.

Thoracic aortic aneurysms

IV DSA provides an alternative to CT and conventional angiography in those patients with findings suggesting the presence of thoracic aortic aneurysms. IV DSA may provide more information than CT in that the branches of the aortic arch are more readily displayed; but, similar to conventional angiography, mural thrombus is better detected by CT.

Pulmonary arteriography

A discussion of the application of DSA for determination of the presence of pulmonary embolism requires separation of the several clinical presentations of such patients: (a) patients suspected of having acute massive pulmonary embolus with compromise of cardiopulmonary parameters, who are being considered for either embolectomy or anticoagulants; (b) patients with less acute presentations who are more likely to have smaller and multiple peripheral pulmonary emboli in whom anticoagulation therapy may be indicated; and (c) a class of patients with progressive

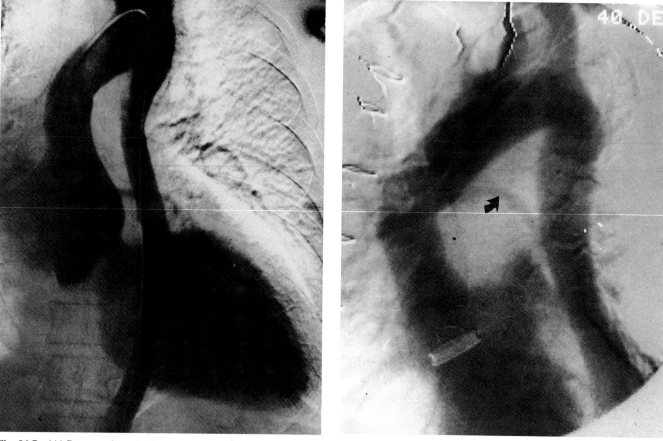

Fig. 96.7 (A) Preoperative selective catheter (film/screen) angiography demonstrating a Type I aortic dissection and marked aortic regurgitation. (B) Postoperative examination (IV DSA) showing the presence of a prosthetic aortic valve, an ascending aortic graft, and a coronary artery bypass graft [arrow].

pulmonary fibrosis in whom small, repeated pulmonary emboli are suspected of being the aetiological factor. The diagnostic approaches to these different categories of patients is significantly different.

Large-field-of-view image intensifiers, 14 to 15 inch, are required to visualize both lungs. The chest presents particular problems due to the wide range of absorbers ranging from small pulmonary arteries in the lung periphery to the main pulmonary arteries located in an area of higher attenuation of photon flux in the mediastinum. As a consequence, the dynamic range of the system is often exceeded in either the peripheral lung fields or the mediastinum, resulting in saturation of the image in either of these two areas, depending upon the initial radiographic technique chosen. Second, pulsation in the pulmonary arteries, particularly in the periphery of the lungs, makes proper registration of mask and contrast frames difficult. Third, again in the periphery of the lungs, the very asset of DSA, namely, high contrast sensitivity, works to the disadvantage of small-vessel digitization because of the thousands of smaller pulmonary arteries and earlier filling pulmonary veins superimposed upon one another from front to back of lung. Reports [13,14] on small numbers of patients have indicated a significant potential

of IV DSA in the diagnosis of pulmonary embolus and possible superiority over radionuclide techniques [15].

Acute pulmonary embolus

The diagnosis of acute massive pulmonary embolus in critically ill patients with compromised cardiopulmonary status represents one of the most difficult group of patients for diagnostic radiologic procedures. The working clinical diagnosis is often not precise and commonly requires a differentiation between pulmonary embolus and acute myocardial infarction. A diagnosis of massive pulmonary embolus is followed by pulmonary embolectomy or anticoagulant therapy instituted immediately depending upon the length of symptomatology. A negative pulmonary angiogram will result in a totally different form of therapy. No reports of an adequate number of patient studies in this category have appeared which allow conclusions of statistical significance. Major pulmonary emboli can be demonstrated by IV DSA. The IV DSA approach is attractive because of the potential lesser burden of fluid volume imposed directly into the pulmonary system. However, the inability to measure pulmonary artery pressure prior to injection may still produce a serious hazard in patients with acute pulmonary arterial hypertension. In patients undergoing IV DSA pulmonary arteriography, the immediate availability of conventional arteriography is a significant asset should the IV DSA be negative or technically unsatisfactory.

Subacute pulmonary embolism

These patients present clinically more stable and are usually suspected of having small or multiple small emboli in secondary or tertiary pulmonary artery branches. In patients with normal chest radiographs, many clinicians prefer radionuclide ventilation and perfusion studies as the initial diagnostic study and, when positive, institute anticoagulation therapy. Pulmonary arteriography is generally required when low-probability diagnoses by radionuclide techniques are found. In this event, accuracy of pulmonary angiographic diagnosis is central to the institution of anticoagulant therapy. For the reasons discussed above relative to technical considerations, visualization of smaller pulmonary emboli by DSA may be difficult. However, it still may be the initial angiographic method of choice because conventional angiographic techniques can be carried out in the instance of a negative pulmonary IV DSA study.

Pulmonary embolus and pulmonary fibrosis

This is a most difficult diagnostic category of patients, because the emboli are generally quite small and may not, in fact, be present at the time an angiographic procedure is performed. If angiography is considered essential to patient management, it is probable that only multiple selective pulmonary angiography with high spatial resolution is appropriate.

Congenital heart disease

Both anatomical and functional imaging in patients suspected of congenital heart disease can be performed with intravenous DSA. Buonocore et al [16] in a study of 54 patients with 90 separate congenital defects found that DSA would have excluded cardiac catheterization in the identification of 67 of the 90 defects. Interatrial septal defects had a high degree of successful identification (Fig. 96.8). Of particular value was the postoperative evaluation of patients in the determination of the success of surgery.

Digital data available from DSA studies make it possible to perform shunt determinations which correlate well with single-pass nuclear medicine techniques and catheter angiography.

Acquired heart disease

IV DSA may be used to evaluate and quantitate left ventricular dimensions and function (Fig. 96.9). Higgins et al [17] found IV DSA to be useful and accurate in quantification of central cardiovascular physiology both in animals and patients. Evaluation of functional parameters required rapid framing. Engles et al [18] have utilized the time-interval difference mode for measuring ejection fraction and wall motion of the left ventricle and found good correlation between conventional left ventriculography and the measurement of

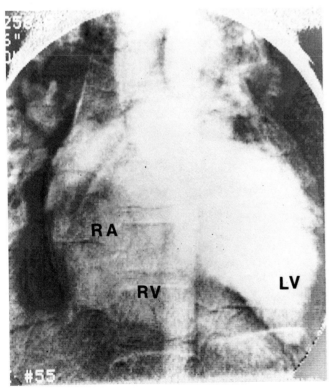

Fig. 96.8 Laevo phase in frontal projection in a patient with inter-atrial septal defect. The right atrium [RA] and right ventricle [RV] reopacify promptly after filling of the left atrium and ventricle [LV].

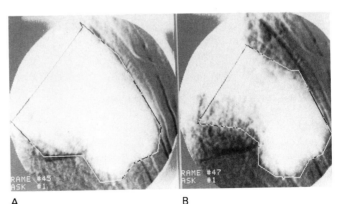

A   B

Fig. 96.9A & B Diastolic (A) and systolic phase (B) of the left ventricle made in the 30° RAO projection in a patient with severe advanced coronary artery disease. A large akinetic segment is present in the inferior wall of the left ventricle adjacent to the apex, characteristic of a left ventricular aneurysm. Regions of interest have been traced about the left ventricle to give quantitative determinations of left ventricular ejection fraction.

ejection fraction and motion of the anterior wall and apex of the heart. These authors found the correlation was not as good for determining motion of the inferior ventricular wall due to difficulties of separating the left ventricular wall from the left hemidiaphragm utilizing the time-interval difference method.

Intra-arterial DSA provides a method for carrying out left ventriculography utilizing about one half to one third of the volumes or concentrations of contrast material.

Coronary artery bypass grafts

Return of symptoms or development of new symptoms suggesting myocardial ischaemia in patients who have previously undergone coronary artery bypass surgery raises clinical questions regarding graft stenosis or occlusion, or development of new disease in native coronaries. Coronary artery bypass grafts can be identified by intravenous DSA. However, identification of the native coronary arteries or the site of anastomosis of the bypass graft to the native coronary artery cannot be identified. Hence, DSA is limited to the establishment of open or closed grafts and is usually not satisfactory to satisfy the clinical questions raised in such patients.

Abdominal aorta

The abdominal aorta can generally be displayed in excellent fashion using IV DSA. Diagnosis of occlusion, stenosis, and aneurysm are readily appreciated. Buonocore et al [19] compared IV DSA to conventional angiography and found an accuracy of 100%. In addition to visualization of the renal arteries, other major branches of the abdominal aorta can be visualized by DSA. These include the origins of the coeliac and the superior mesenteric arteries with the patient in the steep oblique or lateral projection. Similarly, the accuracy in the diagnosis of occlusive, aneurysmal, or stenotic disease of the common and external iliac arteries is very high and generally subject only to motion artifacts caused by movement of intestinal gas projected over the arteries of interest.

Kidney and renal artery disease

With some exceptions [20-22], DSA by intravenous injection has not played a significant role in the evaluation of renal masses. The primary limiting factor has been peristaltic motion of bowel superimposed upon the kidney, producing unacceptable misregistration artifacts. The administration of antispasmodic drugs prior to DSA has reduced or eliminated these artifacts in some patients but not with sufficient consistency as to recommend this application of DSA. The misregistration problem can be markedly reduced by selective intra-arterial contrast injection into the renal artery.

Evaluation of the main renal arteries and portions of the major interlobar arteries can usually be identified by IV

DSA with good technical and diagnostic success in patients suspected of renovascular hypertension. The problem of misregistration artifacts caused by peristaltic motion can usually be reduced or eliminated through external compression devices which, depending on patient size, displace these bowel structures laterally. Because of global opacification resulting from intravenous injection, there is occasional difficulty in visualizing the main renal artery because of overlap of branches of the coeliac or superior mesenteric artery on the renal arteries (Fig. 96.10). Technical artifacts partially obscuring the right renal artery are sometimes seen when a central catheter is placed from the femoral vein. Misregistration of the catheter which moves between the mask and appropriate contrast frames can obscure 0.5 to 1.0 cm of the right renal artery.

Branches of the renal artery are usually not sufficiently identified by intravenous DSA because of problems related to peristaltic motion obscuring extrarenal arteries and limitations of spatial resolution (Fig. 96.11). The search for branch stenosis or occlusion is especially important in young patients suspected of renovascular hypertension.

Another approach to suspected renovascular hypertension has been suggested [23]. The combination of intravenous DSA and selective renal vein sampling with renin determination may be a useful screening procedure. Lack of correlation between successful renovascular surgery for hypertension in patients without measurable renin discrepancies between the two kidneys has been reported to occur in 15 to 25% of patients.

Gomes et al [24] have suggested that IV DSA is a preferable approach to the study of the hypertensive patient than rapid-

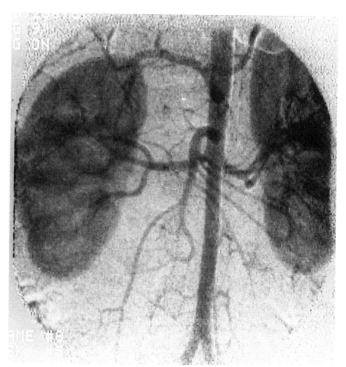

Fig. 96.10 Intravenous DSA of the abdominal aorta and branches showing overlap of the superior mesenteric artery upon the proximal right renal artery inhibiting adequate evaluation for right renal artery stenosis.

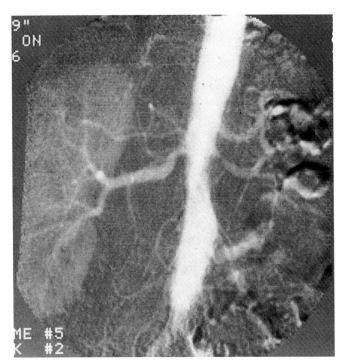

Fig. 96.11 IV DSA of the abdominal aorta and branches showing mild stenosis of the origin of the right renal artery and severe stenosis located in the proximal 1 cm of the left renal artery. Branches of the left renal artery are obscured by peristaltic motion artifact.

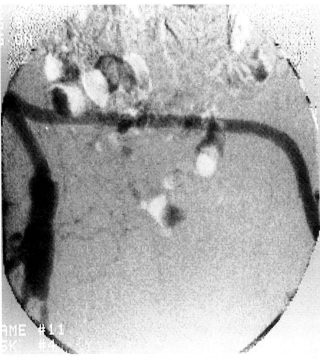

Fig. 96.12 Anteroposterior projection of an IV. DSA examination of the pelvis and proximal thighs showing a patent femoral-femoral bypass graft.

sequence excretory urography, but the latter technique is falling out of favour.

IV DSA provides a convenient method for assessing the effectiveness of renal artery surgery and establishes a baseline should a recurrence of hypertension occur. IV DSA is very useful for demonstrating the integrity of the arterial supply and the state of the renal parenchyma and drainage in the transplanted kidney.

Extremities

The application of digital subtraction angiography to the evaluation of the arterial and venous systems of the upper and lower extremities has been explored only to a limited degree. This is occasioned by the fact that the image intensifier field of view is limited so that multiple arterial or peripheral venous injections would be required to evaluate an entire extremity. As a consequence, DSA has found its greatest use in the postoperative evaluation of patients who have undergone vascular procedures (Fig. 96.12) and where the field of view of the intensifier can be positioned on the basis of previous knowledge [25,26]. In such patients, IV DSA has been applied to the routine postoperative evaluation of vascular reconstruction procedures, serving as both an index of the operative success and a baseline for future evaluations if necessary.

In addition to the evaluation of postoperative occlusive disease, IV DSA of the extremities has proven to be very useful in the follow-up evaluation of arteriovenous malformations of the extremities, in the preoperative evaluation of patients with bone or soft tissue tumours to determine vascularity, and for patients suspected of ischaemic upper extremity disease due to subclavian artery compression.

DSA by intra-arterial injection has been advocated by Crummy et al [27] to determine refilling of major arteries in the lower leg which have not been identified on conventional lower extremity arteriography. Such visualization of patent arteries has permitted attempts at vascular bypass procedures in place of amputation. In this category of patient, DSA has augmented conventional lower extremity arteriography.

A major advantage of intra-arterial DSA of the extremities is the ability to use much smaller amounts of contrast material or diluted contrast material in order to reduce patient discomfort (Fig. 96.13). An important clinical application is the evaluation of the digital arteries of the hands in patients with finger ischaemia.

A relatively recent innovation in DSA equipment has been the development of a moving table. A series of mask exposures is obtained along the entire length of the extremity, the table repositioned, and, following either the intravenous or intra-arterial injection of contrast material, a collection of contrast frames is obtained and subtracted from the appropriate mask image in each area of the extremity. Such equipment obviates the need for a large image intensifier and multiple injections. As a result, the vascular system in the extremities of patients can be evaluated using DSA as the primary imaging technique without previous knowledge of the probable level of

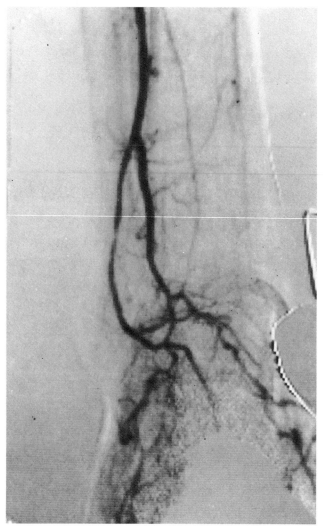

Fig. 96.13 Visualization of the distal arteries in the left leg and ankle by intra-arterial DSA using 10 ml of contrast material diluted 50%.

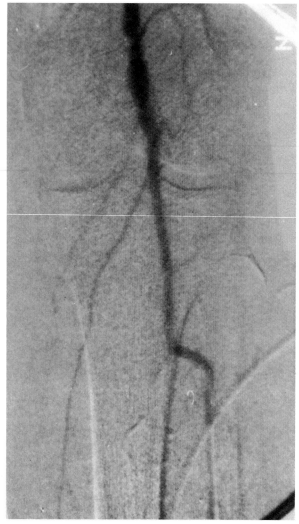

Fig. 96.14 IV DSA examination of the left leg carried out utilizing a moveable table top. Occlusions of the peroneal and posterior tibial arteries are well demonstrated.

disease (Fig. 96.14). Similarly, patients undergoing leg venography can be studied with such equipment, again permitting a decrease in contrast material volume or concentration, with reduction of both pain and the occasional chemical thrombophlebitis following conventional contrast medium venography.

ANTICIPATED CLINICAL UTILISATION

The promised rapid increase in technical design and capability of DSA equipment seems to be occurring. At the time of going to press (March 1985), DSA systems (either integrated or add-on) are becoming available with rapid acquisition rates, very large storage capacity and processing power, broad dynamic range and 512^2 or 1024^2 matrix. These units provide very good subtraction pictures after intra-arterial injection of small quantities of contrast medium. Arteries of 1 mm diameter can be clearly seen and the real-time subtraction facility and contrast enhancement suggest that intra-arterial DSA using state of the art equipment may well replace conventional film-screen arteriography for many clinical applications, particularly in interventional work and in spinal and cerebral angiography.

Enthusiasts suggest that conventional film-screen arteriography may become obsolete in the well-equipped department in the next few years.

BIBLIOGRAPHY

REFERENCES

1. Castellanos A, Pereiras R, Garcia A 1937 La angiocardiografia radioopaca. Arch Soc Estud Clin (Habana) 31:523
2. Robb G P, Steinberg I 1939 Visualization of the chambers of the heart, the pulmonary circulation, and the great blood vessels in man. Am J Roentgenol 41:1–17
3. Strother C M, Sackett J F, Crummy A B et al 1980 Clinical applications of computerized fluoroscopy. The extracranial carotid arteries. Radiology 136:781–783
4. Crummy A B, Strother C M, Sackett J F et al 1980 Computerized intravenous fluoroscopy: Digital subtraction for intravenous angiocardiography and arteriography. Am J Roentgenol 135:1131–1140
5. Chilcote W A, Modic M T, Pavlicek W A et al 1981 Digital subtraction angiography of the carotid arteries: A comparative study in 100 patients. Radiology 139:287–295
6. Meaney T F, Weinstein M A, Buonocore E et al 1980 Digital subtraction angiography of the human cardiovascular system. SPIE 233:272–278
7. Buonocore E, Pavlicek W, Modic M T et al 1983 Anatomic and functional imaging of congenital heart disease with digital subtraction angiography. Radiology 147:647–654
8. Pavlicek W, Weinstein M A, Modic M T, Buonocore E, Duchesneau P M 1982 Patient doses during digital subtraction angiography of the carotid arteries: Comparison with conventional angiography. Radiology 145:683–685
9. Modic M T, Weinstein M A, Pavlicek W et al 1983 Intravenous digital subtraction angiography: Peripheral versus central injection of contrast material. Radiology 147:711–715
10. Crummy A B, Stieghorst M F, Turski P A et al 1982 Digital subtraction angiography: Current status and use of intra-arterial injection. Radiology 145:303–307
11. Weinstein M A, Pavlicek W A, Modic M T, Duchesneau P M 1983 Intra-arterial digital subtraction angiography of the head and neck. Radiology 147:717–724
12. Modic M T, Weinstein M A, Chilcote W A et al 1981 Digital subraction angiography of the intracranial vascular system: Comparative study in 55 patients. AJNR 2:527–534
13. Pond G D, Ovitt T W, Capp M P 1983 Comparison of conventional pulmonary angiography with intravenous digital subtraction angiography for pulmonary embolic disease. Radiology 147:345–350
14. Goodman P C, Brant-Zawadski M 1982 Digital subraction pulmonary angiography. Am J Roentgenol 139:305–309
15. Ludwig J W, Verhoeven L A J, Kersbergen J J, Overtoom T T C 1983 Digital subtraction angiography of the pulmonary arteries for the diagnosis of pulmonary embolism. Radiology 147:639–645
16. Buonocore E, Pavlicek W, Modic M T et al 1983 Anatomic and functional imaging of congenital heart disease with digital subtraction angiography. Radiology 147:647–654
17. Higgins C B, Norris S L, Gerber K H, Slutsky R A, Ashburn W L, Baily N 1982 Quantitation of left ventricular dimensions and function by digital video subtraction angiography. Radiology 144:461–469
18. Engels P H C, Ludwig J W, Verhoeven L A J 1982 Left ventricle evaluation by digital video subtraction angiocardiography. Radiology 144:471–474
19. Buonocore E, Meaney T F, Borkowski G P, Pavlicek W, Gallagher J 1981 Digital subtraction angiography of the abdominal aorta and renal arteries: Comparison with conventional aortography. Radiology 139:281–286
20. Smith C W, Winfield A C, Price R R et al 1982 Evaluation of digital venous angiography for the diagnosis of renovascular hypertension. Radiology 144:51–54
21. Hillman B J, Ovitt T W, Capp M P, Fisher H D, Frost M M, Nudelman S 1982 Renal digital subtraction angiography: 100 cases. Radiology 145:643–646
22. Hillman B J, Ovitt T W, Nudelman S et al 1981 Digital video subtraction angiography of renal vascular abnormalities. Radiology 139:277–280
23. Sos T A, Sniderman D W, Suddekni S et al 1982 Renal vein renin assay and digital intravenous angiography in patients with renovascular hypertension. Presented at the 68th Scientific Assembly and Annual Meeting of the RSNA, Chicago, Illinois, Nov 27–Dec 3, 1982
24. Gomes A S, Pais S O, Barbaric Z L 1983 Digital subtraction angiography in the evaluation of hypertension. Am J Roentgenol 140:779–783
25. Guthaner D F, Wexler L, Enzmann D R et al 1983 Evaluation of peripheral vascular disease using digital subtraction angiography. Radiology 147:393–398
26. Pond G D, Osborne R W, Capp M P et al 1982 Digital subtraction angiography of peripheral vascular bypass procedures. Am J Roentgenol 138:279–281
27. Crummy A B, Strother C M, Lieberman R P et al 1981 Digital video subtraction angiography for evaluation of peripheral vascular disease. Radiology 141:33–37

97 Vascular ultrasound

Hylton B. Meire

Introduction

Vessel imaging
   Static 'B' scanning
   Real-time scanning

Abdominal vessels
   Small parts scanners

Doppler techniques
   Doppler imaging
   Spectrum analysis
   Blood flow measurement

Introduction

It is over 20 years since the abdominal aorta was first imaged by diagnostic ultrasound and there has been a steady progression in the applications of ultrasound in vascular disease since that date. The rate of development has accelerated recently with modern technical developments and an increasing awareness of the value of non-invasive vascular imaging and blood flow measurement techniques.

The applications of ultrasound in modern vascular investigation can be divided into two main categories. Firstly, imaging of the vessel wall and disorders of the wall and secondly, measurements and/or imaging of the blood flowing within the vessel lumen. Special scanners have been devised to perform each of these functions and in the last few years 'Duplex' scanners have been developed which perform both functions.

For the purposes of this chapter I have separated the imaging functions from the physiological measurement techniques and will deal initially with vessel imaging.

Vessel imaging

Static 'B' scanning

This was the earliest technique used for vascular imaging and is still capable of producing very high quality images in the hands of an expert operator and with appropriate transducer selection. As mentioned in the introduction, the abdominal aorta was probably the first major vessel to be imaged [1] but the technique has now been developed for the demonstration of many vessels including the major intra-abdominal vessels and the proximal peripheral vessels [2] (Figs. 97.1 & 97.2).

Real-time scanning

The advent of automatic real-time scanners in the last few

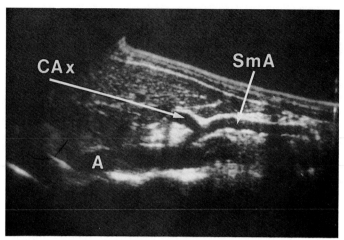

Fig. 97.1 Longitudinal static scan of the abdominal aorta (A) showing an anomalous origin of the coeliac axis (CAx) from the superior mesenteric artery (SmA).

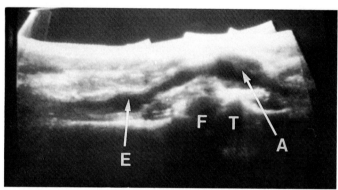

Fig. 97.2 Longitudinal static scan over the lower thigh and popliteal fossa. A small area of ectasia is shown in the lower femoral artery (E) and a frank aneurysm is present in the popliteal artery (A). Femoral condyle (F), Tibial condyle (T).

Abdominal vessels

Within the abdomen the prime function of ultrasound imaging is to detect or exclude the presence of aneurysm formation in the abdominal aorta (Fig. 97.3). The technique must include both longitudinal and transverse scans of the aorta. The information obtained will indicate not only the external diameter of an aneurysmal segment but will also indicate the amount of thrombus within the aneurysm and the site and size of the residual lumen [4]. In this respect the information obtained is greater than that obtained purely by angiography. The major disadvantage of abdominal ultrasound imaging is difficultly in identifying with certainty the site of origin of the renal arteries in patients with abdominal aortic aneurysms. However the very large majority of such aneurysms originate distal to the renal arteries and as techniques and apparatus improve identification of the renal arteries is being achieved with increasing frequency.

Imaging of the inferior vena cava *per se* is seldom of great value since this vessel is not prone to primary disease. Dilatation of the IVC may be seen in patients with venous hypertension [5] and the presence of tumour thrombus within the vessel should be sought in patients diagnosed as having a primary renal carcinoma [6]. A range of other intra-abdominal tumours may also give rise to tumour extension into the IVC.

The coeliac axis and superior mesenteric artery are regularly imaged and are occasionally seen to be aneurysmal or atheromatous. More often, they are used as anatomical landmarks for detection of the pancreas [7] which invariably lies inferior to the origin of the coeliac axis and anterior to the upper few centimetres of the superior mesenteric artery.

The major components of the extra-hepatic portal venous system can also normally be identified (Fig. 97.4A & B). The

years has greatly aided the demonstration of the major vessels. Real-time scanners are in general either linear arrays or sector scanners [3]. The latter systems have the advantage of a small area of contact with the patient and are to be preferred, particularly for examination of the upper abdomen where contact between the patient's skin and a long linear array transducer may prove difficult.

The major advantage of real-time scanners is the speed with which a vessel can be located. In addition, the connections of the major vessels can usually be demonstrated quickly and easily thereby enabling the operator to confirm the identity of a vessel which has been imaged. The image quality from real-time scanners is still somewhat inferior to the better static scanners, but the speed and ease of use of the real-time systems are ensuring that they rapidly replace the manually operated static systems.

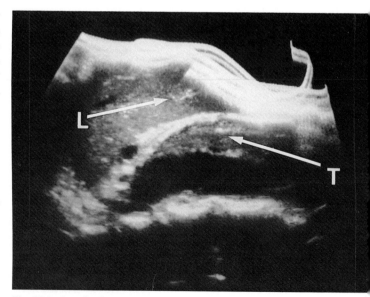

Fig. 97.3 Longitudinal static scan showing a fusiform aneurysm of the aorta with layers of thrombus (T) anteriorly within the aneurysm. Left lobe of liver (L).

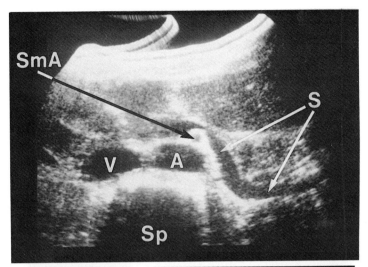

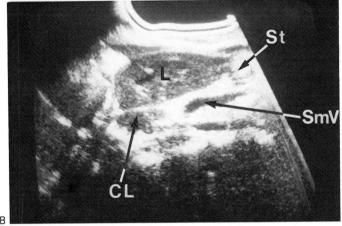

Fig. 97.4 (A) Transverse scan of the upper abdomen showing the splenic vein (S) passing anterior to the superior mesenteric artery (SmA) and aorta (A). Inferior vena cava (V), spine (Sp). (B) Longitudinal scan to the right of the midline showing the superior mesenteric vein (SmV) ascending to join the splenic vein posterior to the left lobe of the liver (L). Stomach (St), caudate lobe of liver (CL).

size and patency of the splenic, superior mesenteric and portal veins can be determined and their normal variation during respiration and after food can be detected [8]. The dimensions of the portal vein have been studied in the hopes that portal venous hypertension could be diagnosed by this technique. In general, this has not been found to be the case, many young women having rather large portal veins with normal tension and a great number of patients with proven portal hypertension having normal diameter vessels.

In children, portal venous thrombosis with cavernous transformation can be identified as a cause for portal hypertension. This diagnosis is relatively straightforward by ultrasound imaging and can be difficult to achieve by other techniques.

Small parts scanners

Ultrasound imaging of the major intra-abdominal vessels can

be achieved with the ordinary general purpose ultrasound scanner. These scanners have ultrasound beams focused in the 5–10 cm range and have poor resolution within the proximal few centimetres of the beam. Imaging of the more superficial vessels, particularly the carotids and femorals, is therefore not easily obtained by general purpose scanners.

The ultrasound beam is attenuated and absorbed as it passes through the patient and the rate of attenuation is proportional to the ultrasound frequency. The resolution obtained from an ultrasound system is also directly proportional to the frequency and one therefore attempts to use as high a frequency as possible consistent with obtaining information from as deep as necessary in any particular application. For imaging the superficial vessels penetration is not a major consideration and the advantage of improved resolution with increase in frequency can be used to obtain very high definition images. These factors have given rise to the advent of 'small parts scanners' [9] which employ frequencies of the order of 7.5–10 MHz, compared with the normal 3.5 MHz for abdominal imaging. The small parts scanners also employ transducers which are focussed to give maximum resolution in the first few centimetres beneath the skin. These systems are now capable of imaging the superficial blood vessels with a resolution of 0.2–0.3 mm. Small parts scanners are now capable of demonstrating the normal thickness of the vessel intima and media (Fig. 97.5) and are thus very sensitive for the detection of small atheromatous plaques.

There are three major disadvantages of small parts scanners. Firstly, calcification within the proximal vessel wall may totally reflect the ultrasound and prevent imaging of vessel segments. Secondly, fresh thrombus within a vessel may not appear significantly different from normal fluid blood and may therefore be entirely undetectable [10]. Thirdly, in common with all other pure imaging systems, small parts scanners produce no functional information concerning the blood flowing within the vessel or the haemo-dynamic significance of any lesions seen.

Despite these significant disadvantages, small parts scanners do permit rapid and accurate assessment of

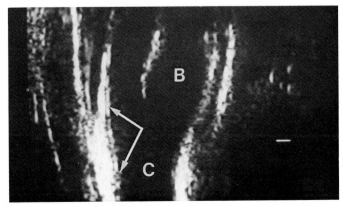

Fig. 97.5 Real time 'small parts' scanner image of a normal carotid bifurcation. The thickness of the proximal arterial wall (arrows) can be resolved. Common carotid artery (C), carotid bulb (B).

accessible vessels, in particular the extra-cranial carotid arteries. Over 80% of carotid arterial disease occurs in the region of the bulb and this area is readily accessible to dedicated small parts scanners. Application of this technique as a screening procedure for disease at this site has gained slow acceptance in the United Kingdom but is widely applied throughout the United States of America and in many European countries. Present experience suggests that ultrasound imaging of the carotid arteries is a valuable technique for the detection or exclusion of arterial disease in patients being considered for vascular surgery at other sites [11], particularly coronary artery surgery. There is a significant morbidity and mortality from cerebro-vascular accidents after coronary artery surgery. It is probably not justifiable to perform invasive vascular studies on the carotid circulation of all coronary artery surgery patients and ultrasound appears to be a suitable technique for selection of patients for further investigation prior to coronary artery surgery.

Small parts scanners have also found a valuable role in the assessment of vascular surgery [12]. The increase in vessel lumen, resolution of an atheromatous plaque and the adequacy of a vascular anastomosis can all be rapidly checked by ultrasound imaging. Many vascular surgeons are now using these scanners to exclude the presence of intimal flaps after vascular surgery before closing the patient's skin.

Doppler techniques

As emphasized above, static and real-time vessel imaging systems do not produce any functional information concerning the haemodynamic significance of any of the lesions detected. The only way in which such information can be obtained is by use of the Doppler technique. Most vascular surgeons currently use simple Doppler apparatus to detect or exclude the presence of significant stenoses in the lower limb arteries. These continuous wave Doppler systems merely give an audible indication of the velocities of the blood flowing within the vessels and its pulsatility. An experienced operator rapidly learns how to detect stenoses and to assess their severity. However, these systems do not produce images of the vessel, though the Doppler information can be processed to produce a 'sonargram' (see Figs. 97.9, 97.10 & 97.12) which gives a graphical representation of the blood velocities against time. Production of the 'sonargram' is achieved by means of spectral analysis which will be discussed later.

One of the disadvantages of continuous wave Doppler ultrasound systems is their inability to separate out signals coming from overlying vessels at different depths. If the vessels are abnormally tortuous or the anatomy unusual, it may be impossible to interpret information obtained from a simple continuous wave system. This problem is overcome by means of employing short pulses of ultrasound similar to those used in conventional imaging systems. Because sound

travels at a constant known velocity the time taken for echoes to return to the surface can be used to calculate the depth from which those echoes arise. Pulsed Doppler systems therefore permit the operator to selectively interrogate or surpress information from overlying vessels at different depths.

Pulsed Doppler systems are sub-divided into single channel and multi-channel systems. Single channel systems are capable of interrogating a single depth at a time whereas multi-channel systems can interrogate multiple adjacent depth increments simultaneously and can therefore be used to measure the velocity profile of blood flowing within a given vessel [13]. The multi-channel systems are in general more complex and expensive than single systems and rely upon precise focusing of the ultrasound beam. It is impossible to obtain fine focusing of an ultrasound beam at a depth of more than 5–6 cm from the skin surface and multi-channel systems are therefore currently confined to investigating superficial vessels such as the femorals and carotids.

The duplex systems referred to above incorporate both a small parts scanner and a Doppler system which may be either continuous or pulsed with either single or multiple range gates. The advantage of duplex systems is their ability to produce instantaneous images of the vessel under investigation and to use the imaging capability to direct the Doppler transducer at a specific area of interest within the vessel (Fig. 97.6). This combination of techniques enables rapid survey of the vessel for stenoses and plaques with subsequent Doppler studies to assess the haemodynamic significance.

Doppler imaging

An alternative to 'duplex' systems is the direct use of the Doppler information to produce a vessel image. Once again the systems can be divided into continuous wave and pulsed [14], the respective advantages and disadvantages be-

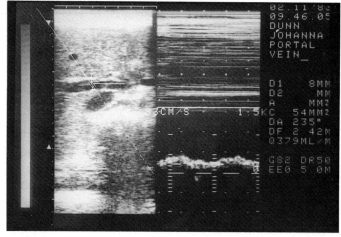

Fig. 97.6 Display from a duplex scanner showing the combination of 2D image and spectrum analysis of the Doppler signal.

ing the same as those for simple Doppler systems. The continuous wave systems contain no range information and can therefore only produce images in a single plane. Overlapping vessels cannot be separated by these systems. Pulsed systems do contain range information and can therefore be used to compile both AP, transverse and lateral views of the area under investigation (Fig. 97.7A & B) [15] and imaging of vessels within a selected depth slice can be achieved thereby

avoiding any ambiguities which may arise as a result of over-lying vessels.

Imaging with Doppler systems is very slow compared with modern small parts real-time scanners. With both continuous and pulsed systems the image is built up over a period of several minutes whilst the operator manually scans the interrogating transducer in a raster fashion over the vessel of interest. The imaging resolution is probably worse than one millimetre, but is nevertheless of considerable clinical value. It must be remembered that these systems produce images only of the column of blood flowing within the vessel and do not image the adjacent vessel wall. Areas of stenosis or obstruction therefore appear as defects in the image and are readily identifiable (Fig. 97.8). Cross-sectional imaging with the pulsed systems at the site of a stenosis will enable the cross-sectional diameter of the vessel at the stenosis to be measured and compared with the normal diameter elsewhere. The percentage stenosis can therefore be calculated directly from this sort of imaging. Continuous wave systems do not permit this facility.

Having obtained a Doppler image the transducer can then be aimed at any selected area of the vessel seen within the image and further information obtained for spectrum analysis of the Doppler signal to permit haemodynamic assessment of any flow disturbance.

Spectrum analysis

All the Doppler systems mentioned above produce information composed of a range of sound frequencies which are proportional to the velocities of the red cells moving within the vessel under interrogation. Within a healthy artery blood flow during systole is normally laminar owing to the viscosity of the blood slowing flow near the vessel walls. A Doppler signal obtained from a system which interrogates the entire vessel lumen simultaneously will therefore contain a wide range of frequencies, the low frequencies corresponding to slow flow near the vessel wall and the higher frequencies to

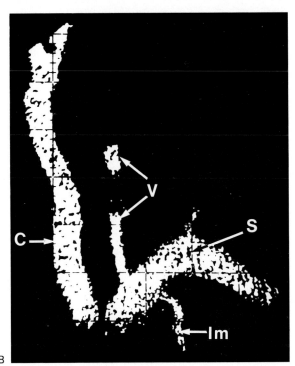

Fig. 97.7 (A) Pulsed Doppler image of the arteries in the left side of the neck. The image has been displayed to give a 'lateral' view. Segments of the vertebral artery (V) are seen where they are accessible in the gaps between the vertebrarterial canals of the cervical vertebrae. Common carotid artery (C). (B) Pulsed Doppler image of the arteries in the left side of the neck displayed to give an 'anterior' view. Common carotid artery (C), vertebral artery (V), subclavian artery (S), internal mammary artery (IM).

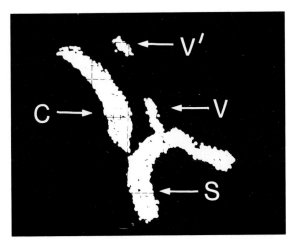

Fig. 97.8 Pulsed Doppler image of the arteries in the left side of the neck in a patient with a major stenosis at the origin of the common carotid artery (C). Vertebral artery (V), subclavian artery (S).

the more rapid flow within the centre of the vessel. Spectrum analysis permits graphical representation of the range of blood velocities and displays their changes with time throughout the cardiac cycle [16]. There is a great deal of information contained within the Doppler spectrum and only part of this is currently used in vascular assessment techniques. The two major features of interest are the pulsatility of the blood within the artery and the spectral width at different points during the cardiac cycle [17].

The pulsatility of blood within a healthy vessel varies with different sites in the arterial tree. Blood flowing into an organ with low vascular resistance, such as the brain or liver, shows continuous forward flow throughout the cardiac cycle with a systolic peak and continuous low velocity flow throughout diastole (Fig. 97.9) [18]. High vascular resistance organs, such as the muscles of the lower limb at rest, exhibit

biphasic flow with forward flow during systole and early diastolic flow reversal followed by further low velocity forward flow in late diastole (Fig. 97.10).

When vascular resistance is reduced after exercise the reverse flow component disappears and flow proceeds in a continuous forward direction. The differences between systolic and diastolic flow can therefore be used to assess the resistance of a vascular bed distal to the examination site.

A wide range of different indices have been described and although none of these is entirely foolproof two have gained wide clinical acceptance. These are the pulsatility index [19] and the A/B ratio (Fig. 97.11A & B) [20]. Both of these figures have different normal values at different sites in the vascular tree. In general the pulsatility will be increased proximal to an area of increased resistance and decreased distal to a significant stenosis. Numerical values can be calculated to assess the degree of pathological change. If the Doppler information is obtained from two sites simultaneously the time taken for transmission of the systolic pulse along a vessel segment can be calculated. This is termed the 'transit time' and will also be found to be prolonged if there is a severe stenosis or obstruction with collateral circulation formation.

The breadth of the Doppler spectrum indicates the range of red cell velocities within a vessel. These vary under different physiological and pathological conditions and at different sites throughout the arterial tree. In a normal healthy vessel there is a relatively narrow range of velocities present at any one site at a given time and the Doppler spec-

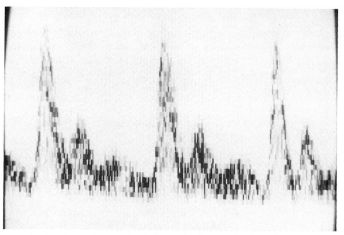

Fig. 97.9 Spectral analysis of the blood flow in the hepatic artery. The low vascular resistance gives rise to continuous forward flow throughout the cardiac cycle.

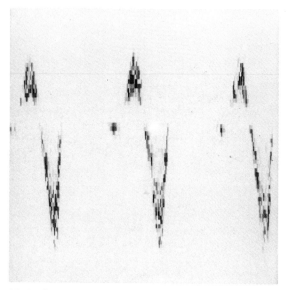

Fig. 97.10 Spectral analysis of the blood flow in a normal brachial artery at rest. The high peripheral resistance gives rise to early diastolic flow reversal.

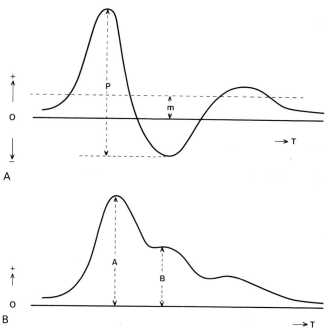

Fig. 97.11 (A) The Pulsatility Index is defined as the 'peak-to-peak' value (P) divided by the mean value (m). This index may be abnormally high proximal to a stenosis or occlusion and will be very low distal to a stenosis or in a segment supplied via a collateral circulation. Time (T), forward flow (+), reverse flow (−). (B) The points of measurement for the A/B ratio on a tracing of the normal internal carotid artery flow pattern. The ratio decreases with age and shows greater reduction in cerebro vascular disease.

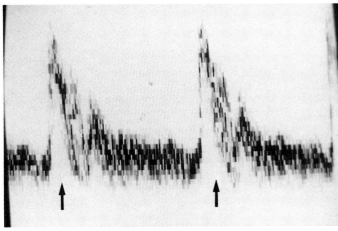

Fig. 97.12 Spectral analysis of the blood flow in a normal common carotid artery. There is a very narrow spectrum during the systolic peak giving rise to a normal 'window' (arrow) in the tracing.

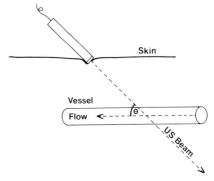

Fig. 97.13 The Doppler frequency shift produced by moving blood is proportional to the cosine of the angle θ between the ultrasound beam and the direction of movement of the blood. If this angle can be measured the Doppler frequencies can be converted to indicate actual blood velocity.

trum is therefore said to be narrow (Fig. 97.12). If there is roughness of the arterial wall or blood flow is disturbed by a plaque or stenosis then the normal laminar flow is disturbed and turbulence may occur. In turbulence blood is passing in a wide range of different directions with a wide range of velocities at any one time. The result is broadening of the displayed spectrum. There is no simple method of allocating a numerical value to the degree of spectral broadening but experienced observers are rapidly able to assess the degree of pathological change by observing the sonargram display. In general the more severe the disturbance in flow the greater the degree of spectral broadening. Caution has to be exercised when using assessment of spectral broadening with pulsed Doppler systems in which the range gate is very narrow. Information may be being obtained from a very limited area of the vessel cross section and the Doppler information will therefore not be representative of the disturbance in blood flow across the entire vessel. This may be advantageous when attempting to detect small changes in blood flow adjacent to very small plaques but if the plaque is not known to be present the technique cannot really be used as a means of determining the presence of this sort of disease.

Blood flow measurement

As described above the frequencies present within the Doppler signal are related to the velocities of the red cells within the blood vessel. The greater the blood velocity the higher the Doppler frequency. The exact Doppler shift frequency produced by blood of a given velocity will be determined by the cosine of the angle between the direction of flow of the blood and the interrogating beam (Fig. 97.13). In 'duplex' imaging systems and pulsed Doppler imaging systems the vessel axis can be identified and the beam vessel angle calculated. The cosine of this angle then permits the Doppler frequencies to be converted to blood velocities and since the vessel diameter can be seen from the images we have in theory all the information we require to calculate the volume of blood flowing through the vessel. In practice, however, there are two major difficulties. Firstly, small errors in measurement of the vessel diameter lead to relatively large errors in calculation of the cross sectional area of the vessel with a consequent effect upon the accuracy of the flow calculations. Secondly a greater degree of error arises from uncertainties about the mean blood velocity within the vessel. Blood does not flow with a uniform velocity across the vessel lumen and the overall velocity varies continuously throughout the cardiac cycle. In practice it is usually impossible to measure the instantaneous velocity at multiple sites across the vessel lumen throughout the cardiac cycle and a range of assumptions has to be made when using Doppler information to calculate volume blood flow.

The most accurate blood flow measurements are obtained from the multi-channel pulsed Doppler systems which do achieve instantaneous measurement of volume blood flow at multiple sites across the vessel throughout the cardiac cycle. Extensive complicated computations are necessary to convert these to a mean velocity and the systems are highly dependent upon operator expertise. Simpler systems interrogate the entire vessel cross-section with a single range gate and use the resulting frequencies to make a fair estimate of the mean value. These estimates may be accurate if blood flow is normal, but when there is any flow disturbance present the inherent assumptions become invalid and flow calculations are therefore much less reliable in pathological situations.

The clinical role of volume blood flow measurement has not yet been fully established; for the present, assessment of the vessel wall by small parts scanners in combination with Doppler spectrum analysis of information obtained from known sites within the vessel, permit the detection of the majority of significant disease with the minimum of effort and error.

REFERENCES

1. Goldberg B B, Ostrum B J, Isard H J 1966 Ultrasonic Aortography. J Am Med Assoc 198:353
2. Leopold G R 1975 Gray Scale ultrasonic angiography of the upper abdomen. Radiology 117:665–671
3. Wells P N T 1982 Real-time scanners. In: Wells P N T (ed) Scientific basis of medical imaging. Churchill Livingstone, Edinburgh, pp 156–161
4. Hassani N, Bard R, von Micsky L 1975 Ultrasonic investigation of the geriatric aorta. Geriatrics 30:154–155
5. Weill F, Maurat R 1974 The sign of the vena-cava: echotomographic illustration of right cardiac insufficiency. J Clin Ultrasound 2:27–34
6. Pussell S J, Cosgrove D O 1981 Ultrasound features of tumour thrombus in the IVC in retroperitoneal tumours. Brit J Radiol 54:866–869
7. Meire H B, Farrant P 1979 Pancreatic ultrasound — a systematic approach to scanning technique. Brit J Radiol 52:562–567
8. Bellamy E A, Bossi M C, Cosgrove D O 1984 Ultrasound demonstration of changes in the normal portal venous system following a meal. Brit J Radiol 57:147–149
9. Leopold G R 1980 Ultrasonography of superficially located structures. Rad Clin N Am 18:61–73
10. Cooperberg P L, Robertson W D, Fry P, Sweeney V 1979 High resolution real-time ultrasound of the carotid bifurcation. J Clin Ultrasound 7:13–17
11. Woodcock J P 1980 Doppler ultrasound in clinical diagnosis. Brit Med Bull 36:243–248
12. Baird R 1982 Diagnosis and monitoring in arterial surgery: the use of ultrasound and related techniques. Ann R Coll Surg Eng 64:91–95
13. Fish P J 1981 Recent advances in cardio vascular Doppler. In: Progress in Medical Ultrasound 2:217–237
14. Atkinson P, Woodcock J P 1982 Doppler flow meters. In: Atkinson P, Woodcock J P (eds) Doppler ultrasound and its use in clinical measurement. Academic Press, London, pp 22–74
15. Fish P J 1975 Multichannel direction resolving Doppler angiography. In: Proceedings of the 2nd European congress on ultrasound in medicine. Excerpta Medica, Amsterdam, pp 153–159
16. Gosling R G, King D H, Newman D L et al 1969 Transcutaneous measurement of arterial blood velocity by ultrasound. J Ultrasonics (USI Conference papers): 16–23
17. Gosling R G 1976 Extraction of physiological information from spectrum analysed Doppler shifted continuous wave ultrasound signals obtained non-invasively from the arterial system. In: Hill D W, Watson B W (eds) IEE medical electronics monographs. Peregrinus, London, p 73
18. Gosling R G, King D H 1975 Processing arterial Doppler signals for clinical data. In: deVlieger et al (eds) Handbook of clinical ultrasound. John Wiley, New York, pp 613–646
19. Gosling R G, King D H 1975 Ultrasonic angiography. In: Harcus A W, Adamson L (eds) Arteries and veins. Churchill Livingstone, Edinburgh, pp 61–84
20. Baskett J J, Beasley M G, Hyams D E, Gosling R G 1977 Screening for carotid junction disease by spectrum analysis of Doppler signals. Cardiovasc Res 11:147–155

98 Interventional radiology

David J. Allison

Biopsy procedures

1. Percutaneous transthoracic biopsy
2. Percutaneous abdominal biopsy
3. Musculoskeletal biopsy
   Bones
   Joint aspiration
   Soft tissue lesions
4. Miscellaneous biopsy techniques

Percutaneous puncture, decompression and drainage
procedures
1. Renal tract
   a. renal cyst puncture
   b. antegrade pyelography
   c. percutaneous catheter nephrostomy (PCN)
   d. ureteric dilatation and stent insertion
2. Biliary tract
3. Other sites

Extraction techniques
1. Percutaneous removal of gallstones
2. Extraction of renal stones
3. Vascular extraction techniques
4. Removal of gastrointestinal foreign bodies

Imaging-guided therapy

Interventional vascular techniques
1. Vascular therapy
   a. vascular infusion of chemotherapeutic agent
   b. vascular infusion of constrictor agents
   c. vascular infusion of dilator agents
   d. regional infusion of thrombolytic agents
   e. vascular extraction techniques
   f. vascular prosthesis insertion

2. Vascular dilatation (transluminal angioplasty)
   Techniques and mechanism of PTA
   Clinical applications of PTA
   a. lower extremity PTA
   b. renal PTA
   c. percutaneous transluminal coronary
      angioplasty (PTCA)
   d. PTA at miscellaneous sites
   Complications of PTA

3. Vascular embolization
   a. embolic materials and techniques
   b. indications for therapeutic arterial embolization
      (i) acute bleeding
      (ii) tumours
      (iii) vascular abnormalities
      (iv) central nervous system
      (v) hypersplenism
      (vi) priapism
   c. Indications for venous embolization
      (i) varices
      (ii) adrenal venous obliteration
      (iii) varicocele
      (iv) arteriovenous malformations
   d. complications of embolization

The impact of interventional techniques on Medicine
and Radiology

Innovations and improvements in imaging techniques during the past two decades have resulted in most of the more unpleasant and hazardous radiological procedures being supplanted by easier and safer methods of investigation. Despite this general trend towards less invasive radiology in the diagnostic field, the same period has witnessed the rapid growth of a new and more intrusive subspeciality known as 'interventional radiology'. This term* was originally used to describe procedures that were in some way therapeutic or curative rather than purely diagnostic, i.e. the radiologist 'intervened' in the natural history of the disease; by general consent, however, 'interventional radiology' has become an umbrella description for all types of procedures that are invasive or surgical in nature, even though some of these serve a purely diagnostic function (e.g. lung biopsy, trans-hepatic portal sampling).

The term 'invasive' is an emotive one and it should be emphasized that although the interventional techniques referred to below may seem invasive in comparison with the methods of diagnostic imaging in general, they are usually performed to obviate alternative surgical techniques that are associated with a much higher morbidity than their radiological counterparts. Compare, for instance, a percutaneous lung biopsy with an exploratory thoracotomy, or a percutaneous nephrostomy in obstructive renal failure with a formal surgical decompression: the advantages of the radiological techniques in both these situations are too obvious to require further elaboration. It would be wrong, however, to imagine from this that interventional radiology is merely a section of diagnosis and therapy that has been transferred from the surgical department to the radiology department. Advances in catheter and instrument technology, together with the development of appropriate radiological expertise and improvements in image monitoring systems, have brought about methods of diagnosis and treatment which simply did not exist previously. It is now possible to cannulate duct-systems and vessels throughout the body and, with the aid of specialised tools, perform a variety of procedures including drainage, extraction of endogenous or exogenous materials, dilatation, occlusion, selective infusion, selective sampling, and the insertion of mechanical devices. With the aid of sophisticated imaging equipment, needles can be accurately positioned deep in organs or tissues to obtain material for cytological or microbiological diagnosis, or to inject therapeutic agents locally.

The variety of diagnostic and therapeutic manoeuvres that these advances have made possible makes it difficult to classify the techniques of interventional radiology in a way that is both logical and comprehensive and the scheme outlined below is no doubt incomplete in many respects. I hope, however, that the procedures described below include most of the important current interventional methods, and give some impression of the wide-ranging applications of this new branch of radiology. Detailed descriptions of the techniques, indications, contraindications, limitations and complications relating to specific procedures have been deliberately avoided; for these the interested reader is referred to the bibliography which has been constructed with this purpose in mind.

BIOPSY PROCEDURES

The accurate positioning of biopsy needles and instruments in areas of interest in the body has been greatly facilitated by the improvements in imaging equipment that have occurred in recent years. The accurate guidance of biopsies by bi-plane or multi-angle fluoroscopy, ultrasound [1,2], or CT [3,4] has made it possible to obtain diagnostic material from sites previously thought to be inaccessible, or accessible only to the surgeon in the operating theatre. Most of these biopsies are obtained by percutaneous puncture using only local anaesthesia and many are performed on an out-patient basis. Some of the principal methods of percutaneous biopsy are considered below.

1. Percutaneous transthoracic biopsy

Transthoracic needle biopsy of pulmonary lesions is not a new technique. Its first use is attributed to Leyden (1883) who employed it to diagnose pneumonia [5], and a few years later Menetrier aspirated lung cancer cells by the same route [6]. These early investigations did not of course have the benefit of imaging guidance for their procedures but they demonstrated that percutaneous biopsy was technically possible. During the 1930s fine needle aspiration was used in several centres for the diagnosis of pneumonia [6,7] but attempts to diagnose lung cancer using larger bore needles (3 mm or more in diameter) resulted in significant complications such as air embolism, haemorrhage, tension pneumothorax and death [6,8].

The modern era of lung biopsy really dates from the work of Dahlgren and Nordenstrom (1966) [9] who showed that fluoroscopically-guided fine needle biopsy could give a high diagnostic yield with a low complication rate. Since that time the technique has become accepted as a standard diagnostic method and is used by radiologists throughout the world. Three important factors in the development of the technique in the past two decades have been improvements in image intensification, improvements in cytological methods for analysing small or fragmentary tissue samples, and an increasing readiness on the part of radiologists to undertake more 'invasive' diagnostic procedures. The commonest indication for lung biopsy is the investigation of an opacity shown on the chest radiograph when sputum culture, sputum cytology and bronchoscopy have failed to establish a diagnosis. The method can also be used to obtain material for microbiological examination from areas of consolidated lung, and to investigate pleural, hilar or mediastinal lesions. Fine needle biopsy techniques are generally unsuitable for the investigation of diffuse lung diseases. Percutaneous trans-

---

* A more facetious explanation for the term 'interventional radiology' is that it is that branch of medicine in which the radiologist *intervenes* between the private surgeon and his bank account!

thoracic biopsy is normally performed under local analgesia using single plane, or preferably, bi-plane fluoroscopic imaging (Fig. 98.1). The technique is most safely performed using a needle with an aspiration or corkscrew action rather than a drilling or cutting action, and suitable needles are readily available commercially. Needles 1 mm in diameter or smaller (18–23 gauge) are now used, the exact size being very much a question of personal preference. The finer needles (20–23 gauge) are probably less liable to produce complications, but the greater rigidity of 18–19 gauge needles gives the operator much greater control when positioning the tip of the needle deep in the chest. Percutaneous lung biopsy has been shown in many series to yield clinically useful information in 80–90% of cases with a surprisingly low incidence of serious complications [6,10,11,12,13]. The commonest *complication* is a pneumothorax which occurs in 15–25% of patients as shown by post-biopsy radiographs (CT shows a much higher percentage); the pneumothorax is usually small and resolves spontaneously, the insertion of a pleural drain being only rarely necessary [13]. Other possible complications include haemoptysis, pulmonary or pleural haemorrhage, subcutaneous or mediastinal emphysema, air or tumour embolism, tumour implantation along the biopsy track, empyema and broncho-pleural fistula. Most of these compli-

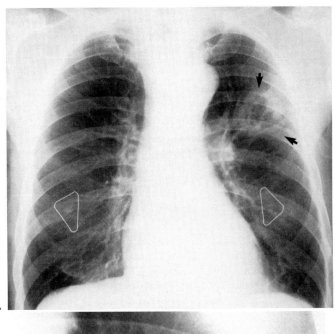

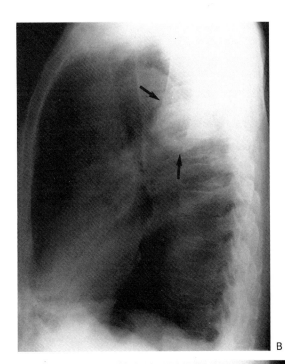

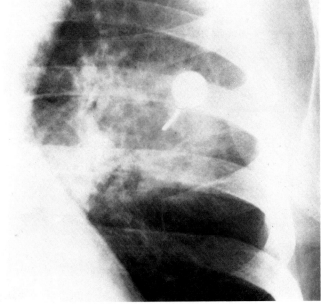

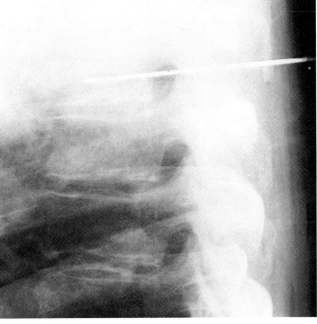

Fig. 98.1A, B, C & D   Percutaneous lung biopsy. (A) An opacity is present in the left upper zone (arrows) (the triangular metallic opacities are nipple markers). (B) The lesion is seen to lie posteriorly in the lateral projection (arrows). (C) and (D) The biopsy needle is inserted under fluoroscopic control.

cations are exceedingly rare and the procedure has a very low mortality rate [12,13,14,15,16]. The *contraindications* to percutaneous biopsy (Table 98.1) are for the most part relative rather than absolute: the value of the diagnostic yield has

Table 98.1 Contraindications to percutaneous lung biopsy

Bleeding diathesis

Anticoagulant therapy

Contralateral pneumonectomy

Seriously impaired lung function

Severe emphysema

Presence of bullae

Suspected vascular malformation

Suspected hydatid cyst

Pulmonary hypertension

Intrathoracic sepsis

Myocardial infarction

Patient's inability to co-operate

Patient's refusal to accept further treatment

to be balanced against the potential risks in each patient and many of the conditions listed in Table 98.1 would not consitute an absolute bar to the procedure in appropriate circumstances.

Percutaneous transthoracic biopsy has proved to be particularly useful in investigating peripheral lung lesions where the results of less invasive methods of diagnosis such as bronchoscopy and transbronchial biopsy often prove negative, and where an exploratory thoracotomy may be the only alternative to percutaneous biopsy. It is important, however, to remember that even in the best hands the procedure carries a false negative rate of approximately 5%. This means that the result of a single percutaneous biopsy can never be used to exclude absolutely the presence of a malignant tumour. If an unexpected negative result is obtained from a biopsy it is common policy to repeat the procedure (if necessary more than once) in an attempt to reduce the risk of a false negative result. In a small number of patients a diagnostic thoracotomy will still be necessary. Percutaneous needle biopsy of the lung is now established as a routine diagnostic procedure in most radiology departments servicing chest and oncology units and it is a valuable technique for the interventional radiologist to learn.

2. Percutaneous abdominal biopsy

The value of percutaneous biopsy in the evaluation of soft-tissue masses in the abdomen, retroperitoneal space and pelvis is now firmly established [17,18,19,20]. The technique may obviate the need for an exploratory laparotomy or peritoneoscopy, and the result frequently has a significant influence on the subsequent clinical management of the patient. The rapid growth in the use of the method has been dependent

on two principal factors: the improvement in imaging techniques, particularly the development of high resolution cross-sectional imaging, and the use of fine flexible needles to obtain aspiration specimens. Fine needle aspiration biopsy (FNAB) permits diagnostic material to be obtained from deep-seated lesions without significant risk. The flexibility of the needle shaft (approximately 22 gauge) permits movement of the needle during respiratory excursions and minimises tissue or organ damage from tearing. The needle is sometimes introduced co-axially through a short wider-gauge needle to provide a stable entry point through the skin and subcutaneous tissue. Despite the potential risks of haemorrhage, sepsis, and tumour seeding, the safety record of FNAB is truly astonishing; there are now several large series of cases reported in the literature with only negligible complication rates [17,20,21,22,23]. Serious complications of the procedure are so rare that FNAB is now routinely performed on an outpatient basis in many centres. In the case of large, superficial, and/or relatively avascular tumours, it is possible to use a larger-bore needle with a cutting or cork-screw action, and in the case of very firm tumours it may be necessary to use such a needle to obtain an adequate biopsy specimen. The increased risks of using a wide-bore needle must clearly be weighed against the potential diagnostic benefits that might accrue in the particular case concerned; the pros and cons of the subject are well-summarised by Mueller et al (1981) [20].

Close co-operation between the cytopathology department and the radiology department is clearly a *sine qua non* for the development of a successful diagnostic biopsy service. The correct handling of aspirated material is critical to the outcome of the procedure, and the successful development of FNAB is due in no small part to advances in cytology (both in technique and refinements of interpretation), that have permitted the accurate evaluation of minute quantities of aspirated material. The method used for localising the lesion to be biopsied and guiding the biopsy instrument to its correct position will depend on a number of factors including the size, site and likely nature of the mass, the availability of different imaging modalities, and the personal preferences and expertise of the radiologist concerned. If a mass is palpable and non-pulsatile it can be biopsied without sophisticated radiological localisation. For small or deep-seated lesions imaging control is necessary, and for masses that can themselves be opacified or are adjacent to structures that can be opacified, simple fluoroscopy is often the most suitable imaging method. The ease with which a needle tip can be positioned in a lesion is obviously greatly increased if biplane fluoroscopy is available. Depending on which organ-system is adjacent to or involved by the mass, accurate localisation may be assisted by one or more opacifying techniques such as lymphangiography, cholangiography (Fig. 98.2), single or double-contrast GI studies, ERCP, intravenous urography, angiography or venography. The possibility that a procedure such as cholangiography or angiography may pin-point a potential biopsy site should be borne in mind when planning these investigations so that facilities for taking a biopsy are available if necessary. If a biopsy is ever performed in conjunction with angiography (e.g. a hepatic lesion) the angiographic catheter should be left *in situ* until the end of the procedure so that any potential bleeding resulting from the biopsy can be embolised if necessary. An example of a fluoroscopically-guided fine-needle biopsy is given in Figure 98.3, which shows the puncture of an opacified lymph node using the transperitoneal approach described by Gothlin (1976) [24].

Many abdominal and retroperitoneal masses cannot be localised fluoroscopically, or even if they can, may be more rapidly and accurately localized by cross-sectional imaging techniques such as ultrasound (US), or computerised tomography (CT). US-guided biopsy or cyst puncture is versatile, usually quick to perform, does not involve ionizing radiation, and is available as a portable technique. It has proved particularly useful for the biopsy of large mass lesions [17,18], hepatic lesions [25], renal lesions [25], gynaecological lesions and amniocentesis [18,26], and cystic lesions in general. For more detailed descriptions of the techniques of US-guided biopsy the reader is referred to the excellent chapter on the topic by Haubek and colleagues (1982) [1].

CT-guided biopsy is usually more time-consuming than US, but has its own advantages: it is uninfluenced by gas shadows (an important consideration in the abdomen and pelvis), it gives good resolution of different tissue components, it produces good anatomical cross-sections, and the precise localization of the needle tip can be ascertained and documented during the biopsy procedure. CT-guided FNAB has proved to be of great benefit in the

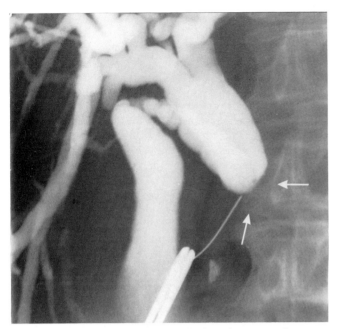

Fig. 98.2 Percutaneus fine-needle aspiration of a suspected cholangio-carcinoma. A PTC has revealed an obstruction in the common bile duct (arrows). A 22-gauge aspiration biopsy needle has been inserted into the lesion using a direct percutaneous approach. The diagnosis was positive for cholangiocarcinoma.

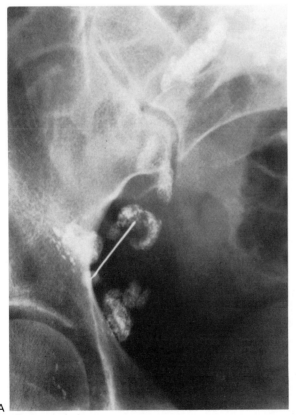

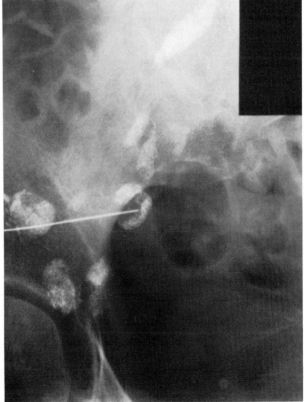

A   B

Fig. 98.3A & B Percutaneous lymph node biopsy. A specimen is obtained from a lymph node in which a previous lymphangiogram has revealed a filling defect. The use of different projections (A, B) enables the position of the needle tip to be precisely determined. This procedure revealed secondary tumour in the node (Figure by courtesy of Dr N. Bowley).

evaluation of pancreatic masses and other retroperitoneal lesions, pelvic lesions, and non-opacified lymph nodes [18,19].

It seems probable that the radiologist will be called upon with increasing frequency to attempt aspiration biopsies of abdominal lesions. The success rate of FNAB in obtaining positive cytology has exceeded 80% in several large series [20,23] and this fact, coupled with its low complication rate, is rapidly making it into a routine diagnostic procedure for the assessment of abdominal tumours. Further details concerning the techniques of fine-needle aspiration biopsy may be found in the article by Doherty (1982) [28].

3. Musculoskeletal biopsy

Bones in the body can be biopsied using a percutaneous approach under fluoroscopic control. The technique is used to investigate areas of abnormality suggestive of tumour or infection, to identify the cell type in the case of tumour, or the micro-organism in the case of infection, and to differentiate these lesions from each other and from abnormalities due e.g. to trauma or metabolic disease. The types of needles available for this procedure are reviewed by Griffiths (1979) [29], the essential feature of most being the incorpor-

ation of a pointed trochar for penetration, and a cutting edge or trephine for obtaining the biopsy by a drill-action. It should be emphasised, however, that in the case of a lytic bone lesion, where there is clear radiographic evidence of cortical penetration, it if often possible to obtain an adequate sample of tissue using a straightforward aspiration technique. Aspiration has also proved valuable in the investigation of suspected disc-space disease in the spine [30]. Bone biopsy is simple to perform and often spares the patient a formal surgical biopsy, which in the case of a deep-seated or relatively inaccessible lesion may be of considerable benefit (Fig. 98.4).

In the case of vertebral or disc-space lesions where an oblique approach is necessary to avoid the pleura and other structures, bi-plane fluoroscopy makes the procedure very much easier and safer, and for the same reason CT-guidance is extremely useful for this type of biopsy. The success rate of bone and joint biopsy is in the order of 70–80% in different series, with only occasional complications [30,31,32,33,34]. As with all types of percutaneous biopsy a negative result does not disprove the suspected clinical diagnosis, and multiple biopsies taken during the same procedure or repeat procedures serve to reduce the sampling errors that lead to false-negative results. In the absence of a clearly positive result it is almost always wise to recommend the surgeon to proceed to an open biopsy.

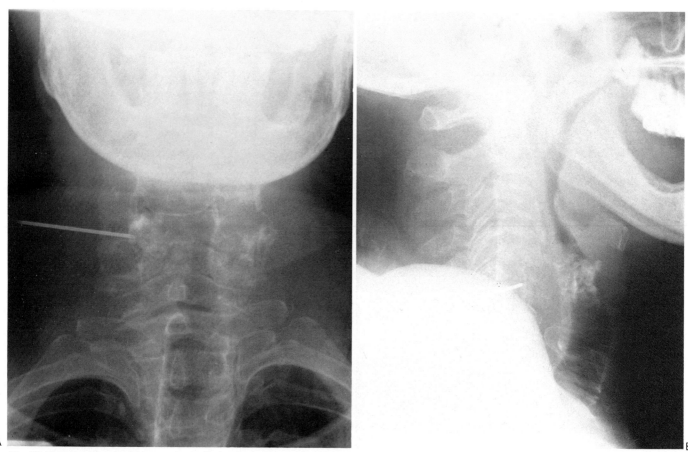

Fig. 98.4A & B   Vertebral biopsy. A needle has been directed into a lytic lesion in C5 using both antero-posterior (A) and lateral (B) projections for guidance. The biopsy, performed under local anaesthesia, showed the lesion to be an osteoclastoma.

The potential complications of bone and joint biopsy include infection, haemorrhage, neurological damage, tumour dissemination along needle tracks, inadvertent puncture of adjacent organs and the production of distal metastases owing to the haematological or lymphatic dissemination of tumour cells dislodged during biopsy. In clinical practice the incidence of serious complications following bone biopsy by an experienced operator is very low [35], and the procedure may yield crucial information with minimal patient inconvenience and discomfort.

Joint aspiration [36] can be performed to help in the evaluation of pain or other features that may indicate possible infection. This is particularly important in the assessment of complications following joint surgery and the insertion of prostheses.

Soft tissue lesions are easily biopsied using percutaneous needle techniques (Fig. 98.5) and if the mass lies in a site where it cannot be easily palpated computerised tomography assists in the accurate positioning of the biopsy needle [29].

4. Miscellaneous biopsy techniques

Percutaneous biopsy techniques are by no means restricted to the more conventional areas of interest outlined above. With the advantage of current imaging technology, and the confidence and experience radiologists have acquired in these methods, there is now virtually no organ or tissue in the body in which percutaneous biopsy or aspiration has not been attempted. The method has been used with success in all compartments of the mediastinum [15,37,38,39], the breast [40,41,42,43],

the thyroid gland [17,44,45,46], the adrenal gland [47], the orbit [48,49], lymph nodes [24,50] and even the central nervous system [51].

Yet another ingenious biopsy method has been the use of a *transvenous* approach to organs or tissues, usually to avoid transgressing mesothelial surfaces such as the pleura or peritoneum. Transvenous biopsies of the endocardium and myocardium have been performed for many years [52,53], and the technique has proved extremely useful in the evaluation of a number of cardiac disorders, including the cardiomyopathies and, more recently, suspected transplant rejection. Nordenstrom [54] has described a transjugular approach to mediastinal biopsy, and the transvenous approach has also been used to biopsy both extra-and intravascular tumours [54,55,56]. A transjugular biopsy instrument can be used to obtain a liver biopsy via the hepatic vein in patients with defective coagulation mechanisms in whom a conventional liver biopsy is considered too dangerous because of the risk of intraperitoneal bleeding [57,58]. A specimen of liver tissue can thus be withdrawn from the neck without transgressing the peritoneal cavity, haemorrhage from the percutaneous jugular puncture site being readily controlled by manual pressure for a few moments. The hepatic venous wedge pressure and a hepatic venogram can be obtained during the same procedure and these may add useful diagnostic information. An example of the technique is shown in Figure 98.6.

More recently percutaneous embolization kits have become available (William Cook, Europe) which allow the percutaneous introduction of embolic material including steel coils through a fine needle system. These kits can be used to occlude biopsy tracks through the same sheath that has been employed to introduce a biopsy needle into an organ such as the liver.

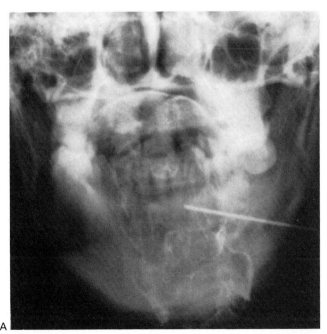
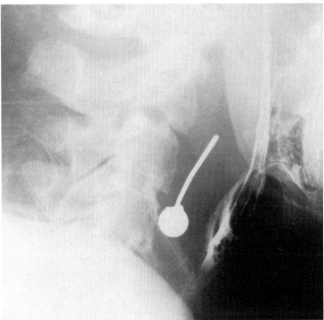

A   B

Fig. 98.5A & B   Biopsy of a soft-tissue mass. A prevertebral mass displacing the pharynx has been biopsied under local anaesthesia using both antero-posterior (A) and lateral (B) projections for guidance. The procedure yielded tuberculous pus and appropriate treatment was instigated immediately.

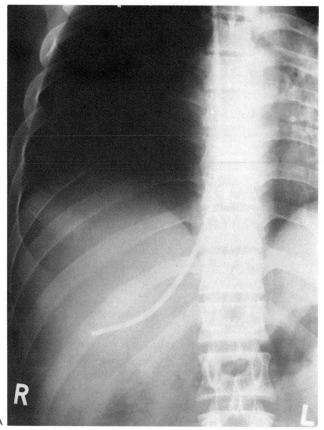

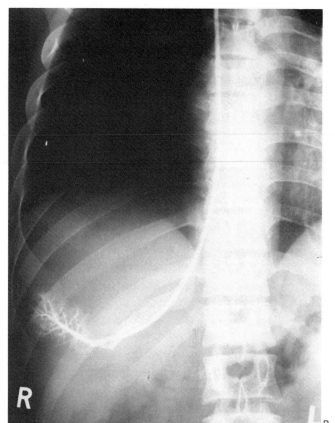

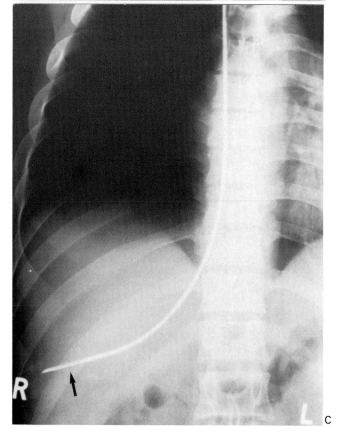

Fig. 98.6A, B & C   Trans-jugular biopsy of the liver in a patient with thrombocytopaenia. (A) A French 9 catheter has been introduced percutaneously into the right internal jugular vein using a standard Seldinger technique and passed down into an hepatic vein. Hepatic venous wedge pressures and a full hepatic venogram were obtained. (B) Injected contrast medium shows the local venous pattern. (C) A flexible biopsy instrument has been passed down the catheter and into the liver parenchyma through the vein wall (arrow). A biopsy was obtained from this and another site in the liver (using a different vein). The catheter was then withdrawn and bleeding controlled in the neck by simple digital pressure.

PERCUTANEOUS PUNCTURE, DECOMPRESSION AND DRAINAGE PROCEDURES

1. Renal tract

a. Renal cyst puncture

Percutaneous needle puncture of cystic renal masses is now a routine diagnostic manoeuvre in the evaluation of such lesions following their demonstration at urography, US, CT, etc, if further investigation is deemed appropriate. Aspiration of the cyst provides material for chemical, cytological and microbiological analysis, and opacification of the cavity allows further radiological assessment of its nature. Benign renal cysts have been treated non-surgically by complete aspiration and the instillation of iophendylate (*Pantopaque, Myodil*) [59], other non-water-soluble contrast media or sclerosing agents [60].

b. Antegrade pyelography

Antegrade pyelography opacifies the collecting system above an obstructing lesion when this cannot be achieved satisfactorily by intravenous urography, and provided that there is no evidence of coagulation abnormality, it is a safe method which offers several advantages over retrograde studies in the obstructed system. It is less likely to introduce infection, is technically easier to arrange and perform, and permits the evaluation of a completely obstructed system in which retrograde passage of a catheter is impossible. Percutaneous pyelography not only gives a method for opacifying the collecting system, but permits direct sampling of the pelvi-ureteric contents for analysis, allows urodynamic studies of the upper urinary tract [61,62,63], and gives valuable anatomical and pathological information in preparation for surgical nephrostomy. Perhaps even more important from the point of view of the interventional radiologist is the fact that percutaneous pyelography is the starting-off point for a number of interventional uroradiological procedures. These include brush biopsy of pelvic and ureteric lesions demonstrated during the study [64], identification of sites for transperitoneal or translumbar fine needle aspiration biopsy, dilatation of ureteric stenoses, percutaneous pyelonephrostomy, stent insertion, balloon occlusion of the ureter, drug irrigation for stone dissolution or chemotherapy, and stone extraction. Some of these procedures (which are reviewed by Pfister et al 1981 [63]) are considered in more detail below.

c. Percutaneous catheter nephrostomy (PCN)

There are many indications for percutaneous catheter nephrostomy [65,66,67] (Table 98.2). Early relief of urinary tract obstruction is desirable to minimize damage to functioning renal tissue and avoid renal failure. Urgent decompression

Table 98.2 Indications for percutaneous catheter nephrostomy

1. Relief of obstruction
2. Drainage of pyonephrosis
3. Assessment of renal function following decompression
4. Diversion of urinary flow
5. As a preliminary to a variety of diagnostic or therapeutic manoeuvres:
   Stone removal or dissolution
   Ureteric stenting
   Ureteric dilatation
   Percutaneous meatotomy
   Ureteric embolization
   Percutaneous irrigation or instillation procedures
   Catheter or stent extraction
   Biopsy procedures
   Nephroscopy

is necessary if the obstructed system is infected, if the obstruction is bilateral, or if a single or transplanted kidney is affected (Fig. 98.7). In many such patients, immediate surgery may be undesirable for a variety of reasons including the presence of renal failure or other severe metabolic disturbances, recent previous surgery, the presence of associated diseases which would increase the risk of surgery in a

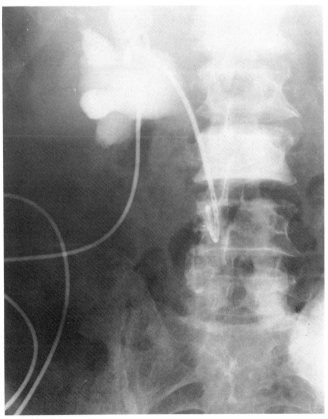

Fig. 98.7 Percutaneous nephrostomy drainage. A pig-tailed catheter with multiple drainage ports has been positioned in the ureter above a complete obstruction.

debilitated patient, and the presence of infection which could jeopardise the success of any definitive urological operation to relieve obstruction. In such cases, a percutaneous catheter nephrostomy performed under local analgesia permits decompression to allow recovery of renal function (and drainage if the obstructed system is infected) cytological and microbiological examination of aspirated urine or pus, and a detailed radiological examination of the collecting system either immediately, or at any time subsequently during the period of free drainage. Percutaneous nephrostomy is also useful in cases of urinary leakage in the early post-operative period following renal or ureteric surgery. PCN, together with ballon tamponade of the ureter if appropriate [63] decompresses the system above the leak and allows it to close.

There are several different techniques described for PCN [63,64,66]; most of them employ a postero-lateral approach through the flank and involve the insertion of catheter with multiple large calibre side-ports, usually pig-tailed in configuration to prevent displacement from the collecting system. The catheter may be passed over a guide-wire following the formation of a suitable track with dilators; alternatively catheters can be passed through a cannula using a trochar-cannula system. The beginner will find the article by McLean et al (1981) [66] to be an excellent practical guide to the different available techniques. Once a percutaneous pyelo-nephrostomy has been established and is draining freely, the necessity for acute surgical intervention is removed. Indeed,

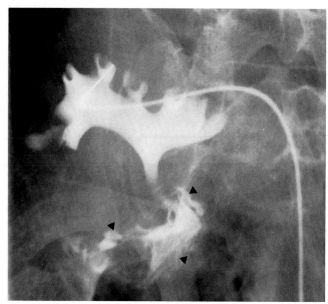

Fig. 98.9 Transplant nephrostomy. Contrast medium was seen to be leaking from the ureteric anastomosis site in a transplanted kidney (arrowheads indicate extravasated contrast medium). The kidney was drained percutaneously for a few days through a catheter after which period the leak sealed off; drainage into the bladder was established and the catheter removed without any further surgical intervention being necessary.

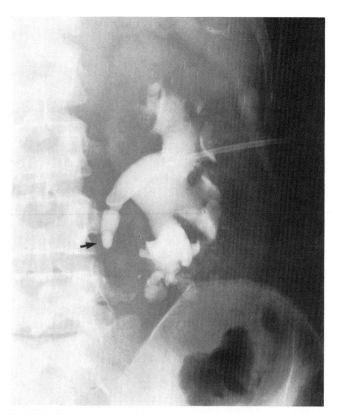

Fig. 98.8 Percutaneous nephrostomy. A single kidney is acutely obstructed by a ureteric calculus (arrow) in a patient with pneumonia. The catheter was left to drain the renal pelvis until the patient was fit for surgery.

some patients may never require subsequent surgery since the cause of the obstruction may disappear in the interim period. Examples of how this might happen include the spontaneous passage of an obstructed calculus or blood clot, or a decrease in the bulk of an obstructing tumour as a result of radiotherapy or chemotherapy during the period of percutaneous drainage.

Other patients will still require definitive surgery but this can be done electively in the absence of renal failure or sepsis, with the benefit of detailed radiological data concerning the anatomy of the collecting system and the obstructive lesion, and with cytological and microbiological information obtained from percutaneous catheter specimens. Examples of the uses of PCN in obstruction and leakage are given in Figs 98.7, 98.8 and 98.9.

d. Ureteric dilatation and stent insertion

Ureteric stenosis may occur from a variety of causes, and in suitable cases it is possible to perform dilatation of the stricture using either balloon catheters or tapered catheters [67,68], from a percutaneous nephrostomy approach. PCN can also be used for internal drainage through an obstruction using a stent [67,69]. A stent catheter is passed through the obstructing lesion using guide wires and dilating catheters as necessary. The stent catheter is furnished with holes above and below the obstruction and allows internal drainage. A double pig-tailed catheter can be sited with its curves in the renal pelvis and the urinary bladder respectively so as to give

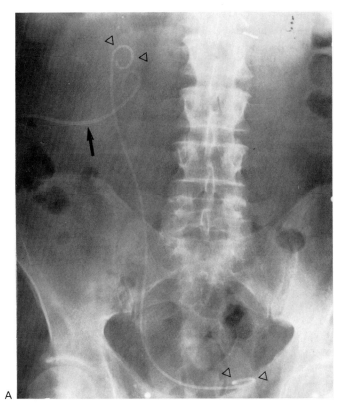

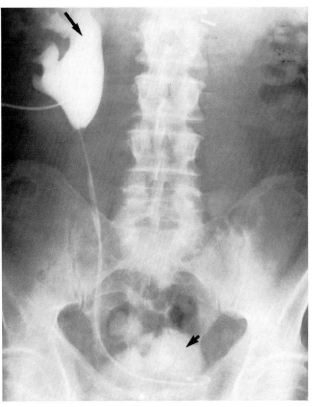

Fig. 98.10A & B Urinary stent insertion. (A) A double pig-tailed stent has been positioned so that one pig-tail lies *above* a ureteric obstruction in the renal pelvis and the other pig-tail *below* the obstruction in the urinary bladder (arrowheads). A second catheter (long arrow) lies in the percutaneous tract used to insert the stent. (B) An injection of contrast medium through the external catheter opacifies the renal pelvis (long arrow) and the urinary bladder (short arrow) showing that a satisfactory communication has now been established between kidney and bladder.

an internal stent across a ureteric obstruction (Fig. 98.10); such an internal stent leaves the patient un-encumbered with an external tube but is then only accessible from below (bladder endoscopy or surgery) in case of displacement or obstruction. An external stent (in which the upper end comes to the skin) allows catheter adjustment, irrigation or replacement, and is a route for repeated percutaneous pyelography to assess the effects of therapy etc. during the ensuing management period. Ureteric *embolization* [70] may be useful in some patients with persistent urinary leakage secondary to malignant disease or surgery.

2. Biliary tract

The past decade has seen a rapid expansion in the application of diagnostic and therapeutic radiological techniques in the hepato-biliary system. Fine-needle cholangiography is now a routine diagnostic procedure in departments serving a hepato-biliary unit, and the same percutaneous transhepatic approach is being employed for a number of more complicated interventional procedures in the biliary and portal systems (Figure 98.11). These diagnostic and interventional biliary techniques are considered in greater detail in Chapter 52 and there are also a number of other excellent review articles to which the reader is referred for further infor-

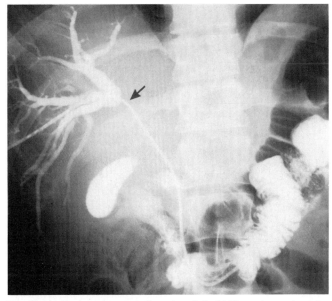

Fig. 98.11 Percutaneous transhepatic relief of biliary obstruction. A catheter has been passed through an obstructing tumour high in the biliary system (arrow) and into the duodenum to provide an internal biliary drainage pathway. In this case there was an additional obstruction at the ampulla which also required bypassing, otherwise the distal end of the drainage catheter could simply have been positioned in the lower common bile duct.

mation [71,72,73]. A treasure-trove of good practical advice on the subject is to be found in the chapter by Oleaga et al (1981) [74].

3. Other sites

Similar techniques to those available for decompressing and draining obstructed visceral duct systems can be applied to the drainage of cysts or abscesses at various sites throughout the body, and the percutaneous drainage of abdominal and retroperitoneal abscess cavities has proved to be a particularly valuable application of this branch of interventional radiology [75,76,77]. For these lesions the initial approach may be facilitated by the use of US or CT guidance, and these modalities may be crucial in defining the extent and anatomical boundaries of the abscess or cyst. For other lesions simple fluoroscopy may suffice: the choice of imaging modality will obviously depend on the site and nature of the pathology and the equipment available. In the abdomen an extra-peritoneal route is preferred to a transperitoneal route for percutaneous drainage whenever possible; it is however, possible to use the transperitoneal route provided the imaging system employed provides sufficient detail to avoid transgressing loops of bowel.

Clearly not every abscess is suitable for percutaneous drainage, and the radiologist should never attempt to do something that can be done more safely or effectively by operative surgery. In appropriate situations, however, the interventional technique offers several advantages: it may obviate difficult or dangerous surgery, and general anaesthesia; it saves time, expense and discomfort; it makes nursing care easier, and reduces post-operative complications; and finally, it may be a valuable temporary expedient in a very sick patient until definitive surgery is possible. Gerzof et al (1981) [77] suggest that percutaneous drainage techniques are applicable to the majority of intra-abdominal abscesses, and it looks as though the interventional radiologist is expanding into yet another area traditionally regarded as being strictly the province of the surgeon. The techniques and applications of abdominal drainage procedures are reviewed by Haaga et al (1979) [75] and Gerzof et al (1981) [77].

In the central nervous system computerized tomography has facilitated the precise positioning of needles in the brain and spinal cord to reduce the mass effect of necrotic or cystic tumours, and to evaluate abscesses or haematomas [78,79]. The development of stereotactic head frames to be used in conjunction with CT, promises to yield more advances in this field in the future [80].

In the *gastrointestinal tract* a number of interventional techniques can be applied and these are for the most part directed towards the relief or prevention of obstruction. The radiologist can assist in the positioning of intraluminal feeding and decompression tubes [74], dilate strictures and tight anastomoses [74], insert stents (Fig. 98.12), and remove foreign bodies [81,82]. *Oesophageal dilatation* is one of the most important gastrointestinal interventional techniques and

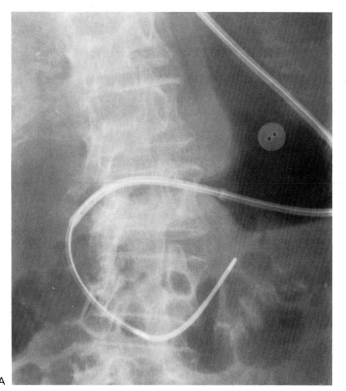
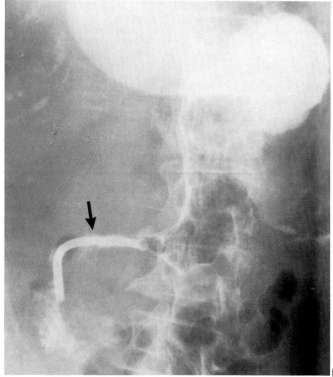

Fig. 98.12A & B Insertion of stent through inoperable malignant stricture of the gastric pylorus. (A) A catheter has been passed through the pyloric stricture into the duodenum. (B) An indwelling stent (arrow) permits the free passage of liquid food through the obstructing lesion. (Figure by courtesy of Dr D. Irving.)

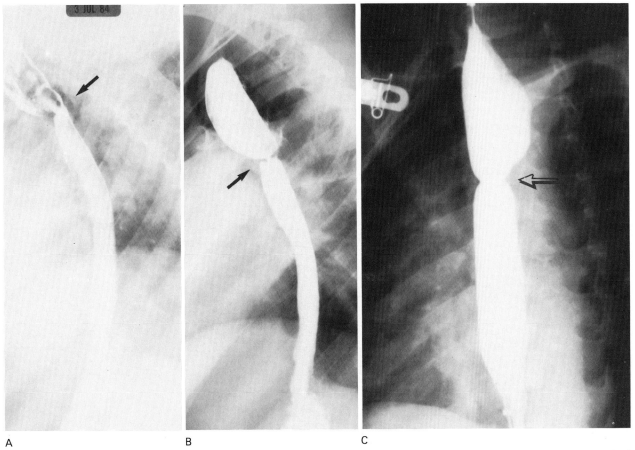

Fig. 98.13A, B & C Balloon dilatation of a post-surgical stricture in the oesophagus of an infant (born with tracheo-oesophageal fistula). (A, B) The tight oesophageal stricture (arrowed) is shown in two different projections. (C) The stricture is dilated with a balloon catheter. Note the 'waisting' of the balloon at the site of the stricture (arrow).

special balloon catheters are available for the procedure. The method seems to be very safe and it is usually technically straightforward; it can of course be easily repeated if necessary. In adults oesophageal dilatation is usually performed under mild sedation, but sometimes the procedure can be moderately painful and an intravenous bolus of analgesic (e.g. opiate) given just before the dilatation of the balloon may be helpful. In infants the technique can be used to relieve post-surgical strictures secondary to operations for tracheo-oesophageal fistula (Fig. 98.13).

EXTRACTION TECHNIQUES

Improvements in catheter technology and imaging systems have brought many extraction procedures that were formerly regarded as strictly operative surgical manoeuvres within the ambit of the interventional radiologist. Some examples of these procedures are considered below.

1. Percutaneous removal of gallstones

Residual biliary calculi are a common problem following surgery in the biliary tract [83]. They pose a serious problem since they may cause further obstruction and surgical re-exploration in this area is a procedure carrying significant morbidity. Techniques for dissolving common duct stones have met with modified success and are only suitable for certain types of calculus [84]. There is no doubt that if a T-tube is present, the most effective method of dealing with retained stones is to remove them through the T-tube track, using a steerable catheter and basket retrieval system [74,85,86,87]. The morbidity of the technique is extremely low and its success rate is in excess of 90%. There are few procedures in therapeutic radiology that are more rewarding, and none that has proved to be so consistently successful in the hands of relatively inexperienced operators.

An example of percutaneous removal of calculi is given in Figure 98.14, and the technique is described in detail in Chapter 52. The interested reader should also refer to the endoscopic techniques for removing calculi described in Chapter 53.

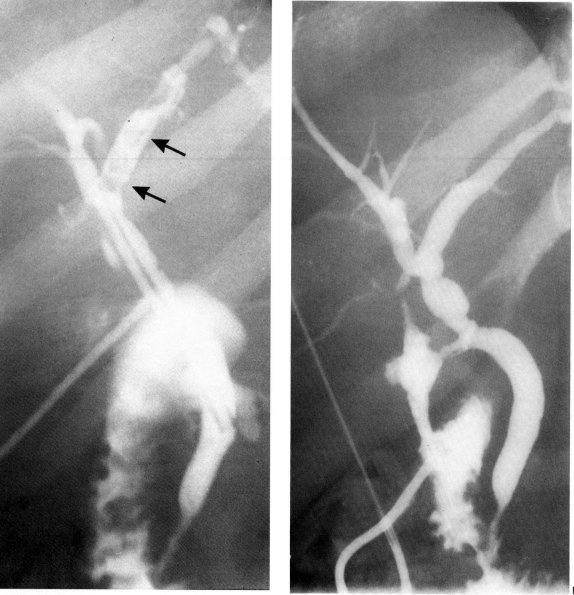

Fig. 98.14A & B Percutaneous removal of gallstones through T-tube track. (A) Several stones are demonstrated in the left hepatic duct on a 10-day post-cholecystectomy T-tube cholangiogram (arrows to stones). (B) The stones have been removed using a percutaneous retrieval technique; no further surgery is required.

2. Extraction of renal stones

Renal or ureteric calculi are a common problem and in many cases it is desirable to remove them because of the risks of urinary tract obstruction and infection. Four types of interventional radiological techniques are available for the elimination of urinary calculi: first, it may be possible to push the stone(s) onwards into the bladder (or conduit loop) using a PCN approach [65,89]. Secondly, using the same route the stone(s) may be dissolved by irrigation with an appropriate solution [88,90]. Thirdly, it may be possible to fragment them mechanically [65] or by ultrasound. Finally it is possible in many cases to extract the stone(s) percutaneously through the loin using either a nephroscope [91] or a stone-basket retrieval system analogous to those used in the biliary system [89,92,93,94]. The track required to extract stones through the loin is large and the procedure is often conducted in two or more stages to allow gradual dilatation of the percutaneous passage. Recently, however, some centres have been performing the procedure in a single stage using a large balloon catheter or mechanical dilator to expand the track to sufficient size. General anaesthesia is normally required for this procedure. Percutaneous stone extraction is particularly useful in patients who have had an ileal or colonic loop diversion, when a retrograde approach to the distal ureter is difficult or impossible.

3. Vascular extraction techniques

These are considered below under Interventional Vascular Techniques.

4. Removal of gastrointestinal foreign bodies

If endoscopic facilities are not available, foreign bodies can be removed from the upper gastrointestinal tract under fluoroscopic guidance using balloon catheters or baskets [81,82].

IMAGING-GUIDED THERAPY

There are a number of forms of therapy that demand the exact positioning of drugs, radio-active particles, etc. in a particular anatomical location using radiological imaging techniques to achieve the required degree of precision. These procedures are conducted in the radiology department either by the radiologist, or by a specialist working in close co-operation with a radiologist whose assistance in guiding the former is indispensable to the technique. Examples of this type of therapy include the technique of percutaneous thermocoagulation of the Gasserian ganglion performed by Thurel et al (1980) [95] for the relief of essential trigeminal neuralgia; puncture of thyroid or renal cysts under US-guidance [96]; the ultrasonically-guided percutaneous implantation of iodine-125 seeds in pancreatic malignancies [97]; the implantation of Iridium-192 wires in cholangiocarcinoma using the percutaneous transhepatic approach [98], and the injection of alcohol into the coeliac ganglion for intractable

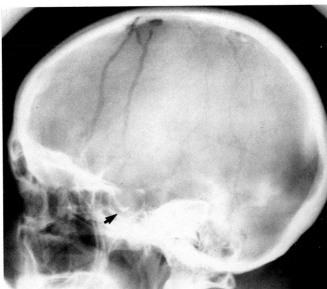

Fig. 98.15 Pituitary implantation. [90]Yttrium seeds (arrowed) have been implanted into a pituitary tumour using a percutaneous approach under fluoroscopic control. This technique has proved to be outstandingly successful in the treatment of certain pituitary conditions such as acromegaly. [99]

pain under the guidance of a previously sited selectively-placed coeliac artery catheter. In the central nervous system the implantation of radioactive seeds into hormonally-active pituitary tumours can be performed under radiological guidance [99] (Fig. 98.15). It seems likely, with current advances in cross-sectional imaging techniques and the increased confidence and expertise radiologists are acquiring in respect of all types of percutaneous instrumentation, that there will be a continued expansion in the use of imaging-guided therapeutic techniques.

INTERVENTIONAL VASCULAR TECHNIQUES

During the past decade the growth in interventional vascular radiology has been such that the subject itself almost comprises a new medical sub-speciality. The percutaneous vascular approaches evolved originally for purely diagnostic imaging purposes have been adapted to a variety of therapeutic manoeuvres which have had a profound impact on many branches of medicine and surgery, and have moved the radiologist to the 'front-line' of patient management. Interventional vascular methods can be considered under three broad headings: vascular therapy, which includes various types of therapeutic techniques conducted via vascular systems under radiological control; vascular dilatation; and vascular embolization.

1. Vascular therapy

a. Vascular infusion of chemotherapeutic agents

It is possible by the use of selective arterial catheterization to deliver a high local concentration of an appropriate chemotherapeutic agent to the feeding vessels of a tumour. The technique has been used with varying degrees of success for a wide range of neoplasms particularly primary and metastatic liver tumours, bone neoplasms, sarcomas, melanomas and pelvic neoplasms [100,101,102,103]. With the use of suitable indwelling catheters, infusion regimens can be continued for up to several weeks if necessary [104,105].

b. Vascular infusion of constrictor agents

The selective arterial or venous infusion of pharmacologically active substances can be used either as a diagnostic aid, to improve the quality of arteriography or venography by altering local flow dynamics, or as a therapeutic manoeuvre for the treatment of various vascular disorders.

The commonest use of constrictor agents has undoubtedly been for the control of gastrointestinal bleeding, and the present agent of choice for this purpose seems to be vasopressin [106,107,108], although adrenaline and nonadrenaline have also been employed [104,109], and prostaglandins are currently under evaluation. Vasopressin in doses of 0.1–0.4iu/min delivered selectively into the vessel supplying the bleeding site is usually an effective means of controlling gastrointestinal haemorrhage and the more selective the infusion the greater the chance of success. Dose rates above 0.4 iu/min appear to increase systemic side-effects without increasing local efficacy. Vasopressin infusion has been used to control bleeding at all levels in the gastrointestinal tract, but is particularly useful in diffuse gastric bleeding (e.g. haemorrhagic gastritis), and in bleeding from sites such as the descending colon where therapeutic embolization is regarded by many radiologists as being hazardous. It has been used with great success in the management of bleeding diverticula [110,111]. Various programmes for the effective and safe use of vasopressin infusions in the control of gastrointestinal bleeding are given by Athanasoulis and co-workers [106,107]. Vasopressin can also be used to control bleeding from varices. The drug may be infused selectively into the superior mesenteric artery in order to reduce splanchnic flow and hence lower portal venous pressure [112]. Simple intravenous infusion however, is probably just as effective as selective intra-arterial administration in this situation [113,114].

The question of whether constrictor therapy or therapeutic embolization is the more appropriate treatment in a given case of gastrointestinal bleeding depends on several factors: these include the site and nature of the pathology; the previous history and treatment; and the preferences and experience of the radiologist. This topic, together with a comprehensive bibliography is considered in some detail in the excellent article by Clark and Colley (1981) [108]; they also review the side effects and possible dangers of vasopressive therapy.

c. Vascular infusion of dilator agents

Dilator agents such as tolazoline, histamine, papaverine, reserpine and prostaglandins, have been selectively infused in attempts to improve the diagnostic yield from arteriographic examinations. Some of these have also been used as therapeutic agents in a variety of ischaemic and vasopastic disorders including mesenteric ischaemia, Raynaud's disease, ergotism, frostbite and atherosclerosis [108,115,116,117]. While occasionally a dramatic improvement results from such treatment, it would be fair to say that the long-term results of this type of therapy are generally disappointing. Vasodilator agents have also been used to combat spasm engendered by transluminal angioplasty; nitroglycerin and nifedipine have proved useful in this context.

d. Regional infusion of thrombolytic agents

The high morbidity and mortality related to vascular thrombosis at different sites in the body has led to considerable interest in the therapeutic effects of the selective regional infusion of thrombolytic enzymes such as streptokinase and urokinase. The latter agent has considerable theoretical advantages over the former including rapid onset of action, a more predictable dose response [118], a higher gel:soluble phase ratio [118] and much lower antigenicity [119]. The principal disadvantage of urokinase is that it is 15–20 times as expensive as streptokinase; a difference worthy of some consideration in most institutions! The agents can be given systemically or, using the services of the radiologist, into a regional vascular bed following selective catheterization.

Local thrombolytic therapy has been used in a variety of clinical situations including pulmonary embolism, deep venous thrombophlebitis, coronary thrombosis, peripheral arterial thrombosis (particularly acute lower limb thrombosis or embolism) and dialysis shunt thrombosis.

Thrombolytic therapy is unfortunately associated with a relatively high morbidity (and mortality). Haemorrhage is a major problem and intracerebral haemorrhage, often fatal, has been noted in 3–13% of patients undergoing therapy with streptokinase or urokinase [118,119]. Pyrexia (50%) and anaphylactic responses (6%) are other problems that may be encountered. A large number of contraindications to thrombolytic therapy exist and the principal ones are listed in Table 98.3.

Table 98.3 Contraindications to thrombolytic therapy (after Gallant and Athanasoulis 1982 [119])

1. Bleeding diathesis
2. Surgery or translumbar aortography during the preceding 14 days
3. History of cerebral haemorrhage
4. History of gastrointestinal haemorrhage
5. Uncontrolled hypertension
6. Severe hepatic or renal disease
7. SLE
8. Active TB
9. Visceral carcinoma
10. Atrial fibrillation or known ventricular thrombus
11. Significant carotid atherosclerosis
12. External cardiac massage during the preceding 10 days
13. Biopsy from an inaccessible site during the preceding 10 days

As local thrombolytic therapy is usually given by continuous pump infusion, the patient must be monitored in an intensive care unit (or similar special care ward) with constant checks for overt or occult bleeding and monitoring of appropriate haematological indices. Because of this intensive monitoring requirement and the high morbidity that exists despite it, thrombolytic therapy has not gained the wide acceptance it might have otherwise achieved by virtue of its theoretical appeal. The future role of this type of treatment remains uncertain.

Readers seeking more detailed information about thrombolytic therapy including treatment protocols and dosage regimens are referred to Gallant and Athanasoulis (1982) [119].

e. Vascular extraction techniques

i. Intravascular foreign bodies

With the growth in intravenous monitoring and parenteral feeding that has occurred in many hospitals in recent years the loss of part of an indwelling venous line is becoming an increasingly frequent occurrence; indeed this complication of intravenous therapy has been the subject of a hazard notice by the Department of Health and Social Security in the UK [120]. Other foreign bodies that may require removal from the vascular system include: guidewire or catheter fragments, ventriculo-venous shunts, Swan-Ganz catheters, pacing wires, angiography needle fragments, Holter valves, angiographic dilators, and misplaced therapeutic embolizing materials such as steel coils or balloons. Fortunately these objects can usually be removed without having recourse to surgery and a variety of different percutaneous retrieval techniques have been described for this purpose [76,121,122,123,124]. These methods include the use of purpose-designed fragment graspers, looped-wire snares, dormia baskets, steerable catheters, balloon catheters, magnets, endoscopy forceps, and biopsy forceps. Figure 98.16 shows how a steel embolization coil (that was originally intended for an aorta-pulmonary communication but lost its way!) was successfully removed from the iliac artery using a biliary stone-basket passed through an arterial sheath. Detailed descriptions of the many different techniques available for the removal of intravascular fragments are available in the literature [76,121,123,124]. Techniques are also described for untying knots in intravascular catheters [76].

Any interventional radiologist undertaking regular vascular work is well advised to become acquainted with the above methods *before* the need arises (it will!) and make sure that the necessary equipment is available in the department.

ii. Parasites

The portal venous system can be entered by the percutaneous transhepatic route either to embolise varices or to obtain selective pancreatic venous samples (see below). This mode of access to the portal system can also be exploited to remove schistosomes from the portal venous blood [125]. The adult worms are mobilised from the splanchnic bed with antimony potassium tartrate, and the portal blood then filtered by means of an extracorporeal portosaphenous shunt.

iii. Intravascular thrombus

Intravascular thrombus can be removed percutaneously using a special suction catheter introduced through a jugular or femoral venotomy. The technique has been used in the management of pulmonary embolism [126]. Alternatively, a catheter can be used to fragment or dislodge a life-threatening centrally-occluding clot in the pulmonary artery so as to redistribute the thrombus peripherally, and reduce overall pulmonary vascular resistance [127].

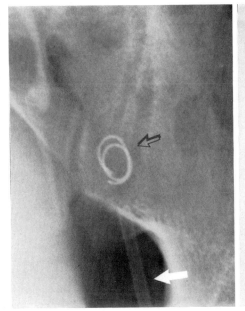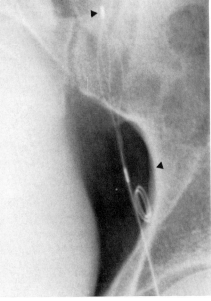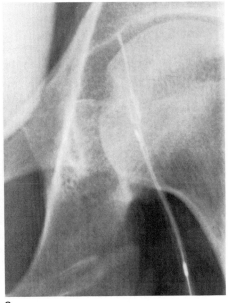

A   B   C

Fig. 98.16A, B & C Extraction of a misplaced embolization coil. (A) The coil (originally intended for a bronchial artery) has escaped and become lodged in the left external iliac vessel (hatched arrow). The hub of the embolizing catheter was cut off, a sheath (white arrow) introduced into the artery over the catheter, and the catheter removed. (B) A biliary stone-removal basket has been introduced through the sheath. The radio-opaque markers (arrowheads) indicate the proximal and distal ends of the basket (see C). (C) The coil has been caught by the basket and is being drawn into the sheath through which it was successfully removed. The original procedure was then resumed and proceeded to a successful conclusion.

f. Vascular prosthesis insertion

i. Vena caval filters

In cases of recurrent or threatened pulmonary embolization from the lower extremities and pelvis, inferior vena caval interruption can be achieved using interventional techniques (venous filters or balloons) that obviate general anaesthesia and abdominal surgery in what may be desperately ill patients. The technique is particularly useful in patients in whom anticoagulation is contra-indicated, has failed, or in whom anticoagulation has already produced complications such as gastrointestinal, retroperitoneal or wound haemorrhage. The preferred route for percutaneous inferior vena caval interruption is a right jugular venotomy, the filter or balloon normally being placed below the renal veins. In some patients a right femoral approach is used. The prosthesis is preceded by inferior cavography to ascertain IVC size, renal vein level and to assess caval abnormalities, such as caval thrombosis, left-sided cava and other potential anomalies. Three principal systems are in general use. The Mobin-Uddin (MU) filter [128], the Kimray-Greenfield (KG) filter [129] and the Hunter detachable occlusion balloon [130]. The complications of inserting such filters include continued recurrent pulmonary embolization, inferior vena caval thrombosis with lower extremity venous stasis phenomena, and migration of the occluding device to the heart or lungs (sometimes with a fatal outcome). Because of these potential complications the procedure should not be undertaken unless there are pressing clinical indications to do so [131]. All three available systems have undergone clinical trials and seem effective in reducing the dangers of recurrent embolism in selected patients [132]. There seems to be a higher likelihood of preservation of IVC patency in patients with the KG filter (95%) than the MU filter (47%), and the former device is probably also more effective in reducing the incidence of recurrent thromboembolism [132]. Devices are currently under development that can be introduced through standard calibre catheters, yet expand to occupy and filter the inferior vena cava. These new filters will not require a formal venotomy procedure for their insertion, and it seems likely that their introduction will result in a more widespread use of these techniques in the future.

ii. Percutaneous closure of congenital vascular defects

One of the most spectacular manoeuvres in interventional radiology must surely be the method described by Portsmann for the percutaneous closure of a patent ductus arteriosus (PDA) using a preshaped conical plug [133]. The technique, which is performed using a loop-system from simultaneous femoral venous and arterial approaches, has been successfully performed in several hundred patients since first introduced in 1966. Unfortunately the transfemoral method is not applicable in those very young infants in whom the majority of PDA closures are required and the procedure has not gained wide acceptance among paediatric cardiologists and cardiac surgeons. It is possible, however, that technological advances may change this situation in the future. Other congenital vascular defects and communications can be treated by the interventional radiologist; among the most useful of these procedures must be included the closure of aorto-pulmonary communications by means of coils or balloons as an alternative or adjunct to surgery [134,135].

2. Vascular dilatation (transluminal angioplasty)

There is probably no field of interventional radiology that has undergone more rapid and successful development in recent years than that of *percutaneous transluminal angioplasty* (PTA). Although Dotter and Judkins (1964) [136] introduced a method for the dilatation of arterial stenoses almost twenty years ago, improvements in technique and catheter technology, introduced by Portsmann, Zeitler, Van Andel, Gruntzig and others, have resulted in an upsurge of interest in this mode of therapy in recent years, and there are now many reported series showing a high success rate with relatively low morbidity [137,138,139,140]. One of the most important developments in the evolution of the present technique was the introduction of the rigid polyvinyl chloride balloon by Gruntzig and Hopff in 1974 [141]; because of its low compliance this balloon could be distended to a predetermined diameter and a high inflation pressure (4–5 atmospheres) applied without fear of over-distension and vessel rupture. Modern balloons can be inflated to much higher pressures, and relatively large dilatation diameters can be achieved using catheters of only conventional calibre, an important factor with regard to the reduction of complications at the arterial puncture site.

The term percutaneous transluminal angioplasty encompasses both the *dilatation* of stenotic lesions and the *recanalization* of occluded vessels. Although atherosclerosis is the underlying vascular pathology in the majority of patients the technique has also been successfully applied to a variety of causes of vascular narrowing including congenital defects, fibromuscular dysplasia, arteritis, and other disorders.

Techniques and mechanism of PTA

The fundamental technique of PTA is to position a balloon catheter in the region of a vascular stenosis and carefully dilate the balloon under fluoroscopic control to distend the stenotic segment and improve flow. Prior to undertaking the procedure good preliminary angiography should have delineated the area of abnormality, together with views of the vessels lying proximal and distal to the lesion. Cases are normally discussed with a vascular surgeon (or other interested party) and a decision taken as to what constitutes the most appropriate treatment for the particular patient concerned. Some patients may require no treatment or only drug therapy, some need surgery, some need angioplasty and yet others may benefit from both angioplasty and surgery. Many radiologists have a working arrangement with their clinical colleagues so that in suitable cases they can proceed directly to angioplasty without further consultation if an appropriate lesion is revealed at arteriography; this saves the patient a return visit and may obviate a further groin puncture. Whatever system is adopted the radiologist should work in close association with the clinician(s) concerned, and this is particularly true when angioplasty is contemplated in difficult or dangerous circumstances (e.g. coronary PTA or PTA of a single kidney).

There are many different techniques for performing angioplasty and the reader is referred to specialist texts for detailed practical information [142,143,144]. The basic method consists of passing a guiding catheter (which will often have been employed for preliminary arteriography) to a site from which a guidewire can be negotiated through the region to be dilated. An injection of contrast medium delineates the exact length and position of the lesion and its proximal and distal limits are defined with radio-opaque markers so the site of the lesion is known thereafter (Fig. 98.17A). The guide-wire and catheter are then manipulated through the stenosis, the wire withdrawn and an injection of contrast medium (preferably low-osmolality!) made to show that the lesion has been safely negotiated and that the 'run-off' remains intact (Fig. 98.17B, C, D). The guidewire (exchange wire) is then replaced so that its tip lies well distal to the abnormal segment, and the original catheter (if not itself an angioplasty catheter) is replaced by a balloon catheter of appropriate dimensions without altering the position of the wire. The balloon is then manipulated into the area of stenosis (defined by the markers) and inflated (Fig. 98.17E, F). The balloon should be fully deflated before any further attempt is made to alter its position. Other methods include the use of small balloon catheters passed co-axially through a larger guiding catheter (the method used in coronary angioplasty), and pre-shaped balloon catheters (e.g. Cobra; Sidewinder) which obviate the requirement for an exchange technique. A very wide variety of guide-wires is available for angioplasty including straight wires, 'mini' J-wires (1.5 mm), 'angioplasty' J-wires (Fig. 98.17), and torque wires, all of which may help to negotiate a diseased arterial segment; and *heavy-duty* wires that are less likely to buckle and become displaced during difficult catheter introductions and exchanges. Many different catheters are available for angioplasty and the catheter selected will depend on the site and nature of the lesion to be dilated: as balloons vary in both their calibre and distensible length, both the length of the stenosis and the estimated 'normal' diameter of the artery in which it is situated must be taken into account.

Radiologists vary in their attitudes towards balloon inflation and pressure monitoring devices. Various pressure pumps are available for mechanically inflating angioplasty balloons which allow for rapid inflation at a pre-selected pressure and rapid and complete deflation; many operators, however, prefer to use manual inflation with a 10 ml syringe loaded with dilute contrast medium. Balloon inflation pressures can be monitored with a pressure gauge interposed between the syringe and the catheter. Inflation can be controlled and kept within the pressure limits recommended by the catheter manufacturer. As with the automatic pumps, however, many operators regard such devices as cumbersome and superfluous and prefer to rely on a combination of manual judgement of resistance to inflation, and the fluoroscopic appearances of the contrast-filled balloon to assess how the procedure should be conducted. There is no general agreement as to the ideal way to inflate an angioplasty balloon: some advocate one or two successive dilatations lasting 30 seconds or more; others rely on multiple short bursts of inflation. With regard to the calibre of dilatation some operators advocate inflation to the size of the predicted 'normal' for the artery concerned; others believe in over-inflation to produce adequate stretching of the arterial wall.

The mechanism whereby angioplasty increases the effective lumen of blood vessels is not fully understood, but it is probable that it involves some change in the mechanical structure of the vessel wall rather than a simple flattening and redistribution of atheroma [139,146]. Desquamation of superficial plaque elements occurs with splitting of the plaque and cracking and dehiscence of the intima and media. The actual increase in calibre that occurs is probably due to overstretching and/or rupture of the tunica intima and tunica media [145]. The disruption of the intima and media accounts for the irregular intraluminal appearance of a vessel on post-angioplasty arteriography (Fig. 98.18, see also Fig. 98.21) and this rather worrying picture should not be mistaken for dissection; it is a 'normal' result of a successful procedure. The restoration of pulsatile flow through a previously stenosed segment often continues the beneficial effect started by the dilatation, and the angiographic appearances may continue to improve for weeks or months after the procedure. It has been suggested that the mechanical disruption of atheroma may even assist in its subsequent removal by the body [104].

Low osmolality contrast media should be used for transluminal angioplasty procedures; they are relatively painless (an important consideration in the 'slow-flow' situations encountered in the technique), and they are less injurious to the endothelium than conventional media. In the case of renal, coronary and cerebral vessels the adverse effects of contrast medium on the organs concerned are also minimized by avoiding the conventional agents.

Digital subtraction angiography is an invaluable aid for transluminal angioplasty. It provides multiple, rapid, subtracted images; allows 'road-mapping' on a second television monitor; and allows good images to be acquired using only small quantities of diluted contrast medium.

When deciding on the possible benefit an angioplasty may confer it can be helpful to attempt some quantitative assessment of haemodynamic parameters such as pressure and flow in the vascular region affected by the procedure. Such measurements are also important clinically and academically for evaluating the effects of an angioplasty procedure, both short-term and long-term. *Non-invasive* techniques for assessing the effects of angioplasty include Doppler ultrasound methods, and pulse-volume recordings. *Direct* pressure measurements can be made proximal and

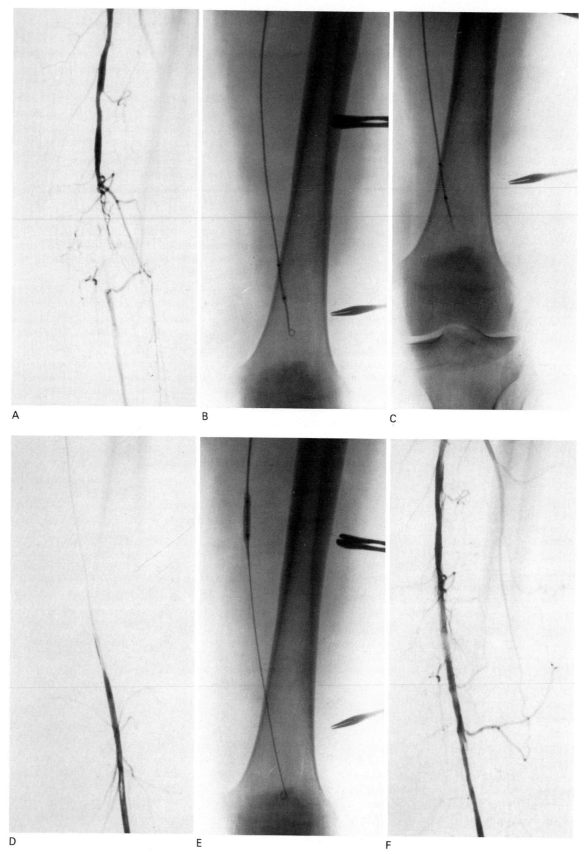

Fig. 98.17A, B, C, D, E & F Percutaneous transluminal angioplasty in a case of superficial femoral artery occlusion. (A) A preliminary arteriogram shows the extent of the occlusion. (B) Radio-opaque markers delineate the proximal and distal limits of the occlusion and an 'angioplasty' J-wire (tip forms complete circle) has been used to guide a catheter through the occlusion without creating a false passage. A wide variety of guide-wires and catheters are available for negotiating such occlusions. (C) The wire has been withdrawn. (D) An injection of contrast medium (iohexol) shows that the occlusion has been safely negotiated and that the 'run-off' is intact. (E) The wire is re-introduced and a balloon catheter used to inflate the area of occlusion. (F) A final arteriogram shows successful re-canalization of the occluded segment.

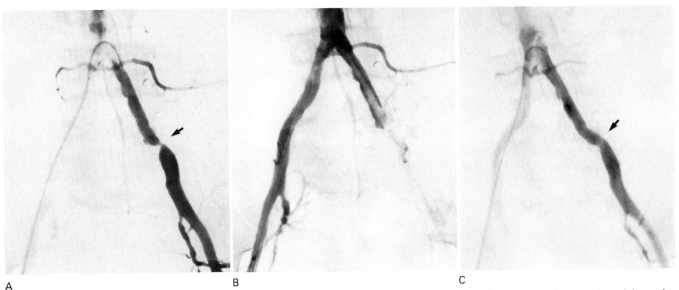

A   B   C

Fig. 98.18A, B & C   Dilatation of an iliac stenosis. (A) The stenosis (arrowed) is delineated by an arteriogram using the contralateral femoral approach. (B) The stenosis is dilated using a balloon catheter introduced from the ipsilateral groin. (C) A post-dilatation study shows some intimal irregularity at the site of the angioplasty (arrow), but the calibre of the vessel at this site is now significantly increased in comparison with (A).

distal to a stenosis before and after angioplasty using two catheters (Fig. 98.18) or a multiple lumen catheter. Providing care is taken not to compromise the pressure readings with the obstruction produced by the catheter itself (which may be difficult or impossible to avoid), this information can provide accurate and objective evidence of the pressure gradient across a stenosis and whether or not it is likely to be haemodynamically significant. Further information can be obtained by using the technique in association with flow augmentation across the stenosis using vasodilator drugs or ischaemic reactive hyperaemia [145]. Following angioplasty direct pressure measurements are more useful than the arteriographic appearances in evaluating the effect of the procedure.

Considerable differences exist in the attitudes of radiologists to the use of antiplatelet, anticoagulant and fibrinolytic drugs as adjunctive treatment to PTA. A typical regimen might include *aspirin* for 24–48 hours prior to the procedure and for several months following (or for life), and *heparin* administered parenterally at the time of the procedure, and for 24–48 hours subsequently. Many radiologists, however, use heparin only rarely, and very few ever use fibrinolytic agents such as streptokinase. Other operators use heparin routinely and put the patient on long-term anticoagulants following the procedure. The interested reader is referred to specialist articles for details of such adjunctive therapy [142,144], and in view of the rapidly changing fashions in this field, would be well advised to consult the current literature on the subject.

Clinical applications of PTA

Transluminal angioplasty has been applied to vessels in most areas of the body and in situations where it is technically safe and feasible, the indications for its use are, broadly speaking, similar to those for surgery. At first angioplasty was often reserved for cases where surgery was contraindicated or might be hazardous (e.g. poor 'anaesthetic-risk' patients), but it is becoming increasingly clear that in many circumstances PTA is to be regarded as the preferred method of treatment because of its competitive success rate, low morbidity and reduced in-patient time.

a. Lower extremity PTA

Vascular occlusive disease in the lower limb is a common clinical problem and PTA has proved to be an invaluable form of therapy in appropriately selected patients. Isolated stenoses of the *iliac vessels* respond well to angioplasty and the technique can be performed from a retrograde ipsilateral approach (Fig. 98.18) or a contralateral approach across the aortic bifurcation. Some radiologists consider total occlusion of the common iliac artery to be a contraindication to PTA. Others report successful cases [144] but there is no doubt that recanalization of an iliac occlusion is likely to be a technically more difficult and dangerous task than the comparable procedure in a femoral artery, and the technique probably should not be attempted unless there are pressing clinical reasons to do so. Localised stenoses of the *superficial femoral, deep femoral origin* or *popliteal* arteries are all suitable for PTA, and occlusions of the superficial femoral artery up to 10 cm in length can usually be successfully dilated (Fig. 98.17); it is technically feasible to traverse even longer occlusions than this, but the long-term results of such procedures are disappointing. Using smaller co-axial balloon catheters even *tibial* arteries can be dilated successfully providing a suitable 'run-off' is present below the stenosis. In a co-operative study of the results of femoro-popliteal

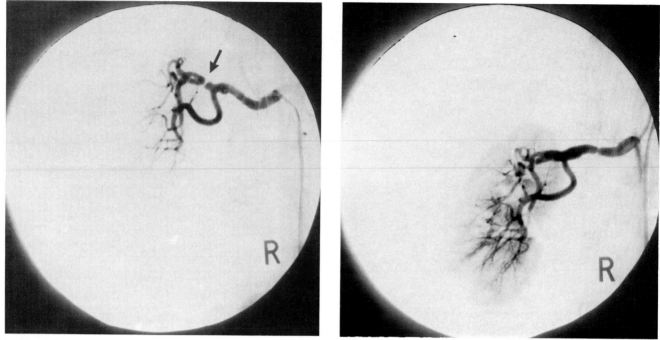

Fig. 98.19A & B   Renal artery angioplasty. The patient (a 40-year-old woman) presented with severe hypertension and a right renal bruit. Selective renal arteriography (A) showed a branch stenosis in the upper pole artery (arrow). Transluminal angioplasty was successful (B), and the patient's blood pressure returned to normal within 24 hours.

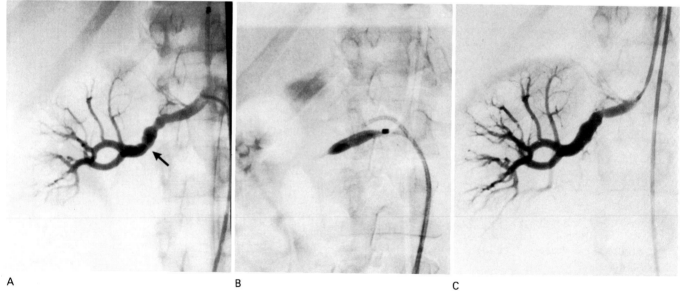

Fig. 98.20A, B & C   Renal angioplasty in a 33-year-old female patient with fibromuscular hyperplasia and severe hypertension. (A) Renal arteriogram showing 'string of pearls' appearance. Arrow indicates site of maximum obstruction as indicated by direct pressure measurements. (B) The stenosis is dilated. (C) Post-dilatation study. The former region of principal obstruction is much wider in calibre. The patient's blood pressure remains normal (off all therapy) three years later.

PTA from several centres the procedure was successful in 74% with a failure rate of 15% and an early re-occlusion rate of 11% [142].

b. Renal PTA

Transluminal angioplasty is an extremely useful technique in the management of renovascular hypertension [137,139,144]. In one large series of 54 procedures an excellent outcome was reported in 44%, a satisfactory outcome in 48% and failure in only 8% [137].

The technique has not only proved successful in cases of atheromatous stenosis (Fig. 98.19) but also in fibromuscular dysplasia (Fig. 98.20) and other disorders. It should be borne in mind that renal function is put at risk by renal artery stenosis, and the preservation of renal function may be an indication in its own for for PTA, irrespective of the effect on blood pressure. Renal angioplasty should always be undertaken with great caution because of the risk of irreversible renal damage, and the procedure should be performed in co-ordination with the vascular or transplant surgeon so that prompt surgical intervention is available in case of disaster.

Stenosis of the artery supplying a *transplanted kidney* is a particularly unfortunate occurrence since it may not only cause hypertension but can compromise the precious function of the transplanted organ. Percutaneous angioplasty of the transplant renal artery is often more difficult than it is in a native kidney, but is usually successsful [144]. A satisfactory outcome earns the undying gratitude of both the patient and the transplant surgeon since re-operation can often be very difficult owing to dense scarring at the site of the previous operation. Transplants anastomosed to the internal iliac artery are best approached from the contralateral groin (Fig. 98.21), while transplants attached to the external iliac artery can often be more easily catheterized using an ipsilateral approach.

c. Percutaneous transluminal coronary angioplasty (PTCA)

The first coronary angioplasty in humans was performed by Gruntzig in 1977 [143] and since then has rapidly become established as one of the standard forms of treatment for coronary artery disease; few methods of therapy in medicine can have become so popular and widely accepted by the medical establishment in so short a period. The technique employs a guiding catheter introduced through the groin or the arm, and an inner balloon catheter which passes co-axially through the guiding catheter into the coronary artery. Details of the technique are given in specialist texts [143], and not considered further here. The potential complications of the technique may be serious and sudden (e.g. complete coronary occlusion) and it should only be performed when a cardiac surgeon and operating theatre are available for immediate intervention. An example of PTCA is shown in Figure 98.22.

d. PTA at miscellaneous sites

Angioplasty has been successfully used in a variety of vascular sites other than the principal areas of application already mentioned. *Aortic* stenoses can be dilated [144] though in the adult this may require the use of two balloon catheters inflated simultaneously (Fig. 98.23)! *Internal iliac PTA* may cure impotence in some patients, and the dilatation of *coeliac* or *mesenteric* vessels can relieve visceral angina in selected cases. Other vessels in which PTA has been performed include the *subclavian* artery and even the basilar artery [147].

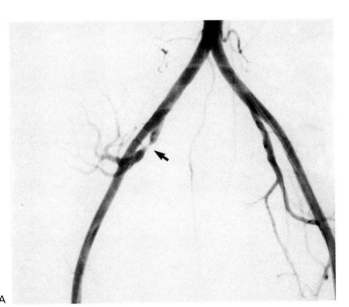 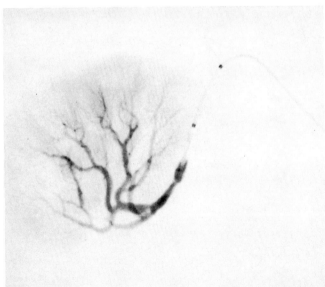

Fig. 98.21A & B Transplant artery stenosis. (A) A severe stenosis is shown in the artery to a transplant kidney (arrow). (B) Post-angioplasty study. The stenosis has been dilated using an approach from the opposite groin across the aortic bifurcation.

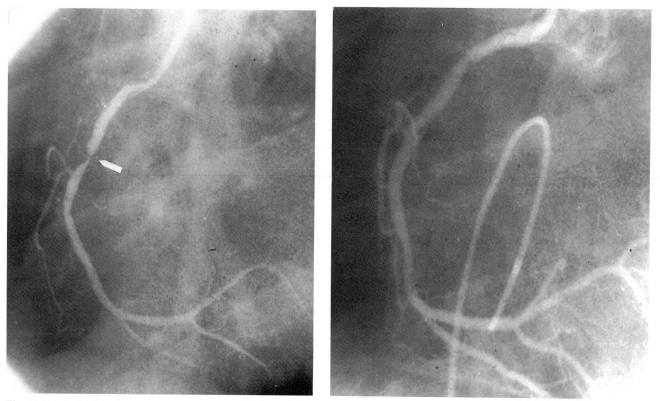

Fig. 98.22A & B   Percutaneous coronary artery angioplasty. (A) A stenosis in the coronary artery is shown by preliminary arteriography. (B) Post-angioplasty appearances. (Figure by courtesy of Dr D. C. Cumberland.)

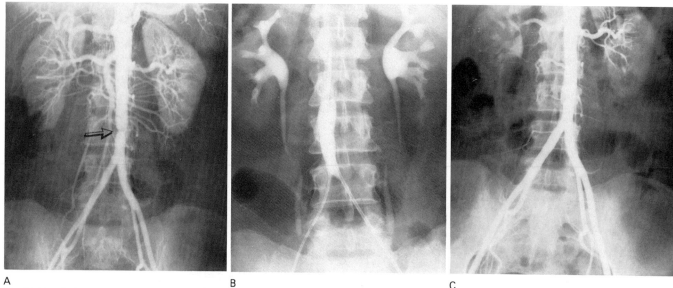

A   B   C

Fig. 98.23A, B & C   Aortic angioplasty. (A) A preliminary aortogram shows a stenosis of the lumbar aorta (arrow). (B) Two 8 mm balloon catheters (one from each groin) have been inflated simultaneously in the stenosis. (C) The procedure was successful arteriographically and clinically. (Figure by courtesy of Dr T. Buist.)

PTA can be used as a pre-operative adjunct to surgery [144] and has also proved valuable as a post-operative technique for the dilatation of graft stenoses and anastomotic stenoses [144].

Complications of PTA

No invasive technique is without its complications and transluminal angioplasty is no exception to this rule. Problems may arise at the puncture site (haemorrhage, thrombosis, pseudoaneurysm); in the target vessel and its distribution territory (embolization, thrombosis, dissection, perforation, occlusion), or with the catheter itself (balloon rupture). Rupture of an angioplasty balloon is not in itself hazardous in most cases; three secondary complications may arise however: firstly, the irregular contours of the ruptured balloon may damage the vessel wall that has just been dilated as the balloon is removed; secondly, a fragment of the balloon may become detached and embolize somewhere in the local vascular tree (uncommon); and thirdly, the balloon may rupture circumferentially, fold over itself or ruck, and then be impossible to remove from the vascular tree without an arteriotomy.

The most feared theoretical complication of PTA — peripheral embolization from atheromatous deposits — seems to be suprisingly infrequent in practice. The incidence of peripheral embolization following femoral artery dilatation is 3–5%, but in the majority of these cases the emboli are not demonstrable angiographically and may not result in clinically apparent ischaemia [144]. The incidence of groin *haematoma* following PTA is probably much higher than a perusal of the literature would suggest (see Fig. 94.9 p. 1999). Personal communications to the author from a number of operators suggest that puncture site bleeding is a not infrequent event following balloon dilatation, and the post-procedural care of PTA patients should include frequent and conscientious inspection of the wound site.

3. Vascular embolization

The deliberate occlusion of arteries, veins or abnormal vascular spaces by embolic material injected through a selectively positioned catheter is one of the major therapeutic applications of interventional radiology. The technique can usually be performed through a percutaneous approach under local analgesia, making it an attractive alternative to surgery in those patients with appropriate lesions in whom general anaesthesia would pose a serious risk. There are also certain lesions amenable to embolization for which no other effective form of medical or surgical therapy exists at present; it thus represents a true advance in our therapeutic capability.

a. Embolic materials and techniques

Many different materials have been used to embolize blood vessels. They range from autologous substances such as fat, blood clot, and chopped muscle fragments, to artificial materials such as wool, cotton, steel balls, plastic or glass beads, tantalum powder, silicone compounds, radioactive particles, sterile absorbable gelatin sponge (Sterispon, Gelfoam), oxidized cellulose (Oxycel), steel coils, alcohol, lyophilised human dura mater (Lyodura), microfibrillar collagen (Avitene), collagen fibrils (Tachotop), polyvinyl alcohol sponge (PVA; Ivalon), Barium-impregnated silicon spheres (Biss), detachable balloons and liquids such as alcohol, acrylates, silicones or polyurethanes.

Ideally an embolic substance should be non-toxic, thrombogenic, easy to inject down vascular catheters, radio-opaque, rapid and permanent in effect, sterile and readily available in different shapes or sizes at the time of the procedure. None of the currently available substances meets all these requirements and the choice of the material is normally determined by the nature of the embolism required, and the preference or experience of the operator [148,149].

Sterispon is a useful, readily available material which is easy and relatively safe to use; it may sometimes produce only a temporary effect, however, and a situation where permanent obliteration of flow is necessary may call for the use of dura mater [148,150,151], PVA, steel coils and other mechanical devices [152,153], balloons [154,155] and iso-butyl-2-cyanocrylate [156,157]. The latter substance sets so quickly in contact with blood that is carries the risk of incorporating the catheter tip in the embolus, and there is no doubt that it should only be used by experienced operators. Various types of resins and polymers with more controllable setting characteristics are currently under development.

Other new developments include the use of electro-coagulation, and the use of direct percutaneous embolization through a needle in areas inaccessible to a vascular catheter. Detailed descriptions of the radiological techniques employed in embolization are unnecessary in this context, but a few important points should be noted:

(i) Embolization should always be preceded by high quality angiography to define precisely the vascular territory under consideration, and its anastomotic communications. Subtraction films may be helpful in areas containing complex bony structures.

(ii) Embolizing catheters should be sited as selectively as possible to avoid the unintentional embolization of adjacent vascular territories. Special catheter systems such as steerable catheters or co-axial catheters may be necessary to achieve the necessary degree of selectivity, and failure to obtain a satisfactory catheter position will require the procedure to be abandoned.

(iii) The likely route of any 'overspill' of emboli should be noted during preliminary angiography. Reflux of emboli into other vessels occurs very easily as flow progressively diminishes in the embolized bed and this hazard is best avoided by injecting emboli in small quantities at a time under constant fluoroscopic control or by the use of a balloon catheter (see below).

(iv) Non-opaque emboli should always be injected in contrast medium so that they are visible as filling defects during the injection sequence. A video-recorder is an added safety precaution if available since the course and destination of the emboli injected in each bolus can be recorded, and then immediately reviewed before the next phase of the embolization is undertaken. If *digital subtraction angiography* is available then subtracted vascular images can be instantly reviewed and a 'road-map' of a selectively catheterized artery can be used to guide the operator on a second TV monitor.

(v) Particular care is necessary in certain areas (e.g. CNS, lower GI tract, peripheral limb vessels); where there has been previous surgery (which may have reduced potential collateral circulation to a region); and where there is pre-existing vascular insufficiency (e.g. atheroma).

(f) It may be necessary to employ a balloon catheter in some situations [158]. This may be used either to reduce flow through the bed to be embolized, or as a temporary obstruction to flow in nearby vessels supplying normal structures when there seems a potential danger of emboli entering such vessels. These balloons can either be employed in vessels distal to those being embolized (e.g. to protect digital vessels when embolizing at the wrist), or at a site proximal to the embolism to prevent the possible reflux of emboli (e.g. in the renal artery to prevent reflux into the aorta) [159].

Catheters with detachable balloons are also available; the effects of inflating such a balloon *in situ* can be observed and if the results of this test inflation are satisfactory the balloon is detached and the catheter withdrawn [160]. Balloons can also be used to 'float' small catheters into vessels which are inaccessible to conventional guidance systems.

b. Indications for therapeutic arterial embolization.

(i) Acute bleeding

Embolization to prevent acute bleeding can be used to obviate surgery in difficult or dangerous situations (particularly in poor-risk patients or those with coagulation disorders), and may be life-saving in cases of massive haemorrhage from surgically inaccessible lesions.

The technique has been used extensively in the management of *gastrointestinal bleeding*. Major branches in the coeliac territory such as the left gastric, hepatic, gastro-duodenal or gastro-epiploic arteries can be individually embolized with very little risk of infarction of normal viscera owing to the rich collateral blood supply in the upper gastrointestinal tract. Ischaemic necrosis can occur, however [161], and the risk of this is greatly increased if multiple simultaneous embolizations are performed, if there is pre-existing arterial disease, or if previous surgery has compromised the available collateral circulation. The method can be used to control acute bleeding from Mallory-Weiss tears, peptic ulcers (see Fig. 94.72), tumours,

trauma (Fig. 98.24), aneurysms, vascular malformations and iatrogenic bleeding due to recent biopsy or surgery [148,162,163,164,165]. Bleeding from varices can also be controlled by embolization, access to the portal venous system being achieved by a percutaneous transhepatic approach [166,167]. Bleeding in the *liver* (post-traumatic, post-operative, post-biopsy) is particularly difficult for the surgeon to locate and control. Therapeutic embolization of an intra-hepatic bleeding source can be a life-saving manoeuvre (Fig. 98.25)

It is more hazardous to embolize lesions in the lower gastrointestinal tract than in the stomach and duodenum. This is because less reliance can be placed on the existence of adequate alternative arterial pathways, particularly in the splenic flexure and descending colon. Although there are case reports of successful colonic embolization, the procedure is probably inadvisable in most cases.

The *renal* arteries are readily catheterised and branch arteries can be selectively embolized to control bleeding. The technique has been used in post-biopsy haemorrhage, post-operative bleeding [168], renal trauma [164], and bleeding tumours. Sometimes embolization provides the only alternative to nephrectomy [169], a particularly important consideration where only a single functioning kidney is present.

Embolization can be used very effectively in other types of bleeding including post-traumatic bleeding [170], especially from pelvic fractures [164,171,172], haemoptysis [173] epistaxis [174,175], gynaecological haemorrhage [176] and post-biopsy bleeding (Fig. 98.26).

(ii) Tumours

Embolization is used in three principal ways to assist in the management of neoplasms.

1. Definitive. Benign tumours can sometimes be successfully treated by embolization alone. Examples include simple tumours of vascular origin (e.g. haemangiomas), endocrine tumours such as parathyroid adenomas [177] and benign bone tumours [178]. Figure 98.27 shows the embolization of a benign hepatic angioma.

2. Pre-operative embolization. This technique has been used extensively in renal adenocarcinoma [148,175,176]. The vascular tumour is embolized hours or days before surgical resection to reduce operative blood loss, shorten the duration of the operation, and reduce the risk of dissemination of viable malignant cells by surgical manipulation of the tumour. Many other types of tumour have been embolized pre-operatively including naso-pharyngeal tumours [175], glomus jugulare tumours [150,179], meningiomas [150], chemodectomas [148] and vagal neuromas (Fig. 98.28). Figure 98.29 shows the pre-operative embolization of an osteoclastoma.

3. Palliative embolization. Embolization can be used as a primary mode of treatment in inoperable malignancy [176], and the embolization of metastatic deposits has been shown to extend survival times in patients with advanced disease [180].

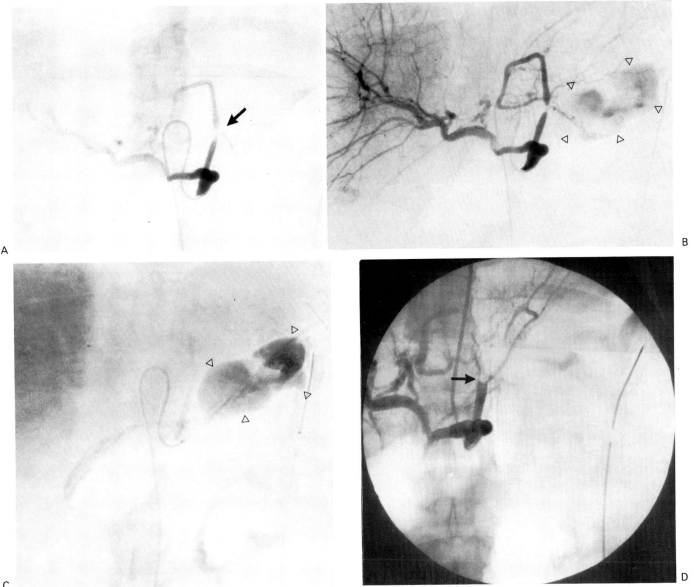

Fig. 98.24A, B, C & D Embolization in post-surgical bleeding. The patient suffered severe trauma to the pancreas, spleen and stomach in a road accident and had a surgical splenectomy. A few hours later he became shocked and a coeliac arteriogram (A) showed active bleeding from the left gastric artery (arrow). The extravasated contrast medium filled a large cavity (B, C, arrowheads). (D) The bleeding point was successfully embolized with a steel coil (arrow).

Embolization can produce a marked improvement in the quality of life of patients with malignant tumours by alleviating unpleasant symptoms such as bleeding (Fig. 98.30), venous obstruction, tracheal compression etc. Radio-active emboli have been used in these circumstances [181], and the embolization can be used as an adjunct to radiotherapy or chemotherapy. The greatest benefit from palliative tumour embolization, however, seems to be derived by patients suffering from the humoral effects of malignant endocrine tumours [148,182]. Metastases from carcinoid tumours and other endocrine neoplasms such as insulinomas and glucagonomas may be slow growing yet cause great distress by virtue of the endocrine syndromes they produce. Such tumours are suit-

able for embolization because they are usually vascular and because they are frequently situated in the liver; this is a favourable site because embolization of the hepatic artery usually deprives the metastases of their principal source of blood, whereas normal liver cells seem able to survive on portal venous blood alone.

Hepatic arterial embolization has several advantages over surgical ligation of the hepatic artery; it can be performed in extremely ill patients under local analgesia; it avoids a laparotomy; the small peripheral arteries can be embolized with showers of tiny emboli making the development of a collateral circulation less likely (a common complication of simple ligation; Sivula and Sipponen 1976); and the

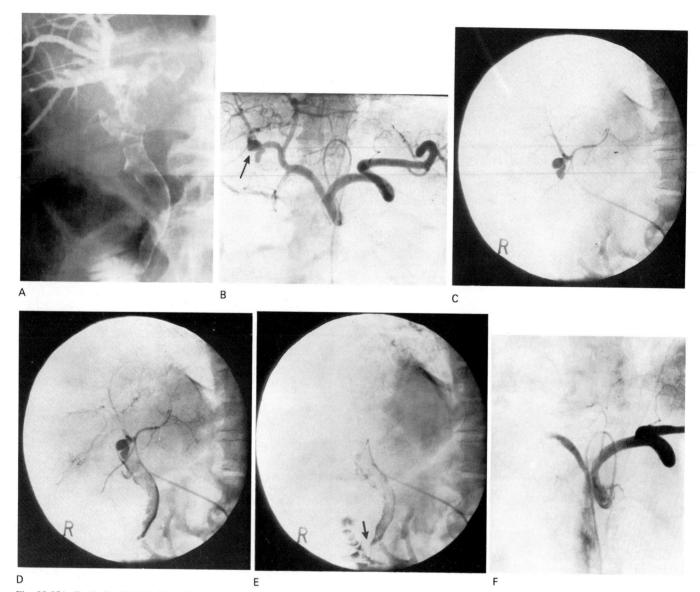

Fig. 98.25A, B, C, D, E & F   Embolization of an intrahepatic aneurysm. The patient had undergone a difficult cholecystectomy three months earlier and now presented after recent jaundice and melaena with active gastrointestinal bleeding. (A) A PTC shows the common bile duct to contain blood clot (filling defects). (B) A coeliac arteriogram shows an aneurysm (presumably post-surgical) in the right hepatic artery (arrow). (C) A selective study shows detail of the aneurysm which is actively bleeding into the biliary tree. (D) and (E) Note the contrast outlining the ampulla and duodenum (arrow) only 12 seconds after the arterial injection of contrast medium. (F) The hepatic artery has been embolized (arrow). The patient was discharged from hospital with no further treatment 1 week after the procedure.

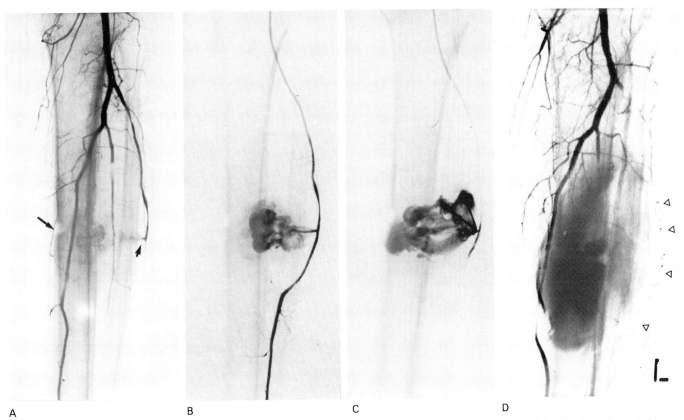

A   B   C   D

Fig. 98.26A, B, C & D Bleeding following an orthopaedic biopsy of the tibia. (A) Popliteal arteriogram showing bleeding from the anterior tibial artery into the tissues of the lower limb (short arrow). Note the bone defect (long arrow) indicated the site of the orthopaedic drill biopsy; the biopsy was clearly not restricted to bony structures! (B, C) Selective anterior tibial arteriogram showing active bleeding into the leg. (D) The anterior tibial artery has been embolized with a series of coils (arrowheads). Note that some emboli have been placed *distal* to the bleeding point to prevent bleeding retrogradely via foot collaterals.

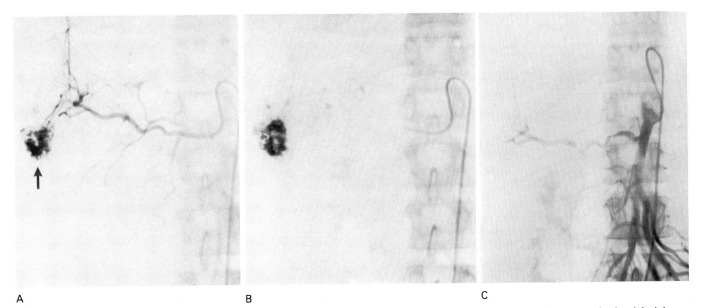

A   B   C

Fig. 98.27A, B & C Embolization of an hepatic angioma. (A) A selective right hepatic arteriogram shows a vascular tumour in the right lobe (arrowed). (B) Late film showing tumour 'blush'.
(C) The lesion has been embolized. Note that the hepatic artery arises anomalously from the superior mesenteric artery — an important technical consideration with regard to the safety of embolization.

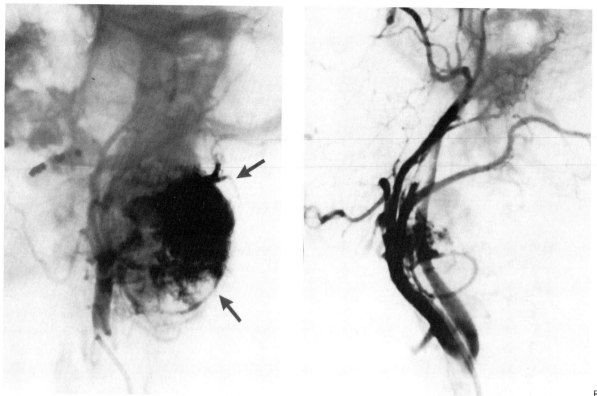

Fig. 98.28A & B Pre-operative embolization of a vagal neuroma. A preliminary external carotid arteriogram (A) shows the very vascular tumour high in the neck (arrows). A common carotid study (B) following embolization shows the tumour circulation to have been occluded. The lesion was successfully removed two days later with minimal intraoperative blood loss.

procedure may be repeated as necessary to deal with fresh tumour growth or the recanalization of prevously embolised vessels. Figure 94.48 p. 2024 shows an example of the therapeutic devascularization of massive hepatic metastases from a malignant glucagonoma, an intervention that produced a striking improvement in the clinical picture owing to the resulting reduction in blood glucagon levels. Figure 98.31 shows the embolization of a liver full of secondary carcinoid tumour. The patient experienced immediate relief from her symptoms, which included persistent flushing and intractable diarrhoea.

(iii) Vascular abnormalities

Vascular malformations, arteriovenous shunts, benign tumours of vascular origin, and aneurysms in certain sites are often treated most appropriately by embolization. They usually present formidable problems to the surgeon by virtue of their vascularity and (in the case of malformations and tumours), their tendency to recur owing to the enlargment of previously undetectable collateral vessels. These lesions may affect the patient in a variety of ways including serious disfigurement, bleeding, pressure symptoms, and (in the case of arterio-venous shunts) cardiac failure. The management

of arteriovenous malformations and fistulae has proved to be one of the most successful applications of the technique of therapeutic embolization and it has been used throughout the body for such lesions [150,151,179,183,184]. Even if embolization is inappropriate as a definitive form of treatment in a particular case, it may be a valuable pre-operative manoeuvre to reduce the vascularity of the lesion before surgical removal.

Figure 98.32 shows a benign tibial haemangioma which had caused extensive bone destruction and fracture of the bone was imminent. Therapeutic embolization has caused complete regression of the lesion and a regrowth of bone into the affected area. Figure 98.33 shows an example of embolization at the base of the skull. The patient suffered from a post-traumatic arteriovenous fistula between the ascending pharyngeal and the jugular bulb which caused tinnitus. The surgical task of closing such a fistula would have been formidable, but embolization was successfully performed under local anaesthesia using a right femoral approach.

Surgery in arteriovenous malformations can be difficult and dangerous. Embolization either alone or in combination with surgery is often a preferable therapeutic option. If a surgeon ligates the feeding arteries to a vascular malformation, collateral vessels will continue to supply the lesion but it may be difficult or impossible for the radiologist to embolize the lesion because of the small calibre or the

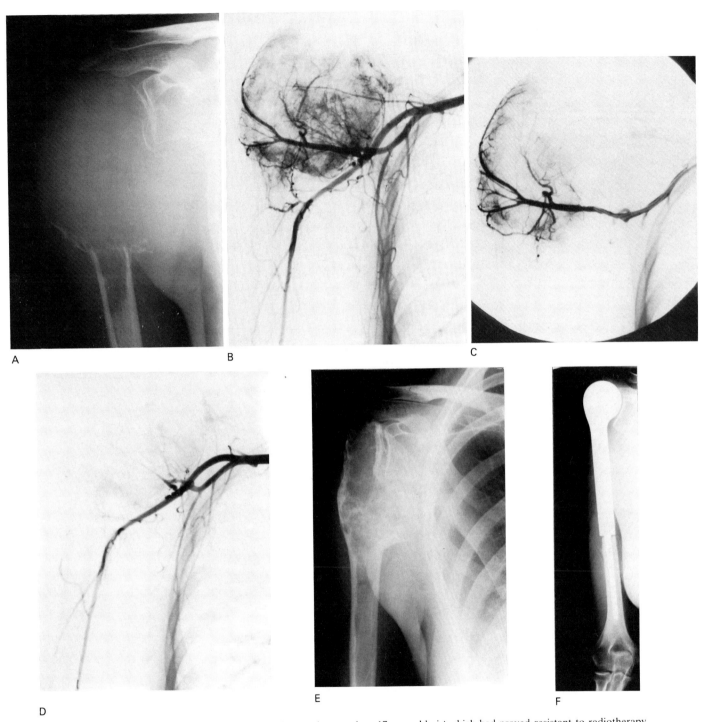

Fig. 98.29A, B, C, D, E & F Embolization of a humeral osteoclastoma in a 17-year-old girl which had proved resistant to radiotherapy. (A) Plain radiography showing soft tissue mass and extensive bone destruction by a giant-cell tumour. (B) Axillary arteriogram showing tumour circulation. (C) Selective catheterization of one of the principal feeding vessels to the lesion. This and the other feeding arteries were occluded. (D) Post-embolization arteriogram. (E) Plain radiograph three months after the embolization. Note the disappearance of the soft tissue mass (cf 98.28A) and the regrowth of bone in the humeral head. (F) The improvement engendered by embolization enabled reconstructive surgery to be performed. A shoulder replacement was successfully carried out.

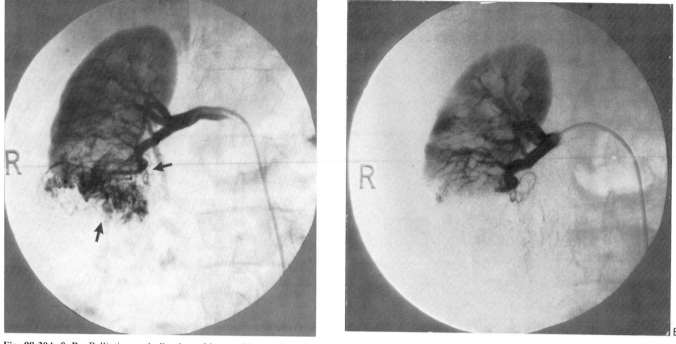

Fig. 98.30A & B   Palliative embolization of inoperable renal carcinoma producing severe bleeding. (A) Renal arteriogram showing tumour circulation (arrows). (B) Post-embolization study: the pathological circulation has been selectively occluded leaving the normal renal circulation intact.

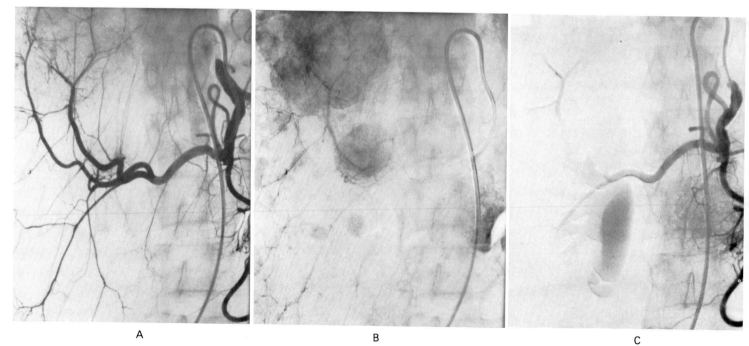

Fig. 98.31A, B & C   Hepatic embolization for secondary carcinoid tumour. (A) Early arterial phase of study. The liver is enlarged. (B) Late arterial/parenchymal phase. Multiple tumour deposits show as vascular densities in the liver substance. (C) The entire lobe has been embolized.

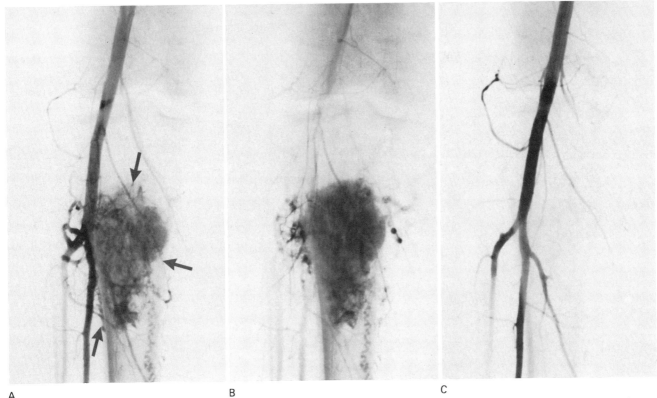

A   B   C

Fig. 98.32A, B & C Embolization of a tibial haemangioma. (A) Early arterial phase of popliteal arteriogram showing vascular tumour in upper tibia (arrows). (B) Late arterial phase; the tumour circulation is much more conspicuous. (C) Post-embolization study: all the branches feeding the haemangioma have been occluded.

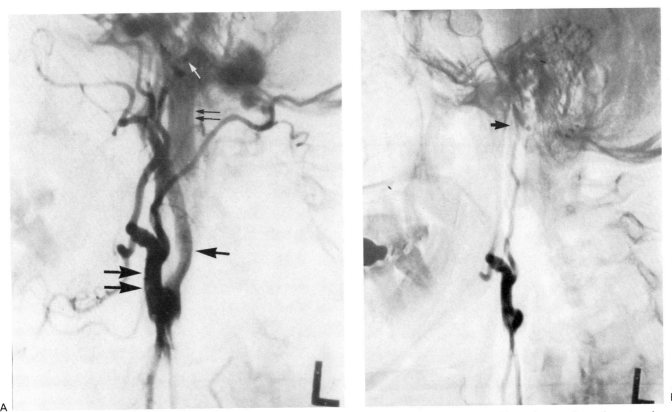

A   B

Fig. 98.33A & B Embolization of an ascending pharyngeal-internal jugular fistula. (A) An external carotid arteriogram shows the external carotid artery (double large arrows), and reflux into the internal carotid artery (single large arrow). A branch of the ascending pharyngeal artery (white arrow) is communicating with the jugular bulb and causing early opacification of the internal jugular vein (double small arrows). This post-traumatic lesion was causing continuous tinnitus in a 24 year-old woman. (B) The distal segment of the ascending pharyngeal artery (arrow) has been embolized from the groin under local anaesthesia) with abolition of the arterio-venous shunt.

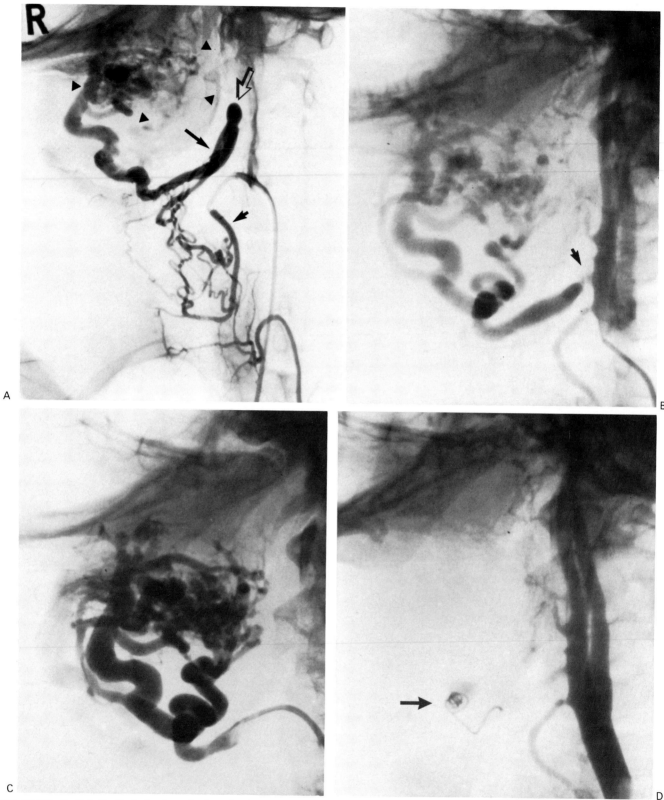

Fig. 98.34A, B, C & D Embolization of a lingual AVM where the lingual artery has been previously ligated. (A) Superior thyroid arteriogram (short arrow) shows collateral vessels feeding into previously ligated lingual artery (long arrow), which continues to feed the arteriovenous malformation (arrowheads). Note the ligated stump of the lingual artery (hatched arrow). Attempted embolization from the superior thyroid artery would simply block the collateral vessels and leave the AVM unaffected. (B) A vascular surgeon has regrafted the lingual artery back on to the external carotid artery. The graft is arrowed. (C) The embolizing catheter can now be passed through the graft and into the malformation. (D) The lesion has been successfully embolized. The steel coil (arrow) was only inserted after complete peripheral occlusion had been achieved.

inaccessibility of the new feeding vessels. Since it is mandatory to embolize the nidus of such a lesion for a permanent cure to be achieved it may be necessary in those cases for a vascular surgeon to create a *new* vascular pathway into the lesion through which the embolizing catheter can be passed (Fig. 98.34).

Pulmonary arteriovenous communications pose a special problem for the embolist. When a *systemic* embolization is performed the operator endeavours to avoid any embolic material passing through the lesion being embolized; if (as sometimes happens) emboli do pass into the venous system, they become trapped in the pulmonary circulation as small pulmonary emboli and usually produce no observable clinical ill-effects. If any embolic material should pass through a *pulmonary* AVM, however, the effects could be disastrous for the emboli might be carried into any systemic vessel including the coronary arteries or the cerebral arteries. Pulmonary embolization should never be performed therefore with fluid or particulate emboli; the only safe agents to

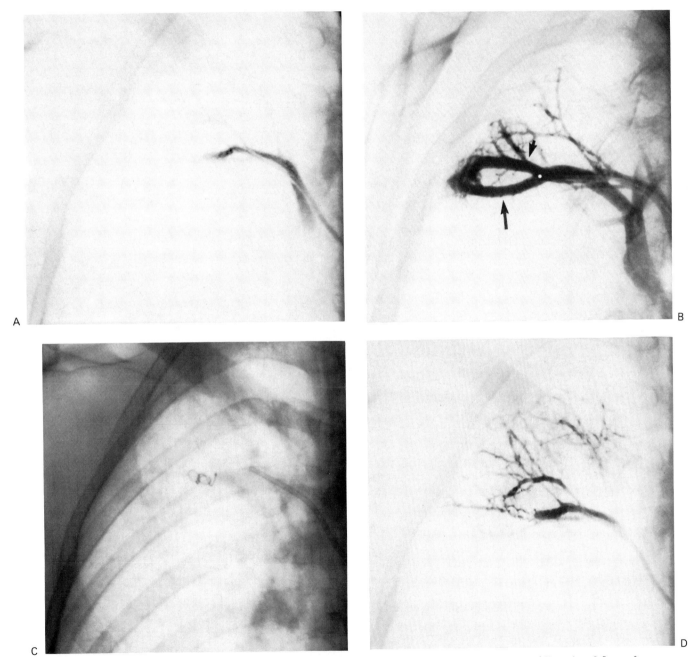

Fig. 98.35A, B, C & D Embolization of a pulmonary AVM. (A) Selective upper lobe pulmonary arteriogram: film taken 0.5 sec after injection of contrast medium. (B) Same study: film taken at 1.5 seconds showing abnormal shunting into large pulmonary vein (artery: short arrow; vein: long arrow). (C) The lesion has been embolized with a steel coil. (D) Post-embolization study: the shunt has been abolished, but considerable flow to the adjacent normal lung has been preserved.

use are detachable balloon catheters [185,186], or steel coils. The balloon or coil should be carefully size-matched to the shunt in question: too small a coil will pass into the systemic system; too large a coil will block an unnecessarily large proportion of the adjacent (normal) pulmonary vascular bed. An example of a pulmonary embolization is given in Figure 98.35.

(iv) Central nervous system

Interventional techniques in the central nervous system constitute a specialised subject that is beyond the scope of this chapter (and certainly this author!). The various methods employed are reviewed in the excellent articles by Berenstein and Kircheff (1981) [18] and Moseley (1983) [188].

(v) Hypersplenism

Splenectomy is indicated in various haematological disorders, but may present a difficult surgical problem owing to the abnormalities of coagulation which are so often a feature of such disorders, or to the presence of other 'poor risk' factors. In these circumstances embolization of the spleen can be performed to obviate surgery [148,153,176,189,190]. In a proportion of patients the procedure produces an abscess in the spleen that subsequently requires surgical drainage. This complication can be minimized by the use of antibiotic prophylaxis, and by performing the embolization in stages separated by suitable intervals.

World experience of this technique is still too limited to form an objective opinion on its clinical value at present. In many patients the procedure obviates surgery, and even in those requiring a later drainage operation embolization has usually improved the haematological status thereby making surgery safer. A cautious summary of the present position would be that splenectomy is the preferred treatment in most patients, but that embolization may be of value in carefully selected cases who present particular problems to the surgeon.

Embolization of the splenic artery has also been performed successfully for the treatment of leaking splenic artery aneurysm. An example of splenic embolization in a young man with idiopathic thrombocytopaenia is shown in Figure 98.36.

Gas may be seen in the spleen (and other embolized organs) following therapeutic embolization (Fig. 98.37). It can be detected on plain radiography, ultrasound or CT scanning and may appear within a few hours of the procedure being performed. The quantities of gas present are extremely variable but may be so large as to give rise to free intra-peritoneal gas [191]. In most cases gas appearing in embolized organs appear to be a relatively benign phenomenon [192,193] and in a large series of hepatic embolizations it was observed to occur in 44% of patients [193], apparently unassociated with any ill effects. There are many different theories as to the origin of this gas: *infection* with gas-producing micro-organisms is obviously a cause in some cases but almost certainly does not account for all the reported instances; introduction of atmospheric gas mixed with particulate emboli at the time of embolization has been postulated but does not account for the occurrence of gas following embolization with liquid materials. Other theories include the production of gas by anaerobic reticulocyte metabolism, or the release of oxygen from haemaglobin trapped in degenerating red cells in the occluded vessels of the embolized organ [191].

(vi) Priapism

Spontaneous priapism is a distressing condition for which medical treatment is ineffective and surgical treatment may result in permanent impotence. Some reports suggest that embolization of the internal pudendal artery is the best treatment for this disorder [194,195]. Early embolization with non-permanent material (e.g. Sterispon) permits detumescence, but allows the prospect of subsequent recovery with restoration of normal sexual function. The procedure should therefore be regarded as a radiological emergency [195].

c. Indications for venous embolization

(i) Varices

Oesophageal and gastric varices can be embolized either to control bleeding in an emergency situation, or as a prophylactic measure to divert blood flow to other collaterals in sites less vulnerable to trauma than the oesophageal or gastric mucosa. The portal vein can be catheterised from the transhepatic, transjugular or transumbilical routes for this purpose; the most commonly used approach is the first of these described by Lunderquist and Vang in 1974 [196], and details of the technique are given in Chapter 52 and in the review article by Keller et al [197]. When medical measures are ineffectual in controlling bleeding from varices therapeutic embolization can be a life-saving procedure [198]. The role of elective variceal obliteration however, is currently the subject of controversy: some groups report good long-term results, while others have experienced a high incidence of recurrent bleeding and other complications [197]. The increasingly successful use of endoscopic variceal injection techniques is a further factor affecting current attitudes to the transhepatic approach for the elective obliteration of varices. The *pros* and *cons* of the method are reviewed in a recent article by Sos [199]. The transhepatic approach to the portal vein can also be used to collect selective blood samples for the localisation of hormonally active tumours [200]; to conduct metabolic studies in the portal circulation [201]; and to perform pancreatic phlebography [202].

(ii) Adrenal venous obliteration

It has been known for many years that the adrenal gland may become infarcted following damage to the vein such as

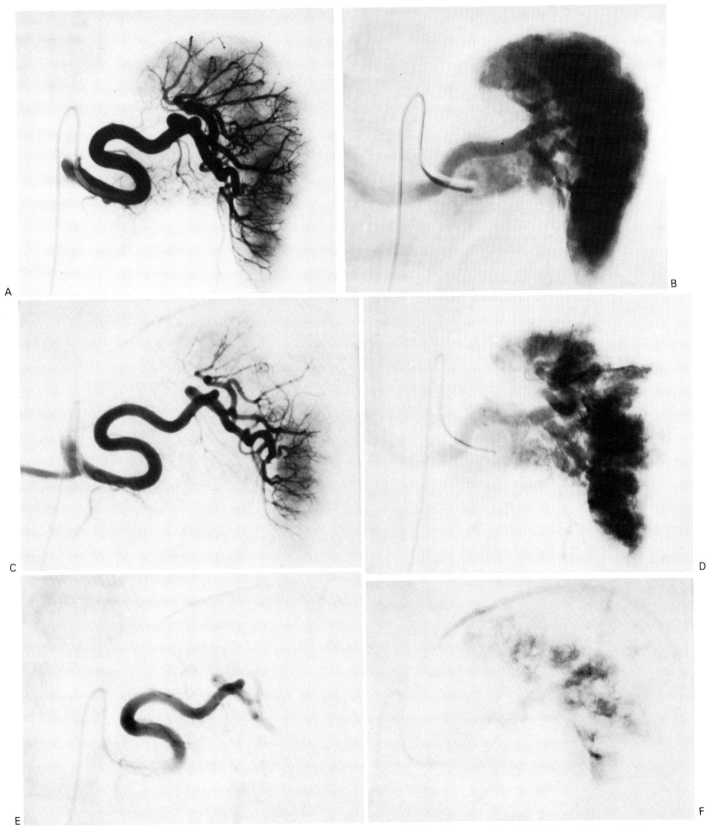

Fig. 98.36A, B, C, D, E & F   Embolization of the spleen in a 25 year-old man with thrombocytopaenia. (A) Splenic arteriogram (pre-embolization). (B) Indirect splenoportogram (pre-embolization). (C) Splenic arteriogram 1 month after partial embolization. (D) Indirect splenoportogram 1 month after partial embolization. (E) Splenic arteriogram after further (final) embolization. (F) Indirect splenoportogram after further (final) embolization. A small proportion of the spleen was left unembolized at the request of the referring physician. This can be embolized subsequently if necessary.

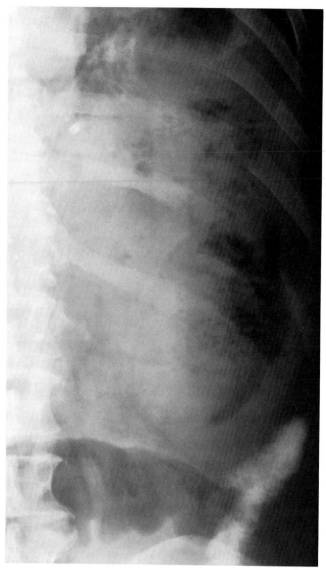

Fig. 98.37 Intraparenchymal gas in a spleen following extensive splenic embolization (not the same patient as in Fig. 98.35).

(iii) Varicocele

Varicocele is associated with sub-fertility and fertility can be restored to a considerable number of patients if the varicocele can be obliterated by embolization of the testicular vein, using the percutaneous approach described in Chapter 95. Embolization is most safely performed using a detachable balloon [208] or a coil, but other embolic agents have also been used. There are a number of important technical and anatomical points to be considered when using the method in order to prevent recurrence of the varicocele; these and other details of technique are discussed by Kaufman et al 1983 [209].

(iv) Arteriovenous malformations

Most arteriovenous malformations and fistulae are embolized using an *arterial* approach for obvious reasons: flow is directed towards the abnormal area; injected emboli impact and are maintained in position by arterial pressure until thrombosis occurs; the risk of venous embolization is small provided due care is observed during the procedure; and repeated arteriograms can be performed to assess the progress of the embolization. Occasionally, however, it may be impossible to embolize a lesion safely using the arterial approach, and it is sometimes possible to achieve success from the venous side because of a more favourable anatomical situation. The risk of pulmonary embolism is obviously very high using the venous approach and the emboli must be safely embedded at the site of the abnormality so that there is no risk of dislodgement (Fig. 98.39). In some circumstances it may even be possible to pass an embolizing catheter from a venous approach *through* a shunt or fistula to the arterial side and embolize from that (more favourable) position.

d. Complications of embolization

The principal complications of embolization are listed in Table 98.4. Details of these complications and techniques for their avoidance are to be found in the specialist texts listed in 'Suggestions for further reading'. The incidence of serious complications following embolization is low provided the procedure is conducted with patience and scrupulous care and that only suitable patients are selected for treatment by the technique.

A *post-embolization syndrome* is commonly experienced by patients who have had an embolization, particularly if a large volume of tissue has been rendered ischaemic. The 'syndrome' is a variable phenomenon but may include fever, discomfort or pain at the site of embolization, leucocytosis, nausea, and a general feeling of being unwell. It may last for only a day or two or up to 10–14 days depending on the nature of the embolization and usually disappears with only symptomatic treatment being required. Care must be taken however, not to dismiss all such symptoms and signs as

rupture or thrombosis and adrenal insufficiency is a well-recognized complication of adrenal phlebography [203]. Deliberate obstruction of the adrenal veins has been used to obliterate adrenal function as an alternative to bilateral surgical adrenalectomy in patients with advanced malignant disease [204,205] and the wedged retrograde injection of contrast medium mixed with sclerosant liquids such as hypertonic dextrose or alcohol has been used in the treatment of Cushings syndromes [206], and primary aldosteronism due to an adrenal adenoma [207]. In some centres patients have undergone severe metabolic crises or died following retrograde adrenal infarction (unpublished personal communications to the author), and the technique should clearly be used only in selected cases with extreme caution, and in co-operation with a skilled medical team.

An example of the venous embolization of a Conn's tumour is shown in Figure 98.38.

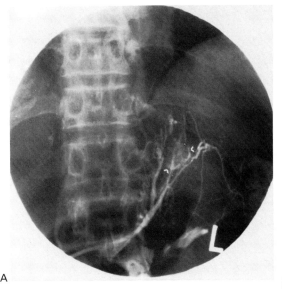

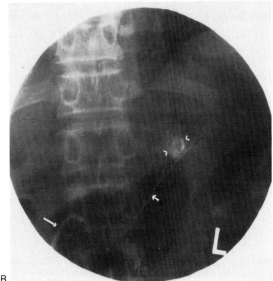

Fig. 98.38A, B & C   Retrograde adrenal venous embolization in a case of primary aldosteronism. (A) Adrenal venogram. The position of the Conn's tumour is indicated by the displacement of veins around it (small arrowheads). (B) A fine (French 3) coaxial catheter (short arrow) has been passed up the adrenal vein from a larger guiding catheter (long arrow). An injection of contrast medium opacifies the tumour retrogradely (arrowheads). (C) The tumour has been ablated with a mixture of contrast medium and ethyl alcohol. This radiograph taken 15 minutes after the injection shows complete stasis in the tumour bed (arrow).

Table 98.4 Complications of embolization

1. **General**
   — usual hazards of superselective arteriography
   — contrast medium reactions

2. **Specific** — *immediate*
   — pain
   — nausea
   — inadvertent embolization of normal structures
   — loss of embolic devices in the vascular system
   — pulmonary embolization through A–V shunts
   — adherence of catheter tip to vessel wall by liquid adhesives
   — reaction to embolic agent (rare)

   — *delayed*
   — pain ⎫
   — fever ⎬ 'post-embolization syndrome'
   — leucocytosis ⎭
   — infection — local
              — systemic
   — tissue necrosis (unintentional)
   — extension of thrombosis beyond embolized area
   — release of humoral substances from infarcted endocrine tissue
   — renal failure (owing to combination of dehydration and massive tissue necrosis)

3. *Death* may occur as a result of one or more of the above complications

simply being part of the syndrome: the same manifestations may be produced by a more serious complication such as infection and the diagnosis of 'post-embolization syndrome' should be made when other treatable causes of the patient's condition have been excluded.

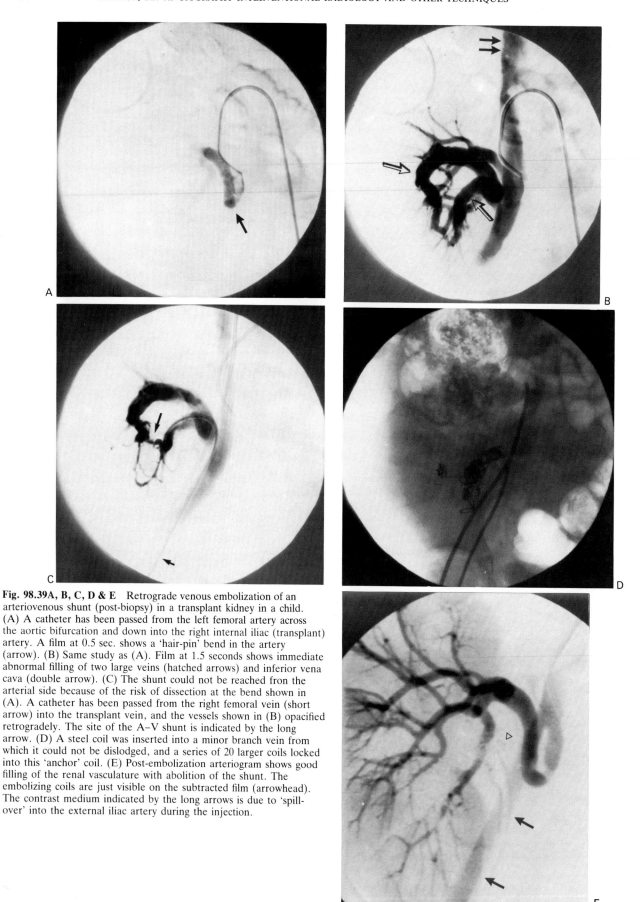

Fig. 98.39A, B, C, D & E Retrograde venous embolization of an arteriovenous shunt (post-biopsy) in a transplant kidney in a child. (A) A catheter has been passed from the left femoral artery across the aortic bifurcation and down into the right internal iliac (transplant) artery. A film at 0.5 sec. shows a 'hair-pin' bend in the artery (arrow). (B) Same study as (A). Film at 1.5 seconds shows immediate abnormal filling of two large veins (hatched arrows) and inferior vena cava (double arrow). (C) The shunt could not be reached from the arterial side because of the risk of dissection at the bend shown in (A). A catheter has been passed from the right femoral vein (short arrow) into the transplant vein, and the vessels shown in (B) opacified retrogradely. The site of the A–V shunt is indicated by the long arrow. (D) A steel coil was inserted into a minor branch vein from which it could not be dislodged, and a series of 20 larger coils locked into this 'anchor' coil. (E) Post-embolization arteriogram shows good filling of the renal vasculature with abolition of the shunt. The embolizing coils are just visible on the subtracted film (arrowhead). The contrast medium indicated by the long arrows is due to 'spillover' into the external iliac artery during the injection.

THE IMPACT OF INTERVENTIONAL TECHNIQUES ON MEDICINE AND RADIOLOGY

The techniques of interventional radiology are now being applied to practically every branch of medicine. The spectrum of techniques ranges from safe effective procedures that have become established as routine methods of management in many centres, to extremely invasive and experimental feats of technical expertise that are still undergoing evaluation in a few specialised units. The discriminating application of interventional methods can bring many benefits; the patient may avoid a general anaesthetic and a surgical operation; alternatively an operation may be postponed until the increased risks imposed by infection, hypovolaemia, or metabolic disturbances have been eradicated or minimized. The surgeon may be saved a difficult or dangerous operation in an unfit patient and, when he eventually operates, his task may be made technically easier by preliminary embolization of an appropriate vascular territory. The physician may be assisted in diagnosis by interventional techniques and treatment may include one of the many therapeutic procedures now available.

There are also considerable potential financial benefits to be derived from interventional radiology. Inpatient time can sometimes be cut drastically — compare for instance the outpatient removal of gallstones with a difficult surgical re-exploration of the biliary system. In many cases where surgery is necessary the preliminary use of an interventional procedure, (for example, percutaneous pyelonephrostomy) may reduce surgical morbidity, and the costs of prolonged post-operative inpatient treatment.

Finally, interventional radiology has played a role in changing the status of radiology itself. It has brought a new dimension of clinical responsibility into radiology which has contributed, together with many other factors, such as the advances in new imaging techniques, towards making radiology into one of the most exciting and rapidly developing branches of modern medicine.

BIBLIOGRAPHY

REFERENCES.

1. Haubek A, Gammelgard J, Gronvall S, Holm H H 1982 Ultrasonically-guided percutaneous puncture and biopsy techniques. In: Wilkins R A, Viamonte M (eds) Interventional radiology. Blackwell Scientific Publications, Oxford, pp 373–408
2. Hancke S, Holm H H, Koch F 1975 Ultrasonically-guided percutaneous fine needle biopsy of the pancreas. Surgery Gynecology and Obstetrics 140:361–364
3. Husband J E, Golding S J 1983 Recent developments in whole body computed tomography. In: Steiner R E (ed) Recent advances in Radiology 7, Churchill Livingstone, Edinburgh, ch 6, pp 88–106
4. Haaga J R, Reich N E, Havrilla T R, Alfidi R J 1977 Interventional CT scanning. Radiologic Clinics of North America 15:449–456
5. Leyden T 1883 Uber infektiose Pneumonie. Dtsch Med Wschr 9:52
6. Greene R E 1981 Transthoracic needle aspiration biopsy. In: Athanasoulis C A, Pfister R C, Greene R E, Roberson G H (eds) Interventional radiology. W B Saunders, Philadelphia, ch 46, pp 587–634
7. Sappington S W, Favourite G O 1936 Lung puncture in lobar pneumonia. Am J Med Sci 191:225
8. Grunze H 1960 A critical review and evaluation of cytodiagnosis in chest diseases. Acta Cytologica IV p 175
9. Dahlgren S, Nordenstrom B 1966 Transthoracic needle biopsy. Year Book Medical Publishers, Chicago
10. Nordenstrom B 1965 A new technique for transthoracic biopsy of lung changes. British Journal of Radiology 38:550
11. Walli A F, McCormackc L J, Zelch M, Reich M E, Elavich C T 1978 Aspiration biopsies of chest lesions. Radiology 127:35–40
12. Sinner W N 1979 Pulmonary neoplasms diagnosed with transthoracic needle biopsy. Cancer 43:1533–1540
13. Allison D J, Hemingway A P 1981 Percutaneous needle biopsy of the lung. British Medical Journal 282:875–878
14. Sargent E N, Turner A F, Gordonson J, Schwinn C P, Pashky O 1974 Percutaneous pulmonary needle biopsy, report of 350 patients. Am J Roentgen 122:758–768
15. House A J S 1979 Biopsy techniques in the investigation of diseases of the lung, mediastinum and chest wall. Radiologic Clinics of North America 17(3):393–412
16. Nordenstrom B 1981 Transthoracic needle biopsy. In: Anacker H, Hullotta U, Rupp N (eds) Percutaneous biopsy in therapeutic vascular occlusion. International Symposium Munchen 1979 Thieme-Stratton, New York
17. Holm H H, Pederson J F, Kristenson A K, Rasmussen S N, Hanke S, Jensen F 1975 Ultrasonically-guided percutaneous puncture. Radiologic Clinics of North America 13:493–503
18. Staab E V, Jaques P F, Partain C L 1979 Percutaneous biopsy in the management of solid intra-abdominal masses of unknown aetiology. Radiologic Clinics of North America 17(3):435
19. Husband J E, Trott P A 1980 CT-guided percutaneous fine needle aspiration of intra-abdominal and pelvic masses. In: Veiga-Pires J A (ed) Intervention radiology. Excerpta Medica, Amsterdam, p 340
20. Mueller P R, Wittenberg J, Ferrucci J T 1981 Fine needle aspiration biopsy of abdominal masses. Seminars in Roentgenology 16:52–61
21. Kline T S, Neal H S 1978 Needle aspiration biopsy: a critical appraisal. Journal of the American Association 239 (1):36–39
22. Lunderquist A 1971 Fine needle aspiration biopsy of the liver. Acta Medica Scandinavica 520:1–28
23. Holm H H, Als O, Gammelgaard J 1978 Percutaneous aspiration biopsy procedures under ultrasonic visualization. In: Taylor K J W (ed) Clinics in diagnostic ultrasound, vol 1. Diagnostic ultrasound in gastrointestinal disease. Churchill Livingstone, New York, pp 137–149
24. Gothlin J H 1976 Post-lymphographic percutaneous fine needle biopsy of lymph nodes guided by fluoroscopy. Radiology 120:205–207
25. Fuchs W A, Vock P, Haertel M 1980 Indications for needle biopsy of abdominal neoplasm guided by ultrasonography and computerised tomography. In: Veiga-Pires J A (ed) Intervention radiology. Excerpta Medica, Amsterdam, pp 335–339
26. Dossetor R S 1980 Use of ultrasound for fluid aspiration and biopsy with particular reference to amniocentesis and renal puncture. In: Veiga-Pires J A (ed) Intervention radiology. Excerpta Medica, Amsterdam, p 402
27. Hancke S, Holm H H, Koch F 1975 Ultrasonically-guided percutaneous fine needle biopsy of the pancreas. Surgery, Gynecology & Obstetrics 140:361–364
28. Doherty F J 1982 Fine needle percutaneous aspiration biopsy of abdominal mass lesions. In: Athanasoulis C A, Pfister R C, Green R E, Roberson G H (eds) Interventional radiology. W B Saunders, Philadelphia, ch 45, pp 568–583

29. Griffiths H J 1979 Interventional Radiology: the musculoskeletal system. Radiologic Clinics of North America 17(3):475

30. Armstrong P, Chalmers A H 1978 Needle aspiration/biopsy of the spine in suspected disc space infection. British Journal of Radiology 51:333–337

31. Deeley T J 1972 The dual biopsy of bone lesions. Clinical Radiology 23:536–540

32. De Santos L A, Lukeman J M, Wallace S, Murray J A, Araya A G 1978 Percutaneous needle biopsy of bone in the cancer patient. American Journal of Roentgenology 130:641–649

33. Legge D, Ennis J T, Dempsey J 1978 Percutaneous needle biopsy in the management of solitary lesions of bone. Clinical Radiology 29:497–500

34. Nordenstrom B 1971 Percutaneous biopsy of vertebrae and ribs. Acta Radiologica Diagnostica 11:113–121

35. Murray W T, Mueller P R 1982 Bone biopsy. In: Athanasoulis C A, Pfister R C, Greene R E, Roberson G H (eds) Interventional radiology. W B Saunders, Philadelphia, ch 56, pp 753–763

36. Mueller P R, Murray W T 1982 Hip aspiration arthrography. In: Athanasoulis C A, Pfister R C, Greene R E, Roberson G H (eds) Interventional radiology. W B Saunders, Philadelphia, ch 57, pp 764–772

37. Nordenstrom B 1967 A para-xyphoid approach to the mediastinum and mediastingraphy and mediastinal needle biopsy. Investigative Radiology 2:141–146

38. Jereb M, Uskrasowec M 1977 Transthoracic needle biopsy of mediastinal and hilar regions. Cancer 40:1354–1357

39. Rosenberger A, Adler O 1978 Fine needle aspiration biopsy in the diagnosis of mediastinal lesions. American Journal of Roentgenology 131:239–242

40. Tabar L, Dean P B 1979 Interventional radiological procedures in the investigation of lesions in the breast. Radiologic Clinics of North America 17(3):607

41. Muller Th J W 1980 Management of benign looking breast lesions. Diagnostic and therapeutic puncture of mammary cysts. In: Veiga-Pires J A (ed) Intervention radiology. Excerpta Medica, Amsterdam, p 361

42. Kopans D B, Meyer J E 1982 Localisation of occult breast lesions. In: Athanasoulis C A, Pfister R C, Greene R E, Roberson G H (eds) Interventional radiology. W B Saunders, Philadelphia, ch 54, pp 745–748

43. Kalisher L 1982 Breast cyst aspiration with air insufflation. In: Athanasoulis C A, Pfister R C, Greene R E, Roberson G H (eds) Interventional radiology. W B Saunders, Philadelphia, ch 55, pp 749–752

44. Einhorn J, Franzen S 1962 Thin needle biopsy in the diagnosis of thyroid disease. Acta Radiologica 58:321–336

45. Gobien R P 1979 Aspiration biopsy of the solitary thyroid nodule. Radiologic Clinics of North America 17(3):543

46. Lutz H, Ehler R, Reichel L 1980 Ultrasound-guided biopsy. In: Veiga-Pires J A (ed) Intervention radiology. Excerpta Medica, Amsterdam, p 331

47. Scheible W, Coel M, Siemers P T, Seigel H 1977 Percutaneous aspiration of adrenal cysts. American Journal of Roentgenology, 128:1013–1016

48. Schyberg E 1975 Fine needle biopsy of orbital tumours. Acta Opthalmologica 125 (Suppl):11

49. Dubois P J, Kerber C W, Heinz E R 1979 Interventional techniques in neuroradiology. Radiologic Clinics of North America 17(3):515

50. Novelline R A 1982 Percutaneous transperitoneal fine needle lymph node biopsy. In: Athanasoulis C A, Pfister R C, Greene R E, Roberson G H (eds) Interventional radiology. W B Saunders, Philadelphia, ch 45, pp 577–583

51. Moran C J, Naidich T P, Gado M H, Marchosky J A 1979 Central nervous system lesions, biopsied or treated with CT-guided needle placement. Radiology 131:681–686

52. Mason J W 1978 Techniques for right and left ventricular endomyocardial biopsy. American Journal of Cardiology, 41:887

53. Kadir S, Miller S W 1982 Percutaneous transvascular biopsy. In: Athanasoulis C A, Pfister R C, Greene R E, Roberson G H (eds) Interventional radiology. W B Saunders Philadelphia, ch 30, pp 391–397

54. Nordenstrom B 1967 Transjugular approach to the mediastinal needle biopsy. Investigative Radiology 2:134–140

55. Coel M N, Chalmers J 1975 Percutaneous catheter transcaval tumour biopsy. Radiology 116:222

56. Mills S R, Doppman J L, Head G L, Javadpour N, Brennan M F, Chu E W 1978 Transcatheter brush biopsy of intravenous tumour thrombi. Radiology 127:667–670

57. Rosch J, Laking P C, Antonovic R, Dotter C 1973 Transjugular approach to liver biopsy and transhepatic cholangiogram. New England Journal of Medicine 289:227–231

58. Gilmore R I, Bradley R D, Thompson R P H 1978 Improved method of transvenous liver biopsy. British Medical Journal 2:249

59. Newhouse J H, Pfister R C 1982 Renal cyst puncture. In: Athanasoulis C A, Pfister R C Greene R E, Roberson G H (eds) Interventional Radiology. W B Saunders, Philadelphia, ch 32, pp 409–425

60. Pfister R H, Schaffer D 1979 Percutaneous ablation of renal cysts. American Journal of Roentgenology 132:1031

61. Whitaker R H 1973 Diagnosis of obstruction in dilated ureters. Annals of the Royal College of Surgeons of England, 53:153–166

62. Michaelson G 1974 Percutaneous puncture of the renal pelvis, intrapelvic pressure and the concentrating capacity of the kidney in hydronephrosis. Acta Radiologica (Suppl) 559:1–25

63. Pfister R C, Yodar I C, Newhouse J H 1981 Percutaneous uroradiological procedures. Seminars in Roentgenology 16:135–151

64. Barbaric Z L 1979 Interventional uroradiology. Radiologic Clinics of North America 17(3):413

65. Gunther R W, Alken P 1982 Percutaneous nephropyelostomy: applications, technique and critical evaluation. In: Wilkins R A, Viamonte M (eds) Interventional radiology. Blackwell, Oxford, ch 23, pp 333–357

66. McLean G K, Gordon R D, Ring E J 1981 Interventional uroradiology. In: Ring E J, McLean G K (eds) Interventional radiology: principles and techniques. Little, Brown, Boston, ch 4, pp 379–410

67. Pfister R C, Newhouse J H 1979 Percutaneous nephrostomy and other procedures. Radiologic Clinics of North America 17:351–363

68. Pingoud E G, Bagley D H, Zeman R K, Glancy K E, Pais O S 1980 Percutaneous antegrade bilateral ureteral dilatation and stent placement for internal drainage. Radiology 134:780

69. Goldin A R 1977 Percutaneous ureteral splinting. Urology 10:165–168

70. Hennessy O F, Gibsdon R N, Allison D J 1984 Therapeutic ureteric embolization. British Journal of Radiology.

71. Pereiras R, Schiff E, Barkin J, Hutson D 1979 The role of interventional radiology in diseases of the hepatobiliary system and the pancreas. Radiologic Clinics of North America 17(3):555

72. Oleaga J A, Ring E J 1981 Interventional biliary radiology. Seminars in Roentgenology 16:116–134

73. Irving J D 1981 Relief of biliary obstruction. British Journal of Hospital Medicine 26:329–338

74. Oleaga J A, McLean G K, Freiman D B, Ring E J 1981 Interventional biliary radiology. In: Ring E J, McLean G K (eds) Interventional radiology: principles and techniques. Little, Brown, Boston, ch 3, pp 245–377

75. Haaga J R, Georges C, Weinstein A J, Cooperman A M 1979 New interventional techniques in the diagnosis and management of inflammatory disease with the abdomen. Radiologic Clinics of North America 17(3):485

76. McLean G K, Rosen R J, Ring E J 1981 Miscellaneous interventional procedures. In: Ring E J, McLean G K (eds) Interventional radiology: principles and techniques. Little, Brown, Boston, ch 5, pp 411–463

77. Gerzof S G, Spira R, Robbins A H 1981 Percutaneous abscess drainage. Seminars in Roentgenology 16:62–71

78. Quencer R M, Tenner M S, Rothman L M 1976 Percutaneous spinal cord puncture and myelocystography. Radiology 188:637–644

79. Moran C J, Naidich T P, Gado M H, Marchosky J A 1979 Central nervous system lesions biopsied or treated by CT-guided needle placement. Radiology 131:681–680

80. Dubois P J, Kerber C W, Heinz E R 1979 Interventional techniques in neuroradiology. Radiologic Clinics of North America 17(3):515

81. Faure C, Brunelle F, Garel L, Montagne J P 1980 Upper gastro-intestinal tract foreign bodies in the child. In: Veiga-Pires J A (ed) Intervention radiology. Excerpta Medica, Amsterdam, p 400

82. Borden S 1982 Removal of oesophageal foreign bodies by balloon catheter. In: Athanasoulis C A, Pfister R C, Greene R E, Roberson G H (eds) Interventional radiology. W B Saunders, Philadelphia, ch 60, pp 780–781

83. Larson R E, Hodgson J R, Priestley J T 1966 The early and long-term results of 500 consecutive explorations of the common bile duct. Surgery, Gynecology & Obstetrics 122:744–750

84. Editorial in the Lancet 1981

85. Burhenne H J 1973 Non-operative retained biliary tract stone extraction: a new roentgenologic technique. American Journal of Roentgenology 117:388–399

86. Bean W J, Smith S L, Calonje M A 1974 Percutaneous removal of residual biliary tract stones. Radiology 113:1–9

87. Mazzariello R M 1976 Residual biliary tract stones. Non-operative treatment of 570 patients. Surgical Annual 8:113–144

88. Dretler S P, Pfister R C, Newhouse J H 1979 Renal stone dissolution via percutaneous nephrostomy. New England Journal of Medicine 300:341–343

89. Pfister R C, Newhouse J H 1982 Percutaneous renal pelvic stone extraction and ureteral stone displacement. In: Athanasoulis C A, Pfister R C, Greene R E, Roberson G H (eds) Interventional radiology. W B Saunders, Philadelphia, ch 39, pp 509–515

90. Newhouse J H, Pfister R C 1982 Percutaneous dissolution of renal stones. In: Athanasoulis C A, Pfister R C, Greene R E, Roberson G H (eds) Interventional radiology. W B Saunders, Philadelphia, ch 40, pp 516–520

91. Wickham J E A, Kellett J 1981 Percutaneous nephrolithotomy. British Medical Journal 283:1971–1972

92. Fernstrom I, Johansson B 1976 Percutaneous pyelolithotomy. A new extraction technique. Scandinavian Journal of Urology and Nephrostomy 10:257–259

93. Smith A D, Reinke D B, Miller R P, Lange P H 1980 Percutaneous nephrostomy in the management of ureteral and renal calculi. Radiology 133:49–54

94. Palestrant A M et al 1980 Post-operative percutaneous kidney stone extraction. Radiology 134:778–9

95. Thurel C, Levante A, Riche M C, Ludena J 1980 Technique and results of percutaneous controlled thermocoagulation in 350 cases of essential trigeminal neuralgia. In: Veiga-Pires J A (ed) Intervention radiology. Excerpta Medica, Amsterdam, p 407

96. Lutz H, Ehler R, Reichel L 1980 Ultrasound-guided biopsy. In: Veiga-Pires J A (ed) Intervention radiology. Excerpta Medica, Amsterdam, p 331

97. Holm H H, Stroyer I, Hansen H, Stodil F 1981 Ultrasonically-guided percutaneous interstitial implantation of iodine 125 seeds in cancer therapy. British Journal of radiology 54:665–670

98. Fletcher M S, Dawson J L, Wheeler P G, Brinkley D, Nunnerley H, Williams R 1981 Treatment of high bile duct carcinoma with Iridium-192 wire. Lancet 2:172–174

99. Joplin G F et al 1978 Treatment of acromegaly by pituitary implantations of 90 Y. In: Fahlbusch R, Werder K (eds) Treatment of pituitary adenomas. Thieme, Stuttgart, p 261

100. Oberfield R A et al 1979 Prolonged and continuous percutaneous intra-arterial hepatic infusion chemotherapy in advanced metastatic liver adenocarcinoma from colorectal primary. Cancer 44:414–23

101. Lunderquist A, Forsberg L, Hafstrom L O 1980 Intra-arterial infusion therapy of liver metastasis. In: Veiga-Pires J A (ed) Intervention radiology. Excerpta Medica, Amsterdam, p 238

102. Jander P H, Balch C M 1980 Some new aspects of percutaneous arterial chemotherapy infusion in localized, non-resectable malignancies. In: Veiga-Pires J A (ed) Intervention radiology. Excerpta Medica, Amsterdam, p 236

103. Chuang V P, Wallace S 1981(b) Arterial infusion and occlusion in cancer patients. Seminars in Roentgenology 16:13–25

104. Thomson K R, Goldin A R 1979 Angiographic techniques in interventional radiology. Radiologic Clinics of North America 17(3):375

105. Wilkins R A, Pevsner P, Spencer J D 1980. Placement of long-term cytotoxic perfusion catheters. In: Veiga-Pires J A (ed) Intervention radiology. Excerpta Medica, Amsterdam, p 245

106. Athanasoulis C A 1976 Angiographic methods for the control of gastric haemorrhage. American Journal of Digestive Diseases 21:174–181

107. Athanasoulis C A et al 1976 Angiography: Its contribution to the emergency management of gastrointestinal hemorrhage. Radiologic Clinics of North America 14:265–280

108. Clark R A, Colley D P 1981 Pharmacoangiography. Seminars in Roentgenology 16:42–51

109. Rosch J, Dotter C T, Rose R W 1971 Selective arterial infusion of vasoconstrictors in acute gastrointestinal bleeding. Radiology 99:27–31

110. Baum et al 1973 Selective mesenteric arterial infusions in the management of massive diverticular haemorrhage. New England Journal of Medicine 288:1269–1272

111. Athanasoulis C A et al 1975 Mesenteric arterial infusion of vaso-pressin for haemorrhage from colonic diverticulosis. American Journal of Surgery 129:212–216

112. Kaufman S L et al 1977 Control of variceal bleeding by superior mesenteric artery vasopressin infusion. American Journal of Roentgenology 128:567–9

113. Barr J W, Lakin R C, Rosch J 1975 Similarity of arterial and intravenous vasopressin on the portal and systemic haemo-dynamics. Gastroenterology 69:13–19

114. Davis G B, Bookstein J J, Hagan P L 1976 The relative effects of selective intraarterial and intravenous vasopressin infusion. Radiology 120:537–8

115. Boley S J et al 1973 An aggressive roentgenologic and surgical approach to acute mesenteric ischaemia. Annals of Surgery 5:355–78

116. Porter J M, Snider R L, Bardana E J, Rosch J, Eidemiller L R 1975 The diagnosis and treatment of Raynaud's phenomenon. Surgery 77:11–23

117. Szczeklik A, Nizankowski R, Skawinski S, Szczeklik J, Gluszko P, Gryghewski 1979 Successful therapy of advanced arteriosclerosis obliterans with prostacyclin. Lancet:1111–4

118. Fletcher A P, Alkjaersig N, Lewis M 1976 A pilot study of urokinase therapy in cerebral infarction. Stroke 7:135

119. Gallant T E, and Athanasoulis C A 1982 Regional infusion of thrombolytic enzymes. In: Athanasoulis C A, Pfister R C, Greene R E, Roberson G H (eds) Interventional radiology. W B Saunders, Philadelphia, ch 28, pp 374–378

120. John G E 1972 DHSS Hazard Notice No 6

121. Kadir S, Athanasoulis C A 1982 Percutaneous retrieval of intra-vascular foreign bodies. In: Athanasoulis C A, Pfister R C, Greene R E, Roberson G H (eds) Interventional radiology. W B Saunders, Philadelphia, ch 29, pp 379–390

122. Davies J, Alvares R, Allison D J 1981 An intracardiac foreign body: diagnosed non-invasively and removed non-surgically. British Journal of Radiology 54:987–989

123. Rossi P 1982 Percutaneous removal of intravascular foreign bodies. In: Wilkins R A, Viamonte M (eds) Interventional radiology. Blackwell, Oxford, ch 24 pp 359–369

124. Dotter C T, Keller F S, Rosch J 1982 Transluminal catheter removal of foreign bodies from the Cardiovascular system. In: Athanasoulis C A, Pfister R C, Greene R E, Roberson G H (eds) Interventional radiology. W B Saunders, Philadelphia, ch 107, pp 2395–2403

125. Pereiras R, Schiff E, Barkin J, Hutson D 1979 The role of inter-ventional radiology in diseases of the hepatobiliary system and the pancreas. Radiologic Clinics of North America 17(3):555

126. Greenfield L J, Peyton M D, Brown P P, Elkins R C 1974 Trans-venous management of pulmonary embolic disease Annals of Surgery 180:461–468

127. Dotter C T 1981 Interventional radiology — review of an emerging field. Seminars in Roentgenology 16:7–12

128. Mobin-Uddin K, Utley J R, Bryant L R 1975 The inferior vena cava umbrella filter. Progress in cardiovascular diseases. 17:391–399

129. Greenfield L J, Zocco J, Wilk J et al 1977 Clinical experience with the Kim-Ray-Greenfield vena caval filter. Am Surg 185:692

130. Hunter J A, Dye W S, Javid H et al 1977 Permanent trans-venous balloon occlusion of the inferior vena cava. Am Surg 186:491

131. Dotter C T 1981 Interventional Radiology — review of an emerging field. Seminars in Roentgenology 16:7–12

132. Dedrick C G, Novelline R A 1982 Transvenous interruption of the inferior vena cava. In: Athanasoulis C A, Pfister R C, Green R E, Roberson G H (eds) Interventional radiology. W B Saunders, Philadelphia, ch 26 pp 355–369

133. Porstmann W, Wierny L 1981 Percutaneous transfemoral closure of the patent ductus arteriosus — an alternative to surgery. Seminars in Roentgenology 16:95–102

134. Szarnicki R, Krebber J H, Wack J 1981 Wire coil embolization of systemic-pulmonary artery collaterals following surgical correction of pulmonary atresia. J Thorac Cardiovasc Surg 81:124–126

135. Yamamoto S, Nozawa T, Aizawa T, Honda M, Mohri M 1979 Transcatheter embolization of bronchial collateral arteries prior to intracardiac operation for tetralogy of Fallot. J Thorac Cardiovasc Surg 78:739–743

136. Dotter C T, Judkins M P, Transluminal treatment of arteriosclerotic obstruction: Description of a new technic and a preliminary report of its appplication. Circulation 30:654–70

137. Schwarten D E, Yune Y Y, Klatte E C, Grim C E, Weinburger M H 1980 Clinical experience with percutaneous transluminal angioplasty (PTA) of stenotic renal arteries. Radiology 135:601–604

138. Dotter C T 1980 Transluminal angioplasty: a long view. Radiology 135:561–564

139. Sos T A, Sniderman K W 1981 Percutaneous transluminal angioplasty. Seminars in Roentgenology 16:26–41

140. Dacie J E 1981 Percutaneous transluminal angioplasty. British Journal of Hospital Medicine. 26:314–329

141. Gruntzig A, Hopff H 1974 Perkutane Rekanalisation chronischer arterieller Verschlusse mit einem neuen Dilaations-Katheter. Dtsch Med Wschr 99:2502

142. Zeitler E 1982 Percutaneous transluminal angioplasty. In: Wilkins R A, Viamonte M (eds) Interventional radiology. Blackwell, Oxford, ch 18, pp 267–278

143. Gruntzig A 1982 Percutaneous transluminal coronary angioplasty. In: Athanasoulis C A, Pfister R C, Greene R E, Roberson G H (eds) Interventional radiology. W B Saunders, Philadelphia, ch 89, pp 2087–2098

144. Freiman D B, McLean G K, Oleaga J A, Ring E J 1981 Percutaneous transluminal angioplasty. In: Ring E J, McLean G K (eds) Interventional radiology: principles and techniques. Little, Brown, Boston, ch 2, pp 117–244

145. Waltman A C, Greenfield A J, Athanasoulis C A 1982 Transluminal angioplasty: general rules and basic considerations. In: Athanasoulis C A, Pfister R C, Greene R E, Roberson G H (eds) Interventional radiology. W B Saunders, Philadelphia, ch 17, pp 253–272

146. Castaneda-Zuniga W R, Formanek A, Tadavarthy M et al 1980 The mechanism of balloon angioplasty. Radiology 135:565–571

147. Sundt T M, Smith H C, Campbell J K, Vlietstra R E, Cucchiara R F, Stanson A W 1980 Transluminal angioplasty for basilar artery stenosis. Mayo Clinic Proceedings 55:673–680

148. Allison D J 1978 Therapeutic embolization. British Journal of Hospital Medicine 20:707–715

149. Berenstein A, Kricheff I I 1981 Neuroradiologic interventional procedures. Seminars in Roentgenology 16:79–94

150. Djindjian R, Merland J J 1978 Superelective arteriography of the external carotid artery (translated by Moseley I F). Springer-Verlag, Berlin

151. Allison D J 1980a Therapeutic embolization and venous sampling. In: Taylor S (ed) Recent advances in surgery 10. Churchill Livingstone, Edinburgh, ch 2, p 27

152. Gianturco C, Anderson J H, Wallace S 1975 Mechanical devices for arterial occlusion. American Journal of Roentgenology, Radium Therapy and Nuclear Medicine 124:428–435

153. Wallace S, Gianturce C, Anderson J H, Goldstein H M, Davis L J, Bree R L, 1976 Therapeutic vascular occlusion utilizing steel coil technique: clinical applications. American Journal of Roentgenology 127:381–387

154. Kerber C 1976 Balloon catheter with a calibrated leak. A new system for super-selective angiography and occlusive catheter therapy. Radiology 120:547–550

155. Pevsner P H 1977 Micro-balloon catheter for super-selective angiography and therapeutic occlusion. American Journal of Roentgenology 128:225–230

156. Dotter C T, Goldman M L, Rosch J 1975 Instant selective arterial occlusion with Isobutyl-2-cyanoacrylate: Radiology 114:227230

157. Zanetti P H, Sherman F E 1972 Experimental evaluation of a tissue adhesive as an agent for the treatment of aneurysms and arteriovenous anomalies. Journal of Neurosurgery 36:72–79

158. Wholey M H 1977 The technology of balloon catheters in interventional angiography. Radiology 125:671–676

159. Greenfield A J, Athanasoulis C A, Waltman A C, Le Moure E R 1978 Trans-catheter embolization: prevention of embolic reflux using balloon catheters. American Journal of Roentogenology 131:651–655

160. White R I, Kaufman S L, Barth K H, De Caprio V, Standberg J D 1979 Therapeutic embolization with detachable silicone balloons: Early clinical experience. JAMA 241:1257–1260

161. Goldman M L, Land W C, Bradley E L, Anderson J 1976 Transcatheter therapeutic embolization in the management of massive upper gastrointestinal tract bleeding. Radiology 120:513–521

162. Rosch J, Dotter C T, Brown M J 1972 A new method for the control of gastrointestinal bleeding. Radiology 102:303–306

163. Reuter S R, Chuang V P, Bree R I 1975 Selective arterial embolization for control of massive upper gastrointestinal bleeding. American Journal of Roentgenology 125:119–126

164. Katzen B T, Rossi P, Passariello R, Simonetti G 1976 Transcatheter therapeutic arterial embolization. Radiology 120:523–531

165. Allison D J 1980 Gastrointestinal bleeding. British Journal of Hospital Medicine 23:358–365

166. Lunderquist A, Vang J 1974 Transhepatic catheterization and obliteration of the coronary vein in patients with portal hypertension and oesophageal varices. New England Journal of Medicine. 291:646–649

167. Keller F S, Rosch J, Dotter C T, Jendrzejewski J, 1981 Embolization in the treatment of bleeding oesophageal varices. Seminars in Roentgenology 16:103–115

168. Lea Thomas M, Lamb G H R 1977 Selective arterial embolization of the management of post-operative renal hemorrhage. Acta Radiologica 18:49–54

169. Allison D J 1979 Arterial embolization in post-biopsy renal haemorrhage. European Journal of Rheumatology and Inflammation 3:125–127

170. Chang J, Katzen B T, Sullivan K P 1978 Transcatheter gelfoam embolization of posttraumatic bleeding pseudoaneurysms. American Journal of Roentgenology 131:645–650

171. Margolies M N, Ring E J, Waltmann A C, Kerr W S, Baum S 1972 Arteriography in the management of haemorrhage from pelvic fractures. New England Journal of Medicine 287:328–331

172. van Urk H, Perlberger R R, Muller H 1978 Selective arterial embolization for control of traumatic pelvic haemorrhage. Surgery 83:133–137

173. Remy J, Voisin C, Dupuis C, Begnery P, Tonnel A B, Dehies J L, Douay B 1974 Traitement des Hemotysies par embolisation de la circulation systemique. Annales de Radiologie 74(1):5–16

174. Sokoloff J, Wickbom I, McDonald D, Brahme F, Goergen T G, Goldberger L E 1974 Therapeutic percutaneous embolization in intractable epistaxis. Radiology 111:285–287

175. Foley W D, Glancy J J, Tulloch A G S 1976 Catheter embolic therapy in vascular tumours. Australasian Radiology 20:380–390

176. Goldstein H M, Wallace S, Anderson J H, Bree R L, Gianturco C 1976 Transcatheter occlusion of abdominal tumours. Radiology 120:539–545

177. Doppman J L, et al 1975 Treatment of hyperparathyroidism by percutaneous embolization of a mediastinal adenoma. Radiology 115:37–42

178. Chuang V P, Wallace S 1981 Arterial infusion and occlusion in cancer patients. Seminars in Roentgenology 16:13–25

179. Hilal S K, Michelsen J W 1975 Therapeutic percutaneous embolization of extra-axial vascular lesions of the head, neck and spine. Journal of Neurosurgery 43:275–287

180. Chuang V P, Wallace S 1981 Hepatic artery embolization in the treatment of hepatic neoplasms. Radiology 140:51–58

181. Lang E K 1971 Superselective arterial catheterization as a vehicle for delivering radioactive infarct particles to tumors. Radiology 98:391–399

182. Blumgart L H, Allison D J 1982 Resection and embolization in the management of secondary hepatic tumours. World Journal of Surgery 6:32–45

183. Kendall B, Moseley I 1977 Therapeutic embolization of the external carotid tree. Journal of Neurology, Neurosurgery and Psychiatry 40:937–950

184. Rizk G K, Atallah W K, Bridi G I 1973 Renal arterio-venous fistula treated by catheter embolization. British Journal of Radiology 46:222–234

185. White R I, Mitchell S E, Barth K H, Kaufman S L, Kadir S, Chang R, Jerry P B 1983 Angioarchitecture of pulmonary arterio-venous malformations: an important consideration before embolotherapy. AJR 104:681–686

186. Terry P B, White R I, Barth K H, Kaufman S L, Mitchell S E 1983 Pulmonary arteriovenous malformations: physiologic observations and results of therapeutic balloon embolization. N Eng J Med 308:1197–1200

187. Berenstein A, Kricheff II 1981 Neuroradiologic Interventional Procedures. Seminars in Roentgenology 16:79–94

188. Moseley I F 1983 Interventional neuroradiology: embolization of the arteries of the head and neck. In: Steiner R E (ed) Recent advances in Radiology 7. Churchill Livingstone, Edinburgh, ch 7, pp 107–137

189. Maddison F E 1973 Embolic therapy of hypersplenism. Investigative Radiology 8:280–281

190. Castaneda-Zuniga W R, Hammerschmidt D E, Sanchez R, Amplatz K 1977 Nonsurgical splenectomy. American Journal of Roentgenology 129:805–811

191. Allison D J, Fletcher D R, Gordon-Smith E C 1981 Therapeutic arterial embolization of the spleen: a new cause of free intraperitoneal gas. Clinical Radiology 32:617–621

192. Sim E, Fleckenstein P 1982 Gas formation following hepatic embolization. British Journal of Radiology 55:926–928

193. Hennessy O F, Allison D J 1983 Intra-hepatic gas following embolization. British Journal of Radiology 56:348–350

194. Wear J B, Crummy A B, Munson B O, 1977 A new approach to the treatment of priapism. Journal of Urology 177:252–4

195. Wafula J M C, Davies P 1981 Treatment of spontaneous priapism by embolization of internal pudendal artery. British Medical Journal 282:363–4

196. Lunderquist A, Vang J 1974 Transhepatic catheterization and obliteration of the coronary vein in patients with portal hypertension and oesophageal varices. New England Journal of Medicine 291:646–649

197. Keller F S, Rosch J, Dotter C T, Jendrzejewski J, 1981. Embolization in the treatment of bleeding oesophageal varices. Seminars in Roentgenology 16:103–115

198. Smith-Laing G, Camilo M E, Dick R, Sherlock S 1981 Percutaneous transhepatic portography in the assessment of portal hypertension. Gastroenterology 78:197–205

199. Sos T A 1983 Transhepatic portal venous embolization of varices: pros and cons. Radiology 148:569–570

200. Ingemansson S, Holst J, Larsson L, Lunderquist A 1977 Localization of glucagonomas by catheterization of the pancreatic veins and with glucagon assay. Surgery Gynecology & Obstetrics 145:509–516

201. Viamonte et al 1975 Selective catheterization of the portal vein and its tributaries. Radiology 114:457–460

202. Gothlin J, Lunderquist A, Tylen U 1974 Selective phlebography of the pancreas. Acta Radiologica (Diagnosis) 15:474–480

203. Jorgensen H, Stiris G 1974 Hypertension crisis followed by adrenocortical insufficiency after unilateral adrenal phlebography in a patient with Cushing's syndrome. Acta Medica Scandinavica 196:141–143

204. Lecky J W, Plotkin D 1971 Adrenal function ablation utilizing the angiographic catheter. Journal of the American Medical Association 218:1438

205. Jablonski R D, Meaney T F, Schumacher O P 1977 Transcatheter adrenal ablation for metastatic carcinoma of the breast. CLeveland Clinic Quarterly 44:57–63

206. Rosenstock J, Allison D J, Joplin G F et al 1981 Therapeutic adrenal venous infarction in ACTH-dependent Cushing's syndrome. British Journal of Radiology 54:912–915

207. Mathias C J, Peart W S, Carron D B, Hemingway Anne P, Allison D J 1984 Therapeutic venous infarction of an aldosterone producing adenoma (Conn's tumour). British Medical Journal 288:1416–1417

208. White R I, Kaufman S L, Barth K H, Kadir S, Smyth J W, Walsh P C 1981 Occlusion of varicoceles with detachable balloons. Radiology 139:327–334

209. Kaufman S L, Kadir S, Barth K H, Smyth J W, Walsh P C, White R I 1983 Mechanisms of recurrent varicocele after balloon occlusion of the internal spermatic vein. Radiology 147:435–440

SUGGESTIONS FOR FURTHER READING

Abrams H L 1983 Vascular and interventional radiology, 3rd edn. Little, Brown, Boston

Athanasoulis C A, Pfister R C, Greene R E, Roberson G H 1982 Interventional radiology. W B Saunders, Philadelphia

Herlinger H, Lunderquist A, Wallace S 1983 Clinical radiology of the liver. Marcel Dekker, New York

Macintosh P K, Thompson K 1979 Symposium on interventional radiology. Radiologic Clinics of North America. W B Saunders, Philadelphia

Ring E J, McLean G K 1981 Interventional radiology: principles and techniques. Little, Brown, Boston

Steiner R E 1983 Recent advances in radiology and medical imaging 7. Churchill Livingstone, Edinburgh

Wilkins R A, Viamonte M 1982 Interventional radiology. Blackwell, Oxford

99 Radiology in oncology

Colin Parsons

T staging
Lymph node staging

Lymphography
    Complications
    Lymphographic interpretation
    Clinical value of radiology

The lymphomas

Systemic malignant metastases
    Skeletal metastases
    Pulmonary deposits
    Hepatic deposits
    Brain metastases
    Metastases from occult pulmonary tumours

The roles which radiology fulfils in oncology are listed in Table 99.1.

Table 99.1 Applications of radiology in cancer.

1. Initial diagnosis
2. Staging
3. Assessment of response to treatment
4. Monitoring for relapse
5. Guided biopsy
6. Radiotherapy planning
7. Demonstrating complications of disease or treatment
8. Interventional procedures

A provisional diagnosis of cancer based on histology of an operative biopsy, fine needle aspiration cytology or compelling radiological or clinical evidence will have been made on virtually all patients by the time of their referral to a specialist Oncology Unit.

Whilst histology is the 'gold standard' for the diagnosis of cancer, it would be wrong to accept the provisional histological opinion as necessarily correct. Error can arise within that speciality in two ways. First, the pathologist of the referring hospital may not be greatly experienced in cancer work, so that particularly the less common tumours may be misdiagnosed. A provisional diagnosis of malignancy is rarely wrong, but, the precise type of tumour may not be identified correctly. Second, whilst histological features may be very definitely in favour of malignancy, it may not be possible to identify the tissue of origin. This is usually because the tumour is so undifferentiated that the pathologist merely finds sheets of small round cells, or because there is a considerable degree of necrosis. Highly undifferentiated tumour is often seen in Ewing's sarcoma, rhabdomyosarcoma, neuroblastoma and oat cell bronchial neoplasms.

When the tissue of origin can not be precisely identified, there may be some feature which will allow further diagnostic effort to be directed to a particular area. For instance, the demonstration of mucin in the tumour or its metastases will suggest an origin within the gastrointestinal tract or ovary. Occasionally, the situation has to be accepted that no precise histological diagnosis can be reached without further tissue sampling.

All the existing evidence must be assessed to insure that it is compatible with the provisional diagnosis. Attention

2167

should be given to the likelihood of the proposed histological diagnosis occurring in a patient of that particular age and sex. A suggestion of osteosarcoma occurring in a middle aged patient with no history of pre-existing bone disease at that site would clearly deserve second thoughts. Furthermore, *common things are common*. Metastases occur from the majority of malignant tumours sooner or later and are frequently the cause of the patient presentation.

Some tumours have such a characteristic radiological appearance that there can be little doubt of the diagnosis on those features alone. One can be very confident when a carcinoma of the breast is demonstrated at mammography as a spiculated soft tissue mass and causing skin retraction (Fig. 99.1A). However, radiology is much less accurate in this regard than histology, so that, however convincing the radiological features, a biopsy must always intervene between radiology and radical treatment. Fat necrosis, sclerosing adenosis and surgical scarring can all closely mimic the radiological features of breast cancer (Fig. 99.1B).

Once a firm histological diagnosis has been made, the disease must be *staged*. This is the process of demonstrating the full extent of disease at presentation in order to permit logical treatment selection, to indicate prognosis and to provide criteria for assessing response to treatment or relapse. Obviously, heroic attempts at local treatment are of no value if there is evidence of dissemination of the tumour. Accurate staging is essential if comparisons are to be made between various treatments or between the 'same' treatment carried out in different hospitals.

In differing clinical circumstances, different levels of quality of radiological information are necessary. Simply identifying that disease is present at a particular site is usually sufficient for staging, but may not be enough for treatment selection. Detailed anatomical information may influence the choice of treatment, for instance, when involved lymph nodes incorporate some vital structure preventing their complete surgical removal.

Staging in a new cancer patient depends upon:

1. A knowledge of the precise histology of the tumour.
2. Experience of its biological behaviour, with particular interest in:

   (a) The potential pattern of spread
   (b) The likelihood of early metastases

Staging is the major time-absorbing occupation in cancer radiology. From experience of the biological behaviour of a particular histological type of tumour, it would be apparent whether one is dealing with a situation in which local infiltration is of major concern, or whether efforts should be diverted to identifying a particular pattern of lymphatic or systemic spread. Some tumours are known to metastasize early, so that they should be considered likely to be systemic at presentation. Nevertheless, the decision whether or not to give systemic therapy, which may be unpleasant to the patient, may depend on the radiological demonstration of secondary deposits. Many medical oncologists prefer to withold treatment until it is shown to be clinically necessary rather than to waste the best chance of the treatment being effective, by giving it as an adjuvant to a patient in whom systemic disease has not been proven.

T Staging

Many metastasizing tumours have now been categorized by the International Union Against Cancer — TNM system. *T* staging refers to the local extent of tumour and in the absence of nodal (*N*) or distant metastases (*M*) this determines the treatability of the tumour by local methods. Of course, this does not always imply *curative* surgery or radiotherapy but may relate to the feasibility of debulking a tumour mass or some palliative procedure. In many tumour situations, the demonstration of nodal or distant metastases will overshadow the importance of local tumour extent.

Treatment selection based on the precise radiological demonstration of the primary tumour can be illustrated by *carcinoma of the maxillary antrum*, in which, radiology demonstrates disease much more precisely than clinical examination. The T staging criteria are based upon routes of spread which directly influence operability [1] (Table 99.2.). Diagnosis is usually delayed because of the similarity in symptoms produced by common benign paranasal sinus

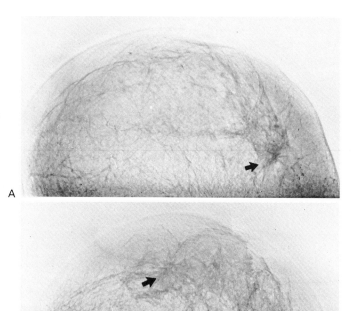

Fig. 99.1 Skin retraction identifies the spiculated soft tissue mass in (A) as a carcinoma. A similar spiculated mass in (B) was due to sclerosing adenosis.

Table 99.2 T staging of maxillary antral tumours.

T1 Confined to mucosa
T2 Bone eroded
T3 Involvement of skin, orbit, ethmoid
T4 Extension to nasopharynx, sphenoid sinus, cribriform plate or pterygoid fossa

disease and that produced by malignancy, so that advanced malignant disease is frequent when the patient is diagnosed. Clinical assessment is hampered by the surrounding bony structures and radiology has always had an important role in assessment.

Computed tomography which allows the soft tissues of the face to be demonstrated and to be distinguished one from another because of the intervening fat-filled fascial planes has brought a sensitivity to local tumour assessment which was not previously available [2]. The demonstration of tumour confined within the maxillary antrum indicates an excellent prognosis with the potential of cure by surgery. Extension forward into the soft tissues of the face, or upward into the anterior part of the orbit or into the ethmoid air cells will not preclude curative surgery. But, a more extensive operation must be planned which will include plastic reconstruction of the face, orbital exenteration or a combined excision of the ethmoid and antrum.

T3 information obviously plays a vital role in the planning and success of surgery and alters the proposed operation in ways which the surgeon will need to discuss with the patient. T4 disease, involving the nasopharynx, pterygoid fossa or skull base, excludes curative surgery; radiotherapy then becomes the treatment of choice (Fig. 99.2).

The same principles as have been outlined for the maxillary antrum can be applied to the local extent of any tumour. Radiological features are particularly important in T staging of laryngeal, bronchial, renal and pelvic malignancies. The benefit of such an approach is the more accurate planning of surgery and the avoidance of operations which are doomed to failure because of the otherwise occult extent of disease.

Lymph node staging

N staging is the demonstration of local, regional or distant lymph node metastases. Such involvement denotes a worse prognosis than completely localized disease. Most imaging techniques detect lymph node abnormality by nodal enlargement, but that does not always imply malignant involvement. Benign lymph node enlargement may coexist with malignant disease. The most frequent example of this is reactive hyperplasia, for which there is often no obvious cause, although, there is commonly a history of recent surgery. Infections, such as pelvic abscess following laparotomy for ovarian carcinoma, or pneumonia distal to a bronchial neoplasm, may be responsible for local benign lymph node enlargement.

Imaging methods such as *ultrasound*, *computed tomography* and *general radiological* procedures such as chest radiographs and IVU may demonstrate enlarged nodes or the effects of enlarged nodes on adjacent structures such as the bronchus or ureters. Ultrasound and computed tomography can show changes within the nodal tissue caused by necrosis. A major advantage of lymphography over these methods is the ability to demonstrate the internal architecture of *normal* size lymph nodes. Table 99.3 compares the advantages of lymphography and computed tomography in lymph node assessment.

Table 99.3 Advantages of lymphography and computed tomography in lymph node assessment.

Lymphography
1. Shows internal architecture of unenlarged nodes.
2. A dynamic process with easy, cheap follow up.
3. The equipment required is generally available.

Computed tomography
1. Assesses all lymph node areas.
2. Defines relationships of nodal areas to adjacent structures.
3. Other viscera examined at a single investigation.
4. Few medical contraindications.

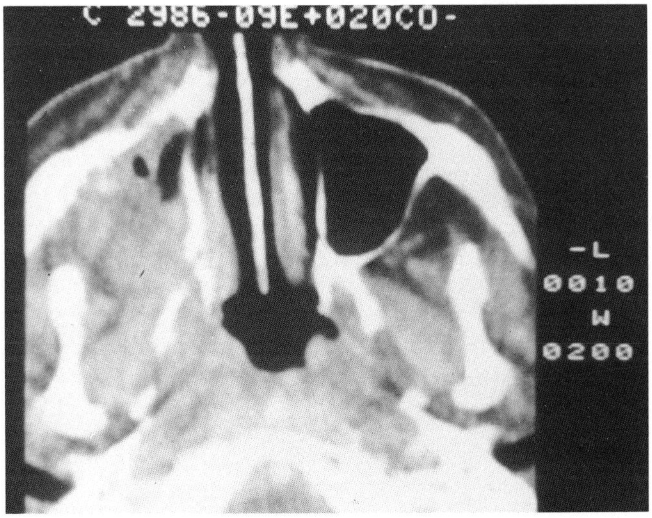

LYMPHOGRAPHY

The technique of lymphography in the assessment of lymph node disease relies on the identification of lymphatic vessels following the subcutaneous injection of a dye, e.g. patent blue V, and the ability of lymph nodes to retain injected oily contrast medium.

The procedure is in two stages, the *lymphangiogram* phase in which the lymph vessels are opacified followed by the *lymphadenogram* in which the lymph nodes are shown.

Patent blue V has a molecular weight of 1158 (as the calcium salt) and readily diffuses through the lymphatic walls. There is persistent blue staining at the site of injection but of the dyes which have been evaluated, patent blue V has the least protein binding. Following the injection of the dye at the base of the toes, lymphatics can be identified and cannulated following a 'cut down' on the dorsum of the foot (Fig. 99.3). Oily contrast medium—ultrafluid Lipiodol is

Fig. 99.2 A T4 carcinoma of the maxillary antrum is extending posteriorly destroying bone and invading the pterygoid muscle.

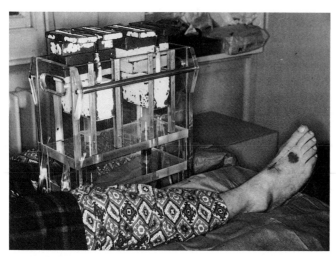

Fig. 99.3 The cut-down procedure of lymphography and the gravitational pump used to inject the oily contrast medium.

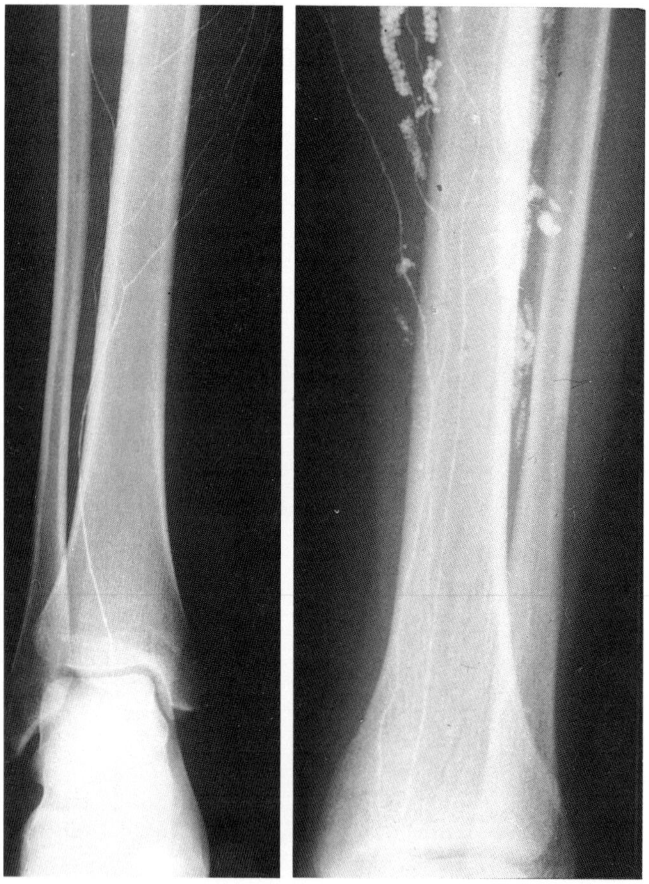

injected into the cannulated lymphatic by a gravitational or electric pump (Fig. 99.3). As soon as the injection is commenced, an X–ray film of the calf is exposed to confirm that the injection is into a lymphatic rather than a vein. Within the lymphatic, the column of contrast medium is continuous, numerous valves can be identified and the vessels branch in an upward direction (Fig. 99.4A). Intravenous injection is recognized by the oil column becoming broken up into numerous globules which have the appearance of caviar, and the venous system branches in both upward and downward directions (Fig. 99.4B). After 5 ml have been injected, a radiograph of the pelvis is taken and the further amount of Lipiodol required for the column of contrast medium to reach the upper border of L4 vertebral body is estimated. In the average adult, a total of 7 ml is usually needed on each side.

As a rule of thumb, babies aged 1 year need 1 ml, and a child of 5 years, 2 ml on each side. The dose is carefully controlled since any excess of contrast medium not taken up by the lymph nodes will pass on to the pulmonary capillaries (Fig. 99.5). Once the injection is complete, the patient walks for 5 minutes and then has a radiograph of the abdomen to show the course of the lymphatic vessels.

In the normal lymphangiogram, three or four lymph channels follow the course of the major vessels around the pelvic side wall, and thereafter a right and left para-aortic chain ascends within a line joining the tips of the lumbar transverse processes [3] (Fig. 99.6). In 65% of individuals, a middle chain arises from the right para-aortic lymph vessels. Numerous, often tortuous, transverse channels unite the three para-aortic lymphatic chains.

A   B

Fig. 99.4 (A) Normal lymphatics of the calf showing a continuous column of oil, branching upwards and with irregularity caused by valves.

(B) An intravenous injection of oily contrast medium recognized by globules having the appearance of caviar, followed by a satisfactory intralymphatic injection.

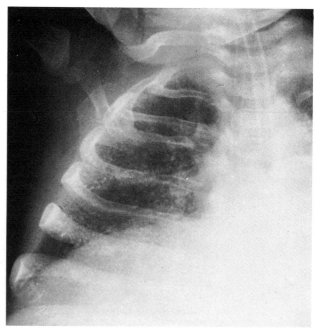

Fig. 99.5 Pulmonary oil embolism in a baby inadvertently injected intravenously with oily contrast medium, at St Elsewheres.

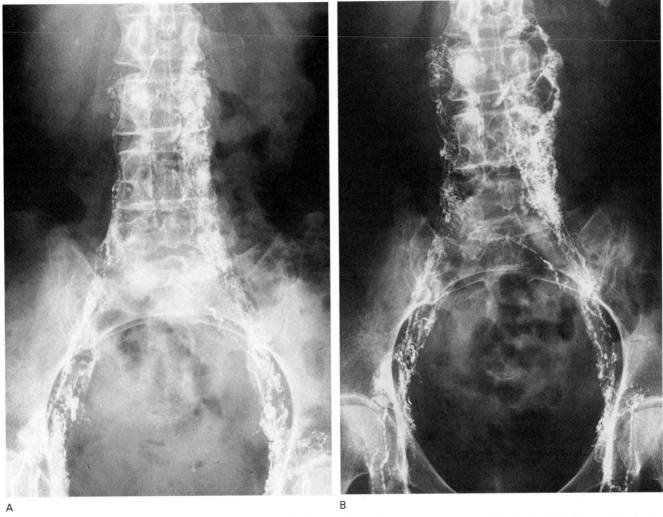

A   B

Fig. 99.6 (A) Normal lymphatic channels follow the course of major vessels and in the para-aortic region lie in the longitudinal axis of the body. (B) 3 years later the para-aortic lymphatics are displaced as a result of Hodgkins disease.

CT shows the lymph vessels and lymph nodes to be randomly distributed circumferentially around the aorta and inferior vena cava.

A major feature of the lymphangiogram phase is the demonstration of the precise position of the afferent and efferent vessels of the lymph node (Fig. 99.7). The course of the lymphatic channels can usually be traced through the nodes and this is extremely helpful in distinguishing fibrofatty filling defects from metastases on the lymphadenogram phase of the investigation (Fig. 99.8). The lymph channels pass through fibrofatty filling defects but are displaced around metastases.

In the event of lymph node replacement by tumour, collateral lymphatic channels may become opacified or there may be lymph stasis [4]. In the presence of extensive metastatic disease or following surgery, lymphaticovenous fistulae may develop to the systemic or portal venous systems (Fig. 99.9). Free spill of contrast medium into the peritoneal cavity may also occur (Fig. 99.7).

On the day following the injection, the lymph nodes will be opacified. These have a fine homogeneous granular appear-

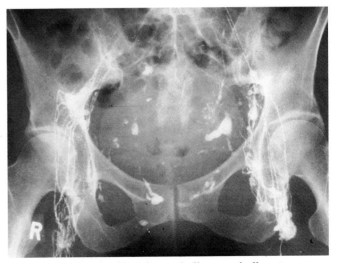

Fig. 99.7 The relationships of normal afferent and efferent lymphatics to the lymph nodes in the groins are demonstrated. There is in addition peritoneal spill as a result of a Wertheim hysterectomy.

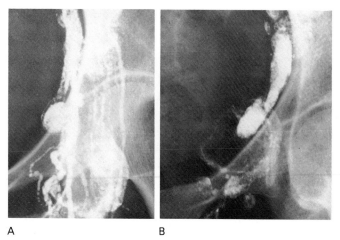

A   B

Fig. 99.8 (A) Abnormal lymphangiogram and (B) abnormal lymphadenogram due to a large metastasis occupying a superficial inguinal lymph node. The lymphatics are displaced around the metastasis.

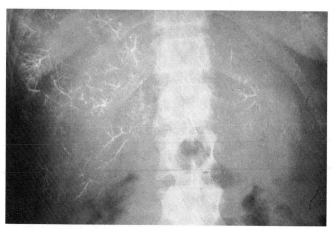

Fig. 99.9 Gross nodal metastases have caused a lymphaticoportal fistula with opacification of the liver.

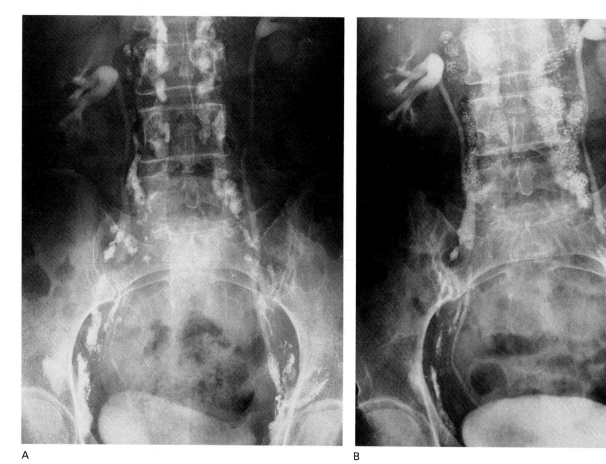

A   B

Fig. 99.10 (A) A normal lymphadenogram in a patient with carcinoma of the cervix. (B) The para-aortic nodes have now become lymphomatous as a result of Hodgkin's disease. The pelvic nodes are unusually small because of the radiotherapy given to treat the carcinoma of cervix. (Same case as Fig. 99.6.)

ance caused by oil trapped in the sinusoidal tissue which is interspersed amongst nonopacified follicles. In the abdomen and pelvis, nodes range in size from a a few millimetres (when they are often spherical) up to 3.5 cm in a longitudinal axis (Fig. 99.10). The longest dimension of the nodes is in the course of the major blood vessels. The right para-aortic chain commonly terminates at the level of L2 as a result of the cisterna chyli. A gap in the chain above this level should not be regarded, on its own, as abnormal. Similarly, there is often a gap in the lower right para-aortic lymph node chain and this is accompanied on the lymphangiogram phase by a bypass vessel [3]. There is never a normal lower lumbar gap on the left.

In the upper left para-aortic region, the lymph nodes are often represented by numerous tiny fragments of lymphoid tissue, the 'upper lumbar clump'. Recognition of this normal feature will avoid the misdiagnosis of malignant involvement.

Complications of lymphography

There are a number of minor complications of lymphography which are unavoidable [5].

The patent blue dye disperses throughout the patient so that the skin has a dusky hue for 24 hours, this resolves as the blue dye is excreted in the urine and faeces.

More serious is the fact that some of the oil which is injected, however small the dose, will pass onward into the lungs [6]. Immediately following the procedure, oil can be identified in pulmonary capillaries, and over the course of the next 24 hours, the oil works its way into the alveolar spaces and thence into the bronchi. If the contrast medium is labelled with radioactive iodine, this can subsequently be identified in sputum. There is a temporary decrease in pulmonary capillary volume, lung compliance and oxygen diffusing capacity, which returns to normal 3 or 4 days following the injection of oil. A general anaesthetic should be avoided throughout this period. If the patient has diminished pulmonary reserve, it may be wise either to avoid lymphography altogether until the patient's clinical position can be improved, or, the procedure should be carried out with an injection into one side at a time, with a 1 week interval between the two injections. A preliminary chest radiograph is mandatory before lymphography, but even more important is the patient's respiratory reserve on simple exercise.

Absolute contraindications to the technique are *allergy* to iodine, right to left cardiac or pulmonary *shunts* and recent thoracic *radiotherapy*. During the 6 weeks following radiotherapy, there is an inflammatory response which sets up small vascular shunts. The majority of patients who died as a result of the early use of lymphography had very large doses of oil injected whilst the patient was undergoing thoracic radiotherapy. Should systemic embolism occur, the iodinated oil may be detectable on a lateral skull film or at ophthalmoscopy and also in the patient's urine.

Relative contraindications to lymphograpy are significant lung disease, previous allergy to patent blue (on a future occasion, the technique can be carried out without using the dye) and previous radical surgery or radiotherapy which may have destroyed the lymph nodes which are intended to be opacified by lymphography.

Lymphographic interpretation

The criteria of metastatic involvement include abnormalities seen in either the lymphangiogram and the lymphadenogram phases [4] (Table 99.4). On the day of the injection, the

Table 99.4 Features of metastatic involvement at lymphography.

Lymphangiogram phase
1. Stasis
2. Displacement from normal course
3. Collateral flow
4. Lymphaticovenous fistulae
5. Intraperitoneal spill

Lymphadenogram phase
1. Spherical filling defects
2. Displacement by unopacified mass
3. Opacification of nodes in unusual sites
4. Increase in size on follow up
5. Differential response to therapy

abnormalities seen are *stasis*, *displacement* of normal channels, filling of *collateral* or unusual channels, lymphaticovenous *fistulae* and peritoneal *spill*.

Thereafter, spherical nodal *filling defects* which expand over time or show a differential response to treatment are evident (Fig. 99.11). A *pseudolymphomatous* pattern of involvement with diffuse foamy enlargement without a clearly defined filling defect is seen occasionally in testicular teratoma and carcinoma of the ovary.

Unopacified lymph node masses may be responsible for displacing nodes filled with contrast medium or causing their axis to turn away from the long axis of the body (Fig. 99.12). Opacification of nodes in an *unusual position* such as the internal iliac region, is a suspicious feature.

A lymphogram should be regarded as a dynamic procedure. Approximately one third of lymphograms are equivocal when injected but by following the appearance of the lymph nodes over the course of the ensuing 4 to 8 weeks, changes may occur which make the diagnosis more certain. Without effective treatment, one would expect metastases not only to look like metastases but behave as tumour by increasing in size. With effective treatment, metastases commonly decrease in size at a greater rate than the surrounding lymphoid tissue. Whilst the nodes are opacified, the lymphogram can be used in fluoroscopically guided fine needle aspiration for cytology. This is useful when the initial lymphogram appearance is equivocal and treatment can not be delayed for the benefit of follow up.

With experience, lymphography is a simple technique. It demonstrates smaller volume disease than any other procedure and has a high accuracy when the lymphangiogram and adenogram phases are considered together and if advantage is taken of follow up radiographs. It provides a cheap and simple method of following the patient's response to treatment and of monitoring for relapse.

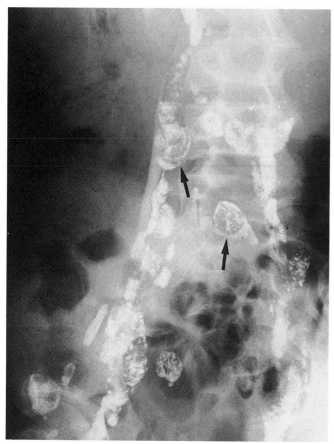

Fig. 99.11 Oblique view of a lymphogram showing the typical spherical filling defects due to metastases [arrows]. In addition there is an unopacified mass compressing nodes in the upper left para-aortic region.

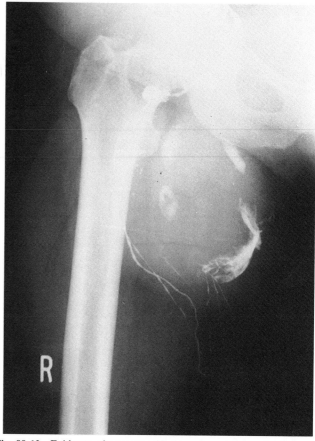

Fig. 99.12 Evidence of an unopacified lymph node mass due to malignant melanoma in the foot. Normal lymphatic vessels and nodes are displaced.

Clinical value of radiology in lymph node assessment

Lymphography and computed tomography provide complementary information so that often both tests are necessary.

Lymphography plays an important part in the staging of metastatic disease and lymphomas. In the first group it is used predominantly for tumours of the pelvis and lower limbs. The incidence of lymphogram positivity, in particular malignant diseases, varies from one centre to another, depending on the treatment available and consequently on the type of caseload.

The incidence of lymph node metastases is directly related to the clinical stage of disease and the histological grade. The *clinical stage* reflects the extent of tumour at presentation and the *histological grade* reflects the degree of differentiation.

Typically, about 34% of all patients presenting with *carcinoma of the cervix* are shown to have lymph node deposits [7]. In the vast majority of these, the pelvis alone, or both the pelvic and para-aortic regions are involved. However, 3% show deposits confined to the para-aortic

region; these are rarely large so that lymphography is essential for their detection.

Endometrial carcinoma produces about 20% lymph node involvement at presentation, of which about 10% are confined to the para-aortic area. 18% of *ovarian carcinoma* patients have lymph node involvement initially and these are distributed fairly equally between the pelvis and para-aortic regions. Rarely, ovarian carcinoma deposits are seen in the superficial inguinal region as a result of spread down the round ligament.

Almost a half of *prostate* and *kidney carcinomas* are accompanied by lymph node metastases at clinical presentation. Although lymphography fails to opacify consistently some groups of pelvic nodes, which are commonly involved early in lymphatic dissemination, the technique is valuable in showing disease which may not be evident in any other way short of surgery. Fibrofatty filling defects are common in pelvic nodes particularly in the elderly and can lead to false positive diagnoses. Such filling defects are usually ill-defined rather than spherical and fail to increase in size with time or to respond to treatment.

The value of lymphography in the management of metastatic disease can be illustrated by the way in which it influences treatment selection in *testicular teratoma* [8,9]. A half of testicular teratoma patients have lymph node deposits at presentation. *Stage 1* is the group in which there is no detectable residual disease after orchidectomy. To come to that conclusion, the patients will have had a negative CT scan of the chest and abdomen and a negative lymphogram.

Since 1979 stage I teratoma patients have received no treatment other than orchidectomy. Approximately 20% subsequently relapse and are cured by chemotherapy.

Stage II patients (abdominal node involvement) receive chemotherapy followed in selected cases by surgery to excise the residual masses.

Whilst lymphography and CT are equally accurate in identifying nodal disease of this type, CT give a better estimation of the precise size. In addition it shows the relationship to important structures such as the renal vessels prior to lymphadenectomy.

In stage III, lymph node metastases are present on both sides of the diaphragm. These patients also procede to chemotherapy, radiotherapy and possibly lymphadenectomy.

Stage IV disease is characterized by systemic metastases usually to the lungs, demonstrated by conventional radiography or CT. Since both pulmonary and lymphatic involvement are common at presentation, the patients undergo chest and abdominal computed tomography and lymphography. CT has the advantage of demonstrating pulmonary metastases and mediastinal lymph node enlargement more sensitively than any other procedure. In the abdomen, whilst CT shows the relationship of massive lympadenopathy to surrounding structures (Fig. 99.13), lymphography is necessary for follow up studies.

The recognition of abnormality by CT relies upon an increase in lymph node size. Nodes greater than 2 cm are considered definitely abnormal: those between 1 and 2 cm equivocal. An asymmetric distribution of nodes of normal size may also be significant, particularly in the pelvis where lymph node metastases are often small and may involve groups of nodes unopacified by lymphography.

CT assessment of the para-aortic region is much easier than the pelvis since the transverse plane of CT cuts perpendicularly across the long axis of the nodes, whilst in the pelvis the nodes run obliquely. The aorta and inferior vena cava are surrounded by a fat plane which facilitates recognition of lymph nodes. A fat plane is not present in the pelvis. Assessment of lymphadenopathy in children and the cachectic (with no fat) is less accurate than in normal adults.

Lymph nodes off the axis normally opacified by lymphography can be shown by CT but this is often difficult. Nodes in the mesentery and splenic hilum, which are most often abnormal due to lymphoma, are frequently obscured by adjacent bowel (Fig. 99.14). The 'advantage' of CT has an important but relatively limited practical application. CT shows lymphadenopathy above the level of L2 which is often the upper limit of lymphogram opacification (Fig. 99.15).

The demonstration of metastatic involvement of *mediastinal lymph nodes* can have an important impact on treatment selection. In carcinoma of the bronchus, a negative radiological assessment would mean that the patient would procede to pulmonary resection, whilst if it were positive, radiotherapy would be the treatment of choice.

In the presence of a normal or equivocal appearance of the mediastinum on a PA chest radiograph, further assessment relies on CT, which is a very sensitive method of showing enlarged mediastinal lymph nodes [11]. It will certainly demonstrate areas which are not visible by conventional methods, such as the pretracheal and internal mammary nodes. Whilst nodes greater than 2 cm in diameter are usually malignant, CT does not provide histology and since lymph nodes may be enlarged as a

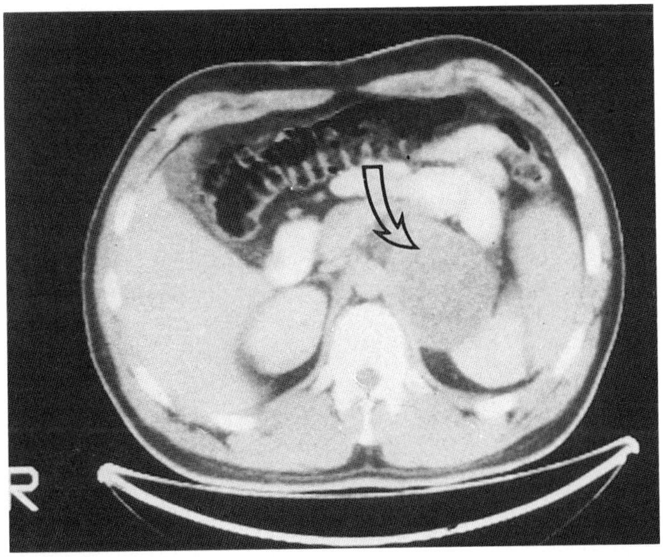

Fig. 99.13 CT scan. A lymph node mass [arrow] in the left para-aortic region lies in contact with the aorta and left crus of diaphragm and is displacing the left kidney laterally. A common appearance in testicular teratoma.

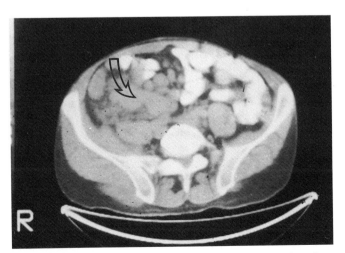

Fig. 99.14 A CT scan through the lower abdomen shows enlarged mesenteric nodes [arrow] displacing opacified loops of bowel.

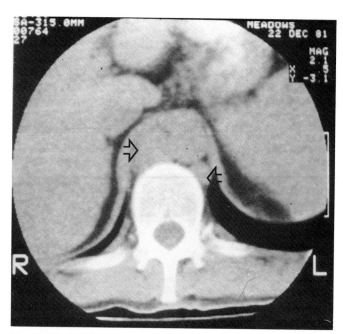

Fig. 99.15 A CT scan at the level of D12 demonstrates retrocrural lymphadenopathy [arrow]. Lymphography is not usually helpful at this level.

THE LYMPHOMAS

The lymphomas are not a homogeneous group of diseases but are a complex group with widely differing cellular origin, natural history and variable response to treatment. No single staging protocol is appropriate to the whole group. Treatment selection however, has to be based on two fundamental factors (a) the *histological* subtype and (b) the *extent* or *stage* of the disease.

Radiology plays a major part in determining the staging criteria in both *Hodgkin's disease* (*HD*) and *non-Hodgkin's lymphoma* (*NHL*) which are defined by the Ann Arbor classification set out in Table 99.5 [13]. This assigns a *clinical stage* determined from the history, physical examination, tissue biopsy, laboratory and radiological investigations. The absence (A) or presence (B) of the specific symptoms of fever, weight loss and night sweats is also noted. A more accurate *pathological stage* is decided on the additional results of bone marrow and liver biopsies, laparotomy and splenectomy.

About a quarter of all lymphoma patients have an abnormal chest radiograph at presentation [14,15]. This is

result of concommitant inflammatory disease in the presence of malignancy, a biopsy procedure may still be necessary. CT may indicate whether this would be best carried out by transcervical mediastinoscopy or anterior parasternal mediastinotomy.

CT allows the assessment of nodal areas which are inaccessible by these operative methods, such as the aortopulmonary window, anterior prevascular space, left tracheobronchial angle and posterior mediastinum. In the presence of a negative CT scan, mediastinoscopy is unneccessary [12].

Whilst AP and 55 degree oblique hilar tomography together have hitherto been accepted as the best method of demonstrating hilar lymph node enlargement, with newer CT scanning machines, a greater amount of accumulated experience and the use of intravenous contrast medium, CT is probably just as accurate.

The criteria for the assessment for cervical lymph nodes by CT are virtually identical to those for other areas. These include nodal enlargement above 2 cm diameter, collections of multiple nodes of normal size, and effacement of tissue planes in clinical circumstances where nodal disease is likely. No other radiological procedure is helpful in this regard. However, CT rarely shows cervical lymph node enlargement which is not evident clinically. One area which may be missed clinically is enlargement of the lymph node of Rouvier, in the nasopharynx, where it can be difficult for the surgeon to recognize that the lateral wall of the nasopharynx is closer to the midline on one side than the other.

CT and clinical assessment are equally difficult in those situations where normal tissue planes have been destroyed either by radical neck dissection or by radiotherapy.

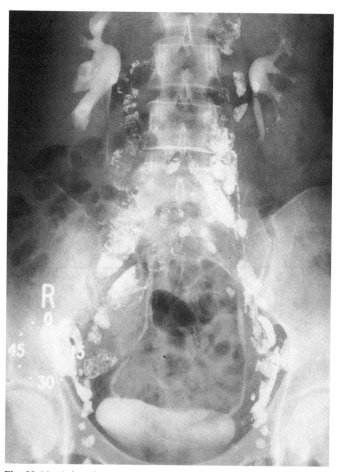

Fig. 99.16 A lymphogram showing the typical foamy lymph node enlargement in lymphoma. There is a minor degree of hydronephrosis on the right and the lower end of the right ureter is displaced medially.

usually due to upper mediastinal lymphadenopathy sometimes extending to one or other hilum. Pulmonary parenchymal disease is rare at presentation in HD and occurs in about 4% of patients with NHL. The most common pattern of pulmonary involvement is by direct extension from

Table 99.5 Ann Arbor staging classification.

Stage I
Involvement of a single lymph node region (I) or single extralymphatic site (IE)

Stage II
Involvement of two or more lymph node regions on the same side of the diaphragm (II), which may also include the spleen (IIS), localized extralymphatic involvement (IIE), or both (IISE), if confined to the same side of the diaphragm.

Stage III
Involvement of lymph node regions on both sides of the diaphragm (III), which may also include the spleen (IIIS), localized extralymphatic involvement (IIIE), or both (IIISE)

Stage IV
Diffuse or disseminated involvement of extralymphatic sites (e.g. bone marrow, liver, or multiple pulmonary metastases)

involved hilar nodes. If mediastinal lymphadenopathy is massive, whole lung tomograms or CT may be necessary before the pulmonary involvement is recognized.

Lymphography demonstrates retroperitoneal lymph node involvement in about 40% of patients with HD. The incidence of positivity in NHL varies with the histological subtype from 57% in diffuse histiocytic lymphoma to 90% in the nodular forms of the disease. The lymphogram is a good predictor of finding NHL in off-axis lymph nodes or extranodal sites at laparotomy. 81% of stage III patients with a positive lymphogram have been shown to have such involvement, whilst it was present in only 18% when the lymphogram was negative [15]. Similarly, in 80% of HD patients in whom the lungs or spleen are involved, the lymphogram is also positive [14].

The characteristic lymphographic abnormality is *nodal enlargement* with a *loose foamy internal pattern* due to promininent follicles (Fig. 99.16). Radiological interpretation, with appropriate experience, is highly accurate. The appearance of the lymph node in HD is identical to that in NHL and the various histological subgroups of each cannot be differentiated. Metastatic malignant disease can produce a pseudolymphomatous lymph node pattern, as may benign conditions such as

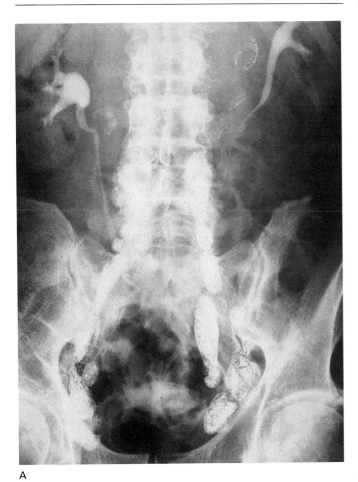

A

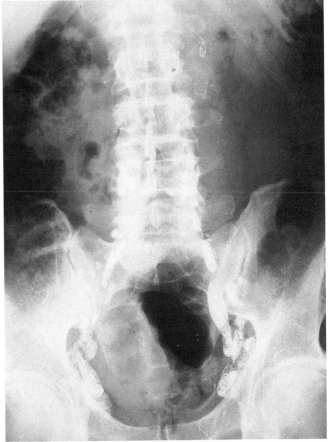

B

Fig. 99.17 (A) The typical lymphogram appearance of a lymphoma with displacement of the upper end of left ureter laterally. The patient was treated with hemicorporeal irradiation, the lower limit of which was the iliac crest.
(B) Not only have the nodes within the treated area responded, but those outside the radiotherapy field have also decreased in size. This is known as the abscopal effect.

reactive hyperplasia, sarcoidosis, tuberculosis and rheumatoid arthritis [16]. Large series comparing lymphography with laparotomy show a true positive score for lymphography in excess of 90%. Patients with a negative lymphography report have about a 25% chance of microscopic involvement being shown by nodal sampling at laparotomy.

The behaviour of the nodes is as important as their appearance. Even normal nodes are slightly swollen immediately after the injection of oil and return to their usual size over a few weeks. Those containing active lymphomatous tissue enlarge without effective treatment, or show a differential rate of volume decrease with treatment (Fig. 99.17).

It is common practice to carry out routine chest and abdominal radiographs throughout follow up in all patients thought to be in remission following treatment for lymphoma. This identifies the first evidence of relapse in about 35% of symptom-free patients who have no clinical evidence of disease [17]. The changes are equally divided between enlargement of opacified retroperitoneal nodes and evidence of mediastinal or lung involvement. A further 30% of relapsing patients produce simultaneous clinical and radiological evidence of disease activity. The need to refill lymphograms by further lymphography and to take routine chest and abdominal radiographs cannot be over emphasized.

Almost half the patients with NHL have mesenteric lymphadenopathy at presentation, which is detectable by CT but not by lymphography. Hodgkins disease only rarely (5%) involves the mesentery and then the nodes are often of normal size. The high incidence of mesenteric involvement coupled with the nodal enlargement permits CT to be more useful in staging non-Hodgkins lymphoma than it is in HD. The incidence of hepatic involvement ranges from 5 to 50% depending upon the histological subgroup in NHL and is only 10% overall in HD.

From these figures, lymphography would seem to be the most useful test in HD and computed tomography in NHL. However, since the information provided by the two tests is different and complementary, both are needed.

SYSTEMIC MALIGNANT METASTASES

The demonstration of dissemination indicates a worse prognosis than localized disease in any tumour type. The primary value in demonstrating metastases in cancer patients is if that knowledge influences the choice of treatment. Haematogenous spread occurs to every organ or tissue at some time and may be diffusely distributed in the terminally ill. The main purpose in carrying out radiological investigations in such circumstances is to identify a complication such as a fracture which is symptomatic and treatable.

The majority of deposits occur first in the *bones, lungs, liver* or *brain*. Occasionally a solitary metastasis or a small group of deposits confined to a single area will precede the development of further spread even by several years. This most commonly occurs in carcinoma of the kidney. In such circumstances it is important to rule out further dissemination, as far as possible, since the single metastasis may be excised at the time the primary tumour is treated.

Whilst in general, dissemination indicates the need for systemic treatment, if such is available, local methods may still be necessary to overcome symptoms caused by the primary tumour such as haemorrhage, pain or obstruction.

Skeletal metastases

Skeletal metastases are particularly common in *carcinoma of the breast, prostate, bronchus, kidney* and *thyroid* and are frequently the first evidence of dissemination. Bone involvement usually occurs at multiple sites but large solitary lytic deposits due to tumours of the kidneys or thyroid occur from time to time.

Breast cancer provides a good model for considering bone involvement. In that disease, the first evidence of metastases occurs in bone in 30%, lung 20%, liver 9% and brain 3% [18]. Radiographic examination is insensitive as 50% of the bone in the line of the X-ray beam must be destroyed before the lesion is visible radiologically.

Scintigraphy is more sensitive and more accurate than radiography for the early detection of skeletal metastases and more accurate even than symptomatology, physical signs or biochemistry. Of the 138 patients with early operable tumours in which there was no other evidence of dissemination, Galasko found 24% to have positive scintigrams. 83% of these patients died of their tumour in 5 years, whilst of those with negative scintigrams, only 26% succumbed. Amongst patients with known dissemination of breast cancer to bone, the scintigram shows additional disease in 72% compared with radiography. In essence, because of the lack of effective treatment, isotope studies merely identify a group of breast cancer patients with a bad prognosis.

If bone scintigraphy is used routinely in all breast cancer patients preoperatively, the positive rate is very low. However, it is now common practice for the patient to undergo biopsy and axillary sampling prior to definitive radical treatment. In those in which the axillary dissection (at biopsy or removal of the breast tumour) identifies four or more histologically involved nodes, the isotope bone scan will be positive in between 10 and 25%. Such an approach confining the investigation to a high risk group is an efficient use of nuclear medicine resources.

The same overall principles will apply in the second most common disease to produce skeletal metastases. In *carcinoma of the prostate*, the skeletal system is involved in about 60% of patients at presentation. Bone scans are the most sensitive method of demonstrating these and will detect involvement in 30 to 50% of patients with negative radiographic studies. Although false negative scans are very uncommon, a radiograph should be obtained of clinically suspicious negative areas. In addition when the isotope scan shows a solitary abnormality, the radiograph must be used to confirm that this actually represents a metastasis and not some other disease.

Bone destruction associated with skeletal metastases is mediated by osteoclasts stimulated by a diffusable activating factor, prostaglandin, secreted by the tumour [19,20]. *New bone formation* similar to callus occurs simultaneously with the destruction. The radiological appearance of the lesion depends on the proportion of each which is present.

Skeletal radiology is enormously useful in showing response to treatment or progression of disease. Progressive disease is recognized by the appearance of new lytic lesions or enlargement of existing deposits. A good response to treatment produces a greater variety of radiological changes. The boundary of a lytic deposit may become better defined as a result of healing in the periphery: continuation of this process may produce a sclerotic rim. The lesions may

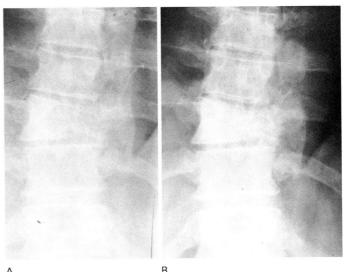

A   B

Fig. 99.19 (A) A metastasis occupying the body of D10 has caused sclerosis on the right but is purely lytic on the left where there is collapse. (B) Following hormone treatment there is re-ossification.

decrease in size and eventually redevelop a trabecular structure, which is often coarser than normal. The healing process may progress to such a degree that homogeneous sclerosis of the whole involved area occurs (Figs 99.18 & 99.19).

Progressive changes on isotope scanning provide the earliest imaging evidence of treatment failure. The most consistent index of response to treatment is symptomatic pain relief which is very rarely experienced by patients with progressive disease [21]. Biochemical evaluation is unreliable, usually because of disease at other sites, particularly the liver.

Pulmonary deposits

The more effort which is put into searching for pulmonary metastases, the more will be found. CT is more sensitive than whole lung tomograms, which in turn is more sensitive than the PA chest radiograph. The greater sensitivity of CT is due to the efficiency of the detector system and the transverse plane of the images [22]. Because of the high contrast of the soft tissue deposits against the surrounding air, very small lesions are detectable (2 to 3 mm) (Fig. 99.20). At CT a metastasis needs to be greater in diameter than the adjacent blood vessels to be recognizable. The sensitivity of CT is about twice that of whole lung tomograms. Either technique is capable of showing more lesions when some are evident on the conventional chest radiograph. However, CT is relatively nonspecific, due to the difficulty of recognizing calcification within soft tissue opacities. To obtain an accurate CT density reading, the metastases must be greater in diameter than the CT slice width. To obtain this, the area containing a suspected metastasis may have to be re-examined using a very narrow slice width such as 2 mm. A CT density reading greater than +100 HU indicates the presence of calcification and the

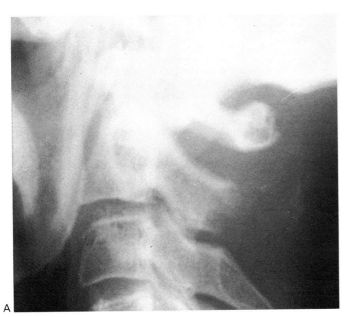

A

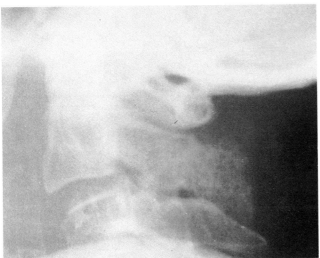

B

Fig. 99.18 (A) A lytic metastasis occupies the spinous process of C2. (B) After radiotherapy, there is re-ossification although not with a normal trabecular pattern.

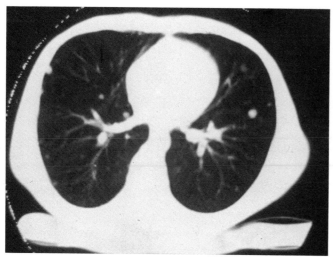

Fig. 99.20 A CT scan through the chest shows numerous small pulmonary metastases. Some of those which lie peripherally would not be demonstrated by conventional methods.

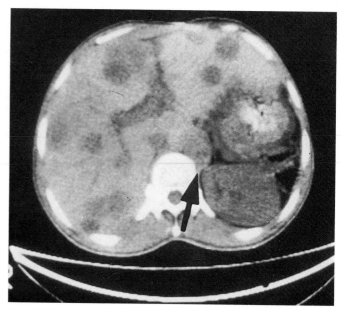

Fig. 99.21 A CT scan shows multiple metastases within the liver even before intravenous contrast medium. In addition there is lymph node enlargement in the left para-aortic region [arrow].

likelihood of a granuloma. A density CT reading in a purely soft tissue range (say 20 to 40 HU) is of course nonspecific.

Routine use of CT or whole lung tomograms is not justifiable in evaluating patients for unsuspected metastases except when there is a high propensity for pulmonary involvement. This occurs predominantly in the *sarcomas* and *testicular teratoma*. CT has been shown to provide additional useful information in about one third more patients with testicular teratoma than is available from whole lung tomograms [23].

Hepatic deposits

Liver scintigraphy is a sensitive method of detecting liver metastases but lacks specificity, so that benign conditions or normal anatomical structures may cause false positive reports (Ch. 100). Lesions less than 2 cm in diameter or those deep within the liver may be missed. If liver biochemical function tests are completely normal, there is a very low positivity rate for liver scintigraphy. As a result of this, the test should be confined to those patients in whom there is clinical evidence of hepatomegaly or when at least one liver function is abnormal. The most commonly used of the function tests is alkaline phosphatase, LDH or SGOT.

A positive liver scintigram should be confirmed by ultrasound which will give increased specificity. Both ultrasound and CT (Fig. 99.21) will show greater than 90% of present liver deposits, but ultrasound has the advantage of being more readily available, cheap and equally sensitive and specific as CT.

Even in those diseases in which liver deposits are particularly common, it is unjustifiable to carry out any radiological procedure in the absence of clinical or biochemical abnormality.

Brain metastases

CT scanning for intracranial metastases is more specific and more sensitive than *radionuclide scanning*. CT is particularly valuable in showing multiple lesions and can usually differentiate benign from malignant. Deposits from breast and lung tumours usually produce irregular areas of decreased density, commonly surrounded by oedema. Enhancement after intravenous contrast medium occurs in 90% of such lesions (Fig. 99.22). In about 10% of these patients, the metastases are only shown after contrast medium. Hyperdense deposits are shown in very vascular metastases particularly from malignant melanoma and occasionally from the bowel.

Routine brain scanning is unjustifiable in neurologically normal patients. The pick-up rate of silent brain deposits is only in the order of 1 in 80 in breast cancer and 1 in 20 in carcinoma of the bronchus.

Metastases from occult primary tumours

3 to 4% of all cancer patients present with a metastasis from an occult primary tumour [24]. 90% of these are in the age range 40 to 80 years but no age is exempt. In only about one third of these patients is the site of origin eventually found, most often at autopsy [25]. About 10% are shown to have second tumours histologically different from the symptomatic metastasis.

The metastatic potential of a tumour does not appear to be related to its size. It is quite possible for early metastatic lesions to themselves produce deposits to other organs. The most common origin of occult primary tumour is the *lung* (40%), after which a wide variety of tissues and *lymphoma*

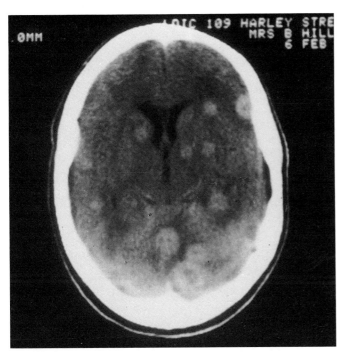

Fig. 99.22 A CT scan after intravenous contrast medium shows multiple cerebral metastases each demonstrating enhancement and some showing surrounding oedema.

account for 1 to 5% each. There is no precise correlation between the presenting clinical features and the site of the primary tumour. The most common clinical presentations are lymphadenopathy, pulmonary or pleural masses and bone or hepatic metastases.

A number of approaches have been advocated in identifying the site of origin. Whichever is used, it should be realised that the median survival is 9 months, with only 10% of patients surviving 5 years, so that investigation should not delay treatment. The most important step is to sample the metastasis to establish histology. Sputum, pleural fluid or ascites should be submitted for cytology.

A thorough investigation using multiple radiological and isotope tests does have the benefit of showing the full extent of disease and indicating prognosis even if the primary tumour is infrequently found. A more rational approach may be to only look for those primary tumours for which there is a useful treatment.

There are reports of successfully using a CT scan of the whole trunk as a single examination to search for the tissue of origin. That approach does have the merit of producing a lot of information without unduly taxing the patient or relatives.

But, a more thoughtful approach using carefully selected tests having regard to the histology of the metastasis and the pattern of spread is this author's preferred approach. Squamous carcinoma in cervical lymph nodes would for instance lead to a chest radiograph and an examination under anaesthesia (EUA) of the larynx and pharynx only.

BIBLIOGRAPHY

REFERENCES

1. Harrison D F N 1978 Critical look at the classification of maxillary sinus carcinomata. Ann Otol Rhinol Laryngol 87:3–9
2. Parsons C, Hodson N 1979 Computed tomography of paranasal sinus tumours. Radiology 132 (3):641–645
3. Jackson B T, Kinmonth J B 1974 The normal lymphographic appearances of the lumbar lymphatics. Clin Radiol 25:175–186
4. MacDonald J S 1982 Lymphography in lymph node disease. In: Kinmonth J B (ed) The lymphatics. Edward Arnold, London
5. Macdonald J S 1976 Lymphography. In: Ansell G (ed) Complications in diagnostic radiology. Blackwell, Oxford
6. Wallace S 1967 Alterations in pulmonary function secondary to oil embolism during lymphography. In: Ruttiman A (ed) Progress in lymphology; Proceedings of International Symposium on Lymphology. George Thieme Verlag, New York
7. Nuttall J, Macdonald J S 1978 Lymphography in tumours of the urogenital tract. J Roy Soc Med 71:41–43
8. Hendry W F, Tyrrell C J, Macdonald J S, McElwain T J, Peckham M J 1977 The detection and localisation of abdominal lymph node metastases from testicular teratomas. Br J Urol 49:739–745
9. Husband J E, Barrett A, Peckham M J 1981 Evaluation of computed tomography in the management of testicular teratoma. Br J Urol 53:179–183
10. Peckham M J, Barrett A, Horwich A, Hendry W F 1983 Orchiectomy alone for Stage I testicular non-seminoma. Br J Urol 55:754–759
11. Osborne D R, Korobkin M, Ravin C E et al 1982 Comparison of plain radiography, conventional tomography and computed tomography in detecting intrathoracic lymph node metastases from lung carcinoma. Radiology 142 (1):149–162
12. Goldstraw P, Kurzer M and Edwards D 1983 Preoperative staging of lung cancer: accuracy of computed tomography versus mediastinoscopy. Thorax 38:10–15
13. Rosenberg S A, Boiron M S, DeVita V T 1970 Report of the committee on Hodgkin's disease staging procedures. Cancer Res 31:1862–1880
14. Jones S E 1980 Importance of staging in Hodgkin's disease. Semin Oncol VII (2):38–47
15. Clabner B A, Fisher R I, Young R C, DeVita V T 1980 Staging of non-Hodgkin's lymphoma. Semin Oncol VII (3):193–199
16. Parker B R, Blank N, Castellino R A 1974 Lymphographic appearance of benign conditions simulating lymphoma. Radiology III:267–274
17. Castellino R A, Blank N, Cassady J R, Kaplan H S 1973 Roentgenologic aspects of Hodgkin's disease: role of routine radiographs in detecting initial relapse. Cancer 31:316–323
18. Galasko C S B 1977 Screening for the potentially curable patient. In: Stoll B A (ed) Breast cancer management. Heinemann, London
19. Galasko C S B 1976 Mechanisms of bone destruction in the development of skeletal metastases. Nature 263:507–508
20. Galasko C S B 1976 Relationship of bone destruction in skeletal metastases to osteoclast activation and prostaglandins. Nature 263:508–510
21. Coombes R C, Dady P, Parsons C, Powles T J 1980 Assessment of response of bone metastases to systemic treatment in patients with breast cancer. Eur J Cancer Supp 1 (1):131–135
22. Sagel S S 1983 In: Lee J K T, Sagel S S, Stanley R J (eds) Computed Body Tomography. Raven Press, New York
23. Husband J E, Peckham M J, Macdonald J S, Hendry W F 1979 The role of computed tomography in the management of testicular teratoma. Clin Radiol 30:243–252
24. Gaber A O, Rice P, Eaton C, Pietrafitta J J Spatz E, Deckers P J 1983 Metastatic malignant disease of unknown origin. Am J Surg 145:493–497
25. Didolkar M S, Fanons N, Elias E G, Moore R H 1977 Metastatic carcinoma from occult primary tumours. Ann Surg 186 (5):625–630

SUGGESTIONS FOR FURTHER READING

Alfonso A E, Gardner B 1982 The practice of cancer surgery. Appleton-Century-Crofts, New York

Coltman C A, Golomb H M 1980 Hodgkin's and non-Hodgkin's lymphomas. Grune and Stratton, New York

Galasko C S B 1977 Screening for the potentially curable patient. In: Stoll B A (ed) Breast cancer management. Heineman, London

Kinmonth J B 1982 The lymphatics. Arnold, London

Smalley R V, Malmud L S, Ritchie W G M 1980 Pre-operative scanning, evaluation for metastatic disease in carcinoma of the breast, lung, colon, bladder and prostate. Semin Oncol 7 (4):358–369

Steckel R J, Kagan A R 1976 Diagnosis and staging of cancer: a radiological approach. Saunders, Philadelphia

100 Nuclear medicine in oncology

William D. Kaplan

Radionuclide liver imaging
  Tumour detection and cell type
  Topography of lesions
  Liver metastases correlated with liver size and liver
    function tests
  Abnormal scintigraphic patterns
  Comparing imaging modalities

Radionuclide bone imaging
  Rationale
  Technical factors
    Radiopharmaceuticals
    Instruments
  Lesion distribution
  Bone scans and serum phosphatase levels
  Bone scans and bone pain
  Bone scans and cell type and clinical stage
  Scan Interpretation

Gallium imaging
  Technical factors
    Instrumentation
    Administered patient dose
    Patient preparation
    Time of imaging
  Mechanism of action
  Scan findings and tumour histology
    Lymphomas
    Pulmonary Malignancies
  Defining the effects of therapy

Dynamic studies
  Venous studies
    Superior vena cava
    Inferior vena cava
    Peripheral venous studies
  Arterial studies
    Hepatic artery infusions

Internal mammary lymphoscintigraphy
  Technical considerations
  Interpretation
  Localization

Radio-immunodetection

Macroscopic tumours can be reliably detected by a number of procedures, including many that use radionuclides. Because so many neoplasms show a propensity to spread to the liver and skeletal system, hepatic and bone scintigraphy have assumed a major role in the identification of metastases and in the evaluation of the cancer patient.

RADIONUCLIDE LIVER IMAGING

For the purpose of this discussion, radionuclide liver imaging implies the use of technetium-99m (^{99m}Tc) sulphur colloid, 85% of which distributes to the liver within 2 to 3 minutes of intravenous administration. Localization of the radiocolloid within this organ is thought to represent sequestration within the Kupffer cells lining hepatic sinusoids. A normal scan demonstrates a pattern of homogenous radiocolloid distribution throughout the liver with any perceptible extrahepatic tracer localized to the spleen (Fig. 100.1).

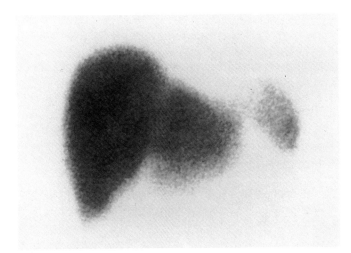

Fig. 100.1 Normal anterior liver-spleen scan. Homogeneous distribution is seen throughout a liver and spleen which are normal in size. The liver accumulates the majority of the radiocolloid.

Tumour detection and cell type

Detection of liver metastases depends largely on the cell type of the primary tumour, as well as on the pathways of spread. A study of more than 1000 patients who were undergoing radiocolloid liver-spleen scans and in whom 17 different tumour cell types were represented, showed an obvious correlation between the scan findings and the specific primary tumour under evaluation [1]. Liver metastases were correctly diagnosed with 84 to 91% accuracy in patients with carcinoma of the testis, ovary, colon, and sarcoma; between 75 to 81% of liver metastases were correctly diagnosed when carcinoma originated in the pancreas, lung, breast, prostate, and in the lymphomas and leukaemias. Least accurate were the liver scan results obtained in patients with upper gastrointestinal tract tumours and malignant melanoma metastatic to the liver.

Up to one third of patients with colon carcinoma will demonstrate liver metastases at the time of initial diagnosis and surgery [2], whereas breast malignancy appears less frequently to involve the liver at the time of initial clinical presentation [3]. Therefore, the anticipated yield from performing a radionuclide liver scan must be adjusted to the specific tumour under investigation.

Topography of lesions

In one series of 450 consecutive autopsies, gross liver involvement by tumour was evident in one third of all cases [4]. Although the right lobe was more commonly affected than the left, the most frequent pattern was bilobar (77% of cases). Approximately one third of the cases with metastases showed involvement by lesions of less than 2 cm in diameter.

Liver metastases correlated with liver size and liver function tests

In the study described above, 31% of the postmortem examinations demonstrated intrahepatic metastases within a liver which was *normal* in size [4].

Although a positive radionuclide scan might seem unlikely in a patient with normal liver function tests, normal liver function tests have been reported in 10 to 40% of patients with liver metastases. Hepatomegaly and/or elevated liver function test results are not the only forerunners of abnormal findings on the liver-spleen scan [5]. Liver metastases may exist with both a normal liver size and normal liver function tests.

Abnormal scintigraphic patterns

The classic pattern for an abnormal liver scan is one of multiple, large, focal abnormalities. Early in the course of metastasis, malignancies such as small cell carcinoma of the lung, carcinoma of the stomach and breast, and the lymphomas may demonstrate only sinusoidal infiltration, so that they resemble diffuse liver disease in scintigraphic appearance (Fig. 100.2). Drum and Beard [6] showed that

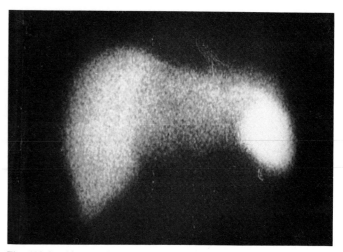

Fig. 100.2 Abnormal anterior liver-spleen scan. Minimal heterogeneity and a shift of radiocolloid uptake to the splenic reticuloendothelial system is seen in the liver and spleen of this patient with carcinoma of the breast metastatic to liver.

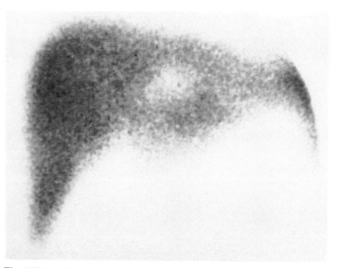

Fig. 100.3 Abnormal anterior liver scan. A solitary focal defect seen in the mid-aspect of the left hepatic lobe in this patient with colon cancer was shown on ultrasound examination to be an echolucent defect due to a dilated hepatic vein.

defining focal defects alone would allow detection of only 67% of hepatic metastases from breast tumours. By adding the criteria of heterogeneity or hepatomegaly, they increased their ability to diagnose liver metastases to 87% without affecting overall accuracy.

Comparing imaging modalities

Three imaging modalities are currently used in the search for liver metastases: radionuclides (RN), ultrasound (US), and computerized tomography (CT) (Table 100.1). Each has advantages and disadvantages. Comparative studies have attempted — unsuccessfully — to define the best single test for this purpose.

Table 100.1 Relative merits of radionuclide (RN), computerized tomographic (CT) and ultrasonographic (US) studies of the liver.

	RN	CT	US
Patient preparation	No	No	No
Contrast required	No	Yes	No
Costly	No	Yes	No
Operator dependent	No	No	Yes
Image affected by:			
bowel gas	No	No	Yes
abdominal wounds	No	No	Yes
metal clips	No	Yes	Yes
patient cooperation	No	Yes	Yes
breathing	No	Yes	Yes
Extrahepatic information	No	Yes	Yes
Specific	No	Yes	Yes
Routinely sensitive to:			
focal defects <1 cm	No	Yes	Yes
focal defects >1 cm	Yes	Yes	Yes
mild diffuse disease	Yes	No	No
Radiation exposure	Yes	Yes	No
Usually easy to schedule	Yes	No	Yes

The CT scanner is the newest and most sophisticated imaging tool to be incorporated in the diagnostic work-up; therefore, the image interpreter tends to be more critical in his appraisal of the CT image [2]. Contiguous 1 cm CT slices taken before and after oral and intravenous contrast are frequently compared to standard ultrasound studies and to radionuclide scans performed with round-hole, low-energy, all-purpose collimators as opposed to one with hexagonal holes and high resolution [7].

Alderson and his colleagues [7] analysed the data by both the usual 'sensitivity and specificity' approach and by receiver operating characteristic (ROC) curves. They found that CT had a slightly higher sensitivity $\frac{TP}{(TP + FN)}*$ (0.93) than RN (0.86) or US (0.82), with specificities $\frac{TP}{(TN + FP)}*$ of 0.88, 0.83, and 0.85, respectively. These differences were not statistically significant.

Analysis of ROC curves indicated that CT demonstrated a higher true positive rate for every rate of false positive. The overall performance of CT, however, did not differ significantly from that of scintigraphy.

Additional metastatic findings (e.g. ascites, pleural effusions), although related to the primary neoplastic process, were not critical in patient management.

In a similar study by Smith et al [8], a lesion-by-lesion analysis of 82 metastatic foci in 18 patients showed that although CT could best define small metastatic deposits followed by US and RN, none of the three current techniques could be expected to detect *routinely* lesions smaller than 2 cm in size. A research technique involving prior intravenous injection of emulsified iodinated oil will show smaller hepatic metastases on CT scanning.

Summary The radionuclide approach is sensitive and cost-effective and serves as a reasonable and acceptable first step when liver images are required in malignant disease.

* TP = true positive FP = false positive
  TN = true negative FN = false negative

Ultrasound should be utilized to answer questions about specificity i.e. extrinsic compression, a prominent porta-hepatis or solitary focal defects (Fig. 100.3).

RADIONUCLIDE BONE IMAGING

Rationale

The advantages of evaluating the skeletal system with radionuclides lies in the exquisite sensitivity of this test for defining regions of increased blood flow and bone turnover. Before a lytic lesion is apparent on plain radiograph, approximately 50% of the bone mineral content must be lost. Bone scan findings may precede X–ray changes by months or even years.

Skeletal scintigraphy is the screening examination of choice in the search for bony metastases among cancer patients. Radiographs are then indicated to clarify (a) any abnormal sites defined on bone scan or (b) clinically symptomatic foci which show no scintigraphic evidence of tumour. Table 100.2 summarizes the results of five series comparing the yield of bone scans and radiographs [9].

Table 100.2 Correlation of scan and X–ray findings (%) in skeletal evaluations of 2282 patients [9]

Scan findings	+	+	−	−
X–ray findings	+	−	+	−
	33	25	2	40

Technical factors

Radiopharmaceuticals

Use of a technetium-99m (^{99m}Tc) labelled phosphate compound for bone imaging combines the physical characteristics of (a) a 140 keV photon, (b) a 6-hour half-life and (c) a 555 to 740 MBq dose to produce a remarkably sensitive test for defining early skeletal metastases.

The selection of a 'best' ^{99m}Tc labelled phosphate compound is however a matter of continued debate. It would appear that the diphosphonates allow more rapid blood clearance than the pyrophosphates [10], providing greater bone to soft-tissue ratios earlier in time. Recently, a number of chemical substitutions on the central carbon atom of the diphosphonates have shown potential for providing superior clinical images.

Instrumentation

We recommend use of a gamma camera as opposed to a rectilinear scanner: (a) the tomographic effect of a focused collimator precludes optimal resolution of skeletal structures close to the crystal; (b) it is frequently difficult to set the margins of a rectilinear scanner so that the entire body is included; (c) it is difficult to monitor the collimator-to-patient distance continually during the imaging procedure when using a rectilinear scanner with the probe above the table; and (d) the information density (counts per cm[2] of film) is two to four times greater with the gamma camera.

Lesion distribution

Skeletal metastases most commonly involve the axial skeleton [11] but the extremities should also be imaged.

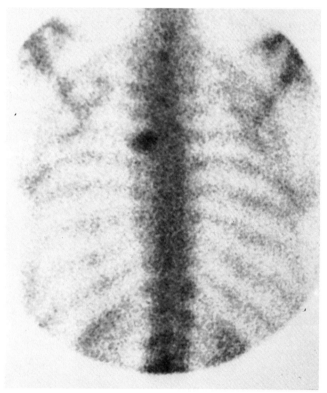

Fig. 100.4   Abnormal posterior thoracic bone scan. A solitary focus of increased uptake is seen to the left of the vertebral body at the approximate level of T5 in this patient with early breast cancer.

Without baseline information about the whole skeleton prior to treatment, one cannot be sure of the patient's response to chemotherapy. In approximately 6 to 8% of patients, the abnormal skeletal metastasis will appear as a solitary focus on scan [12] (Fig. 100.4); of these solitary foci, approximately 20% will occur in the extremities.

Relationship of bone scan findings and serum phosphatase levels

Cowan and Young [13] reviewed the serum alkaline phosphatase determinations in 100 patients with bone scans positive for metastatic disease. 38% of these had *normal* enzyme levels. It has been reported that up to 90% of the alkaline phosphatase elevations in Hodgkin's patients are hepatic (rather than skeletal) in origin [14].

Serial acid phosphatase levels are sometimes used to monitor skeletal metastases in patients with prostatic carcinoma. Paulson et al [15] reviewed the implications of bone scan results on the staging of 425 such patients. Of 190 individuals with negative radiographs and *normal* serum acid phosphatase levels, 30 (16%) evidenced positive RN bone scans. Schaffer and Prendergrass [16] showed that 39% of patients with positive bone scans had *normal* acid phosphatase determinations.

The clinician should not therefore rely solely upon the serum phosphatase (alkaline and/or acid) determination when screening patients for suspected bony metastases.

Relationship of bone scan findings and bone pain

Although pain is a nonspecific finding, its presence in a patient with a known primary malignancy must raise the suspicion of skeletal metastases. However, the absence of bone pain in such patients should not be construed as indicating an absence of skeletal metastases. From 20 to 50% of patients with proven metastases may be symptom-free at the site of bony involvement [9,16].

Relationship of bone scan findings to cell type and clinical staging

Not all of the tumours encountered in clinical practice will commonly involve the skeletal system (Table 100.3) [17]. For

Table 100.3 Incidence of bone metastases at postmortem examination [17].

Primary tumour	Involvement of bone (%)
Breast	50–85
Hodgkin's Disease	50–70
Lung	30–50
Prostate	50–70

instance, metastases from gynaecological malignancies [18] and those originating from tumours of the head and neck [19] uncommonly disseminate to the bones.

Of equal importance is the stage of disease at the time of obtaining the bone scan. In patients with bronchogenic carcinoma, Harbert [20] found a clear correlation between bone scan findings and the presence of certain clinical factors: bone pain or an elevated serum alkaline phosphatase level (Table 100.4). Patients with breast carcinoma however,

Table 100.4 Relationship of clinical signs and symptoms to bone scan results in patients with lung cancer [20]

Clinical signs and symptoms	No. of Patients	True positive bone scans (%)
Absent	90	5.5
Present	116	41.0

Table 100.5 Correlation of clinical stage of breast cancer and bone scan results in 1507 patients [20].

Stage of disease	I	II	III
Number of patients	533	696	278
Percentage of true-positive scans	3	7	25

provide the best demonstration of the relationship between clinical stage of disease and bone scan findings. Table 100.5 presents a summary of 12 studies evaluating bone scan results in over 1500 patients with carcinoma of the breast [20]. The yield of positive scans increases dramatically in patients with clinical stage III disease.

Scan interpretation

Relationship to radiographs

Conventional bone radiographs are frequently of little value for detecting focal (metastatic) lesions in trabecular bone, and in demonstrating changes secondary to metastatic disease which occurs slowly. Citrin et al [21] noted that 29% of patients with breast cancer demonstrated persistently normal bone radiographs in spite of documented and unequivocal scan evidence for skeletal metastases.

Both healing and progression of disease can produce similar radiographic findings (Fig. 100.5). An osteolytic lesion which converts to a sclerotic lesion on radiographic evaluation usually represents a response to therapy.

A meticulous and orderly evaluation of *both* the bone scan and the bone radiographs is therefore mandatory for accurate diagnosis. In evaluating bone scans for the effects of therapy for skeletal metastases, we routinely review at least two preceding studies of the entire skeleton.

The diagnostic criteria commonly utilized for interpreting a bone scan as 'abnormal' are summarized in Table 100.6.

Table 100.6 Diagnostic criteria for interpreting bone scan as abnormal [22].

Resolution of disease
   decreased uptake in known lesions
   disappearance of known lesions

Progression of disease
   increased uptake in, and increased size of known lesions
   new lesions

Healing or 'flare' response to therapy
   increased uptake in known lesions
   new lesions seen
   occurrence within months of commencing therapy
   repeat scan (2 to 3 months) shows decreased uptake in known lesions
   with no change in therapy.

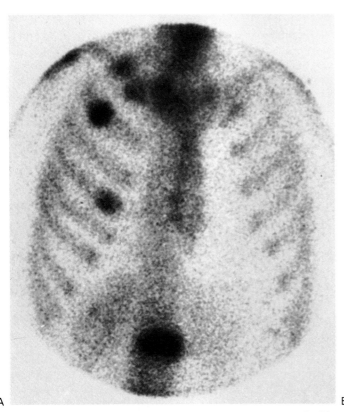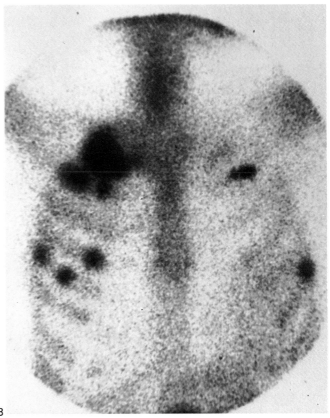

A   B

Fig. 100.5 (A) Abnormal baseline anterior thoracic bone scan. In this patient who failed hormonal therapy for breast cancer, abnormal uptake is seen in the right anterior first, second, and fourth ribs, as well as in a posterior lesion in the lumbar spine and the left anterior first rib.
(B) Abnormal follow-up anterior thoracic bone scan. A follow-up scan 3 months later showed a marked increase in the abnormal uptake involving the right first rib, as well as more extensive involvement of the second and fourth ribs. New lesions are seen in the right fourth and left sixth ribs.
Radiograph showed destruction of distal right first rib at time of (A). Follow-up radiography at time of (B) showed marked sclerosis of the distal first right rib indicating healing.

A decrease of focal tracer accumulation, or its complete disappearance on bone scan, is generally considered to indicate resolution of disease. Progression of skeletal disease is generally manifested as an increase in either the degree or the size of abnormal RN uptake, or the appearance of new lesions.

In patients with breast cancer, however, it is probable that increased RN uptake in a previously defined abnormal focus (Fig. 100.5) or the appearance of new RN lesions may also represent healing, probably due to a positive response to therapy, which initiates an osteoblastic reaction and an increase in bone turnover[22]. Pollen and Shlaer[23] have reported similar findings in a series of patients with prostate cancer, 44% of whom demonstrated an osteoblastic response as part of the healing reaction. The initial worsening of the bone scan was thought to be an example of a 'flare' effect of healing.

Sclerosis of a previously lytic bone lesion does qualify as radiographic evidence for healing; but Bitran[24] showed that recalcification of lytic lesions occured infrequently (11%). Correlation of scan findings and median survival in months from both the Citrin and Bitran series[21,24] suggests that the scintigrapher may be able to provide a broad estimate of prospective survival (Table 100.7).

Table 100.7 Survival correlated with bone scan findings in patients with breast cancer.

Scan interpretation	Median survival	months
Progression	9[†]	7.8[*]
Stable	19[†]	17.7[*]
Improved	30[†]	—

† Citrin[21]
* Bitran[24]
— Not reported

Summary The bone scan is an extremely sensitive technique for defining sites of skeletal metastases. Meticulous attention to detail during the film interpretation is mandatory. High-resolution, static views of the axial skeleton must be correlated with radiographs of all abnormal areas as well as areas which are normal on scan but are clinically symptomatic.

GALLIUM IMAGING

Although many radiopharmaceuticals have been used to define neoplastic tissue, gallium-67 (^{67}Ga) as the citrate has been the tracer most widely applied for this purpose.

In any discussion of gallium imaging, a number of key technical factors must be considered. These include instrumentation, patient dose, patient preparation, time of imaging, mechanism of action, histology of the tumour under study, and the effects of therapy on ^{67}Ga tumour uptake.

Technical factors

Instrumentation

Until the last few years, ^{67}Ga imaging was commonly performed with a rectilinear scanner, utilizing a 5-inch focused collimator and a wide-window energy setting encompassing two or three of the four ^{67}Ga photopeaks. This approach was used in a number of cooperative studies which evaluated the efficacy of ^{67}Ga imaging in patients with Hodgkin's and non-Hodgkin's lymphoma, lung cancer, and genitourinary cancer[25,26,27].

Studies have shown that the best ^{67}Ga images are obtained with a large field gamma camera with triple peak window capability (approximately eight times more efficient than the dual probe-5-inch rectilinear scanner, using a single 93 keV photopeak window). This appears true for ^{67}Ga images obtained from either planar or tomographic gamma cameras.

The ^{67}Ga energy spectrum (four photopeaks in the range of 93 to 394 keV) dictates collimator selection; therefore, even if the photopeak selected for imaging is at the lower range of energies (i.e. 93 or 185 keV), a thick septa collimator is required to eliminate high-energy photon interactions with the crystal. A low-energy, technetium-99m collimator *cannot* be used to image a gallium patient.

Administered patient dose

The recommended injected dose for the adult population has been in the range of 1300 to 1850 KBq/kg. Over the past few years, larger doses (111 to 222 MBq) have been utilized routinely, with up to 370 MBq given to patients with a known malignancy. The increased number of photons available with these larger doses provides an increase in both resolution and sensitivity, both of critical importance in tumour staging and follow up. The increase in photon flux of larger administered doses should not result in decreased imaging time, but should provide an increased count density for the same imaging time.

Patient preparation

Novetsky et al[28] evaluated four separate regimens designed to optimize abdominal gallium imaging: they found that failure of patients to follow instructions was a significant impediment to success.

Time of imaging

Patients are usually studied between 48 and 72 hours after tracer administration. This delay allows greater tumour to background ratios and, therefore, greater sensitivity in defining sites of neoplastic tissue. Images obtained at 96 to 120 hours allow the clinician to differentiate physiological versus pathological focal accumulations of the tracer. Beal and Chaudhuri[29], who investigated sequential images performed over a 1-week time interval, showed that no studies negative at day 3 became positive at day 7, and that positive exams, abnormal at 72 hours, remained positive over the 1-week imaging interval. On the other hand, there were some examples of findings questionable at 72 hours (especially in the abdominal area) which became normal with delayed views.

Mechanism of action

Gallium-67 sequesters in tissue which is well vascularized and viable; accumulation is much less avid in regions of necrosis or fibrosis. [67]Ga uptake appears to be related to rapid tracer binding to transferrin. The gallium-transferrin unit then serves as the active radiopharmaceutical, thought to interact with specific transferrin receptor sites on the wall of the tumour cell. Binding to the cell wall allows incorporation of the radiogallium into the cell. Once inside, the gallium is thought to be deposited within lysosomes and then further distributed to intracellular ferritin, microvesicles, and the rough endoplasmic reticulum. Hoffer et al indicate that ^{67}Ga is primarily associated with lactoferrin which is normally found in breast milk, bone marrow, and nasopharyngeal, salivary, and genital secretions [30]. Lactoferrin binds gallium more avidly than does transferrin and can account for the common sites of ^{67}Ga uptake seen during routine imaging.

Relationship of scan findings to tumour histology

Certain malignancies appear to be delineated more successfully than others by gallium-67. These include Hodgkin's disease, diffuse histiocytic and Burkitt's lymphoma, hepatomas, melanomas, and leukaemias. There appears to be no major application for gallium imaging in patients with tumours of the head and neck, gastrointestinal tract, genitourinary system, and breast.

Those malignancies in which gallium may prove useful include the non-Hodgkin's lymphomas, testicular cancers, mesotheliomas, and carcinoma of the lung. We have selected lymphomas and pulmonary malignancies for further discussion.

Lymphomas

In general, Hodgkin's lymphomas appear to show the greatest degree of ^{67}Ga uptake. Nodular sclerosing type of lymphoma sequesters gallium to a greater degree than does the lymphocyte predominant type [25] (Fig. 100.6).

Gallium-67 shows a sensitivity of nearly 90% for identifying tumour foci in Hodgkin's patients. With non-Hodgkin's lymphoma, sensitivity is lower — approximately 75% — and again it varies according to cell type, being highest for histiocytic lymphoma and lowest for well differentiated lymphocytic lymphoma [26]. A review [31], by histological classification and tumour location of all lymphoma cell types in patients undergoing gallium scanning, looked at disease sites versus scan sensitivity. They found a range of 0.53 to 0.78. This

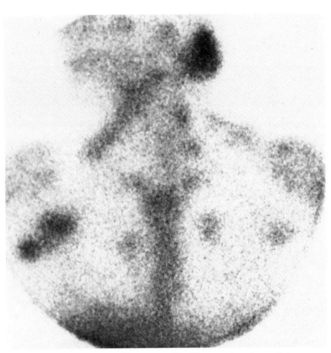

Fig. 100.6 Abnormal gallium scan. In this anterior view of the thorax obtained 72 hours following administration of 8 mCi of ^{67}Ga-citrate, we see abnormal tracer accumulation in the neck, perihilar and axillary areas bilaterally. This patient, with nodular sclerosing Hodgkin's disease, presented for restaging.

suggests that with a negative test result, if there continues to be suspicion of persistent disease, the clinician *must* pursue the work-up of occult lymphomatous disease.

The specificity of gallium imaging in lymphoma patients approaches 95%. The false positive rate is only 5%. This suggests that an abnormal scan *must* be interpreted as representing disease until proven otherwise. The sensitivities quoted should be considered the least that ^{67}Ga can provide as suboptimal techniques were used to generate the data.

Superficial lesions and those located within the thorax are more readily defined (sensitivity of 0.83 and 0.96, respectively) than those located in the abdomen or pelvis (sensitivity of approximately 0.50) [31].

We suggest that, although a negative study may not exclude the presence of disease, demonstration of an abnormal focus strongly suggests that the site in question does, in fact, represent tumour until proven otherwise.

Pulmonary malignancies

Because ^{67}Ga is not normally found within the thorax, it is highly suitable for defining sites of pulmonary tumour. Its usefulness in this area does not appear to have a major relationship to cell type, and its overall sensitivity for defining lung tumours approaches 0.90.

Candidates for gallium imaging include the patient with positive sputum cytology and patients with a hydrothorax, in whom standard radiological techniques and bronchoscopy are unrewarding.

When the gallium image is positive in the mediastinum, or when radiographic changes within mediastinal nodes are present, mediastinoscopy is indicated. Should the mediastinum show no gallium-67 uptake, and the chest radiographs and computed tomography are normal, mediastinoscopy can be avoided and the patient can be assumed to be free of mediastinal metastases.

Data comparing gallium-67 to preoperative chest radiographs, linear tomography and computed tomography for the staging of patients with primary lung cancer, indicate that gallium scintigraphy is extremely sensitive for defining hilar and/or mediastinal disease, while computed tomography appears to be most effective for the evaluation of paramediastinal masses.

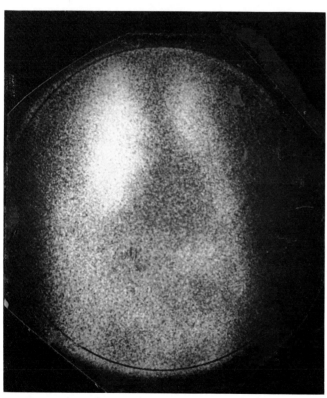

Fig. 100.7 Abnormal gallium scan. Diffuse uptake is seen throughout both lungs in this 96-hour anterior image of the thorax and abdomen in a patient proven to have Bleomycin lung toxicity.
(Activity recorded as white spots on blackground).

A positive gallium scan is helpful in defining the extent of disease and predicting whether or not a surgical cure is possible. Caution must be exercised, however, since many benign inflammatory lesions may cause either focal or diffuse pulmonary uptake of the radiotracer (Fig. 100.7). A normal gallium scan is also important, since the false-negative rate for pulmonary malignancies approximates 0.05.

Defining the effects of therapy

Among cancer patients, gallium-67 is chiefly used to monitor the effects of radiation or chemotherapy, and to search for recurrent disease. There is experimental evidence from animal studies to indicate that *whole body* irradiation will decrease ^{67}Ga uptake within tumour foci, a finding not seen when radiation therapy is directed to the *tumour site alone* [32]; some investigators also suggest that irradiation or chemotherapy will produce changes in whole body retention of [67]Ga. Whether this data will be supported in humans remains to be determined. Certainly, evidence that steroids suppress gallium uptake in brain tumours is sufficient to make negative imaging results highly questionable in a cancer patient with a CNS neoplasm who has been receiving steroid drugs. The most important finding, however, is persistent radiogallium concentration within a tumour site which has been previously irradiated or exposed to chemotherapy. This finding is highly indicative of residual or recurrent disease (Fig. 100.8). Recurrent malignancy is most likely when a scan that appeared normal following treatment, then becomes positive on later follow-up.

We have recently evaluated 52 consecutive lymphoma patients (21 with Hodgkin's disease and 31 with non-

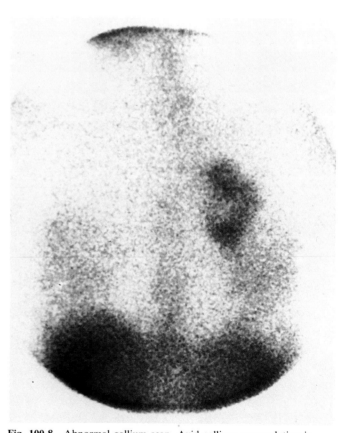

Fig. 100.8 Abnormal gallium scan. Avid gallium accumulation is seen in the mid-aspect of the left lung in a site of active Hodgkin's disease which recurred outside the radiation field. The scan was ordered to differentiate chest radiographic changes of radiation fibrosis or recurrent tumour. Diffuse uptake in the both lower lung fields represents tracer accumulation in the breasts.

Hodgkin's lymphoma) who were seen for staging and/or post-treatment follow-up [33]; a total of 99 gallium scans were obtained.

Gallium-67 imaging in defining or excluding sites of active lymphoma had an accuracy of 0.96 with a sensitivity and specificity of greater than 0.90 for both Hodgkin's and non-Hodgkin's patients. There were no false-positive scans in our series. Although pneumonia, a *potential* source of false-positive results, occurred in four patients, the pattern of abnormal gallium uptake within the lung along with radiographic findings correctly defined the nonmalignant aetiology.

There was a single false-negative result in the Hodgkin's group in a patient with biopsy-proven liver metastases. In three patients with non-Hodgkin's lymphoma, the technique failed to identify subsequent progression of disease. The gallium scan proved more accurate than other contemporaneous radiological studies in defining the clinical course of this group of patients (Table 100.8).

Table 100.8 ^{67}Ga scan results compared with contemporaneous radiological studies [33]

| | Tests agree | | Tests disagree | |
	Both +	Both −	^{67}Ga correct	^{67}Ga incorrect
Abdominal CT	10	6	5	0
Lymphangiogram	3	2	0	1
Ultrasound	12	13	6	2
Liver-spleen scan	15	18	0	1
Chest radiograph	26	23	5	0
Chest CT	1	2	1	0
Bone scan	7	9	1	0
Totals	74	73	18	4

^{67}Ga = gallium^{67}

Summary We suggest that with larger administered tracer doses, dual or triple peak Anger camera imaging and careful attention to both technical details and clinical correlation, for selected tumours, ^{67}Ga will offer the clinician accurate information about the status of his patient.

DYNAMIC STUDIES

The use of radiopharmaceuticals makes it possible for the clinician to evaluate dynamically both the peripheral and central venous system, by rapid sequence image collection during tracer injection. The study is physiological in nature since (a) only small injected volumes are necessary to delineate vascular anatomy, (b) the material is injected in a vehicle of normal saline, and (c) slow flow rates can be used as opposed to the bolus injections needed for radiological contrast studies. The patient can be injected while supine, seated or standing and imaged from the anterior, posterior, or lateral position; any region of the body can be evaluated.

Venous studies

Radionuclide studies of the venous anatomy have generally centred about evaluations of the superior vena cava (SVC) and inferior vena cava (IVC) following upper and lower extremity injections, respectively.

Superior vena cava

The thin-walled SVC is confined to a relatively small and rigid space, with the ascending aorta situated posteromedially, and perivenous lymph nodes laterally. Extrinsic compression from either enlarging lymph nodes or adjacent tumour can result in compromised venous return, with subsequent development of collateral circulation.

Malignancies, mainly bronchogenic carcinoma and lymphoma, are the most common causes of SVC compression and obstruction, accounting for 80% and 10% of cases, respectively.

Radionuclides provide a useful tool for the investigation of potential SVC obstruction and the assessment of collateral flow [34].

Collateral venous structures include the azygos, internal mammary, vertebral, and lateral thoracic systems. The level of obstruction will determine which route will predominate (Fig. 100.9).

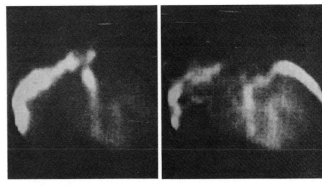

Fig. 100.9 Abnormal SVC flow study. On the left, a unilateral flow study demonstrates dilatation of the right subclavian vein with marked narrowing at the junction of the subclavian vein and the superior vena cava. On the right, a follow-up study performed approximately 3 weeks later shows occlusion of the right innominate vein with marked collateral formation. A simultaneous left-sided injection demonstrates persistent patency of the superior vena cava.

Technical considerations

When patients present with clinical signs suggesting SVC syndrome, and unilateral upper extremity oedema, we suggest that every attempt should be made to inject *both* arms. Concomitant injection of the normal arm will allow evaluation of the SVC should the inlet to that structure on the oedematous side be occluded.

Use of a small-gauge needle, slow infusion as opposed to bolus administration, and attention to achieving haemostasis by applying external compression at the puncture site for 15 minutes will ensure no haemorrhagic complications.

Interpretation of SVC studies

Miyamae [34] has summarized the radionuclide results in 92 patients and documented a range of normal anatomical variants. These include:

(a) Nonpathological abnormalities involving the innominate vein, especially on the left when viewed anteriorly, since the injected radionuclide travels in a horizontal course posterior to the sternum

(b) Attenuation of gamma rays from overlying skeletal absorption which can artifactually produce a region of apparent 'decreased flow'

(c) A normal narrowing of the axillary vein because of compression by adjacent muscles and ligaments (particularly prominent during marked supination of the forearm or with compression of the axillary vein by the humeral head)

(d) A normal 'filling defect' as the superior vena cava enters its intrapericardial portion.

Inferior vena cava (IVC)

Compromised blood flow in the IVC is seen less frequently than in the SVC: malignancy is the most common single aetiology. The usual radionuclide method of evaluation involves bipedal tracer injection. The normal lower extremity radionuclide venogram does not outline secondary and tertiary channels of the venous circulation but when the inferior vena cava is obstructed, some of the smaller tributaries assume the function of the cava. The major venous collateral channels that may be visualized include the ascending lumbar veins, the azygos and hemiazygos systems, the paravertebral venous plexus, the anterior parietal veins, as well as caval-portal anastomoses [35]

Interpretation of IVC studies

Visualization of the IVC as well as the common and external iliac veins in an inverted Y configuration is characteristic of a normal examination. Arrival time of the radioactive injectate in the region of the external iliac veins can vary by several seconds between the two sides and is related to injection technique. Asymmetry of initial tracer appearance, therefore, is not necessarily indicative of venous obstruction [35]. The appearance of venous collaterals in the region of the azygos-hemiazygos veins is a characteristic and early feature of caval obstruction during the radionuclide study.

The radionuclide approach should be considered an acceptable alternative to other radiological modalities in assessing patients suspected of IVC obstruction.

Peripheral venous studies

During the bipedal administration of radiotracer, venography of the lower extremities can be performed. Results from numerous series indicate that the tracer technique allows adequate identification of the deep venous system; the popliteal, femoral, common femoral, and iliac veins are those most frequently visualized. Venous thrombosis is indicated by the presence of defects, collateral venous flow, and complete occlusion.

Arterial studies

Hepatic artery therapeutic infusions

Without treatment, the median survival of 390 patients with hepatic metastases was 75 days, with only 7% alive at one year [36]. For patients in whom the liver was shown to be the major site of tumour involvement, direct infusions of chemotherapeutic agents into the hepatic artery allowed four times the amount of drug to reach the tumour than reached it via peripheral intravenous administration. With this mode of therapy, liver metastases have regressed in patients in whom systemic treatment with the same drug had been previously unsuccessful, and the improved response rate has in some series been associated with increased survival.

Rationale

The selectivity of hepatic drug infusions requires that the chemotherapeutic agent is injected into the afferent blood supply of the tumour, reaching the lesion on the first pass through the liver. A technique capable of accurately defining intra-arterial patterns of drug flow at the time of catheterization would allow more precise catheter positioning thereby ensuring delivery of maximal drug to tumour bearing areas; it would also allow identification of those patients who, based on perfusion patterns, would be most likely to benefit from infusion chemotherapy. It has been shown that 'slow-flow' intra-arterial infusion of ^{99m}Tc sulphur colloid (SC) was a better indicator of hepatic drug distribution than was contrast medium angiography [37]. This study suggested the potential advantages of utilizing ^{99m}Tc-macroaggregated albumin (MAA) as a radiotracer, since deposition of this agent reflects capillary blockade rather than phagocytosis. In a prospective study based on the scintigraphic distribution patterns of ^{99m}-Tc-MAA introduced into the liver as an hepatic artery infusion, the response of liver tumours to intra-arterial chemotherapy was predicted.

Interpretation

19 patients with biopsy-proven primary or metastatic hepatic tumours were evaluated. Catheters were placed in the common hepatic artery, either by percutaneous route or intraoperatively. Baseline ^{99m}Tc-SC liver-spleen scans were obtained on all patients, and intra-arterial infusions of ^{99m}Tc-MAA were performed within 48 hours of catheter placement. Approximately 148 MBq of the radiopharmaceutical in a volume of less than 0.2 ml were introduced into the arterial line via a 3-way stopcock. A portable infusion pump was attached to the distal end of the catheter, and the radioaggregates were infused at a flow rate of 10 to 21 ml per hour (the actual flow rate utilized for chemotherapy

infusions). Following initial infusion, a 500 000 count anterior image of the liver was obtained.

Prediction of response to chemotherapy was based upon the slow-flow distribution of radiolabelled macroaggregates to those locations where focal defects had been identified on baseline ^{99m}Tc-SC liver-spleen studies. When the tracer was shown to have reached the tumour site, a response to chemotherapy was predicted (Fig. 100.10). If post-infusion images indicated extrahepatic activity (i.e. extravasation, gastric, or splenic uptake) or absence of perfusion to a tumour-bearing area of the liver, a predictive statement of 'no response' was made.

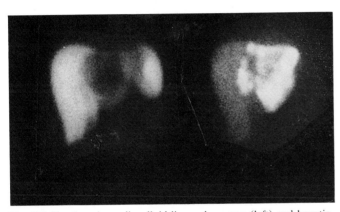

Fig. 100.10 Anterior radiocolloid liver-spleen scan (left) and hepatic artery infusion (right). A large focal defect is seen in the left hepatic lobe on the liver-spleen scan (left) of this patient with colon cancer metastatic to the liver. On the right, is seen an image obtained immediately following the slow hepatic artery infusion of technetium-99m labeled MAA. The preferential flow of aggregates to the tumour-involved left lobe would predict response to infusion chemotherapy.

Follow-up ^{99m}Tc-SC images were used to evaluate the effectiveness of chemotherapy. A response to treatment was equated with a decrease in overall liver size and/or a decrease in the size of perfused focal defects.

When the presence of ^{99m}Tc-MAA within focal hepatic defects or tumour involved hepatic lobes was used as a guideline, the response to intra-arterial chemotherapy was correctly predicted in 18 of 19 patients.

The radionuclide technique described above has been adapted to a totally implanted drug delivery system for hepatic arterial chemotherapy [38].

Summary Hepatic artery infusion can easily be adapted to the angiography suite, using a portable gamma camera for both percutaneously and surgically placed catheters. Visualization of extrahepatic radioaggregates at the slow drug infusion flow rates may be the most sensitive indicator of potential toxic episodes and serves as an accurate indicator of optimal catheter placement.

INTERNAL MAMMARY LYMPHOSCINTIGRAPHY

The trend in patients presenting with carcinoma of the breast is for less invasive surgery; 'lumpectomies', and simple and modified radical mastectomies are now more routinely utilized than is the classical radical mastectomy. These surgical approaches, however, usually include axillary lymph node dissections for staging the disease and for selecting candidates for chemotherapy. Unfortunately, even in the absence of axillary tumour, a significant percentage of patients will develop distant metastasis during the course of their disease.

Although lateral breast lesions are more likely to metastasize to the axilla, and medial lesions more commonly involve the internal mammary lymph node chain, experimental information shows that the internal mammary chain can be involved by lesions originating in any quadrant of the breast. Identification of the position and status of the internal mammary nodes is extremely important, partly because radiation therapy portal planning attempts to include these nodes in the treatment beam.

In the 1950s and 1960s, investigators were able to visualize the lymphatic system following interstitial injection of radiocolloids utilizing gold-198 as the gamma emitter. With ^{99m}Tc available for use as a radiolabel for antimony trisulphide colloid*, it remained for Ege [39] to place internal mammary lymphoscintigraphy in perspective.

Technical considerations

The technique involves a subcostal radiocolloid injection of 37 MBq in a volume of 0.2 ml into the posterior rectus sheath at a point approximately 3 cm inferior to the xyphoid process and 1 to 2 cm medial to the midclavicular line on the side of the tumour-involved breast. 3 hours following injection, the patient returns for imaging. This includes anterior and cross-table lateral views for a minimum of 100 000 counts each.

Interpretation

Two important pieces of information are available from the images:

(a) The relative degree of uptake of radiocolloid within the nodes

(b) The position of the lymph nodes. Lymph nodes infiltrated by tumour show a compromised ability to sequester and phagocytoze radiocolloid shown as either decreased or absent nodal uptake and, on occasion, visible collateral lymphatic channels (Fig. 100.11).

Radionuclide lymphoscintigraphy has been shown in several series to be both sensitive and specific for identifying

---

* Cadema Medical Inc, PO Box 250, Middletown, NY 10940, USA

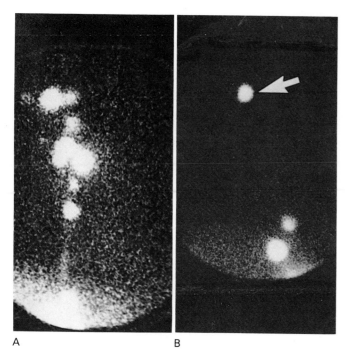

A   B

Fig. 100.11A & B Internal mammary radionuclide lymphoscintiscans. (A) Normal progression of radiocolloid from a right subcostal injection site is noted with normal filling of the internal mammary nodes to the level of the supraclavicular fossae.

(B) There is abrupt termination of radiocolloid migration from the left subcostal injection site with nonvisualization of internal mammary nodes due to replacement by metastatic tumour cells. The level of the superior sternal notch has been noted by a cobalt marker [arrow].

early nodal tumour involvement. Abnormal scan findings carry prognostic implications. Ege [40] demonstrated a two-fold increase in local recurrence and a three-fold increase in distal metastases in such patients.

Localization

A review of the lymphoscintiscans of 400 consecutive patients revealed that a minimum of 14% of nodes located between the second and fifth interspace were positioned at a distance greater than 3 cm deep to the sternum and off the midline.

A method for precisely defining three-dimensional nodal position using a scintillation camera, a parallel hole collimator, and a series of three cobalt-57 disc markers has been described. The data generated allows the radiotherapist to define the position of a node with respect to the sternal notch, distance from the midline, and its depth. Using this information, Rose et al [41] retrospectively analysed the treatment plans of 68 patients. They found that 13% of the nodes (40% of treatment plans) in the second to fifth interspace would have been inadequately treated had lympho-scintigraphic data not been available.

Stereolymphoscintigraphic techniques which achieve the same information by using unilateral and bilateral slant hole collimators have been reported. The spatial relationship of the lymphatic chain obtained with these collimators can be

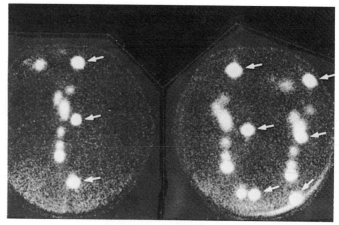

Fig. 100.12 Parallel and slant hole collimator views of normal internal mammary lymph nodes. On the left is the normal internal mammary lymph node chain viewed with a parallel hole collimator. Arrows denote cobalt markers at the superior sternal notch, midsternum, and xyphoid.

On the right the lymph node chain has been viewed at 0 and 180° using a 30° slant hole collimator. The 'duplicated' information allows computer analysis of the lymph nodes with respect to the cobalt markers for three-dimensional localization.

used to generate three-dimensional information from simple geometric functions (Fig. 100.12).

Summary The unique utility of this technique resides with its ability to visualize nodes of 3 to 5 mm in size. Ultrasonic and computerized tomographic techniques have not proven as useful. Tracer evaluation of the lymphatic system may become the method of choice.

RADIO-IMMUNODETECTION

One of the most exciting areas of diagnostic cancer investigation centres about the immunological approach to tumour definition. Initial tracer techniques reported in 1948 used rabbit antibodies, radiolabelled with iodine-131, which were raised against non-rabbit (human) tissue; this allowed sites of antigen-antibody reaction to be identified by scintillation detectors [42].

Tumour cells which show the capacity to express distinct cell-surface antigens provide a method for differentiating neoplastic from normal tissue.

A monoclonal antibody can be radiolabelled for external imaging experiments. The intravenously administered antibody readily allows external detection of a subcutaneously implanted tumour in a mouse model.

Clinicians will no doubt be able to choose specific radioactive labels with physical and biological half-lives optimally suited to the time of imaging and the route of administration i.e. intravenous versus interstitial injection [43].

There are a multitude of problems that must be addressed before this new radiolabelled monoclonal antibody diagnostic technique will be ready for routine clinical use, but preliminary results have been extremely encouraging and promise well for the future.

BIBLIOGRAPHY

REFERENCES

1. Lunia S, Parthasarathy K L, Bakshi S, Bender M A 1975 An evaluation of ^{99m}Tc-sulfur colloid liver scintiscans and their usefulness in metastatic workup: a review of 1424 studies. J Nucl Med 16:62–65
2. Finlay H G, Meek D R, Gray H W, Duncan J G, McArdle C S 1982 Incidence and detection of occult hepatic metastases in colorectal carcinoma. Br Med J 284:803–805
3. Haid M, Singh J, Nevinny H B 1980 Liver scanning in newly diagnosed breast cancer. J Surg Oncol 13:265–268
4. Ozarda A, Pickren J 1962 The topographic distribution of liver metastases. Its relation to surgical and isotopic diagnosis. J Nucl Med 3:149–152
5. Cedermark B J, Schultz S S, Bakshi S, Parthasarathy K L, Mittelman A, Evans J T 1977 The value of liver scan in the follow-up study of patients with adenocarcinoma of the colon and rectum. Surg Gynecol Obstet 144:745–748
6. Drum D E, Beard J M 1976 Scintigraphic criteria for hepatic metastases from cancer of the colon and breast. J Nucl Med 17:677–680
7. Alderson P O, Adams D F, McNeil B J et al 1983 Computed tomography, ultrasound and scintigraphy of the liver in patients with colon or breast carcinomas: a prospective comparison. Radiology 149:225–230
8. Smith T J, Kemeny M M, Sugarbaker P H et al 1982 A prospective study of hepatic imaging in the detection of metastatic disease. Ann Surg 195:486–491
9. Brady L W, Croll M N 1979 The role of bone scanning in the cancer patient. Skel Radiol 3:217–222
10. Davis M A, Jones A G 1976 Comparison of ^{99m}Tc-labeled phosphate and phosphonate agents for skeletal imaging. Semin Nucl Med 6:19–31
11. Tofe A J, Francis M D, Harvey W J 1975 Correlation of neoplasms with incidence and localization of skeletal metastases: an analysis of 1355 diphosphonate bone scans. J Nucl Med 16:986–989
12. Corcoran R J, Thrall J H, Kyle R W, Kaminski R J, Johnson M C 1976 Solitary abnormalities in bone scans of patients with extra-osseous malignancies. Radiology 121:663–667
13. Cowan R J, Young K A 1973 Evaluation of serum alkaline phosphatase determinations in patients with positive bone scans. Cancer 32:887–889
14. Aisenberg A C, Kaplan M M, Reider S V, Goldman J M 1970 Serum alkaline phosphatase at onset of Hodgkin's disease. Cancer 26:318–326
15. Paulson D F and Uro-oncology research group 1979 The impact of current staging procedures in assessing disease extent of prostatic adenocarcinoma. J Urol 121:300–302
16. Schaffer D L, Pendergrass H P 1976 Comparison of enzyme, clinical, radiographic and radionuclide methods of detecting bone metastases from carcinoma of the prostate. Radiology 121:431–434
17. McNeil B J 1978 Rationale for the use of bone scans in selected metastatic and primary bone tumors. Semin Nucl Med 8:336–345
18. Harbert J C, Rocha L, Smith F P, Delgado G 1982 The efficacy of radionuclide liver and bone scans in the evaluation of gynecologic cancers. Cancer 49:1040–1042
19. Belson T P, Lehman R H, Chobanian S L, Malin T C 1980 Bone and liver scans in patients with head and neck carcinoma. Laryngoscope 90:1291–1296
20. Harbert J C 1982 Efficacy of bone and liver scanning in malignant diseases: Facts and opinions. In: Freeman L M, Weissmann H S

(eds) Nuclear medicine annual. Raven Press New York. pp 373–401
21. Citrin D L, Hougen C, Zweibel W et al 1981 The use of serial bone scans in assessing response of bone metastases to systemic treatment. Cancer 47:680–685
22. Rossleigh M A, Lovegrove F T A, Reynolds P M, Byrne M J, Whitney B P 1984 The assessment of response to therapy of bone metastases in breast cancer. Aust NZ J Med 14:19–22
23. Pollen J J, Shlaer W J 1979 Osteoblastic response to successful treatment of metastatic cancer of the prostate. Am J Roentgenol 132:927–931
24. Bitran J D, Bekerman C, Desser R K 1980 The predictive value of serial bone scans in assessing response to chemotherapy in advanced breast cancer. Cancer 45:1562–1568
25. Johnston G, Go M F, Benua R S, Larson S M, Andrews G A, Hübner K F 1977 ^{67}Ga-citrate imaging in Hodgkin's disease: Final report of cooperative group. J Nucl Med 18:692–698
26. Andrews G A, Hübner K F, Greenlaw R H 1978 Ga-67 citrate imaging in malignant lymphoma: final report of cooperative group. J Nucl Med 19:1013–1019
27. Sauerbrunn B J L, Andrews G A, Hübner K F 1978 Ga-67 citrate imaging in tumors of the genito-urinary tract: Report of a cooperative study. J Nucl Med 19:470–475
28. Novetsky G J, Turner D A, Ali A, Raynor Jr W J, Fordham E W 1981 Cleansing the colon in gallium-67 scintigraphy: a prospective comparison of regimens. Am J Roentgenol 137:979–981
29. Beal W H, Chaudhuri T K 1978 One week post injection gallium-67 scan — is it of any added advantage? J Nucl Med 19:733 (abstr)
30. Hoffer P B, Huberty J, Khayam-Bashi H 1977 The association of Ga-67 and lactoferrin. J Nucl Med 18:713–717
31. Turner D A, Fordham E F, Ali A, Slayton, R E 1978 Gallium-67 imaging in the management of Hodgkin's disease and other malignant lymphomas. Semin Nucl Med 8:205–218
32. Bradley W P, Alderson P O, Eckelman W C, Hamilton R G, Weiss J F 1978 Decreased tumor uptake of gallium-67 in animals after whole body irradiation. J Nucl Med 19:204–209
33. Anderson K C, Leonard R C F, Canellos G P, Skarin A T, Kaplan W D 1983 High dose gallium imaging in lymphoma. Am J Med 75:327–331
34. Miyamae T 1973 Interpretation of ^{99m}Tc superior vena cavograms and results of studies in 92 patients. Radiology 108:339–352
35. Dhenke R D, Moore W H, Long S E 1982 Radionuclide venography in iliac and inferior vena caval obstruction. Radiology 144:597–602
36. Jaffee B M, Donegan W L, Watson F, Spratt J S 1968 Factors influencing survival in patients with untreated hepatic metastases. Surg Gynecol Obstet 127:1–11
37. Kaplan W D, D'Orsi C J, Ensminger W D, Smith E H, Levin D C 1978 Intra-arterial radionuclide infusion: a new technique to assess chemotherapy perfusion patterns. Cancer Treat Rep 62:699–703
38. Yang P J, Thrall J H, Ensminger W D et al 1982 Perfusion scintigraphy (Tc-99m MAA) during surgery for placement of chemotherapy catheter in hepatic artery: concise communication. J Nucl Med 23:1066–1069
39. Ege G N 1976 Internal mammary lymphoscintigraphy. The rationale, technique, interpretation and clinical application: a review based on 848 cases. Radiology 118:101–107
40. Ege G N, Clarke R M 1980 Internal mammary lymphoscintigraphy in the conservative management of breast carcinoma. Clin Radiol 31:559–563
41. Rose C M, Kaplan W D, Marck A, Bloomer W D, Hellman S 1979 Parasternal lymphoscintigraphy: Implications for the treatment of internal mammary lymph nodes in breast cancer. Int J Radiat Oncol Biol Phys 5:1849–1853
42. Pressman D, Keighley G 1948 The zone of activity of antibodies as determined by the use of radioactive tracers: the zone of activity of nephrotoxic antikidney serum. J Immunol 59:141–146
43. Weinstein J N, Parker R J, Keenan A M, Dower S K, Morse III H C, Sieber S M 1982 Monoclonal antibodies in the lymphatics: toward the diagnosis and therapy of tumor metastases. Science 218:1334–1337

101 Paediatric nuclear medicine

H. Theodore Harcke

Techniques
  Bone imaging
    Infection
    Vascular disorders
    Trauma
    Neoplastic disease
    Systemic disease
    Special techniques
  Urinary tract imaging
    Visualization of functioning tissue
    Assessment of relative function
    Obstructive uropathy
    Vesico-ureteric reflux
    Renal transplantation
  Gastrointestinal imaging
    Liver and spleen
    Hepatobiliary
    Meckel's diverticulum and gastrointestinal bleeding
    Reflux and motility
  Central nervous system imaging
  Thyroid imaging
  Cardiopulmonary imaging
    Nuclear angiocardiography
    Blood pool imaging
    Myocardial imaging
    Pulmonary ventilation and perfusion imaging

The development of low radiation dose tracers and improvements in gamma imaging systems have enabled radionuclide imaging to become a practical diagnostic tool in paediatrics, demanding special knowledge and techniques to ensure sound diagnostic results.

The interpretation of paediatric imaging studies poses additional challenges for the physician, since normal growth and development alter the appearance and function of body organ systems during childhood.

This chapter will review paediatric radionuclide imaging from the perspective of its differences from adult procedures. Attention will focus both on technical aspects of performing studies and guidelines for recognizing disorders common to the paediatric population.

TECHNIQUES

Although the basic principles of gamma scintigraphy apply to both children and adults, the approach in children differs considerably.

The types of equipment and medication used for adult emergencies are not suited for children.

Patient examination should be performed by a technologist who relates well to children. Young patients should be attended constantly by one person while another operates the equipment.

Equipment selection and position are important. Even a cooperative child may have difficulty remaining still for the long periods of time required for whole body scans. With individual gamma camera images, on the other hand, the time required for each image is relatively short and the child is able to relax briefly between imaging periods. When multiple views are required, as many as possible should be obtained with the camera detector under, rather than over, the patient. Lying beneath the detector can be frightening to the child, particularly when it approaches the body, and views in this position should be reserved for the last.

To obtain a satisfactory gamma image, it is essential that the child remain still. Paediatric laboratories find that sedation is rarely necessary. Extra hands, sandbags, and discarded lead aprons provide excellent alternatives to sedatives. When sedation is necessary, it is best to consult the referring physician, taking into account the expected duration of the study.

Oral premedication with potassium perchlorate to minimize uptake of free technetium by the thyroid gland is advocated by some radiologists before technetium pertechnetate and Tc-labelled compounds are administered. The recommended dose of 3 to 6 mg/kg is given 30 to 60 minutes before injection. Perchlorate must not be given for thyroid imaging or abdominal imaging for ectopic gastric mucosa (Meckel's diverticulum). Three drops of Lugol's solution (5% iodine/20% potassium iodide) are given orally 30 to 60 minutes before studies with ^{131}I-labelled tracers [1].

Whereas the dose of tracer used in adults is generally the same for each patient, the dose to be used in a child must be individually determined and reduced to a minimum. It is most common to calculate the dose of a radiopharmaceutical proportionally from the adult dose on the basis of body weight. For some tracers, the manufacturer's packaging insert suggests a dose/weight relationship (e.g. μCi/Kg). Alternative methods for scaling the dose use relationships such as age; for example, a fraction $\dfrac{x+1}{x+7}$ of the adult dose, where x represents age in years (modified Young's rule) [2].

In small infants a practical minimum dose is required to obtain adequate counting statistics, particularly for flow studies. This seems to be about 2.0 mCi for ^{99m}Tc and ^{99m}Tc-labelled compounds. (Note: Thyroid imaging with ^{99m}Tc is an exception, as will be discussed later.) Doses recommended on the basis of body weight may be reduced when flow studies are not necessary and when a limited area of the body is to be imaged. This increases the time required to obtain an adequate image, but decreases the absorbed radiation dose. Adequate hydration and frequent micturition can appreciably decrease the dose to the bladder and gonads.

In infants and young children, the antecubital veins are not as accessible as in adults and veins on the dorsum of the hands and feet are preferable. When cardiac studies requiring a defined injection bolus are performed, injection into an external jugular vein of the neck is preferred. Special considerations for injections will be discussed later. In laboratories where personnel have limited experience with paediatric and especially neonatal venepunctures, it can be requested that inpatients arrive with an indwelling intravenous line. One specific technique ensuring correct intravenous injection has been widely adapted in paediatrics (Fig. 101.1). The syringe containing the dose is connected to a disposable three-way stopcock turned off to the dose. A syringe containing normal saline is connected to the second site on the stopcock. The stopcock is connected to a scalp vein needle (usually 23 or 25 gauge). The venepuncture is made and tested with the saline flush. After confirmation of proper positioning, the stopcock is turned off to the flush and the dose of radiopharmaceutical is injected. In paediatrics, the volume of the dose is often so small that it will only fill the tubing of the scalp vein needle and the saline syringe is pushed to clear the tubing. The dose syringe can be flushed to ensure that the complete dose has been administered.

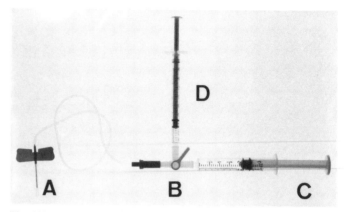

Fig. 101.1 Apparatus for radionuclide injection in paediatric patients. (A) Butterfly needle with flexible tubing. (B) 3-way stopcock. (C) Syringe with saline flush. (D) Syringe with radiopharmaceutical dose. (Syringe shield has been removed for clarity.).

The equipment and collimation selected follow adult principles with little exception. Large field of view cameras make most organ imaging quite simple, since a substantial portion of the body can generally be included within the field. Because of the small size of infants and young children, meticulous attention must be given to positioning. It is essential to have the patient as close as possible to the collimator face. Small patients can be placed directly on the collimator, which is covered by a thin plywood board and plastic sheet. Frequently, (e.g. in imaging of the hips) pinhole or converging collimator images are necessary to visualize adequately the area. It is hoped that the foregoing section has sensitized the reader to the need for treating children differently both before and during the acquisition of radionuclide images.

Bone imaging

Discovery of the ^{99m}Tc-phosphate compounds in 1971 made bone imaging practical for routine diagnostic use in children. Tracers available prior to this time (^{85}Sr, ^{87m}Sr, ^{18}F) delivered too high a radiation dose to be considered for nononcologic paediatric applications. The diphosphonate group of compounds is now most commonly used in paediatrics (dose range 4–15 mCi). Selection of one compound over another remains an open issue. There have been no reported differences between children and adults in the physiological and imaging properties of generally available bone agents.

Images of the normal growing skeleton, which appear differently from one age group to another, provide many pitfalls for the careless interpreter. In growth plate regions, increased tracer activity is normal. This persists until closure, at which time the activity gradually decreases until maturation at the site is complete. The best way to evaluate activity in the growth plate areas is to compare bone activity in the paired structures. Meticulous attention must be given to symmetric positioning however, since even minor differences may simulate unilaterally increased activity. To obtain adequate detail of the small bones in infants and children, it is usually necessary to supplement high resolution images with magnification images obtained by using a pinhole or converging collimator. Computer processing of images may also clarify detail.

Infection

The most important contribution made by bone imaging is to identify skeletal abnormalities which cannot be seen radiographically. Infectious conditions are common in paediatrics and the differentiation of osteomyelitis from cellulitis and septic arthritis is a frequent problem. Early in the course of these disorders, radiographic changes are limited to subtle, nonspecific soft tissue changes. Bone imaging performed in two (or three) phases has reliably provided differential diagnosis in most cases [3,4]. Early imaging (blood pool 5 to 15 minutes, with or without a flow study) characterizes the *soft tissue perfusion*; delayed imaging (2 to 3 hours post injection) shows *bone uptake*.

In *cellulitis* and *septic arthritis*, blood pool images demonstrate increased activity and hyperaemia at the affected site. Delayed bone images may be normal or may show a mild increase in bone uptake and some persistence of soft tissue activity. When this occurs, the pattern is diffuse and lacks the focal bone tracer localization characteristic of osteomyelitis. Since any process causing hyperaemia in and around a joint will appear the same on blood pool and bone images, it is not possible to differentiate septic arthritis from other arthritides or trauma.

The hallmark of *osteomyelitis* is intense focal uptake of bone tracer at the site of involvement. Local hyperaemia accompanies bone infection and flow and blood pool images reveal increased local bone and soft tissue activity. Focal accumulation of the tracer in the bone becomes more apparent on the delayed images as the soft tissue activity wanes (Fig. 101.2).

The pattern of intense focal tracer increase is not the only manifestation of osteomyelitis [5-7]. Early in the course of the illness, there can be a temporary occlusion of small blood

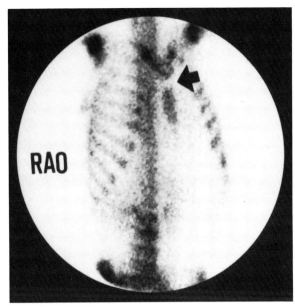

Fig. 101.3 'Cold' osteomyelitis of the sternum. The defect in the sternum [arrow] of this 6 year old child with leukaemia was due to a focus of staphlococcal osteomyelitis.

vessels and a degree of oedema sufficient to reduce the amount of bone tracer reaching the affected area. A bone image may show either normal or decreased activity (Fig. 101.3). 'Cold' osteomyelitis is easily overlooked when interpretation is based on delayed bone images alone and blood pool, flow images and magnification views are necessary.

There has been some disagreement regarding the sensitivity of Tc-phosphate bone imaging in diagnosing osteomyelitis. In paediatric institutions, accuracy with this procedure has been reported in the 90% range, although others find scintigraphy less reliable [8-10]. The frequent occurrence of false negative images in neonates with osteomyelitis has been recognized [11]. The resolving power of the camera is such that increased activity of the growth plate cannot be separated from that of the infection in the small bones of the neonate. The pathophysiology of osteomyelitis in the neonate differs from that of the older infant and child.

Infection of the intervertebral disc space (discitis) causes increased isotope uptake in contiguous vertebral bodies before radiographic changes occur.

Gallium (^{67}Ga) is often advocated in the diagnosis of inflammatory bone and joint disease. It can be useful in revealing infection that is bilaterally symmetric and in infection in areas of bone which are undergoing repair and therefore show increased ^{99m}Tc-phosphate localization. ^{67}Ga is valuable to supplement the unsuccessful ^{99m}Tc-phosphate scan [12]. However, the higher radiation burden and undesirable imaging characteristics associated with gallium reduce its value.

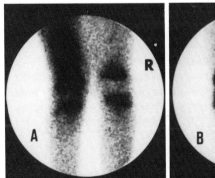
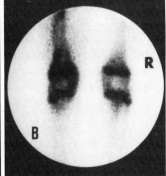

Fig. 101.2 Acute osteomyelitis (A) Blood pool and (B) delayed (2 hour) images. Increased soft tissue uptake is most marked in the region of the distal left femur (A). Focally increased bone activity is seen in the distal left femoral metaphysis on the bone images (B).

Vascular disorders

By means of isotope bone imaging, it is possible to diagnose *aseptic necrosis* of an epiphysis, as in Legg-Calvé-Perthes' disease, before the appearance of radiographic changes[13,14]. The region of the epiphysis which has lost its blood supply will appear as a photon-deficient area (Fig. 101.4). In paediatric patients, imaging must be performed using magnification techniques, preferably with pinhole collimation. Computer techniques may also be useful in improving resolution. Both hips should be examined with careful attention to symmetric positioning and equal imaging time.

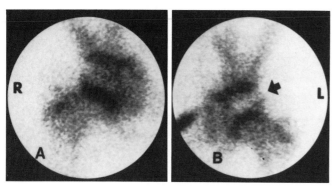

Fig. 101.4 Aseptic necrosis of the left hip. (B) Decreased tracer activity is apparent in the capital femoral epiphysis [arrow]. The normal right hip is presented for comparison (A). These images were obtained using a pinhole collimator.

Bone infarctions in children are most often related to sickle cell haemoglobinopathies, steroid therapy, or storage disorders such as Gaucher's disease. Vascular compromise will usually result in an area of decreased bone uptake on ^{99m}Tc-phosphate imaging. As healing occurs, the uptake will increase with respect to normal bone. The appearance of an infarct, therefore, is dependent upon its age. As previously noted, a photon-deficient area may also be seen on delayed bone images in the early stages of osteomyelitis. Therefore, a clear distinction between osteomyelitis and bone infarction may not be possible on the basis of bone isotope imaging alone [15]. Bone imaging cannot distinguish between a sterile infarct and an infected one. Bone marrow imaging with ^{99m}Tc-sulphur colloid and ^{67}Ga imaging may be employed when phosphate imaging is not definitive [12,16].

Trauma

Bone scintigraphy may identify fractures not visible radiographically and is useful when child abuse is suspected [17]. The soft tissues and several organs can be evaluated from a single injection [18]. Flow studies of the brain can be obtained during injection; kidney images appear in the early minutes and excretion can be evaluated. The skeletal images at 2 to 3 hours will show not only fractures, but even injury to the periosteum alone. One must be careful about relying solely on bone scans for child abuse screening, since epiphyseal fractures and fractures near the growth plates may be difficult to detect due to normally increased growth plate activity. Skull fractures are also difficult to visualize on bone images.

When children and adolescents experience athletic injuries such as stress fractures, bone scintigraphy can lead to prompt diagnosis. Imaging has also been used in cases of spondylolysis; the lesion is judged to be old or recent on the basis of normal or increased bone uptake.

Neoplastic disease

Bone isotope imaging cannot be used in children to differentiate a benign lesion from a malignant one. While the common primary bone malignancies, osteosarcoma, Ewing's sarcoma, and reticulum cell sarcoma usually show an intense increase in tracer localization, so do osteomyelitis, osteoid osteomas, fibrous dysplasia, and traumatized bone cysts. Conversely, a lesion with decreased or normal activity may be malignant, as has been observed in cases of metastatic neuroblastoma and histiocytosis. When a bone lesion is identified on the radiograph, a bone isotope scan is very useful to survey the skeleton for other occult lesions, rather than to assess the degree of neoplasia.

In the identification of *skeletal metastases*, bone imaging has been successful for neuroblastoma, lymphoma, osteosarcoma, and Ewing's sarcoma [19]. Only in patients with histiocytosis has there been difficulty in identifying bone lesions [20]. In addition to focal uptake at the site of a neoplastic lesion, there is often increased uptake in the normal adjacent bones. This 'extended pattern' of increased uptake should not be misinterpreted as an extension of the neoplasm.

Since bone images are altered by radiation and/or chemotherapy, they must be interpreted very carefully after such treatments. Children are always experiencing minor trauma, and those undergoing treatment for malignancy are particularly susceptible to both occult trauma and infection. Since either may result in increased bone tracer accumulation, they can simulate neoplastic uptake. A solitary site of abnormal uptake on a metastatic bone survey is strongly suggestive of trauma.

Benign bone neoplasms in children display variable activity patterns. Osteoid osteomas, osteoblastomas, chondroblastomas, and fibrous dysplasia show focally increased activity. The osteoid osteomas (particularly in the spine or hip) may be difficult to visualize radiographically. A bone scan should be performed if osteoid osteoma is considered in the child with local bone pain and no identifiable lesion on radiography.

Although eosinophilic granuloma may exhibit increased activity on a bone image, the increased uptake is not always marked. Several types of uptake patterns can be observed in osteochondroma, enchondroma, aneurysmal bone cyst, and simple bone cyst; a mild increase in uptake is usual at the margins. In benign cortical defects or bone islands, the bone scan will usually be normal but minimal to mildly increased uptake has been noted.

Injury to a benign lesion will cause the lesion to exhibit an increase in tracer uptake.

Systemic disease

There have been only limited applications of bone scintigraphy to the diagnosis and management of systemic paediatric disorders. Results have been variable [21,22]. The *collagen vascular diseases* which occur in children frequently involve joints and this may be detected by gamma imaging before the onset of clinical symptoms. Two (or three) phase bone imaging is essential; the blood pool phase appears to be the best phase for identifying synovial hyperaemia and associated soft tissue inflammation. The pattern cannot be distinguished from traumatic or septic arthritis. Since chronic joint disease affects adjacent bone, increased tracer accumulation will be seen, usually symmetrically about the joint.

Systemic bone disorders which alter metabolism are likely to produce symmetric alterations of bone images, making detection of the abnormality difficult. Changes in rickets, for example, lead to symmetric increases in growth plate activity. Quantifying activity within bones is being investigated.

Special bone imaging techniques

Computer processing of bone images not only permits contrast enhancement and magnification, but allows relative quantification of activity in such key regions as growth plates and capital femoral epiphyses. Single photon emission computed tomography (SPECT) may have applications in paediatric bone imaging if the resolution proves to be adequate.

Bone imaging can also be used in conjunction with several paediatric orthopaedic procedures [23], including nonunion of fractures, localization of focal bone lesions, identification of pseudarthroses, and evaluation of prostheses.

Urinary tract imaging

Radionuclide studies are used to provide morphological as well as physiological information. The ability to visualize functioning renal tissue, which cannot be adequately imaged radiographically, is a key advantage; the inability to show precise anatomic detail is a disadvantage. In practice, ultrasonography and renal scintigraphy complement each other nicely; ultrasound evaluates structure while radionuclides depict function.

There are virtually no reports of allergic reactions to radioisotopes and one indication for radionuclide evaluation of the urinary tract is a previous reaction to iodinated contrast material.

Most children who require radionuclide urinary tract studies will be re-examined one or more times and these studies have become one of the preferred methods for patient follow up. While analogue imaging alone provides considerable information, it is now common to acquire and process renal studies using a digital computer.

Visualization of functioning renal tissue

Renal morphology may not be adequately defined by some imaging modalities because of anatomical location or inadequate function. Both congenital and acquired conditions may result in such poor function that excretory urography is unsuccessful. In the immediate neonatal period, the glomerular filtration rate is low because of physiological immaturity of the kidneys. Radionuclide imaging in conjunction with ultrasound has been superior to urography in evaluating cystic/dysplastic conditions, obstructive uropathies, and renovascular disturbances [24,25]. ^{99m}Tc-DMSA is accumulated and retained by functional renal parenchyma. ^{99m}Tc-DTPA is filtered by the glomeruli like radiological contrast medium and visualises the collecting system. An enlarged fluid-filled kidney is seen as a photon-deficient region on renal images obtained soon after injection. Delayed imaging at intervals during the next 24 hours may be required to establish the diagnosis. In obstructive conditions, gradual isotope accumulation occurs, and a pattern of activity proximal to the obstruction is usually established within 2 hours. Multicystic kidneys typically show no early function; however, by 24 hours some evidence of tracer accumulation can be observed within the kidney. Renovascular conditions exhibit variable patterns of diminished perfusion and impaired function. Renal venous thrombosis, which can be unilateral or bilateral, most commonly results in decreased perfusion and filtration without holdup of activity in the collecting system. In patients with renal arterial occlusion and renal cortical necrosis, renal perfusion and function are absent.

Large intrarenal masses are generally detected by contrast urography but small masses can be missed. In such cases renal imaging can be helpful, since nonfunctioning tissue will be seen as a defect in the nephrogram phase of a renal study. The images are nonspecific as to the nature of the defect (tumour, cyst, abscess), but effectively distinguish between pathology and a hypertrophied column of Bertin, congenital hump, or lobulation.

Assessment of relative renal function

In instances where a discrepancy in renal size or function has been established by urography or ultrasound, it is useful to quantify the differences. Quantification by nuclear techniques provides objective criteria upon which to base management decisions and permits a more accurate comparison of serial studies [26]. Figure 101.5 illustrates the regions selected to compare a small, scarred kidney with its less severely affected counterpart. The techniques are particularly effective when kidney size is decreased, as in chronic pyelonephritis. In cases of duplication, the upper and lower poles of the same kidney can be compared. The usefulness of the technique diminishes when one of the kidneys is markedly hydronephrotic and has only a thin rim of functioning parenchyma. Renal perfusion is an aspect of kidney 'function' which can be independently assessed by radionuclides. Computer analysis of the renal flow can be made independent of the relative function estimates described above. Most flow comparisons are made by generating time/activity curves for regions of interest over the abdominal aorta and kidneys. Although not perfect, the renal scan is employed as a screening test in children with

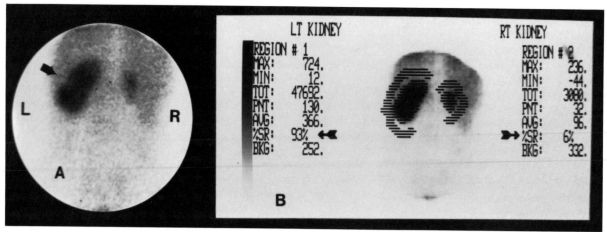

Fig. 101.5   Analysis of relative renal function in chronic pyelonephritis. (A) The ^{99m}Tc-DTPA image obtained one minute post-injection shows a small right kidney and a scar in the left kidney [arrow]. (B) Using computer-selected regions to define kidney and background activity, relative activity in each kidney can be calculated. This determination [arrow] has correlated well with glomerular filtration measurements and is indicative of relative renal function.

hypertension because it evaluates several aspects of kidney function with one study. The follow up of children who have had balloon angioplasty for renal artery stenosis is under evaluation.

Obstructive uropathy

Diuretic renography, the noninvasive counterpart of the measurement of renal pelvic perfusion pressure/flow studies (Whitaker Test), is a technique that is suitable for children as well as adults [27]. The technique may require some modification, however, since children will usually be studied in the supine or prone position. To insure adequate hydration, oral fluids must be given, but if intake is not adequate, an intravenous infusion can be maintained during the study. The recommended dose of intravenous frusemide (furosamide) ranges from 0.3 to 1.0 mg/kg. Some institutions study all children with an indwelling bladder catheter and, any child with known or suspected vesico-ureteric reflux or neurogenic bladder should be catheterized for diuretic renography.

Children who have had surgery to relieve ureteropelvic junction obstruction or ureterovesical junction obstruction may show little anatomical change in the appearance of the dilated system on postoperative urography. After successful surgery, however, diuretic isotope renography will demonstrate prompt wash-out from the dilated renal pelvis in response to the diuretic challenge.

Children with severe, long standing obstruction may have insufficient kidney function to sustain diuresis and the lack of diuretic response may be incorrectly attributed to obstruction.

Vesico-ureteric reflux

Radionuclide cystography provides an alternative to conventional radiographic cystography with iodinated contrast agents. In the evaluation of vesico-ureteric reflux and quan-

tification of bladder function, isotope cystography is quite accurate but lacks the anatomical detail obtained with radiography. A significant advantage of the radionuclide cystogram is the reduction in radiation exposure of 50 to 100 times that produced by a radiographic study using fluoroscopy [28].

One suggested approach is to perform a child's first cystogram radiographically to define the anatomy of the bladder and urethra as well as to determine the presence or absence of ureteric reflux. When follow up studies are required (e.g., to follow the course of reflux) these studies should be done with radionuclides in order to reduce radiation exposure. Most young children will show resolution of their reflux as they grow older.

Radionuclide cystography is performed in a manner comparable to contrast cystography. Following catheterization of the urinary bladder, the bladder is filled with a saline

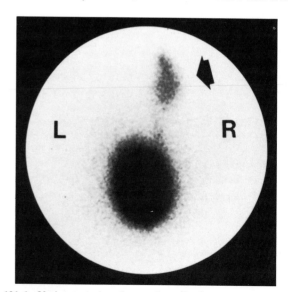

Fig. 101.6   Vesico-ureteric reflux to the collecting system of the kidney [arrow] is demonstrated by radionuclide cystography. This image was obtained during passive filling of the bladder with a ^{99m}Tc pertechnetate/saline solution.

solution containing 1.0 mCi of ^{99m}Tc (or ^{99m}Tc-compound). During this filling, the patient is monitored by a technologist or physician who views the bladder activity on the scintillation camera display oscilloscope. Serial films and/or computer images are obtained as well. Ureteric reflux is seen as linear activity extending vertically above the dome of the bladder (Fig. 101.6).

Since vesico-ureteric reflux may occur during passive bladder filling or at the time of micturition, the cystogram must include evaluation during voiding. After bladder filling, the catheter is removed and monitoring continues as the patient voids in a bedpan or urinal. This can most easily be done in the sitting position by placing the child's back against the vertically oriented detector head of the camera. With simple volumetric measurements and pre- and postvoid bladder counts, objective estimates of residual bladder volume can be made.

Radionuclide cystography documents the resolution or progression of ureteric reflux in children. If surgical intervention becomes necessary, the isotope study can also be used for postsurgical assessment.

Renal transplantation

Isotopic techniques are the preferred method for post-transplant management. The techniques employed are similar to those used in adults, employing both filtration and tubular agents. Perfusion and filtration are assessed with a ^{99m}Tc renal agent, and tubular function is assessed with iodine-labelled Hippuran. As it becomes available, ^{123}I-Hippuran should replace ^{131}I-Hippuran.

The post-transplant schedule of study should be flexible to avoid unnecessary examinations. In the immediate postoperative period, frequent studies are required but can be reduced after 2 to 3 weeks when management of rejection is the major consideration.

Gastrointestinal imaging

As imaging techniques in adults develop and prove clinically beneficial, they are modified and applied to paediatric problems. There is widespread experience in liver/spleen imaging with ^{99m}Tc-sulphur colloid and abdominal imaging with ^{99m}Tc to identify ectopic gastric mucosa (Meckel's diverticulum). Hepatobiliary imaging with ^{99m}Tc-IDA agents and scintigraphy for gastro-oesophageal reflux are increasingly used.

Liver and spleen

The normal range of liver size in childhood has been established [29]. Congenital abnormalities of the liver and spleen are often associated with abnormalities in other organ systems. A horizontal (or transverse) liver position, which can be accompanied by asplenia, is associated with congenital

cardiac abnormalities. With abnormal liver situs, it may not be possible to identify the spleen. Repeat imaging with labelled red blood cells that have been heat-damaged can establish splenic presence [30]. Polysplenia may be difficult to diagnose scintigraphically since several spleens may be clumped together and appear as a single organ. Small splenic implants contiguous with the liver may also escape detection. Storage diseases which affect the liver and spleen usually result in marked organomegaly. In such cases, colloid distribution is typically homogeneous, but appears reduced in intensity because of the organ bulk.

Infants with vascular malformations of the liver often present in cardiac failure. Combined flow and static imaging are the keys to diagnosis. Increased flow to the area of the malformation is noted in a radionuclide angiogram, but no colloid deposition (liver defect) will be found on static liver images because of the absence of reticuloendothelial cells.

Since physiological processes are similar, acquired liver diseases in childhood show the same patterns as in adults. Hepatitis is seen as decreased liver activity in an enlarged liver, with a compensatory increase in splenic size and uptake. Cirrhosis of the liver is also found in paediatrics, often as a sequela of hepatitis, but also in patients with cystic fibrosis. Tumours of the liver (either benign or malignant) are rare in childhood; the presenting feature is often hepatomegaly. While imaging establishes the location as a photon-deficient region on scan, it cannot distinguish the benign (haemangioma, haemangioendothelioma) from the malignant (hepatoblastoma, hepatoma) [31]. Metastatic disease to the liver in childhood is uncommon; if it does occur, it is usually in conjunction with neuroblastoma. It should be noted that extrahepatic masses, such as a Wilms' tumour involving the right kidney or a neuroblastoma arising from the right adrenal, may markedly distort the appearance of the liver without actually invading the organ.

Liver imaging is commonly used to screen for metastatic disease, and the effects of chemotherapy and/or radiation therapy.

A child's spleen function responds to liver insult in the same manner as the adult organ by increasing its size and reticuloendothelial activity. Splenomegaly may be secondary to liver disease, infection, collagen disease, and the haemolytic anaemias. Primary splenic lesions are rare; cysts and hamartomas occur. Septic emboli may seed to the spleen and abscess development must be considered in immune-suppressed children. Functional asplenia (i.e. physical presence of the spleen without ^{99m}Tc-sulphur colloid uptake) is associated with sickle cell anaemia and its variants and develops in children between the ages of 2 and 6 years.

Radionuclide imaging is effective in traumatic lesions of the liver and spleen. In children, splenectomy is not recommended for splenic trauma, since it increases the risk for pneumococcal septicaemia. Conservative management of splenic laceration and/or haematoma is encouraged when the clinical situation permits [32].

Hepatobiliary

In an infant, the differentiation between obstructive jaundice caused by hepatocellular disease and that due to congenital anatomic abnormality of the biliary tree is difficult. Neonatal hepatitis and alpha-1 antitrypsin deficiency can lead to prolonged, essentially complete obstruction to the passage of bile and, thus, are not easily distinguishable from biliary atresia by radionuclide imaging. For more than two decades, radio-iodinated (^{131}I) rose bengal was used in such studies with, at best, limited success [33]. The ^{99m}Tc-labelled immino diacetic acid (IDA) agents offer an attractive alternative and are now being evaluated for sensitivity and specificity. While both agents are handled in a similar manner physiologically, the physical characteristics of the ^{99m}Tc-labelled agents make them more desirable. The large number of IDA derivatives has caused some confusion, however, since reports of sensitivity and specificity may vary with the particular agent used.

Following intravenous injection, the hepatobiliary agents are, under normal circumstances, excreted into the biliary system with subsequent passage into the gastrointestinal tract. In the presence of hepatocellular disease and/or biliary obstruction, the urinary tract provides an alternate pathway of excretion. In the usual clinical situation, the jaundiced neonate has significant impairment of hepatocellular function (total bilirubin > 8 mg per cent) and rapid appearance of tracer occurs in the urinary tract. Serial imaging is performed to establish the presence of activity in the gastrointestinal tract. With ^{131}I rose bengal, these images could be performed over a 72 hour period; the shorter half life of the ^{99m}Tc-IDA derivatives makes imaging impractical after 24 hours.

Stool collection and radio-isotope assay for 72 hours (uncontaminated by urine) is an essential part of the ^{131}I rose bengal evaluation. When less than 5% of the administered dose is recovered in the stool, biliary atresia is suspected. Recovery of more than 15% indicates a patent biliary system. Values in the 5 to 15% range are considered inconclusive. The use of rose bengal requires scrupulously performed stool collections, since contamination with urine causes false negative results. False positive results occur in patients whose biliary tracts are anatomically intact but who have severe cholestasis.

Reports of the use of ^{99m}Tc-IDA derivatives show variable results [34-36]. While several studies report the superiority of the Tc-IDA analogues over ^{131}I rose bengal, there is documentation of severe cases of neonatal hepatitis in which ^{131}I rose bengal images after 24 hours showed bowel activity which had not been visible with a ^{99m}Tc-labelled agent [34]. The results of ^{99m}Tc-IDA scintigraphy are also affected by pretreatment of the neonate with phenobarbitone. Phenobarbitone (5 mg/kg daily for at least 5 days prior to the examination) is reported to enhance biliary excretion in some infants from an undetectable to a visualized amount [35]. Conclusions concerning the accuracy of this test must, therefore, consider these factors.

In neonates without hepatobiliary disease, hepatic extraction is rapid. The gallbladder may be seen 10 to 20 minutes post-injection without visualization of the ducts. Small bowel activity is noted between 20 and 30 minutes. The pattern of excretion in neonatal hepatitis varies with the severity of cholestasis. When there is delayed and/or decreased intestinal activity, gallbladder visualization will also be delayed. Lateral images are helpful in distinguishing gut activity from activity in the urinary tract. Decreased hepatic extraction is frequently noted with hepatitis, and serves to distinguish it from biliary atresia (in which hepatic extraction remains efficient). In biliary atresia, there is no visualization of the gallbladder and bowel. Severe cholestasis with an anatomically intact biliary system, however, will also fail to show gallbladder and intestinal excretion. Choledochal cysts may show delayed accumulation of the radiopharmaceutical.

Meckel's diverticulum and gastrointestinal bleeding

Abdominal imaging with ^{99m}Tc pertechnetate has proven to be reliable for detecting symptom-producing ectopic gastric mucosa in children e.g. in Meckel's diverticulum, gastric or enteric duplications and the oesophagus. Acid secretion by parietal cells can lead to ulceration of the adjacent bowel mucosa, resulting in bleeding. The mucoid surfaces of gastric mucosa selectively accumulate and subsequently secrete the pertechnetate anion, permitting visualization on abdominal images.

When several studies are contemplated for the diagnostic evaluation of *GI bleeding*, it is preferable to do radionuclide imaging first. Both barium studies and endoscopy may adversely affect interpretation and should follow scintigraphy. The child should fast for several hours prior to injection, and should not be given potassium perchlorate. Administration of drugs or hormones to enhance visualization is suggested in several reports. Cimetidine (300 mg/kg for 2 days prior to imaging) [37] and glucagon (50 mg/kg intravenously 10 minutes after tracer injection) [38] appear to delay removal of pertechnetate from gastric mucosa [38]. Pentagastrin (6 mg/kg subcutaneously prior to ^{99m}Tc injection) [39] is believed to stimulate pertechnetate uptake in the gastric mucosa [39].

Imaging should begin at the time of injection and continue at intervals of up to an hour. It is convenient to image the abdomen with the child supine under the detector. While most images can be anterior views, periodic lateral and erect views and images after micturition are helpful to distinguish the structures of the urinary tract.

Pertechnetate concentration in the stomach serves as a reference for other focal accumulations. Gastric concentration begins, usually 5 to 10 minutes post-injection, and then increases in intensity; ectopic mucosa shows the same pattern (Fig. 101.7). Activity can normally be seen in the proximal small bowel during the latter part of the study. A focal collection of pertechnetate in a pattern which parallels the stomach activity suggests ectopic gastric mucosa e.g. in a Meckel's diverticulum or bowel duplication. Most Meckel's diverticula are in the right lower quadrant.

Focal accumulations mimicking ectopic gastric mucosa can occur with localized hyperaemia and inflammation, and have been reported with intussusception, intestinal obstruction, inflammatory bowel disease, and vascular lesions, such as haemangiomas, tumours, and arteriovenous malformations. These may be differentiated from gastric mucosa by their appearance early in the blood pool phase before increased stomach activity is noted. The above 'false positives' may lead to a correct diagnosis. Other 'false positive' cases caused

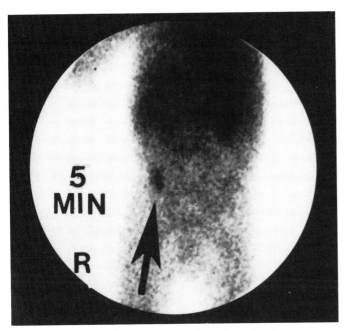

Fig. 101.7 Heterotopic gastric mucosa. The abdominal image obtained 5 minutes after ^{99m}Tc pertechnetate injection shows focally increased accumulation in the right lower quadrant. A Meckel's diverticulum was removed at surgery.

by urinary tract abnormalities such as hydronephrosis, hydroureter, extrarenal pelvis, ectopic kidney, or ureteral reflux are truly misleading. An awareness of urinary tract conditions causing localized accumulation, coupled with proper imaging technique (lateral views, erect views, post-void views, etc.), will minimize this group of potential errors.

False negative studies occur if the mass of gastric mucosa is insufficient to permit visualization against background. Rapid wash-out or bowel hypersecretion may dilute localized activity. Overlapping organs such as the proximal small bowel and bladder may obscure a localization.

In paediatrics, pertechnetate imaging for gastrointestinal bleeding has a reported accuracy of over 90% in a large series of patients[38]. With the assistance of drugs and hormones, it would appear that a good test has the potential for being even better.

Localization of gastrointestinal bleeding with ^{99m}Tc-sulphur colloid can be applied to children when imaging for Meckel's diverticulum is not appropriate.

Gastro-oesophageal reflux and gastrointestinal motility

There is considerable disagreement concerning the significance and management of gastro-oesophageal reflux in infancy. Since reflux has been linked to a number of clinical problems (e.g., oesophagitis, failure to thrive, anaemia, recurrent pulmonary disease, allergy, and apnoea), the radiologist is often asked to evaluate patients for reflux.

The barium swallow has been the conventional technique and is the best study for a first examination. It provides good anatomical detail, an evaluation of swallowing function, and

the opportunity to detect gastro-oesophageal reflux. The scintigraphic method, however has been shown to be a more sensitive detector of gastro-oesophageal reflux and permits delayed evaluation for evidence of pulmonary aspiration.

The infant's customary type and volume of liquid (milk, formula, juice) is divided into two equal parts. ^{99m}Tc-sulphur colloid is mixed with one part and this is fed first; the second part (unlabelled) is given to clear the oropharynx and oesophagus. A dose of 5 µCi of ^{99m}Tc-sulphur colloid/ml of liquid is recommended; but can be reduced appreciably and 100 µCi–300 µCi is adequate even with larger volume feedings. Total body radiation exposure is less from scintigraphy than from the traditional barium study[40]. Feeding should simulate as closely as possible what is normal for the child; the parent can do the feeding but must be instructed to avoid spilling labelled formula on the infant's neck, chest, or clothing. After burping, the face is wiped and the infant is put to bed on the scintillation camera. While any position (prone, semi-erect, lateral, etc.) is acceptable, several laboratories have standardized their study and decided to place all infants supine.

Infants or children with known swallowing dysfunction may receive the colloid/liquid mixture by way of a nasogastric tube. The tube should be rinsed with unlabelled liquid and then removed because of its effect on the oesophago-gastric junction.

Data collection must begin as soon after feeding as possible. While analogue images can be made, it is more important to acquire data continuously by computer. A rate of 1 frame per minute for 60 minutes is recommended. One hour of observation following feeding is sufficient for reflux evaluation. Some infants who show no reflux during the first 30 minutes post-feeding may show reflux after 30 minutes. Delayed imaging (5 1-minute anterior frames; 5 1-minute posterior frames) of the chest and abdomen 2 hours post-feeding permits assessment of gastric emptying and pulmonary aspiration. It may be useful to obtain some additional delayed images to detect aspiration if the stomach still shows activity 2 hours after feeding.

Computer processing of the acquired data is mandatory. While analogue images may show reflux, much reflux activity will be evident only after computer enhancement. The individual 1-minute frames should be viewed following contrast enhancement of low-level activity. The upper threshold should be set at 5 to 10% of the peak activity in the image; the lower threshold should be set at 1 to 2% to clear background activity. This technique permits visualization of small amounts of material refluxed into the oesophagus and/or small amounts of aspirated material in the lungs (Fig. 101.8). Time/activity curves can be generated using a region of interest over the oesophagus and will show spikes of activity during reflux. The computer enhancement technique should be applied to all delay images in order to show lung activity secondary to aspiration.

Interpretation of reflux studies involves identification of the frequency and extent of reflux and detection of pulmonary aspiration. By viewing the processed images sequentially, it is usually apparent whether oesophageal activity on a frame represents a new episode of reflux or the residual from a prior episode.

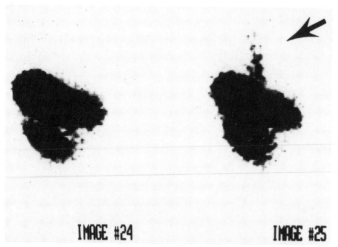

Fig. 101.8 Gastro-oesophageal reflux [arrow] is present on the computer-enhanced 25 minutes image of this [99mTc] sulphur colloid study. The 24 minute image is provided for comparison. Viewed posteriorly, the details of the stomach and small bowel become obscured when contrast is adjusted to enhance low level oesophageal activity.

There is still disagreement as to whether one or more episodes of reflux into the distal oesophagus is abnormal.

The diagnosis of pulmonary aspiration is made by identifying colloid activity in the lung. This requires computer enhancement, since the amount will be minimal in comparison to gastric and oesophageal activity. A false positive diagnosis of aspiration may result from a few drops of the labelled feeding contaminating the skin or clothing. If this projects over the thorax during imaging, it can be mistaken for aspiration. Residual material in the oesophagus or in an oesophageal diverticulum can also simulate aspiration. It is especially important to make the distinction between aspiration during feeding, which is secondary to a swallowing dysfunction, and lung activity which is secondary to a tracheo-oesophageal fistula [41].

The reported percentages of examinations which show reflux scintigraphically, in the absence of reflux on barium swallow, vary [40,42]. It is commonly noted, however, that a higher detection rate is found in nuclear studies. Barium swallow is somewhat traumatic for the infant and may provoke reflux that would not occur under normal physiologic conditions. More recently ultrasound has been used to detect gastro-oesophageal reflux.

A logical extension of the feeding of labelled liquids to evaluate gastro-oesophageal reflux is the examination of gastric emptying by computer techniques.

Central nervous system imaging

The use of radionuclide imaging has declined as a result of computerized cranial tomography and ultrasound which provide greater anatomical detail. Current applications of radionuclide studies in children are primarily related to identifying physiological changes which are not visible on CT because they are isodense with normal brain. The two major categories of disease where this occurs are vascular and inflammatory.

Evaluation of cerebrospinal fluid dynamics by radionuclide cisternography also has paediatric applications. Some special studies with isotopes are used to evaluate the patency of diversionary CSF shunts. The development of single photon emission tomography and positron emission tomography is likely to lead to new paediatric applications. The application of magnetic resonance imaging (MRI) imaging has yet to be determined.

Brain imaging may be performed with [99mTc] pertechnetate; but [99mTc]-DTPA and [99mTc]-glucoheptonate have also become popular agents. When [99mTc]-pertechnetate is used, the patient must receive potassium perchlorate orally 15 to 30 minutes prior to injection in order to block choroid plexus accumulation. Flow images are recommended routinely; static blood pool images following the angiogram can also yield information about localized hyperaemia. Delayed static images in at least four views, 2 to 3 hours post-injection are used to evaluate the integrity of the blood-brain barrier. It is now common to acquire and store these images in a digital computer.

Vascular abnormalities can be seen in children secondary to hypoxia, asphyxia, and thrombosis. Newborns who experience hypoxia in the perinatal period have shown classic patterns of arterial and watershed infarction [43]. Cerebrovascular accidents also occur in association with congenital heart conditions with right to left shunts or sickle cell anaemia. Congenital arteriovenous malformations of the brain may rarely present as congestive cardiac failure in the neonatal period. The radionuclide flow study is also being used in paediatrics as an adjunctive test for documenting cerebral death [44]. Computer processing of cerebral radionuclide angiograms may be helpful, especially as it is possible to compare regional perfusion by generating time/activity curves with the computer.

Cerebral inflammatory diseases are not uncommon in paediatrics. Early in their course, these processes may not cause sufficient density alteration to be visualized with CT. Radionuclide imaging, on the other hand, has been found to be sensitive to early changes in meningoencephalitis. A detection rate superior to that provided by CT has been reported [45]. Temporal lobe involvement is suggestive of herpes encephalitis.

Subdural haematomas may occur in association with cerebral inflammatory disease and trauma. CT will occasionally miss these lesions when they are isodense and/or bilateral. In young infants, ultrasound imaging through the fontanelles does not reliably detect subdural collections over the convexities of the brain. A child suspected of having a subdural collection who has a negative CT or ultrasound examination is a candidate for a nuclide study.

While CT is superior to radionuclide imaging in defining the size and configuration of the ventricular system, it is limited in evaluating *CSF dynamics*.

Radionuclide cisternography complements CT in this respect. A CT study showing mild ventricular dilatation with widening of the subarachnoid space can reflect either cerebral atrophy or communicating hydrocephalus. Cisternography distinguishes between these entities.

In children with *recurrent meningitis* or suspected CSF rhinorrhoea or otorrhoea, cisternography is performed with nasal or ear canal packing to detect CSF leaks.

Cisternography can be performed in children using either 99mTc-DTPA or 111In-DTPA. The more rapid dynamics found in children permit use of the shorter lived 99mTc label in cases where imaging beyond 24 hours is not required. If 48 or 72 hour imaging is anticipated, the 111In label should be used. Following lumbar intrathecal injection, the tracer will reach the basilar cisterns within 30 minutes in young children. It is advisable to image the back and head immediately after injection. Multiple views of the head should be obtained between 30 and 60 minutes post-injection as well as between 2 and 4 hours. Retrograde filling of the ventricular system is most likely to occur between 1 and 4 hours following injection. Later images at 6 and 24 hours should be obtained to assess ventricular emptying (if this occurs) and resorption over the convexities.

When a leak test is performed, packing (of ear or nose) causes considerable discomfort and a child may not tolerate the packs for more than a few hours. These packs may be placed 30 minutes after injection and removed after 4 to 6 hours. Packing should be carefully labelled when removed and counted in a well counter. A plasma sample is recommended as a standard part of this procedure.

Diversionary CSF shunts used in children to relieve hydrocephalus are prone to blockage. Most are placed with a cranial reservoir under the scalp to which the intra- and extracranial portions are connected. When a shunt malfunction is suspected, the reservoir can be injected with 0.5 to 1.0 mCi 99mTc-pertechnetate or 99mTc-DTPA in a small volume. Serial imaging of the head and trunk will document movement of the tracer through the distal tubing and systemic absorption in less than 30 minutes.

The future of radionuclide imaging of the brain lies in the development of new tracers and techniques which demonstrate regional brain physiology and metabolism. Single photon emission computed tomography (SPECT) units are now in clinical use but their usefulness has yet to be established. Such techniques will have to prove superior to both CT and MRI. Positron emission tomography (PET) in combination with labelled biological compounds is hoped to be the forerunner of a new series of developments which will result in paediatric applications.

Thyroid imaging

Thyroid imaging is usually performed in paediatric patients to identify localization or morphology. Thyroid function is assessed by in vitro studies. The ubiquitous 99mTc is quite suitable for thyroid imaging, which should be performed in children using a converging or pinhole collimator. 99mTc gives

a lower dose of radiation to the thyroid than the iodine isotopes [46], is administered intravenously, and permits imaging minutes after injection. Of the available iodine isotopes, 123I offers advantages in both dosimetry and imaging, but is not as readily available as 99mTc, must be given orally, and is imaged 4 to 24 hours after administration. Because of its high radiation dose, use of 131I in children is seldom warranted for diagnostic imaging. Potassium perchlorate should obviously not be given prior to thyroid imaging.

Neonatal metabolic screening programs for congenital hypothyroidism identify patients whose treatment is not dependent upon the establishment of aetiology. The aetiology, however, has implications for genetic counselling. Absence of the thyroid gland (athyreosis) and ectopia are sporadic occurrences. Defects in the synthesis of thyroid hormone, on the other hand, are inherited as autosomal recessive traits. Ectopic thyroid glands are usually visualized adequately with 99mTc (0.7 mCi) or 123I(30 µCi), especially in the neonatal period when salivary gland activity is normally diminished (Fig. 101.9). When the infant is already receiving thyroid replacement, thyroid stimulating hormone (TSH) should be given. When a high level of TSH is documented in untreated infants this is unnecessary. When no thyroid tissue is visualized, suppression by exogenous iodine, maternal antithyroid therapy, and hypopituitarism must be excluded. Hypothyroidism secondary to defects in hormone synthesis shows avid radionuclide trapping by a gland which is generally enlarged [47,48].

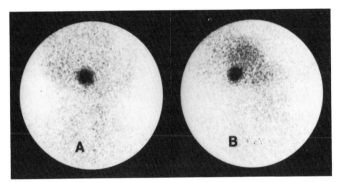

Fig. 101.9 99mTc pertechnetate accumulation in an ectopic thyroid gland. Magnification images of the neck in anterior (A) and lateral (B) views were obtained using pinhole collimation.

Older infants and children presenting with neck masses should have thyroid imaging before surgery to establish that the mass does not contain the patient's only functioning thyroid tissue.

Thyroid nodules can be evaluated with a scan, as in adults, to determine activity. Discordance between the uptake of 99mTc and 131I by nodules has been documented, so a 'hot' nodule detected on a 99mTc scan should be re-imaged with 123I. 'Cold' nodules should be pursued in children as they are in adults, since malignancy may occur.

Lymphocytic thyroiditis, which occurs most frequently in girls between the ages of 6 and 15 years, presents with glandular enlargement. Most commonly, images show a patchy, nonhomogeneous pattern of tracer uptake, which, like the functional status in thyroiditis, is variable. The pattern may range from homogeneous to multinodular with defects that are quite discrete.

With technetium imaging, the diagnosis of a diffuse hyperfunctioning gland is made by comparing thyroid activity to soft tissue background and salivary gland activity. Computerized region of interest analysis or slice profiles provide confirmation.

Cardiopulmonary imaging

The emphasis in paediatric cardiopulmonary scintigraphy is quite different from that in adults. The emphasis in paediatric nuclear cardiology is on congenital heart disease. Pulmonary embolic disease, the most frequent indication for lung imaging in adults, is uncommon in childhood. Paediatric pulmonary imaging is usually performed to investigate regional lung function.

A decade ago, nuclear medicine procedures were being developed as a partial substitute for cardiac catheterization. Echocardiography has evolved in the interim and now offers an alternative. The role of digital subtraction angiography in paediatric cardiology is still being assessed. Both of these techniques have narrowed the use of radionuclides in paediatric cardiology to specific physiological problems.

Nuclear angiocardiography

The nuclear angiocardiogram is simple to perform, and once the data obtained are stored in a computer they become the basis for anatomical and physiological determinations. Serial images can be evaluated for morphological relationships, although the anatomical detail is limited, especially in infants. More important is the physiological information derived from the radionuclide angiogram, (i.e., the calculation of left to right shunts and ventricular ejection fractions).

Good technique is absolutely essential in paediatric nuclear cardiology. All aspects of image interpretation and computer manipulation are dependent upon a 'tight' injection bolus, high count rates, and precise positioning. ^{99m}Tc in a dose of 200 mCi/kg should have a high enough specific activity to keep the injection volume between 0.2 and 0.5 ml. A minimum dose of 2 mCi should be used in infants.

To perform the bolus injection, a three-way stopcock setup or piggyback syringe apparatus is connected to a short intravenous angiocatheter. Another option is to thread a longer catheter through the vein and position the tip close to the superior vena cava. Injection of the external jugular vein in the neck will give the most compact bolus; the medial antecubital vein (basilic) is acceptable.

A high sensitivity parallel hole or converging collimator is used. The anterior view shows the lungs well, but superimposes the chambers; it is acceptable for shunt studies. The anterior view can be modified to a left anterior oblique by tilting the collimator 30 to 45 degrees to the left and 30 degrees caudally. This separates the ventricular chambers, which is essential for calculating ejection fractions. Acquisition at a rate of 0.5 to 1.0 frames per second is suitable if serial mode is not used.

The normal radionuclide angiocardiogram shows a clear progression through the chambers of the right heart and pulmonary outflow tract to the lungs. While the bolus becomes dispersed in the lungs, there is sufficient concentration to show the left ventricle and aorta in the laevophase. The left atrium is not well visualized because of its deep position and masking by pulmonary activity.

Abnormalities such as transposition, dextrocardia, and severe obstructions in the pulmonary artery or aorta can be recognized. Intracardiac shunts can be recognized by alterations in the filling and emptying sequence of the chambers. A left to right shunt at ventricular level will produce early recirculation to the right ventricle and persistence of activity in the lungs during the laevophase. Visual impressions may be confirmed by using a computer to designate regions of interest over the chambers and to generate time/activity curves.

Children who have had palliative or corrective cardiac surgery for congenital heart disease can be monitored by radionuclide angiocardiography.

A quantitative estimate of left to right cardiac shunting can be obtained from the angiocardiogram using a digital computer. The most accurate technique uses gamma variate function approximations over segments of the pulmonary transit curve [49]. This method provides an approximation of the pulmonary to systemic flow ratio (Qp:Qs) by identifying the area of the curve that results from early pulmonary recirculation due to the shunt. The method can accurately quantify left to right shunts in the Qp:Qs range between 1.2:1 and 3.0:1 [50]. The success of this technique is dependent upon a 'tight' injection bolus. It is hoped that computer programs using deconvolution analysis will be successful in correcting for poor bolus injections [51].

Right to left shunts may be identified on angiocardiograms by the early appearance of tracer activity in the aorta. Documentation is more easily accomplished with ^{99m}Tc macroaggregated albumin (MAA). In the normal circulation, no particles are detected outside the lungs (Fig. 101.10). If extrapulmonic activity is noted and the radionuclide preparation was correctly performed, a right to left shunt is present. A number of congenital lesions, such as the tetralogy of Fallot, pulmonary atresia with septal defect, tricuspid atresia, and Ebstein's anomaly, can show right to left shunting.

Blood pool imaging

Gated blood pool imaging is now being performed in children to evaluate both left and right ventricular function. As in adults, several indices of ventricular function can be obtained, including ejection fractions, rates of ventricular filling and emptying, and systolic-diastolic time intervals. In vivo labelling of red blood cells with ^{99m}Tc is accomplished by first injecting stannous pyrophosphate. Using an

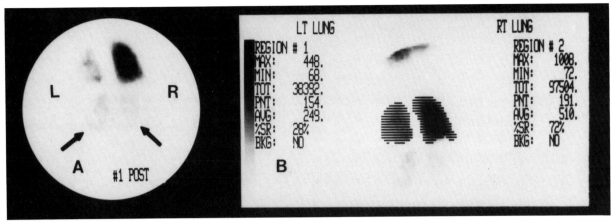

Fig. 101.10 Congenital heart disease. ^{99m}Tc macroaggregated albumin was used to quantitate relative pulmonary blood flow in this child with tetralogy of Fallot and a hypoplastic left pulmonary artery. (A) Posterior image of the body shows decreased activity in the left lung and activity in the abdomen [arrows]. The presence of extrapulmonary activity is evidence of a right to left shunt. (B) Computer approximation of pulmonary activity. The activity is directly proportional to relative pulmonary blood flow.

electrocardiographic gate, several hundred cardiac cycles can be collected in 10 to 15 minutes.

Potential indications for serial monitoring of ventricular function include children who have undergone cardiac surgery, paediatric oncology patients being treated with cardiotoxic drugs such as adriamycin, and patients with cardiomyopathies. In chronic pulmonary conditions such as cystic fibrosis, right ventricular ejection fraction monitoring may be of clinical use.

Myocardial imaging

Ischaemic cardiac disease is rare in children, but is associated with congenital anomalies of the coronary arteries [52] and acquired conditions such as cardiomyopathies.

Thallium (^{201}Tl) imaging has also been used to study children with aortic stenosis and left ventricular hypertrophy, and may play a role in postoperative evaluation. A scaled dose proportionate to adults, 30 µCi/kg, will not provide adequate studies in infants and a practical minimum of 500 µCi is suggested for a ^{201}Tl study. Myocardial imaging should begin 10 to 20 minutes post-injection and should involve multiple 300 to 600 K images (anterior, 45 degrees LAO, and 60 degrees LAO at minimum). More views may be necessary and computer acquisition and processing should also be considered.

While most attention has been given to ^{201}Tl imaging of the left ventricular myocardium, it has been shown that a good correlation exists between right ventricular uptake of ^{201}Tl and right ventricular hypertension. This may be of use in evaluating children at risk for pulmonary hypertension, congenital heart lesions, and chronic pulmonary disease (e.g. cystic fibrosis) [53,54].

Pulmonary ventilation and perfusion imaging

Studies for assessment of regional ventilation are usually performed immediately preceding a perfusion study. If one wishes to assess air trapping, the longer lived xenon tracers (^{131}Xe, ^{127}Xe) must be used. The short lived ^{81m}Kr is useful in identifying regional ventilation defects and in evaluating ventilation-perfusion matching.

Xenon delivery in the cooperative child (generally 5 years of age or older) can be performed with a mouthpiece and nose clip as in adults. With such patients, one can accomplish single breath (30 to 60 seconds), equilibration (1 to 3 minutes), and wash-out images (3 to 8 minutes). The use of xenon in children under 5 years of age or uncooperative older children requires a mask delivery system. In these instances, the study consists of serial wash-in and wash-out images.

Xenon studies require trapping and venting equipment. The ease of ^{81m}Kr use makes this an attractive choice for paediatric use when assessment of air trapping is not mandatory. Placing the generator outflow tube under the child's nostrils is sufficient; a nasal cannula can also be used.

It is possible to study children with endotracheal and tracheostomy tubes using xenon, but it is difficult to avoid leakage and the use of krypton is preferable. Multiple views are easy to obtain with ^{81m}Kr; Xenon imaging is limited to one view, usually posterior.

The ^{99m}Tc-labelled particles (macroaggregated albumin or human albumin microspheres) are injected intravenously. The pulmonary vascular bed is not fully developed in young infants and a number of conditions requiring study are associated with shunting of blood from the right side (pulmonary) circulation to the left (systemic). Care should be taken to ensure that the total number of injected particles is less than 100 000. This is no problem with standard dose preparation and there are no significant risks associated with perfusion studies in children. Perfusion imaging using ^{133}Xe dissolved in saline is possible, but the technique has not been widely used.

While much information can be obtained from imaging alone, the application of computer quantification and graphic display greatly enhances pulmonary studies. Serial evaluations also become more objective when quantitated. Ventilation studies are suited to the display of wash-out by time/activity curves generated from a lung or portion of a lung. Perfusion images can be analyzed by region of interest comparisons of relative activity. Particulate distribution is directly proportional to the blood flow to the region. When perfusion imaging is performed in children with congenital heart disease, it is essential that quantification be employed since these studies will often be repeated to detect physiological changes (Fig. 101.10).

Congenital pulmonary conditions include lung hypoplasia (often secondary to diaphragmatic hernia), lobar emphysema, cystic adenomatoid malformation, and sequestration. A matching defect on ventilation and perfusion images is usually encountered in all of these entities. Wash-out ventilation images in lobar emphysema, however, will show delayed accumulation and trapping in the abnormal lung. A technique for diagnosing a sequestration using a combination of lung perfusion imaging with ^{99m}Tc-MAA and ^{99m}Tc angiography has been described. Following perfusion imaging, the patient is placed in front of the gamma camera in a position which optimizes visualization of the defect. A bolus injection of ^{99m}Tc is administered, and, during the laevophase as the aorta fills with tracer, a sequestration with aberrant blood supply arising from the aorta will fill in with activity.

Ventilation/perfusion (V/Q) imaging in patients with acquired lung disease is performed to assess a region of the lung. When one region is radiographically abnormal due to infection or atelectasis, radionuclide imaging may be performed to identify additional abnormal areas not radiographically apparent. Emphysema from any cause and post-infectious bullae may show perfusion deficit and delayed ventilation with focal trapping on wash-out. Pneumonia and pulmonary infarctions show matched V/Q abnormality and cannot be differentiated by scan. Chronic pulmonary disease and acute asthma at a single point in time can mimic each other with diffuse V/Q abnormalities and trapping. Asthma, however, often shows considerable changes even over short time intervals. Matching V/Q defects are noted in cystic fibrosis[54] when single breath ventilation is compared to perfusion. Focal areas of xenon trapping are seen on wash-out: areas of ventilation/perfusion mismatch also occur. Obliterative bronchiolitis shows a persistent match of V/Q defects.

Paediatric patients with scoliosis and chest wall deformities have been evaluated by V/Q imaging to determine the effects of the deformity on regional lung function.

Pulmonary embolic disease is unusual in children.

Perfusion imaging alone can be quite helpful in any condition which results in right to left shunting by the appearance of lung agent outside the lungs. The brain and kidneys are seen more prominently than the liver. The degree of right to left shunting can be quantitated.

Differential pulmonary perfusion may occur in pulmonary stenosis, patent ductus arteriosis and pulmonary artery anomalies. Palliative surgical shunts are employed to improve pulmonary blood flow e.g. in Fallot tetralogy. These left to right shunts are readily assessed by lung perfusion imaging and can be quantitated.

SUMMARY

Radionuclide studies have proven to be a safe and effective imaging modality in paediatrics. They contribute primarily physiological information, but are often also used to provide morphological data.

Unnecessary studies can be avoided by knowing how to use selected radionuclide imaging in conjunction with the other imaging modalities.

The use of nuclear studies to the best advantage of each patient requires understanding of the differences in technique between paediatric and adult studies, as well as a knowledge of childhood disease processes.

As with all imaging modalities, it is essential that nuclear studies be viewed in conjunction with the other available radiographic studies and a knowledge of the patient's medical history and physical examination.

The digital computer/scintillation camera combination has given a new dimension to paediatric nuclear studies. Current improvements in equipment are being evaluated for effectiveness in paediatrics where count rates are lower and greater resolution is essential. Much of the future of paediatric nuclear medicine also depends upon the development of new radiopharmaceuticals.

BIBLIOGRAPHY

REFERENCES

1. Composite based upon recommendations appearing in: James A E, Wagner H N Jr, Cook R E (eds), Pediatric nuclear medicine. Saunders, Philadelphia
2. Webster E W, Alpert N M, Brownell G L 1974 Radiation doses in pediatric nuclear medicine and diagnostic X-ray procedures. In: James A E, Wagner H N Jr, Cook R E (eds), Pediatric nuclear medicine. Saunders, Philadelphia, pp 34–58
3. Gilday D L, Paul D J, Patterson J 1975 Diagnosis of osteomyelitis in children by combined blood pool and bone imaging. Radiology 117:331–335
4. Maurer A H, Chen D C P, Camargo E E, Wong D F, Wagner H N, Alderson P O 1981 Utility of three-phase skeletal scintigraphy in suspected osteomyelitis: Concise communication. J Nucl Med 22:941–949
5. Trackler R T, Miller K E, Sutherland D H, Chadwick D L 1976 Childhood pelvic osteomyelitis presenting as a 'cold' lesion on bone scan: case report. J Nucl Med 17:620–622
6. Russin L D, Staab E V 1976 Unusual bone scan findings in acute osteomyelitis: case report. J Nucl Med 17:617–619
7. Murray I P C 1982 Photopenia in skeletal scintigraphy of suspected bone and joint infection. Clin Nucl Med 7:13–20
8. Sullivan D C, Rosenfield N S, Ogden J, Gottschalk A 1980 Problems in the scintigraphic detection of osteomyelitis in children. Radiology 135:731–736
9. Handmaker H 1980 Acute hematogenous osteomyelitis: has the bone scan betrayed us? Radiology 135:787–789
10. Gilday D L 1980 Problems in the scintigraphic detection of osteomyelitis. Radiology 135:791
11. Ash J, Gilday D L 1980 The futility of bone scanning in neonatal osteomyelitis: Concise communication. J Nucl Med 21:417–420
12. Lisbona R, Rosenthall L 1977 Observations on the sequential use

of ^{99m}Tc-phosphate complex and ^{67}Ga imaging in osteomyelitis. Cellulitis and septic arthritis. Radiology 123:123–129

13. Danigelis J A, Fisher R L, Ozonoff M B, Sziklas J J 1975 ^{99m}Tc-polyphosphate bone imaging in Legg-Perthes' Disease. Radiology 115:407–413

14. Fasting O J, Langeland N, Bjerkreim I, Hertzenberg L, Nakken K 1978 Bone scintigraphy in early diagnosis of Perthes' disease. Acta Orthop Scand 49:169–174

15. Gilfand M J, Harcke H T 1978 Skeletal imaging in sickle-cell disease. J Nucl Med (abstract) 19:698

16. Chung S M K, Alavi A, Russel M D 1978 Management of osteo-necrosis in sickle-cell anemia and its genetic variants. Clin Orthop 130:158–174

17. Sty J R, Starshak R J 1983 The role of bone scintigraphy in the evaluation of the suspected abused child. Radiology 146:369–375 and 148:573

18. Gilday D L, Ash J M, Green M D 1980 Child abuse — its complete evaluation by one radiopharmaceutical. J Nucl Med (abstract) 21:10

19. Gilday D L, Ash J M, Reilly B J 1977 Radionuclide skeletal survey for pediatric neoplasms. Radiology 123:399–406

20. Parker B R, Pinckney L, Etcubanas E 1980 Relative efficacy of radiographic and radionuclide bone surveys in the detection of the skeletal lesions of histiocytosis x. Radiology 134:377–380

21. Harcke H T 1978 Bone imaging in infants and children: A review. J Nucl Med 19:324–329

22. Gulenchyn K Y, Gildiner M, Ash J M 1982 Pediatric arthritides and useless joint scans. J Nucl Med (abstract) 23:7.

23. Silberstein E B 1980 Nuclear orthopaedics (teaching editorial) J Nucl Med 21: 997–999

24. Harcke H T, Williams J L 1980 Evaluation of neonatal renal disorders: A comparison of excretory urography with scintigraphy and ultrasonography. Ann Radiol 23:109–113

25. Harcke H T, Williams J L, Popky G L, Pollack H M, Parker J A, Capitanio M A 1982 Abdominal masses in the neonate: A multiple modality approach to diagnosis. Radio Graphics 2:69–82

26. Ash J M, Gilday D L 1980 Renal nuclear imaging and analysis in pediatric patients. Urol Clin North Am 7:201–214

27. Koff S A, Thrall J H, Keyes J W 1980 Assessment of hydro20uretero-nephrosis in children using diuretic radionuclide urography. J Urol 123:531–534

28. Conway J J, King L R, Belman A B, Thorsen T Jr 1972 Detection of vesicoureteral reflux with radionuclide cystography. Am J Roentgenol 115:720–727

29. Holder L E, Strife J, Padikal T N, Perkins P J, Kereiakes J G 1975 Liver size determination in pediatrics using sonographic and scintigraphic techniques. Radiology 117:349–353

30. Spencer R P 1980 Role of radiolabeled erythrocytes in evaluation of splenic function. J Nucl Med 489–490

31. Gates G F, Miller J H, Stanley P 1978 Scintiangiography of hepatic masses in childhood. JAMA 239:2667–2670

32. Fischer K C, Eraklis A, Rossello P, Treves, S 1978 Scintigraphy in the followup of pediatric splenic trauma treated without surgery. J Nucl Med 19:3–9

33. Hayden P W, Rudd T G, Christie D L 1979 Rose bengal sodium I-131 studies in infants with suspected biliary atresia. Am J Dis Child 133:834–837

34. Collier B D, Treves S, Davis M A, Heyman S, Subramaniam G, McAfee J G 1980 Simultaneous ^{99m}-Tc-P-butyl-IDA and ^{131}-I-rose bengal scintigraphy in neonatal jaundice. Radiology 134:719–722

35. Madj M, Reba R C, Altman R P 1981 Effect of phenobarbital on ^{99m}-Tc-IDA scintigraphy in the evaluation of neonatal jaundice. Semin Nucl Med 11:194–204

36. Sty J R, Starshak R J, Thorp S M 1982 Preliminary clinical experience with ^{99m}Tc disofenin as a biliary imaging agent in pediatrics. Clin Nucl Med 7:210–212

37. Petrokubic R J, Baums S, Roher G V 1978 Cimetidine administration resulting in improved pertechnetate imaging of Meckel's diverticulum. Clin Nucl Med 3:385–388

38. Sfakianakis G N, Conway J J 1981 Detection of ectopic gastric mucosa in Meckel's diverticulum and in other abberations by scintigraphy: I. pathophysiology and 10-year clinical experience. J Nucl Med 22:647–654. II. Indications and methods — a 10-year experience. J Nucl Med 22:732–738

39. Treves S, Grand R J, Eraklis A J 1978 Pentagastrin stimulation of technetium -99m uptake by ectopic gastric mucosa in a Meckel's diverticulum. Radiology 128:711–712

40. Boonyaprapa S, Alderson P O, Garfinkel D J, Chipps B E, Wagner H N 1980 Detection of pulmonary aspiration in infants and children with respiratory disease: Concise communication. J Nucl Med 21:314–318

41. Rudd T G, Christie D L 1979 Demonstration of gastroesophageal reflux in children by radionuclide gastroesophagography. Radiology 131:483–486

42. Heyman S, Kirkpatrick J A, Winter H S, Treves S 1979 An improved radionuclide method for the diagnosis of gastroesophageal reflux and aspiration in children (milk scan). Radiology 131:479–482

43. Savage J P, Gilday D L, Ash J M 1977 Cerebrovascular disease in childhood. Radiology 123:385–391

44. Ashival S, Smith A J K, Torres F, Loken M, Chou S N 1977 Radionuclide bolus angiography: A technique for verification of brain death in infants and children. J Pediatr 91: 722–728

45. Kim E E, DeLand F H, Montebello J 1979 Sensitivity of radionuclide brain scan and computed tomography in early detection of viral meningoencephalitis. Radiology 132:425–429

46. Task force on short-lived radionuclides for medical applications 1978 Evaluation of diseases of the thyroid gland with the in vivo use of radionuclides. J Nucl Med 19:107–112

47. Bauman R A, Bode H H, Hayek A, Crawford J D 1976 Technetium 99-m-pertechnetate scans in congenital hypothyroidism. J Pediatr 89:268–271

48. Kim E E, Domstad P A, Choy Y C, DeLand F H 1981 Avid thyroid uptake of (Tc-99m) sodium pertechnetate in children with goitrous cretinism. Clin Pediatr 7:437–439

49. Maltz D L, Treves S 1973 Quantitative radionuclide angiocardiography: Determination of Qp:Qs in children. Circulation 47:1049–1056

50. Askinazi J, Ahnberg D S, Korngold E, LaFarge C G, Maltz D L, Trevess 1976 Quantitative radionuclide angiocardiography: Detection and quantitation of left to right shunts. Am J Cardiol 37:382–387

51. Ham H R, Dobbeleir A, Viart P, Piepsz A, Lenaers A 1981 Radionuclide quantitation of left-to-right cardiac shunts using deconvolution analysis: Concise communication. J Nucl Med 22:688–692

52. Rabinovitch M, Rowland T W, Castaneda A R, Treves S 1979 Thallium-201 scintigraphy in patients with anomalous origin of the left coronary artery from the main pulmonary artery. J Pediatr 94:244–247

53. Matthay R A, Berger H J, Davies R A, Loke J, Mathier D A, Gottschalk A, Zaret B L 1980 Right and left ventricular performance in ambulatory young adults with cystic fibrosis. Br Heart J 43:474–480

54. Piepsz A, Wetzburger C, Spehl M, Machin D, Dab I, Ham H R, Vandevivere J J, Baran D 1980. Critical evaluation of lung scintigraphy in cystic fibrosis: Study of 113 patients. J Nucl Med 21:909–913

SUGGESTIONS FOR FURTHER READING

Alderson P O, Gilday D L, Wagner H N, Jr 1978 Atlas of pediatric nuclear medicine. Mosby, St Louis

Gilday D L 1976 Pediatric neuronuclear medicine. In: Harwood-Nash D C, Fitz C R (eds) Neuroradiology in Infants and Children. Mosby, St Louis, pp 505–608

Handmaker H, Lowenstein J M (eds) 1975 Nuclear medicine in clinical pediatrics. Society of Nuclear Medicine, New York

James A E, Wagner H N Jr, Cooke R E (eds) 1974 Pediatric nuclear medicine. Saunders, Philadelphia

Treves S, Fogle R, Lang P 1980 Radionuclide angiography in congenital heart disease. Am J Cardiol 46:1247–1255

102 Paediatric ultrasonography

Constantine Metreweli

Practical considerations

Ultrasound of the newborn and infant brain

The chest
  Opaque hemithorax
  Juxtadiaphragmatic masses

The liver
  Hepatoblastomas and hepatomas
  Hamartomas
  Haematomas
  Haemangiomas
  Adenomas
  Granulomas
  Hydatid disease

The gallbladder and biliary system
  Gallstones
  Biliary sludge
  Gallbladder wall thickening
  Hydrops
  Choledochal cyst
  Biliary atresia

The pancreas

The portal venous system
  The splenic vein

The spleen

The gastrointestinal tract

Aorta and inferior vena cava

The adrenal glands
  Neonatal adrenal haemorrhage
  Neuroblastoma
  Adrenal adenomas

The urinary tract
  The renal parenchyma
  Renal calculi
  Renal cystic disease
  Multicystic kidney
  Infantile polycystic disease
  Microcystic conditions
  Renal mass lesions
  Hydronephrosis and hydroureter

This chapter is not intended to be an exhaustive description of ultrasound as applied in paediatrics but a systematic selection of those features that differ from the adult experience with descriptions of the commoner abnormalities seen in each particular organ. The aim is to assist the general radiologist rather than the paediatric specialist.

Practical considerations

Children should be examined without sedation, without fasting and with short and medium focus 5 MHZ probes, attached to equipment of sufficient quality to make the best of the probes.

In babies a dummy soaked in honey often ensures cooperation, failing which re-examination immediately after a feed is often rewarding. If a child is found to be extremely 'gassy' then a re-examination should be scheduled for the first thing in the morning, preferably before the child's breakfast. The amount of bowel gas increases progressively throughout the day and a starving child seems only to swallow more gas, hence the reason for trying to take advantage of the natural tendency of the abdomen to be fairly free of gas in the morning.

With patience and gentleness it is possible to examine virtually all children successfully. When examining the abdomen or chest always start by gently examining the epigastrium with the child supine. The child can see the examiner, its parents or nurse and the equipment and soon gains confidence. Always leave examination of the kidneys in the prone position to the very end. Real-time equipment is a boon but not essential except for the examination of the newborn brain. The particular advantage of the B scanner lies in the wider range of more appropriate transducers which are available compared with most real-time units, in addition to a better demonstration of anatomy than is possible with the 'keyhole' views of real-time equipment.

Ultrasound of the newborn and infant brain

This topic is considered separately in Chapter 103.

The chest [2]

A child's ribs are thinner and relatively more widespread than an adult's and do not present such a significant barrier to echographic examination. Also, from the subdiaphragmatic approach, the larger area of liver contact with the diaphragm in the child gives better access to parts of the left hemidiaphragm as well as to the whole of the right hemidiaphragm. Generally ultrasound examination is indicated because of the discovery of an opacity on a chest radiograph, a completely opaque hemithorax, a juxtadiaphragmatic or juxtapleural mass, or mediastinal enlargement which can be studied from the suprasternal notch (or through the manubriosternal joint) as well as from the subxiphisternal approach. Sometimes unsuspected posterior mediastinal involvement may be diagnosed when an abdominal retroperitoneal mass can be seen to be extending through the retrocrural space.

Opaque hemithorax

The aetiology of an opaque hemithorax can be difficult to identify on a simple chest radiograph. However, ultrasound can demonstrate a consolidated, collapsed lung with fluid-filled bronchi (hence no air bronchogram), characterized by tramline streaks converging on the hilum of the lung on the echogram. Other causes are massive pleural effusion, massive pericardial effusion reaching to the pleural border, a tumour (Ewing's or neuroblastoma) which will be revealed by its tissue texture echo pattern, or herniation of the liver through a diaphragmatic defect of variable size [1,2].

Juxtadiaphragmatic masses

Ultrasound will quickly distinguish whether a juxtadiaphragmatic mass is truly supradiaphragmatic or is due to herniation of liver or kidney through a diaphragmatic defect (Fig. 102.1). Bowel rarely presents a radiological problem because of the presence of gas [2].

The liver

The child's liver is relatively larger than the adult's. This is said to be due partly to the relatively slower growth of the left lobe. However, careful evaluation of the true embryological left lobe which is made up of the 'surgical left lobe' and the quadrate lobe of the liver, suggests that the whole liver becomes smaller and rotates anticlockwise relative to the spine. In judging hepatic size, ultrasound is superior to clinical estimation of size when the liver is small but only improves clinical estimation of hepatomegaly when the liver is being displaced by a low, flattened diaphragm in chronic lung disease, by other organs such as a large tumour of the adrenal or kidney, or by interposed normal bowel [3]. *Hydrops of the gallbladder* [4] can be mistaken for hepatomegaly. A fair number of palpable livers in children seem to be echo-

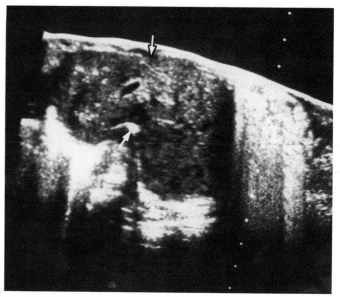

Fig. 102.1 Longitudinal scan. Right paramedian. Large anterior diaphragmatic hernia between the arrows, through which has prolapsed the liver. At the level of the hiatus the gallbladder can be seen within the liver.

graphically normal and in these cases further signs of abnormality must be sought, two major signs being blunting of the lower edge of the liver and increased brightness of the liver parenchyma compared with the adjacent kidney (when the kidney is known clinically to be normal [3]). Unfortunately, the differential diagnosis of diffuse homogenous hepatomegaly is wide and includes:

All causes of hepatitis
Chronic active hepatitis
Haemosiderosis
Parenteral feeding liver ('intralipid liver').
Inborn errors of metabolism, such as glycogen storage disease (Fig. 102.2).
Tyrosinosis
Diffuse infiltration by neuroblastoma or leukaemia

Most often the diagnosis is made by liver biopsy. Conditions causing discrete liver abnormalities, such as liver masses, can be either solitary or multiple. Those which are usually solitary are hepatoblastoma, hepatoma, haematoma, hamartoma, hydatid cyst and focal nodular hyperplasia. Those which are usually multiple are haemangiomas, adenomas, granulomas and metastases.

Hepatoblastomas and hepatomas

These are usually large, disrupt the overall shape of the liver and have an echo pattern which is fairly similar to normal liver echoamplitude but usually with more heterogeneity. [5] Histologically there is considerable similarity between the two tumours but hepatoblastomas tend to occur before the age of four [6]. The identification and tracking of the hepatic venous and portal vessels is most important in the planning

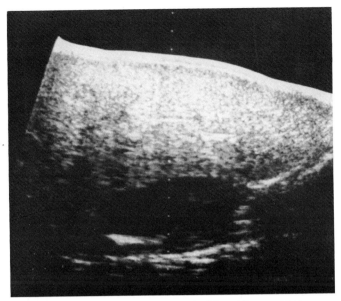

Fig. 102.2 Longitudinal scan of the right lobe of liver and kidney. The liver is enlarged and extremely echogenic with poor penetration at depth and a remarkable difference in echogenicity between the liver and the right kidney which is virtually black behind it. This appearance is characteristic of storage diseases in general but the commonest would be glycogen storage disease.

of surgery and best done in the company of the surgeon contemplating the approach. The finding of multiple tumours in both lobes, or tumour thrombus in the vessels or inferior vena cava precludes surgery (Fig. 102.3) [7].

Hamartomas

The majority of hamartomas are fairly characteristic with cystic areas solid areas and multiple septations. These are invariably benign but because of their size, still need to be removed (Fig. 102.4) [7].

Haematomas

Haematomas are found in a patient with a history of trauma or a haemorrhagic disorder. As is the case anywhere else the appearances are variable depending on the age of the haematoma, its size and the distribution of fibrin debris. The clinical history is therefore of paramount importance in suggesting the diagnosis, as it is also for hepatic abscess or abscesses which are usually accompanied by pyrexia, malaise and leucocytosis. The role of ultrasound in this situation is extended to guiding needles for aspirating pus for microbiological examination [3,8].

Haemangiomas

These may be of several histological types. They can be large

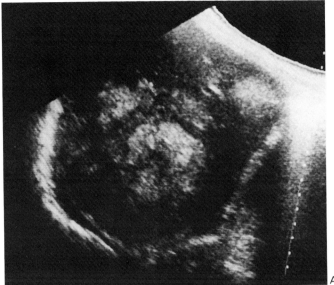

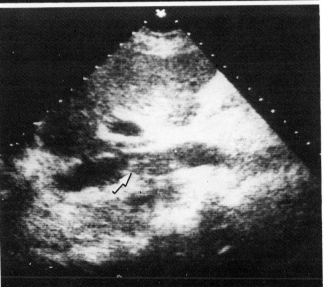

Fig. 102.3 (A) Longitudinal scan of the liver showing a huge hepatoblastoma.
(B) Longitudinal scan of the inferior vena cava reveals tumour thrombosis within the cava [arrow].

and solitary, or multiple, and may cause hyperdynamic heart failure in the child. Although in adults the majority tend to be highly echogenic, in children the pattern is mixed and unless accompanied by signs of external haemangiomas, heart failure or bruits within the liver, can be mistaken for multicentric metastatic malignancy in the liver. In such cases further investigations such as angiography, dynamic CT or MRI may be necessary [9].

It has always been held that needle biopsy is fraught with the danger of torrential haemorrhage, but this view has been called into question and therefore biopsy of a potentially accessible lesion should also be considered.

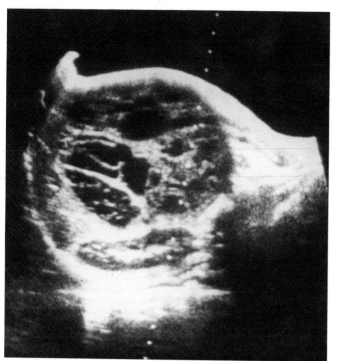

Fig. 102.4 Longitudinal scan of the liver showing a large, loculated mass with thickened septae squashing the right kidney posteriorly. The appearance is highly characteristic of a hamartoma of the liver.

Gallstones [11]

These are much less frequently seen than in adults but are found in children with congenital haemolytic anaemias and cystic fibrosis.

Biliary sludge [11,12]

Seriously ill children, particularly those with congenital haemolytic anaemias and primary renal problems, are often found to have considerable quantities of biliary sludge within the gallbladder which manifests itself by a layering of fine echoes. Occasionally this sludge can inspissate and become highly echogenic suggesting the presence of calculi. Unlike true calculi, however, sludge gives only poor acoustic shadowing. If this process also occurs within the biliary ducts of the liver, inspissated bile syndrome with jaundice will result. Usually the sludge clears even though this may take a few weeks. Transformation to a calculus is a rare occurence (Fig. 102.5.)

Gallbladder wall thickening [13]

Thickening can be striking in children and may cause difficulty in identifying the gallbladder. The thickest gallbladder wall the author measured in a child was 10 mm in a 4 year

Adenomas [3]

In adults these tend to have an increase in echogenicity over the normal accompanying liver. In children adenomas usually occur in conditions of inborn errors of metabolism such as *glycogen storage disease* and *tyrosinosis* in which the liver parenchyma is made abnormally echogenic by the storage of precursor substances. In these cases the adenomas tend to be relatively more echolucent.

Granulomas

Granulomas from either *tuberculosis* or *histiocytosis* tend to be large and sometimes surprisingly echogenic.

Hydatid disease [10]

Solidary cysts in the liver are rare in children and the findings of a cyst in a child, particularly from an endemic area, should suggest the possibility of hydatid disease.

The gallbladder and biliary system

Because of the relative size of the liver, the gallbladder is easy to see in all children.

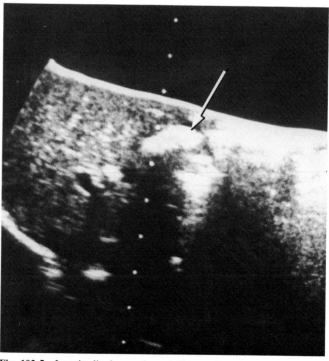

Fig. 102.5 Longitudinal scan through liver and gallbladder. The gallbladder is filled with a highly echogenic white mass [arrow]. This is inspissated bile sludge. Despite its strong echogenicity it tends to cast very poor shadows. Follow-up examinations invariably show disappearance and only very rarely progression to calculus formation.

old boy. The two usual causes are inflammation, the commonest of which seems to be a viral cholecystitis accompanying a hepatitis (in which case the gallbladder wall tends to be fairly homogeneously echogenic), and hypo-albuminaemia which can accompany liver disease and the nephrotic syndrome, which is usually accompanied by a characteristic triple layer 'sandwiching' of the gallbladder wall.

Hydrops of the gallbladder [3,4]

As other parts of the gastrointestinal tract can become inactive during severe illness, so too can the gallbladder and it can distend to its maximum capacity. In children it is a more easily distensible structure than in adults and may attain a large size, when it becomes a palpable mass often confused with the liver and rapidly diagnosed with ultrasound.

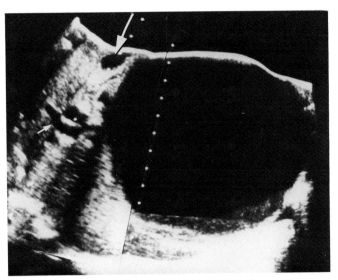

Fig. 102.6 Longitudinal paramedian scan. Huge choledochal cyst communicating with dilated intrahepatic bile ducts [small arrow]. The gallbladder can still be seen above the cyst [large arrow].

Choledochal cyst [14]

Developmental abnormality of the biliary tree can cause cystic swellings anywhere along the common bile duct and common hepatic ducts. These may either be fusiform or saccular. The classical clinical features of recurrent jaundice and fever occur in less than half of all cases and most will present with an abnormal mass. Echography is characteristic showing a cystic swelling within the *porta hepatis* so that the mass is always partly intrahepatic with marked dilatation of the intrahepatic bile ducts, (the commonest reason for this finding in children). The gallbladder is invariably present but small (Fig. 102.6).

Biliary atresia [3,15]

As already stated biliary duct obstruction causing dilatation is rare in children and ultrasound in a jaundiced child usually reveals a normal, undilated biliary tree, unlike the situation in adults where dilatation is frequently found owing to a variety of causes. Biliary atresia is essentially a progressive obliterative inflammatory condition affecting all or any part of the biliary tree. Dilated ducts are rarely found in apparently unaffected regions. Ultrasound demonstrates the lack of the intrahepatic, common hepatic and common bile ducts, usually surrounded by a highly echogenic portal inflammatory reaction. A gallbladder is sometimes present so its discovery does not invalidate the diagnosis (Fig. 102.7).

The pancreas [16,17]

The pancreas is easily visualized in children but is rarely the site of significant disease. The commonest disorder is traumatic haemorrhagic pancreatitis, usually a 'bicycle handlebar' injury. This history will set the diagnostic scene

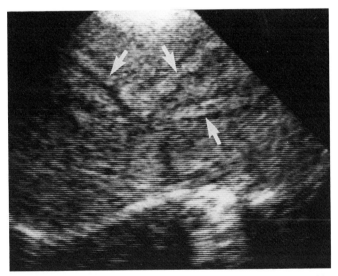

Fig. 102.7 Transverse tilted scan through the liver of a neonate with biliary atresia. The portal venous system has been totally obliterated by the inflammatory reaction and is now represented by white starfish-like cords [arrows].

in such cases but beware of traumatic pancreatitis in nonaccidental injury!

The normal pancreas in the child is usually larger and relatively more echolucent than the adult organ (using the liver as a standard) (Fig. 102.8). The pancreas becomes more echogenic and sometimes enlarges from a variety of causes, such as viral infection, drugs, (particularly steroids and oncolytic agents), chronic debilitating illness, and many other conditions. The criteria for diagnosis of acute pancreatitis, as established in adults i.e. enlargement and increased lucency, do not apply in children and unless

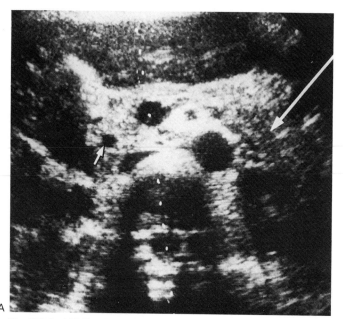
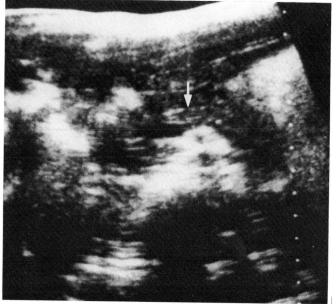

Fig. 102.8   (A) Pancreas of a 60-year-old adult female. Small arrow head shows the CBD in the pancreatic head, long arrow indicates the tail of the pancreas.
   (B) Pancreas of a 4-year-old girl. Arrow indicates the pancreatic duct. Note the relative size and echolucency compared with the adult.

there are gross signs of enlargement or complications such as pseudocysts and free fluid, the diagnosis is very difficult to make. Chronic pancreatitis results in a small echogenic organ which looks like that of a normal middle aged adult. It is most commonly seen in cystic fibrosis but the changes occur too late in that condition to be of diagnostic value.

The portal venous system [18,19]

The major components of the portal venous system, both extrahepatic and intrahepatic, can be easily identified with ultrasound and rare abnormal pathways are sometimes found. *Portal hypertension* can be confidently diagnosed by the presence of variceal collaterals seen either on the medial aspect of the inevitably enlarged spleen or in the upper pre-aortic area, where either a large tortuous coronary vein or multiple small gastro-oesophageal varices may be seen. Alternatively there may be echogenic thickening of the lesser omental root. As a rough guide this area occupying the space between the anterior aspect of the aorta and the posterior aspect of the left lobe of the liver is rarely more than 2 aortic diameters at the same level. Portal hypertension causing the development of small collaterals running through the omental root thickens the omental root (Fig. 102.9B). Changing to a higher frequency, a more appropriate focus and reducing the sensitivity often reveals fine tortuous vessels running in this echogenic mass. A further sign which is most useful in indicating the possibility of portal hypertension is the presence of vessels running cephalad from the splenic vein in this area. The appearance causes the superior mesenteric vein to appear as if it is overshooting the splenic vein, so for convenience this sign is called the 'shoot through'

sign. In children there are two major groups of diseases causing portal hypertension. The first is similar to the situation found in the adult where disease primarily affects the liver, such as cirrhosis and congenital hepatic fibrosis. The second consists of obliterative disorders of the portal vein itself, usually given the title 'portal vein thrombosis' but only some of these cases are actually caused by neonatal umbilical sepsis. In this condition the portal vein is replaced by a leash of small tortuous vessels creating an echogenic mass in the porta hepatis [19]. This is termed cavernous transformation of the portal vein (Fig. 102.9A).

The splenic vein

The splenic vein acts as an excellent indirect marker for retroperitoneal disease. It usually lies transversely across the abdomen above the SMA and aorta, describing a circum-spinal orbit to about the region of the left kidney. The left upper quadrant of the abdomen has always been a difficult area for the echographer and in children one is anxious that a left adrenal, renal, or retroperitoneal nodal mass could be missed. Careful attention to the orbit of the splenic vein is often rewarding as anterior deviation of the portion to the left of the spine indicates displacement, usually by a mass lesion. When this sign is seen, further views such as coronal views, prone views and repeat examinations are indicated to establish the reason for the appearance. The splenic vein is similarly useful in distinguishing a left upper quadrant mass as being the normal enlarged pancreatic tail of childhood rather than a retroperitoneal mass; in the case of the pancreas the splenic vein can be seen running *posteriorly* to the pancreatic tail, i.e. the suspected mass.

The spleen [20,21]

The commonest abnormality of the spleen is splenomegaly resulting from a multitude of causes. Ultrasound is useful in demonstrating or confirming that the palpable mass is in fact spleen and in a small number of cases, it may be able to point to the cause. Generally the aetiology may be identifiable by attention to extrasplenic abnormalities such as varices in portal hypertension, gallstones in congenital haemolytic anaemia, and retroperitoneal lymph node enlargement in lymphoma. Rarely is there any intrinsic splenic abnormality but the commonest of these will be splenic cyst [21] (Fig. 102.10), either congenital or following trauma, splenic haematoma, and relatively transonic patches within the spleen which are often found in cases of lymphoma.

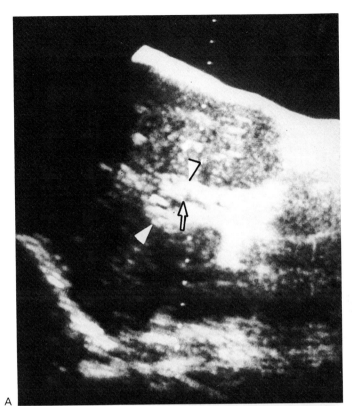

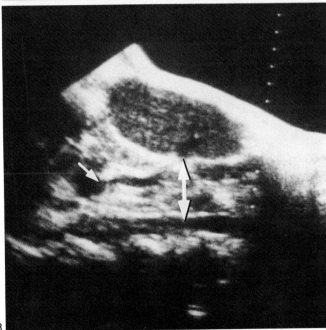

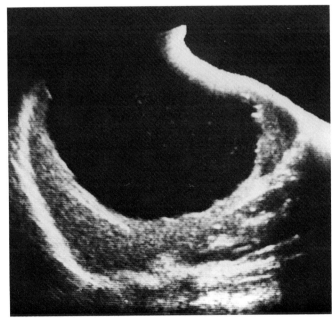

Fig. 102.10 Longitudinal scan through the spleen. The bulk of the spleen consists of a huge cyst with splenic tissue around the outside and a squashed left kidney posteriorly.

Fig. 102.9 (A) Longitudinal scan through the porta hepatis. The normal large echolucent portal vein has been replaced by an echogenic mass (between arrow heads) indicating the presence of cavernous transformation of the portal vein. Sometimes small tortuous vessels can be seen within this [small arrow].

(B) Longitudinal scan over the aorta demonstrating thickening of the root of the lesser omentum between aorta and left lobe of the liver [double arrow] and a large gastro-oesophageal varix [small arrow].

The gastrointestinal tract

Although the gastrointestinal tract itself often interferes with good visualization in the abdomen many intrinsic conditions are nevertheless demonstrable and ultrasound can provide useful information. Cysts of mesenteric and lymphangiectatic origin and duplication cysts are readily identified [22] and ascites can be subdivided into transudates (clear fluid) and exudates (multiple fibrin strands within the fluid) [23]. Particularly useful is the ability of ultrasound to see bowel wall thickening which may be the result of congenital hypertrophy, pyloric stenosis (Fig. 102.11), lymphoma, tuberculosis, haematoma and granulomas (e.g. Crohn's disease) [24]. At the other end of the gut the length of the atretic segment

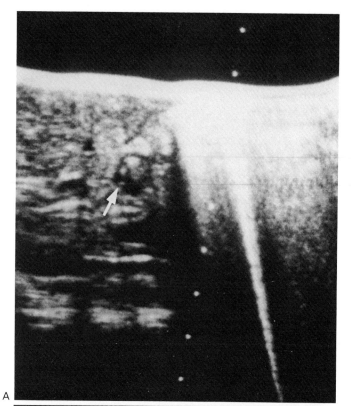

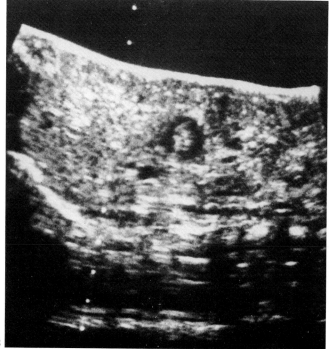

Fig. 102.11 (A) Longitudinal scan above the region of the inferior vena cava showing a normal pyloric region of the stomach [arrow]. Note the white-out of echoes inferior to this representing gas within the bowel.

(B) A 4-week-old boy with a prominent target lesion in the region of the pylorus representing congenital hypertrophic pyloric stenosis. Note the relative absence of gas inferior to this.

in anorectal atresia can be measured from the perineum to the cystic dilated distal portion of the bowel.

The aorta and inferior vena cava

The great vessels rarely suffer intrinsic disease but their demonstration is important in the study of cases of malignancy in childhood. Elevation of the aorta by a retroperitoneal mass is common in invasive neuroblastoma (Fig. 102.12) and this feature is very important as an indicator of inoperability. Demonstration of this simple point will save an unnecessary exploratory laparotomy. The inferior vena cava may be invaded by Wilms' tumour or hepatoblastoma (see Fig. 102.3B).

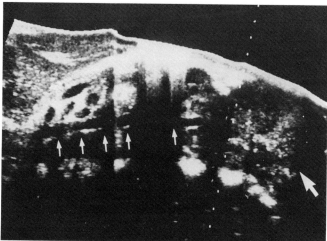

Fig. 102.12 There is a huge retroperitoneal mass seen particularly clearly just above the pelvis [large arrow] but the marked elevation of the aorta from the spine [small arrows] indicates widespread retroperitoneal infiltration highly characteristic of the more aggressive forms of neuroblastoma.

The adrenal glands [25]

There is no doubt that in adults CT is generally very successful in demonstrating the adrenal glands because both sides are equally visible, whereas ultrasound has difficulty on the left because of gastric gas. However, the adult body has more fat between organs, enhancing delineation by CT. In children the lack of fat and small body size actually improves ultrasonic penetration and resolution and it is much easier to identify the adrenals, particularly on the right (Fig. 102.13). Also, masses tend to be relatively large in children at the time of presentation and the vast majority of them should be demonstrable echographically.

The three commonest adrenal abnormalities found in the paediatric age group are neonatal adrenal haemorrhage, neuroblastoma and adrenal adenomas.

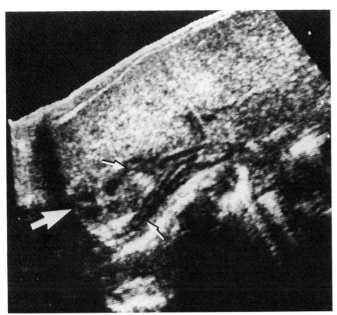

Fig. 102.13 An oblique scan through the right upper abdomen of a 1-day-old newborn, through the upper pole of the right kidney [large arrow] and showing a relatively enlarged right adrenal gland, the lower limbs of which are indicated by small arrows. Distinction between echogenic medulla and echolucent cortex is clearly seen and the relatively large size of the gland in comparison with that in the adult is also easily appreciated.

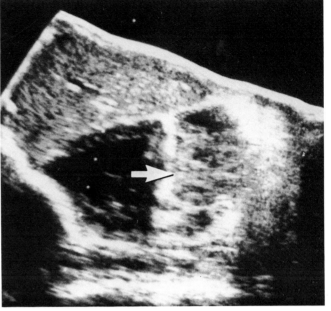

Fig. 102.14 Longitudinal scan through a newborn abdomen. The large triangular, mainly echolucent mass is a right adrenal haemorrhage which is pushing down and rotating about its horizontal axis the right kidney [arrow].

Neonatal adrenal haemorrhage [26,27]

This is found not only in newborns with the classical history of perinatal stress but also as a palpable mass in an otherwise healthy newborn, with a normal perinatal history. It is found more often on the right and more often in males. The echo pattern is very variable. The commonest appearance is of an upper retroperitoneal mass displacing the kidney downwards. The mass is of mixed echo character with a relatively more transonic centre and a ragged echogenic edge (Fig. 102.14). However, the spectrum can vary from a predominantly cystic to predominantly solid appearance. There are only two pathognomonic echographic features. Firstly, haemorrhage occasionally bursts through the adrenal capsule and surrounds the kidney. The crescentic perirenal haematoma shrinks in size but it may take up to 6 weeks for this to be clearly demonstrated [27]. The differential diagnosis most feared is neonatal neuroblastoma but at this age the prognosis is usually good and time is available to watch for shrinkage. In the waiting period urine collections for VMA estimation and measurement of systemic blood pressure will probably ensure that a neuroblastoma is not missed.

Neuroblastoma [7,25]

This is one of the commonest solid tumours of childhood. The prognosis under 1 year of age is good but in older children it is poor because of resistance to available treatment.

The tumour does have a tendency to spontaneously mature and become benign. To the echographer, a neuroblastoma can present in four different ways:

1. Adrenal enlargement of variable size, usually large at the time of presentation with some degree of infiltration of the local structures and displacement of the kidneys downwards.
2. An extensively infiltrating retroperitoneal mass undermining the aorta and encasing the major vessels (Fig. 102.12).
3. A tumour remote from the adrenal region.
4. Infiltration of the liver with no evidence of tumour elsewhere.

When a discrete mass is demonstrable two features are strongly suggestive of neuroblastoma. Firstly, the tendency to infiltrate surrounding organs and tissue planes and secondly a marked heterogeneity of echo amplitudes with very bright irregular echo clusters. Some of these may indicate the presence of calcification not appreciated radiographically. The appearances can be very variable however; relatively homogeneous smooth walled masses are particularly misleading and measurement of the systemic blood pressure and urinary vanillyl mandelic acid (VMA) excretion are particularly important initial investigations in all children with mass lesions suspected of being malignant.

Adrenal adenomas [25]

Functioning endocrine tumours such as *virilizing adrenal adenomas* or *phaeochromocytomas* (Fig. 102.15) always

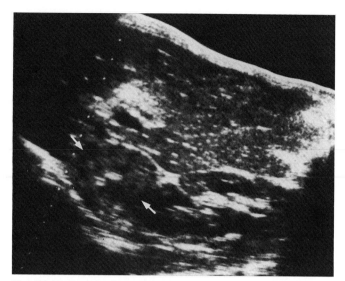

Fig. 102.15 Longitudinal scan through liver and right kidney above which is a 3 × 4 cm adrenal tumour [arrows]. There was clinical and biochemical evidence of phaeochromocytoma. The ultrasound here just confirmed the site.

present with their hormonally induced abnormalities rather than as mass lesions. Therefore the diagnosis has often been made before the child presents to the radiologist and the radiologist's brief is to identify the location of the mass and exclude any possibility of malignant spread. The one difficult condition is Cushing's disease because the fat hypertrophy induced by that disorder seems to be particularly echoreflective and there can be a great problem in providing adequate penetration coupled with adequate resolution. Fortunately in this situation CT is likely to be successful.

The urinary tract

The echography of the paediatric urinary tract provides a wealth of information unobtainable by any other means of imaging. It documents the presence, position and size of the kidneys, and hydronephrosis of the whole kidney or part of the kidney in duplex conditions. It can demonstrate the presence of hydroureter, renal cysts, renal masses, parenchymal crystal deposits, calculi and parenchymal scars.

In children the kidney is much nearer to the surface than it is in adults and the echographer can take full advantage of 5- and 7.5-MHZ frequency probes with close focus to obtain superb renal parenchymal detail of the glomerular-bearing cortex, the medullae, and vessels within the parenchyma. The kidneys can be studied adequately from the front in children and all studies should be accompanied by a search for the ureters and an examination of the bladder.

The renal parenchyma

The normal echo nephrogram (ENG) shows the renal cortex

to be less echogenic than the liver and the renal medullae to be less echogenic than the cortex. The corticomedullary distinction (CMD) is clear, sometimes so marked that a mistaken diagnosis of polycystic kidneys may be made (Fig. 102.16A). In fact if the CMD cannot be resolved in a child, this is strong evidence that the parenchyma is unhealthy (or that the equipment being used may be

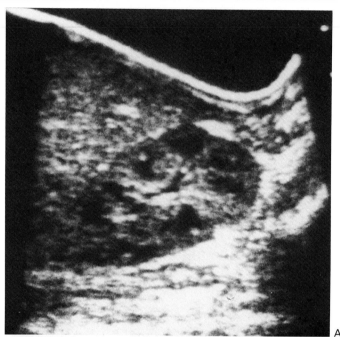

A

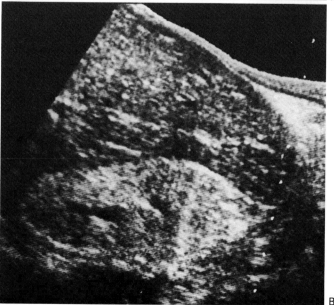

B

Fig. 102.16 (A) Longitudinal scan through the right kidney of the normal 3-week-old newborn. Note the relative brightness compared with adjacent liver, the triangular echolucent medullae with small, bright dots representing the arcuate arteries.

(B) Kidney of normal size and shape without dilatation of the collecting system but the cortex is highly echogenic and featureless suggesting the presence of a crystallopathy or microcystic dysplasia (in this case the latter).

unhealthy). The majority of parenchymal abnormalities are accompanied by increased echogenicity of the cortex ('bright ENG') and variable loss of the CMD. In many of these other abnormalities are prominent and suggest a diagnosis but there are a few disorders in which the ENG is abnormal while the kidneys may remain normal in size and shape; the characteristics of some of these conditions are listed below:

Bright ENG with CMD
Normal in the first 2 weeks of life [28].
Infective nephritis
Immune nephritis (acute glomerulonephritis)
Nephrotoxic myoglobinuria
Nonspecific effects of septicaemia

Bright ENG without CMD (Fig. 102.16B)
Congenital nephrotic syndrome
Medullary cystic disease
Hyperuricaemia
Hyperoxaluria (some)
Reversed ENG (bright medulla with normal or bright cortex) (Fig. 102.17)
Nephrocalcinosis
Hyperoxaluria

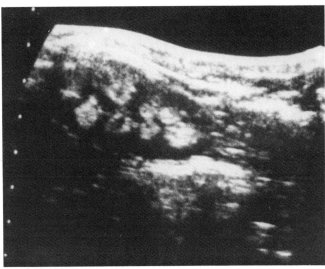

Fig. 102.17 Prone longitudinal scan of right kidney in a 6-year-old girl. The medullary areas are replaced by highly echogenic echo clusters indicating the presence of nephrocalcinosis.

These lists are not exhaustive but are intended to give an idea of the importance of studying the echonephrogram carefully. As nephrocalcinosis is easily diagnosable in the paediatric kidney and a radiograph taken at the same time may not show any abnormality, the echonephrogram is the method of choice in diagnosing this condition.

Renal calculi

A standard radiograph may miss urinary tract calculi when they are radiolucent, small or obscured by overlying gas, and bowel shadows sometimes falsely suggest the presence of a calculus. Ultrasound will reveal the presence of a true calculus by its acoustic shadow providing care is taken not to misinterpret shadows from overlying ribs or bowel. Real-time examination is particularly useful as the shadow of a calculus can be seen to move with the kidney rather than with surrounding structures.

Renal cystic disease

Solitary cysts are rare in children but many of the renal dysplasias are accompanied by cysts of variable size. Echography is superior to other methods because dysplastic kidneys may function poorly and give poor quality IVU and because some of the cysts may be relatively small and cause no calyceal distortion. In extreme cases the kidneys may be nonfunctioning and there will be no morphological information at all on an IVU.

Multicystic kidney (Fig. 102.18)

This is the commonest abnormality in this category and

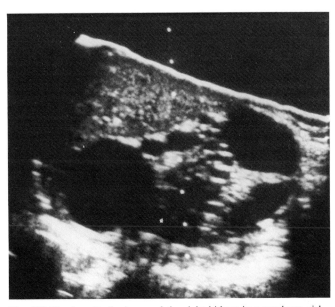

Fig. 102.18 Longitudinal scan of the right kidney in a newborn girl demonstrating a multicystic kidney.

usually presents as a unilateral mass in the neonate [29]. The mass consists of a collection of cysts which may be mistaken for hydronephrosis unless one looks carefully for two particularly valuable signs [30,31]. Firstly, in multicystic disease, the cysts are of various size so that in addition to the large lesions there may be small ones which could not possibly be a dilated calyx. Secondly, in transverse cuts the presence of the 'Mickey Mouse' sign suggests the diagnosis of hydronephrosis. In this sign the dilated calyces, (the ears) communicate with the dilated renal pelvis (the head) (Fig. 102.19). These appearances are not seen in the case of

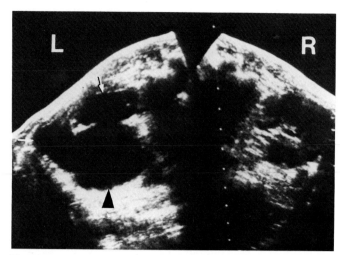

Fig. 102.19 Transverse prone scan showing a normal kidney on the right side but a hydronephrotic kidney on the left side. This shows a characteristic Mickey Mouse sign in which the calyces [small arrows] represent the ears and the renal pelvis [arrow head] represents the head.

multiple cysts in which no communication is found as the walls of the cysts are always between fluid areas in whichever plane the scan is performed [31]. The contralateral kidney must also be carefully studied in cases of multicystic kidney because of a 25% incidence of abnormalities, the most common being pelvi-ureteric junction obstruction (PUJO).

Infantile polycystic disease [32] (Fig. 102.20)

This is a bilateral condition, usually of recessive inheritance. The kidneys are always enlarged and highly echogenic with an obscured collecting system. Most of the cysts are microcysts below 1 mm diameter) and cannot be resolved but cause the marked increase in echogenicity. In

a fair proportion of cases, some cysts are above the 1 mm level and can be demonstrated. The degree of abnormality seen is not proportional to the severity of the prognosis. Adult type polycystic disease with obvious large cysts occurs in children but is relatively rare [13].

Microcystic conditions

See 'Bright ENG without CMD'.

Renal mass lesions

Palpable hydronephrosis and cystic abnormalities account for most of the renal mass lesions in childhood. The commonest solid lesion of the paediatric kidney however is *Wilms' tumour*; this is almost equal in incidence to *neuroblastoma* and these two conditions form the bulk of the solid tumours of childhood [29].

The characteristic appearance of Wilms' tumour is a large mass with a general echogenicity that is usually lower than that of the liver or spleen. The medial border is well defined (the lateral borders of both neuroblastoma and Wilms are virtually always well defined because they are pressed smooth against the abdominal wall). A variable size and number of echolucent lakes will be found within the mass [7,34] (Fig. 102.21).

In contrast, neuroblastoma is generally brighter than the liver and contains echogenic clusters, most of which correspond to calcium deposits which may not be appreciable on radiographs. The propensity of neuroblastoma to invade locally is demonstrated by the poorly defined medial edge. There is however, a significant proportion of tumours in which the diagnosis of either neuroblastoma or Wilms' tumour cannot be made simply from the ultrasonographic

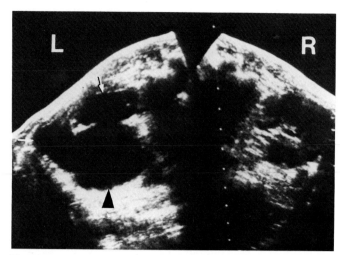

Fig. 102.20 Tranverse supine scan of a newborn abdomen showing 2 huge echogenic masses replacing the kidneys. Characteristic appearance of infantile polycystic disease.

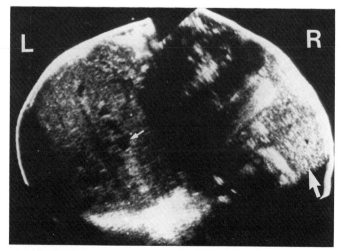

Fig. 102.21 Prone transverse scan of a child with Wilms' tumour. The mass can be seen on the left side. It is generally less echogenic than the liver on the right [large arrow]. There are many small characteristic echolucent lakes, one of which is indicated by an arrow.

appearances [7] and it must be remembered that an estimation of VMA in the 24 hour urine collection is mandatory in all such cases.

There are other conditions that enter the differential diagnosis; *mesoblastic nephroma* is a mass found in the newborn which is in the hinterland between malformation and malignancy and needs surgical removal. *Xanthogranulomatous pyelonephritis* is almost always mistaken for a tumour prior to surgical removal. *Renal abscesses* are usually fairly echolucent and homogeneous and present with malaise, fever and leucocytosis. The urine is often unremarkable and the mass is rarely larger than the kidney, unlike a Wilms' tumour.

Hydronephrosis and hydroureter

Hydronephrosis is an excessive volume of urine in the drainage system of the kidney in relation to the function of that kidney. Empirically, in children, dilatation of the calyceal fornix and dilatation of the ureter to a diameter greater than 3 mm is abnormal. The pelvis is suspicious if dilated beyond 10 mm but is so variable in its original size, its distensibility and the degree of hydration that measurement is unreliable. It follows that 'severity' cannot be judged on the echographic size of the collecting system. The thickness of the cortex that remains can give some clue but does not take the place of a functional study and here echography and scintigraphy go hand in hand providing the complete picture.

Documentation of hydronephrosis is not enough. It is essential to demonstrate whether or not the ureter is also dilated in order to establish the level of the abnormality [35]. The dilated ureter can be seen behind the filled bladder in transverse and longitudinal views (Fig. 102.22) but it is much

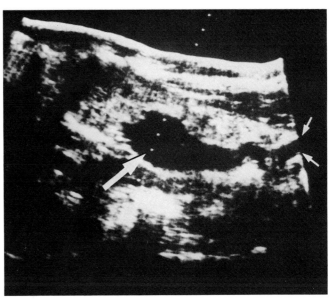

Fig. 102.23 Prone longitudinal oblique tilted view of the left kidney to show the dilated ureter [small arrow] leaving the dilated renal pelvis [large arrow].

more fruitful to seek the upper ureter in the prone position, remembering that the ureter runs a course along a line that transects the long axis of the kidney by some 45° medially. Also the probe must be tilted in order to 'see under' the transverse processes (Fig. 102.23).

Causes

Pelviureteric junction obstruction (PUJO) [36] The pelvicalyceal system is dilated but the ureter is normal. The condition is often intermittent and 10 to 15% will be bilateral but not necessarily at the same time. Therefore long term surveillance of the unaffected side will be necessary. Most cases are idiopathic but occasionally there is a tumour or granuloma at the PUJ which may be demonstrable by ultrasound.

Mid-ureteric obstruction In children this is often an extrinsic mass such as a retroperitoneal lymphoma, pelvic tumour metastases or a neuroblastoma. It is rare that these are not large enough to be demonstrable by ultrasound.

Vesicoureteric junction obstruction (VUJ) [28,35] This can either be VU reflux or VUJ obstruction from malformation, ectopic insertion, ureterocele or rarely calculus or tumour. It is not possible to establish the difference between obstruction and reflux without a classical micturating cystogram.

Outflow obstruction [28,35] This can be a physical obstruction, the commonest being posterior urethral valves (PUV) in males; functional, such as neurogenic bladder, or a mixture of the two as occurs in prune belly syndrome. Invariably hydronephrosis and hydroureter are bilateral and there are likely to be bladder abnormalities: either a thick-walled,

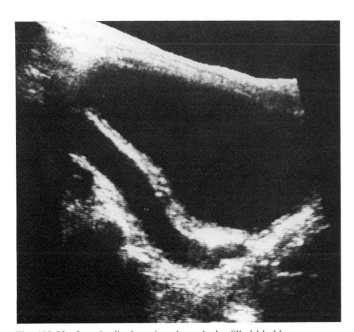

Fig. 102.22 Longitudinal section through the filled bladder demonstrating a dilated ureter behind the bladder terminating at the VUJ.

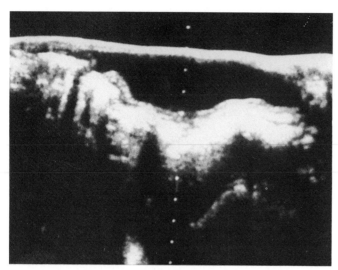

Fig. 102.24 A thin-walled elongated but extremely 'floppy' bladder seen in prune belly syndrome and occasionally in some children with neurogenic disabilities.

trabeculated bladder (sometimes with a visible dilatation of the posterior urethra) in PUV or neurogenic bladder, or a large flaccid bladder in the prune belly syndrome and some neurogenic conditions (Fig. 102.24).

Dysplasia and malformation The commonest example is prune belly syndrome. The entire urinary tract is affected with marked dilatation and tortuosity of the ureters, a floppy bladder, and less marked hyronephrosis of the kidneys, the cortex of which may show dysplastic changes such as brightening of the ENG and cysts.

Ultrasound is very sensitive in revealing such abnormalities in the paediatric urinary tract but do not forget that the child will still need scintigraphic studies to quantify function and establish whether urine is draining from an apparently large system because not all hydronephrosis is caused by obstruction.

BIBLIOGRAPHY

REFERENCES

1. Haller J O, Schneider M, Kassner E G et al 1980 Sonographic evaluation of the chest in infants and children. Am J Roentgenol 134:1019–1027
2. Moccia W A, Kaude J V, Felman A H 1981 Congenital eventration of the diaphragms: diagnosis by ultrasound. Pediatr Radiol 10:197–200
3. Madigan S M, Teele R L 1984 Ultrasonography of the liver and biliary tree in children. Seminars in Ultrasound, CT and MR Vol 5 No 1:68–84
4. Barth R A, Brasch R C, Filly R A 1981 Abdominal pseudotumor in childhood: Distended gallbladder with parenteral hyperalimentation. Am J Roentgenol 136:341–343
5. Kaude J V, Felman A H, Hawkins I F 1980 Ultrasonography in primary hepatic tumours in early childhood. Pediatr Radiol 9:77–83
6. Miller J H 1981 The ultrasonic appearance of cystic hepatoblastoma. Radiology 138:141–143
7. Gates G F, Miller J H 1977 Combined radio-nuclide and ultrasonic assessment of upper abdominal masses in children. Am J Roentgenol 128:773–780
8. Chusid M J 1978 Pyogenic hepatic abscess in infancy and childhood. Paediatrics 62:554–559
9. Abramson S J, Lack E E, Teele R L 1982 Benign vascular tumors of the liver in infants: sonographic appearances. Am J Roentgenol 138:629–632
10. Niron E A, Ozer H 1981 Ultrasound appearances of liver hydatid disease. Br J Radiol 54:335–338
11. Sarniak S, Slovis T L, Corbett D P et al 1980 Incidence of cholelithiasis in sickle cell anaemia using gray scale technique. J Pediatr 96:1005–1008
12. Gard L, Lallemand D, Montagni J P L et al 1981 The changing aspects of cholelithiasis in children through a sonographic study. Pediatr Radiol 11:75–79
13. Patriquin H B, DiPietro M, Barber F E, Teele R L 1983 Sonography of thickened gallbladder wall: Causes in children. Am J Roentgenol 141:57–60
14. Kangarloo H, Sarti D A, Sample W F et al 1980. Ultrasonographic spectrum of choledochal cysts in children. Pediatr Radiol 9:15–18
15. Abramson S J, Treves S, Teele R L 1982 The infant with possible biliary atresia: evaluation by ultrasound and nuclear medicine. Pediatr Radiol 12:1–5
16. Harkanyi Z, Vegh M, Hittner I, Popik E 1981 Gray scale echography of traumatic pancreatic cysts in children. Pediatr Radiol 11:81–82
17. McCain A H, Berkman W A, Bernardino M E 1984 Panceatic sonography, past and present. J Clin Ultrasound 12:325–332
18. Sassoon C, Domiller P, Cronfalt A M et al 1980 Ultrasonographic diagnosis of portal carcinoma in children: a study of twelve cases. Br J Radiol 53:1047–1–51
19. Grand M P, Remy J 1979 Ultrasound diagnosis of extrahepatic portal vein obstruction in childhood. Pediatr Radiol 8:155–159
20. Mittlestaedt C A, Partain C L 1980 Ultrasonic-pathologic classification of splenic abnormalities. Gray scane patterns. Radiology 134:697–705
21. Daneman A, Martin D J 1982 Congenital epithelial splenic cysts in children. Pediatr Radiol 12:119–125
22. Teele R L, Henschke C I, Tapper D 1980 The radiographic and ultrasonographic evaluation of enteric duplication cysts. Pediatr Radiol 10:9–14
23. Newman B, Teele R L 1984 Ascites in the fetus and neonate and young child: emphasis on ultrasonographic evaluation. Seminars in Ultrasound, CT and MR Vol 5 No 1:85–101
24. Fakhry J R, Berk R N 1981 The 'target' pattern: characteristic sonographic feature of stomach — bowel abnormalities. Am J Roentgenol 137:969–972
25. Mitty H A, Yeh H C 1982 Radiology of the adrenals with sonography and CT. Saunders, Philadelphia
26. Mittlestaedt C A, Volberg F M Jr, Merten D F 1979 Sonographic diagnosis of neonatal adrenal haemorrhage. Radiology 131:453–457
27. Pery M, Kaftori J K, Bar-Maor J A 1981 Sonography for diagnosis and follow up of neonatal adrenal haemorrhage. J Clin Ultrasound 9:397–401
28. Barth R A, Mindell H J 1984 Renal masses in the fetus and neonate: ultrasonographic diagnosis. Seminars in Ultrasound, CT and MR Vol 5, No 1:3–18
29. Griscom N T 1965 The Roentgenology of neonatal abdominal masses. Am J Roentgenol 93:447–463
30. Bearman S B, Hine P L, Sanders R C 1976 Multicystic kidney: a sonographic pattern. Radiology 118:685–688
31. Ralls P W, Esensten M L, Boger D et al 1980 Severe hydronephrosis and severe renal cystic disease: Ultrasonic differentiation. Am J Roentgenol 134:473–475
32. Boal D K, Teele R L 1980 Sonography of infantile polycystic kidney disease. Am J Roentgenol 135:575–580
33. Kaye C, Lewy P R 1974 Congenital appearance of adult type (autosomal dominant) polycystic kidney disease. J Pediatr 85:807–810
34. D'Angio G J, Beckwith J B, Breslow N E et al 1980 Wilms' tumour: an update. Cancer 45:1791–1798

35. Lebowitz R L, Griscom N T 1977 Neonatal hydronephrosis: 146 cases. Radiol Clin North Am 15:46–59
36. Alton D J 1977 Pelviureteric obstruction in childhood. Radiol Clin North Am 15:61–70

SUGGESTION FOR FURTHER READING

Canty T G, Leopold G R, Wolf D A 1982 Ultrasonography of Pediatric Surgical Disorders. Grune and Stratton, New York
Best English text available. Wider in its appreciation than the title suggests. Its practical flavour is particularly useful.
Haller J O, Shkolnik A, eds. Ultrasound in Pediatrics. Churchill Livingstone, Edinburgh
Chapters on chest, high resolution, real-time, antenatal diagnosis and the pelvis are particularly recommended.
Kalifa G (ed) 1983 Echographie pediatrique. Vigot, Paris
The best all round text available. Worth learning French for! English translation in preparation.
Mitty H A, Yeh H C 1982 Radiology of the adrenals with sonography and CT. Saunders, Philadelphia
Raymond H W, Zwiebel W J (eds) 1984 Seminars in Ultrasound, CT and MR Vol 5 No1

103 Ultrasonography of the infant brain

Keith Dewbury

Technique
Indications for ultrasound scanning
Normal appearances
Hydrocephalus and cystic lesions
Haemorrhage
Conclusion

Ultrasound examination of the brain in infants has become established over the past few years as an important new use for ultrasound, replacing computed axial tomographic scanning (CT) in many instances. In fact this is not a new area for ultrasound investigation. The brain was one of the first organs to be systematically examined by ultrasound using A-mode echoencephalography [1]. Initial attempts at two-dimensional B-scan imaging of the brain met with variable success as a result of poor resolution and failure to penetrate the thick adult calvarium [2]. Detailed cross-sectional images of the infant brain were first published by Kossoff et al in 1974 [3]. These studies were carried out using an automated water-path scanner, the Octoson. The importance of this imaging technique was not well appreciated, and until 1980 the most widely accepted method for evaluating intracranial abnormalities in infants was CT. Clearly this is an accurate method but not without significant disadvantages in the neonate and young infant.

In 1979 Pape et al [4] first reported the demonstration of haemorrhage by ultrasonography, in the pre-term infant. A linear array real-time scanner was used, applied to the side of the infant's head, so producing transverse slices similar in orientation to those produced by CT, with which it was compared. In 1980 Dewbury and Aluwihare [5] and Babcock et al [6] first reported using the anterior fontanelle as a bone free window through which to image the brain using B-mode static ultrasound. In the short time since these first descriptions of transfontanellar ultrasound, it has become a widely used technique now widely regarded as the primary imaging procedure for the neonatal and infant brain.

Technique

The ideal equipment for the examination of the infant brain is a high resolution sector real-time scanner, fitted with a 5 MHz transducer (or higher frequency). The scan head should ideally be as small and manoeuvrable as possible. The sector field of view is particularly well suited for showing the maximum area of information through a small acoustic window. This type of equipment is usually mobile and taken to the infant and the transducer applied to the head via a port-hole in the incubator. In this way the baby is almost undisturbed by the examination.

If this type of equipment is not available, it is possible and reasonable to examine the brain with either static equipment or linear array real time, provided that a suitable high frequency transducer is available (5 MHz). The quality of image that can be obtained with static scanners remains excellent, the disadvantage being that the infant has to be brought to the machine and removed from its incubator or cot for the examination. With very sick patients this may pose problems.

The linear array transducer has a long scan head and rectangular field of view. The shape and size of the scan head do not optimize the small acoustic window of the fontanelle, and the rectangular field of view is far from ideal to image a round structure such as the brain. These features are illustrated diagramatically in Figure 103.1.

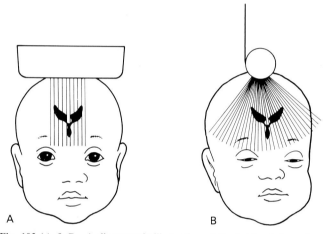

Fig. 103.1A & B A diagramatic illustration of the fields of view of a linear array scanner (A) and a sector scanner (B).

In each examination a series of closely spaced scans are made in both the coronal and sagittal planes, by altering the angulation of the transducer to the fontanelle; the aim being to include as much as possible fo the brain on each scan. More limited access may also be possible through the posterior fontanelle and through the sutures. Occasionally it may be of value to image directly through the skull vault.

The larger the fontanelle and therefore the freer the access, the better will be the images. As the fontanelle begins to decrease in size the access becomes more limited and the visualization of the brain less complete. Therefore ultrasound studies of the brain are most valuable in the first 6 months of life.

Indications for ultrasound scanning

The two most common abnormalities of the neonatal brain requiring confirmation or exclusion by imaging techniques are hydrocephalus and intracranial haemorrhage. These are the major indications for an ultrasound scan in the neonatal period. Ultrasound reliably and accurately demonstrates the size of the lateral ventricles and also sensitively detects the presence of intracerebral haemorrhage.

Hydrocephalus may result from congenital malformation. Haemorrhage into the ventricles or subarachnoid space may also cause hydrocephalus. It may develop following intra-uterine infection such as toxoplasmosis. The definitive surgical management of hydrocephalus is to perform a shunt procedure of some type. The position of the shunt and the early complications such as shunt failure may also be monitored by ultrasound.

The incidence of intracerebral haemorrhage is considerably increased in premature infants [7]. With the growth of high risk nurseries, allowing the survival of very premature infants, this complication is increasingly frequently seen and needs evaluation. The diagnosis of intracerebral and/or intraventricular haemorrhage may be made with ultrasound.

Normal appearances

Ultrasound is able to demonstrate the normal brain structure in considerable detail. The coronal sections are particularly valuable for showing focal abnormalities, as advantage may be taken of the brains symmetry. Recently, Cremin et al [8] have described a series of landmarks in both coronal and sagittal planes. These allow recognition of the position at which the scan has been taken and subsequently the acquisition of standard reproducible sections. These levels are illustrated diagramatically in Figure 103.2.

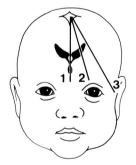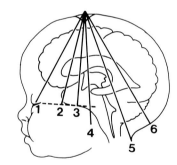

Fig. 103.2 A diagramatic representation of the positions of the six standard coronal sections and three sagittal sections.

Within the brain, structures containing cerebro-spinal fluid (CSF) such as the ventricles and cisterns appear anechoic, normal brain tissue generates low to mid-level echoes and higher level echoes are generated from the cerebellum, the sulci and vascular structures. It is likely that a great deal of the internal echo reflection in the brain is due to the collagen content of the pia ependyma and the vascular sheaths. One of the most echogenic intracerebral structures seen with ultrasound is the choroid plexus. This stretches around the floor of the lateral ventricles from the foramen of Monro into the temporal horns, enlarging at the level of the glomus in the trigone before sweeping down into the temporal horn. The bones of the vault also produce highly echogenic reflections and so may be useful as landmarks.

In the *first coronal plane* described by Cremin [8], the transducer is angled anteriorly in the fontanelle producing a section through the frontal lobes, which are seen separated centrally by the interhemispheric fissure and the falx. The lateral ventricles will not be seen in this section. The far field landmark is the high amplitude echoes from the orbital roofs and the central echoes from the ethmoid complex extending downwards to a lower level.

As the transducer is angled slightly back to the *second position* the far field landmark changes so that the lesser wings of the sphenoid with the greater wings of the sphenoid behind forming the anterior floor of the temporal fossa, are seen. The anterior horns of the lateral ventricles may be seen in this section as small slit like spaces on either side of the central midline echo.

Angling the transducer slightly further back so it is now almost vertical, produces the *third coronal section* where the most prominent landmark is the sylvian fissures. These are seen just behind the lesser wings of the sphenoid and run laterally and outward becoming Y-shaped between the temporal and frontal lobes. Within this echo complex, pulsation from branches of the middle cerebral artery will be readily seen. This section lies just anterior to the foramen of Monro, and between the lateral ventricles, the echo free box like structure of the cavum septum pellucidum may be seen (Fig. 103.3). This is present during fetal life where it is used as a landmark to optimize a biparietal diameter measurement of the fetus, and it is also present in about a half of all full term infants. It is seen more commonly in premature infants. Its incidence decreases sharply with age so that by 6 months its incidence compares with the 15 to 20% reported in adults [9]. The roof of the lateral ventricle is formed by the corpus callosum which is echogenic, and the floor by the head of the caudate nucleus with lower level echoes.

With the transducer angled vertically, the *fourth coronal plane* passes through the third ventricle which is not usually resolved in this plane when of normal size. A very prominent

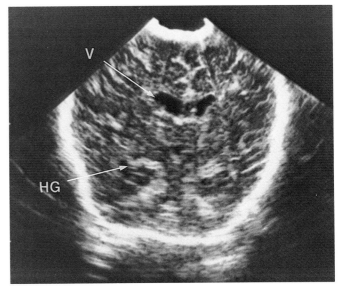

Fig. 103.4 A coronal section in the fourth positon showing the prominent landmark of the parahippocampal gyri ([HG]) [V = lateral ventricles].

far field landmark is formed by the paired C-shaped echoes from the parahippocampal gyri and medial surface of the temporal lobes (Fig. 103.4). Part of the Sylvian fissure will again be seen in this section. The bodies of the lateral ventricles now lie more horizontally and reflections from the choroid plexus may be seen in the floor of the ventricles.

Angling the transducer posteriorly on the fontanelle leads to the *fifth coronal section* where the prominent landmark is the highly echogenic tentorium and cerebellum shaped like an inverted V.

Slight further angulation will bring into view the echogenic divergent bands characteristic of the glomus of the choroid plexus. These are the landmarks for the *sixth section*. In the

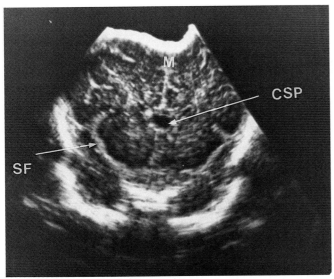

Fig. 103.3 A coronal section in the third position showing the Sylvian fissures [SF] and midline structures [M] lying between the lateral ventricles is the cavum septum pellucidum [CSP].

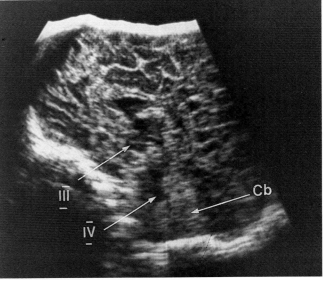

Fig. 103.5 A sagittal section in the midline showing 3rd and 4th ventricles [Cb = cerebellum].

normal infant the choroid plexus will always be seen in this section although the fluid filled ventricles will not always be separately distinguished around the choroid.

Rotating the transducer through 90° into the sagittal plane, the *first sagittal section* is taken in the midline. The sulcal detail is usually prominent and the cingulate sulcus, containing the branches of the anterior cerebral artery can be identified. The echogenic cerebellum is seen posteriorly, and anterior to this the fourth ventricle can be recognized. Above this the third ventricle and the massa intermedia are demonstrated and often the Aqueduct of Sylvius is outlined. The clivus forms the far field landmark (Fig. 103.5).

The *second parasagittal section* is angled about 15° away from the midline and shows almost the full sweep of the lateral ventricle containing the echogenic choroid plexus. Within the sweep of the ventricles, the rounded mass is formed by the thalamus and caudate nucleus (Fig. 103.6). The far field landmark is the floor of the middle fossa.

The *third parasagittal section* is angled outward about 30°, lateral to the ventricle and through the sylvian fissure.

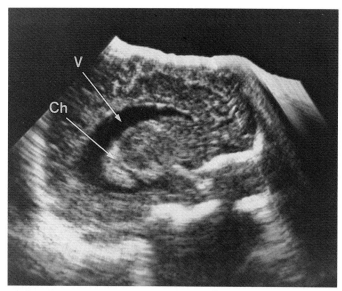

Fig. 103.6 An angled sagittal section showing the full sweep of one lateral ventricle [V] enclosing the thalamic nucleus. [Ch = choroid plexus].

Hydrocephalus and cystic lesions

The lateral ventricles in the normal neonate may be small and even difficult to accurately define. The mean width of the lateral ventricle in the full term infant is 12 mm and in the 30 week premature infant 9 mm [10], measured at the level of the body of the lateral ventricle (coronal section 3). In the past the measurement of the lateral ventricle has usually been expressed as a ratio of the skull vault. In axial CT scanning, deviation of the medial walls of the lateral ventricle is an early sign of dilatation but the normal ratio of 30% appears large when measured in the coronal plane and the ratio may not be valid in this circumstance.

The occipital poles of the lateral ventricles are generally the largest part of the entire ventricular system, however no convenient landmark exists to monitor accurately changes in size, and in any event there may be considerable variation in the shape of this structure. However, early dilatation is often most prominently featured in the trigone, occipital and temporal horns, possibly reflecting the lesser compliance of the supporting structures in this region.

Ultrasound has proved to be accurate and reliable in detecting and grading the severity of hydrocephalus and is ideally suited to following progress. Figure 103.7 is a coronal section at the level of the bodies of the lateral ventricles showing the appearances of established hydrocephalus. Further evaluation of hydrocephalus to establish a precise aetiology may require diagnostic procedures in addition to ultrasound. However, in certain instances ultrasound may provide most or all of the answers. In addition to the diagnosis and follow-up of hydrocephalus, ultrasound may also be helpful following shunt procedures particularly in the evaluation of complications.

Besides hydrocephalus, other cystic lesions within the brain may show a dramatic appearance. In hydranencephaly no brain parenchyma is present above the level of the mid brain and no cortical mantle is seen.

The *Dandy Walker syndrome* has a characteristic appearance where cystic dilatation of the fourth ventricle can be recognized (Fig. 103.8). This condition must however be distinguished from a retrocerebellar *arachnoid cyst* which may produce a similar appearance. In the latter instance however a normal fourth ventricle is identified compressed anteriorly by the cyst. The development of *porencephalic cysts* after periventricular haemorrhage has now been well documented with ultrasound (Fig. 103.9). A wide variety of other cystic lesions has also been described [11,12].

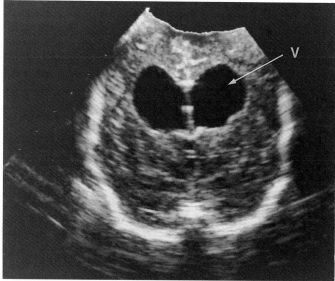

Fig. 103.7 A coronal section showing the typical appearance of hydrocephalus, with the lateral ventricles [V] measuring 22 mm.

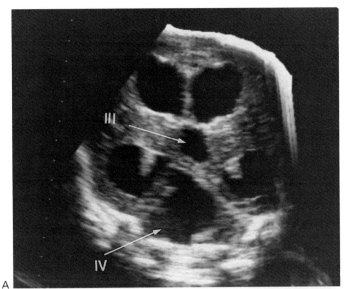

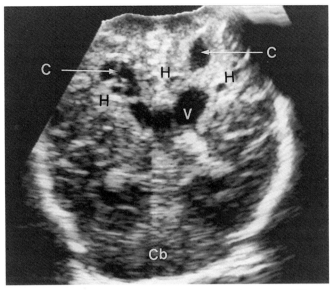

Fig. 103.9 In this coronal section cystic areas are developing [C] within an area of patchy high reflectivity around the ventricles. This represents haemorrhage [H], and shows the sequence of development of porencephalic cysts.

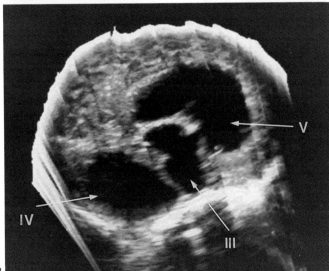

Fig. 103.8A & B Dandy Walker Syndrome. (A) A coronal section; (B) a sagittal section showing the characteristic findings. There is cystic dilatation of the 4th ventricle [IV]. The 3rd ventricle [III] and the lateral ventricles are also markedly dilated.

White matter haemorrhage occurs in both pre-term and full term infants. In the former it is associated with *periventricular leucomalacia*. This lesion is attributed to under perfusion of the boundary zones between different arterial territories within the periventricular white matter: it may develop during episodes of hypotension. Ultrasound may show a periventricular increase in echo amplitudes with follow up studies showing formation of cystic spaces [13]. In full term neonates, intraparenchymal haemorrhage may be diffuse and petechial in the cortical areas. The diagnosis of intracerebral, periventricular and intraventricular haemor-

Haemorrhage

The germinal matrix is a vascular tissue in the fetus which has normally involuted by term. It is situated subependymally in the ventricles and is prominent in the grove between caudate nucleus and thalamus. This is a frequent site for haemorrhage in premature infants (Fig. 103.10). The vascular choroid plexus is also an important site for cranial haemorrhage in infants.

The shape of the choroid plexus as it surrounds the caudate nucleus and thalamus is fairly constant so that any irregular increase in size is suspicious of haemorrhage. The symmetry of the two sides may also be of value in detecting abnormality.

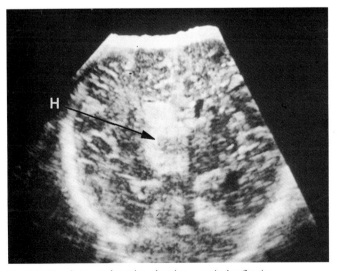

Fig. 103.10 A coronal section showing a typical reflective haemorrhage in a premature infant from the germinal matrix. A mass effect from the haemorrhage is distorting and elevating the lateral ventricle on this side.

rhages may be reliably made using ultrasound where the haemorrhage shows as a brightly reflective area. This is mainly due to the fibrin mesh formed which produces multiple reflecting interfaces for the ultrasound beam.

Subarachnoid haemorrhage is not reliably demonstrated using ultrasound. Subdural haemorrhage is usually shown as a crescentic echo poor region separating brain from skull vault [14]. Haemorrhage, particularly in premature infants may rupture into the lateral ventricles. This may enlarge the ventricles either due to brain tissue loss and atrophy, or to hydrocephalus due to CSF flow obstruction. The combination of both may occur and monitoring to show progress or stablization is important in these circumstances.

Conclusion

Over the past 3 to 4 years the technique of transfontanellar ultrasound of the infant brain has clearly emerged as a major new application for ultrasound. It has a high degree of accuracy and reproducibility in demonstrating and assessing hydrocephalus, cystic lesions of the brain and intracerebral haemorrhage. The correlation with CT is excellent. For the purpose described, ultrasound has to a large extent replaced the use of CT in the neonate, certainly as the primary imaging procedure. CT is able to image the entire brain and is undoubtedly more accurate than ultrasound in certain conditions, for example, delineation of brain turmours particularly in the posterior fossa and the demonstration of subarachnoid haemorrhages.

At present ultrasound reveals relatively little detail of the cerebral substance and is unable to detect ischaemic damage in the early stages. It may be that ischaemic cerebral damage following hypoxia provides the more significant permanent brain damage, and that haemorrhage is only an associated finding, possibly of less significance, although more prominent from the imaging view point. It is not yet known if the readily detectable sonographic haemorrhage parallels the ischaemic damage, thereby enabling some prediction of the likely clinical outcome.

It has therefore been suggested that it may still be appropriate to perform CT scans in such infants until this matter is resolved [15]. There can be little doubt that in the meantime, ultrasound will continue to play an important role.

BIBLIOGRAPHY

REFERENCES

1. Leksell L 1955 Echo encephalography. Acta Chi. Scand 110:301
2. Brinker R A, Taveras J N 1966 Ultrasound cross sectional pictures of the head. Acta Radiol (Diag) (Stockh) 5:745–753
3. Kossoff G, Garrett W J, Radovanovich G 1974 Ultrasonic atlas of normal brain of infant. Ultrasound Med Biol 1:259–266
4. Pape K E, Blackwell R J, Kusic G, Sherwood A et al 1979 Ultrasound detection of brain damage in pre-term infants. Lancet 1261–1264
5. Dewbury K C, Aluwihare A P R 1980 The anterior fontanelle as an ultrasound window for study of the brain. Br J Radiol 53:81–84
6. Babcock D S, Hann B K, Lequesne G W 1980 B mode grey scale ultrasound in the head of the newborn and the young infant. Am J Roentgenol 134:457–468
7. Burnstein J, Papille L, Burnstein R 1979 Intraventricular haemorrhage and hydrocephalus in premature newborns: a prospective study with CT. Am J Roentgenol 132:631–635
8. Cremin B J, Chilton S J, Peacock W J 1983 Anatomical landmarks in anterior fontanelle ultrasonography. Br J Radiol 56:517–526
9. Farrugia S, Babcock D 1981 The cavum septum pellucidum: its appearance and incidence with cranial ultrasonography in infancy. Radiology 139:147–150
10. Levene M I 1981 Measurement of the growth of the lateral ventricles in pre-term infants with a real time ultrasound. Arch Dis Child 56:900–904
11. Mack L A, Rumack C M, Johnson M L 1980 Ultrasound evaluation of cystic intracranial lesions in the neonate. Radiology 137:451–455
12. Chilton S J, Cremin B J 1983 Ultrasound diagnosis of CSF cystic lesions in the neonatal brain. Br J Radiol 56:613–620
13. Levene M I, Wigglesworth J S, Dubowitz V 1983 Haemorrhagic periventricular leucomalacia in the neonate: a real time study. Paediatrics 71:794–797
14. Dewbury K C, Bates R I 1983 Neonatal intracranial haemorrhage: the cause of the ultrasound appearances. Br J Radiol 56:783–789
15. Harwood-Nash D C, Floodmark O 1982 Diagnostic imaging of the neonatal brain: review and protocol. Am J Neuro radiol 3:103–115

Index

Index

The principal reference for a subject is indicated by bold type; references to figures are in italic type

Abdomen, abdominal
  aneurysms, 2010, *2011*
  biopsy, percutaneous, **2124–2126**
    CT-guided, 2125
    fine needle aspiration, 2124, 2126
    needles, 21
  compression, investigative, 1046
  CT scan, *42, 48, 49*
  magnetic resonance imaging, *9, 83*
  maternal, radiography, **1589**
    risks of exposure, 1589
  plain radiography, **719–742**, 1045
    abscess, intra-abdominal, 736–738
    gynaecology, 1593–1594
      abnormal appearances, 1593
    inflammatory conditions, 734–736
    kidney injuries, 1171
    mesoblastic nephroma, 1102
    in neuroblastoma, 1206
    normal appearances, 720
    paediatric, 1180
    renal masses, 1089–1090
    renal parenchyma, normal, 1116
    technique, 719
  postoperative, 734
  tumours, magnetic resonance imaging, *9*
Abortion
  criminal, 1622
  recurrent, hysterosalpingography, 1595
  sonography, 1557, *1558*
    incomplete, 1557
    missed, 1557
  surgical, 1622
Abscess
  alveolar, 1932
  appendix, 1083
  brain, 1739–1740
  Brodie's, of bone, 1353
  definition, 367
  drainage, CT-guided, 53
  fungal, magnetic resonance imaging, 76, *77*
  intra-abdominal, 736–738
  intrahepatic, 980
  liver, **948**
    CT scanning, 938
    scintigraphy, 934
    ultrasound, 930, *931*
  lung, 205
    differentiation from bronchopleural fistula, 164 (*table*)
    primary, 202, *203*
    pyaemic, 289
  mediastinum, *194*

pancreatic, 735, *736*
paracolic, 737, *738*
pericolic, 878
renal, 1099
  in transplantation, 1147 (*table*)
spleen, 1015
subphrenic, 736, *737*
Absorption, ultrasound, 26
Acanthosis nigricans, oesophageal involvement, 769
Accordion artery, 2017
Acetabulum
  accessory centres, and trauma, 1464
  fractures, **1244–1245**
    central, 1245
    classification, 1245
    CT scan, 1245
    single column, 1245, *1525*
    two column, 1245
  roofs, irregularity, 1452, *1454*
Achalasia
Achilles tendon injuries, 1268, 1269
Achondrogenesis, **1423–1424**
Achondroplasia, 1416, **1417–1418**, *1420, 1421*
  affecting facial bones, 1915
  differential diagnosis, 1418, *1420, 1421*
  maternal, 1418
  neonatal, *1418*
  and tooth eruption, 1930
Acinus, 119, 367
Acoustic impedance, 26
Acoustic neuroma, **1733–1734**
  air meatography, 1702
  angiography, 1733–1734
  CT, 1702, 1733
  diagnosis, 1962
  8th cranial nerve, 1962
  magnetic resonance imaging, 69, *73*
  petrous bone, 1961
  pneumoencephalography, 1733
Acquired immunodeficiency syndrome (AIDS), lung disease, 287
Acromegaly, 1020, **1389–1392**
  eosinophil tumour, *1021*
  facial bones, 1916
  hand findings, *1391*
  heart involvement, 640
  heel pad thickness, *1391*
  radiological diagnosis, 1389
    pathological considerations, 1389–1392
  skull findings, *1390*
  soft tissue thickness measurement, 1509
  spinal changes, *1390*

Acromioclavicular
  joints, rheumatoid arthritis, *1478*, 1479
  separation, **1251–1252**
    types of injury, 1251–1252
Acromium process, fractures, 1250
Acro-osteolysis, 1443
Acropachy, 1025, **1408–1409**
Actinomycosis, 216
  affecting bone, 1363
  cholecystitis, 976
  mandible, 1914
  small bowel, 847
Acute tubular necrosis
  or acute rejection in renal transplantation, 1145–1146
  diagnosis, 1141
  features, 1119
  urography, 1119
Adamantinoma of long bones, 1324–1325
Addison's disease, 1033
  delayed skeletal maturation, 1396
  heart involvement, 640
Adenocarcinoma
  Fallopian tubes, 1619
  maxillofacial region, 1910
  oropharynx, 1970
  renal *see* Renal cell carcinoma
  submandibular gland, 1921
Adenoids, 1967
Adenoma
  gallbladder, 977
  liver, ultrasound, children, 2216
  parathyroid, detection, 1026
  provoking factors, 1040
  renal, 1102
  sebaceum, 1779
  villous, gastric, 799
  visualization methods, 1039
Adenomeloblastoma, maxillo-facial, 1908
Adenomyomatosis (cholecystosis), 977
Adenomyosis, 1617
Adenosis, benign, breast, 1633
  microcalcifications, 1633
  sclerosing, 1633, 1639
Adhesions
  intrauterine, 1617–1618
  pleural, 158
Adrenal glands, **1033–1036**
  arteriography, 2053, *2054*
  carcinoma, 1035, *1036*
  CT scan, target, *42*
  haemorrhage, neonatal, children, 2221
  investigation methods, 1035

Adrenal glands (*cont.*)
  magnetic resonance imaging, 84, *85*
  tumours, investigative methods, 1035
  ultrasound, children, 2220–2222
    adenomas, 2221–2222
    haemorrhage, 2221
    neuroblastoma, 2221
  venography, 2094
    contraindication, 2094
  venous obliteration, 2156–2158, *2159*
Adrenogenital syndrome, children, **1464**
Aggressive fibromatosis, 1292
Agnogenic myeloid metaplasia, **1333**
AIDS (acquired immunodeficiency syndrome),
    lung disease, 287
Ainhum affecting bone, **1364**
Air
  in bile ducts, 960
  bronchogram, 144
  definition, 367
  embolism complicating venography, 2064
  extrapulmonary, post-operative, 320
  leak, pulmonary, in infants, 351–355
  meatography, CT, in acoustic neuroma,
    1702–1703
  myelography in syringomelia, 1829
Airspace, definition, 367
Airway(s)
  definition, 367
  in primary tuberculosis, 207
  large airway obstruction, 221–232
  obstruction, in infants and young children,
    340–344
Albers-Schönberg disease, **1427**, *1428*
  see also Osteopetrosis
Albright's syndrome, 1438
Albumen
  macroaggregated, contraindications, 23
  99mTc human serum, 423
Alcoholic heart disease, 640
Alcoholism, 1745
Aldosteronism, primary and embolization,
    2158, *2159*
Algorithms
  evaluation, renal masses, 1091
    employing CT, 1096
    non-cystic renal masses, *1093*
    pseudotumour, renal, 1091, *1093*
  radiologic valuation in kidney injuries, 1172
Alkaptonuria, 1496
Alpha-chain disease, 845
Alpha decay, 14
Alphafetoprotein, amniotic fluid elevation,
    causes, 1569
Altitude, pulmonary oedema, 265
Alveolar
  abscess, 1932
  fractures, 1934
  pore, definition, 367
Alveolarization, definition, 367
Alveolitis, extrinsic allergic, 267, *268*
  fibrosing, 272–274
    distinction from asbestosis, 270
Ameloblastic fibroma, maxillo-facial, 1908
Ameloblastoma (adamantinoma), maxillo-
    facial, 1908
Amelogenesis imperfecta, 1927
Amenorrhoea, 1036
Amniocentesis
  placental localization prior to, 1563–1564
  second trimester, fetal anomalies detected,
    1569
Amniography, **1580–1583**

indications, 1580–1581
  atresia upper alimentary tract, 1581
  gastroschisis, 1581
  iniencephaly, 1581
  monoamniotic twins, 1581
  neural tube defects, 1580
  prune belly, 1581
technique, 1581
  radiation exposure, 1582
  radiographic exposure, 1582–1583
  risks, 1581
  with ultrasound, 1583
    and amniotic fluid analysis, 1583
Amniotic fluid
  analysis with sonography and amniotic fluid
    analysis, 1583
  aspiration, 347, *348*
Amoebiasis
  biliary, 986
  colitis, 890
  pulmonary, 217
Amu, definition, 14
Amyloid disease
  heart, 639
  lung, 275
Amyloidosis
  infiltrating kidneys, 1121
  oesophagus, 776
  orbital involvement, 1889
  small bowel, 855
  stomach, 797
Anaemias, **1327–1334**
  chronic haemolytic, **1328–1332**
  Fanconi's, **1333**
  heart involvement, 641
  iron deficiency, **1332**
  polycythaemia, **1333**
Anaesthesia in arteriography, 1992–1993
Anal fistulae in Crohn's disease, *887*
Analgesic nephropathy, papillary necrosis,
    1121, 1122
Anaplastic sarcoma, 1324
Anasarca, fetal, sonography, 1577
Androgens
  deficiency, 1038
Android pelvis, 1587
Anencephaly, fetal detection, sonography,
    1569, 1570, 1575
Aneurysm
  aortic, 308, **705–708**
    abdominal, digital subtraction
      angiography, 2105
    leaking, 740
    causes, 705 (*table*)
    distribution, 708 (*table*)
    false, 705
    mycotic, 712–713
    plain radiography, 604
    radiology, 706–708
    signs and symptoms, 706
    sinus of Valsalva, 713
    thoracic, 179–181, *182, 183, 184*, **705–712**
      digital subtraction angiography, 2105
    traumatic, 713–714
  arteriography, 941, **1749–1751, 2009–2014**
    abdominal, 2010
    cirsoid, 2014
    congenital, 2009
    curvilineal calcification, 2010
    degenerative, 2010
    dissecting, 2010–2012
    ectasia, 2009
    false, 2009

  infective, 2009–2010
  post-inflammatory, 2013–2014
  post-stenotic, 2012–2013
  syphilitic, 2009
  traumatic, 2012
  true, 2009
cardiac, dilatation of left atrium, 555
  false, 650
  left ventricular, 627–628
    CT scanning, 444
    echocardiography, 629
    of myocardial infarction, 627–628
    magnetic resonance imaging, 87, *88*
cerebral, magnetic resonance imaging, 74, *75*
coronary artery, 613
embolization, 2150
hepatic artery, arteriography, 941
intracranial, 1746–1749
  angiography, 1749–1751
  CT, 1746–1748
intra-orbital, 1890
pseudoaneurysm, left ventricular, 629
pulmonary artery, 580–582
renal, 1100
  CT, 1100
renal artery, arteriography, 2035
subclavian artery, 699, *700*
Aneurysmal bone cyst, **1287–1288**
  juvenile, 1458
Angel-Shiley valve, 664
Angina pectoris, 620
Angiocardiography, **382**
  aortic valve disease, 605
  aortic valve stenosis, 697
    fixed, 698
  atrial septal defect, 484–486
  CO2, in pericardial effusion, 682
  congenital diseases, 470–473
  constrictive pericarditis, 687
  contrast media, adverse reactions, 107
    limitations, 429
  dextrocardia, 543, 545
  Ebstein's anomaly, 530
  mitral valve disease, 594–596
  nuclear, children, 2208–2209
  patent ductus arteriosus, 493
  pericardial effusion, 682
  persistent truncus arteriosus, 515, *516*
  pulmonary infundibular stenosis, 532, *533*
  pulmonary valve stenosis, 531
  right ventricular, enlargement, *559*
    pulmonary artery absence, congenital, 534
  sequential chamber identification and
    analysis, 473–475
  tetralogy of Fallot, 500
  tricuspid atresia, 499
  tricuspid valve disease, 598
  tumours, heart, 650
  ventricular septal defect, 489
  ventriculoarterial discordance, 520, 523
Angiodysplasia, arteriography, 2042
Angiofibroma, juvenile, 1967–1968
  angiography, 1968
  arteriography, 2030
  CT, 1968
  radiography, 1968
Angiography
  acoustic neuroma, 1733–1734
  angiofibroma, juvenile, 1968
  aorta, 605
  biliary tract, 973–974
  with catheterization, liver, pre-embolization,
    995

Angiography (*cont.*)
cerebral haemorrhage, 1755–1756
cerebral ischaemic disease, 1759–1762
chordoma, 1736
choriocarcinomas, 1609
coronary, contrast media, 109
digital *see* Digital
duodenum, 817
encephalitides, 1743
endocrine disease, 1020
endometrial carcinoma, 1609
extracerebral haemorrhage, 1786
fibroids, 1606
glomus jugulare tumours, 1960
hilar tumours, 979–980
intracranial arteriovenous infections, 1752–1755
kidney, transplanted, 1144–1145
liver, *958*
meningioma, 1731–1732
neurofibromatosis, 1778
orbit, 1877–1880
ovarian cysts, 1610
pancreas, 1001
parathyroid, 1027
pulmonary, 135, 300
cor triatum, 538
pulmonary artery sling, 534
renal cell carcinoma, 1103
renal, in arteriovenous fistula, 1158
in kidney injuries, 1172
masses, 1099
paediatric, 1182
in renal artery aneurysm, 1158
in renal artery stenosis, 1152, 1154
in renal infarction, 1156
in small renal vessel disease, 1156
selective, in renal vein thrombosis, 1161
transplantation, 1141
small bowel, 836
spine, **1811–1813**
arteriography, 1811–1812
see also Arteriography, spine
contraindications, 1811
cord compression, 1841–1843
phlebography, 1812–1813
trauma, 1850
vascular lesions, **1852–1853**
spleen, 1011
Sturge-Weber disease, 1778
subarachnoid haemorrhage, 1749–1751
subdural empyema, 1741
thoracic systemic arteries, 135
in urinary obstruction, 1078
urinary tract, 1048
see also Arteriography:
Angiocardiography: Venography
Angioma
bone, **1293**
capillary, orbital, 1890
cerebral, radionuclide scanning, 1866
choroidal, 1896
intracranial, 1751–1755
magnetic resonance imaging, 74, *75*
nasal cavity, 1946
plexiform, arteriography, 2006–2008
spinal, **1852–1854**
Angiomatosis, cystic, **1293–1294**
Angiomyolipomas, renal, 1100–1101
arteriography, 2034
Angioplasty
percutaneous transluminal *see* Percutaneous
transluminal angioplasty

renal artery in renovascular hypertension, 1155
Angiosarcoma, **1324**
Aniridia, 1880
Anisakiasis, 848
Ankle, joint injuries, **1264–1266**
eversion, 1264–1265
fifth metatarsal base, 1266, *1267*, 1271
inversion, 1264–1265
posterior tibial lip fracture, 1266
rheumatoid arthritis, **1479**, *1480*
trimalleolar fracture dislocations, 1266
Ankylosing spondylitis, **1486–1488**, 1490
associated with sialectasis, 1920
complications, 1487–1488
differential diagnosis, 1488
enthesitis, 1486
large and small joints, 1487
lungs, 283
radionuclide bone scanning, 1543
sacroiliac joints, 1486
spine, 1486
Ann Arbor staging classification of
lymphomas, 2177
Annuloaortic ectasia, 705, *706*
Anodontia, 1929
complete, 1929
partial, 1929
Anophthalmia, 1880
Anorectal atresia, ultrasound, children, 2220
Antacids, cause of calculus disease, 1059
Antegrade pressure studies *see* Whitaker test
Anterior commissure, tumours, 1977
Anterior segment, lesions, 1894
Anthropoid pelvis, 1587
Antibiotics, associated colitis, 890
Anticoagulant therapy and arteriography, 1992
Anticonvulsant drugs and osteomalacia, 1378
Antigon, 1621
Antrochoanal polyps, 1946
Anus
atresia, neonatal, 910–912
imperforate, neonatal, 910–912
Aorta, 473, **691–715**
abdominal, digital subtraction angiography,
2108
anatomy, 691
aneurysm *see* Aneurysm, aortic
angiography, 605
annuloaortic ectasia, 705, *706*
arch, 691
cervical, 695, *697*
congenital anomalies, 693–703
double, 695, *697*
interrupted, 494, 703
right, 694–695
arteritis syndromes, 704–714
ascending, 691
atresia, 703
bicuspid valve, 698
branch disease, aortography, 2031
bulb, 691
coarctation, 699–702
pseudo-, 702, *703*
congenital conditions, 469
arteriography, 2003–2004
CT scanning, 446
cusp disease, 600–603
descending, 692
displacement, in heart enlargement, 555
disease, echocardiography, 416
dissection, 708–712
classification, 708

clinical findings, 709
CT scanning, 445
DeBakey classification, *708*
digital subtraction angiography, 2105
magnetic resonance imaging, 448
prognosis, 711
radiology, 709–711
hypoplastic, 540, 703
incompetence, 600–602
isthmus, 692
knob, definition, 367
normal, 691–693
occlusion, 2018, *2019*
pseudocoarctation, 702, *703*
pulmonary medastinal stripe, 127
puncture, translumbar *see* Translumbar
aortography
regurgitation, left ventricular enlargement,
558
rupture, 308, 713–714
sinus fistula, 495
stenosis, **598–600**
calcific, 598–599
congenital, *556*
differentiation from hypertrophic
cardiomyopathy, 642
fixed, 698
rheumatic, 599–600
supravalvar, 698
transluminal angioplasty, 2143
valvular, congenital, 695, 697
tetralogy of Fallot, 501
thoracic, CT scanning, 445
displacement of oesophagus, 779
ultrasound, children, 2220
valve, atresia, 538
disease, **598–603**
pulmonary vascularity, 573
wall, disease, 603–607
Aortitis
arteriography, 2031
arthritis, 713
giant cell, 705
plain radiography, 604
syphilitic, 705
Aortoduodenal fistula, 825
arteriography, 2037
Aortography, 445
arch, 2027
contrast media, 109
dissection, 709–711
renal paediatric, 1182
rupture, 714
thoracic, 701, **2030**
translumbar *see* Translumbar aortography
Aortopulmonary
shunt, 492–495
window, 367, 495
Apatite depositions, clacification, 1517, *1518*,
1519
Apert's syndrome, 1881
Apical dental cyst, 1932
Apophyseal joint osteoarthritis, 1501
Appendicitis
acute, 734, *735*, 894
causing pelvic inflammatory disease, 1603
Appendicular skeleton, trauma, **1246–1271**
see also specific bones
Appendix, 894
abscess, causing obstruction, 1083
Apudoma, 1032
arteriography, **2053–2054**
magnetic resonance image, *9*

Aqueduct stenosis, *1707*, **1793**
Aqueduct of Sylvius, in
 pneumoencephalography, 1699
Arachnodactyly (Marfan's syndrome), **1424**
Arachnoid cyst, 1772, **1773–1774**, 1825, *1826*
 ultrasound, neonate, 2232
Arachnoiditis
 complication of myelography, 1806
 post-traumatic, 1851
Arcuate uterus, 1600
Arm
 arteriography, 2046–2047, *2048*
 venography, 2086–2087
Armillifer armillatus infection, calcification,
 1516
Arnold-Chiari malformation, 1825–1826
Arrhythmias, complicating venography, 2063
Arteriography, **1989–2058**
 aftercare, 1996–1997
 anaesthesia, 1992–1993
 aneurysms, 2009–2014
 arterial puncture, 1993
 arteriotomy, 1996
 arteritis, 2015–2017
 atheroma, 2014–2015
 biliary tract, 973–974
 bronchial, 2030
 cardiovascular system, contrast media, 108
 catheters, 2000–2001
 catheterization, 1993–1996
 cerebral *see* Cerebral arteriography
 cine radiography, 1991
 complications, 1999–2002
 contraindications, 1992
 contrast media, 1991–1992
 coronary, myocardial infarction, 622
 digital subtraction *see* Digital subtraction
  angiography
 dilators, 1991
 embolism, 2019–2020
 endocrine organs, 2053
 gastrointestinal, **2037–2045**
 in gynaecological conditions, 1598
 haemangiomas, 1102
 haemorrhage, 2021
 hand and neck, 2027–2030
 hilar tumours, 981–982
 intravascular contrast media, adverse
  reactions, 107
 ischaemia, 2020
 liver, 939–941
 lower extremity, **2048–2053**
 lumbar, 2031–2032
 magnification, 1998
 methods, **1992–1998**
 orbit, 1877, *1879*, 1880
 patient preparation, 1992
 pelvic, 2032–2033
 pharmacoangiography, 1997–1998
 pyelonephritis, 1120
 radiographic considerations, 1997
 regional, 2026–2057
 renal, **2033–2037**
  contrast media, 108
  masses, 1094
 sheaths, 1991
 spine, 1811–1812
  anatomy, 1811–1812
  contraindications, 1811
  indications, 1811
  procedure, 1811
 stenosis, 2017–2018
 subtraction technique, 1997

 see also Digital subtraction angiography
 Takayasu's arteritis, 704
 thoracic, 2030
 thrombosis, 2018–2019
 transitional cell carcinoma, 1105
 trauma, 2025
 tumours, **2021–2025**
  see also Tumours, arteriography : and
   specific names
 upper extremity, 2046–2048
 uterine arteriovenous malformations, 1619
 vascular disorders, 2002–2056
  congenital abnormalities, 2003–2006
  malformations, 2006–2008
 vasoconstrictor agents, 1998
 vasodilator agents, 1998
 videorecorder, 1992
Arterioportography, 941, 974, **2082–2084**
 indications, 2082–2084
 techniques, 2082
Arteriotomy, 1996
Arteriovenous fistula, 367, 579
 arteriography, 2008, *2009*
 complicating hysterectomy, 1623
 complicating renal trauma, 1177
 complicating venography, 2063
 cranial, traumatic, **1789**
 intrarenal, 1158–1159
  causes, 1158
  radiology, 1158
 lung, congenital, 361, *362*, 363
 orbital, 1890
 pharyngeal-internal jugular, embolization,
  2150, *2153*
Arteriovenous malformation, *147*
 arteriography, 2006, 2030, 2035
 cerebral radionuclide scanning, 1866
 embolization, arterial, 2150, *2154*
  venous, 2158
 hand arteriography, 2047
 intracranial, **1751–1755**
  angiography, 1752–1755
  CT, 1752
 pulmonary system, 524
 renal, 1100
Arteriovenous shunts
 arteriography, 2053
 embolization, 2150, *2160*
Arteritis
 arteriography, **2013–2014, 2015–2017**
  giant cell, 2106
  infective, 2016
  necrotizing, 2016
  Takayashu's syndrome, 579, **704**, 705, **2016**
  thrombangiitis obliterans, 2017
  young female, 2016
 intracranial, **1765–1766**
 pulmonary, 579
 Takayasu's, 579, 704, *705*
Artery (arteries)
 calcification, 1514
 infusion chemotherapy, liver, 941, *942, 943*
 stenosis, 2017
 see also specific arteries under Pulmonary
  system
Arthritis
 aortitis, 713
 candida (septic) in the neonate, **1352–1353**
 gonococcal, 1356
 infective, 1356
 pyogenic (septic), children, **1452–1455**
 radionuclide bone scanning, **1542–1543**
 rheumatoid *see* Rheumatoid arthritis

 rubella, 1366
 tuberculous, **1358–1359**
  children, **1455**
Arthrography, **1505–1506**
 hip, 1506
 knee, 1505–1506
 shoulder, 1506
 temporomandibular joint, 1506
Arthropathies
 crystal deposition, **1491–1496**
 enteropathic, **1488**
 neuropathic, **1498–1499**
 psoriatic, 1488–1490
  see also Psoriatic arthropathy
 pyogenic, 1504–1505
Arthus type II reaction, 267
Artificial insemination, hysterosalpinography
 before, 1595
Ary-epiglottic tumours, 1977, *1978*
Asbestosis, 269–272
 differential diagnosis from fibrosing
  alveolitis, 270
Ascariasis, biliary tract, 985
Ascending
 lumbar venography, 2074–2075
  anatomy, 2074
  indications, 2075
  technique, 2075–2076
 urethrogram, 1047
 urethrogram combined with micturating
  cysto-urethrogram, 1049
Ascites
 maternal, *1578*, 1580
 and ovarian carcinoma, radiography, 1594
Aseptic necrosis, children, bone imaging, 2200
Aspergillosis, 216
 bronchopulmonary, 233
  allergic, 217, 267
   eosinophilia, 285
 invasive, 216
Asphyxia syndrome, in the newborn, 347
Asphyxiating thoracic dystrophy, **1422**
Aspiration
 pneumonitis, following laparotomy, 315, *316*
 syndrome, perinatal, 347
Asthma, 233–234
 differentiation from emphysema, 236
 occupational, 267
 radiographic abnormalities, 234 (*table*)
 simulating conditions, 234
Astrocytoma, *55, 68*
 CT, 1709
  cerebellar, 1711, *1712*
 cystic, radionuclide imaging, 1861
 intramedullary, *1847, 1848*
Atelectasis *see* Lungs, collapse
Atheroma
 arteriography, 2014–2015
 coronary artery, 613
 renal, causing hypertension, 1151
  renal angiography, 1156
 see also Atheromatous : Atherosclerosis
Atheromatous
 aneurysms, arteriography, 2010
 disease, arteriography, 2018
 ulcers, cerebral, 1760
Atherosclerosis
 arteriography, 2014–2015
 carotid artery, digital fluorogram, *7*
 lumbar aortography, 2031
 magnetic resonance imaging, 448
 premature, arteriography, 2003
 see also Atheroma

Atlantoaxial rotary displacement *see* Torticollis
Atom, structure, 13
Atresia
    anal, neonatal, 910–912
    biliary, in infants, 985
        neonatal, 945
    bronchial, 358
    duodenal, fetal, 905
    oesophageal, infants, 906–908, *909*
    posterior choanal, in infancy, 340
    pulmonary artery, 494
    pyloric, infants, 908
    small bowel, infants, 909–910
    tracheal, congenital, 357
    tricuspid, 497–499
    ureteric, 1083
Atrial septal defect, 478–486
    see also Heart, atrial septal defect
Atrophy *see* specific headings
Attenuation, ultrasound, 26
Auger electrons, 14
Autoimmune disease, hypoadrenalism, 1033
Avascular necrosis, radionuclide bone
        scanning, **1543–1545**
Aviator's astragalus, 1268
Avulsion
    elbow, in children, 1461
    fracture, triquetral, 1259
    injuries, pelvis, 1243, *1244*
    medial epicondylar apophysis, 1253
    tibia, in children, 1462
Axial loading fractures
    cervical, 1228–1229
    thoracolumbar, 1237
Axillary skin folds, 128
Azygo-oesophageal recess line, 127
Azygos
    lobe fissure, 114
    vein, 368, 391
    venography, 2074–2075
        anatomy, 2074
        causes of vein enlargement, 2075
        indications, 2075
        techniques, 2074–2075

Back pain, **1830–1854**
    acute, and chronic, presentation, 1817, 1818
    CT scanning, *56*
Back pressure atrophy, 1069, 1126
    differential diagnosis, 1128 (*table*)
Bacterial infection and calcification, 1515
Baker's cyst, 1506
Barium examination
    biliary tract, 973
    complete reflux, 834
    duodenum, 816, 821
    enema, **862–866**
        cervical carcinoma, 1608
        colonoscopy, 900–902
        ovarian cysts, 1610
    filled radiography, 786
    follow-through, 834
    gastrointestinal bleeding, 2041
    infusion (enteroclysis, small bowel enema),
        834–835, *836*
    large bowel, 862–866
    liver, 928–930
    oesophagography, 132, 342
    per oral pneumocolon, 834
    small bowel, 834–835
        intubation, 835
        obstruction, 850
    stomach, 784–787

thyroid, 1024
    versus endoscopy, 829
Barrett's oesophagus, 753, *754*, **755**, 762
Barton fracture, wrist, 1257
Barytosis, 272
Basal
    cell naevi syndrome, 1915
    ganglia, calcification, 1791, *1792*
    ganglia disease, magnetic resonance
        imaging, 77
Baseball (mallet) fractures, 1261
Basilar invagination, 1776
Basophil tumours, pituitary, 1722
Battered child *see* Child abuse
Bead phenomenon, 2017
Beall valve, 664, 666, 668, *669*, *670*, *672*
Becquerel (Bq), definition, 16
Bedside radiography, 313
'Beer drinker's syndrome', 1075
Behçet's disease, 284, 889
    arteriography, 2017
        aneurysms, 2014
    oesophagitis, 758, 759
    small bowel, 855
Belsey transthoracic procedure, 780
Bending injuries, thoracolumbar spine, 1237
Benign prostatic hypertrophy, causing
        obstruction, 1085
Bennett fracture dislocation, 1260
Benzoic acid molecule, *100*
Beri beri, heart involvement, 640
Berylliosis, 272
Beta decay, 15
Beta-blocking drugs, heart myopathy, 640
Bicornuate uterus, 1599
Bilateral interfacetal dislocation, 1225–1226
    radiographic features, 1225–1226
Bile ducts, **978–986**
    abscess, 980
    anatomy, 956
    atresia, in infants, 985
    Caroli's disease, 985
    endoscopy, 1007
    exploration during cholecystectomy,
        indications, 966
    infection, 980
    perforation, spontaneous, in infants, 985
    trisegmentectomy, 980
    tumours, **979–982**
        angiographic assessment, 979–980
        arteriography, 981–982
        extension of neoplasm, 980
        ultrasound, 968–970
Bile leaks, scintigraphy, 972
Bile reflux, 972
Bilharzia (urinary schistosomiasis), 1130
    calcification, 1130
Biliary
    atresia, neonatal, 945
    drainage, percutaneous, 991–993
    sludge, 976
        ultrasound, 968
            children, 2216
    tract, **955–987**
        anatomy, 955–958
        angiography, 973–974
        arteriography, 973–974
        barium studies, 973
        calculi, 966–967
        CAT scanning, 970
        computer diagnosis, 959
        dyskinesia, 978
        ERCP, 1006

fistulography, 967
history-taking and examination, 959
interventional technique, 2131
investigation, methods, 959–973
magnetic resonance imaging, 83
obstruction, malignant, endoscopy, 1007
operative and therapeutic planning,
        angiography, 973
paediatric problems, 981–985
parasite infestation, 985–986
plain abdominal radiography, 959–961
strictures, benign, 983–984
trauma, angiography, 973
tumours, angiography, 973
    children, 983
ultrasound, children, 2216
    atresia, 2217
Billroth operative procedures, 807–808
Binswanger's disease, magnetic resonance
        imaging, 79
Biological Effects of Ionizing Radiation III
    report, 1657
Biopsy
    biliary system, 974
    CT-guided, 52
    lung, 136, 289
    pancreas, percutaneous, 1002
    percutaneous, hepatobiliary system, 989–991
    procedures, **2122–2228**
        embolization, 2127
        musculoskeletal, 2126–2127
        percutaneous abdominal, 2124–2126
        percutaneous transthoracic, 2122–2124
            complications, 2123
            contraindications, 2124
        transjugular, liver, *2128*
        transvenous approach, 2127, *2128*
Bi-plane fluoroscopic unit, 4
Bird fancier's lung, 267 (*table*)
'Bird of prey' sign, 729
Birnberg bow, 1621
Bismuth poisoning, 1408
Bjork-Shiley valve, 664, 666, *669*, *670*, 671
Bladder
    abnormalities causing ureteric obstruction,
        1085
    carcinoma, magnetic resonance imaging, *86*
        intravenous urography, 1110
        plain radiography, 1110
        staging, 1113
    complications, following hysterectomy, 1623
        following radiotherapy, 1624
    congenital abnormalities, 1183–1185
    injuries, 1166–1168
        anatomy, 1166–1167
        cystography, 1168
        evaluation, 1167–1168
        mechanism of injury, 1167
        ruptures, 1168
    instability, urodynamics, 1212–1214
    neck contracture causing obstruction, 1086
    neuropathic, urodynamics, 1216
    outflow obstruction, urodynamics, 1215
    paediatric, anomalies, 1196–1198
        epispadias, 1196
        exstrophy, 1196
        neurogenic, 1198
        prune belly syndrome, 1198
    residual volume, dynamic scanning, 1055
    tumour, CT scan, *54*
        magnetic resonance imaging, *86*
    ultrasound, children, 2225–2226
Blalock anastomosis, in tetralogy of Fallot, 503

Blalock-Taussig shunt, 575
Blastomycosis
    bone infection, 1364
    North America, 215
Bleb, definition, 368
Bleeding
    biliary tract, 973
    diatheses and arteriography, 1992
    diverticular, 879
    embolization, 2146, *2148*
    gastrointestinal, hepatic arteriography, 940
        radionuclide studies, 836
        see also Gastrointestinal haemorrhage
    mediastinal, 195
    oesophageal varices, portal embolization, 997
    portal hypertension, radiological investigation, 950
    rectal, colonoscopy, 901
    small bowel, intramural, 851
Blood
    circulation *see* Circulation
    flow in kidney transplantation, 1143
        measurement, Doppler ultrasound, 2119
        measurement by magnetic resonance imaging, 67, 448
    pool imaging, children, 2208–2209
    ^{99m}Tc labelled red cells, 423
    transfusion, pulmonary oedema following, 165
Blount's disease, 150
Blow-out fractures, orbital floor, **1901–1902**
Bochdalek hernia, 170, *171*, *333*, 334
Boerhaave's syndrome, 769
Bolus, contrast medium injection, thoracic aorta, 445
Bone
    biopsy, **2126–2127**
    cyst, aneurysmal, **1287–1288**
        juvenile, 1458
        spinal cord, 1841
    dental, 1906–1907
    solitary, 1285–1287
    unicameral, juvenile, 1458
    density *see* Metabolic disease
    dysplasias, **1415–1445**
        apophyses, 1424–1427
        chromosomal disorders, 1444–1445
        diaphyses, 1431–1432
        epiphyses, 1424–1427
        growth plate, 1416–1424
        metaphyses, 1427–1431
        miscellaneous, 1435–1444
        mucolipidoses, 1432
        mucopolysaccharidoses, 1432–1435
    growth, normal, **1416**
    inborn errors of formation, thoracic cage, 333
    imaging, children, 2198–2201
        infection, 2199
        neoplastic disease, 2200
        special, 2201
        systemic disease, 2200–2201
        trauma, 2200
        vascular disorders, 2199–2200
    infarction, in sickle cell disease, 1330–1332
        in polycythaemia, 1333
        children, bone imaging, 2200
    infection, **1349–1367**
    irradiated, sarcoma arising, **1315**
    lesions, radiolucent/radio-opaque, differential diagnosis, 1914–1915
    marrow aplasia in sickle cell disease, 1330

    in metabolic and endocrine disease, **1369–1414**
        anatomy, 1369–1371
        calcium homeostasis, 1371–1373
        density, decrease, 1373–1396
            disorders associated with, 1374
        effects of vitamin D and metabolites, 1371–1373
        hormones, 1373
        physiology, 1371–1373
        resorption, 1371
            intracortical, in osteomalacia, 1379
        see also specific diseases
    metastases, from female genital tract tumours, 1594
        radionuclide bone scanning, **1538–1540**
    mineral analysis, using CT, 1532
    mineral integrity in evaluation of arthritis, 1477
    pain, undiagnosed, radionuclide bone scan, 1545
    radionuclide imaging, **2185–2188**
        and bone pain, 1545, 2186
        and cell type, 2186
        and clinical staging, 2186–2187
        interpretation, 2187–2188
        lesion distribution, 2186
        rationale, 2185
        and serum phosphate levels, 2186
        technical factors, 2185–2186
    resorption in hyperparathyroidism, 1385, 1392
        primary, 1384, 1385
        subperiosteal, in renal dystrophy, 1382, *1383*
    sclerosis (bone islands), 1909
    tumours, **1273–1326**
        benign, **1273–1300**
            see also specific names
        CT, 1524–1526
        general characteristics, **1273–1276**
            age of patient, 1274
            benign, characteristics, 1275
                metastases from, 1275
            diagnostic considerations, 1273–1274
            histological typing, 1273–1274
            malignant, primary characteristics, 1275
                secondary characteristics, 1275
            'moth-eaten' appearance, 1275–1276
            permeative pattern, 1276
            rate of growth, 1275–1276
            regularity of margin, 1276
        magnetic resonance imaging, 89
        malignant, **1301–1326**
            children, 1306–1307, 2200
            investigation, management by radiologist, 1305–1306
            metastatic spread, **1301–1303**
                diagnosis in bone, 1303–1305
                differential diagnosis, 1305
                skeletal distribution, 1303
            primary, 1307–1324
            see also Metastases, bone : specific names
            primary, radionuclide bone scan, 1540
Bourneville's disease, 1779
Bowel
    calibre, 720, 722
    dilatation, 721–731
    duplication, in infants, 913
    inflammatory disease, colonoscopy, 901
    large, 859–895
        anatomy, 859–860, *861*

    atresia, infants, 909
    barium enema, 862–866
    carcinoma, *822*, 902
        and diverticular disease, 880
        see also Colorectal carcinoma : Rectal carcinoma
    clinical presentation of disease, 861
    endometriosis, 892
    function, 861
    ganglion cells, absent (Hirschsprung's disease), 916
    immaturity, in infants, 916, *918*
    inflammatory disease, *see* Colitis
    lipomatous disorders, 892
    lymphoma, 876
    megacolon, 893
    metastases, 875, *876*
    necrotizing enterocolitis of the newborn, 920
    neonatal small left colon, 916
    obstruction, 879
    polyposis syndromes, 871–872
    polyps, 866–871
    preparation, for barium enema, 862
    radiological investigation, 862–866
    sigmoid volvulus, 894
    solitary ulcer syndrome, 893
    strictures, 891
    taeniae coli, 859, *860*
    tumours, 866–876
    volvulus, 728–729
    wall, configuration, 881
    see also Colonoscopy
loop protrusion, fetal, sonography, 1577
obstruction, fetal, sonography, 1577
    infants, 906, *907*
    large bowel, mechanical, 726–729
    small bowel, 722–725
    strangulating, 723
    opacification, for CT scan, 48
    preparation, for colonoscopy, 899
    rotation abnormalities, 912, *914*
    small, **833–858**
        actinomycosis, 847
        adenomatous polyp, 842
        amyloidosis, 855
        angiography, 836
        anisakiasis, 848
        atresia, infants, 909–910
        barium studies, 834–835
        Behçet's disease, 855
        'blind loop' syndrome, 852
        carcinoid, 843–845
        carcinoma, primary, 845, *846*
        Crohn's disease *see* Crohn's disease
        diverticula, 851–852
        endoscopy, 830
        giardiasis, 848
        graft-versus-host disease, 855
        haemangioma, 843
        hamartomatous polyp, 843
        infections, 847
        infestation, 847–849
        intramural haemorrhage, 851
        ischaemia, 851
        leiomyoma, 842, *844*
        leiomyosarcoma, 845, *846*
        lipoma, 843
        lymphangiectasia, 854
        lymphoma 845–847
        mastocytosis, 855
        metastases, 846
        mucosal oedema, 853

Bowel (*cont.*)
  small (*cont.*)
    nodular lymphoid hyperplasia, 853
    normal, 833
    obstruction, mechanical, 849–851
    plain radiographs, 834
    progressive systemic sclerosis, 853
    radiation enteritis, 849
    radiological investigation, 833–857
    radionuclide imaging, 836
    secondary tumours, 846
    South American blastomycosis, 848
    strictures, 839–841
      ischaemic, 851
      radiation, 849, *850*
    strongyloidiasis, 848
    tapeworm infestation, 849
    tuberculosis, 847
    tumours, 842–847
    ulcer, coexisting portal hypertension, 929
    ulcerative enteritis, idiopathic, 855
    varices, *1012*
      barium study of liver disease, 929, *930*
    Waldenström's macroglobulinaemia, 855
    Whipple's disease, 853, *854*
    yersiniosis, 847
Boxer's fracture, 1260
Brachiocephalic vein, 126
Brain
  abscess, 1739–1740
    CT, 1739–1740
    radiography, 1739
  arteriography *see* Cerebral arteriography
  cerebral disorders, 1703
  coma, 170
  computed tomography, **1678–1682**
    anatomy, 1681–1682
    contrast media, 1678–1681
      indications, 1679–1680
      intrathecal, 1679–1681
      ischaemic lesions, 1679
    craniocervical junction, 1679
    pituitary loss, 1679
    posterior cranial fossa, 1678
    technique, 1678
  cranial nerve palsies, 1701
  developmental problems, 1703
  endocrine disturbances, 1703
  fetal sonography, 1577
  head injuries, 1700–1701
  headache, 1701, 1702
  hemisyndromes, 1701
  infections, **1739–1767**
    degenerative disorders, 1744–1745
    demyelinating disorders, 1745–1746
    parasitic, 1743–1744
  loss of consciousness, 1701
  magnetic resonance imaging, *9, 65*
  meningitis, 1703
  metastases to, 1717–1718
    CT, 2180
  nerve disorders, 1702
  neurological disorders, radiology, **1700–1703**
  otorrhoea, 1703
  phlebography, 1693–1695
  plain radiography, **1671–1678**
    see also Skull
  pneumography, **1694–1700**
    see also Pneumoencephalography and
      specific disorders
  radionuclide scanning, **1857–1871**
    blood-brain barrier, 1857–1858
      diffusible, 1858

non-diffusible tracers, 1858
    cerebral angiogram, radionuclide, 1859–
      1860
    cerebrovascular accidents, 1864
    children, **2206–2207**
    cisternography, **1866–1871**
    comparison with CT, 1862–1863
    cystic lesions, 1863
    demyelinating lesions, 1863
    inflammatory lesions, 1863
    radiopharmaceuticals, 1857
      properties, 1867
    scan interpretation, 1859
    skull lesions, 1863–1864
    trauma, 1863–1864
    tumours, 1860–1863
  rhinorrhoea, 1703
  stem, deficit, acute, 1702
    angiography, 1702
    CT, 1702
    glioma, CT, 1710–1711
    infarcts, 1757
    radiography, 1702
  trauma, **1780–1789**
    see also Head injury
  tumours, **1708–1721**
    CT, 1702, 1703
    incidence, 1708
    radiography, 1701, 1702, 1703
    scanning, radionuclide, 1860–1863
    see also Glioma
  ultrasound, 1682
    infant, **2229–2234**
      cystic lesions, 2232–2233
      equipment, 2229–2230
      haemorrhage, 2230, 2233–2234
      hydrocephalus, 2230, 2232–2233
      indications, 2230
      normal appearances, 2230–2232
      technique, 2229–2230
    vascular occlusion, 1787–1788
    see also Cerebral
Branchial cysts causing laryngeal displacement,
  1981
Branham's sign, 2008
Braunwald-Cutter valve, 664
Breast, 89, 151
  abscess, 1639
  benign dysplasias, 1631–1633
  biopsy scarring, 1638
  cancer, 1637–1643
    circumscribed, 1639–1640
      differential diagnosis, 1240
    gelatinous (mucinous, colloid), 1640
    histology, 1637
    internal mammary lymphoscintigraphy,
      2193–2194
    'knobby', 1639
    location, 1637
    malignant calcifications, 1641–1643
      differential diagnosis, 1642–1643
      idiopathic skin, 1642
      pseudocalcifications, 1643
      vascular, 1642
    medullary, 1639
    metastases to oesophagus, 766
    papillary, 1639
    scirrhous, 1637–1638
      differential diagnosis, 1637–1638
    screening, **1657–1659**
      comparison of risk, 1659
      criteria for benefit, 1657–1658
      Detection Demonstration Projects,

1658–1659
      evidence of benefit, 1658
      Health Insurance Plan Study, 1658
      see also Mammography
    'simplex', 1639
    thermography, 1660–1661
      see also Thermography
  computed tomography, 1664–1665
  cysts, 1634
  fat necrosis, traumatic, 1639, 1640
  fibrous mastopathy, 1639
  hyalinized fibroadenoma, 1639
  magnetic resonance imaging, 1665
  mammography *see* Mammography
  microcalcifications, 1633
  normal anatomy, 1631–1633
  parenchymal patterns and cancer risk, 1635–
    1636
    D2 and PY patterns, 1635–1636
  parenchymal scarring, 1638
  sclerosing adenosis, 1633, 1639
  transillumination light scanning, 1665–1666
  ultrasound, **1661–1664**
    abscess, 1663
    accuracy, 1663
    appearance, 1661, 1662 (*table*)
    carcinoma, 1662
    compared with mammography, 1663, 1664
    cyst, 1661, *1662*
    diagnostic criteria, 1661
    fibroadenoma, 1661–1662
    general purpose equipment, 1661
    haematoma, 1663
    indications, 1663–1664
    simple and compound scans, 1663
Brodie's abscess, **1353**, 1453
Bronchi, *115*, 116
  anatomy, *120, 471*
  left main, elevation, in heart enlargement,
    553, *554*
  obstruction, in infants and young children,
    342
  rupture, 308
Bronchial
  adenoma, 250
  arteries, 567
  arteriography, 2030–2031
  carcinoma, **241–249**
    adenocarcinoma, 248
    alveolar cell, 249
    cell type, radiographic patterns, 248
    central, 243
    concomitant with tuberculosis, 211
    CT, *1528*, 247
    differentiation from silicosis, 269
    with emphysema, *235, 238*
    large cell, 248
    metastases, 246
    oat cell (small cell), 249
    peripheral, 242
    rate of growth, 243
    secondary pneumonia, 246
    small cell (oat cell), 249
    squamous cell, *244, 245, 247*, 248
  circulation, enhanced, in congenital heart
    disease, 466
  isomerism, left, *543*, 545
Bronchiectasis, 230–232
  allergic bronchopulmonary aspergillosis, 285
Bronchio-alveolar carcinoma, 249
Bronchiolar carcinoma, 249
  systemic sclerosis, 282
Bronchioles, 119

Bronchioles (*cont.*)
  obstruction, infants and young children, 342
Bronchiolitis
  children, 336, *338*
  obliterans, 230, 238
Bronchitis, chronic, 235
Bronchocele, *147*, 229, 285
Bronchocentric granulomatosis, 286
Bronchogenic
  carcinoma, magnetic resonance imaging, *88*
  cyst, 188, *189*
Bronchography, *119*, 135
Bronchomalacia, congenital, 358
Bronchopleural fistula, 163
  differentiation from lung abscess 164 (*table*)
Bronchopleurocutaneous fistula, 321, *322*
Bronchopneumonia
  definition, 200
  tuberculous, 210
Bronchopulmonary dysplasia, in infants and
    young children, 344
Bronchostenosis
  isolated, congenital, 358
  of sarcoidosis, 278
Brown opalescent dentine, 1926–1927
Brown tumour
  of hyperparathyroidism, **1298**, 1386
    jaws, 1910
  radionuclide bone scanning, 1539
Brucellosis, 1361–1362
  melitensis, abortus and *suis*, 1361
Brunner's gland hyperplasia, 820, *821*
Budd-Chiari syndrome, 945, 950, 2071, 2073,
    2079
Buerger's disease *see* Thromboangiitis
    obliterans
Bulb ureterography in ureteric tumours, 1111
Bulla, definition, 368
Burkitt's lymphoma, **1338**
  maxillofacial region, 1911
Bursae, **1511**
  iliopsoas, CT scan, *1525*
Burst(ing) fracture
  CT scan, 1228–1229, 1524
  Jefferson, 1228–1229
  lower cervical spine, 1229
Byssinosis ('Monday morning fever'), 267

Caecum
  deformity following appendicectomy, 894
  volvulus, 728, 894
Caesarean section
  hysterosalpingography following, 1595
  lower segment, changes following, 1618
Caffey's disease, **1408**, **1431–1432**
  mandible, 1914
Calcaneal (calcaneus)
  cyst, simulated, *1461*
  injuries, **1268–1269**
    fractures, 1269
      classification, 1269
  normal irregularity, simulating trauma, 1464,
    1465
Calcification
  acute abdomen, 740
  adrenals, 1033
  aortic stenosis, aortography, 605
  bladder tumour, 1110
  defective, 1926–1927
  eggshell nodes, causes, 277, *279*
  Eisenmenger reaction, 507
  gallbladder, 959–960, 976, 977
  heart, 380

constrictive pericarditis, 686, *687, 688*
  mitral ring, 593
  rheumatic mitral valve disease, 587, *588,
    589*
  liver, 927, 928 (*table*)
  pancreas, 960
  patent ductus arteriosus, 492
  provisional, dense zones, 1470
  pulmonary artery wall, 466
  renal, parenchymal disease, 1119
    tuberculosis, 1124
    tumour, 1065
  soft tissue, 1513–1520
    generalized conditions, 1513
    infection, 1515–1517
    local conditions, 1513
    metabolic conditions, 1513–1514
    vascular conditions, 1514–1515
  thyroid nodules, 1024
  see also specific headings throughout
Calcified papillae, 1060
Calcifying epithelial odontogenic tumour, 1908
Calcinosis, tumoral, 1512
Calcitonin, 1025, 1026
Calcium
  deficiency and osteomalacia, 1378
  homeostasis, **1371–1373**
  ipodate, 963
  oxalate, stone, 1060
  phosphate, stone, 1058
  pyrophosphate dihydrate crystal deposition,
    disease, 1494–1495
  serum, estimation, in hyperparathyroidism,
    1039
  see also Parathyroids
Calculi, **1059–1063**
  anatomical causes, 1060
  bile duct, 966–967
    endoscopic sphincterotomy, 1006
  bladder, causing obstruction, 1082
    postoperative complicating hysterectomy,
    1623
  clinical features, 1060
  complicating renal trauma, 1177
  computed tomography, 1062
  differential diagnosis from urothelial
    tumours, 1112
  gallbladder, **975**
    children, 985, 2216
    cholesterol, 975
    complications, 976–977
    ileus, 724, 976
    mixed, 975
    nonoperative removal, 993–995
    pigment, 975
    radioisotopes, 977–978
    ultrasound, *34*, 2216
  intravenous urography, 1063
  kidney (nephrocalcinosis), **1062–1064**
    causes, 1063, 1064
    cortical, 1062
    medullary, 1063
    ultrasound, children, 2223
  periodontal, 1933
  pulmonary alveolar microlithiasis, 275
  radiology, **1060–1061**
  salivary glands, 1919–1920, 1922
  staghorn, 1059
  ultrasound, 1062, 2223
  ureteric, causing urinary obstruction, 1069,
    1070, 1081–1082
    in pregnancy, 1074–1075
  urethral, causing obstruction, 1082

  urinary, **1059–1062**
    aetiology, 1059
    causing obstruction, 1069, *1070*, 1081–
    1082
      oedema, distant ureter, 1081–1082
    structure, 1059
    vaginal, 1616
Calyces (caliceal)
  crescents, 1072–1073
  renal parenchyma, 1117–1118
    misleading views, 1118
    normal appearances, 1117–1118
    vascular impressions, 1118
Camurati-Engelmann disease, 1407
  see also Engelmann's disease
Candida albicans infection
  oesophagus, 755, **756**, *757*
  urinary tract, 1130, 1131
Candida arthritis in the neonate, **1352–1353**
  osteomyelitis in the neonate, **1352–1353**
Capillary
  malformations, arteriography, 2006–2008
  telangiectasia, radionuclide scanning, 1866
Caplan's syndrome, 269, 280
Carcinogenesis, radiation risks, 1590
Carcinoid tumours, metastases, embolization,
    2147, *2152*
Carcinoma *see* Tumours and specific organs,
    regions and names
Cardiac
  arrhythmias, fetal sonography, 1577
  incisura, definition, 368
Cardiomegaly in thalassaemia, 1329
Cardiophrenic fat pads, 193
Cardiopulmonary disease, postoperative and
    critically ill patients, 313–321
Cardiopulmonary imaging in children, 2208–
    2210
Cardiovascular system
  changes, in pulmonary thromboembolism,
    299
  contrast media, 108
  CT scanning, 56
  radionuclides, 21 (*table*)
Caries, dental, 1931–1932
  radiation, 1931
Carina, splaying, in heart enlargement, 553,
    554
Caroli's disease, 985
Carotid
  angiography in cranial nerve disturbances,
    1702–1703
    in intracranial brain tumours, *1720, 1721*
  artery, atherosclerosis, digital fluorogram, *7*
    common, arteriography, 2027, *2028*
    external, arteriography, 2027–2028
    internal, arteriography, 2030
    puncture, cerebral arteriography, 1682–
    1683
  system, anatomy, 1684–1689
    anastomotic pathways, 1689
    anterior cerebral, 1686
    external carotid, 1687–1689
    internal, 1684–1687
    left common, 1684
    middle cerebral, 1686
    right common, 1684
  -cavernous fistula, radionuclide scanning,
    1863
Carpal bones, injuries, **1257–1259**
  fractures, 1259
    radionuclide bone scan, 1541
  instability, 1257, 1259

Carpal bones, injuries (*cont.*)
  perilunate dislocation, 1257, **1258**
  rotary subluxation of lunate, 1258
  rotary subluxation of scaphoid, 1257
Carpentier-Edwards valve, 664, *665*
Cartilage
  -capped exostosis *see* Osteochondroma
  costal, 153
  space, in evaluation of arthritis, 1477
Castleman's disease, 187
Cataract, congenital, 1880
Catecholamines, 1033
Catheters and catheterization
  angiographic, removal of gallstones, 991
  for arteriography, **1990–1991, 1993–1996**
    balloon, 1990
    co-axial, 1990
    cobra, 1990
    complications, 2001–2002
    percutaneous arterial, 1994–1996
    percutaneous needle puncture, 1993–1994
      complications, 1999–2001
    pigtail, 1990
    selective, 1996
    sidewinder, 1990
    size and shapes, 1990
  balloon, rectal, complications, 863
  cardiac, 382
    aortic valve disease, 605, 697
    congenital disease, **470–473**
    congestive myopathy, 637–638
    hypertrophic myopathy, 643–645
    left atrial myxoma, 648
    mitral valve disease, 594–596
    pacemaker, malposition (dislodgement),
      656, *657*
    patent ductus arteriosus, 493
    restrictive myopathy, 646
    tricuspid valve disease, 597
  duodenum, 816
  Foley, with balloon, in intussusception, 919
    peroperative cholangiography, 966
  liver, and arteriography, 939
  nephrostomy, percutaneous, 2129–2130
    indications, 2129
    techniques, 2130
  percutaneous femoral arterial, 609
  portal embolization, 997
  pulmonary intravascular, *316, 319*, 324
  steerable, removal of gallstones, 994
Cavernous
  angiomas, cerebral, radionuclide scanning,
    1866
  haemangiomas, arteriography, 2008
  orbital effects, 1891
Cavity
  definition, 368
  pseudocavity, definition, 371
  ultrasound, 31
Cavography *see* Inferior vena : Superior vena
Cellulitis
  bone imaging, children, 2199
  caused by contract medium extravasation,
    2088
  CT, 1887
  differential diagnosis from gas gangrene,
    1521
  orbital effects, 1887
Cementomas, 1908, 1928
Cementum hypoplasia, 1928
Central nervous system
  embolization, 2156
  radionuclides, 21 (*table*)

children, 2206–2207
Cephalhaematoma, 1783
Cerebellar tonsillar ectopia myelography, 1703
Cerebellopontine angle tumours, 1862
Cerebral (cerebrum)
  abscess complicating sinusitis, 1943
  angiography, intra-axial brain tumours,
    suspected, **1719–1721**
    pituitary tumours, **1724–1725**
  arteriography, **1682–1693**
    anastomotic pathways, 1689
    apparatus, 1683–1684
    arch aortography, 1682
    arteries, anatomy, 1684–1689
    brain stem deficit, acute, 1702
    cerebral hemisyndromes, acute, 1701
    coma, 1701
    contraindications, 1684
    direct puncture of vertebral artery, 1683
    femoral artery catheterization, 1683
    head injuries, 1701
    loss of consciousness, 1701
    preparation of patient, 1683
    puncture of carotid artery, 1682
    retrograde brachial angiography, 1683
    subclavian artery puncture, 1683
    suspected subarachnoid haemorrhage,
      1701˙
    technique, 1684
    transaxillary artery catheterization, 1683
    transient ischaemic attacks, 1701
    veins, anatomy, 1689
    vertebrobasilar arteries, 1690–1692
    vertebrobasilar veins, 1692–1693
  arteritis, 1765–1766
  atrophy, **1744–1745**
    magnetic resonance imaging, 77
    radionuclide scanning, 1868–1869
  degenerative disorders, magnetic resonance
    imaging, 77
  embolism, CT, 1701
  haemorrhage, spontaneous, **1755–1756**
    angiography, 1755–1756
    CT, 1755
    ultrasonography, 1756
  infarction, **1756–1757**, 1787
    angiography, 1759–1762
    contrast enhancement, 1758–1759
    haemorrhagic, 1758
    late results, 1759
    magnetic resonance imaging, 73
    radionuclide scanning, 1864–1865
    venous, 1758–1759
  ischaemia, **1756–1766**
    angiography, 1759–1762
      postoperative, 1762
    arteritis, 1765–1766
    infarction, features, 1756–1757
      contrast enhancement, 1759
    intracranial abnormalities, 1763–1764
    Tolosa Hunt syndrome, 1766
    vertebrobasilar insufficiency, 1762–1763
  malformations, **1769–1777**
  swelling, 1787
    angiography, 1787
  tumours *see* Brain tumours
  veins, anatomy, 1689–1690
  venography, 2064
  see also Brain
Cerebrospinal fluid
  circulation disturbances, 1793–1795
  CT, 1703
    cisternography, 1703

leakage, in ear trauma, 1963
  otorrhoea radiography, 1703
    cisternography, 1703
    CT, 1703
  post-traumatic, 1788–1789
  in radionuclide cisternography, 1866–1867
    tracers, properties, 1867
  radionuclide scanning, 1870–1871
  radiography, 1703
  rhinorrhoea, 1963
Cerebrovascular accidents
  CT, 1679
  digital subtraction angiography, 2102
  radionuclide scanning, **1864–1866**
    haemorrhage, 1865–1866
    hypoperfusion syndromes, 1865
    infarction, 1864–1865
  see also Cerebral infarction: Strokes:
    Transient ischaemic attacks
Cervical
  carcinoma, 1607–1608
    barium enema, 1608
    CT, 1608, 1625
    distant metastases, 1608
    isotope imaging, 1608
    lymph node metastases, 2174
    lymphography, 1607
    pelvic urography, 1608
    radiotherapy complications, 1624
    ultrasonography, 1608
    ultrasound, 1625
    urography, 1608
  dysphagia *see* Dysphagia, cervical
  spine, trauma, **1223–1234**
    classification, 1224–1232
    degree of stability, 1224 (*table*)
    dens fractures, 1233–1234
    examination, 1223–1224
    extension-rotation injuries, 1227–1228
    hyperextension, 1229–1232
    hyperflexion injuries, 1224–1226
    mechanism of injury, 1224 (*table*)
    paediatric, 1232–1233
    torticollis, 1232
    vertical compression, 1228–1229
Cervicitis, 1604
Cervicothoracic fractures, 1236
Cervix, carcinoma, arteriography, 1598
Chagas' disease, 638, 773, 890
  megacolon, 893
Chamberlain's line, 1776
Chance fracture, lumbar spine, **1237, 1239**
Chemodectomas
  causing laryngeal displacement, 1981
  middle ear, 1959
Chemotherapeutic
  agents, vascular infusion, 2135
  infusions, *see* Infusion techniques
Cherubism, 1913
Chest
  corona radiata, 242
  CT scanning, *42, 44*
  expiratory filming, 132
  infection, bronchial wall thickening, 234
    fungal, infants and young children, 338
    virus, in children, 336
  mimicking of acute abdomen, 720
  normal, 113–129
    infants and young children, 330
  opacities, abnormal, radiograph, 142–148
  ossification centres, appearance and fusion,
    330 (*table*)
  pulmonary nodule, CT scan, *46*

Chest (*cont.*)
  radiograph, abnormalities, detection and
      descriptions, 140–149
    bone, 141
    constrictive pericarditis, 686–688
    generic diagnosis, 149
    in gynaecology, 1594
    inspiration, degree of, 140
    interpretation, 139–150
    lateral, 379
    newborns, 562
    normal heart variations, 390–391
    oblique views, 380
    overpenetrated frontal, 379
    penetration, 140
    posture, 140
    projection, 139
    rotation, 140
    side marker, 139
    silhouette sign, 140
    soft tissue, 141
    specific diagnosis, 150
    standard frontal, 379
    transradiancy, 141
    tube-film distance, 140
    tuberculosis, 212
  radionuclide imaging, 133–135
  techniques, 131–137
  tomography, 132
  trauma, 305–311
  ultrasound, 135
    paediatric, 2213
      juxtadiaphragmatic, 2214
      opaque hemithorax, 2214
  wall, 151–156
    carcinomatous invasion, 247
    loculation against, 163
    soft tissues, 152
  see also Hila : Lungs : Mediastinum : Pleura :
      Pulmonary system
Chiari malformation, **1772–1773**, 1826, *1828*,
    1829
Chicken pox *see* Varicella
Chilaiditis syndrome, 733
Child abuse, fractures, radiography, 1248
Children, *see* Paediatric; and specific
    conditions
Chlamydial
  pneumonia, 204
  trachomatis, 337, *338*
Choanal atresia, **1941**
  radiological appearances, 1941
'Chocolate cysts', 1620
Cholangiocarcinoma, interventional
    radiograph, *8*
Cholangiography
  fine needle, 2131
  hilar tumour assessment, 979
  intravenous, 963
  percutaneous transhepatic, 963–965
  peroperative, 966–967
  transtubal, 967
Cholangitis, primary sclerosing, 984
Cholecalciferol *see* Vitamin D
Cholecystectomy
  exploration of bile duct during, indications,
      966
  postoperative problems, 978
Cholecystitis
  actinomycotic, 976
  acute, 734
    acalculous, in children, 983
    calculous, 975–976

gangrenous, 976
  radionuclide imaging, 971
  scintigraphy, 972
chronic, 976
complications, 974–975
emphysematous, 739, 960
  arteriography, 976
glandularis proliferans, 977
non-calculus, 976
typhoid, 976
Cholecystogram, oral, 961–963, 976
Cholecystokinin, 972
Cholecystosis, 977
Choledochal cyst, childhood, 984
  ultrasound, 2217
Choledochopancreatography, endoscopic
    retrograde (ERCP) *see* Endscopy,
    retrograde choledochopancreatography
Choledochoscopy, stone removal, 1007
Cholelithiasis *see* Calculi, gallbladder
Cholesteatoma
  ear, 1956–1958, 1961
    acquired, 1957–1958
    congenital (epidermoid), 1958
  implantation, **1296**
  intracranial, 1734–1735
    CT, 1714
  paranal sinuses, 1946, 1948
  and urinary tract infection, 1131, *1132*
Cholesterol stones, 975
Cholesterosis (strawberry gallbladder), 977
Cholinesterase inhibitors and idiopathic
    achalasia, 773
Chondroblastoma, **1280–1281**
  clinical presentation, 1280
  pathology, 1280
  radiological features, 1280–1281
Chondrocalcinosis, **1494–1495**
  in hyperparathyroidism, primary, 1386, *1387*
Chondrodysplasia, metaphyseal, **1430–1431**
  types, 1430–1431
Chondroectodermal dysplasia, **1422**
Chondroma, 1276, **1277–1278**
  clinical presentation, 1277
  differential diagnosis, 1277
  enchondromatosis, 1278
    with haemangiomas, 1278
  juxtacortical, 1278
  larynx, 1979
  maxilla, 1907
  multiple, 1278
  radiological features, 1277–1278
Chondromatosis, synovial, 1501
Chondromyxoid fibroma, **1281–1282**
  appearance, 1275
  clinical presentation, 1281
  pathology, 1281–1282
  radiological features, 1282
Chondrosarcoma, 1277, **1307–1309**
  clear cell, 1309
  clinical presentation, 1307–1308
  juxtacortical, 1309
  larynx, 1979
  mesenchymal, 1309
  pathological considerations, 1308
  radiological features, 1308–1309
Chordoma, **1322–1323**, 1735–1736
  clinical presentation, 1322
  myelography, *1841*
  nasopharyngeal, 1968–1969
  radiological features, 1323
Choriocarcinomas, 1609–1610
  angiography, 1609

metastases, 1609
  ultrasonography, 1610
Choristoma, 1723
Choroid(al)
  angiomas, 1896
  lesions, 1896
  plexus, papilloma, CT, 1716–1717
Christmas disease, **1345**
Chromium-51 EDTA, 1052
  glomerular filtration rate in renal
      transplantation, 1141
Chromophobe adenoma, 1021
Chromosomal disorders and bone dysplasias,
    1444
Churg-Strauss syndrome, 282
Chylothorax, 163, 306
  infants and young children, 335
Cigarette smoking, peptic ulcer, 817
Cine-radiography
  in arteriography, 1991
  cardiac, 382
Circadian rhythms, 1018
Circulation
  bronchial, enhanced, in congenital heart
      disease, 466
  changes, with intravascular contrast media,
      107
  fetal, 459–460
    persistence of, in infants, 347, 351
  newborn infants, 351, 460
  pulmonary system, **565–583**
    congenital conditions, radiological
        assessment, 464–468
  see also Pulmonary system, arteries
Circulatory disorders and oral contraception,
    1622
Circumscribed, definition, 368
Cirrhosis, 949
  Laennec's, 853
  in osteomalacia, 1378
  scintigraphy, 935
Cirsoid aneurysm, arteriography, 2014
Cisterna magna, large, 1772
Cisternography
  metrizamide, empty sella syndrome, 1594
  positive contrast, 1695, 1697–1698
  water soluble, CT, cranial nerve
      disturbances, 1702–1703
    CSF rhinorrhoea/otorrhoea, 1703
    meningitis, recurrent, 1703
Cisterns, subarachnoid, in
    pneumoencephalography, 1699–1700
Clavicles, 155
  injuries, 1251–1252
    acromioclavicular separation, 1251
    radiographic examination, 1251
Clay shoveller's fracture, 1225
Clear cell chondrosarcoma, 1309
Cleft palate, 1915
  effect on tooth eruption, 1930
Cleidocranial dysostosis, **1429–1430**, 1915
  effect on teeth, 1930
Cloaca, persistent, 1601
Clonorchiasis, biliary, 985
Clostridium welchii, gas formation, 739
Clot, definition, 368
Club foot, 1452
Coagulation defects, and arteriography, 1994
Coalescent, definition, 368
Coalworker's pneumoconiosis, 268
Coarctation of the aorta, 699–702
  arteriography, 2003, 2004
  pseudo-, 702, *703*

Coccidioidomycosis, 215
bone, **1364**
Coeliac
axis, angioplasty, 2143
arteriography, 2037–2039
ganglion block, CT-guided, 53
ultrasound, 2114
disease, **841**, *843*
malignant histiocytosis, 845
Colic
oesophageal, 749
renal, 739, *740*
Colitis, 800, **881–891**
acute, 729, 887, *888*
amoebic, 890
antibiotic-associated, 890
complications, 881
cystica profunda, 893
distribution of lesions, 881
herpetic, 890
infectious, 889
ischaemic, 730, 888–889
lymphogranuloma venereum, 891
mucosal abnormality, 881
parasitic infestation, 890
radiation, 889
schistosomiasis, 891
tuberculous, 890, *891*
ulcerative, and Crohn's disease, 881–888
differential features, 886
extent of colitis, 886
radiological features, 882–886
ulceration, 882–885
carcinoma, 887
Yersinia enterocolitis, 890
Collagen diseases
heart involvement, 638
vascular, children, gamma imaging, 2200–2201
lung, 279–284
see also specific names
Colles fracture, wrist, 1257
Collimators, radionuclide imaging, 18
Colloid cysts, CT, 1712, *1713*
Colobomatous cyst, 1881
Colon, *see* Bowel
Colonoscopy, **897–903**
and barium enema, 900–902
complications, 899
first-line, 901
instrument, 897
paediatric, 902
preparation and sedation, 899
technique, 898
Colorectal carcinoma, **872–876**
advanced, 874
complications, 875
radiological features, 872–874
recurrent, 875
unusual forms, 875
Coma
angiography, 1701
CT, 1701
radiography, 1701
Comet sign, in atelectasis, 228
Communication, clinician-radiologist, 10
Composite, definition, 368
Compression filming, stomach, 784
Compton interaction, 17
Computed tomography
abscess drainage, CT-guided, 53
acetabular fracture, 1245
acoustic neuromas, 1733, 1962

adrenals, 1035
angiofibroma, juvenile, 1968
angiomas, intracranial, **1752–1755**
aortic dissection, 711
arachnoid cyst, 1773–1774
aertfacts, 46
astrocytoma, 1709
cerebellar, 1710
biliary tract, 970
biopsy, CT-guided, 52
bladder tumours, 1113
brain, **1678–1682**
abscess, 1739–1740
compared with radionuclide scanning, 1863
scanning, 2180
stem, 1710
deficit, acute, 1702
breast, 1664–1665
calculi, 1062
cardiovascular, future prospects, 447
cellulitis, 1887
cerebellar disturbance, acute, 1702
cerebral developmental problems, 1703
cerebral haemorrhage, 1755
cerebral hemisyndromes, 1701
cervical carcinoma, 1608, 1625
chest, 133
Chiari malformations, 1772–1773
chordoma, 1323, 1734–1735
nasopharyngeal, 1969
clinical use, 55
coeliac axis ganglion block, 53
colloid cyst, 1712
coma, 1701
compared with radionuclide scanning in hydrocephalus, 1869
constrictive pericarditis, 687
corpus callosum defects, 1771
cranial nerve disturbances, 1702–1703
cranial nerve palsies, 1701
craniopharyngioma, 1726–1727
cryptorchidism, 1037
CSF rhinorrhoea/otorrhoea, 1703
dacryocystitis, 1887
Dandy-Walker syndrome, 1771
data storage, 46
development, 5
duodenum, 817
dynamic scanning, 42, 441
dysphasia, 1701
eighth nerve tumours, 1961, 1962
emission (ECT), 20
positron transaxial, 440
SPECT (single photo emission computerized tomography), 2201
liver, 933
empty sella, 1725–1726
encephalitides, 1743
endocrine disease, 1020
endometrial carcinoma, 1609, 1625–1626
enhancement, 45
ependymoma, 1711
epidural abscess, 1943
future of, *57*
glioblastoma multiforme, 1710
glioma, **1709–1712**, 1720
malignant, 1709–1710, *1720, 1721*
neurohyphysis, 1723
glomus jugulare tumours, 1960
-guided biopsy, 52–53, 2125
percutaneous drainage, 53, 2132
therapy, 2135

gynaecology, **1598–1599, 1624–1626**
haemangioblastoma, 1714, *1715*
head injuries, 1700
headache, 1701
facial or occipital, 1702
heart, 440–447
clinical applications, 443–447
gating techniques, 441–443
motion, 440
technical considerations, 441
hemianopia, 1701
hemiplegia, 1701
historical background, 39
holoprosencephaly, 1770
Hounsfield scale of numbers, 43
hydranencephaly, 1771
hydrocephalus, 1869
hypothalamic pituitary axis lesions, 1703
image, 43–45
influencing factors on values, 44
intracranial aneurysms, 1746–1748
Jefferson bursting fracture, 1228–1229
kidney, injuries, 1172
transplanted, 1144
larynx, 1975
lesion size, *57*
liposarcoma, 1324
liver, **936–939**
compared with nuclear imaging and ultrasound, 2184–2185
scanning, 2180
loss of consciousness, 1701
lymph node metastases, 1626, **2175–2176**
machine parameters, 47
magnification, 45
malignancy, 56
medulloblastoma, 1714
melanoma, malignant, choroidal, 1896
meningioma, 1730–1731
meningitis, 1743
recurrent, 1703
metastases to brain, 1717–1718
microadenomas, 1723, *1724*
millisecond cine scanner, 5
mineral measurements, bone, 1410–1411
quantitative, 1411
mucoceles, 1943–1944
musculo-skeletal system, **1523–1534**
bone mineral analysis, 1532
clinical applications, 1524
infection, 1524
low back pain syndrome, 1529–1532
neoplasms, 1524–1529
technical advances affecting, 1523–1524
trauma, 1524
myelography, 51
in neuroblastoma, 1207–1208
neurofibromatosis, 1778
occult spinal dysraphism, 1823
oesophagus, 748
oligodendroma, 1710
orbit, 1877, *1878*
foreign bodies, 1886
trauma, 1882
osteosarcoma, 1311–1312
ovarian carcinoma, 1626
paediatric, 1182
examinations, 54
Paget's disease, 1790
pancreas, 1001
pancreatitis, 736
papilloma, choroid plexus, 1716–1717
paranasal sinus carcinoma, 1948–1950

Computed tomography (*cont.*)
  parasitic brain infections, 1743–1744
  parathyroid adenoma, 1027
  parietal lobe dysfunction, 1701
  partial volume effect, 45
  patient examination, technique, 47–55
  patient factors, 48
  pearly tumours, 1734–1735
  in pelvic rhabdomyosarcoma, 1210
  percutaneous procedures, CT-guided, 52
  pericardial effusion, 683–684
  physical principles, 39–47
  pineal region tumours, 1712–1714
  pituitary, *1021*
    adenoma, 1723–1724
    fossa, 1594
  positron emission transaxial, 440
  pulmonary arterial sling, 535
  pulmonary thromboembolism, 303
  pyelonephritis, acute, 1120
  radiation dose, 47
  radiotherapy planning, 53
  reading difficulties, 1703
  renal cysts, 1190
  renal masses, 1091, 1095
    abscess, 1099
    adenoma, 1102
    angiomylipomas, 1101
    cysts, 1097, 1098, *1100*
    lobar nephronia, 1099
    lymphoma, 1105
    renal cell carcinoma, 1103
    sinus lipomatosis, 1101
    transitional cell carcinoma, 1106
    Wilm's tumour, 1104
  in renal vein thrombosis, 1161
  resolution, 45
  retarded mental development, 1703
  retroperitoneal fibrosis, 1083
  scan times, 47
  scanner, 40–42
  single photon emission (SPECT), 2201
    liver, 933
  skull fractures, growing, 1782, 1783
  slice, 47
    interval, 47
    thickness, 47
    width, 46
  in spinal trauma, 1849–1850
  spinal vascular lesions, 1852–1853
  spine, 1799–1801
  spleen, 1011
  Sturge-Weber disease, 1778
  subarachnoid haemorrhage, 1747–1749
  subdural empyema, 1740
  suspected subarachnoid haemorrhage, 1701
  in syringomelia, 1829
  thalassaemia, *1329*
  thymoma, 1027
  thyroid mass, 1024–1025
  tissue specificity, lack of, 57
  transient ischaemic attacks, 1701
  transmission, 440
  tuberculomas, 1742
  tuberculosis, cranial, 1741–1742
  tuberous sclerosis, 1779
  in tumour diagnosis, 56, 2169 (*table*), 2171
    clinical value, 2175–2176
    metastatic involvement, 2175–2176
      from occult primary tumours, 2180
      systemic, 2178–2181
  in urinary obstruction, 1069, 1077–1078
  urinary tract, 1048

  uterine sarcoma, 1626
  whole body, 39–59
  in Wilm's tumour, 1205
  windowing system, 43, *44*
  see aslo Tomography
Computer assisted thermography, 1660
Conception, retained products, 1617
Congenital
  abnormalities, radiation risks, 1590
  dislocation of the hip, **1450–1452**
    CT scan, 1533
    radiographic assessment, 1451–1452
  heart disease, digital subtraction
    angiography, 2107
  see also Heart; and individual congenital
    conditions
Congestive heart failure, 316–318
Conn's syndrome, 1034
Conn's tumour, embolization, 2158, *2159*
Connective tissue diseases, **1484–1488**
  and arteriography, 1992
  associated with sialectasis, 1920
  calcification, 1517–1518
  mixed, *1484*, **1485**
  oesophagus, 775
Conradi's disease, **1424–1426**
Consciousness, loss
  angiography, 1701
  CT, 1701
  radiography, 1701
Constrictor agents, vascular infusions, 2135–
  2136
Contraception
  devices, plain radiography, 1594
  see also Intrauterine contraceptive devices ;
    Oral contraception
Contrast media
  in arteriography, 1991
    coronary, 610
    injection apparatus, 1991
    radiographic apparatus, 1991–1992
  CT, heart, 440
  definition, 368
  development, 5
  enema, water-soluble, 866
  intracardiac injections, 109
  intravascular, **99–110**
    adverse reactions, 104–107
      predisposing factors, 106
        specific radiological procedures, 107
    allergic reactions, 105
    anaphylactic reactions, 105
    characteristics, 101 (*table*)
    chemotoxic reactions, 104
    complications, 105
    CT scanning, 49
    death from, 106
    ionic monomeric, conventional, 100
    low osmolar, 102
    osmolality, 101, 102 (*fig.*)
    osmolar reactions, 104
    specific clinical areas, 107–109
    structural formulae, 102 (*fig.*)
    toxicity, 104 (*table*)
  intravenous cholangiography, 963
  intravenous urogram, 1046
    paediatric, 1181
      adverse reactions, 1181
      findings, 1181
      technique, 1181
  magnetic resonance imaging, 9, 67
  oral cholecystographic, 961
  osmolality, methods of reducing, 102–104

  paramagnetic, 5
  perforation, abdominal, 733
  -related complications, arteriography, 1999
    inadvertent intramural or perivascular
      injection, 2000
  ultrasound, 36
  water-soluble duodenography, 817
    stomach, 787
Contusion, pulmonary, 306
Cooley's anaemia *see* Thalassaemia
Cooley-Cutter valve, 664
Cor pulmonale, definition, 368
Cor triatum, 537
Coracoid process, fractures, 1250
Corneal opacity, ultrasound, 1894
Coronary arteriography, **609–619**
  indications, 625–627
  therapeutic, 625
  see also Arteriography
Coronary artery
  anatomy, normal, *610*, 611–613
  aneurysm, 613
  angiography, 595
  anomalous, 614–616
  arising from pulmonary artery, 495
  atheromatous disease, 613
  bypass grafts, arteriography, 625
    CT scanning, 443
    digital subtraction angiography, 2108
    post-operative radiograph, 323
  congenital anomalies, 612, 614–616
  digital radiograph, *459*
  disease, diagnosis, 625
    echocardiography, 415
    postoperative investigations, 626
    prognosis, 625
    radionuclide ventriculography, 425
    transluminal angioplasty, 626
    treatment, 625
  fistula, 616
  left, aberrant, 541
  muscle bridge, 614
  narrowing, non-atheromatous, 614
  spasm, 620
  trauma, 651
Coronary endartarectomy, 625
Corpus callosum
  agenesis, magnetic resonance imaging, 79
  defects, **1770–1771**
Corpus luteum
  cysts of pregnancy, sonography, 1567
  ultrasonography, in infertility, 1038
Corrosive gastritis, 797, *798*
Corrugated artery, 2017
Cortical bone measurements, **1409–1411**
  appendicular, 1410
    radiogrammetry, 1410
    single photon absorptiometry, 1410
Cortical
  buckling fracture, 1248
  desmoid, post traumatic, 1292
  hyperostosis, infantile, **1431–1432**
  infarction, radionuclide bone scanning, 1544
  necrosis, acute, 1119–1120
  tunnelling in Sudeck's atrophy, 1401–1402
Cortisol, 1033
  Cushing's syndrome, 1034
Costal cartilages, radiograph, 153
Coulomb/kilogram (C/kg), definition, 16
CPPD crystal deposition disease, 1494
Cranial
  foramina and canals, 1676 (*table*)
  malformations, **1769–1777**

Cranial (*cont.*)
  nerve, disturbances, chronic, angiography,
    1702–1703
      CT, 1702–1703
      radiography, 1702–1703
    palsies, angiography, 1701
      CT, 1701
      radiography, 1701
  sutures, abnormalities, **1775–1776**
  trauma, magnetic resonance imaging, 74, *76*
Craniodiaphyseal dysplasia, **1432**
Craniofacial dysostoses, 1881, 1915
Craniolacuna, 1775
Craniopharyngioma, 1022, 1707, 1723, 1726–
  1727
  CT, 1726–1727, *1727*
  nasopharyngeal, 1969
  pneumoencephalography, *1727*
Craniostenosis in children, **1448–1449**
Craniosynostosis, 1775
  classification, 1775–1776
Cranium bifidum occultum, 1769
Crescents, caliceal, 1072–1073
Cretinism, 1023, 1025
Cricopharyngeus spasm, 1972
Critically ill patients, pulmonary aspects, 313–
  327
  support and monitoring apparatus, 324
Crohn's disease, **837–841**
  anal fistulae, *887*
  asymmetry, 840, *841*
  clinical features, 837
  cobblestoning, 838, *840*
  colonoscopy, 902
  differentiation from anisakiasis, 848
  differentiation from gastrointestinal
    tuberculosis, 847
  and diverticula, 880, *881*
  duodenal involvement, 823, *824*
  featureless outline, *842*
  incidence, 881
  causing obstruction, 1083
  oesophagitis, 758
  radiological appearances, 837–841
  stomach, 796
  and ulcerative colitis, 881–888
    differential features, 886
    extent of colitis, 886
    radiological features, 882–886
    see also Colitis, ulcerative
Crona radiata, definition, 368
Cronkite-Canada syndrome, 872
Cross-Jones valve, 668
Croup, airway obstruction, *341, 342,* 343
Crouzon's disease, 1881, 1915
Crown, tooth, fracture, 1934
CRST syndrome, calcification, 1518
Cruciate ligaments, tears, CT scan, 1533
Cryptococcosis (torulosis), 214, *215*
  bone, **1364**
Cryptorchidism, 1038
Crystal deposition arthropathies, **1491–1496**
CT *see* Computed tomography
Cuboid fractures, 1269
Cuneiform fractures, 1269
Curie, definition, 16
Cushing's disease (endogenous and exogenous),
  1020, 1034, **1376–1378**
  arteriography, contraindicated, 1992
  and embolization, 2158
  heart involvement, 640
  mediastinal lipomatosis, 193
  radiological diagnosis of bone, 1376–1377

  differential diagnosis, 1377–1378, 1380
  pathological considerations, 1377
Cyanosis, central, and anteriovenous
  malformation, 524
Cyanotic congenital heart disease, 461–463
Cyclopia, 1880
Cyst(s)
  brain, children, ultrasound, 2232
  bronchogenic, 188, *189*
  choledochal, of childhood, 984
  definition, 368
  dental, benign, 1904–1906
  duplication, gastric, 800
  enteric, 188
  foregut, 188–190
  gastrointestinal, ultrasound, children, 2219
  giant, large bowel, 879
  hydatid, 217
    ultrasound, 930
  liver, **948**
    CT scanning, 938
    ultrasound, children, 2216
  neurenteric, 188
  oesophageal, 762
  ovarian, 1036–1038
  pancreas, 1000, 1003
  pancreatic pseudocyst, 736
  parasitic, cardiac, 649
  pericardial, 677–678, *679*
  pleuropericardial, 190
  polycystic disease in neonates, 945
  pulmonary, congenital, 363
  recurrence, ovarian carcinoma, CT scan, 51
  renal, **1097–1099**
    adult polycystic, 1098
    amniography, 1583
    arteriography, 2034
    children, ultrasound, 2223
    complicated, 1097
    hydatid, 1099
    multicystic dysplasia, 1098
    multilocular (benign cystic neoplasm),
      1098
    parapelvic, 1098
    puncture, 2129
    serous, 1097
    ultrasound, children (poly-, solitary and
      multi-), 2223–2224
  thymus, 1029, *1030*
  thyroid, 1025
  ultrasound, children, 2216
  see also Cystic and specific names
Cystadenocarcinoma, mucinous and serous,
  ovarian, 1612
  CT, 1613
  ovarian, 1593
  radiology, 1612–1613
  ultrasound, 1613
Cystadenoma, mucinous and serous, 1612
  CT, 1613
  during pregnancy, sonography, *1566,* 1567
  ovarian, 1593
  radiology, 1612–1613
  ultrasound, 1613
Cystic
  adenomatoid malformation, differentiation
    from congenital lobar emphysema, 365
  pulmonary, congenital, 363
  angiomatosis, **1293–1294**
  disease of the kidney, 1188–1190
    adult polycystic, 1188
    infantile polycystic, 1188
    multicystic dysplastic, 1189

    multiocular cysts, 1189–1190
    simple, 1190
  duct variations, 956
  fibrosis, bronchiectasis, 230
    respiratory disease, 344
  hygroma, 192, *193*
    fetal detection, sonography, 1569, 1570,
      1571
  pneumatosis, 738
  rhabdomyosarcoma, CT scan, *51*
  teratomas (dermoid cysts), 1614
    ovarian, 1593
    see also Dermoid cysts
Cysticercosis
  calcification, 1515–1516
  CT, 1743–1744
Cystine stones, 1060
Cystitis
  emphysematous, 739, 1131
  haemorrhagic, 1202
Cystocele causing obstruction, 1086
Cystography in bladder injuries, 1168
Cystourethrography in stress incontinence,
  1624
Cytomegalovirus
  of AIDS, 287
  pneumonia, 289
Cytoscopy, bladder tumours, 1110
  ureteric tumours, 1111
Cytotoxic drugs
  heart myopathy, 640
  lung effects, 287

Dacryocystitis, 1887
Dacrocystography, 1880
Dactylitis in yaws, 1361
Dalkon Shield, 1621
Dandy-Walker syndrome, 1706, **1771–1772**
  neonate, 2232, 2233
DeBakey, classification of dissecting aortic
  aneurysm, *708*
Debakeys-Surgitool valve, 664, 668, *670*
De Morsier's disease, 1770
Deafness
  congenital, 1965
  post-traumatic, 1963
Death, prenatal, radiation risks, 1590
Decay mechanisms and radioactivity, 14–16
Deceleration injuries, arteriography, 2025
Decubitus radiography, 313
Delivery, conditions affecting, sonography,
  1579
Dementia
  angiography, 1703
  CT, 1703
  radiography, 1703
Dens fractures, **1233–1234**
  types, 1234
Dens invaginatus (dens indente) *see*
  Odontomes, dilated composite
Density differences of soft tissues, 1509–1510
Dental
  cyst, apical, 1932
    benign, 1904
      apical, 1904
      lateral (periodontal), 1904
      residual, 1904
  infection, periapical, 1927, 1932
    see also Teeth
  radiology, **1925–1935**
    anatomy, 1925–1926
    developmental anomalies, 1926–1930
      abnormally shaped teeth, 1927–1929

Dental (*cont.*)
  radiology (*cont.*)
    defective calcification, 1926–1927
    periapical infection, 1932–1933
    periodontal disease, 1933–1934
    pulpitis, 1932–1933
    radiography, 1925
      cassette, 1925
      non-screen, 1925
      panoramic, 1925
    see also Teeth
Dentigerous cysts, 1905–1906, 1945
Dentinogenesis imperfecta, 1926–1927
Dentinomas, 1908
Dermatomyositis, *1484*, **1485**
  calcification, 1518
  children, **1457**
  lungs, 283
  oesophagus, 775
Dermoid cysts, **1614–1615**
  intracranial, 1734–1735
  lacrimal gland effects, 1892
  during pregnancy, sonography, 1567, *1566*
  radiology, 1614
  spinal, 1823–1824
  spinal cord, 1846
  ultrasonography, 1614–1615
Desmoid tumours
  cortical, post-traumatic, 1292
  extra-abdominal, 1292
Desmoplastic fibroma, 1292
Dextrocardia, 542–545
Di George syndrome, 1026, 1027
Diabetes mellitus, 1031
  associated with periodontal disease, 1934
  delayed skeletal maturation, 1396
  emphysematous pyelonephritis, 1131
  gas-forming infections, 739
  gastroparesis, 806
  papillary necrosis, 1121, 1122
  radiological features, 1031 (*table*)
Diaphanography, breast, 1666
Diaphanoscopy, breast, 1666
Diaphragm, 141, 167–173
  eventration, 169, *334*, 335
  hernias, 170–172, 190
  height, 168
  infants and young children, 333–335
  movement, 170
  neoplasma, 173
  paralysis, 170, 335
  rupture, 310
  screening, for subphrenic abscess, 737
  traumatic tears, 171
Diaphyseal
  aclasis (multiple exostoses), **1437–1438**
  dysplasia, **1431**
    progressive, 1407
  fractures, 1248
Diasternatomyelia, *1823*
Diastrophic dwarfism, **1423**
Digastric line, 1776
Digital arteritis, *2046*
Digital radiography, **93–98**
  central diagnostic centre, 452
  control centre, 96 (*fig.*), 97
  development, 7
  examination room, 95
  future prospects, 459
  heart, 449–452
    advantages, 449 (*table*), 450 (*table*)
    quantitation methods, 459
  image processing and storage, 96

  pulmonary thromboembolism, 302
  receptors, 94
  spleen, 1011
  subtraction angiography, 7
  technologies involved, 94 (*fig.*)
Digital subtraction angiography, 1996–1997, **2099–2111**
  abdominal aorta, 2108
  acquired heart disease, 2107–2108
  advantages, 2099–2100
  aortic dissection, 2105
  apudomas, 2054
  clinical applications, 2102–2110
  congenital heart disease, 2107
  contrast medium and delivery, 2101
  coronary artery bypass grafts, 2108
  embolization procedures, 2102
  equipment, 2101
  extracranial vascular studies, 2102–2103
  extremities, 2104–2110
  framing rate, 2102
  future designs, 2110
  intracranial vascular studies, 2104–2105
  kidney disease, 2108
  and left ventriculography, 2108
  liver, 940
  mediastinal masses, 2105
  motion artefacts, 2101
  moving table, 2109–2110
  new designs with rapid acquisition rates, 2110
  parathyroid tumours, 2053
  and percutaneous transluminal angioplasty, 2139
  pulmonary arteriography, 2105–2107
  renal artery disease, 2108
  renal artery stenosis, 1154
  strokes, 2102
  subtraction methods, and delivery, 2101
  thoracic aortic aneurysms, 2105
  transient ischaemic attacks, 2102
1,25-Dihydroxyvitamin D, 1371–1373
Dilatation
  bowel, 721–731
    distinction between small and large bowel, 721, 722 (*table*)
Dilator agents
  in arteriography, 1991
  vascular infusion, 2136
Diphtheria, heart failure, 638
Disappearing bone disease, 1403
Disc
  lumbar, intervertebral, CT scan, 1529
  protusion and prolapse, **1830–1838**
    lumbar spinal canal, stenosis, 1833
    myelography, functional, 1835
      postoperative, 1835
    phlebography, 1832
Discitis, lumbar, 1355, *1356*
Discography, 1813
Dislocations, CT, 1524
Dissecting aneurysms, arteriography, 2010–2012
Disuse osteoporosis, 1400–1401
Diuresis, dynamic renal scanning, 1053
Diverticula, **877–879**
  colonoscopy, 901
  differentiation from adenomatous polyps, 880
  fundus, 956
  pericardial, 678
  pharyngeal, posterior (Zenker's), 1972
  pseudodiverticula, 853, 884, *885*

  small bowel, 851–852
  stomach, 804
Diverticular disease, **876–881**
  coexistent disease, 879
  complications, 877–879
  Crohn's disease superimposed, 880, *881*
Diverticulitis, 877
  causing pelvic inflammatory disease, 1603
Diverticulosis, Fallopian tubes, 1604
  oesophageal, 778
Doppler principle, 29, 394
  safety, 31
Doppler techniques *see* Ultrasound, Doppler techniques
Dorsum sellae, truncation, 1708
Double-contrast radiology, stomach, 786
Double outflow right ventricle, 512, *513*
Doubling time, definition, 368
Down's syndrome, **1444**
  amniography, 1583
  dental anomalies, 1928
  heart malformations, 469
Dracunculosis, and calcification, 1516–1517
Drainage, biliary, percutaneous techniques, 991–993
Dressler syndrome, 621, 685
Drip infusion, rapid, CT of aorta, 445
Drowning, pulmonary oedema, 263, *264*, *571*
Drugs
  abuse, endocarditis, 597
    pulmonary oedema, 263
  heart myopathy, 640
  lung disease induced by, 289–291
  reactions in arteriography, 1997
  role in pulmonary radiation reaction, 325
Dual photon absorptiometry in cortical bone measurement, 1410
Duke's classification of bowel carcinoma, 872
Dumb-bell tumours, 190
Duodenum, **815–826**
  aortoduodenal fistula, 825
  atresia, fetal, 905–906
    sonography, 1577
    infants, 909
  barium infusion, 835, *836*
  barium studies, 816
  cap, double-contrast view, *816*
  carcinoma, primary, 821
    secondary, 822
  hypotonic duodenography, 816
  intramural haematoma, 824
  intubation, 816
  involvement in Crohn's disease, 823, *824*
  involvement in pancreatitis, 823
  leiomyosarcoma, *822*
  loop, double-contrast view, *817*
  normal anatomy, 815
  obstruction, in infants, 985
  peptic ulceration, 817–820
  progressive systemic sclerosis, 824
  radiation damage, 824
  radiological investigation, 816
  rupture, traumatic, 825
  superior mesenteric artery compression syndrome, 825
  tuberculosis, 823
  tumours, benign, 820
    malignant, 821
    secondary, 822
  ulcer, endoscopy, 828
  varices, 825
Duplex kidney, excretion urography, 1118
Dura mater, thickening, 1843

Dwarfism
  diastrophic, **1423**
  fetal, sonography, 1577 (*table*), 1578 (*table*)
  long-limbed, **1424**
  metatropic, **1422–1423**
  short-limbed, 1416, **1417–1424**
  thanatophoric, **1419**, *1420, 1421*
  see also Achondroplasia
Dysautonomia, familial, oesophagus, 776
Dyschondroplasia, **1436–1437**, 1438
  see alo Enchondromatosis
Dyschondrosteosis, **1435**
Dysgerminoma, ovarian, 1615
Dysostosis
  cleidocranial, **1429–1430**
  facial, 1915
  multiplex, **1434**
Dysphagia, 748
  cervical, 1971–1973
    cricopharyngeus spasm, 1972
    pharyngeal protusions, 1972
    postcricoid carcinoma, 1970, 1971
    postcricoid web, 1972–1973
    posterior pharyngeal diverticula, 1972
  CT, 1701
  goitrous, 1025
  radiography, 1701
Dysplasia epiphysealis hemimelica, **1426**
Dysraphism, occult spinal, **1822–1824**
  CT, 1823
  myelography, 1823
  radiography, 1823

Ear, **1951–1965**
  anatomy, 1951–1954
    external, 1951
    facial nerve canal, 1953–1954
    inner, 1953
    internal auditory meatus, 1954
    mastoid arcello, 1953
    middle, 1953
  cholesteatoma, 1956–1958
  congenital abnormalities, 1964–1965
  infections, 1955–1959
  inflammatory diseases, 1955–1959
  nose and throat, 1937–1983
  otitis media, 1955–1956
  post-traumatic deafness, 1963
  radiological investigation, 1951, 1952 (*table*)
  temporal bone, radiology, 1952 (*table*)
  tomography, 1954–1955
  trauma, 1962–1964
  tumours, **1959–1962**
    benign, 1959
    external ear, 1959
    middle ear, 1959–1961
  see also specific headings
Ebstein's anomaly, 528–530
Echinococcosis (hydatid disease), 217
  bone infection, 1364–1365
Echo production, ultrasound, 27
Echocardiography, 381, **393–417**
  amyloid heart disease, 639
  anatomy, 395–408
  angina pectoris, 621
  aorta, 693
    aneurysm, mycotic, 712
      sinus of Valsalva, 713
    coarctation, 702
    dissection, 711
    incompetence, acute, 601–602, *603*
    stenosis, calcific, 599
      fixed, 698

  supravalvar, 698
  atrial septal defect, 481–484
  bicuspid aortic valve, 603
  Chagas disease, 638
  clinical applications, 414–416
  coarctation of the aorta, 702
  congenital conditions, 470
  congestive cardiomyopathy, 636
  constrictive pericarditis, 686
  contrast, 408, *409*
  contrast media, 5, 36
  cor triatum, 538
  coronary artery disease, 617
  dextrocardia, 542–545
  Doppler technique, 394
  Ebstein's anomaly, 530
  endocardial fibroelastosis, 641
  enlarged heart, 553
  examination, 395
  global evaluation, 394
  hypertensive heart failure, 641
  hypertrophic myopathy, 642
  intraventricular thrombus, 629
  ischaemic heart disease, left ventricular
      function, 619–620
  left atrial enlargement, 556
  left atrial myxoma, 647
  left ventricular, aneurysm, 629
    enlargement, 557
    pseudoaneurysm, 629
  mitral valve prolapse, 591
  M-mode, 393, **408–414**
  myocardial structure, 629
  myopathic trauma, 650
  patent ductus arteriosus, 492
  pericardium, 446
    effusion, 684
  persistent truncus arteriosus, 515
  primary dextrocardia, 542
  principles, 393
  prosthetic valves, 666–668
  pulmonary, artery absence, congenital, 534
    infundibular stenosis, 532
    total anomalous venous drainage, 512
    valve absence, 532
    valve stenosis, 531
  quantitative analysis, 394, 408
  rheumatic mitral valve disease, 589–590
  right atrial enlargement, 561
  right ventricular enlargement, 560
  spatial orientation, 394
  Taussig-Bing deformity, 514
  tetralogy of Fallot, 500, *501*
  tricuspid valve disease, 597
    atresia, 498
  tumours, 649
  two-dimensional, 394
  ventricular septal defect, 489
    post-infarction, 629–632
  ventriculo-arterial discordance, *519*, 520,
      521, 523
Ectopic pregnancy, sonography, **1557–1562**
  abdominal, *1559*, 1561
  conditions mimicking, *1560*, 1562
  interstitial and with decidual cast, *1559*, 1561
  pregnancy tests, 1559–1560
  ruptured, *1559*
  sonographic findings, 1558 (*table*), 1560
  unruptured, *1559*
Eggshell nodal calcification, 277, *279*
Ehler's Danlos syndrome, 1922
  calcification, 1517
Eighth cranial nerve tumours, 1961–1962

Eisenmenger reaction (pulmonary arteriolar
      obstruction), 466, **505–507**, 567, *575*, 580
  complicating patent ductus arteriosus, 492
Elbow
  injuries, **1252–1254**
    adult injury, 1253–1254
    dislocations, 1253–1254
    fractures in children, 1461
    Monteggia fracture-dislocation, 1254
      reversed, 1254
    olecranon fat pad signs, 1252
    paediatric injury, 1252–1253
    radial head fractures, 1254
  rheumatoid arthritis, **1478–1579**
    juvenile, 1482
Electrodes, cardiac pacemakers, 655
  complications, 656
Electromagnetic radiation, 17
Electrons, 14
Ellis-Van Creveld syndrome
      (chondroectodermal dysplasia), **1422**
  dental abnormalities, 1928, 1929
  heart anomalies, 470
Emboli, lower limb arteriography, 2051
Embolism
  air, vascular, diffuse, in infants, 355
  aneurysm, 2150
  arteriography, 2019–2020
  cardiac valve prosthesis causing, 671
  definition, 368
  fat, pulmonary, 307, *308*
  left atrial myxoma, 647
  pacemaker poppet, 668
  portal, 997
  pulmonary, cardiac pacemaker causing, 660
    complicating venography, 2065
    oedema, at autopsy, 264
    postoperative, 318
    see also Thromboembolism, pulmonary:
        Thrombosis
Embolization
  arterial, ateriography, 2027
  in arteriovenous fistulae, 1158
  biopsy procedures, 2127
  catheter thrombus, 2001
  definition, 368
  digital subtraction angiography, 2102
  liver, 941
    bleeding, 2146, *2148*, 2149
    hepatic arterial, 995–997
  peripheral, in arteriography, 2001
  portal, 997–998
  renal cell carcinoma, 1103
  renal masses, 1095
  spleen, 1015
  tumours, **2146–2150**
    see also Tumours
  ureteric, 2131
  see also Vascular embolization: Venous
      embolization
Embolus, definition, 369
Embryo, radiation risks, 1590
Embryonal cell carcinoma, CT, 1714
Emphysema, 235–238
  cholecystitis, arteriography, 976
  congenital lobar, 364
  differentiation from asthma, 236
  gastric, intramural, 797
  interstitial, 738
  mediastinal, 195
  obstructive, 237, *238*
  pulmonary, interstitial, cystic, differentiation
      from congenital lobar emphysema, 364

Emphysema (*cont.*)
  pulmonary, interstitial, cystic (*cont.*)
    infants, 353–355
    post-operative, 320
    surgical, 1521
Emphysematous
  cholecystitis, 739, 960
  cystitis, 1131
  pyelonephritis, 1131
  vaginitis, 1604
Empty sella syndrome, 1594
  CT, **1725–1726**
  pneumoencephalography, *1725*
Empyema, 202, 205
  paranasal sinus, 1944
Enamel, teeth, anomalies, 1926–1927
Enameloma, 1908
Encephalitis, **1742–1743**
  acute disseminated, 1742
  acute haemorrhagic leukoencephalopathy, 1742
  herpes simplex, 1742
  progressive multifocal leukoencephalopathy, 1743
  subacute sclerosing panencephalitis, 1743
Encephaloceles, **1769–1770**
  fetal, amniography, *1582*, 1583
  fetal detection, sonography, *1571*, 1576
  nasal cavity, 1948
Enchondromatosis (Ollier's disease), **1436–1437**, 1438, 1278
  with haemangiomas (Maffucci's syndrome), 1278
Endobrachial infection in postprimary tuberculosis, 210
Endocardial fibroelastosis, 641
Endocarditis
  in drug abuse, 597
  infective, 668, 670, 671, *713*
Endochondrial growth plate, axis, 1233
Endocrine
  disease, 1017–1042
    of bone, **1369–1414**
      anatomy, 1369–1371
      physiology, 1371–1373
      see also specific diseases: Bone
    cerebral effects, CT, 1703
      radiography, 1703
    children, **1466**
    pathophysiology, 1019
    radiological examination, 1019–1020
  organs, arteriography, 2053–2057
    venography, 2093–2095
  system, historical background, 1018
  see also Hormones
Endometrial
  carcinoma, 1608–1609
    angiography, 1609
    arteriography, 1598
    CT, 1609, **1625–1626**
    distant metastases, 1609
    hysterosalpingography, 1608
    lymph node metastases, 2174
    lymphography, 1608
    ultrasound, 1609
    urography, 1609
  polyps, 1616, 1619
Endometriosis, 1620
  large bowel, 892
Endomyelography, 1805
Endoprostheses, biliary, 991–992
Endoscopy
  biliary tract obstruction, malignant, 1005

lower gastrointestinal *see* Colonoscopy
  oesophageal carcinoma, 765
  pancreatitis, 1007
  papillotomy, 965
  retrograde choledochopancreatography, 830, *965*, **1005–1007**
    biliary tract disease, 1004
    obstructive jaundice, 979
    pancreas, 1000, **1005–1007**
      indications, 1006
    post-cholecystectomy, 978
  sphincterotomy, 1006
  upper gastrointestinal, 830
    complications, 828
    diagnostic accuracy, 828
    equipment, 827
    in relation to radiology, 827–831
    routine methods, 828
    special circumstances, 829
    therapeutic, 829
    who should do it? 830
Endosteal hyperostosis (van Buchem's disease), 1432
Endotracheal tube, 325
Engelmann's disease *see* Camurati-Engelmann's disease
Enostosis, 1909
Enteric cysts, 188
Enteritis
  radiation, 849
Enterocolitis
  emphysematous, 739
  necrotizing, of the newborn, 920
Enteropathic arthropathies, 1488
Enterouterine fistula, 1618
Eosinophil tumours, pituitary, 1722
Eosinophilia, pulmonary, 284–286
Eosinophilic
  gastritis, 796
  gastroenteritis, 854
  granuloma (histiocytosis X), 274, **1342–1344**
    in children, **1458–1459**, 2216
    clinical features, 1342
    liver, children, 2216
    maxillofacial region, 1910
    orbital manifestations, 1889
    petrous bone, 1961
    radiological features, 1343–1344
Ependymal cysts, 1774–1775
Ependymoma
  CT, 1711
  intramedullary, 1847, *1848*
  radionuclide imaging, 1861
Epidermoid *see* Cholesteatoma
Epidermolysis bullosa dystrophica, oesophagus, 768
Epidural abscess, complicating sinusitis, 1943
Epidurography, 1816
Epiglottis, carcinoma, 1977
  obstruction, 340
Epiglottitis, *341*, 343
Epilepsy
  angiography, 1703
  CT, 1703
  radiography, 1703
Epiloia, 1779
Epiphyses, disorders mainly affecting, 1424–1427
  see also specific names
  dysplasia, hemimelica, **1426**
    multiple, **1424**, **1425**
    punctate, **1424–1426**
    spondylo-, **1426–1427**

-metaphyseal injuries, 1247
Epispadias, 1196
Epistaxis, arteriography, 2030
Epithelial tumours, ovarian, 1612–1614
  angiography, 1613
  barium studies, 1612
  radiology, 1612
  urography, 1612
  see also specific names
ERCP *see* Endoscopy, retrograde cholangiopancreatography
Erlenmeyer flask appearance, 1328
Eruption of teeth
  abnormal, 1930–1931
  normal, 1930
Erythroblastosis fetalis, 1470
Escherichia coli
  gas formation, 738
  urinary tract infection, women, 1135
Ethmoid sinuses
  anatomy, 1939
  carcinoma, 1949
    CT, 1949
  mucocele, 1944
  osteoma, 1946
  see also Paranasal sinuses
Eunuchoidism, 1399–1400
Ewing's sarcoma, **1317–1320**
  appearance, 1276
  in children, 1459–1460
  clinical presentation, 1317
  CT, *55*
  development in mass, 1319
  maxillofacial region, 1911
  'onion peel' appearance, 1318
  pathological considerations, 1317–1318
  prognosis, 1319
  radiological features, 1318–1320
  therapy, 1319–1320
Exophthalmos
  endocrine, eyes, 1887
  thyroid, 1025
Exostoses
  benign, external ear, 1159
  multiple (diaphyseal aclasis), **1437–1438**
External ear
  auditory meatus, anomalies, 1964
    atresia, *1964*, 1965
  congenital anomalies, 1965
  tumours, 1959
  see also Ear anomalies
Extraction techniques, 2133–2135
  gallstones, percutaneous, 2133
  gastrointestinal foreign bodies, 2135
  renal stones, 2134
Extradural haemorrhage, acute, **1783–1784**
  chronic, 1784
Extravasation, contrast medium, 1063
  adrenal venography, 2094
  causing cellulitis, 2088
Exstrophy, bladder, 1196
Extension-rotation injuries of cervical spine, **1227–1228**

Facial
  arteries, calcification, 1922
  bones, abnormalities, 1915
  malformations, **1769–1777**
  nerve canal, anatomy, 1953
  nerve injury, 1963–1964
  paralysis, 1963–1964
Fallopian tubes
  hysterosalpingography, 1595–1597, 1619

Fallopian tubes (*cont.*)
  plastic operations, 1620
  pregnancy, 1619
  sterilization, 1620
  tumours, 1619–1620
  ultrasonography, 1619
Fallot's tetralogy, *see* Heart, tetralogy of Fallot
Fanconi's syndrome and osteomalacia, 1378
Fascioliasis, biliary, 985
Fat
  embolism, pulmonary, 307, *308*
  lines, abdominal, 721
  measurement, techniques, 1509–1510
  mediastinal mass, 193
Fatigue fractures, foot, 1271
Femoral
  anteversion, CT scan, 1533
  arteriography, 1993
    leg, 2048–2051
  artery catheterization, cerebral
      arteriography, 1683
    thrombosis, 2018, *2019*
  head viability, radionuclide bone scanning,
      1544
  see also Perthes' disease
Femur injuries, **1261–1264**
  distal fractures, 1263–1264
  fractures in children, **1462**
  head, fractures, 1262
  intertrochanteric fractures, 1262
    types I–IV, 1262
  neck, fractures, 1262
  proximal, 1261–1262
    radiographic examination, 1261
  shaft fractures, 1263
  slipped epiphyses, 1462
  subtrochanteric fractures, 1262
Fetus
  circulation, 459–460
  demise, amniography, 1581
    sonography, 1569
  duodenal atresia, 907–908
  position, determination, 1554–1556
  structural anomalies detectable, second
      trimester, 1569–1572
  ultrasonogram, *8*
  viability, evaluation, 1556
  well-being, impaired, amniography, 1583
Fibre-endoscopy *see* Colonoscopy : Endoscopy
Fibrinogen, radionuclide studies of venous
      thrombosis, 296
Fibroadenoma
  breast, 1633–1634
    ultrasound, 1661–1662
  hyalinized, 1639
Fibrodysplasia ossificans progressiva, **1435**
  calcification, 1517
Fibroids (fibromyomata), **1605–1607**
  angiography, 1606
  barium enema, 1606
  hysterosalpingography, 1605–1606
  IVU, 1606
  plain radiography, 1605
  ultrasonography, 1606–1607
  uterine, arteriography, 1598
    calcification, 1593
  see also Leiomyomas
Fibroma
  ameloblastic, maxilla-facial, 1908
  cardiac, 649
  chondromyxoid, appearance, 1275
  desmoplastic, 1292
  intraorbital, 1893

larynx, 1979
maxillofacial, 1907
non-ossifying, **1291–1292**
  clinical features, 1291
  juvenile, 1458
  pathology, 1291
  radiological features, 1291–1292
ossifying of jaws, 1907
  of Kempson, 1297
ovarian, 1615
paranasal sinuses, 1948
pericardial, *680*
pleural, 161, *162*
Fibromatosis, aggressive, 1292
Fibromuscular dysplasia
  carotid arteries, 1765
  in renovascular hypertension, 1151, 1152
Fibromuscular hyperplasia, arteriography,
    2017
Fibromyoma, vagina, 1616
Fibromyxoma, dental, 1907
Fibroplasia, media, renal artery, 1154
Fibrosarcoma, **1315–1317**
  appearance, 1275, 1276
  clinical presentation, 1315–1316
  larynx, 1978
  nasopharynx, 1969
Fibrosing alveolitis *see* Alveolitis, fibrosing
Fibrosis
  lung, 268, **272–276**
    radiation, 326
  pulmonary, and pulmonary embolism, digital
      subtraction angiography, 2107
  retroperitoneal, and ureteric obstruction,
      1083
Fibrous
  cortical defect, **1291**
  dysplasia, **1296–1297**, **1438**, **1439**
    maxillofacial region, 1912
    petrous bone, 1961
    radionuclide bone scan, 1545
    skull, **1789–1790**
      cystic form, 1790
      sclerotic form, 1789–1790
  histiocytoma, malignant, 1316, *1317*
Filariasis, lungs, 284
Film
  contrast factor, definition, 368
  definition, 369
Filter, definition, 369
Filtration, definition, 369
Fine needle
  aspiration biopsy, abdominal, 2124, 2126
  cholangiography, 2131
First arch dysplasia, 1915
First branchial arch syndrome, 1881
Fissural cysts, 1906
  globulomaxillary cyst, 1906
  incisive canal, 1906
Fistula
  anal, in Crohn's disease, *887*
  aortic sinus, 495
  aortoduodenal, 825
  arterioportal, 982
  arteriovenous, definition, 367
  bronchopleural, 163
    differentiation from lung abscess, 164
      (*table*)
  bronchopleurocutaneous, 321, *322*
  choledochoduodenal, iatrogenic, 983
  colovesical, 879
  coronary, 616
  cysto-enteric, 976

oesophagus, infants, 906–908, *909*
pulmonary arteriovenous, 579
  congenital, 361, *362*, 363
tracheo-oesophageal, 308
  infants, 907–908
vaginal, 1616
Fistulography, biliary, 967
Fitzgerald-Gardner syndrome *see* Gardner's
    syndrome
Fleischner line, 148
Fleischner's plate atelectasis, 314
Flexion injuries, thoracolumbar spine, 1236
Flexion teardrop fracture, 1226, *1227*
Fluid
  abdominal, 720
  collections in renal transplantation, 1146–
      1147
  intraperitoneal, **734**
  level, definition, 369
  restriction, before intravenous urogram, 1046
  small bowel, causes, 722, 723 (*table*)
Fluoroscopy
  chest, 132
  heart, 380
    calcification, 587
  liver, 928
  pericardial effusion, 681
  valvular prosthetic implantation, 665–666
Fluorosis, **1406–1407**
  bone changes, 1405, 1406
  radiological diagnosis, 1406
    pathological considerations, 1406–1407
  and tooth enamel, 1927
Focal cortical abscess, CT scan, *1525*
Focal reflux nephropathy, 1126–1127
Follicle-stimulating hormone, 1036
  males, 1038
Follicular cysts, ovary, 1610
Follicular hyperplasia, thymus, 1028
Foot
  in gout, 1491–1492
  injuries, **1266–1271**
    calcaneus, 1268–1269
    fatigue (march) fractures, 1271
    Lisfranc injuries, 1270–1271
    mid- and forefoot, 1269–1271
    talus, 1266–1268
  in Reiter's syndrome, 1490
  in rheumatoid arthritis, **1479**, **1481**
Forearm
  fractures in children, 1462
  Galeazzi fracture dislocation, 1254, *1255*
  injuries, 1254
Forefoot injuries, 1269–1271
Foregut cysts, 188–190
Foreign body
  ear, 1963
  gastrointestinal removal, 2135
  inhaled, 343
  intranasal, 1950
  intraorbital, **1883–1887**
    CT, 1886
    localization techniques, 1883–1887
    radiography, 1883
    ultrasound, 1885, 1886
  intravascular, extraction techniques, 2137
  oesophageal, 771–772
  pacemakers as, 659–661
  paranasal sinuses, 1950
  pharynx, 1973
  radio-opaque radiography, 1594
Fractures
  basic tenets, 1246

Fractures (*cont.*)
　burst, *see* Burst(ing) fractures
　in children, **1461–1465**
　　see also specific bones
　CT, 1524, 1525
　osteogenesis imperfecta, 1393
　pacemaker lead, 657–658
　pathological, in myelomatosis, 1340
　radiographic examination, 1246
　radionuclide bone scanning, *1539*, 1540–1541
　Salter-Harris classification, 1247
　terms and conventions, 1246–1248
　valvular prosthesis, 668, *669, 670*
　see also specific bones
Fragilitas ossium, **1441–1442**
Frankl, white line, in scurvy, 1383
Frauenhofer zone, 29
Free induction decay, 63
Freiberg's infraction, 1502
Fresnel zone, 29
Frey's classification, external and middle ear
　deformities, 1964
Frontal sinuses
　anatomy, 1939
　carcinoma, 1950
　mucocele, 1943
　osteoma, 1944
　see also Paranasal sinuses
Frusemide, dynamic renal scanning, 1053
Fumes, inhalation, pulmonary oedema from,
　264
Fundoplication, 808, *809*
Fungus
　balls causing obstruction, 1082
　　differential diagnosis from urothelial
　　　tumours, 1112
　cause of extrinsic allergic alveolitis, 267
　　(*table*)
　infections, bone, **1363–1364**
　　chest, infants and young children, 338
　　lungs, 213–217, 289
　　urinary tract, 1130
Fusiform abdominal aneurysm, 2010

Gadolinium DTPA, 67
Galeazzi, fracture dislocation, forearm, 1254,
　1255
Gallbladder
　absence (agenesis), 955
　adenoma, 977
　anomalous ducts, 956
　bilobed, 955
　calcification ('porcelain'), 959–960, 976, 977
　carcinoma, 977
　double, 955, *956*
　folded, 956
　function, quantitation, 973
　inflammation, 976
　intrahepatic, 956
　left-sided, 956
　nonvisualization, 962–963
　papilloma, 977
　'porcelain', 959–960, 976, 977
　radionuclide imaging, 970
　strawberry (cholesterosis), 977
　tumours, 977
　ultrasound, *32*, 968
　　children, 2216
　　hydrops, 2217
　　wall thickening, 2216–2217
Gallium
　citrate, 134
Gallium (⁶⁷Ga) imaging, 2188–2191

administered patient dose, 2188
defining effects of therapy, 2190–2191
inflammatory disease, 1541
instrumentation, 2188
lymphomas, 2189
mechanism of action, 2189
mechanisms, 1536
patient preparation, 2188
pulmonary tumours, 2189–2190
renal infection, 1057
sarcoidosis, 278
scan findings/tumour histology, relationship,
　2189
technical factors, 2188–2189
time of imaging, 2188–2189
Gallstones, ultrasound, children, 2216
　see also Calculi, gallbladder
Gamekeeper's thumb, 1260
Gamma-ray radiation, definition, 14
Gamma scintigraphy, children, 2197–2198
　see also Bone imaging: Cardiovascular
　　imaging: Central nervous system
　　imaging: Gastrointestinal imaging:
　　Thyroid imaging: Urinary tract imaging
Ganglioneuroma, 190, *191*
　maxillofacial, 1907
Gangliosidoses, CT, 1745
Gangrene
　ischaemic colitis, 889
　pulmonary, 205
Gardner's syndrome, 871, **1282**
　affecting facial bones, 1916
Gargoylism *see* Hurler's disease
Garre's osteomyelitis (subperiosteal sclerosing),
　1354, 1453, 1914
Gas
　abdominal, normal appearances, 720
　biliary tree, 724, 960–961, *976, 977*
　gallbladder wall, 960, *961*
　infections forming, 739
　inhalation, pulmonary oedema from, 264
　intra-abdominal abscess, 736
　　free, 731
　intramural, 738
　liver, 928
　shadow, definition, 369
　in soft tissues, 1521–1522
　　air insufflation, 1522
　　formed within, 1521–1522
　　introduced from without, 1522
Gas gangrene, 1521
　differential diagnosis from cellulitis, 1521
　uterine, 1604
Gastrectomy, total, 808
Gastrinoma, 1032
Gastritis *see* Stomach, inflammatory conditions
Gastroduodenal arteriography, *2038*, 2039,
　2141
Gastroenteritis, eosinophilic, 854
Gastrografin, 48
　duodenography, 817
Gastrointestinal tract
　arteriography, **2037–2045**
　　bleeding, 2040–2045
　　　see also Gastrointestinal bleeding,
　　　　arteriography
　　coeliac axis, 2037–2039
　　hepatic, *2038*, 2039
　　mesenteric, 2037, *2038*, **2039–2040**, *2043*,
　　　2044
　bleeding, arteriography, **2040–2045**
　　active, 2041
　　angiodysplasia, 2042, *2044*

barium studies, 2041
chronic, 2041–2042
embolization, 2146
endoscopy, 2041–2042
isotope studies, 2041
portal hypertension, 2042
radionuclide imaging, children, 2204–2205
gynaecological conditions, 1597
malabsorption in osteomalacia, 1378
motility, radionuclide imaging, children,
　2205–2206
radionuclide imaging, 21 (*table*)
　children, 2203–2204
tumours, 1032
ultrasound, children, 2219–2220
upper, endoscopy *see* Endoscopy, upper
　gastrointestinal
Gastro-oesophageal reflux
　and hiatus hernia, in infants, 915
　radionuclide imaging, children, 2205–2206
Gastroschisis, fetal, amniography, 1580, 1583
Gaucher's disease, 1331, **1344–1345**, **1435**
　differential diagnosis, 1345
　Erlenmeyers flask, 1328, **1344**
　pathological considerations, 1344
Gemination, 1927, 1928
Genitography, intersex states, 1601
Genitourinary tract
　injuries, 1163–1178
　　bladder, 1166–1168
　　kidney, 1170–1177
　　ureter, 1168–1170
　　urethra, 1163–1166
　radionuclide, 22 (*table*)
Gerbode defect, 487, 491
Germ cell tumours, 179
Germinomas, CT, 1714
Gestational age, sonographic determination,
　1552–1554
Giant cell aortitis *see* Takayashu's syndrome
Giant cell arteritis, arteriography, 2016
Giant cell tumour, **1289–1290**
　benign status, 1289
　clinical presentation, 1289
　dental, 1907
　pathology, 1289
　radiological features, 1289–1290
　radionuclide bone scan, 1540
Giardiasis, 848
Gierke's (glycogen storage) disease, 541, 639
Gigantism, 1020, 1022, **1389–1392**
　pathological considerations, 1389–1392
　radiological diagnosis, 1389
Glaucoma, congenital, 1881
Glenn procedure, 575
Glenohumeral joint, rheumatoid arthritis, **1478**
Glenoid fractures, 1249, 1250
Glioblastomas
　multiforme, CT, 1710
　radionuclide imaging, 1861
Glioma, **1708–1712**
　astrocytoma, 1709
　　cerebellar, 1711, *1712*
　brain stem, 1710–1711
　CT, 1709–1712
　malignant, 1709–1710
　optic chiasma, 1727–1728
　optic nerve, 1892
　radionuclide imaging, **1860–1861**
Globulomaxillary cyst, 1906
Globus
　hystericus, oesophagus, **748**, 1971
　oesophagus, 1971

Glomerular filtration rate, transplanted kidney, 1143
Glomerulonephritis
  chronic, renal angiography, 1156
  urography, 1119
Glomus tumour
  bone, 1295
  jugulare, middle ear, 1960
Glossary of radiological terms, 367–373
Glottic tumours, 1976–1977
Glucagonoma, 1032
  embolization, 2147
Gluteal arteriography, 2033
Gluten-sensitive enteropathy (coeliac disease), 841, *843*
Glycogen
  plaques, oesophageal, 769
  storage cardiomyopathy, 541, 639
Goitre, 1040
  intrathoracic, 1024
Gonadal venography, 2084–2086
  anatomy, 2084
  indications, 2085–2086
  technique, 2084–2085
Gonadoblastoma, ovarian, 1593, 1615
Gonadotrophin, 1036
  -releasing hormone, 1036
    males, 1038
Goodpasture's syndrome, 266
Gorham's disease, **1293**
Gorlin's syndrome, 1915, 1922
Gortex graft, 575
Gout, **1491–1494**
  articular, 1492
  differential diagnosis, 1492–1494
  feet, 1491–1492
  hand, 1491–1492
  other joints, 1492
  tophaceous, 1492
Graft vs host disease
  oesophageal involvement, 769
  small bowel, 855
Granuloma
  eosinophilic *see* Eosinophilic granuloma
  extradural, 1849
  giant cell reparative, 1907
  idiopathic orbital (psuedo-tumour), 1888–1889
  periapical, 1932
  syphilitic, 1360
  tuberculous, liver, ultrasound, children, 2216
  Wegener's, orbital manifestations, 1889
Granulomatous disease, chronic, **1354**
Graphic stress telethermography, 1660
Gravigard (Copper 7), 1621
Gray (Gy), definition, 16
Greig's ocular hypertelorism, 1915
Greig's syndrome, 1881
Growth
  hormone, 1022
    in hyperpituitarism, 1389–1390
    releasing factor, 1022
  plate, changes in scurvy, 1388
    disorders, 1416–1424
    in metabolic and endocrine diseases, 1369–1370
    see also specific names
  retardation, intrauterine, sonography, 1567–1569, 1575
    amniography, 1583
  see also Acromegaly: Dwarfism
Guillain-Barré syndrome in spinal cord enlargement, 1849

Guinea worm *see* Dracunculosis
Gummas, syphilitic, 1360
Gunshot injury
  arteriography, 2025
  kidney, 1170
Gynaecoid pelvis, 1587
Gynaecology, **1593–1629**
  acute abdomen, 740
  computed tomography, 1594
  hysterosalpingography, 1595–1597
  pituitary fossa, 1594
  plain radiography, 1593–1594
  skeleton, 1594
Gyne T (Copper T), 1621

Haemangioblastoma
  cerebellar, CT, 1714–1715
  spinal, **1854**
Haemangioendothelioma, **1324**
  orbital effects, 1891
Haemangioma
  bone, **1293**
  cavernous *see* Cavernous haemangiomas
  cranial vault, 1791, *1792*
  with enchondromatosis, 1278
  larynx, 1979
  liver, CT scanning, 937
    ultrasound, 931
      children, 2215
  mandible, 1907
  paranasal sinuses, 1948
  renal, 1102
  small bowel, 843
  spinal cord, 1841, 1842, *1843*
  tibia, arteriography, 2052
Haemangiopericytoma, **1294**
  orbital effects, 1891
Haematocolpos, 1036
  ultrasonography, 1601–1602
Haematologic disorders, with osteosclerosis, 1404
Haematoma
  calcification, 1519
  complicating hysterectomy, 1622
  epidural (extradural) spontaneous, **1783–1786**, 1841
  extracranial, **1783–1786**
  intracerebral, magnetic resonance imaging, 69, *73*
  intramural, duodenum, 824
    oesophageal, *770*, 771
  intrarenal, 1100, 1159
  liver, ultrasound, 930
    children, 2215
  perirenal, 1160
  pulmonary, 306
  subdural, **1783–1786**
  subscapular, 1159–1160, 1173, *1174*
Haematopoiesis, extramedullary, 192
Haematuria, angiography, 1048
  and calculi, 1060
  post-traumatic, 1171, 1177
Haemobilia, 940
Haemochromatosis, **1495–1496**
  heart involvement, 638
Haemodialysis, prolonged, causing erosions, mandibular condyle, 1917
Haemoglobinopathies, **1328–1332**
Haemolytic anaemia
  chronic, **1328–1332**
  congenital, 1468–1470
Haemophilia, 1345, 1346
  arthropathy, 1498

  articular haemorrhages, 1457
  pseudotumour, 1347
Haemopneumothorax, 306
Haemopoiesis, extramedullary, 1334
Haemorrhage
  arteriography, 2021
  brain, ultrasound, neonate, 2230, 2233
  complicating portography, 2081
  complicating splenoportography, 2080
  intracerebral, radionuclide scanning, 1865
  intracranial traumatic, 1783–1786
  lung, 256–266, 287, 294
  puncture site, arteriography, 1999–2000
  renal, spontaneous, 1159–1160
  subretinal, 1894
  uterine, arteriography, 1598
  see also other specific types
Haemorrhagic
  bone cyst, 1906
  infarction, 1758
Haemosiderosis, idiopathic, 266
Haemostasis
  endoscopic, 830
  techniques, 830
Haemothorax, 158, 163
Hall-Kaster valve, 664
Hamartomas, liver, ultrasound, children, 2215
  lung, 250, *251*
Hampton's hump, 319
Hampton's line, *790, 791*
Hancock valve, 664, *665*
Hand
  arteriography, *2046*, 2047
  -foot syndrome of sickle cell anaemia, 1469
  in gout, 1491–1492
  injuries, bones, **1259–1261**
    baseball ('mallet') fracture, 1261
    Bennett fracture-dislocation, 1260
    boxer's fracture, 1260
    Rolando fracture, 1260
    skier's (gamekeeper's) thumb, 1260
    volar plate fracture, 1261
  in Reiter's syndrome, 1490
  in rheumatoid arthritis, **1478**
    juvenile, 1482
Hand-Schuller-Christian disease, 274, 1342, 1459
Hangman's fracture, 1231
Harken valve, 664, 668
Hashimoto's thyroiditis, 1025
Hassall's corpuscles, 1027
Haustra, 772, 859, *860, 888*
Head
  injury, angiography, 1701
    CT, 1700–1701
    late effects, 1788
    radiography, 1700
    radionuclide scanning, 1863–1864
    see also Brain trauma: Skull trauma
  and neck arteriography, 2027–2030
  size, abnormal, radiography, 1703
    ultrasound, 1703
Headache
  angiography, 1701
  CT, 1701
  radiography, 1701
Heart
  acquired disease, **551–715**
  advanced imaging modalities, 439–453
  alcoholic disease, 640
  amyloid disease, 639
  anatomy, echocardiography, 395–408
    normal, 382–392

Heart (*cont.*)
  aneurysm *see* Aneurysm, cardiac
  angiography, 382
    see also Catheters and catheterization
  arrhythmia complicating catheterization, 611
  arteries, abnormal connections, congenital, 463
    identification, 474
    transposition *see* Transposition
    see also Coronary artery
  atrial appendages, apposition, 528
    enlargement, 555
  atrial isomerism, right, 545
  atrial septal defect, **478–486**
    angiocardiography, 484–486
    associations, 484
    before and after closure, *480*
    echocardiography, 481–484
    Eisenmenger reaction, 505, *506*
    endocardial cushion, 479, *480*, 481
    ostium primum, *486*
    ostium secundum, 479, *480*
    radiology, 481
    sinus venosus, 479
    types, 479
  atrial situs, determination, 474
  atrioventricular concordance, 517
  atrium, common, 508–512
  bicuspid aortic valve, 602–603
  calcification *see* Calcification, heart
  catheterization *see* Catheters and cardiac catheterization, cardiac
  central cyanosis, 497–525
  chambers, **384–390**
    abnormal connections (discordance), 517–524
    common, cause of central cyanosis, 508–517
    congenital anomalies, angiography, 471–473
    orientation, 382
    sequential identification and analysis, 473–475
    see also Heart, enlargement
  chordal rupture, 592–593
  CT *see* Computed tomography, heart
  congenital conditions, **457–548**
    anatomical deformity, cause of cyanosis, 463
    chamber identification, 471–473
    classification, principles, 473–475
    cyanosis, central, 461–463
    diagnosis, 461–463
    echocardiography, 470
    infantile heart failure due to, 545–546
    left heart, 527–535
    pulmonary arterial hypertension, obstructive, 466
    pulmonary oedema and venous congestion, 465, *466*
    pulmonary perfusion, 462, *464–466*
    radiography, conventional, 463–470
      diagnostic features, 464–470
    right heart, 527–535
    shape, 468
    situs abnormalities, 542–545
    size, 468
    skeletal features, 469
    terminology, 473–475
    types of abnormality, 461
    see also individual conditions
  congestive heart failure, **316–318**

  congestive myopathy, **635–641**
    differential diagnosis, 638–641
    familial, 641
  dextrocardia, primary, 542–545
  dextroversion (dextrorotation), 544–545
  diastolic volume overload, 468
  digital subtraction radiography *see* Digital radiography, heart
  double outflow right ventricle, 512, *513*
  double shadow, 555
  Ebstein's anomaly, 528–530
  echocardiography *see* Echocardiography
  Eisenmenger reaction (pulmonary arteriolar obstruction), 466, 492, **505–507**, 567, *575*, 580
  embryonic development, 457–459
  endocardial fibro-elastosis, 541
  endocarditis, 597, *713*
  enlargement, **551–563**
    biventricular, 561
    congestive myopathy, 636
    displacement of oesophagus, 779
    echocardiography, 553
    mitral disease, 556
    rheumatic disease, 586
    selective chamber, 553–562
      left atrial, 553–556
      left ventricular, 556–558
      right atrial, 560
      right ventricular, 558–560
  failure, congestive, 316–318
    definition, 369
    diphtheria, 638
    hypertensive, 641
    infantile, 545–546
  Fallot's tetralogy *see* Tetralogy of Fallot
  fluoroscopy, 380
  Gerbode defect, 487, 491
  glycogen storage myopathy, 541
  high cardiac output states, pulmonary vascularity, 574
  hypertrophic myopathy, **642–645**
    pulmonary vascularity, 573
  hypoplastic left heart syndrome, 495, **538–540**, 703
    cause of central cyanosis, 524
  infantile myopathy, 541
  infections, 638
    pacemaker as cause of, 660, *661*
  infective endocarditis, 668, *670*, 671, *713*
  inferior vena cava, infrahepatic interruption, 528
  infiltrations, 638
  intracardiac injections, contrast media, 109
  intraventricular thrombus, 629
  inversed relationship, 475
  ischaemic disease, **609–633**
    clinical syndromes, 620–625
    CT scanning, myocardial ischaemia, 444
    echocardiography, left ventricular function, 619–620
    isotopes, 380
    ventriculography, 381
  laevoversion, 545
  left atrial myxoma, 647–649
  left atrial thrombus, differentiation from LA myxoma, 647
  loop rule of van Praagh, 542
  magnetic resonance imaging, 87, *88*, 381, **447–449**
  mass, echocardiography, 416
  millisecond cine CT scan, *7*
  murmur, rheumatic mitral valve disease, 586

  muscle diseases, 635–646
  myopathy, congestive, pulmonary vascularity, *569*, 573
    echocardiography, 416
    hypertrophic, 642–645
      pulmonary vascularity, 573
    infantile, 541
    radionuclide ventriculography, 426–428
    restrictive, endomyocardial fibrosis, 646
  paediatric conditions, echocardiography, 414
    heart failure, 545–546
    see also Heart, congenital conditions
  papillary muscle dysfunction, 593
  patent ductus arteriosus, Eisenmenger reaction, 506
  performance, echocardiography, 413
  pericardium *see* Pericardium
  post-cardiotomy syndrome, caused by pacemaker, 660
  pulmonary vascularity in heart disease, 568–575
  pump failure, 468, 542
  radiograph, 142
  radiography techniques, 382
  radiology techniques, 379–382
  right atrial obstruction, central cyanosis, 497–499
  right ventricular obstruction, central cyanosis, 499–505
  rupture, myocardial infarction, 627
  shape, congenital conditions, 468
  shunt, aorto-pulmonary, 492–495
    cyanotic congenital disease, 461–463
    left-to-right, 477–496
      infancy, 546
      radiological features, 478
      pulmonary vascularity, 574–575
      radionuclide imaging, 419
      ventriculography, 428
    systemic arteriovenous, 546
  situs, congenital anomalies, 542–545
    inversus, 542, *543*
    solitus, 542, *543, 544*
  size, cardio-thoracic ratio, 551, *552*
    cause of pulmonary oedema, in the newborn, 350, *351*
    congenital conditions, 468
    echocardiography, M-mode, 410–413
    left-to-right shunt, 478
    transverse cardiac diameter, 551
    see also Heart, enlargement
  skeletal abnormalities in heart disease, 562
  stenosis, in tetralogy of Fallot, 501
  superior vena cava, left, persistence of, 527, *528*
  surgery, post-operative radiograph, 323
    trauma, 651
  Taussig-Bing deformity, 514
  technetium-labelled polyphosphate, 381
  thallium scanning, 381
  thromboembolism, 294
  transposition of great arteries *see* Transposition
  traumatic injury, 310, 650
  tumours, 647–650
  Uhl's anomaly, 530
  valves, disease, acquired, **585–607**
    echocardiography, 416
    radionuclide ventriculography, 428
    disruptions, 651
    insufficiency, pacemaker causing, 660
    motion, echocardiography, *411*, 414
    prostheses *see* Valves, prostheses

Heart (*cont.*)
  valves, disease, acquired (*cont.*)
    see also Mitral: Tricuspid: Valves
  venoatrial concordance, 517
  ventricle(s) see Left ventricles: Ventricles
  viral myocarditis, 638
  volume, 552
  wall dynamics, CT scanning, 444
  see also Aorta: Cardiovascular system:
    'Coronary' entries
Heartburn, 748
Heavy chain disease, 1341
Heavy metal poisoning, **1408**
Heel in rheumatoid arthritis, 1479, *1480*
Hemianopia
  angiography, 1703
  CT, 1703
  radiography, 1703
Hemiatrophy, traumatic, 1788
Hemiazygos venography, 2074–2075
Hemiplegia
  CT, 1701
  radiography, 1701
Hemithorax
  hypertransradiant causes, 238 (*table*)
  opaque, ultrasound, children, 2214
Hepatic
  arteriography, 2021, 2039, *2042*
  artery embolization, 2147, *2148*, *2149*
    infusions, 2192–2193
    see also Liver metastases
    therapeutic infusions, 2192–2193
  deposits, liver scintigraphy, 2180
    CT, 2180
  venography, 945, **2078–2079**
    anatomy, 2078
    indications, 2079
    technique, 2078
    thrombosis causes, 2079
  see also Liver
Hepatitis
  neonatal, 945
  in osteomalacia, 1378
  scintigraphy, 936
  ultrasound, children, 2214
Hepatobiliary disease in children, radionuclide
  imaging, 2203–2204
Hepatoblastomas, ultrasound, children, 2214
Hepatolenticular degeneration see Wilson's
  disease
Hepatomas, ultrasound, children, 2214
  see also Liver tumours
Hepatomegaly, ultrasound, children, 2214
  see also Liver, enlarged
Hernia
  Bochdalek, 170, *171*, *333*, 334
  definition, 369
  diaphragmatic, 170–172, 190
  gut, following diaphragmatic rupture, 310
  hiatus, 172, 190, **749–750**, *805*
    and gastro-oesophageal reflux, in infants,
      915
  Morgagni, 170, *171*, 190, 334
  strangulated, 723
Herpes
  colitis, 890
  oesophagitis, 756–757
  simplex encephalitis, 1742–1743
Hiatus hernia, 172, 190, **749–750**, *805*
  and gastro-oesophageal reflux, in infants, 915
HIDA see Radioisotope scanning
Hila, **116–119**
  adenopathy, in sarcoidosis, 276

atelectasis, 222
  blood vessels, *115*, 116
  CT scans, *118*
  definition, 369
  enlargement, unilateral, in bronchial
    carcinoma, 243, *245*
  lymph node metastases, 246
  lymphadenopathy, 186, *187*, 291
  radiograph, 142
Hilar tumours see Bile duct tumours
Hill gastropexy, 780
Hill-Sachs fracture, humeral head, 1249
Hip
  arthrography, **1506**
  avascular necrosis, in haemophilia, 1347
  congenital dislocation (infantile hip
    dysplasia), **1450–1452**
    radiographic assessment, 1451–1452
  dislocation, **1243–1244**
  fractures in children, 1462
    CT scan, *1525*
  injuries, **1261–1264**
    see also Femur
  prostheses, radionuclide bone scan, 1542
  rheumatoid arthritis, **1479**
    juvenile, 1482
^{123}-Hippuran
  kidney transplantation, 1143
  in renal artery stenosis, 1153
Hirschsprung's disease, 916, *917*
  megacolon, 893
Histiocytic lymphoma, lung involvement, 254
Histiocytoma, fibrous, malignant, 1316, *1317*
Histiocytoses (non-lipoid histiocytoses), **1341–
  1344**
  malignant, 845
  see also Eosinophilic granuloma
Histology, tumour, and radiological findings,
  2167–2168
  and gallium imaging, relationship, 2189–
    2190
Histoplasmosis affecting bone, 1364
  gastric, 796
  mediastinal effects, 187
  pulmonary, 213
HLA-B27 antigen in ankylosing spondylitis,
  1486, 1488
Hodgkin's disease, **1336–1337**
  causing laryngeal displacement, 1981
  clinical features, 1336
  cysts following thymic irradiation, 177
  differential diagnosis, 1337
  gallium imaging, 2189
  infiltrating kidneys, 1121
  lung involvement, 253, *254*
  radiological features, 1336–1337
  radionuclide bone scan, 1336–1337
  staging, radiology, 2176
Holoprosencephaly, 1770
Holt-Oram syndrome, heart anomalies, 470
Homeokinesis, 1017–1018
Homeostasis, 1017–1018
Homogeneous, definition, 369
Homovanillic acid in neuroblastoma, 1206
Hormonal disorders
  associated with oesophagus, 776
Hormones, 1017
  abbreviations, 1018 (*table*)
  ectopic, 1020
  feed-back mechanisms, 1018
  first use of term, 1018
  half-life, 1018
  see also specific names and disorders

Horner's syndrome, 248
Horseshoe kidney, 1187
  and calculi, 1061
Hounsfield scale, CT numbers, 43
  unit, definition, 369
'Housemaid's knee', 1511
Hufnagle value, 668
Human chorionic gonadotrophin
  radioimmunoassay in ectopic pregnancy,
    1559–1560, 1562
Humeral condyle, lateral, fracture, 1252–1253
  epiphyseal line, not a fracture, 1464
  head fractures, 1249–1250
    Hill-Sachs, 1249
  notches, simulating neoplasia, 1460
Hunter's syndrome, **1434**
Huntington's chorea, 1745
Hurler's syndrome, *1433*, **1434**, 1452, *1453*,
  1918
  heart involvement, 639
Huygen's principle, 30
Hyaline membrane disease, 346
Hydatid cysts (echinoccocosis), 217
  CT, 1744
  kidney, 1099
    CT, 1099
    ultrasound, 1099
  liver, CT scanning, 938
  pulmonary, 217
  ultrasound, 930
Hydatid disease
  biliary tract, 985
  of bone, **1364–1365**
  ultrasound, children, 2216
Hydatiform mole, sonography, **1562–1563**
Hydramnios, sonography, 1564, **1575–1576**
  causes, 1574 (*table*)
Hydranencephaly, **1771**
  fetal, sonography, 1576–1577
Hydrocalycosis, 1125
  obstructive, 1068
Hydrocephalus
  CNS shunts, radionuclide imaging, 2207
  communicating, **1793–1794**, *1795*
    and atrophy, 1794 (*table*)
      external, **1794**
    neonatal, 1794
    ultrasound, 1794
    ventricular shunting procedures, 1795
  CT, 1869
  fetal, sonography, 1576
  magnetic resonance imaging, 76, *77*
  radionuclide cisternography, **1867–1870**
    compensated, 1868
    non-obstructive, 1868
    normal pressure versus cerebral atrophy,
      1868–1869
    obstructive, 1867–1868
    paediatric, 1869
    shunt patency studies, 1869–1870
  following subarachnoid haemorrhage, 1748
  ultrasound, neonate, 2230, 2232
  ventriculography, 1703
  water soluble CT cisternography, 1703
Hydronephrosis
  complicating renal trauma, 1177
  obstructive, 1068
    grading, 1068
    intravenous urography, 1073
  simulating kidney mass, 1101
  transient, complicating hysterectomy, 1623
    radiotherapy complication, 1624
  ultrasound, children, 2225

Hydropneumothorax, 205
Hydrops fetalis
    amniography, 1581
    sonography, 1577
        anatomical and functional anomalies, 1577
Hydrosalpinx, **1602–1603**, 1619
    hysterosalpingography, 1602–1603
    ultrasonography, 1603
Hydroureter
    obstruction, 1068
    transient, complicating hysterectomy, 1623
    ultrasound, children, 2225–2226
Hydroureteronephrosis of pregnancy, 1074
Hydroxyapatite deposition disease (HADD)
    calcification, 1496, 1517, *1518*, *1519*
25-Hydroxyvitamin D, 1371–1373
Hymen, imperforate, and vaginal atresia, 1600
    ultrasonography, 1601
Hyperaemia, definition, 369
Hyperaldosteronism, 1034
    venography, 2094
Hypercalcaemia, infantile
    idiopathic, soft tissue calcification, 1514
    peripheral pulmonary artery stenosis, 532
Hypercementosis, 1928
Hyperextension
    fracture-dislocation, **1231–1232**
    injuries of cervical spine, **1229–1232**
        dislocation, 1229–1231
        extension teardrop fracture, 1231
        fracture dislocation, 1231–1232
        hangman's fracture, 1231
Hyperflexion injuries of cervical spine, **1224–1226**
Hypernephroma *see* Renal cell carcinoma
Hyperostosis
    cortical bone disorders associated, **1407–1408**
    infantile, 1408
    skeletal, idiopathic, *1499*, 1500
Hyperoxaluria, calculus, 1064
Hyperparathyroidism, 1026
    and atherosclerosis, 2014, *2015*
    brown tumour, **1298**
    and periodontal disease, 1934
    primary, **1384–1387**
        differential diagnosis, 1386–1387
        PTH secretion, 1384
        radiological diagnosis, 1385
            pathological considerations, 1385–1386
        venography, 2093
    secondary and renal osteodystrophy, 1382, 1384
    soft tissue calcification, 1514
Hyperphosphatasia, **1395–1396**, **1432**
Hyperpituitarism, 1022, **1389–1392**
    in children, **1466**
    see also Acromegaly: Gigantism
Hypersplenism, embolization, 2156, *2157*, *2158*
Hypertelorism, 1915
Hypertension
    complicating renal trauma, 1177
    definition, 369
    heart failure, 641
    portal *see* Portal hypertension
    pulmonary *see* Pulmonary hypertension
    in renal transplantation, 1146–1147
    renovascular *see* Renovascular hypertension
Hyperthyroidism, **1392**
    in children, **1466**
Hypertrophic
    gastritis, 794, *795*
    pyloric stenosis, 805
        in infants, 913, 915, *916*

Hypertrophy, benign prostatic *see* Benign prostatic hypertrophy
Hypervitaminosis A, **1409**
Hypervitaminosis D, **1407**
Hypochondroplasia, 1419
Hypogammaglobulinaemia, bronchiectasis, 230
Hypogonadism, **1399–1400**
    see also Eunuchoidism: Turner's syndrome
Hypoparathyroidism, 1026, **1405–1406**
    effect on tooth enamel, 1927
    and periodontal disease, 1934
    radiological diagnosis, 1405
        pathological considerations, 1406
    soft tissue calcification, 1514
Hypoperfusion syndromes, 1865
Hypopharynx, malignant tumours, 1970–1971
Hypophosphataemia, x-linked and osteomalacia, 1378
Hypophosphatasia, 1495–1496
    and osteomalacia, 1378
    effect on tooth enamel, 1927
Hypopituitarism, 1023, **1397**
    in children, **1466**
Hypoplastic left heart syndrome, 495, 524, **538–540**, 703
Hypotelorism, 1880
Hypothalamic-pituitary axis, 1018
Hypothalamus/median eminence, 1020
Hypothyroidism, 1023, **1397–1399**
    delayed maturation, 1396
    infants, newborn, 1025
    radiological diagnosis, 1397
        pathological considerations, 1398–1399
Hypotonic duodenography, 1000
Hysterectomy, complications, 1622–1624
Hysterography, retained products of conception, 1617
Hysterosalpingography, 1038, **1595–1597**
    complications, 1596
    contraindicated in ectopic pregnancy, 1619
    contraindications, 1595
    endometrial carcinoma, 1608
    in endometriosis, 1620
    fibroids, 1605–1606
    hydrosalpinx, 1602
    indications, 1595
    normal variants, 1596–1597
    ovarian cysts, 1610
    radiological anatomy, 1596
    Stein-Leventhal syndrome, 1611
    technique, 1595
    in tubal plastic operations, 1620

[131]I-meta iodobenzyl guanidine, 1040
    phaeochromocytoma, 2095
[123]I-orthoiodohippurate, dynamic renal scan, 1052
Idiopathic juvenile osteoporosis, 1395
Ileal pouch, colonoscopy, 901
Ileocaecal valve, lipomatous infiltration, 892
Ileosigmoid knot, 729
Ileostomy, colonoscopy, 901
Ileum
    atresia, infants, 909, *910*
    gallstone, 724, 974
    meconium, 917–918
    paralytic, **730**, *731*
        causes, 726 (*table*)
Iliac artery stenoses, transluminal angioplasty, 2141, 2143
Iliac occlusion, 2018, *2019*
Iliopsoas abscess, CT scan, *1525*

Iliopsoas bursa, CT scan, *1525*
Imaging
    algorithmic system integration, 10
    cost-effectiveness, 10
    developments, 3–11
    equipment, 17–20
    -guided therapy, 2135
    techniques, 2125, 2132
    historical background, 3
Immobile cilia syndrome, 544
Immobilization
    of infants and young children for examination, 329
    prolonged, thromboembolism caused by, 294
Immune deficiency disease, thymus, 1028
Immune system, 1027
Immunoblastic lymphadenopathy, 188
Immunocompromised host, pulmonary disease, 296–289
Immunoglobulin deficiency, nodular lymphoid hyperplasia, 853
Immunology, radio-, in tumour detection, 2194
Implantation epidermoid, **1296**
Impotence, 1039
113m-In-DTPA (diethylene triamine pentaacetic acid), in brain scanning, 1858, 1858 (*table*)
Incontinence
    stress, radiological investigation, 1624
    urinary, urodynamics, 1214–1215
Incudomallear joint dislocations, 1963
Incudostapedial joint dislocations, 1963
Indium-111-labelled autologous white cells, in brain scanning, 1858, 1858 (*table*)
    in renal infection, 1057
Infant, brain, ultrasound, 2229–2234
    see also Brain, ultrasound, infant: Paediatric conditions: and under specific condition
Infantile cortical hyperostosis, **1408**, **1431–1432**
Infarct, definition, 369
Infarction
    cerebral, *see* Cerebral infarction
    definition, 370
    focal, in renal parenchymal disease, 1121
    liver, scintigraphy, 935
    myocardial *see* Myocardial infarction
    pulmonary, 294
        embolism, 576–578
    renal, 1155–1156
        radiology, 1156
    small intestine, 725
Infection and calcification, 1515–1517
    cardiac pacemaker causing, 660, *661*
    cardiac valve prosthesis causing, 668, *670*, 671
    children, bone imaging, 2199
    gas-forming, 739
    heart involvement, 638
    musculoskeletal, CT, 1524
    splenomegaly, 1012
    see also specific oragnisms and specific parts of the body
Infective arthritis, **1356**
Infective endocarditis, 668, *670*, 671, *713*
Inferior vena cava, 128, 303
    cavography, 945, **2067–2074**
        abnormal venous drainage, 2067
        absent, 2069
        anatomy, 2069–2070
        compression, 2071
        embryology, 2069
        extrinsic obstruction, 2071–2073
        following surgery or therapeutic

Inferior vena cava (*cont.*)
  cavography (*cont.*)
      obstruction, 2073–2074
    hepatic tumours causing, 2073
    hilar tumour, 982
    indications, 2070
    intrinsic obstruction, 2071–2073
    persistent left, 2069
    technique, 2070
    tumours, 2074
    in Wilms' tumour, 1204
  infrahepatic interruption, 528
  tumours, radionuclide studies, 2192
  ultrasound, 2114
    children, 2220
Infertility, hysterosalpingography, 1595
  male, 1038
Inflammatory conditions
  CT scanning, 56
  radionuclide, 22 (*table*)
  radionuclide bone scan, **1541–1542**
  spinal cord, 1848–1849
    intraspinal abscess, 1848–1849
    myelography, 1848
    tuberculous, 1849
Influenza A pneumonia, 203
Infusion techniques
  chemotherapy, arterial, liver, 941, *942, 943,* 2135
    hepatic metastases, 2192–2193
  constrictor agents, 2135–2136
  dilator agents, 2136
  thrombolytic agents, 2136
Iniencephaly, fetal, amniography, 1581
Injection accidents, arteriography, 2000, 2002
Inner ear
  auditory meatus, dilatation, 1965
  congenital anomalies, 1965
Insulinoma, 1031
  embolization, 2147
Interface, definition, 370
Interfacetal dislocation, bilateral, 1225–1226
  unilateral, 1226–1227
Intersex states, genitography, 1601
Interstitium, definition, 370
Intervention radiology, 8, **2121–2165**
  definition, 2122
  hepatobiliary system, 989–998
  impact, 2161
  see also Biopsy: Embolization:
      Percutaneous: Transluminal: Vascular
      techniques: and other procedures
Intervertebral disc, osteomyelitis, 1355–1356
Intervertebral fusions, 1798
Intracardiac injections, contrast media, 109
Intracerebral
  haematoma, magnetic resonance imaging, 69, *73*
  haemorrhage, traumatic, **1786–1787**
    ultrasound, neonate, 2230, 2233–2234
Intracranial
  arteriovenous infections, 1751–1755
  arteritis, 1765–1766
  CT scanning, 56
  haemorrhage, traumatic, **1783–1786**
  infections, **1739–1767**
    magnetic resonance imaging, 76, *77*
  pressure, raised, adults, 1707–1708
    children, 1705–1707
  pulmonary oedema, 265
Intracranial tumours, **1705–1737**
  angiography, 1719–1721, 1719 (*table*)
  CT, 1709–1712

effects of radiation therapy, 1718–1719
  incidence, 1708 (*table*)
  magnetic resonance imaging, 68, 70, *71*
  raised intracranial pressure, 1705–1708
  see also Brain tumours and specific names
Intramedullary
  abscess, 1849
  vascularity, 99m-Tc-sulphur colloid scan, 1544
Intraperitoneal fluid, 734
Intrarenal
  haematoma, 1159
  reflux, paediatric, 1200
  transit time in kidney transplantation, 1144
Intraspinal abscess, 1849
Intrauterine
  adhesions, 1617–1618
  contraceptive devices, 1620–1622
    complications, 1621–1622
    pregnancy with, sonography, *1562,* 1563
    ultrasonography, 1622
  growth retardation, amniography, 1583
    sonography, 1567–1569, 1575
Intravenous urography, 107, **1042–1047**
  bladder exstrophy, 1197
  bladder tumours, 1110
  calculi, 1062
  fibroids, 1606
  generalised small renal vessel disease, 1156
  in gynaecological conditions, 1597
  interpretation of findings, 1085
  in kidney injuries, 1171
  kidney, transplanted, 1142
  neuroblastoma, 1206
  paediatric, 1180–1181
    contrast media, 1181
    cystic disease of the kidney, 1188–1190
    renal pelvis, 1190–1196
    ureter, 1190–1196
  pelvic rhabdomyosarcoma, 1209
  prostatic carcinoma, 1085–1086
  prune belly syndrome, 1197
  in renal artery aneurysm, 1158, *1159*
  renal artery stenosis and renal hypertension, 1152, 1155
  renal infarction, 1156
  renal masses, 1090, *1092*
    with tomography, 1090
  renal transplantation, 1141
  in renal vein thrombosis, 1161
  stones, 1081–1082
  stress incontinence, 1624
  in ureter injuries, 1169
  ureteric, 1081–1082
    tumours, 1110–1111
  ureterocele, 1194
  urinary obstruction, **1069–1076**
    acute, 1069–1072
      dilatation, 1071
      increasingly dense, 1069–1071
      parenchymal rupture, 1072
      pyelosinus extravasation, 1071–1072
    benign, 1083
    infravesical obstructions, 1085–1086
    nonopaque filling defects, 1082
    urothelial tumours, 1082–1083
  Wilms' tumour, 1203, 1205
Intussusception, 724
  complicating colorectal carcinoma, 875
  infants, **918–920**
Iodine, as intravascular contrast medium, 99
Iodipamide, 963
Iodoxamate, 963

Ioglycamide, 963
Iohexol, formula, *103*
  myelography, 1802, 1805
Ionescu-Shiley valve, 664, *665*
Ionization, definition, 14
Iopamidol, formula, *103*
  myelography, 1802, 1805
Iothalamate, iodine-125 labelled, 1052
Iotroxinate, 963
Ioxaglic acid, formula, *103*
Iron deficiency anaemia, 1332
Ischaemia
  and arteriography, 2021
  cerebral, **1756–1766**
    see also Cerebral ischaemia
  heart disease *see* Heart, ischaemic disease
  small bowel, 851
Ischaemic colitis, 730
  complicating colorectal carcinoma, 875
Ischiopubic synchondrosis
  incompletely fused, 1240
  simulating neoplasia, 1460
Islets of Langerhans, 1031
Isobar, definition, 14
Isobaric transition, 15
Isolated heterotaxy, stomach, 805
Isomer, definition, 14
Isomeric transitions, 15
Isotone, definition, 14
Isotopes, 20–23
  clinical applications, 22–23 (*table*)
  definition, 14
  radioactive, heart, 380
  scanning, endocrine disease, 1020
    gastrointestinal bleeding, 2041
      paediatric, 1182
    parathyroid adenoma, 1027
    thyroid mass, 1024, 1025
  ventriculography, 381, 636
Isthmus, uterine, incompetence, 1618
IUDS *see* Intrauterine contraceptive devices
Ivemark syndrome, 545
Ivory osteomas, maxilla/mandible, 1907

Jaccoud's arthropathy, 1485
Jansen type of metaphyseal chondrodysplasia, 1430
Jaundice, **978**
  CT scanning, 970
  infants, 984
  obstructive, children, radionuclide imaging, 2203–2204
    flow chart, *992*
  ultrasound, 968
Jaws
  cysts, benign, 1904–1906
    nonepithelial bone, 1906, *1907*
    odontogenic keratocyst, 1906
  familial intra-osseous swellings (cherubism), 1913
  tumours, 1909–1910
    malignant, 1910–1912
      metastases, 1911–1912
  see also Mandible: Maxillofacial radiology
Jefferson bursting fracture, 1228–1229
  CT scan, 1228
Jejunum
  atresia, infants, 909, *910*
  diverticulosis, 851, *852*
  retrograde jejunal intussusception, 808
Jeune's syndrome, **1422**
Joint
  alignment in evaluation of arthritis, 1477

Joint (*cont.*)
　arthroplasty, CT scan, 1533
　biopsy, 2127
　disease, **1473–1508**
　　arthrography, 1505–1506
　　articular metaplasia, 1501–1505
　　connective tissue diseases, 1484–1491
　　crystal deposition arthropathies, 1491–
　　　1496
　　degenerative diseases of spine, 1500–1501
　　degenerative joint disorders, 1496–1500
　　in haemophilia, 1347
　　inflammatory (synovial), 1477–1484
　　　see also Rheumatoid arthritis and other
　　　　specific diseases
　　neoplasia, 1501–1505
　　organized observation, approach, 1477
　　osteochondrosis, 1501–1505
　　pathophysiological concepts, **1473–1477**
　　　bone erosions, 1476
　　　cartilage loss, multifactorial, 1475–1476
　　　generalised osteopenia, as chronic stage,
　　　　1476
　　　periarticular osteopenia, as acute stage,
　　　　1476
　　　soft tissue, first recognition, 1474–1475
　　　summation of mechanisms, 1473–1474
　　　synovial beginnings, 1474
　　infection, **1349–1367**
　see also specific joints
Jones fracture, fifth metatarsal base, 1266,
　1267, 1271
Joule/kilogram (J/kg), definition, 16
Judet projection of the hip, 1245
Jugular venography, 2064
Juvenile
　benign cortical defect *see* Fibroma, non-
　　ossifying
　chronic polyarthritis (Still's disease), **1481–
　　1484**
　　complications, 1484
　　differential diagnosis, 1484
　　radiological findings, 1482–1484
　rheumatoid arthritis, **1456–1457**
Juxtacortical chondroma, 1278
Juxtacortical chondrosarcoma, 1309
Juxtadiaphragmatic masses, ultrasound,
　children, 2214

Kallikrein conversion test, 106
Kartagener's syndrome, 230, *543*, 544
Kay-Shiley valve, 664, 668
Kay-Suzuki valve, 664
Kempson, ossifying fibroma, 1297
Keratosis obturans, external ear, 1959
Kerley lines, 146, 147, 317, **568–570**
Kidneys
　anatomical causes of calculi, 1060, 1063
　calculi *see* Calculi, kidney
　colic, 739, *740*
　contrast media, intravascular, 107
　cysts, 1097–1099, *1100*
　　see also Cysts, renal
　disease, digital subtraction angiography,
　　2108
　　and osteomalacia, 1378
　duplex, excretion urography, 1118
　effective renal plasma flow, 1052
　failure, *see* Renal failure
　function, tests, after contrast medium, 108
　glomerular filtration rate, 1052
　infection, gallium-67, 1057

indium-111-labelled autologous white
　cells, 1057
injuries, **1170–1177**
　aetiology, 1070
　angiography, 1172
　classification, 1173–1177
　complications, 1177
　contused, 1173
　CT scans, 1172
　evaluation, 1070–1073
　　algorithm, 1072
　haematuria, 1170–1171
　intravenous urography, 1171–1172
　laceration, 1173–1174
　pedicle injuries, 1176
　plain radiography, 1171
　shattered, 1175
　therapy, 1173–1177
　ultrasound, 1173
　uretero-pelvic junction disruption, 1175
magnetic resonance imaging, 85
masses, **1089–1108**
　abscesses, 1099
　acute lobar nephronia, 1099
　algorithms, 1091, *1093, 1096*
　angiomyolipomas, 1100–1101
　arteriography, 1094–1095
　computed tomography, 1093, 1095, 1097
　differentiation from cysts, 1090
　hydronephrosis, 1101
　intravenous urography, 1090, *1092*
　malakoplakia, 1100
　metastases, 1105
　needle aspiration, 1094
　neoplastic, 1102–1106
　　benign, 1102
　　malignant, 1102–1106
　　see also specific headings
　non-cystic, algorithm, evaluation, *1093*
　non-neoplastic, 1096–1102
　non-renal, 1101
　plain abdominal radiography, 1089–1090
　pseudotumour, algorithm, evaluation,
　　1091, *1093*
　pseudotumours, pathological, 1096–1102
　radionuclide imaging, 1091
　retrograde pyelography, 1094, *1096*
　sinus lipomatosis, 1101
　ultrasonography, 1091–1094
　　children, 2224–2225
　vascular, 1100
　xanthogranulomatous pyelonephritis, 1099
nuclear medicine, 1051–1057
obstruction, 1067–1087
　chronic partial, 1069
　intravenous urography, 1069–1076
　　acute, 1069–1072
　　chronic, 1072–1076
　　crescents, 1072
　　hydronephrosis, 1073
　　hydroureteronephrosis of pregnancy,
　　　1074
　　increasingly dense, 1069–1071
　　intermittent, 1075
　　nephrogram, 1072
　　non-obstructive dilatations, 1075
　　parenchymal rupture, 1072
　　parenchymal thickness, 1072
　　postobstructive atrophy, 1069, 1073
　　pyelosinus extravasation, 1071–1072
　　renal size, 1072
　　rims and shells, 1073, *1074*
　see also Urinary obstruction

paediatric abnormalities, **1185–1190**
　cystic disease, 1188–1190
　ectopy, 1187
　embryonic, 1183
　fusion abnormalities, 1187
　horseshoe, 1187
　malrotation, 1187
　pancake, 1188
　pelvic, 1187
　renal agenesis, bilateral, 1186
　　unilateral, 1185–1186
　thoracic, 1187
solitary, *1140*
static renal scan, 1055, *1057*
tomography, 1045
total renal function, 1052
transplantation *see* Transplantation, kidney
tumour, CT scan, *51*
　see also Kidney masses
ultrasound, children, 2222–2226
　see also Renal: Urinary tract
Kienbock's disease, 1502
Killian's dehiscence, 1972
Klebsiella aerogenes, gas formation, 739
Klebsiella pneumoniae pneumonia, 202
Klinefelter's syndrome, 1400
Klippel-Feil syndrome, **1449–1450**
Klippel-Trenaunay syndrome, 2091
Knee(s)
　arthropathy, **1505–1506**
　bowing, physiological, 1452, *1454*
　injuries, **1264**
　　epiphyseal fractures, 1264
　　patella fractures, 1264
　joints, rheumatoid arthritis, **1479**
　　juvenile, 1482, *1483*
　prostheses, radionuclide bone scan, 1542
Knife injuries, kidney, 1170
Köhler's disease, tarsal scaphoid, children,
　1463
Krukenberg tumours, ovarian, 1615
KUB *see* Abdomen, plain radiography
Kyphiscoliosis, 156
Kyphosis, juvenile *see* Scheuermann's disease
Kyphotic angulation, localized, 1224

Labour, conditions affecting, sonography, 1579
Labyrinth, fractures involving, 1963
　congenital deformity, 1965
Lacrimal
　gland tumours, 1891–1892
　　CT, 1892
　system, contrast examination, 1880
　　radionuclide, 22 (*table*)
Lacunar
　infarcts, 1757, *1758*
　skull, 1775
Ladd's bands, 912–913
Laennec's cirrhosis, 853
Lamina
　dura, erosion, 1707
　fracture, *5*
　necrosis, radionuclide scanning, 1865
Lap seat-belt injuries, 1237, *1239*
Laparoscopic sterilisation,
　hysterosalpingography following, 1595
Laparotomy, cardiopulmonary disease
　following, 314–321
Laryngocele, 1979–1980
Laryngography, 1974–1975
Laryngotracheobronchitis (croup), obstruction,
　341, 342, 343
Larynx, **1973–1981**

Larynx (*cont.*)
  anatomy, 1975
  carcinoma, 1975–1976
  chondrosarcoma, 1978
  cine radiography, 1975
  CT, 1975
  cysts, 1978–1979
  extrinsic displacement, 1981
  fibrosarcoma, 1978
  Hodgkin's disease, 1981
  infections, 1979
  inflammatory disease, 1979
  laryngocele, 1979–1980
  laryngography, 1974–1975
  obstruction, 340
  papilloma, 1978
  polypoid tumour mass, 1978
  radiography, 1973
  recurrent laryngeal paralysis, 1981
  sarcoma, 1978
  stenosis, 1979
  thyroid tumours, 1981
  tomography, 1974
  trauma, 1979
  tumours, 1975–1979
    benign, 1978–1979
    malignant, 1975–1978
  xerography, 1973–1974
Lateral humeral condyle fracture, 1252–1253
Le Fort fractures, **1899–1900**
  radiography, 1902
Lead
  poisoning, **1408**
    in children, **1467**
  -zirconate-titanate (PZT), 26
Left ventricular
  ejection fraction, digital subtraction
    angiography, 2107–2108
  function, echocardiography, 619–620
    prostheses, effects, 673
  wall motion, digital subtraction angiography,
    2107–2108
Left ventriculography, 617–619
  and digital subtraction angiography, 2108
  myocardial infarction, 623–625
Leg
  arteriography, 2048–2053
  fractures in children, 1462
  see also specific bones
Legg-Perthes disease, 1502, *1503*, 1504
Legionella pneumophila, 202
Leiomyomas
  during pregnancy, *1566*, 1567
  gastric, 799, *800*
  oesophageal, 761
  small bowel, 842, *844*
  vascular, orbital effects, 1891
Leiomyosarcoma
  duodenum, *822*
  gastric, malignant, 804
  small bowel, 845, *846*
  ultrasonography, 1610
Lenticular opacity, ultrasound, 1894
Leontiasis ossium, 1947
Leprosy, 1362–1363
  and calcification, 1515
  calcification of peripheral nerves, 1363
  neuropathic changes, 1362–1363
  nose involvement, 1946
  osteitis, 1362
Leptomeningeal cysts, 1782–1783
Leriche syndrome, arteriography, 2019–2020
Letterer-Siwe disease, 274, **1341**, *1342*

in children, 1458–1459
Leukaemias, **1334–1335**
  acute, childhood, *1469*, 1470
    lymphocytic, 1334
    myeloblastic, 1334
  clinical features, 1334
  diffuse destruction of bone, 1334
  infiltrating kidneys, 1121
  and malignant lymphoma, 187, *188*
  metaphyseal lesions, 1334
  mixed lesions, 1334
  osteoblastic lesions, 1334
  osteolytic lesions, 1334
  periosteal lesions, 1334
  radiological features, 1334–1335
Leukoagglutinin transfusion reaction, lung
    effects, 287, *288*
Leukodystrophies, congenital, 1745
Leukoencephalopathy
  acute haemorrhagic, 1742
  progressive multifocal, 1742
Leukoplakia
  differential diagnosis from urothelial
    tumours, 1112
  and urinary tract infection, 1131
Leukoria, 1881
Ligaments, pulmonary, inferior, 119
Lillehei-Kaster valve, 664
'Limey bile', 960, 976
Line
  definition, 370
  shadow, barium, 865
Lingual arteries, calcification, 1922
Linitis plastica, 802
Lipodystrophy, fat measurement, 1509, *1510*
Lipoma, *1512*, 1513
  chest wall, *152*
  CT scan, 1526, *1528*
  intracranial, CT, 1714
  intraosseous, **1295–1296**
    CT scan, 1296
  large bowel, 892
  maxillofacial, 1907
  small bowel, 799, 843
  spinal, 1823–1824
  spinal cord, 1846, *1847*
  subperiosteal, **1295–1296**
    CT scan, 1296
  xeroradiography, *1511*
Lipomatosis
  mediastinal, 193
  pelvic, causing obstruction, 1083, *1084*
  sinus, renal, 1101
Liposarcoma, **1324**
  CT scan, 1526, *1528*
  mediastinal, 192
Lippes loop, 1620
Liquid crystal thermography, 1660
Lisfranc injuries, 1270–1271
Lithium, cardiac pacemakers, 654
'Little leaguer's elbow', 1253
Liver, **925–953**
  abnormalities, 945–951
  abscess, **948**
    CT scanning, 938
    scintigraphy, 934
    ultrasound, 930, *931*
  anatomy, segmental, 957 (*table*)
  arterial embolization, 995–997
  arteries, 940
  arteriography, 940–941, 2021, 2039, *2040*
  atrophy, 981
  barium studies, 928–930

bleeding, embolization, 2146, *2148*, *2149*
bright liver pattern (ultrasound), *932*
calcification, 927, 928 (*table*)
cirrhosis, causing portal hypertension, 949
  scintigraphy, 935
congenital lesions, 945
CT scanning, *44*, **936–939**, 2180
  artefacts, *47*
  examination technique, 936
  intravenous contrast medium, 50
cysts, **948**
  CT scanning, 938
dark liver pattern (ultrasound), *933*
deposits, scintigraphy and CT, 2180
diffuse disease, CT scanning, 939
  scintigraphy, 935–936
  ultrasound, 932
embolization, 941, 995, 997
  bleeding, 2146, 2147, *2148*, *2149*
enlarged, 927, *929*
  barium studies, 928
  children, ultrasound, 2214
fatty infiltration, CT scanning, 939
fluoroscopy, 928
focal disease, CT scanning, 936–939
  nodular hyperplasia, 947
  scintigraphy, 934–935
  ultrasound, 930
function, biochemical tests, 959
gas within, 928
gross anatomy, 925–927
haemangioma, CT scanning, 937
  ultrasound, 931
haematoma, ultrasound, 930
hydatid cyst, *51*
imaging, children, 2203
  see also specific techniques
infarction, scintigraphy, 935
infusion chemotherapy, arterial, 941, 2192–
    2193
investigation, methods, 927–945
magnetic resonance imaging, 83, 939
metastases, **948**
  arteriography, infusion, *939*, 940
  infusion chemotherapy, *942*, *943*, 2192
  scintigraphy, 934, 948, 2180, 2184
  survival, 2192
    chemotherapeutic infusions, 2192
  ultrasound, 948
neonatal disorders, 945
normal, scintigraphy, 933–934
  variants, scintigraphy, 934
in osteomalacia, 1378
plain film diagnosis, 927–928
polycystic disease in neonates, 945
radionuclide imaging, 2183–2185
  comparison with CT and ultrasound,
    2184–2185
Riedel's lobe, 945
scintigraphy, 933–936
  in hepatic metastases, 934, 948, 2180, 2184
subtraction techniques, 945
trauma, **949**
  CT scanning, 938
  scintigraphy, 936
tumours, 945–948
  adenoma, 947
  arterial embolization, 995–997
  arteriography, 2021
  assessment by arteriography, 940
  carcinoma, hepatocellular, 947
  children, 985
  CT scanning, *42*, 937–938

Liver (*cont.*)
  tumours (*cont.*)
    haemangioma, cavernous, 945–947
    investigation, **951**
    magnetic resonance imaging, 83, *84*
    and oral contraception, 1622
    scintigraphy, 934, 935, 2180, 2184
    ultrasound, 931, *932*
  ultrasound, 930–933
    children, 2214–2216
    gain settings, *35*
    linear scan, *28*
    malignant, 931, *932*
    mass lesions, 931
    metastases *see* Liver, metastases
    normal, *32*
    sector scan, *28*
    shadowing, *34*
  vascular studies, 945
  vascular interventional techniques,
    arteriography, 941
  vascular supply, 957–958
  venography, 945, 2078–2079
    see also Hepatic venography : Portal
      hypertension : Portography
Loa-Loa, calcification, 1516
Lobar nephronia, acute, 1099
Lobe, definition, 370
Lobectomy, post-operative radiograph, 321
Lobule, definition, 370
Local, definition, 370
Localized kyphotic angulation, 1224
Loeffler's syndrome, 282, 284
Loopography, paediatric, 1182
'Looser's zones', 1373
  in osteomalacia, 1379, 1380
Lorain dwarfism, 1023
Lotasul, chemical structure, *103*
Low back pain syndrome, CT scan, 1529–1532
Lower limb, arteriography, *2026*, 2048, 2053
  emboli, 2051
  femoral, 2048–2051
  indications, 2049–2050
  percutaneous transluminal angioplasty,
    2141–2143
  tumours, 2051
  vascular malformations, 2053
  vascular occlusive disease, 2141
  venography, 2088–2091
    anatomy, 2088
    artefacts, 2089
    complications, 2088–2089
    contraindications, 2088
    deep venous thrombosis, 2089–2090
    indications, 2089–2091
    post-phlebitic syndrome, 2090
    technique, 2088
      ascending, 2088
      descending, 2088
    varicose veins, 2090–2091
Lumbar
  aortography, 2031–2032
    atherosclerosis, 2031
    congenital lesions, 2031
    tumour, 2031–2032
  discitis, 1355, *1356*
  intervertebral discs, CT scan, 1529
  spine, injuries, **1237–1239**
    in myelomeningocele, *1450*
Lunate
  dislocation, 1259
    volar, 1259
  rotary subluxation, 1258

Lung
  abscess, 205
    differentiation from bronchopleural fistula,
      164 (*table*)
    primary, 202, *203*
    pyaemic, 289
  agenesis, 359
  air leak, in infants, 351–355
  air-trapping, 149
  alveolar microlithiasis, 275
    proteinosis, 275
Lung
  alveolitis, fibrosing, 272–274
  amyloid, 275
  arterial pressure, 295
  arteriovenous fistula, congenital, 361, *362*,
    363
  atelectasis, *see* Lung, collapse
  biopsy, 136, 289, **2122–2124**
    complications, 2123–2124
    contraindications, 2124
    indications, 2123
    needles, 2123, 2124
  blood flow redistribution, definition, 371
  bullae, in emphysema, 236
  carcinoma, *see* Bronchial carcinoma
  cavitation, bronchial carcinoma, 242, *244*
    postprimary tuberculosis, 209
  collagen vascular diseases, 279–284
  collapse (atelectasis), 222–228
    atypical forms, 228
    bronchiectasis causing, 230–232
    bronchocele causing, 229
    definition, 368
    disc, 148
    entire lung, 227
    following laparotomy, 314
    foreign body obstruction, 344
    general features, 222
    individual lobes, 222–227
    nonobstructive lobar, 228
    pneumonia, 206
    rapid re-expansion, 264
    sarcoidosis, 278
    segmental, 228
    signs, 222
  congenital anomalies, 357–365
  consolidation, primary tuberculosis, 207
    radiograph, 143
  cystic adenomatoid malformation, 363
    differentiation from congenital lobar
      emphysema, 365
  cysts, congenital, 363
    differentiation from congenital lobar
      emphysema, 365
  dermatomyositis, 283
  diffuse disease, 259–292
    infants and young children, 344
    radiographic patterns, 260 (*table*)
  drowned, 228, *264*, *571*
  drug-induced disease, 287, 289–291
  embolism *see* Embolism, pulmonary
  emphysema *see* Emphysema
  fibrosing alveolitis, differentiation from
    asbestosis, 270
  fibrosis, 268
    ankylosing spondylitis, 283
    diffuse, 272–276
    sarcoidosis, 278, *279*
  fissures, radiograph, 142
  gallium-67 scintiscanning, 278
  gangrene, 205
  'ground glass' appearance, 273

  haemorrhage, 287
    diffuse, 265–266
    thromboembolism, 294
  haemosiderosis, idiopathic, 266
  hyperinflation, 149
    obstructive, 229
  hypertension *see* Pulmonary hypertension
  hypogenetic (scimitar) syndrome, 136, **361**,
    535, *537*, *574*
  hypoplasia, 359–361
    infants, 353
  immunocompromised host, 286–289
  infarction, 294
  infection, **199–219**
    fungal, 213–217, 289
      infants and young children, 338
    gram negative, 289
    infants and young children, 336–340
    virus, of childhood, 336
  interstitial disease, rheumatoid arthritis, 280
  intracavitary body, causes, 146 (*table*)
  Kerley lines, 146, 147, 317, **568–570**
  large airway obstruction, 221–232
  line and band shadows, 145–148
  lobar expansion, 206
  lymphangiomyomatosis, 275
  lymphoma, malignant, 253
  malformations, congenital, 359–365
  magnetic resonance imaging, 88
  metastases, 251–253
    CT scanning, 253
    endobronchial, 253
    miliary, 253
    rate of growth, 252
    techniques, 253
  myocardial infarction, 621
  neoplasms, 241–257
    benign, 249–251
    malignant, 241–249, 251–253
    see also Lungs, tumours
  neurofibromatosis, 275
  nodular opacities, 144
  normal, 113
    fissures, (CT scan), 113, *114*
  oedema, *see* Oedema, pulmonary
  overinflation, emphysema and chronic
    bronchitis, 235
  parenchyma, inorganic material inhalation,
    268–272
    organic dust disease, 267
    sarcoidosis, 277
    thromboembolism, radiography, 298
  particle inhalation, disease due to, 267
  perfusion, definition, 371
  polymyositis, 283
  post-operative radiography, 321–324
  radiotherapy reactions, 325
  rheumatic mitral valve disease, 589
  rheumatoid disease, 280
  ring shadows, 145
    causes, 146 (*table*)
  scimitar (hypogenetic) syndrome, 136, **361**,
    535, *537*, *574*
  segments, positions, *121*
  septal lines, 147, 262, **568–570**
    drug-induced disease, 290
  sequestration, 361, *362*
  Sjögren's syndrome, 283
  systemic sclerosis, 281
  thromboembolism *see* Thromboembolism,
    pulmonary
  tuberose sclerosis, 275
  tumours, benign, 249–251

Lung (*cont.*)
  tumours, benign (*cont.*)
    CT scan, *1528*
    growth rates, 256
    hamartoma, 250, *251*
    magnetic resonance imaging, 88
    malignant, 241–249, 251–253
    solitary mass, 255
  varix, congenital, 363
  veins *see* Veins, pulmonary
  vessels, assessment, 149
  emphysema, 235
    'marker', 236
    radiograph, 142, 144, *145*
  see also Pleura: Pulmonary system
Lutein cysts, ovary, 1610
Luteinizing hormone, 1036
  males, 1038
Lutembacher syndrome, associated with atrial
    septal defect, 484, *486*
Lye ingestion, cause of oesophageal stricture,
    758
Lymph node
  calcification, 1922
  metastases, 2167–2177
    CT, 2175–2176
    radiology, value, 2173, 2174–2176
Lymphadenoma *see* Hodgkin's disease
Lymphadenopathy
  causing laryngeal displacement, 1981
  definition, 370
  immunoblastic, 188
  mediastinal, 183–186
  primary tuberculosis, 207
Lymphangiectasia, intestinal, 854
Lymphangioma, 192, *193*
  bone, **1293**
Lymphangiomyomatosis, lung involvement,
    175
Lymphangitis carcinomatosa, *161*, 252
Lymphatics
  chest, 121
  radionuclide, 22 (*table*)
Lymphoblastic lymphoma, 1338
Lymphoceles in renal transplantation, 1147
Lymphocysts complicating hysterectomy, 1624
Lymphocytes, 1027
Lymphoepithelioma, nasopharynx, 1969
Lymphogranuloma venereum, colitis, 891
Lymphography in cancer staging, **2169–2173**
    (*table*), *2174*
  cervical carcinoma, 1607
  clinical value, 2174–2176
  complications, 2173
  contraindications, 2173
  endometrial carcinoma, 1608
  in gynaecological conditions, 1598
  interpretations, 2173
  metastatic involvement, 2167–2177
  ovarian carcinomas, 1612–1613
  in pelvic cancer metastases, 1626
Lymphoma, **1336–1338**
  Burkitts, **1338**
    maxillofacial region, 1911
  cerebral (microglioma), 1718
  gallium imaging, 2189
  gastric, 802–804
  gastric pseudolymphoma, 796
  Hodgkin's, **1336–1337**
  lung metastases, 253, 1320
  malignant, mediastinal, 187, *188*
    primary, bone, 1320, *1321*
      maxillofacial region, 1912

  Mediterranean, 845
  nasopharynx, 1969
  non-Hodgkin's, **1338**
    CT scan, *56*
    orbital, 1893
    renal, 1104
      CT, 1105
    small bowel, 845–847
    spinal cord, 1841
    spleen, 1015
    staging, radiology, 2176
Lymphomatoid granulomatosis, 283
Lymphoreticular hyperplasia (gastric
    pseudolymphoma), 796
Lymphosarcoma
  of bone, 1338
  maxillofacial region, 1911
Lymphoscintigraphy, mammary *see* Mammary
    lymphoscintigraphy

MacGregor's line, 1776
McKusick type of metaphyseal
    chondrodysplasia, 1430
MacLeod's (Swyer-James') syndrome, 229,
    238–239, 337
Macrodystrophia lipomatosa, *1511*
Macroglobulinaemia, Waldenström's, **1341**
Madelung deformity, 1444
Madura foot, 1363
Maffucci's syndrome, 1278, 1437, 2008
  calcification, 1515
Magnetic resonance imaging (MRI), 5, 9, **61–
    91**, 447
  adrenals, 1035
  aorta, 693
  breast, 1665
  components of system, 64
  contrast media, 67
  current developments, 67–90
  data presentation, storage and interrogation,
    64
  echo-planner imaging, 66
  heart, 87, *88*, 381, **447–449**
    ECG gated, 448
  high resolution techniques, 66
  historical background, 61
  image interpretation, 66
  liver, 939
  localization of signal, 64
  multi-slice imaging, 66
  pancreas, 1000
  paradoxical enhancement, heart, 448
  physical principles, 62
  position and thickness of plane, selection, 64
  production of signal, 62
  relaxation times, 63
  safety considerations, 67
  scanner, *62*
  spectroscopy, 90
  spine, 1817
  spleen, 1009
  steady state free precession sequence, 64
  timing of sequences, 64 (*table*)
  tissue characterization, 67
  variations on basic methods, 66
Magovern valve, 668
Majzlin spring, 1621
Malacoplakia, renal, 1100
  urinary tract, 1132
Malgaigne fracture, pelvis, 1242
Malignancy *see* Tumours: and specific names,
    organs and regions, and radiological
    techniques

Mallet (baseball) fractures, 1261
Mallory-Weiss syndrome, 769
Mammary
  arteriography, phaeochromocytoma, *2055*
  lymphoscintigraphy, internal, 2193–2194
    interpretation, 2193–2194
    localization, 2194
    technical considerations, 2193
Mammography, 1631–1668
  accuracy, 1643–1644
    clinical information, 1643–1644
    technical quality, 1643
  benign dysplasias, 1633–1635
  biopsy method for non palpable lesions,
    1645–1646
    alternative techniques, 1646–1647
    lesion localization, 1645
    needle insertion, 1646
    technical requirements, 1647
  compared with ultrasonography, 1663, 1664
  comparison of screen film systems, 1648–
    1649
  dedicated units, 1650–1652
    focal spot size-breast surface distance,
      1650
    grids, 1650–1652
    low energy beam and compression, 1650
  direct film, 1648
  exposure factors, 1649
  indications, 1645
  low-dose, 1648
  normal anatomy, 1631–1633
  parenchymal patterns and cancer risk, 1635–
    1636
  see also Breast
  positioning and compression, 1649–1650
  questionnaire for patients, *1644*
  risk from, 1656–1657
    high dose, 1656
    hypothetical, 1657
    possible low dose, 1656–1657
  versus physical examination, 1644–1645
  xeromammography, 1652–1654
    exposure factors, 1652–1654
    imaging processing, 1652
    positioning and compression, 1654
    positive and negative mode, 1652
    receptors, 1654–1656
    versus screen film mammography, 1652–
      1654
Mandible
  cysts, benign, 1904–1906
    median, 1906
    median palatal, 1906
  fractures, **1902–1904**
    radiography, 1904
  osteomyelitis, **1354**, **1913–1914**
  see also Maxillofacial region
Mandibular condyle
  asplasia, 1918
  erosions, 1918
  Hurler's syndrome, 1918
  hypoplasia, 1918
Mandibulofacial dyostosis, 1915
Marble bones, **1427**, *1428*
  see also Osteopetrosis
March fractures, foot, 1271
Marfan's syndrome (arachnodactyly), 562, 713,
    1424
Margulies coil, 1621
Mason-Sones cutdown technique, 1996
Mass number, nuclear, 14
Massive osteolysis, **1294**

Mast cell reticulosis, **1335–1336**
Mastocytosis, 855, **1335–1336**
Mastoiditis, acute, 1955–1956
  chronic, 1956
Maternal
  abdomen, radiography, **1589**
    risks of exposure, 1589
  disorders occurring during pregnancy, *1578*,
    1580
Matter, structure, 13
Maturation, skeletal, delayed, disorders, **1396–**
  1400
Maxillary
  antra, anatomy, 1938
    carcinoma, 1948–1949
      CT, 1949
  fractures, **1899–1900**
    indirect signs, 1902
    radiography, 1902
Maxillofacial radiology, **1899–1923**
  adenomeloblastoma, 1908
  ameloblastoma, 1908
  benign cysts, 1904–1906
  benign tumours, 1907
  bone lesions, non-neoplastic, 1909
  development abnormalities, 1915–1916
  duct strictures, 1920
  fibro-osseous lesions, 1912
  fractures, 1899–1904
  growth abnormalities, 1915–1916
  infections, 1913–1914
  malignant tumours, 1910–1911
  odontogenic tumours, 1908
  odontomes, 1908–1909
  osteomyelitis, 1913–1914
  radiolucent lesions, jaws, 1909–1910
    differential diagnosis, 1914–1915
  salivary glands, 1918–1920
  sialectasis, 1920
  soft tissue calcification, 1922
  temporomandibular joint, 1916–1918
  trauma, 1922
  tumours, 1921–1922
Measles, pneumonia, *204*
Meckel's diverticulum, 852
  radionuclide imaging, children, 2204–2205
Meconium
  aspiration syndrome, 347, *348*
  ileus, 917–918
    sonography, 1577
  plug syndrome, 916
Medial
  epicondylar apophysis, avulsion, 1253
  fibroplasia, renal artery, 1154
  sclerosis, arteriography, 2015
Mediastinitis, 194
Mediastinum, 122–128, **175–196**
  adenopathy, 246, *247*
  carcinoma, 187, 247
  CT scanning, 122, *123*
  dilatation of veins, 181
  emphysema, 195
  germ cell tumours, 179
  haemorrhage, 195
  infants and young children, 331
  junction lines, 122–125
  lymph node metastases, 246, *247*
  lymphadenopathy, **183–186**
  masses, **175–194**
    CT scan, *57*
    digital subtraction angiography, 2105
    magnetic resonance imaging, 89
    parathyroid, 177

  techniques, 175
  metastases, 187
  pleuro-oesophageal stripe, 125
  pneumomediastinum, post-operative, 320
  pseudomediastinum, 234
    definition, 371
    result of pulmonary air leak, in infants,
      352
  radiograph, 142
  teratoma, 179, *180*
  thyroid mass, 176
  trauma, 308–310
  tuberculosis, nodal, 207
  veins, dilatation, 181
Mediterranean lymphoma (alpha-chain
  disease), 845
Medullary sponge kidney, calculi, 1060, 1063
Medulloblastoma, CT, 1714
  cerebellar sarcoma, 1714
  desmoplastic, 1714
  post-operative, 1714
  radionuclide imaging, 1861
Megacalices, congenital, non-obstructive
  dilatation, 1075
Megacolon, 893
Meglumine, 101
Megaureter, primary (megaloureter) non-
  obstructive dilatation, 1075–1076
Meig's syndrome, 1615
Melanoma
  external ear, 1959
  malignant, choroidal, 1896
Melorheostosis, **1436**
Mendelson's syndrome, 263
Ménétrièr's disease, 795
Menière's disease, 1959
Meningioma, **1728–1732**
  angiography, 1731–1732
  CT, 1730–1731
  magnetic resonance imaging, 69
  optic nerve sheath, 1892–1893
  petrous bone, 1961, 1962
  plain film manifestations, 1728–1730
  radionuclide imaging, 1861, *1862*
  spinal cord, myelography, **1844–1846**
Meningitis, 1743
  recurrent, CT, 1703
    cisternography, 1703
    radiography, 1703
    radionuclide imaging, children, 2207
  tuberculous, 1741
Meningoceles, **1769–1770**, 1821
  anterior sacral, **1821–1822**
    CT, 1822
  lateral thoracic, 192, **1822**
  nasal cavity, 1948
  post-traumatic, 1851
Meningomyelocele
  amniography, *1582*, 1583
  fetal detection, sonography, 1569, *1570*, 1576
  and neurogenic bladder, 1198
Meniscus sign, colonic polyp, 867, *868*
Menstrual cycle, 1036
Mental retardation, CT, 1703
Mesenchymal tumours, 192–194
  chondrosarcoma, 1309
Mesenteric
  arteriography, 2037, *2038*, 2039–2040, *2043*,
    2044
  artery angioplasty, 2143
    superior, compression syndrome, 825
    ultrasound, 2114
  infarction, 725

Mesothelioma
  of asbestosis, 271
  pericardial, 679, *680*
Metabolic disease
  of bone, **1369–1413**
    anatomy, 1369–1371
    children, **1464–1468**
    generalized increase in bone density,
      1404–1407
    generalized loss of bone density, 1396–
      1400
    localized increase in bone density, 1407–
      1409
    localized loss of bone density, 1400–1404
    physiology, 1371–1373
    quantitative bone mineral analysis, 1409–
      1410
    skeletal maturation, delayed, 1396–1400
    see also specific diseases: Bone
  heart anomalies, 470, 640
  oesophagus, 776
  with osteosclerosis, 1404
  soft tissue calcification, 1513–1514
Metacarpophalangeal joints, rheumatoid
  arthritis, 1478
  juvenile, 1482
Metaphysis
  bands, dense, conditions associated with,
    1407–1409
  disorders mainly affecting, **1427–1431**
  distal femoral, posterior, irregularity, *1461*
  dysplasia, **1427–1429**
    chondrodysplasia, **1430**–1431
      Jansen type, 1431
      McKusick type, 1430
      Schmid type, 1430
  fibrous defect *see* Fibrous cortical defect
  radiolucency, of newborn, 1470
Metaplasia, squamous, and urinary tract
  infection, 1131
Metaplastic polyposis, 872
Metastases
  adrenals, *1033*, 1034, 1040
  from benign tumours, 1275
  bone, **1301–1307**
    radionuclide bone scanning, **1538–1540**
    spread, 1301–1302
      commonest sites, 1302
      diagnosis, 1303–1304
      differential diagnosis, 1305, 1306
      distribution, 1303
      frequency, from different tumours, 1303,
        1304
      from bladder, 1305
      from breast, 1304, *1306*
      from gastrointestinal tract, 1305
      from kidney, 1304–1305
      from lung, 1304
      from medulloblastoma, *1307*
      from melanoma, 1305
      from pancreas, 1305
      from thyroid, 1305
      from uterus, 1305
      incidence, 1302
      investigation, by radiologist, 1305–1306
      paradoxical embolism, 1302
      pulmonary lesions, 1301
      radiographic features favouring
        metastases, 1305
      retrograde venous embolism, 1302
      transpulmonary passage, 1302
  to brain, CT, 1717–1718
    radionuclide imaging, 1861

Metastases (*cont.*)
  to brain, CT (*cont.*)
    from cervical carcinoma, 1608
    duodenum, 822
    endometrial carcinoma, 1609
    liver, 932
      chemotherapeutic infusions, 2192–2193
      CT scanning, 938
    lung, 251–253
    lymph node from pelvic cancer, 1626
    lymphography, 2173–2175
      CT, 2176
      from occult primary tumours, 2180–2181
      systemic, radiology, 2178–2181
  to maxillofacial region, 1911
  mediastinal, 187
  pericardial, 680
  renal, *1140*
  skeletal, CT scan, 1527, *1528*
  small bowel, 846
  'super scan', 1545
  thyroid carcinoma, 1025
  to ureter, causing obstruction, 1083
  urothelial, 1112
  from vulval carcinoma, 1615
Metatarsal, fifth, base, Jones fracture, 1266, *1267*, 1271
Metatarsophalangeal joint, rheumatoid arthritis, 1479
Metatropic dwarfism, **1422–1423**
Metazoal infection, pulmonary, 217
Meteorism, 720
Methylcholine test, 774
Methylene diphosphonate, labelled, whole body dosage, 1536
  clearance, 1538
  imaging protocol, 1536–1537
Metrizamide
  cisternography, empty sella syndrome, 1594
  formula, *103*
  myelography, spine, **1801–1802**, 1805, **1824–1825, 1827–1828**
Metropathia haemorrhagica, 1617
Microadenomas, **1721**, *1724*
  CT, 1723
  radiography, 1721
Microaneurysms, arteriography, 2014
Microcalcifications, benign adenosis, breast, 1633
  malignant, 1641–1643
Microencephaly, fetal detection, sonography, 1570
Microphthalmia, 1880
Micturating cysto-urethrogram, 1047
  combined with ascending urethrogram, 1049
  in vesico-ureteric reflux, children, 1075
Middle ear
  congenital anomalies, 1965
  otitis media, 1955–1956
  tumours, 1959–1961
  see also Ear: Otitis media
Midfoot injuries, 1269–1271
Midgut volvulus, 912
Midline lethal granuloma, 1950–1951
Migraine, radiography and CT, 1702
Miliary pattern, definition, 370
Milk alkali syndrome, 1060
Millisecond cine CT scanner, 5
Mineral measurements, bone, axial, 1410–1411
  CT, 1410–1411
    quantitative, 1411
  dual photon absorptiometry, 1410
Mirrizzi syndrome, 956

Mitral
  regurgitation, 592
    non-rheumatic, 595–596
      differentiation from hypertrophic myopathy, 642
    post-infarction, 632
  ring calcification, 593
  valve atresia, 538
    disease, **585–596**
      non-rheumatic, 591–594
      pulmonary vascularity, 572
      rheumatic, 586–590
    parachute, 540
    prolapse, 591
Mixed connective tissue disease, *1484*, **1485**
Molar pregnancies, 1562–1563
Monckeberg's medial calcific sclerosis, 1514, 2015
Monday morning fever (byssinosis), 267
Monteggia fracture-dislocation, 1254
  reversed, 1254
Morgagni hernia, 170, *171*, 190, 334
Morquio's syndrome, **1434–1435**
Morquio-Brailsford syndrome, 1927
Movements, involuntary, 1703
  angiography, 1703
  CT, 1703
  radiography, 1703
Moyamoya, 1765–1766
MRI *see* Magnetic resonance imaging
Mucocele
  appendix, 894
  paranasal sinuses, **1943–1944**
    empyema, 1944
    ethmoid, 1944
    frontal, 1943
    maxillary, 1943
    orbito-ethmoidal, *1944*
Mucoid impaction, definition, 370
Mucopolysaccharidoses, 1745
  and mucolipidoses, **1432–1435**
    principle conditions, **1432**
    see also specific conditions
Mucosal-relief
  examination, oesophageal, 747
  radiographs, stomach, 785
Mucus inspissation, 365
Mueller manoeuvre, 132, 181, 363
  definition, 370
Müllerian duct fusion, failure, 1599–1600
Multicentric reticulohistiocytosis, 1485
Multiformatting, 4
Multiple
  epiphyseal dysplasia, **1424, 1425**
  pregnancy, sonography, 1564–1565
  sclerosis, 1746
    magnetic resonance imaging, 77
Mundini deformity, 1965
Muscle bridge, coronary artery, 614
Muscle diverticular disease, 876
Muscular dystrophies, fat measurement, 1509
Musculoskeletal system
  biopsy, **2126–2127**
    bones, 2126–2127
    joint, 2127
    soft tissue, 2127
  children, **1447–1471**
    congenital anomalies, 1448–1452
    development, 1447
    maturation, 1447
    disorders, 1448 (*table*), 1447
  CT, **1523–1534**
    see also Computed tomography

magnetic resonance imaging, 89
Myasthenia gravis, 1028, *1029*, 1030
  oesophagus, 776
Mycetoma, 211
  pulmonary, 216
Mycobacterial infection
  M.kansasii, pulmonary, 212, *213*
  non-tuberculous, 212
Mycoplasma pneumoniae pneumonia, 202, *203*
  infants and young children, 338
Mycoses, affecting bone, 1363–1364
Mycotic aneurysm, 2010
  aortic, 712–713
Myelination process, magnetic resonance imaging, 79, *80*, *81*
Myelitis, in spinal cord enlargement, 1849
Myelography
  Arnold-Chiari malformation, 1826
  cerebellar tonsillar ectopia, 1703
  contrast media, 108
  CT scanning, 51
  in disc protrusion, 1830–1832
  functional, disc protrusion, 1835
  haemangioblastomas, spinal, 1854
  in myelopathy, 1837–1838
  occult spinal dysraphism, 1823, 1824
  postoperative, 1835–1836
  in radiculopathy, 1837–1838
  spine, **1801–1811**
    anatomy, 1806–1811
      cervical region, 1809
      lumbar region, 1806–1808
      thoracic region, 1808
    arachnoiditis, 1806
    cisternal puncture, 1804, 1805
    complications, 1805–1806
    contrast media, 1801–1803
      choice, 1803
      gaseous contrast, 1802–1803
      oily contrast, 1802, *1825*, *1826*, *1827*
      water soluble, 1801–1802, 1805
    cord, compression, **1840–1848**
      inflammatory lesions, 1848
    endomyelography, 1805
    haemangioblastoma, 1854
    hyperexcitation states, 1805–1806
    interpretation, 1811
    lateral cervical puncture, 1804, 1805
    lumbar puncture, 1803, 1805
    marker films, 1805
    meningeal reaction, 1806
    puncture site, 1803–1805
    radicular effects, 1806
    technical considerations, 1804–1805
    trauma, 1850
    vascular lesions, 1853–1854
  suspected subarachnoid haemorrhage, 1701
  syringomelia, 1827–1829
Myeloid metaplasia, **1333**
Myelolipoma, adrenal, 1035
Myelomatosis, **1339–1341**
  clinical features, 1339
  differential diagnosis, 1341
  mandible, 1911
  pathological considerations, 1339–1340
  prognosis, 1341
  radiological features, 1340–1341
Myelomeningocele, **1450**, *1451*, 1821
Myelopathy, spondylotic, **1837–1838**
Myeloproliferative syndromes, **1327–1348**
  coagulation disorders, 1344–1347
  haemophilia, 1344
  histiocytoses, 1341–1344

Myeloproliferative syndromes (*cont.*)
   red cell disorders, 1327–1334
   white cell disorders, 1334–1341
   see also specific disorders
Myelosclerosis, **1333**
Myoblastoma, intraorbital, 1893
Myocardial
   imaging, children, 2209
   infarction, **621–625**
      CT scanning, 443
      Dressler syndrome, 685
      heart size, 621
      lung, 621
      mechanical complications, 627–628
      post cardiotomy-post myocardial
         infarction syndrome, 685
      pulmonary vascularity, *569, 573*
      radionuclide imaging, 419, 436
      thallium imaging, 436
   mass, CT scanning, 444
   perforation, by pacemaker, 658, *659*
   perfusion, radionuclide imaging, 419
   stricture, echocardiographic, 629
Myositis ossificans progressiva, 1435
   calcification, 1517
   radionuclide bone scan, 1541
Myotonic dystrophy, oesophagus, 776
Myxoedema, 1023, 1025
   heart involvement, 640
   juvenile, 1023
Myxoma
   intraorbital, 1893
   left atrial, 647–649

Naegele pelvis, 1587
Nail-patella syndrome, **1442–1443**
Nasopharynx tumours, benign, 1967–1969
   malignant, 1969–1971
Navicular
   fractures, 1269
   multipartite, simulating trauma, 1464, *1465*
Neck and head, arteriography, 2027, 2030
Neck root, radiograph, 141
Necrotizing enterocolitis of the newborn, 920
Needle
   aspiration, renal masses, 1094, 1097
   percutaneous biopsy, 987–988
   puncture, percutaneous, for arteriography,
      1993–1994
Negatron, definition, 15
Nelson's syndrome, 1022
Neonate
   brain, ultrasound, 2229–2234
      see also Brain, ultrasound, infant
   chest radiography, 562
   see also Paediatric conditions
Neoplasms, musculoskeletal, CT scan, 1523–
      1529
   bony, 1524–1526
      locally recurrent, 1527
      skeletal, metastases, 1527–1529
      soft tissue, 1526–1527
   with osteosclerosis, 1404
   radiotherapy-induced, 326
   splenomegaly, 1012
   see also Tumours : and specific organs, names
      and regions
Nephritis, lung haemorrhage (Goodpasture's
      syndrome), 266
   see also Kidney : Renal
Nephroblastoma *see* Wilms' tumour
Nephrocalcinosis *see* Calculi, kidney

Nephrography
   differential diagnosis, renal parenchymal
      disease, 1127–1229
   renal failure, 1137–1141
   in urinary obstruction, 1069–1076
      see also Intravenous urography
Nephrolithiasis, 1062
Nephropathy, acute obstructive, 1068
Nephrosclerosis, renal angiography, 1156
Nephrostomy
   catheter, percutaneous, 2129–2130
      indications, 2129
      techniques, 2130
   see also Percutaneous
Nephrotomography, renal mass, 1090, *1091*
Nervous system, contrast media, 108
Neural foramina, patency, CT scan, 1530–1531
Neural tube defect, fetal detection,
      sonography, 1569
   amniography, 1580
Neuralgia, occipital, radiography and CT, 1702
Neurenteric cysts, 188
Neurilemmoma
   associated with bone, 1295
   dental, 1907
Neuritis, optic, 1889
Neuroblastoma
   adrenal, 1036
      ultrasound, 2221
   childhood, **1205–1208**
   clinical features, 1206
   epidemiology, 1206
   intra-abdominal, CT scan, *55*
   malignant, **1321–1322**
   metastatic, maxillofacial region, 1911
   myelography, *1841*
   pathology, 1206
   radiographic evaluation, 1206–1208
   renal, ultrasound, 2224
Neuroectodermal tumours, classified, *1706*
Neurofibroma
   chest wall, *153*
   dental, 1907
   intraosseous, 1295
   larynx, 1979
   nasal cavity and paranasal sinuses, 1946,
      1948
   optic nerve, 1893
   spinal cord, **1844–1846**, *1846*
Neurofibromatosis, **1438–1441**
   affecting facial bones, 1915
   CT, *1528*
   lungs, 275
   skeletal changes, 1440
   skull films, 1777–1778
      angiography, 1778
      CT, 1778
Neurofibrosarcoma, 190, *191*
Neurogenic
   bladder, 1198
      ultrasound, children, 2225–2226
   tumours, 190, *191*
Neurological disorder, paediatric, magnetic
      resonance imaging, 79
Neuroma
   acoustic *see* Acoustic neuroma
   vagal, embolization, 2146, *2150*
Neuromuscular disorders
   heart involvement, 641
   oesophagus, 776
Neuropathic
   arthropathy, 1498–1499
   bladder, urodynamics, 1216

Neutron, 14
Nezelof syndrome, 1027
Nidus, definition, 1283
Niemann-Pick disease, **1345**
Niopam *see* Iopamidol
Nissen fundoplication, 779
Nitrofurantoin, lung disease caused by, 284,
      290
NMR *see* Magnetic resonance imaging
Nocardiosis, pulmonary, 214
Nodular lymphoid hyperplasia, small intestine,
      853
Nodular pattern, definition, 370
Nodules, thyroid, 1040
Nonepithelial bone cyst, 1906, *1907*
Non-Hodgkin's lymphoma, **1338**
   radionuclide bone scan, 1538
   staging radiology, 2176
Non-lipoid histiocytoses, **1341–1344**
Nonossifying fibroma *see* Fibroma,
      nonossifying
Noonan's syndrome, heart anomalies, 470
North American blastomycosis, 215
Nose and paranasal sinuses, **1937–1951**
   allergy, 1941
   anatomy, 1938–1940
      nasal cavity, 1940
   infection, 1941
   inflammation, 1941, 1946
   polyposis, 1945–1946
   radiology, 1937, 1938
   septum, displacement, 1941
   trauma, 1950
   tumours, 1946–1950
      benign, 1946–1948
      malignant, 1950
   ultrasound, 1941
   see also Paranasal sinuses
Nuclear
   magnetic resonance *see* Magnetic resonance
      imaging
   medicine,
      paediatric, 2197–2211
         bone imaging, 2198
            see also Bone imaging
         cardiopulmonary imaging, 2208–2210
         central nervous system imaging, 2206–
            2207
         gastrointestinal imaging, 2203–2205
         techniques, 2197–2198
         thyroid imaging, 2207–2208
         urinary tract imaging, 2201–2203
      renal disease, 1051–1057
      thyroid carcinoma, 1040
      tumours, 2183–2195
         bone, 2185–2188
         dynamic studies, 2191–2193
            arterial, 2192–2193
            venous, 2191–2192
         gallium imaging, 2188–2191
         hepatic artery infusion, 2192–2193
         internal mammary lymphoscintigraphy,
            2193
         liver, 2183–2185
         radio-immuno detection, 2194
         urinary obstruction, 1078–1079
      particles, 13
      see also other specific techniques
Nucleons, 14
Nuclide, definition, 14

Obesity, thromboembolism, 294
Obstetrics, 1551–1592

Obstetrics (*cont.*)
  radiology, **1580–1589**
    amniography, 1580–1583
      see also Amniography
    sonography, **1551–1580**
      conditions affecting labour and delivery, 1579
      date-size discrepancy, 1552–1554
      fetal condition, assessment, 1579
      fetal position, determination, 1554–1556
      fetal viability evaluation, 1556
      first trimester, 1556–1563
        abortion, 1557, *1558*
        bleeding, *1557*
        blighted ovum, 1557
        ectopic, 1557–1562
          see also Ectopic pregnancy
        estimation of gestational duration, 1556 (*table*)
        molar, 1562–1563
        normal features, 1556–1557
        scanning techniques, 1556–1557
        with IUCDs, *1562*, 1563
      general applications, 1552–1556
      indications, 1551 (*table*)
      patient preparation, 1552
      placenta, localization and evaluation, 1554
      real-time scanners, 1552
      scanning methods, 1552
      second trimester, 1563–1572
        fetal structural anomalies detectable, 1569–1572
        intrauterine growth retardation, 1567–1569
        multiple gestation, 1564–1565
        normal features, 1563
        pelvic masses, 1565–1567
          sonographic features, 1567 (*table*)
        placental localization prior to amniocentesis, 1563–1564
        scanning techniques, 1563
      third trimester, 1573–1579
        fetal anomalies detectable, 1574–1578
        maternal anomalies detectable, *1578*
        normal features, 1573
        placenta praevia, 1573–1574
        placental abruption, 1573–1574
        scanning techniques, 1573
      throughout pregnancy, 1552–1556
      transducers, 1552
      unknown dates, 1552–1554
Obstruction
  biliary tract, malignant, endoscopy, 1007
  bowel, pseudo-, 731
  duodenal, in infants, 985
  gastrointestinal, infants, 905–908, *909*
  kidneys in renal failure, 1138
    further procedures, 1140
    high dose urography, 1138
    in transplantation, 1146
    ultrasound, 1140
  large bowel, 879
    mechanical, 726–729
  urinary, **1067–1087**
    see also Urinary obstruction
Occipitalization of the atlas, 1777
Ochronosis, 1496
Odontogenic keratocyst, 1906
Odontomes, 1908–1909
  cementoma, 1908
  complex composite, 1908
  compound composite, 1908
  dentinomas, 1908

dilated composite, 1909, 1927–1928
enameloma, 1908
geminated composite, 1909
Odynophagia, 748
Oedema
  and calcification, 1515
  pleural, re-expansion, 158
  pulmonary, **261–265**
    aetiology, 261
    asymmetrical, causative factors, 570 (*table*)
    batswing distribution, 262, *263*, 264
    causes, 318 (*table*)
    clinical features, 261
    high altitude, 265
    neonatal, 350
    non-cardiogenic, causative factors, 570 (*table*), *571*
    paraphysiology, 261
    postoperative, 316–318
    radiology, 262
Oesophagitis, 751–759
  bacterial, 757
  Behçet's syndrome, 758, *759*
  chemically induced, 757
  Crohn's disease, 758
  development, contributory factors, 753
  differentiation of common causes, 758
  eosinophilic, 758
  herpetic, 756–757
  motility, candidiasis, 756
  peptic (reflux), 751–756, 776
    differential diagnosis, 758
  reflux *see* Oesophagitis, peptic
  secondary to infection, 756–757
Oesophagography, barium, 342
Oesophagus, **743–781**
  atresia, fetal amniography, 1581
    infants, 906–908, *909*
  barium radiography, 746–748
  Barrett's, 753, *754*, **755**, 762
  candidiasis, 755, **756**, *757*
  columnar-lined (Barrett's), 753, *754*, **755**
  compression, extrinsic, 779
  cricopharyngeal impression, 744
  CT scanning, 748
  dermatological conditions, associated with lesions of, 768
  diffuse spasm, 774, *775*
  disease, symptoms, 748
  displacement, 1981
  diverticulosis, 778
    pseudo, intramural, 755, *756*
  duplication, in infants, 913
  endoscopy, therapeutic, 829
  'feline', 776
  filming sequence, 747
  fistula, infants, 906–908, *909*
  inflammatory polyps, 755
  intramural haematoma, *770*, 771
  intramural pseudodiverticulosis, 755, *756*
  lacerations, 769–771
  left atrial enlargement, 553
  lye-induced stricture, *758*
  malignant neoplasm, differential diagnosis, 773
  morphological examination, 746–747
  motility disorders, 773–778
    barium investigation, 747
  normal anatomy, 743–746
    motility, 746
  oesophageal-pleural stripe, 125
  peptic strictures, 754
  perforations, 769–771

plain radiography, 746
post-cricoid impression, 744
postoperative changes, 779
presbyoesophagus, 774
radiological investigation, 746–749
rings, 745–746, 773
rupture, 308
scintigraphy, 748
  motility, 776–778
systemic sclerosis, 773, *775*
tumours, **760–766**
  adenocarcinoma, 765
  benign neoplasms, 761
  carcinoma, argyrophil, 766
    primary, 762–766
    spread, 765
    ulcerative, 764
  carcinosarcoma, 766
  leiomyosarcoma, 766
  lymphoma, 766
  malignant neoplasms, *761*, 762–766
  melanoma, malignant, 766
  rhabdomyosarcoma, 766
  secondary neoplasms, 766
  squamous cell carcinoma, *760*, 762–764
    verrucous, 766
varices, 767
  barium study of liver disease, 928, *929*
  portal embolization, 997
vestibule, 745
wall, thickening, 754
webs, 772
Oestradiol, 1036
Oil myelography, spinal, 1802, *1825*, *1826*, *1827*
Olecranon fat pad sign, 1252
Oligaemia, definition, 370
Oligodendrogliomas, radionuclide imaging, 1861
Oligodendroma, CT, 1710, *1711*
Oligohydramnios, fetal detection, sonography, 1570, 1575–1576
Olivopontocerebellar degeneration, 1745
Ollier's disease, 1278, **1436–1437**, 1438
  calcification, 1515
Omphaloceles, fetal, sonography, 1577
Oncology, radiology, **2167–2182**
  nuclear imaging, 2183–2195
  see also Tumours and specific names of tumours, organs or regions and individual techniques
Opacity
  small irregular, definition, 372
  small rounded, definition, 372
Opisthorciasis, biliary, 986
Optic
  angiography, 1702–1703
  chiasm, 1702
  CT, 1702–1703
  glioma, **1727–1728**
    CT, 1728
    features, 1727–1728
  nerve, disturbances, angiography, 1702–1703
    CT, 1702–1703
    radiography, 1702–1703
    glioma, 1892
    meningioma, 1892–1893
    shearing injuries, 1883
  neuritis, 1889
  radiography, 1702–1703
Oral contraception, 1622
  circulatory disorders, 1622
  liver tumours, 1622
  thromboembolism, 294

Orbit, **1875–1897**
  amyloidosis, 1889
  anatomy, 1875–1877
    contents, 1876–1877
    wall, 1875–1876
  angiography, 1877–1880
  anterior segment lesions, 1894
  arteriography, 1877, *1879*, 1880
  choroidal lesions, 1896
  CT, 1877, *1878*, 1882, 1886
  dacryocystography, 1880
  endocrine exophthalmos, 1887
  floor, blow-out fractures, **1901–1902**
  foreign bodies, 1883–1887
  granuloma (pseudotumour), 1888
    Wegener's, 1889
  infections, 1887–1888
  inflammatory diseases, 1887–1889
  magnetic resonance imaging, 81
  malformations, 1880–1882
  melanoma, malignant, 1896
  neuritis, optic, 1889
  phlebography, 1877
    in cranial nerve disturbances, 1702
  radiography, 1877, 1883
  retinal lesions, 1894–1896
  sarcoidosis, 1889
  tomography, *1876*, 1877
  trauma, 1882–1883
  tumours, 1890–1892
  ultrasound, 1877, 1879, 1882, 1885
  varices, 1889–1890
  venography, 2064
  vitreous, 1894
Oropharynx, malignant tumours, 1970
Os calcis, fractures, 1268, *1269*
Osgood-Schlatter's disease in children, **1463**
Osler-Weber-Rendu disease, 361
Ossification
  soft tissues, 1513
  in paraplegia, 1520
  in trauma, 1520
Osteitis
  condensans ilii, **1355**
  in congenital syphilis, 1360
  deformans (Paget's disease), **1443–1444**
  fibrosa in primary hyperparathyroidism, 1385
  Garré's sclerosing, **1354**
Osteoarthritis, **1496–1498**
  apophyseal joints, 1500–1501
  erosive, 1498
  primary, 1496–1498
  secondary, 1498
  temporomandibular joint, 1917
Osteoarthropathy, hypertrophic pulmonary
  'super scan', 1545
Osteoblastoma, **1283–1285**
  clinical presentation, 1284
  pathological considerations, 1284
  radiological features, 1284
  spinal cord, 1841
Osteochondral fractures, 1268
Osteochondritis dissecans, 1504
Osteochondroma (cartilage-capped exostosis), **1279–1280**
  in children, 1458
  clinical features, 1279
  maxilla/mandible, 1907
  paranasal sinuses, 1946, 1948
  radiological features, 1279–1280
Osteochondromatosis, synovial, **1298–1299**
Osteochondrosis, 1501–1504

in children, **1463–1464**
  dissecans, in children, 1464
Osteoclastoma
  dental, 1907
  embolization, 2146, *2151*
  paranasal sinuses, 1946
  see also Brown tumours : Giant cell tumour
Osteodystrophy, renal, **1382–1384**
  see also Renal osteodystrophy
Osteofibrous dysplasia, 1297
Osteogenesis imperfecta (fragilitas ossium), **1392–1395, 1441–1442**
  differential diagnosis from rickets, 1381–1382
  fetal, sonography, 1578 (*table*)
  radiological diagnosis, 1392
    pathological considerations, 1393
Osteogenic sarcoma, maxillofacial region, 1911
Osteoid osteoma
  CT, *1525*
  juvenile, 1458
  paranasal sinuses, 1946
  radionuclide bone scan, 1540, 1545
Osteolysis, primary syndromes, **1402–1404**
  carpotarsal (idiopathic multicentral), **1403**
  massive of Gorham, **1403**
  transient regional, **1403–1404**
Osteoma, **1282**
  cranial vault, 1791, 1792
  ivory, maxilla/mandible, 1907
  osteoid, **1282–1283, 1284**
    clinical features, 1282
    giant *see* Osteoblastoma
    nidus, definition, 1283
    pathology, 1282–1283
    radiological features, 1283
    paranasal sinuses, 1946
    petrous bone, 1961
Osteomalacia, **1378–1380**
  anticonvulsant drugs, 1378
  calcium deficiency, 1379
  differential diagnosis, 1380
  gastrointestinal malabsorption, 1378
  hypophosphatasia, 1379
  liver disease, 1378
  radiological diagnosis, 1379
    pathological considerations, 1379–1380
  and renal osteodystrophy, 1382, 1384
  renal tubular disorders, 1378
  rickets, 1378, 1381
    vitamin D dependent, 1378
    vitamin D deficiency, 1378
Osteomyelitis
  acute, **1350–1352**
    abscess formation, 1351
    definition, 1350
    in the neonate, **1351–1352**
    radiological features, 1351
  bone imaging, children, 2199
  candida, in the neonate, 1352–1353
  chronic, **1353–1356**
    Brodie's abscess, 1353
    chronic granulomatous disease, 1354
    Garré's sclerosing osteitis, 1354
    intervertebral disc(discitis), 1355–1356
    mandible, 1354
    pubis, 1354–1355
    spine, 1355
    differential diagnosis, 1355
  complicating sinusitis, 1943
  pyogenic, mandible, 1913
    actinomycosis, 1914
    acute, 1913

chronic, 1913–1914
  Garré's, 1914
  in infants, 1914
  osteoradionecrosis, 1914
  tertiary syphilis, 1914
  tuberculosis, 1914
radionuclide bone scan, 1541–1542, 1545
rib lesions, 154
secondary, in sickle cell disease, 1332
pyogenic, **1452–1455**
tuberculous, children, **1455**
Osteo-onychodysplasia, **1442–1443**
Osteopenia, 1373
  generalized in myelomatosis, 1340
  and hyperparathyroidism, primary, 1385–1386
  in osteomalacia, 1379
    in renal dystrophy, 1382
    in rickets, 1381
  pathophysiology, 1476
  in rheumatoid arthritis, 1478, 1479, 1480
Osteopetrosis, **1427,** *1428*
  facial bones, 1916
  with osteosclerosis, 1404
  and periodontal disease, 1934
Osteopoikilosis, **1435–1436**
Osteoporosis, **1373–1376**
  associated with postmenopausal or senile states, 1373, *1376*
  circumscripta, **1790**
  disuse, 1400–1401
    reflex sympathetic distress syndrome, patchy, 1402
    spotty, 1402
  in eunuchoidism, 1399
  in hyperthyroidism, 1392
  in hypothyroidism, 1390
  idiopathic juvenile, **1395**
  osteopenia, 1373
  radiological diagnosis, 1373–1374
    advanced, 1375
    cortical thinning, 1375, *1377*
    differential diagnosis, 1375–1376
    and pathological considerations, 1374–1375
    'picture-framing', *1374*, 1375
  in renal dystrophy, 1382
  in scurvy, 1388
  in Turner's syndrome, 1399
Osteoradionecrosis, maxillofacial region, 1914
Osteosarcoma, **1309–1315**
  age, 1309
  appearance, 1276
  clinical presentation, 1309–1310
  CT scan, 1311–1312
  extraosseous, 1315
  parosteal, 1313
  pathological considerations, 1310
  periosteal, 1315
  primary multifocal, 1315
  prognosis, 1312, 1313
  radiological features, 1310–1315
  sarcoma in Paget's disease, 1314
  site, 1310
  teliangiectatic, 1311
Osteosclerosis
  diffuse, **1404–1407**
    associated disorders, 1404
      haematologic, 1404
      metabolic, 1404
      neoplastic, 1404
      primary osseous, 1404
  in fluorosis, 1406

Osteosclerosis (*cont.*)
 in hyperparathyroidism, primary, 1386,
  1387, 1404
 in hypervitaminosis D, 1407
 in hypoparathyroidism, 1405
 in renal osteodystrophy, 1382, 1384, 1404
Otitis media, acute, 1955–1956
 chronic suppurative, 1956
Otorhinolaryngology, **1937–1983**
 see also specific headings
Otorrhoea, CSF
 CT, 1703
  cisternography, 1703
 radiography, 1703
Otosclerosis, 1958–1959
Ovary (ovarian), **1036–1038**
 abscess, 1603
 carcinoma, and ascites, 1594
  CT, 1626
 cysts, 1610–1611
  angiography, 1610
  barium enema, 1610
  CT, 1613
  during pregnancy, ultrasound, 1567
  hysterosalpingography, 1610
  radiology, 1610
  ultrasonography, 1611, 1613
  urography, 1610
 endocrine disorders, 1036
 epithelial tumours during pregnancy, 1567
 function, 1036
 lesions, calcification, 1593
 non-endocrine disorders, 1038
 size, normal, 1036
 tumours, 86, 87, **1036–1038, 1612–1614**
  arteriography, 1598
  magnetic resonance imaging, 86, *87*
  see also specific name
 vein syndrome, 1133
 venography, 2084–2086
Ovulation, 1036
 premature, following ultrasonography, 1038

Pacemaker(s), 324, **653–662**
 as foreign body, 659–661
 circuit failure, 658
 complications, radiology, 656–661
 electrodes, 655
 energy sources, 654
 implantation, 654
 indications, 653
 lead fracture, 657–658
 pulmonary embolism caused by, 660
 thrombosis caused by, 660
Pachydermoperiostosis, 1408, **1431**
Pachymeninges, thickening, 1843
Paediatric conditions
 biliary tract, 984–985
 cervical spine, **1232–1233**
 chest, 329–356
 cisternography, 1869
 colonoscopy, 902
 echocardiography, 395, 414
 gastrointestinal tract, 905–921
 heart conditions, 414
  failure, 545–546
 kidney, congenital abnormalities, 1183,
  1185–1190
 liver, 945
 musculoskeletal system, **1447–1471**
 nuclear medicine, 2197–2211
  see also Nuclear medicine, paediatric

pulmonary venous congestion and oedema,
  546
 radionuclide imaging, 2197–2111
  see also Nuclear medicine, children
 raised intracranial pressure, 1705–1707
 tumours, 54
 ultrasound, **2213–2227**
  see also Congenital anomalies
Paediatric uroradiology, 1179–1210
 approach, 1180
 congenital abnormalities, 1183–1199
  bladder, 1196–1198
  embryology, 1183–1185
  renal, 1185–1190
  renal pelvis, 1190–1196
  ureteric, 1190–1196
  urethra, 1198–1199
 CT scans, 1182
 infection, 1199–1202
 intravenous urography, 1180–1181
 isotope studies, 1182
 loopography, 1182
 major clinical indications, 1179–1180
 neoplasia, 1202–1210
 plain abdominal films, 1180
 radiologist's role, 1180
 renal angiography, 1182
 retrograde pyelography, 1182
 retrograde urethrography, 1182
 techniques, 1180–1182
 ultrasound, 1182
 voiding cysto-urethrography, 1181–1182
 Whitaker test, 1182
 see also specific names
Paget's disease (osteitis deformans), *1440, 1441,*
  1443–1444
 CT, 1790
 juvenile, **1432**
  see also Hyperphosphatasia
 maxillofacial region, 1912
 with osteosclerosis, 1404
 petrous bone, 1961
 radionuclide bone scan, 1545
Pain during venography, 2084
Palatal cysts, median, 1906
Pancake kidney, 1188
Pancoast tumour, 154, 164, *248*
Pancreas, **999–1008**
 aberrant, 800
 abnormalities, 1002–1005
 anatomy, 999–1000
 aneurysm, arteriography, 2013
 angiography, 1001
 arteries, 1000
 arteriography, *2038, 2039, 2053–2054, 2055,*
  2056
 calcification, 960
 carcinoma, *822*
  CT scan, *56*
 cell types, 1031
 congenital abnormalities, 1002
 CT scanning, *49,* 1001
  cysts, 1002, 1005
  divisum, 1006
  embryology, 999–1000
  endocrine disorders, 1005
 ERCP, 1000, **1005–1007**
  indications, 1006
 functioning tumours, 1031
 hormonal aspects, 1031–1032
 hypotonic duodenography, 1000
 investigation, methods, 1000–1002
 magnetic resonance imaging, 84, 1002

percutaneous biopsy, 1002
percutaneous transhepatic cholangiography
  (PTC), 1001
plain film, abdomen, 1000
polypeptidoma, 1032
scintigraphy, 1001
surgery, 1005
trauma, 1005
tumours, 983, **1002–1005**
 carcinoma, *822*
 functioning, 1031
ultrasound, 1001
 children, 2217–2218
veins, 1000
venography and venous sampling, 1002, 2095
Papilla(e)
 accessory, differential diagnosis from
  urothelial tumours, 1112
 calcified, 1060
 carcinoma, breast, 1639–1640
 ducts of Bellini, 1073
 necrosis, 1121–1124, 1128 (*table*)
  acute, 1123–1124
  acute renal failure, infancy, 1121
  aetiology, 1121
  causing obstruction, 1082
  chronic, 1122
  clinical features, 1121
  complicating candidiasis, 1130
  differential diagnosis, 1128 (*table*)
  differential diagnosis from urothelial
   tumours, 1112
  infection, 1121, 1123
  papillary/calyceal abnormality, 1121–1122
  pathology, 1121
  radiology, 1121–1122
 renal parenchyma,
  normal appearances, 1117–1118
   blush, 1117
   flat or small, 1117
   large, 1117
 of Vater, 999
  carcinoma, *821*
Papilloedema, skull films, 1702
 CT, 1702
Papilloma
 breast, 1634
 gallbladder, 979
 larynx, 1978
 nasal cavity, 1946
  epithelial (converted), 1946, **1947**
Papillomatosis, 1634
Paragonimiasis, 217
Paralytic ileus, 721, 730, *731*
Paramagnetic contrast media, 5
Paranasal sinuses, **1937–1951**
 allergy, 1941–1946
 anatomy, 1938–1940
 carcinoma, 1948
  CT, 1949
 choanal atresia, 1941
 CT, 1938
 cysts, 1944
 empyema, 1945
 infection, 1941–1946
 inflammation, 1941–1946
 mucocele, 1943
  ethmoid sinus, 1944
  frontal sinus, 1943
 polyposis, 1945–1946
 radiography, 1937, 1938
 sinusitis, 1942–1943
 tomography, 1937, 1938

Paranasal sinuses (*cont.*)
 tumours, 1946–1950
  benign, 1946–1948
  malignant, 1948–1950
 underdevelopment, 1940
Paraovarian cysts during pregnancy,
  sonography, *1566*, 1567
Paraplegia, ossification, 1520
Parasitic infection
 affecting bone, 1364–1365
 biliary tract, 985–986
  and calcification, 1515
 colitis, 890
Paraspinal lines, 128
Parathormone, 1026
Parathyroids, **1025–1027**, 1039
 adenomas, arteriography, 2030, 2053
 glands, arteriography, 2053
  venography, 2093–2094
 hormone, in osteomalacia, 1380
  secretion in primary hyperparathyroidism,
   1384
 mass, mediastinal, 177
Parenchyma
 definition, 370
 lung, 267, **268–272**, 277, 298
 malacoplakia, 1100
 renal *see* Renal parenchyma
Parietal
 foramina, 1452, *1454*
 lobe dysfunction, CT, 1701
  radiography, 1701
Parosteal
 chondroma, 1278
 osteosarcoma, **1313**
Parotid glands
 calcification, 1922
 trauma, 1922
 see also Salivary glands
Pars interarticularis defect, 1500
Patella
 dislocations, 1264
 fractures, 1264
Patello-femoral tracking abnormalities, CT
  scan, 1533
Patent ductus arteriosus, 492–494, 506
Pearly tumours, 1734–1735
 CT, 1734–1735
PECT *see* Computed tomography, emission
Pectoralis, absence of, 152
Pelken's sign in scurvy, 1388
Pelvis (pelvic)
 CT scan, *48*
 arteriography, 2032–2033
  aorto-iliac-femoral series, 2033
  haemorrhage, 2033
  phaeochromocytoma, 2033
 cancer, lymph node involvement, 1626
 infection and IUCD, 1621
 inflammatory disease, acute, ultrasound,
   1602
  chronic, 1603
  of extragenital origin, 1603
   appendicitis, 1603
   diverticulitis, 1603
 kidney, 1187
 lipomatosis, 892
  causing obstruction, 1083, *1084*
 magnetic resonance imaging, *9*, 86
 masses during pregnancy, sonography, **1565–
  1567**
 plain radiography, 1593
 pneumography, 1597

Stein-Leventhal syndrome, 1611
 rhabdomyosarcoma, paediatric, 1208–1210
 sepsis, complicating hysterectomy, 1623
 trauma, **1240–1245**
  acetabular fractures, 1244–1245
  avulsion injuries, 1243, *1244*
  caudal-angled arterioposterior view, 1240,
   1245
  classification of injuries, 1241–1242
  hip, dislocation, 1243–1244
  Judet projection, hip, 1245
  Malgaigne fracture, 1242
  normal anatomy, 1240
  oblique projections, 1240, 1245
  pelvic ring disruptions, *1241*, **1242–1243**
   radiography, 1242, 1243
  radiographic examination, 1240–1241
  shear injuries, 1243
 venography, 2091
Pelvicalyceal system, tumours, 1110
Pelvimetry, 1583–1589
 android pelvis, 1587
 anthropoid pelvis, 1587
 exposure, 1584
 gynaecoid pelvis, 1587
 indications, 1583–1584
 interpretation, 1586–1587
 Naegele pelvis, 1587
 pattern of moulding, 1588
 platypelloid pelvis, 1587
 projections, 1585
 Roberts pelvis, 1581
 technique, 1584–1586
Pelvi-ureteric junction
 congenital obstructions, 1083
 obstruction, 1195
  intermittent, 1075
  ultrasound, children, 2225
Pemphigoid, oesophageal involvement, 768
Percutaneous methods, 2129–2133
 antegrade pyelography, 2129
 biliary tract, 2131
 catheter nephrostomy, 2129–2130
  indications, 2129
  techniques, 2130
 CT-guided, 52
 coronary angioplasty (PTA), 2143, *2144*
 extraction techniques, 2133–2135
 imaging-guided, 2135
 nephrostomy in urinary obstruction, 1076
 renal cyst puncture, 2129
 splenoportography, 2080
  complications, 2080
  indications, 2080
 transhepatic cholangiography, 963–965
  hilar tumour, *979*, 980
  obstructive jaundice, 979
  pancreas, 1001
  post-cholecystectomy syndrome, 978
 transluminal angioplasty, 2139–2145
  adjunctive drug treatment, 2141
  clinical applications, 2141–2145
   coronary, 2143
   lower extremity, 2141–2143
   miscellaneous sites, 2143–2145
   renal, 2143
  complications, 2145
  digital subtraction angiography, 2139
  mechanisms, 2139–2141
  techniques, 2139–2141
  with ultrasound, 2139–2140
 ureteric dilatation and stent insertion, 2130–
  2131

Perforation
 acute colitis, 730
 complicating diverticulitis, 878
 spontaneous, complicating colorectal
  carcinoma, 875
 ulcerative colitis, 888
 viscus, 731
Perfusion
 scanning, radioisotope, 296–298
 scintigraphy, 134
Pergolide mesylate, 1039
Periapical granuloma, 1932
Pericarditis, 684–685
 aetiology, 685 (*table*)
 constrictive, 686–688
Pericardium, 675–689
 absence, congenital, 677
 congenital anomalies, 677–679
 CT scanning, 446
 cyst, 677–678, *679*
 diverticulum, 678
 echocardiography, 415
  pulmonary vascularity, 573
 effusion, 681–684
 normal, 675–676
 pneumopericardium, 355, 371
 tamponade, 651
 tumours, 679–680
Perilunate dislocation, 1257, *1258*
Perineural (Tarlov) cysts, 1825, *1827*
Periodontal disease
 abscess, acute and chronic, 1933
 associated with systemic disease, 1934
Periodontitis, atrophic (periodontosis), 1934
Periosteal
 elevation in scurvy, 1389
 new bone infancy, 1349–1350
 osteosarcoma, **1314**
Periostitis, **1349–1350**
 in adult (acquired) syphilis, 1360
 in congenital syphilis, 1359
 in scurvy, 1389
Peripheral venous studies, radionuclide, 2192
Perirenal haematoma, 1160
Peritoneum, reflections and spaces, *737*
Perlschnuraterie, 2017
Persistence of fetal circulation, 347, 351
Perthes' disease in children, **1463**
Pertussis, 338
Petrous bone, tumours, 1961
 fractures, 1963
Peutz-Jegher's syndrome, 843, *844*, 872
Phaeochromocytoma, 1034
 arteriography, *2055*
 CT scanning, 1035
 pelvic arteriography, 2033
 venography, 2094
Phakomatoses, **1777–1779**
 affecting eyes, 1881–1882
Phantom tumour
 definition, 370
 pleural effusion, *162*, 163
Pharmacoangiography and magnification, in
  renal artery stenosis, 1155
Pharyngeal abscess, 1967
Pharynx, 1965–1973
 anatomical features, 1966
 cervical dysphagia, 1971–1973
 cricopharyngeus spasm, 1972
 diverticula, 1972
 foreign bodies, 1973
 inflammatory and related lesions, 1967
 postcricoid web, 1972–1973

Pharynx (*cont.*)
  protrusion, 1972
  radiology, 1965–1966 (*table*)
  tumours, benign, 1967–1969
    malignant, 1969–1971
Phlebolith, *1061*
  arteriography arm, 2047, *2048*
  pelvic, 1593
Phlebography, 1702–1703, 1705
  brain, 1693–1695
  disc protrusion, 1832
  lumbar spinal cord stenosis, 1833, 1834
  orbital, 1877
  peripheral, 107
  pulmonary thromboembolism, 302
  spine, 1812–1813
  uterine, 1598
  see also Venography
Phosphorus poisoning, **1408**
Photoelectric interaction, 17
Photoelectron, 17
Photons, 17
  absorptiometry, single, in cortical bone
    measurement, 1410
  definition, 14
  dual, in axial mineral measurement, 1410
  interaction with matter, 15, *17*
Phrenic nerve, carcinomatous invasion, 247
Phrenic palsy, 170
Phrygian cap deformity, 956
Physics, basic, 13–17
Phthisis bulbi, 1883
Physopyometra, 1604
Pierre Robin syndrome, 1915, 1918
Pigeon chest, 155
Pigment stones, 977
Pigmented villonodular synovitis, 1298–1299,
  1501
'Pillar' fracture, **1227–1228**, *1229*
Pilonidal sinus, sonography, 1569
Pineal region tumours (pinealomas), CT, 1712–
  1714
  raised intracranial pressure, 1705, *1706*
Pineoblastomas, CT, 1714
Pinna, deformities, 1964
Pituitary, 1020–1023
  adenomas, **1021–1022**, 1022 (*table*)
    cerebral angiography, 1702, 1703
    chromophobe, CT, *45*
    CT, 1703, **1723–1724**, *1725*
    orbital phlebography, 1702
  gland, arteriography, 2053
  hyperpituitarism, 1022
  hypopituitarism, 1023
  implantation, 2135
  snuff taker's lung, 267
  tumours, 1721–1723
    angiography, 1724–1725
    choristoma, 1723
    craniopharyngioma, 1723
    CT, 1723–1724
    diffusely invasive, 1722–1723
    enclosed, 1721–1722
    glioma, 1723
    locally invasive, 1722
    magnetic resonance imaging, 69, *72*
    microadenomas, 1721
    radiography, 1701, 1721–1723
    radionuclide imaging, 1861–1862
    see also Pituitary adenomas
Pixel, definition, 43
Placenta
  abruption, sonography, 1573–1574

localization and evaluation, sonography,
  1554, *1555*
    prior to amniocentesis, 1563–1564
  praevia, sonography, 1573–1574
Plasma cell disorders, **1338–1341**
Plasmacytoma, **1338–1339**
  extramedullary, larynx, 1978
  petrous bone, 1961
Platelike atelectasis, definition, 370
Platybasia, differential diagnosis from basilar
  invagination, 1776
Platypelloid pelvis, 1587
Pleonaemia, definition, 370
Pleura, **156–165**
  asbestosis, *270*, 271
  calcification, 165
  effusion, **159–163**
    bronchial carcinoma, 248
    complicating pneumonia, 205
    free fluid, 159–161
    lamellar, 161
    loculated fluid, 161
      fissural (interlobar), *162*, 163
    post-operative, *320*, 321
    post-primary tuberculosis, 210
    post-radiotherapy, 326
    primary tuberculosis, 209
    radiological signs, 159
    round atelectasis, 228
    subpulmonary, 160, *161*
    systemic lupus erythematosus, 279
  hemithorax, opacification, 160
  infants and young children, 335
  local mass lesions, *162*, 165
  normal, radiograph, 156
  oedema, re-expansion, 158
  pathology, 156
  'phantom' tumour, *162*, 163
  pressure, 158 (*fig.*)
  sarcoidosis, 278
  thickening, 164, *165*
  thromboembolism, radiography, 298
  trauma, 306
  ultrasound, 135
Pleuropericardial cysts, 190
Plexiform angiomas, arteriography, 2008
Pneumatocoele, 205
  definition, 371
Pneumatosis coli, 738, 893
  cystoides intestinalis, 738
Pneumoconiosis
  coalworker's, 268
  silicate, 269–272
Pneumocystitis carinii infections, lung, 289
Pneumoencephalography, **1694–1700**
  acoustic neuroma, 1733
  anatomy, 1698–1700
  arachnoid cyst, 1774
  complications, 1698
  cranial nerve disturbances, 1702–1703
  empty sella, *1725*
  in endocrine disease, 1020
  equipment, 1695
  interpretation, 1700
  pelvic *see* Pelvic pneumography
  pituitary tumours, 1725
  preparation of patient, 1695
  technique, 1695–1696
Pneumomediastinum, 176, 1521
  definition, 371
  post-operative, 320
    radiograph, 321
Pneumonias, 199–206

anaerobic, 202, *203*
associated features, 204
atelectasis, 206
bacterial, 289
  infants and young children, 337, *339*
childhood, bacteriological aetiologies, 336
  (*table*)
Chlamydial, 204
complications, local, 204
cryptococcal, 214, *215*
cytomegalovirus, 289
definition, 371
diffuse interstitial, 272–274
eosinophilic, 284
Gram-negative, 200, *201*
influenza A, 203
lobar, definition, 200
localized, transradiancies, 205
measles, *204*
Mycoplasma pneumoniae, 202, *203*
  infants and young children, 338
neonatal, 350
pneumocystis carinii, in infants and young
  children, 340
post-operative, 318
residual scarring, 206
resolution, 206
Rickettsial, 204
secondary to bronchial carcinoma, features,
  246
Staphylococcus aureus, 200, *201*
Streptococcus pneumoniae, 200, *201*
varicella, 203, *204*
viral, 203
  childhood, 337
Pneumonitis
  lupus, 280
  obstructive, 228
  radiation, 325
Pneumopericardium
  definition, 371
  infants, 355
Pneumoperitoneum, plain radiography, **731–
  734**, 1594
  simulating conditions, 733
  supine radiography, 732
  without peritonitis, 733
Pneumothorax, **156–159**
  artificial, 323
  causes, 157 (*table*)
  complicating asthma, 234
    pulmonary bullae, 236
  complications, 158
  definition, 371
  diagnosis, 157
  differentiation from pneumomediastinum,
    196
  infants, 352
  post-operative, 320
  radiology, 156
  spontaneous, post-radiotherapy, 326
  tension, differentiation from congenital lobar
    emphysema, 364
    post-operative, *316, 319*, 320, 325
  traumatic, 306
  underlying lung disease, 158
Poisoning, heavy metal, 1408
  see also substance causing
Poland's syndrome, 152
Polyarteritis nodosa
  associated with sialectasis, 1921
  lungs, 282
  microaneurysms, *2014*

Polyarteritis nodosa (*cont.*)
  small renal vessels, 1156
    subtraction angiogram, 1158
Polychondritis, relapsing, 284
Polycystic
  disease, infantile, ultrasound, 2224
  ovarian disease, 1036, 1038
Polycythaemia, 1333
Polymyositis, lungs, 283
Polypectomy, colonoscopy, 902
Polyps
  adenomatous, large bowel, 879
    polyposis, fibresigmoidoscopy, 901
  colon, colonoscopy, 902
  colorectal, malignant, early, 872
  diffuse polypoid malignancy, 872
  gastric, 798–799
  large bowel, **866–871**
    adenomatous, differentiation from
      diverticula, 880
    barium diagnosis, 865
    diffuse polypoid malignancy, 872
  oesophageal, 762
  small bowel, **842–843**
  stomach, **798–799**
  ulcerative colitis, **885–886**
Polyposis
  antrochoanal, 1946
  juvenile, 872
  lymphomatous, of large bowel, 876
  maxillary, *1945*, 1946
  metaplastic, 872
  nasal, 1945–1946
  syndromes, large bowel, 871–872
Polytomography in external and middle ear
  anomalies, 1964
Pompe's (glycogen storage) disease, 541, 639
Poppet embolization, 668
Porencephalic cyst, ultrasound, neonate, 2232
Porencephaly, fetal, sonography, 1576, 1577
Portal hypertension, **949–951**
  arteriography, 2042
  embolization, 995
  post-hepatic, 950
  splenomegaly, 1012
  surgery, 951
  venography, 2079
Portal vein, 'streaming', 2082, *2083*
Portal venography, **2079–2084**
  anatomy, 2079
  direct, 2080–2082
    percutaneous splenoportography, 2080
    transhepatic portography, 2080–2082
  indirect (arterioportography), 2082–2084
    indications, 2082–2084
    technique, 2082
  techniques, 2080–2084
Portal venous system, ultrasound, children,
  2218, *2219*
Portography, 941–945
  biliary tract, 974
  direct, 941, 944, *945*
  hilar tumours, 982
  indications, 944
  indirect, 941
  transhepatic, 974, **2080–2082**
Positioning of infants and young children, 329
Positron, definition, 15
Postcricoid
  carcinoma, 1970
    and dysphagia, 1970, 1971
  web, 1972–1973
Posterior

fossa mass, 1706
  tracheal stripe, definition, 371
  urethral valves, 1198–1199
Postoperative
  abdomen, 734
  patients, pulmonary aspects, 313–327
  support and monitoring apparatus, 324
Postpartum
  cardiomyopathy, 641
  disorders, sonography, 1580
Post-phlebitic syndrome, 2090
Post-phlebographic syndrome, 2088
Post-stenotic aneurysms, arteriography, 2012–
  2013
Potts shunt, 575
Pouch of Douglas, lesions, 892 (*table*)
Preduodenal portal vein, 985
Pregnancy
  contraindication to arteriography, 1992
  ectopic, hysterosalpingography
    contraindicated, 1595
    ultrasonography, 1619
  hydroureteronephrosis, 1074
  and IUCDs, 1621
    sonography, 1563
  magnetic resonance imaging, 86, *87*
  and periodontal disease, 1934
  sonography, ectopic, **1557–1562**
    see also Ectopic pregnancy
    molar, 1562
    multiple, 1564–1565
  thromboembolism, 294
  ultrasound, **1551–1580**
    see also Obstetrics, sonography
  ureter, dilatation, 1132–1133
    with infection, 1133, *1134*
  ureteric calculus, 1074–1075
Prepyloric web, 804
Priapism, 1039
  embolization, 2156
Probe renography in renal artery stenosis, 1153
Profusion, definition, 371
Progestasert, 1621
Progesterone, 1036
Progressive system sclerosis,
  duodenum, 824
  small bowel, 853
Prolactinoma, CT scan, *1021*
Prolapse
  gastric mucosa, 805, *806*
  mitral valve, 591
Propyliodone, 135
Prostate
  carcinoma, causing obstruction, 1085–1086
    lymph node metastases, 2174
  hypertrophy, magnetic resonance imaging,
    86
Prostheses
  hip or knee, radionuclide bone scanning,
    1542
  insertion, vascular, 2138
    congenital vascular defects, 2138
    vena caval filters, 2138
Proton(s), 14
  in magnetic resonance imaging, 447
Protozoal infections, pulmonary, 217
  infants and young children, 340
Prune belly syndrome, 1196–1198
  amniography, 1580, 1583
  fetal detection sonography, 1570
  ultrasound, children, 2226
Pseudoachondroplasia, **1419**, *1421*
  form of spondylo-epiphyseal dysplasia, **1419**

Pseudoaneurysm
  left ventricular, 629
  post-traumatic, complicating renal trauma,
    1177
Pseudocavity, definition, 371
Pseudocoarctation of the aorta, 702, *703*
Pseudohermaphrodite, female, genitography,
  1601
Pseudohypoparathyroidism, 1026, **1405–1406**
  differential diagnosis, 1406
  radiological and pathological diagnosis,
    1405–1406
  soft tissue calcification, 1514
Pseudolymphoma, gastric, 796
Pseudomediastinum *see* Mediastinum
Pseudomonas pyocyanea, *202*
Pseudo-pseudohypoparathyroidism, 1026,
  1405–1406
  differential diagnosis, 1406
  radiological and pathological diagnosis,
    1405–1406
Pseudotruncus, 502, 503
Pseudotumour, renal
  algorithm, evaluation, 1091, **1093**
  arteriography, 2034
  cysts, 1096–1099
  description, 1097
  pathology, 1097–1102
Psoriatic arthropathy, **1488–1490**
  differential diagnosis, 1489
  feet, 1488
  hands, 1488
  large joints, 1489
  sacroiliac joints, 1489
  spine, 1489
PTC *see* Percutaneous transhepatic
  cholangiography
Pubis, osteomyelitis, **1354–1355**
Pulmonary embolism
  acute, 2106–2107
  chronic, 2107
  complicating venography, 2064
  digital subtraction angiography, 2105–2106
  and fibrosis, 2107
Pulmonary hypertension, 253, 575
  and incompetence, *560*
  venous, 568–571
Pulmonary system
  arteries, 116, 120, 473, **565–567**
    abnormalities, radiographic appearance,
      576–582
    absence (interruption), congenital, 533–
      534
    aneurysms, 580–582
    atresia, 494, 504
    central, 565, *566*
    congenital heart conditions, 469
    coronary artery arising from, 495
    hypertension, 575
      obstructive ventricular septal defect, 491
      radiographic features, 576
    idiopathic dilatation, 579–580
    left, anomalous origin (pulmonary artery
      sling), 534
    poststenotic dilatation, 579–580
    proximal interruption, 360
    ring, 494
    segmental, 565–567
    stenosis, 580, *581*
      peripheral, 532
    tetralogy of Fallot *see* Tetralogy of Fallot
    truncus, 517
      hemitruncus, 517

Pulmonary system (*cont.*)
  arteries (*cont.*)
    truncus (*cont.*)
      Type IV, *516*, 517
  arteriolar obstruction *see* Eisenmenger
    reaction
  arterioles, 567
  arterio-venous communications,
    embolization, 2155–2156
  arteriovenous fistula, 579
  arteriovenous malformations, cause of
    central cyanosis, 524
    see also Arteriovenous malformations
  arteritis, 579
  circulation, **565–583**
    congenital conditions, radiological
      assessment, **464–468**
    congestion and oedema, 541, *542*
      infancy, 546
    cor triatum, 537
    Eisenmenger reaction (pulmonary arteriolar
      obstruction), 466, **505–507**, 567, *575*, 580
    heart disease, **568–575**
      congenital, vascularity, 574
    infundibular stenosis, 504, 532
    metastases, CT, 2179–2180
    oedema *see* Oedema, pulmonary
    oligaemia (undercirculation), 572
    plethora (arterial overcirculation), 571
    radionuclide, 22 (*table*)
    shunt vessels, 571
    specific acquired cardiac lesions, vascularity,
      572–575
    thromboembolism *see* Thromboembolism,
      pulmonary
    tumours, gallium imaging, 2189–2190
      see also Lungs, tumours: Bronchial
        carcinoma
  valve, absence of, 532, **579–580**
  valvular stenosis, associated with atrial
    septal defect, 484
    congenital heart disease, **530–532**
    tetralogy of Fallot, 501, 504
    ventriculo-arterial discordance,
      uncorrected, 520
  vascular anatomy and physiology, 565–568
  veins, 116, 120
    anomalous drainage, 535–537
      total, **508–512**, *536, 537*
        infradiaphragmatic, 511
        mixed patterns, 512
    associated with atrial septal defect, 484
    embryological development, *536*
    obstructed, 537
      in the newborn, 350
    varicosities, 537
  ventilation and perfusion, radionuclide
    imaging, children, 2209
  see also Heart: Lungs
Pulp stones, 1933
Pulpitis, 1932
Pulseless disease *see* Takayashu's syndrome
Punctate epiphyseal dysplasia, **1424–1426**
Puncture site complications in arteriography,
  1999–2001
Pyknodysostosis, 1427, *1429*
  with osteosclerosis, 1404
Pyelocaliectasis, massive, 1073
Pyelography
  antegrade, 2129
    in urinary obstruction, 1069, 1076
  retrograde, in urinary obstruction, 1069, 1076
  urinary tract, 1049

Pyelonephritis
  acute, 1120
    CT, 1120
      suppurative, 1120
      ultrasound, 1120
  atrophic, chronic, 1126–1127
    clinical features, 1126
    differential diagnosis, 1128 (*table*)
    radiology, 1126–1127
  chronic, renal angiography, 1156
  emphysematous, 739, 1131
  xanthogranulomatous, 1099, 1130
Pyelosinus extravasation, 1071–1072
Pyeloureteritis cystica, 1132, *1133*
  differential diagnosis from urothelial
    tumours, 1112
Pyle's disease, **1427–1429**
Pyloric stenosis, hypertrophic, in infants, 913,
  915, *916*
Pyloroplasty, 808
Pyogenic
  arthritis, children, **1452–1455**
  arthropathy, 1504–1505
  infection, CT scan, *1525*
  osteomyelitis, children, **1452–1455**
Pyosalpinx, 1602, 1603
PZT (lead-zirconate-titanate), 26

Rachischisis, 1821
Radial head, fracture, 1254
Radiation
  and breast cancer, 1656–1657
  colitis, 889
  exposure, during amniography, risks, 1582
  gamma-ray, definition, 14
  risks, in utero, **1590**
  therapy *see* Radiotherapy
Radicular cysts, 1945
Radiculopathy, cervical spondylotic, **1837–
  1838**
Radioactive
  decay, 15
  material, activity, 16
    specific, 17
  seed implantation, 2135
Radioactivity
  and decay mechanisms, 14–16
  definition, 14
Radiogrammetry in cortical bone
  measurements, 1410
Radiography
  (entries here are not exhaustive. *See also*
    specific conditions and techniques)
  abdomen *see* Abdomen, plain radiography
  aortic, aneurysm, 604
    coarctation, 701
    fixed aortic stenosis, 698
    supravalvar stenosis, 698
    trauma, 714
    valvular stenosis, 695
  aortitis, 604
  asthma, 233–239
  bedside, 313
  bilharzia (urinary schistosomiasis), 1130
  bladder carcinoma, 1110
  brain, abscess, 1739
    stem deficit, 1702
  cerebral hemisyndromes, acute, 1701
    chronic, 1703
  cerebrospinal fluid, rhinorrhoea, 1703
    otorrhoea, 1703
  chest, constrictive pericarditis, 686–688
    interpretation, 139–150

    trauma, 305–311
    wall, 151–156
  coma, 1701
  computed (scout view, topogram), 41
  contrast, definition, 371
  cost-effectiveness, 4
  cranial nerve disturbances, chronic, 1702–
    1703
  cranial nerve palsies, 1701
  critically ill patient, 313–327
  decubitus, 313
  dental, 1925
  diaphragm, 167–173
  digital *see* Digital radiography
  emphysema, 235–239
  head injury, 1701
  headache, acute, 1707
    chronic, 1702
  infants, 329–355
  large airway obstruction, 221–232
  liver, 927–928
  loss of consciousness, 1701
  maternal abdomen, **1589**
    risks of exposure, 1589
  mediastinum, 175–196
  meningioma, **1728–1732**
  meningitis, recurrent, 1703
  in neurological disorders, 1700–1703
  occult spinal dysraphism, 1823
  optic nerve, 1702
  orbit, 1877
  pancreas, plain film, 1000
  pericardial effusion, 681
  pituitary tumours, **1721–1723**
  quality, definition, 371
  pleura, 156–165
  post-operative patient, 313–324
  post-thoracotomy, 321–324
  pulmonary, congenital conditions, **357–365**
    diffuse disease, 259–291
    infection, 199–219
    neoplasm, 241–257
    thromboembolism, 298–300
  renal artery aneurysm, 1158
  renal failure, 1137
  spinal cord compression, 1839–1840
  spine, 1798
  spleen, 1009, 1010
  suspected subarachnoid haemorrhage, 1701
  Takayashu's arteritis, 704
  tricuspid valve disease, 596
  young children, 329–355
Radio-immunodetection of tumours, 2194
Radioisotope
  definition, 14
  see also Isotopes: Radionuclide
Radiological sign, definition, 371
Radionecrosis, skull, CT, 1718–1719
Radionuclide imaging, 20–23
  bone scanning, **1535–1547**
    in Hodgkin's disease, 1336–1337
    mechanisms of localization, 1535–1537
      see also 99m-Technetium
    in myelomatosis, 1340
    normal bone scan, 1537–1538
    radiopharmaceuticals, 1535–1537
    special applications, 1538–1545
      arthritis, 1542
      avascular necrosis, 1543–1545
      inflammatory disease, 1541–1542
      metastases, 1538–1540
      miscellaneous lesions, 1545–1546
      primary bone tumours, 1540

Radionuclide imaging (*cont.*)
  bone scanning (*cont.*)
    special applications (*cont.*)
      prostheses, 1542
      trauma, 1540–1541
  cardiovascular, 419–438
    standard views, *420*
    technicalities, 421
  central nervous system, **1857–1872**
    see also Brain scanning, radionuclide
  chest, 133–135
  children, 2197–2211
    see also Children and specific techniques
  cisternography, **1866–1871**
    compared with CT, 1869
    in CSF imaging, children, 2206–2207
    CSF physiology, 1866
    CSF rhinorrhoea, 1870–1871
    hydrocephalus, 1866–1869
      normal pressure versus cerebral atrophy,
        1868–1869
    paediatric, 1869
    shunt patency studies, 1869–1870
    techniques, 1866
    ventriculography, 1871
  definition, 14
  gastric emptying, 810–813
  general principles, 13–23
  hepatobiliary, 970–973
  kidney, transplanted, 1143–1144, 1145
  pericardial effusion, 683
  in renal artery stenosis, 1153
  in renal infarction, 1155–1156
  renal masses, 1091
  renal tract, 1052–1057
    clearance techniques, 1052
    dynamic renal scan, 1052–1055
  renal vein thrombosis, 1161
  small bowel, 836
  spleen, 1010
  tumours, **2183–2195**
    see also Tumours, nuclear imaging: and
      other techniques in urinary
      obstruction, 1078
  ventriculography, 381, **421–429**, 636
    see also Ventriculography
  in Wilms' tumour, 1205
Radiopharmaceuticals, 20–23, 1535–1537
  adverse reactions, 23
  in bone imaging, 2185
  clinical applications, 22–23 (*table*)
  definition, 13
  in endocrine disease, 1040
  quality control, 23
  ventriculography, 423
    see also Ventriculography
  see also 99m-Technetium
Radiotherapy
  causing osteoradionecrosis, 1914
  cerebral tumours, effects, CT, 1718–1719
  chest, 325
  duodenal damage, 824
  effect on teeth, 1928, 1929, 1931
    and dental caries, 1931
  enteritis induced by, 849
  -induced neoplasms, 196
  oesophagitis induced by, 758
  pericarditis induced by, 685
  treatment planning, CT, 53
  see also Radiation
Rasmussen aneurysm, 580
Rat handler's lung, 267
Raynaud's phenomenon, 2046

arteriography, 2046
oesophagus, 775
Reactive hyperplasia, 187
Rectilinear scanners, 20
Rectovaginal fistulae, 1616
Rectum
  bleeding, colonoscopy, 901
  carcinoma, 874
    CT scan, *57*
    see also Bowel, large
Red cell disorders, **1327–1334**
Reflection, ultrasound, 27
Reflex sympathetic dystrophy syndrome, **1401–1402**
Reflux
  ileitis, *882*, 884
  intrarenal, 1200
  nephropathy, 1202
  radiography, 1202
  see also Vesico-ureteric reflux
Regurgitation, 749
Reiter's syndrome, 1356, **1490**, 1491
  associated with sialectasis, 1921
Rejection, acute, in renal transplantation, 1145
Relapsing polychondritis, 284
Renal
  agenesis, bilateral, 1185
    fetal detection, sonography, 1570, *1571*,
      1575
    radiographic findings, 1186
    unilateral, 1185–1186
  angiography *see* Angiography, renal
  arteriography, 2033–2037
    cysts, 2034
    malignant, 2035
    trauma, 2037
    tumours, 2034
    vascular abnormalities, 2035
      renal transplantation, 2036–2037
  artery, aneurysm, radiology, 1158, *1159*
    angioplasty in renal artery stenosis, 1155
    anomalies, arteriography, 2004–2006
    avulsion, 1176
    disease, digital subtraction angiography,
      2108
    embolization, 2146
    in hypertension, **1151–1158**
    occlusion in transplantation, 1146
    stenosis, arteriography, **2035–2036**
      causing hypertension, 1151
      clinical features, 1152
      digital subtraction angiography, 1154
      intravenous urography, 1152–1153
      pharmacoangiography and
        magnification, 1155
      radionuclide imaging, 1153
      renal artery angioplasty, 1155
      renal vein renin ratio, 1154
      split renal function studies, 1155
      in transplantation, 1146
    thrombosis, intravenous urography, 1176
  carcinoma, embolization, *2152*
    lymph node metastases, 2174
  cell carcinoma, 1102
    abdominal plain radiography, 1103
    arteriography, 2035
    CT, 1103
    embolization, 1103
    ultrasound, 1103
  collecting system, duplication
  cysts, *see* Cysts, renal
    puncture, 2129

ultrasound, children (poly-, solitary and
    multi-), 2223–2224
  disorders, ultrasound, children, **2222–2226**
  duplication, **1190–1196**
  failure, **1137–1141**
    CT, 1140, 1141
    collecting systems, dilatation, 1138, *1139*,
      1140
    diagnosis, 1140–1141
      acute, 1141
      chronic, 1141
      obstruction/non-obstruction, 1140–1141
      vascular causes, 1141
    high dose urography, 1137–1139
      findings, 1138–1139
        obstructed/non-obstructed kidney,
          1138
      patient preparation, hazards, 1138
      risk factors, 1138
      technique, 1138
    plain films, 1137
    pulmonary oedema, 264
    renal size, 1137
    ultrasound, 1139–1140, 1141
      findings, 1140
  function in obstruction, 1079
    99m-Tc-DMSA scan, 1079
  haemorrhage, spontaneous, 1159–1160
  infarction, 1155–1156
    radiology, 1156
  masses *see* Kidney masses
  osteodystrophy, **1382–1384**, *1385*
    brown tumours, 1383, *1384*
    in children, 1467
    delayed skeletal maturation, 1397
    development, 1382
    differential diagnosis, 1384
    radiological diagnosis, 1382
      pathological considerations, 1382–1384
  parenchyma, anatomy, 1115
    carcinoma, differential diagnosis from
      urothelial tumours, 1112
    disease, 1119–1134
      back pressure atrophy, 1126
      differential diagnosis, 1127–1129
      focal infarction, 1121
      with/without papillary/calyceal
        abnormality, 1128–1129
      see also specific diseases
    normal appearances, 1116–1119
      excretion urography, 1116
      plain film, abdomen, 1116
      renal sinus fat, 1118
    rims and shells, 1073
    rupture, 1072
    thickness, in obstruction, 1072
    transit time of tracers in obstruction, 1079
    tumours, 1102–1105
    ultrasound, children, 2222–2223
  pelvis, paediatric anomalies, **1190–1196**
    duplication, renal collecting system, 1190–
      1196
      embryology, 1191–1192
      ureteric ectopy, 1192
      ureterocele, 1193–1195
      vesico-ureteric reflux, 1192
  radionuclide imaging, children, 2201–2203
    assessment of function, 2201–2202
  transluminal angioplasty (percutaneous),
    2142, 2143
  transplantation *see* Transplantation, renal
  tuberculosis, 1124–1126, 1128 (*table*)
    see also Tuberculosis, renal

Renal (*cont.*)
 tubular acidosis, calculi, 1063
  disorders and osteomalacia, 1378
 tumours, angiography, 1048
  venography, 2077
 vascular calcification, 1065
 vein, renin ratio in renal artery stenosis, 1154
  thrombosis, 1160–1161
   causes, 1160, 1161 (*table*)
   pathogenesis, 1160–1161
   radiology, 1161
   sequelae, 1161
   in transplantation, 1147 (*table*)
   venography, 2076–2077
    causes, 2077
  venography, 2076–2077
   anatomy, 2076
   causes of thrombosis, 2077
   indications, 2076–2077
   non-functioning kidney, 2077
   technique, 2076
   tumours, 2077
   vein assessment, 2077
  see also Kidney : Urinary tract
Renin-angiotensin system in renovascular
  hypertension, 1151
Renovascular hypertension, **1151–1155**
 aetiology, 1151–1152
 angiography, 1048, 1152, 1154
 causes, 1152 (*table*)
 digital subtraction angiography, 1154
 intravenous urography, 1152, 1155
 management, 1152
 radionuclide imaging, 1153
 renal vein renin ratio, 1154
 transluminal angioplasty, 2143
Resolution, definition, 372
Resorption
 bone, 1371
 in hyperparathyroidism, primary, 1384, 1385
 subperiosteal, in renal dystrophy, 1382, *1383*
 of teeth, 1935
Respiratory distress syndrome, 346
 adult, associated diseases, 319 (*table*)
  postoperative, 319
  pulmonary oedema, 265
  traumatic, 307
 of the newborn, 345
  mechanical problems, 352
  transient, 347, 349
 therapy, complications, 351–355
 type II, 347, 349
Respiratory failure, definition, 372
Respiratory phase, in infants and young
  children, 330
Respiratory syncytial virus pneumonia, 336
Reticuloendothelial disorders, 1341–1342
 splenomegaly, 1012
Reticulohistiocytosis, multicentric, 1485
Reticuloses, orbital, 1893
Reticulum cell sarcoma, 1276
 of bone, **1320**, *1321*
  lung metastases, 1320
  maxillofacial region, 1912
Retinal detachment, 1894
Retinoblastoma, 1894–1896
 metastatic, maxillofacial region, 1911
Retrograde
 brachial angiography, 1683
 pyelography, paediatric, 1182
  renal masses, 1095, *1096*, 1105, 1106
 ureterography, in renal infarction, 1156
 in renal vein thrombosis, 1161

 in urethral injuries, anterior, 1164
  posterior, 1165–1166
 paediatric, 1182
Retroperitoneal
 air insufflation, 1522
 fibrosis causing obstruction, 1081
  CT, *1139*
  ultrasound, *1139*
  and ureteric obstruction, 1083, *1084*
Retropharyngeal abscess, 1967
Retrosternal stripe, 128
Reversible ischaemic neurological deficit, 1756
Rhabdomyoma, 649
Rhabdomyosarcoma
 bile duct, in children, 985
 cystic, *51*
 pelvic, paediatric, 1208–1210
Rheumatic fever, 585
Rheumatic mitral valve disease, 556, **586–591**
Rheumatoid arthritis, **1477–1481**
 associated with sialectasis, 1920
 complications, 1480, 1481
 differential diagnosis, 1480–1481
 hand, 1478
 juvenile, 1456–1457
  see also Juvenile rheumatoid arthritis
 lower extremity, 1479
 pathophysiological concepts, 1473–1477
  see also Joint disease
 spine, 1479
 upper extremity, 1478–1479
 wrist, 1478
Rheumatoid arthropathies, pathophysiological
  concepts, 1473–1477
 see also Joint disease
Rheumatoid disease, pleuropulmonary disease,
  280
 'look-alikes', 1491
Rhinorrhoea, cerebrospinal fluid, 1963
 CT, 1703
  cisternography, 1703
 radiography, 1703
 radionuclide scanning, **1870–1871**
Rhomboid fossa, simulating neoplasia, 1460
Ribs
 carcinomatous destruction, 247, *248*
 fracture, 305
 malignant lesions, 154, *155*
 metastases, radionuclide bone scanning,
  1539
 notching, *153*
  causes, 154 (*table*), 700 (*table*)
  congenital heart disease, 469
 superior marginal defects, 154
 tumours, 154, *155*
Rickets, **1381–1382**
 in children, **1466–1467**
 delayed skeletal maturation, 1397
 differential diagnosis, 1381–1382
 effect on tooth enamel, 1927
 hypophosphataemic, soft tissue calcification,
  1514
 neonatal, 1381
 in osteomalacia, 1378
  vitamin D dependent, 1378
 radiological diagnosis, 1381
  pathological considerations, 1381
 tumour associated, 1381
Rickettsial pneumonia, 204
Riedel's lobe, 945
Riedel's struma, 194
Right ovarian vein syndrome, 1083, 1133
Rim nephrogram, 1073

Ring
 epiphyses, thoracic spine, 1235
 shadow, barium, 865
  large bowel, *867*
Road traffic accidents, aortic rupture, 713
 see also Trauma : and specific injuries
Roberts pelvis, 1587
Rokitansky-Aschoff sinuses, 961, *962*, 977
Rolando fracture, 1260
Root fragments, retained, 1909
[131]I-Rose Bengal, 970
Rotational injuries, thoracolumbar spine, 1237
Round cell tumours of bone, malignant, **1317**
Rubella
 arthritis, 1366
 congenital eye and optic nerve
  malformations, 1880, *1881*
 embryopathy, *1365*, 1456
 maternal, pulmonary artery stenosis,
  peripheral, 532
'Rugger jersey' spine
 in hyperparathyroidism, primary, 1387
 in renal osteodystrophy, 1382, 1383
Rupture
 aorta, 308, **713–714**
 diaphragm, 310
 duodenum, traumatic, 825
 mediastinum, 308–310
 spleen, 1015
Ruptured membranes, *1578*

Saccular abdominal aneurysms, 2010, *2011*
Saccular aneurysm, arteriography, 2010
Sacral cysts, **1824**
Sacroiliac joints
 in ankylosing spondylitis, 1486
 in psoriatic arthropathy, 1489
 in Reiter's syndrome, 1490
Sacroiliitis, early, CT scan, 1533
Saf-T-coil, 1620
St Jude valve, 664, 666
Salicylates, lung disease induced by, *290*
Salivary glands, 1918–1920
 calculi, 1919–1920
 duct strictures, 1920
 sialography, 1918–1919
 trauma, 1922
 tumours, 1920
  CT, 1922
  isotope scanning, 1922
  ultrasound, 1922
Salmonella, bone infection, **1363**
Salpingitis
 acute, 1602
  plain radiography, 1602
 tuberculous, 1604–1605
Salter-Harris classification of fractures, **1247–1248**
Santorini, duct of, 999
Sarcoidosis, 186, *187*, **276–279**
 affecting bone, **1366–1367**
 heart involvement, 639
 lymphadenopathy, 276
 nasal involvement, 1946
 orbital manifestation, 1889
 ring shadows, *146*, 149
Sarcoma, *55*, 649
 anaplastic, **1324**
 arising in previously irradiated bone, **1315**
 Ewing's *see* Ewing's sarcoma
 larynx, 1978
 orbital, 1893
 in Paget's disease, **1314**

Sarcoma (*cont.*)
  renal, 1104
  reticulum cell, 1276
  synovial, **1323**
Scalene syndrome, 2013
Scaphoid, carpus, fracture, 1259
Scapulae, 128
  injuries, **1250–1251**
    fractures, 1250–1251
Scarring
  breast biopsy, 1638–1639
  renal cortical, 1126
Scars, and ossification, 1520
SCDK-Cutter valve, 668
Scheuermann's disease, 1502
  children, 1464
Schistosomiasis, 986
  colitis, 893
  and nephrocalcinosis, 1065
Schmid type of metaphyseal chondrodysplasia,
    1430
Schmorl's nodules, 1235
  in Scheuermann's disease, 1464
Schwannomas, optic nerve sheath, 1893
Scimitar syndrome, 136, **361**, 535, *537, 574*
Scintigraphy, 133–134
  adrenals, 1035
  gamma, children, 2197–2198
    see also Bone imaging
  gastric, dual isotope, 811
  gastro-oesophageal, 748, 751–752
  hepatobiliary, 970–973
  liver, 933–936
  oesophageal motility, 776–778
  pancreas, 1001
Scintillation camera, 17
Sclerodactyly, oesophagus, 775
Scleroderma, **1484–1485**
  associated with periodontal disease, 1934
  associated with sialectasis, 1921
  calcification, 1518, *1519*
  gastroparesis, 807
  small renal vessels, radiography, 1156
    see also Sclerosis
Sclerosing stromal cell tumour of ovary, 1615
Sclerosis
  idiopathic, 1909
  medial, calcification, 1514
  in myelomatosis, 1340
  systemic, lungs, 281
    oesophagus, 773, **775**
    see also Scleroderma
Sclerosteosis, **1432**
Scurvy, 1387–1389
  in children, **1446**, *1467*
  radiological diagnosis, 1388
    pathological considerations, 1388
Seat-belt injuries, lap, 1237, *1239*
Sedation, for colonoscopy, 899
Segment, definition, 372
Seldinger catheterization, cardiac, 382
  in cerebral arteriography, 1684
Sella turcica
  empty sella, 1708
  erosion, 1706
Sepsis, local, in arteriography, 2001
Septal lines, 568–570
Septate uterus, 1600
Septic arthritis
  bone imaging, children, 2199
  radionuclide bone scan, 1541–1542
Septicaemia
  neonatal, 350

pulmonary oedema, 264
Septo-optic dysplasia, 1770, 1881
Sequestration, pulmonary, 136
Serum calcium estimation, 1039
Sheaths in arteriography, 1991
Shell nephrogram, 1073
Shoulder
  arthropathy, **1506**
  injuries, **1248–1250**
    dislocations, 1249
    fractures, 1249
      Hill-Sachs fracture, 1249
    rheumatoid arthritis, 1478–1479
Shunts
  aorto-pulmonary, **492–495**
  infancy, 546
  left-to-right, **477–496**
  pulmonary vascularity, 574–575
  radionuclide imaging, 419, 428
    see also Hearts, shunts
SI units, definition, 16
Sialectasis, 1920–1921
  childhood, 1921
  connective tissue diseases, 1920–1921
  infective, 1920
  Sjögren's syndrome, 1920, *1922*
Sialography, 1918–1919
  cannulaton, 1918
  contrast medium, 1918
  delayed radiography, 1919
  sialectasis, 1921
  trauma, 1922
  tumours, 1921–1922
Sickle cell anaemia, 1469
Sickle cell disease, **1329–1332**
  clinical features, 1330
  papillary necrosis, 1121, 1122
  pathological features, 1329–1330
  radiological features, 1330–1332
    bone infarction, 1330–1332
    marrow aplasia, 1330
    secondary osteomyelitis, 1332
Siderosis, 272
Sievert (Sv), definition, 16
Sigmoid volvulus, 728–729, 894
Sigmoidovaginal fistulae, 1616
Silhouette sign, definition, 372
Silicate pneumoconioses, 269–272
Silicosis, 269
Simple cyst, 1285
Single photon
  absorptiometry in cortical bone
    measurements, 1410
  emission computed tomography, 2201
Sinography
  brain and skull, 1694
  skull, 1694
Sinus
  lipomatosis, renal, 1101
  paranasal *see* Paranasal sinuses
  venosus defect, 535
Sinusitis, 1942–1943
  chronic, 1943
  complications, 1943
    epidural and cerebral abscess, 1943
    osteomyelitis, 1943
Sipple's syndrome, 1025, 1035
Situs, cardiac, definition, 471
  inversus, 542, *543*
  solitus, 542, *543*, 544
Sjögren's syndrome, 1921, *1922*
  lungs, 283
Skeletal system

abnormality, in heart disease, 562
  in gynaecological radiography, 1594
  hyperostosis, idiopathic, *1499*, 1500
  metastases, bone imaging, 2200
    CT scan, 1527, *1528*
    radionuclide bone scanning, 1538
  radionuclides, 22 (*table*)
  trauma, **1223–1272**
    see also specific parts of skeleton
Skier's thumb, 1260
Skin, oesophageal lesions causing conditions
    of, 768
Skull
  anatomy, 1675–1676, 1676 (*table*)
  base, deossification, 1708
  computerised tomography, 1678–1682
    see also Brain, computed tomography
  developmental anomalies, 1775–1777
  fractures, **1780–1783**
    growing (leptomeningeal cysts), 1782
  intracranial calcification, 1676–1678
    causes, 1678 (*table*)
  lesions, traumatic, radionuclide scanning,
    1863–1864
  phlebography, 1693–1695
    anatomy, veins, 1693–1694
    general considerations, 1693
  plain radiography, projections, 1671–1678
    general considerations, 1671–1673
    half-axial (Towne's), 1673, *1674*
    jugular foramen, 1674
    lateral, 1673
    optic canal, 1674
    pituitary fossa, 1674, *1675*
    posteroanterior, 1673
    submentovertical, 1674, *1675*
  pneumography, 1694–1700
    see also Pneumoencephalography
  radionecrosis, CT, 1718–1719
  in raised intracranial pressure, 1705–1708
    adults, **1707–1708**
    children, 1705–1707
  sinography, 1694
  trauma, 1780–1789
    see also Head injury
  tumours, **1791–1792**
    secondary, 1791, *1792*
  ultrasound, 1682
Smallpox, affecting bone, 1365
Smelloff-Cutter valve, 664, 669
Smith fracture, wrist, 1257
Snake bite, and adrenal cortical necrosis, *1063*
Sodium hydroxide, cause of oesophagitis, 757
Sodium iodide (NaI) crystal, 17
Soft tissues, 1509–1522
  biopsy, 2127
  calcification, 1513–1520
  density differences, 1509–1510
  edge enhancement (Mach effect), 1509–1510
  gas in, 1521–1522
    gangrene, 1521
    surgical emphysema, 1521
  local lesions, 1511–1513
  necrosis, 1519
  ossification, 1513–1520
  in pathophysiology of joint disease, 1474–
    1475
  radionuclide bone scan, 1545, 1546
  subcutaneous fat thickness, 1509
  trauma, 1519
  tumours, 1519
    CT scan, 1526–1527
  xeroradiography, 1510–1511

Solitary bone cyst, dental, 1906
Somatotropin *see* Growth hormone
Sones technique, arteriotomy, 609
Sonography, with amniography, 1583
   and amniotic fluid analysis, 1583
South American blastomycosis, 848
Spastic ataxia, hereditary, oesophagus, 776
SPECT *see* Computed tomography, emission
Sphenoid sinuses
   anatomy, 1939–1940
   carcinoma, 1950
   see also Paranasal sinuses
Spherocytosis, hereditary, 1332, 1469
Sphincterotomy, endoscopic, 1006
   malignant biliary obstruction, 1007
Spina bifida, **1450**, 1798, 1821
   fetal detection, sonography, 1569
Spinal canal
   contents, CT, 1801
   lumbar, stenosis, **1833–1834**
   magnetic resonance imaging, 81, *82*
Spinal cord
   acute lesions, presentation, 1817, 1818
   compression, **1839–1851**
      abscess, 1848–1849
      angiography, 1841–1843
      inflammatory lesions, 1848–1849
      myelography, 1840
      radiography, 1839–1840
      tumours, 1840–1848
         extradural lesions, 1840–1842
         intradural extramedullary lesions, 1843–1844
         intramedullary lesions, 1844–1848
         metastases, 1840, 1846, *1847*
         see also Spinal cord compression, and specific names of tumours
Spine
   angiography, 1811–1813
   in ankylosing spondylitis, 1486
   back pain, acute, 1817
      chronic, 1818
   cervical, degenerative disease, **1837–1838**
      trauma, 1223–1234
      see also Cervical spine
   CT, 1799–1801
      contents of spinal canal, 1801
      vertebral column, 1799–1801
   cysts, **1824**
   degenerative diseases, 1500–1501
   discography, 1813
   disease, mediastinal mass, 193
   epidurography, 1817
   intervertebral fusions, 1798–1799
   lumbar, injuries, **1237–1239**
   magnetic resonance imaging, 1817
   methods of examination, **1797–1819**, 1797 (*table*)
   myelography, 1801–1811
      see also Myelography, spine
   normal bone-in-bone appearance, 1452, *1454*
   pathology, **1821–1855**
   in psoriatic arthropathy, 1489
   radiograph, 156
   in Reiter's syndrome, 1490
   rheumatoid arthritis, **1479**, **1481**
   root syndromes, acute, 1817
      compression, 1817
   spinal cord, acute lesions, 1817
      chronic lesions, 1818
   stenosis, CT scan, 1531–1532
   thoracic, injuries, **1234–1236**
   thoracolumbar, injuries, **1236–1237**

transitional vertebrae, 1798
trauma, **1849–1851**
tumour, CT scan, *52*
   magnetic resonance imaging, *82*
   sternum, 155
   ultrasound, 1817
vascular lesions, 1851–1854
   angiography, 1852–1853
      arteriovenous malformations, spinal cord, 1852
      arteriovenous malformations, spinal dura mater, 1852
      complications, 1853
   CT, 1852
   haemangiomas, 1854
   myelography, 1853–1854
Spironolactone, 1039
Spleen, 1009–1015
   abscess, 1015
   angiography, 1011
   arteriogram, *2056*
   asplenia, 545
   congenital conditions, 1012
   CT scanning, 1011
   embolization, 1015, **2156**, *2157*, *2158*
   enlarged, 1012–1015
   functional studies, 1010
   haemorrhage, CT scan, *56*
   imaging, children, 2203
   investigation methods, 1009–1011
   isotope studies, 1008
   magnetic resonance imaging, 1011
   pathology, 1011–1015
   plain radiography, 1009, *1010*
   polysplenia, *543*, 545
   rupture complicating splenoportography, 2080
   space occupying lesions, 1015
   trauma, 1015
   ultrasound, 1010
      children, 2219
   vein, ultrasound, children, 2218
Splenomegaly
   blood disorders, 1012
   ultrasound, children, 2219
Splenoportogram, 'direct', *945*, 974
Splenoportography, *958*, 1011, *1012*, 2080
   complications, 2080
   indications, 2080
Split renal function studies in renal artery stenosis, 1155
Spondylo-epiphyseal dysplasia, **1426–1427**
Spondylolisthesis, **1836–1837**
   of axis, traumatic, (hangman's fracture), 1231
Sponge kidney, calculi, 1060, 1063
Squamous cell carcinoma
   excretory urogram, 1106
   maxillofacial region, 1910
   nasopharynx, 1969
   oropharynx, 1970
   renal, 1106
   retrograde pyelography, 1106
Squamous metaplasia and urinary tract infection, 1131
Stafne bone cavity, 1909–1910
Staghorn calculi, *1061*, *1133*
   and ureteric colic, 1060
Standing waves, 2017, *2018*
Stannosis, 272
Staphylococcus aureus pneumonia, 200, *201*
Starling's equation, 261
Starr-Edwards valve, 664, 665, 666, 668

Static shock phenomenon, 2017
Stationary arterial waves, 2017
Stein-Leventhal disease (polycystic disease), 1036, 1038, 1611
Sterilization, tubal, techniques, 1620
Sterispon in embolization, 2145
Sternum, 154
   dehiscence, post-operative, 323, *324*
   depressed, in heart disease, 563, *564*
   disease, mediastinal mass, 193
   fracture, 306
Steroid treatment and arteriography, 1992
Still's disease, **1456–1457**
   see also Juvenile chronic polyarthritis
Stomach, 783–814
   afferent loop syndrome, 809
   amyloidosis, 797
   anastomotic leak, 808
   antral, gastritis, 794
   areae gastricae, 783, *784*
   atrophic gastritis, 794, *795*
   barium examination, 784–787
   corrosive gastritis, 797, *798*
   Crohn's disease, 796
   diabetic paresis, 806
   dilatation, 721
   diverticula, 804
   duplication cyst, 800
   emphysematous gastritis, 739
   emptying, radionuclide evaluation, 810–813
      scintigraphy of disorders, 812
   enterogastric reflux, scintigraphy, 812
   eosinophilic gastritis, 796
   erosion, 793
   erosive gastritis, 794
   extrinsic masses, 807
   filling defects, small, 786
   functional abnormalities, 804–807
   functional disorders, 806–807
   fundoplication, 808, *809*
   histoplasmosis, 796
   hypertrophic gastritis, 794, *795*
   hypertrophic pyloric stenosis, 805
   inflammatory diseases, 787–798
      emphysematous, 797
   isolated heterotaxy, 805
   leiomyosarcoma, malignant, 804
   linitis plastica, 802
   lymphoma, 802–804
   normal anatomy, 783
   operative procedures, types, 807
   outlet obstruction, 806
   plication, 808, *809*
   polyps, 798–799
   postoperative, 807–810
   prepyloric web, 804
   prolapse, mucosal, 805, *806*
   pseudolymphoma (lymphoreticular hyperplasia), 796
   radiology, 784–787
   scleroderma, paresis, 807
   structural abnormalities, 804–807
   surgery, complications, 808–810
   syphilis, 797
   thick folds, causes, 797 (*table*)
   tuberculosis, 796
   tumours, 798–804
      benign, 798–800
      carcinoid, 799
      carcinoma, advanced, 801
         Japanese morphological classification, *801*
      primary, 800–804

Stomach (*cont.*)
 tumours (*cont.*)
  carcinoma, advanced (*cont.*)
   recurrent postoperative, 809
   localized malignant-appearing lesions, 802
     (*table*)
  malignant, 800–804
   mesenchymal, 804
   mesenchymal origin, 799
   metastatic carcinoma, *803*, 804
  varices, 806
  villous adenoma, 799
  volvulus, 721, 805
Stones *see* Calculi
Storage diseases, **1432–1435**
Strawberry gallbladder (cholesterosis), 977
Streptococcus pneumoniae pneumonia, 200, *201*
Streptomyces affecting bone, 1363
Stress fractures
 foot, 1271
 radionuclide bone scan, 1541
Stress incontinence, 1624
Stricture
 biliary, benign, 983–984
 large bowel, 891
 ulcerative colitis, 884
String of beads sign, 723
 arteriography, 2017, *2018*
String of sausages
 appearance, renal artery, 1154
Stripe, definition, 372
Stroke
 angiography, 1701
 completed, 1756
 CT, 1679, 1701
 in evolution, 1756
 see also Cerebrovascular accidents:
    Infarction, cerebral: Transient
    ischaemic attacks
Strongyloidiasis, 848
Strongyloides stercoralis, colitis, 890
Struvite stone, 1060
'Student's elbow', 1511
Sturge-Weber syndrome, 1778, 1882
 angiography, 1778
 CT, 1778
Stuttering lesions, 1756
Subarachnoid
 cisterns in pneumoencephalography, 1699–
    1700
 haemorrhage, **1746–1756**
  aneurysms, 1746–1749
  angiography, 1749–1751
  arteriovenous malformations, 1751–1755
  CT, 1747–1749
  hydrocephalus, 1748
  ischaemic infarction, 1748
  radiography, 1746
  radionuclide scanning, 1865–1866
  suspected, angiography, 1701
   CT, 1701
   myelography, 1701
   radiology, 1701
  trauma, 1746
  traumatic, **1787**
  ultrasound, neonate, 2230, 2234
Subscapular haematoma, 1159–1160
Subchondral synchondrosis, axis, 1233
Subclavian artery
 aneurysm, 699, *700*
 congenital aberrations, 693–695
 puncture in cerebral arteriography, 1683
 right, pressure on oesophagus, 779

steal phenomenon, arteriography, 2020, 2027
Subdural
 empyema, 1741
  angiography, 1741
  CT, 1741
 haematomas, acute, **1784–1785**
  chronic extracerebral collection, 1785
  radionuclide scanning, 1863, *1864*
   children, 2206
  subacute, **1784**
 haemorrhage, **1783**
  ultrasound, neonate, 2234
Subglottic tumours, 1977–1978
Subject contrast, definition, 372
Sublingual glands *see* Salivary glands
Subluxation
 axis, physiological, paediatric, 1233
 of the lens, 1880
 traumatic, 1882
Submandibular glands, calcification, 1922
 see also Salivary glands
Subperiosteal chondroma, 1278
Subphrenic infection, ultrasound, 135
Subretinal haemorrhage, 1894
Subsegment, definition, 372
Subtraction techniques, liver, 945
Sudeck's atrophy, **1401–1402**
 radionuclide bone scan, 1541
 'super scan', 1545
'Super scan', radionuclide bone scan, 1545
Superior vena cava
 cavography, 2064–2067
  indications, 2064
  persistent left superior vena cava, 2067
  technique, 2064
 left, persistence, 527, *528*
 syndrome, 2065–2067
  causes, 2065
 tumours, radionuclide studies, 2191–2192
Supracondylar fracture, children, 1252
Supraglottic tumours, 1977
Surgery
 heart abnormality following, 470
 thromboembolism, 294
Sutures, cranial, premature closure, **1448–1449**
Swan-Ganz catheters, *319*, 324
Swyer syndrome, 1036
Swyer-James (MacLeod's) syndrome, 229, **238–
    239**, 337
Synchodrosis
 ischiopubic, incompletely fused, 1240
 subchondral, axis, 1233
Synechiae, 1617–1618
Synovial
 chondromatosis, 1501
 osteochondromatosis, 1298–1299
 sarcoma, **1323**
Synovioma, **1323**
Synovitis
 in juvenile chronic polyarthritis, 1482, 1484
 radionuclide bone scanning, 1543
 villonodular, pigmented, **1298–1299**, 1501
Syphilis
 adult (acquired), **1360**
 aneurysm, 2009
 aortitis, 705
 congenital, **1359–1360**, 1456
  effect on teeth, 1928
 gastric, 797
 nose involvement, 1946
 tertiary, maxillofacial region, 1914
Syringomelia, **1827–1829**
 differential diagnosis from tumour, 1846, **1848**

Syrinx, post-traumatic, 1851
Systemic lupus erythematosus, **1484**
 associated with sialectasis, 1920
 lungs, 279, 281
 microneurysms, 2014
 subclavian arteriogram, 2046
Systemic vasculitides, lung, 282

Tachypnoea of the newborn, transient, 347, 349
Taenia echinococcus, in bone, 1364
Takayasu's arteritis, 579, **704**, *705*
 arteriography, 2016
Talipes equinovarus (club foot), **1452**
Talus injuries, **1266–1268**
 complete dislocation, 1266–1267
 head, 1268
 linear fractures of the body, 1268
 neck, 1268
 osteochondral fractures, 1268
 subtalar (peritalar) dislocation, 1267–1268
 vertical, congenital, **1452**
Tantalum, 135
Tapeworms, 849
'Tarlov' cysts, 1925, *1827*
Tarsal scaphoid, Köhler's disease, children,
    1463
Tarsometatarsal dislocation, 1270
 fracture-dislocation, 1270
Taussig-Bing deformity, 514
Tay-Sachs' disease, 1432, 1745
Technetium-99m (^{99m}Tc), 20–23
 blood pool phase, 1537, *1540*
 characteristics, **1536–1538**
 clearance of radiopharmaceuticals, 1538
 delayed scan, 1537, *1540*
 flow phase, 1537, *1540*
 ^{67}Gallium citrate, 1536
 imaging protocol, 1536–1537
 intensity of uptake, 1536
 labelled methylene diphosphonate, whole
    body dosage, 1536
 mechanisms in bone uptake, 1536
99m-Tc-DMSA, renal masses, 1091
99m-Tc-diethylene triamine pentaacetic acid,
    1052
 in brain scanning, 1858, 1858 (*table*)
  interpretation, 1859
 CNS imaging, children, 2206–2207
 kidney, transplanted, 1143–1144, 1145
  in obstruction, 1147
 in renal infarction, 1156
 renal masses, 1091
 in urinary obstruction, 1078, *1080*
99m-Technetium
 -glucoheptonate, in brain scanning, 1858,
    1858 (*table*)
 -immino diacetic acid in hepatobiliary
    studies, children, 2204
 -labelled N-substituted iminodiacetic acid
    compounds (^{99m}Tc-HIDA), 970
 -labelled polyphosphate, heart, 381
 -labelled red cells, 837
 -macroaggregated albumin, tracer in hepatic
    metastases, chemotherapy, 2192–2193
 -methylenediphosphate, dynamic renal scan,
    1052
  arthritis imaging, 1542, 1543
 -MMA, cardiopulmonary imaging, children,
    2208
 -pertechnetate, in brain scanning, 1858, 1858
    (*table*)
  interpretation, 1859
  thyroid imaging, children, 2207–2208

99m-Technetium (*cont.*)
  -pyrophosphate scan of knee, 1264
  -sodium pertechnetate, arthritis imaging, 1542, 1543
  -sulphur colloid, 836
    in gastro-oesophageal reflux in children, 2205–2206
    in intramedullary vascularity, 1544
    tracer, in hepatic metastases chemotherapy, 2192, 2193
Teardrop fracture, extension, 1231
  flexion, 1226, *1227*
Teeth
  abnormally shaped, 1928–1930
  anodontia, and partial, 1929–1930
  caries, 1931–1932
  defective calcification, 1926–1927
  developmental anomalies, 1926–1930
  enamel, anomalies, 1926–1927
  eruption, normal and abnormal, 1930–1931
  fractures, 1934–1935
  impacted, 1930–1931
  in newborn, 1929
  periodontal disease, 1933–1934
    associated with systemic disease, 1934
  resorbtion, 1935
  root dilaceration, 1928
    fractures, 1934
  supernumerary, 1929
  supplemental, 1929
  see also Dental
Telethermography, 1660
Temporal
  arteritis *see* Giant cell arteritis
  bone, radiology, 1952 (*table*)
    fractures, 1963
  resolution, radionuclide imaging, 19
Temporomandibular joint, 1916–1918
  anatomy, 1916
  arthritis, 1916–1917
  arthropathy, 1506
  developmental abnormalities, 1918
    arthrotomography, 1916–1917
    degenerative (osteoarthritis), 1917
    effect of prolonged haemodialysis, 1917
    inflammatory, 1917
    pain-dysfunction syndrome, 1916
  injury, 1917–1918
    ankylosis, 1917
    dislocation, 1917–1918
    fractures, 1917
Teratogenesis, radiation risks, 1590
Teratoid tumours, 1614–1615
  benign cystic (dermoid cysts), 1614
Teratoma
  malignant, ovarian, 1615
  mediastinal, 179, *180*
Testes, 1038–1039
  function, 1036, 1038
  tumours, 1039
  undescended, 1037
    venography, 2084–2086
  venography, 2085
Testosterone, 1038
Tetralogy of Fallot, 499–504
  pseudotruncus, 502, 503
  pulmonary infundibular stenosis, 532
  radiology, 500
  surgical repair, 503
  variants, 502
  ventricular septal defect, 491
Thalamic tumour, *1720*
Thalassaemia, **1328–1329**

in children, **1468–1469**
  clinical features, 1328
  radiological features, 1328
Thalidomide toxicity, heart anomalies, 470
Thallium imaging
  -201, 429
  defects, 428
  exercise stress testing, 432–434
  heart, 381, 432
    interpretation, 434
  myocardial infarction, 436, 2209
  myocardial perfusion, 429–436
  rest studies, 432
Thanatophoric dwarfism, **1419**, *1420*, *1421*
  differential diagnosis, 1418, *1420*, *1421*
Thecoma, ovarian, 1615
Thecotympanic fistula, *1963*
Thermography
  computer assisted, 1660
  guidelines, 1661
  limitations, 1660
  liquid crystal, 1660
  prediction of breast cancer risk, 1661
  telethermography, 1660
    graphic stress, 1660
Thoracic
  aortic aneurysms, digital subtraction angiography, 2105
  aortography, 2030
  cage, infants and young children, 333
  dystrophy, asphyxiating, **1422**
  kidney, 1187
  outlet syndromes, arteriography, 2046
  spine, fractures, **1234–1236**
    cervicothoracic, 1236
    compression, 1234–1235
      old healed, 1235
    ring epiphyses, 1235
    Schmorl's nodules, 1235
Thoracolumbar spine, injuries, **1236–1237**
  bending, 1237
  flexion, 1236
  fractures, 1236–1237
  fracture-dislocation, 1236
  rotational, 1237
  shear forces, 1237
  vertical compression, 1237
Thoracoplasty, 212
Thoracotomy, post-operative, radiograph, 321–324
Thorax
  magnetic resonance imaging, 87
  trauma, 305
  see also Chest
Thorium dioxide, 99
Thromboangiitis obliterans, arteriography, 2016
Thromboembolism
  intraventricular, echocardiography, 629
  malignancy, 294
  pulmonary, **293–304**, 576–578
    anatomy, 293
    angiography, 300
    chest radiography, 298
    diagnosis, 295–303
    imaging, 296–303
    pathology, 293
    pathophysiological disturbances, 294
    predisposing conditions, 294
    radionuclide studies, 296–298
    therapy, 303
    traumatic, 294
  see also Embolism, pulmonary

Thrombolytic agents, infusion, regional, 2136
  contraindications, 2136
  indications, 2136
Thrombophlebitis complicating venography, 2063
Thrombosis
  arterial, arteriography, 2018–2019
  cardiac valve prosthesis, 671
  deep venous, venography, 2089–2090
    causes, 2090
  definition, 372
  hepatic vein venography, 2079
    causes, 2079
  mesenteric, 725
  post-venographic, 2088
  renal vein, 1160–1161
    see also Renal vein thrombosis
    venography, 2076–2077
  vascular, in arteriography, 2000
  venous, arm, venography, 2087
    cardiac pacemaker as cause of, 660
    leg, venography, 2089–2090
    radionuclide studies, 296
Thrombus, definition, 372
  embolism, catheter, 2001
  intravascular, percutaneous, removal, 2147
Thymic tumours, 177–179
Thymolipoma, 1030
Thymoma, 1028
Thymopoietin, 1027
Thymosin, 1027
Thymus, 1027–1031
  disorders, 1028
  infants and young children, 331–332
  normal, 1027
    radiology, 1029
  radiology, 1029–1031
  regression, 1028
  status thymico lymphaticus, 1028
  tumours, 177–179, 1028, *1030*
Thyroid, 1023–1025, 1040
  acropachy, 1025, **1408–1409**
  arteriography, 2029
  cartilage, erosion and tumour, 1976–1977
  ectopic lingual, 1025
  eye disease, 1887
  hormone deficiency *see* Hypothyroidism
  hypofunction, 1025
  masses, 1024
  mediastinal mass, 176
  nodules, 1025
  normal, 1023–1024
  radionuclides, 22 (*table*)
    imaging, children, 2207–2208
  -stimulating hormone, national screening of the newborn, 1025
  tumours, 1025, 1040
    causing laryngeal displacement, 1981
  see also Parathyroids
Thyroiditis, lymphocytic, radionuclide imaging, children, 2207–2208
Thyrotoxicosis, 1023
  heart involvement, 640
  oesophagus, 776
Thyroxine, 1023
Tibia
  adamantinoma, 1325
  fractures, in children, **1462**
  haemangioma, embolization, 2150, *2153*
  tubercle, in children, **1463**, *1465*
Tibiotalar joint, rheumatoid arthritis, 1479
Tic doloreux, radiography and CT, 1702

Tinnitus
  CT, 1702
  radiography, 1702
Tissue enhancement, CT, 50
Toe, big, dense epiphysis, simulating trauma, 1465
Tolosa Hunt syndrome, 1766
Tomography
  chest, 132
  in cranial nerve disturbances, 1702–1703
  heart, 380
  hypocycloidal, 1022
  larynx, 1974
  orbit, *1876, 1877*
Tonsil, calcification, 1922
Tonsillar
  ectopia, 1848
    cerebellar, myelography, 1703
  herniation, pneumoencephalography, *1695*
Torticollis, **1232**
Toru palatinus, 1909
Torulosis, bone, **1364**
Torus mandibularis, 1909
Toxic megacolon, 730, 887, *888*
  gangrenous ischaemic colitis, 889
Toxins, heart involvement, 640
Toxoplasmosis, 1743
  eye defect, 1880
Trachea, 125, *126*
  agenesis, 357
  carcinoma, 190
  cervical, obstruction, 340
  displacement, 1981
  infants and young children, 331
  radiograph, 141
  rupture, 308
  stenosis, congenital, 357
  stripe, 125, 371, 372
  tumour, 190
Tracheobronchial tree, 267
  congenital anomalies, 357–359
Tracheomalacia, congenital, 358
Tracheo-oesophageal fistula, 308
  infants, 907–908
Tracheostomy, 325
Transaxillary artery catheterization in cerebral arteriography, 1683
Transhepatic portography, 2080–2082
Transient ischaemic attacks, 1756
  angiography, 1701
  CT, 1679, 1701
  radiography, 1701
Transillumination lightscanning, breast, 1665
Transitional cell carcinoma
  differential diagnosis, 1128 (*table*), 1129
  renal, 1105–1106
Translumbar aortography
  contraindicated in coagulation defects, 1992
  lower limbs, 2049
  puncture, 1993–1994
  technique, 1993–1994
Transluminal angioplasty, coronary, 626
  percutaneous, 2027
Transplantation, renal, 1141–1149
  arteriography, 2036–2037
    artery stenosis, 2036
    donor, 2034
    recipient, 2036–2037
  artery stenosis, transluminal angioplasty, 2143
  dynamic scanning, 1054
  flush aortography, 1048
  magnetic resonance imaging, 85

  preoperative evaluation of recipient, 1141–1142
  pulmonary tuberculosis following, *288*
  radionuclide imaging, children, 2203
  rejection, acute, 1145
    chronic, 1147, *1148*
  surgical technique, 1142
  transplanted kidney, 1142–1147
    acute rejection v. ATN, 1145
    complications, 1145–1147
    investigations, 1142–1145
      angiography, 1144–1145
      computed tomography, 1144
      GFR, 1143–1144
      intravenous urography, 1142–1143
      radionuclide imaging, 1143–1144
      ultrasound, 1144, 1145
  urological complications, 1146–1147
  vascular complications, 1146
Transposition of great arteries (ventriculo-arterial concordance), 475
  associated with tricuspid atresia, 499
  corrected, 521–524
    operative procedures, 521
    radiology, 519, 521, *522*
  uncorrected, 517–521
Transthoracic needle biopsy, **2122–2124**
  complications, 2123–2124
  contraindications, 2124
  indications, 2122
  needles, 2123, 2124
Transvenous biopsies, 2127, *2128*
Trauma
  arteriography, 2025
  bone, 1540–1541
  bone cyst, dental, 1906
  bone scintigraphy, children, 2200
  and calcification, 1519
  chest, 305–311
  ear, 1962–1963
  heart, 650
  larynx, 1979
  liver, 936, 938, **949**
  maxillofacial, 1922
  mediastinum, 308, 310
  and nephrocalcinosis, 1064
  nose and paranasal sinuses, 1950
  orbital, 1882–1883
  and ossification, 1520
  pancreas, 1005
  parotid duct, 1922
  pelvis, **1240–1245**
  pleura, 306
  pneumothorax, 306
  radionuclide bone scan, **1540–1541**
  renal, arteriography, 2037
  skeletal, 1223–1272
  skull, 1780–1789
  spinal, **1849–1851**
    cervical, 1223–1234
  spleen, 1015
  thorax, 305
  thromboembolism, 294
Treacher-Collins syndrome, 1918
  ear deformities, 1965
Treitz ligament, 912–913
Treponematosis, **1359–1361**
  see also specific disorders
Tricuspid atresia, 498
  heart, 497–499
    associated transposition of great arteries, 499
Tricuspid stenosis, right atrial enlargement, *561*

Tricuspid valve disease, 596–598
Trimalleolar fracture-dislocations, ankle, 1266
Triodothyronine, 1023
Triquetrum, carpus, fracture, 1259
Trisomy chromosome 21 *see* Down's syndrome
Trophoblastic tumours, arteriography, 1598
Tropical ulcer, **1361**
Trough filter, definition, 372
Trummerfeld zone in scurvy, 1388
Truncus arteriosus, 514–517
  persistent common, 514–517
Tubal pregnancy, 1619
Tuberculoma, 211
  CT, 1741, 1742
Tuberculosis
  bone, **1356–1359**
    arthritis, **1358–1359**
    dactylitis, *1357*, 1358
    elbow, *1357*
    greater trochanter, 1358
    radiological appearances, 1357
    spine, 1357–1358
  duodenal, 823
  female genital tract, 1604
    salpingitis, 1604–1605
    uterine, 1605
  gastric, 796
  intracranial, 1741–1742
    CT, 1741–1742
    meningitis, 1741
    tuberculomas, 1741
  and nephrocalcinosis, 1064
  nose involvement, 1946
  pericarditis, 685
  pulmonary, **206–217**
    chest radiography, 212
    children, 338, *339*
    clinical features, 206
    concomitant with bronchial carcinoma, 211
    following renal transplantation, *288*
    incidence, 206
    infective organisms, 206
    mediastinal effects, 187
    miliary, 208, 210
    postprimary, 209–212
      surgical treatment, 212
    primary, 206–209
    radiological manifestations, primary and postprimary compared, 207 (*table*)
    response to therapy, 211
    silicosis associated with, 269
    surgical collapse of lung, 323
  renal, 1124–1126, 1128 (*table*)
    hydrocalycosis, 1125
    pathology, 1124
    radiology, 1124–1126
    tuberculous autonephrectomy, 1124
  small bowel, 847
  spinal cord, 1848, 1849
  ulcerative colitis, 890, *891*
Tuberculous
  arthritis, **1358–1359**
    children, **1455**
  autonephrectomy, 1124
  disease, Fallopian tubes, 1593
  osteomyelitis, children, 1455
    and dental extraction, 1914
  salpingitis, 1604–1605
Tuberous sclerosis, 1779, 1882
  lungs, 275
Tubo-ovarian abscess, 1603

Tumours
arteriography, **2021–2025**
 blush, 2021
 diagnosis, 2021–2023
 localization, 2023
 lower limb, 2051
 lumbar aortography, 2031–2032
 operability, 2024
 site of origin, 2023–2024
 treatment, 2025
embolization, **2146–2150**
 definitive, 2146
 palliative, 2146–2150
 pre-operative, 2146
radiology, **2167–2182**
 applications, 2167
 CT, 2169 (*table*), 2171–2173
  clinical value, 2174–2176
 histological evidence, 2167–2168
  relationship to gallium imaging findings,
   2189–2190
 lymphangiogram, 2171, 2172, *2174*
 lymphography, 2169 (*table*)-2173
  see also Lymphography
 metastases, lymphography, 2173–2175
  CT, 2175–2176
  systemic, 2178–2181
  see also Metastases
 staging, 2168–2169
  lymph node (N), 2169
  T, 2168–2169
radionuclide, 22 (*table*)
ulcerative colitis, carcinoma, 887
see also Metastases: specific names, organs
 and regions
Tumoral calcinosis, 1512
Turcot's syndrome, 871
Turner's syndrome, 470, 700, 1036, **1399–1400**
 dental anomalies, 1928
 fetal detection, sonography, 1569, 1570
Twining's line, 114
Twin pregnancy
 monoamniotic, amniography, 1580
 sonography, 1564–1565
  dizygotic, 1565
  monozygotic, 1565
Typhoid cholecystitis, 974

Uhl's anomaly, 530
Ulcer
 Crohn's disease, 837–839
 duodenal *see* Ulcer, peptic
 gastric, *784*, **787–792**
  benign, distribution, 788
   versus malignant, 791
  'collar', 788
  diseases presenting as, 791 (*table*)
  en face signs, 788, *789*
  Hampton's line, *790*, 791
  malignant, 801
   versus benign, 791
  'mound' ('halo'), 788
  'niche', 788
  profile signs, 788, *790*
  scars, *785*, 791, *792*
 gastroduodenal, coexisting portal
  hypertension, 929
 large bowel, solitary, 893
 oesophageal, *754*, 755
 peptic, 817
  complications, 819
  endoscopy, 828
  giant size, 818, *819*

postbulbar, 819
recurrent postoperative, *807*, 808
 tropical, **1361**
 see also Colitis, ulcerative
Ulcerative enteritis, idiopathic, 855
Ultrasonography (ultrasound), **25–37**
 abdominal vessels, 2114–2115
 adenoma, hyperparathyroid, 1026
 adrenals, 1035
  children, 2221–2222
 aorta, children, 2220
 artefacts, 32–34
 'B' scan, 28
 beam shapes, 30
 beam width, effects, 32
 bidimensional scan, 28
 bile ducts, 968–970
 biliary system, children, 2216–2217
 bladder tumours, 1113
 brain, 1682
  infant, 2229–2234
 breast, 1661–1664
  see also Breast, ultrasound
 calculi, 1062
 cerebral haemorrhage, 1755–1756
 cerebral hemisyndromes, acute, 1701
 cervical carcinoma, 1608, 1625
 chest, 135
  paediatric, 2213
 choice of probe, and scanning technique, 36
 cholecystitis, 735
 choriocarcinoma, 1610
 clinical uses, 25 (*table*)
 condition in tissue, 26
 contrast media, 36
 dermoid cysts, 1614
 developments, 37
 Doppler, 29, 394
  safety, 31
 duodenum, 817
 duplex scanning, 29
 dynamic range control, 30
 in ectopic pregnancy, 1619
 electronic ('dynamic') focussing, 30
 electronic sector (phased array) scanning, 30
 endometrial carcinoma, 1609
 in endometriosis, 1620
 enhancement, 34
 equipment, 30
 fibroids, 1606–1607
 follicular development, in infertility, 1038
 future prospects, 8
 gain settings, 35
 gallbladder, 968
  cholecystitis, 975–976
 gastrointestinal tract, 2219–2220
 genital tract, congenital anomalies, 1601–
  1602
 grey-scale, 28
  in gain settings, 35
 -guided biopsy, 2125
  percutaneous drainage, 2132
  therapy, 2135
 in gynaecological conditions, 1598
 head growth/size abnormal, 1703
 head injury, suspected, children, 1700
 heart *see* Echocardiography
 hydrosalpinx, 1603
 interpretation, 32–34
 in IUCD management, 1622
 kidney, children, 2222–2226
  injuries, 1173
  transplanted, 1144, 1145

in obstruction, 1146
 see also Ultrasound, renal masses
leiomyosarcoma, 1610
linear scan, 28
liver, 930–933
 children, 2214–2216
 compared with CT and nuclear imaging,
  2184–2185
M-mode display, 28
in neuroblastoma, 1207
obstetrics, **1551–1580**
 see also Obstetrics, sonography
obstructive jaundice, 979
orbit, 1877, 1879, 1880
 trauma, 1882
ovarian cysts, 1611
ovaries, 1036
paediatric, 1182, **2213–2227**
 practical considerations, 2213
pancreas, 1001
 children, 2217–2218
pelvic inflammatory disease, acute, 1602
 chronic, 1603
 extragenital origin, 1604
pelvic rhabdomyosarcoma, 1210
phased array (electronic sector) scanning,
 30
physical principles, 26
pleura, 135
portal hypertension, children, 2115
portal venous system, children, 2218, *2219*
positioning of patient, 36
pyelonephritis, acute, 1120
real-time scanning, 28, 394
 advantages, 29 (*table*)
 artefacts, 34
 role in interventional procedures, 36
 safety, 31
renal masses, **1091–1094**
 abscesses, 1099
 adenoma, 1102
 angiomyolipomas, 1100–1101
 hydatid cyst, 1099
 mesoblastic nephroma, 1102
 renal cell carcinoma, 1103
 sinus lipomatosis, 1101
 transitional cell carcinoma, 1106
 see also Ultrasound, kidney
repeat echoes, 33
reverberation, 33
ringdown, 33
safety, 31
scanning techniques, 35
scattered echoes, 32
search mode, 29
sector movements, 36
sector scan, 28
shadowing, 34
simple renal cysts, 1190
skull, 1682
spatial resolution, 29
specular echoes, 32
spine, 1817
spleen, 1010
 children, 2219
splenic vein, children, 2218
stand-off, 33
storage of image, 31
swept gain settings, 35, *36*
technology, 30
time-gain control amplifier, 30
tissue characterization, 37
in urinary obstruction, 1077

Ultrasonography (ultrasound) (*cont.*)
  urinary tract, 1048
    children, 2222–2226
  vascular, **2113–2119**
    abdominal vessels, 2114–2115
    Doppler techniques, 2116–2119
      blood flow measurement, 2119
      imaging, 2116–2117
      spectrum analysis, 2117–2119
    real-time scanning, 2113–2114
    small parts scanners, 2115–2116
    static B scanning, 2113
    vessel imaging, 2113–2114
  in Wilms' tumour, 1205
Unicameral bone cyst, 1285, 1906
  juvenile, **1458**
Unicornuate uterus, 1600
Unilateral interfacetal dislocation, 1226–1227
Upper limb, digital subtraction angiography,
    2109
  arteriography, **2046–2048**
  venography, **2086–2087**
    anatomy, 2086
    gangrene, digits, 2087
    indications, 2087
    technique, 2086
    thrombosis, 2087
      causes, 2087
Uraemic pericarditis, 685
Ureters
  calculus *see* Calculus, ureteric
  colic and calculi, 1060
  dilatation and stent insertion, 2130–2131
  ectopy, 1192
  embolization, 2131
  injuries, **1168–1170**
    causes, 1168–1169
    intravenous urography, 1169
    radiation therapy hazards, 1169
    strictures, 1169
    surgical trauma, 1169
    therapy, 1170
    unsuspected, 1169
  obstruction, benign strictures, 1081
    bladder abnormalities, 1085
    calculi *see* Calculi, ureteric
    congenital obstructions, 1083–1085
    distal, 1195–1196
    extraperitoneal causes, 1083
    fibrosis, retroperitoneal, 1081
    infravesical obstruction, 1085–1086
    non-opaque filling defects, 1083
    tumours, 1082
    ultrasound, children, 2225
  associated with uterine prolapse, 1624
  paediatric, congenital anomalies, **1190–1196**
    distal ureteric obstruction, 1195–1196
    duplication, 1190
    ureterocele, 1193–1195
    uterocele, 1193–1195
    vesico-ureteric reflux, 1192
  severance during hysterectomy, 1623
  stricture, after hysterectomy, 1623
    radiotherapy complication, 1624
  transitional cell carcinoma causing
    obstruction, 1082
  tumours, **1110–1111**
    cystoscopy, 1111
    intravenous urography, 1111
Ureterocele, 1193–1195
  and calculi, 1060
  ectopic, 1193–1195
  simple, 1193

Ureterography, bulb in ureteric tumours, 1111
  renal metastases, *1140*
Ureteropelvic junction disruption, *1175*
Ureterosigmoidostomy, 901
Ureterovaginal fistula, 1616
  complicating hysterectomy, 1623
Urethra
  congenital abnormalities, 1183–1185
  injuries, 1163–1166
    anterior, 1163–1164
      retrograde ureterography, 1164
    posterior, 1164–1166
      retrograde ureterography, 1165–1166
  paediatric, 1198–1199
    congenital anomalies, 1198–1199
    posterior valves, 1198
  strictures causing obstruction, 1086
  'syndrome', following hysterectomy, 1623
  valves, posterior, causing obstruction,
    children, 1086
  obstruction, ultrasound, children, 2225–
    2226
Urethrovaginal fistulae, 1616
Uric acid calculi, 1060, *1062*
  differential diagnosis from urothelial
    tumours, 1112
Urinary tract, **1045–1049**
  complications following hysterectomy, 1623
  infection and calculi, 1060
    paediatric, 1199–1202
      and intrarenal reflux, 1200
      nephropathy, 1202
      radiography, 1202
      and vesico-ureteric reflux, 1200
    recurrent, women, **1133–1135**
      reinfection, 1133–1134
      urography, 1134–1135
    lower, urodynamics, **1211–1216**
      applications, 1212–1216
      bladder instability, 1212–1214
      bladder outflow obstruction, 1215
      incontinence, 1214–1215
      neuropathic bladder, 1216
      technique, 1211–1212
    obstruction, **1067–1087**
      acute, 1069–1072
      acute obstructive nepyropathy, 1068
      angiography, 1078
      antegrade pyelography, 1076
      chronic partial, 1067
      classification, 1067
      computed tomography, 1077–1078
      definitions, 1068
      diagnosis, 1069
      dilatation, 1069–1071
      intravenous urography, **1069–1076**
        see also Intravenous urography
      nuclear medicine techniques, 1078–1079
      obstructive atrophy, 1069
      pathophysiology, 1068–1069
      percutaneous nephrostomy, 1076
      post-obstructive atrophy, 1069
      renal function, 1079
        benign, 1083
          tumours, 1082
        causes, 1079–1086
        congenital, 1082
        extraperitoneal, 1083
      retrograde pyelography, 1076
      ultrasonography, 1077
      Whitaker test, 1075, 1076–1077
  opacification, CT, 51
  radionuclide imaging, children, 2201–2203

obstructive uropathy, 2202
  vesico-ureteric reflux, 2202–2203
  retention following hysterectomy, 1623
  stent insertion, 2130–2131
  ultrasound, 1048
    children, 2222–2226
  upper, urodynamics, 1217–1219
    indications for antegrade pressure studies,
      1217–1218
    interpretation of results, 1217
    technique, 1216–1217
    see also Whitaker test
Urinoma, 739, *740*
  as extrarenal mass, 1102
  perinephric, *1174*
  in renal transplantation, 1147 (*table*)
Urodynamics, 1211–1220
Urogenital sinus, persistent, 1601
Urography
  cervical carcinoma, 1608
  endometrial carcinoma, 1609
  excretion, renal parenchyma, normal, 1116
    calices, 1117–1118
    papillae, 1117–1118
    position, 1117
    size, 1117
    squamous cell carcinoma, 1106
  high dose, renal failure, 1137–1139
    findings, 1138–1139
    risks, 1138
    technique, 1138
  intravenous *see* Intravenous urography
  ovarian cysts, 1610
    tumours, 1612–1613
  pelvic cervical carcinoma, 1608
  in recurrent urinary tract infection, women,
    1134–1135
  renal parenchymal disease, 1119
    see also specific diseases
Uropathy, obstructive, radionuclide imaging,
    children, 2202
Uroradiology, paediatric *see* Paediatric
    uroradiology
Urothelial tumours, **1105–1106, 1109–1113**
  aetiology, 1109
  arteriography, 2035
  bladder, 1110
  causing obstruction, 1082
  clinical presentation, 1109–1110
  conservative surgery, 1112
  diagnosis, 1110–1113
  differential diagnosis, 1111–1112
  pathology, 1109
  pelvicalyceal system, 1110
  staging, 1112
  transitional cell, 1105–1106
    CT, 1106
    retrograde pyelouterography, 1105
  ureteric, 1110
  see also specific names
Urticaria pigmentosa, **1335–1336**
Uterus
  arcuate, 1600
  arteriovenous malformations, 1618
  bicornis bicollis, 1599
  bicornuate, 1599–1600
  bleeding, abnormal, hysterosalpingography,
    1595
  Caesarean section, changes following, 1618
  didelphys, hysterosalpingography, 1599
  fistulae, 1618
  haemorrhage, arteriography, 1598
  hypoplasia, 1599

Uterus (*cont.*)
  infections, 1604–1605
  intrauterine adhesions, 1617–1618
  isthmus, incompetence, 1618
  neoplasms, malignant,
      hysterosalpingography, 1595
  perforation, IUCD, 1621–1622
  phlebography, 1598
  prolapse, associated with ureteric
      obstruction, 1624
  retained products of conception, 1617
  sarcoma, CT, 1626
  septate, 1600
  subseptus, *1578*
  tumours, 1605–1610
    see also specific names
  unicornuate, 1600
Uterovesical fistula, 1618

Vaccinia, affecting bone, 1365
Vagina
  aplasia, 1600
  atresia and imperforate hymen, 1600
  calculi, 1616
  fibromyoma, 1616
  foreign bodies, 1616
Vaginitis, 1604
  emphysematous, 1604
Vaginography, 1597, 1616
  fistulae, 1616
  foreign bodies, 1616
Vagotomy
  postoperative dysphagia, 776
Valsalva manoeuvre, 132, 181, 363
  definition, 372
  sinus, aneurysm, 713
Valves, heart
  prostheses, 663–674
    complications, 668–673
    fluoroscopic evaluation, 665–666
    infection, 668, *670*, 671
    radiological studies after implantation,
        663–665
    regurgitation caused by, 671, *672*
    strut fracture, 668, *669*, *670*
    types, 664–665
    ultrasonic evaluation, 666–668
    variance, ball or disc, 668, *669*, *670*
Valves, urethral, posterior, 1198–1199
Valvulae conniventes, 722
  thickened, 854
Van Buchem's disease, 1407, **1432**
Vanillylmendelic acid in neuroblastoma, 1206
Vanishing bone disease, 1293, **1403**
Variants
  anatomic, normal, causing inflammatory
      lesions, 1457
  simulating congenital anomalies, 1452
  simulating neoplasia, 1460
  simulating systemic disease, children, 1470
  simulating traumatic lesions, 1464
Varicella
  affecting bone, 1365
  pneumonia, 203, *204*
Varices
  bleeding, embolization, 2146
  duodenal, 825
  gastric, *1012*
    barium study of liver disease, 929, *930*
    embolization, 2156
  oesophageal, 767
    barium study of liver disease, 928, *929*
    portal embolization, 997, 2156

orbital, 1889–1890
  stomach, 806, 929, *930*, *1012*, 2156
Varicocele
  embolization, 2158
  testis, 1038
Varicography, 2091
Varicose veins, venography, 2090
Vas deferens, obstruction, 1038
Vascular
  complications in arteriography, 2000, 2001
  disorders, aneurysms *see* Aneurysms
    arteriovenous, malformations,
        arteriography, 2006
      see also Arteriovenous
    children, bone imaging, 2199–2200
    congenital, arteriography, 2003–2006
    impotence, 1039
    soft tissue calcification, 1514–1515
  embolization, **2145–2156**
    in acute bleeding, 2146
    central nervous system, 2156
      hypersplenism, 2156
      priapism, 2156
    complications, 2159
    indications, 2146–2156
    liver, 995–997
      bleeding, 2146, *2148*, *2149*
    oesophageal varices, 997
    palliative, 2146–2156
    portal hypertension, 995
    pre-operative, 2146
    pulmonary arteriovenous communication,
        2155–2156
    renal artery, 2146
    spleen, 1015, **2156**, *2157*, *2158*
    techniques, **2145–2146**
      balloon catheters, 2146
      digital subtraction angioplasty, 2146
      non-opaque emboli, 2146
      radiological techniques, 2145
      reflux of emboli, 2145
      siting of catheters, 2145
    tumours, **2146–2150**, *2151*, *2152*
    vascular abnormalities, 2150–2156
  enhancement, CT, 49
  extraction techniques, 2137
  intravascular foreign bodies, 2137
  intravascular thrombus, 2137
  lesions, magnetic resonance imaging, 69, 73
    intrinsic, 74
  occlusive disease, percutaneous transluminal
      angioplasty, 2141
  parasites, 2137
  techniques, interventional, 2135–2160
    dilatation (transluminal angioplasty),
        2139–2145
      see also Transluminal angioplasty
    extraction techniques, 2137
    infusions, chemotherapeutic agents, 2135
      constrictor agents, 2135–2136
      dilator agents, 2136
      thrombolytic agents, 2136
    prosthesis insertion, 2138
  ultrasound, 2113–2119
    see also Ultrasound, vascular
Vasculitis, necrotizing, arteriography, 2013–
    2014
Vasoconstriction, definition, 372
Vasoconstrictor agents, in arteriography, 1998
Vasodilatation, definition, 372
Vasodilator agents in arteriography, 1998
Veins *see* Venous: and specific veins and regions

Venography, **2061–2097**
  ascending lumbar, 2074–2075
  azygos, 2074–2075
  brain, 1693–1695
  cerebral, 2064
  complications, **2063–2064**
    local, 1063
    systemic, 2063–2064
    vascular, 2063
  contrast media, 109
  cranial nerve disturbances, 1702–1703
  in disc protrusion, 1832
  endocrine disease, 1020
  endocrine glands, 2093–2094
  extremities, **2086–2091**
    see also Lower limb: Upper limb
  gonadal, 2084–2086
  in gynaecological conditions, 1598
  inferior vena cavography, 2067–2074
  jugular, 2064
    glomus tumours, 1736
  liver, 945
  in lumbar spinal canal stenosis, 1833, *1834*
  orbit, 1817
  orbital, 2064
  pancreas, 1002
  pelvic, 2091
  peripheral, adverse reactions to intravascular
      contrast media, 107
  portal, 2079–2084
  pulmonary thromboembolism, 302
  regional, 2064–2086
  renal, 1048, 2076–2077
    transitional cell carcinoma, 1105
    vein thrombosis, 1161
  spine, 1812–1813
  superior vena cavography, 2064
  technique, 2061–2062
    contrast media, 2062
    digital subtraction angiography *see* Digital
        subtraction angiography
    direct, 2062
    equipment, 2061–2062
    imaging, 2062
    indirect, 2062
    intraosseous, 2062
    venous access, 2062
  uterine, 1598
  venous sampling, 2092–2093
  see also Phlebography
Venous
  calcification, 1514–1515
  embolization, **2156–2158**
    adrenal venous obliteration, 2156–2158
    arteriovenous malformations, 2158
    complications, 2159
    indications, 2156
    varices, 2156
    varicocele, 2158
  haemangiomas *see* Cavernous
      haemangiomas
  sampling, **2029–2093**
    adrenals, 1035
    anatomical sites, 2092
    complications, 2092–2093
    pancreas, 1002, 2095
    sources of error, 2092
    technique, 2092
    transhepatic portal, 2093
    see also Venography
  thrombosis, arm venography, 2087
    intracranial, 1764
    leg, venography, 2089–2090

Ventilation
　assisted, 325
　infant disorders, 346–351
　　hypoventilation, in the newborn, 347
　/perfusion imaging, children, 2209–2210
　radio-isotope scanning, 296–298
　scintigraphy, 134
　/perfusion, 133
Ventricles, ventricular
　aneurysm, CT scanning, 444
　cerebral, in pneumoencephalography, 1699–
　　1700
　common, 512–514
　function, radionuclide imaging, 419
　septal defect, 486–491
　　angiocardiography, 489
　　associations, 491
　　echocardiography, 489, 629–632
　　Eisenmenger reaction, 506
　　membranous, 487
　　muscular (Maladie de Roger), 487, *489*
　　pulmonary stenosis, tetralogy of Fallot,
　　　504
　　supracristal, 486
　　types, 487
　septal perforation, 650
　shunting procedures, **1795**
　　complications, 1795
　situs, determination, 474
Ventriculoarterial concordance, 517
　see also Transposition
　connections, 474
Ventriculography, 381, **421–429**, 636, **1694–
　1700**
　anatomy, 1698–1700
　in cerebral disorders, 1703
　complications, 1698
　gas, technique, 1695, 1696
　interpretation, 1700
　radionuclide, **423–428**, **1871**
　　data analysis, 423
　　disease, findings, 425–428
　　ECG gating, 423
　　ECG stress testing, 432, 433
　　equilibrium studies, 422
　　interpretation, 423, *425, 426, 427*
　　left, 617–619
　　　myocardial infarction, 623–625
　　normal equilibrium studies, 424, *426*
　techniques, 1696
　with water soluble contrast medium, 1696
Vertebra, metastases, CT scan, *45*
Vertebral
　artery puncture, in cerebral arteriography,
　　1683
　biopsy, 2127
　column, CT, 180
　　trauma, **1849–1851**
　epiphyses, Scheuermann's disease, children,
　　1464
Vertebrobasilar
　arterial system, 1690–1692
　insufficiency, 1762–1763
　venous system, 1692–1693
Vertical compression injuries of cervical spine,
　1228–1229
Vertical talus, congenital, **1452**
Vertigo
　CT, 1702
　radiography, 1702
Vesicoureteric junction obstruction, children,
　2225

Vesicoureteric reflux
　dynamic scanning, 1054, **1055**, *1056*
　non-obstructive dilatation, 1075
　paediatric, with duplication, 1192
　　radiography, 1202
　　voiding cysto-urethrogram, 1200
　radionuclide imaging, children, 2202–2203
　in renal transplantation, 1146, *1147*
Vesicovaginal fistula, 1616
　complicating hysterectomy, 1623
Vestibular folds, tumours, 1977, *1978*
Video cysto-urography, 1212
Video cystourethrography, in stress
　incontinence, 1624
Videorecorder in arteriography, 1992
Villonodular synovitis, pigmented, **1298–1299**
Virchow's triad, 294
Virus disease of bone, 1365–1366
Virus infections, chest, in children, 336
Visceral situs, in congenital heart disease, 470
Vitamin C deficiency, 1387
　see also Scurvy
Vitamin D (cholecalciferol)
　deficiency, in osteomalacia, 1378
　　and rickets, 1381
　intoxication, soft tissue calcification, 1514
　and metabolic disease of bone, **1371–1373**
Vitreous haemorrhages, 1882
Vitreous, scanning, 1894
Vocal folds, tumours, 1977
Voiding cysto-urethrography, paediatric, 1181–
　1182
　findings, 1182
　procedure, 1181–1182
　in vesico-ureteric reflux, 1199, 1200, 1202
Volar plate fracture, 1260–1261
Volvulus
　caecal, 894
　large bowel, 728–729
　sigmoid, 728–729, 894
　small bowel, 723
　stomach, 805
Von Hippel-Lindau disease, 1779, 1882
Von Recklinghausen's disease *see*
　Neurofibromatosis
Von Willebrand's disease, **1345–1347**
　arthropathy, chronic, 1346–1347
　complications, 1347
　haemarthrosis, acute, 1345
　radiological features, 1345–1346
Voxel, definition, 43
Vulva, carcinoma, 1615
Vulval varices, 1615–1616

Wacker's triad, 295
Wada-Cutter valve, 664
Waldenström's macroglobulinaemia, 275, 855,
　1341
Wangensteen-Rice projection, 910
Water, relaxation behaviour in biological
　tissue, 67
Watershed infarction, radionuclide scanning,
　1865
Waterson-Cooley anastomosis, 504
Waterson shunt, 575
'Weaver's bottom', 1511
Wedge fracture, simple
　cervical spine, 1224, 1225
　thoracic spine, 1235
Wedge vertebrae in hyperthyroidism, 1392
Wegener's granulomatosis, lungs, 282
　nose and paranasal sinuses, 1950–1951

orbital manifestations, 1889
Weight reduction surgery, 808
Werner's syndrome arteriography, 2014
Westermark's sign, 319
Wet lung disease, 347, 349
Wheat weevil lung, 267
Whipple's disease, 853, *854*
Whitaker test, 1075, 1076–1077, **1216–1218**
　in children, 1182
　indications, 1217–1218
　interpretation of results, 1217
　technique, 1216–1217
White cell disorders, **1334–1341**
White matter disease, magnetic resonance
　imaging, 77
Whole body computed tomography *see*
　Computed tomography
Wilms' tumour, **1103–1104, 1202–1205**
　aortography, 2030
　clinical features, 1202–1203
　CT scan, *55*, 1104
　pathology, 1203
　radiographic evaluation, 1203–1205
　staging, 1203
　ultrasound, 2224
Wilson's disease, 1745
Wilson-Mikity syndrome, 344
Wimberger's sign in scurvy, 1388
Wirsung, duct of, 999
Wolffian duct remnants, disorders, 1600
Wormian bones in osteogenesis imperfecta,
　1393
Wrist
　injuries, **1255–1257**
　　adult injury, 1256–1257
　　Barton fracture, 1257
　　Colles' fracture, 1257
　　paediatric injury, 1256
　　radiographic views, 1255–1256
　　Smith fracture, 1257
　rheumatoid arthritis, **1478**
　　juvenile, 1482
Wry neck *see* Torticollis

X-linked hypophosphataemia and
　osteomalacia, 1378
X-ray quality, definition, 373
Xanthogranulomatous pyelonephritis, 1099,
　1130
[131]Xenon imaging, cardiopulmonary, children,
　2209–2210
Xerography
　larynx, 1973–1974
　technique, **1510–1511**
XO syndrome *see* Turner's syndrome

Yaws, **1360–1361**
　nose involvement, 1946
Yersinia enterocolitis, 890
Yersiniosis, 847

Zenker's diverticula, 1972
Zollinger-Ellison syndrome, **792**
　gastrinoma, 1032
　and retained gastric antrum, 810
Zuckerkandl, organ, arteriography, 2033
Zygoma fractures, 1900–1901
　radiography, 1902